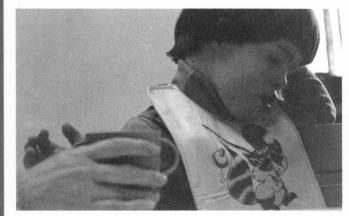

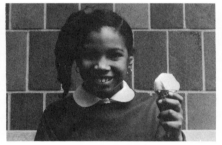

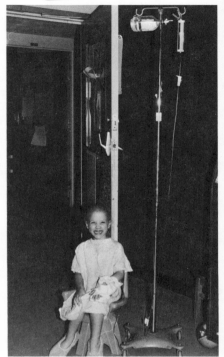

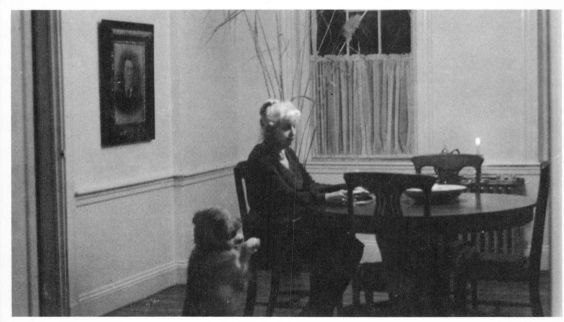

NUTRITION IN CLINICAL CARE

NUTRITION
IN CLINICAL CARE

SECOND EDITION

ROSANNE BEATRICE HOWARD, M.P.H., R.D.

Director of Nutrition Training in the
Developmental Evaluation Clinic
Children's Hospital Medical Center
Boston, Massachusetts

NANCIE HARVEY HERBOLD, M.S., R.D.

Assistant Professor of Foods and Nutrition
Department of Nutrition
Simmons College
Boston, Massachusetts

McGRAW-HILL BOOK COMPANY

New York St. Louis San Francisco Auckland Bogotá Hamburg
Johannesburg London Madrid Mexico Montreal New Delhi Panama
Paris São Paulo Singapore Sydney Tokyo Toronto

NUTRITION IN CLINICAL CARE

Copyright © 1982, 1978 by McGraw-Hill, Inc. All rights reserved. Printed in the United States of America. Except as permitted under the United States Copyright Act of 1976, no part of this publication may be reproduced or distributed in any form or by any means, or stored in a data base or retrieval system, without the prior written permission of the publisher.

2 3 4 5 6 7 8 9 0   DODO   8 9 8 7 6 5 4 3 2

ISBN 0-07-030514-5

Supported in part through the U.S. Department of Health and Human Services, Maternal and Child Health Service (Project 928).

This book was set in Baskerville by University Graphics, Inc. The editors were Anna R. Ferrera, Mark W. Cowell, and Susan Gamer; the designer was Anne Canevari Green; the production supervisor was Leroy A. Young. The drawings were done by Gail L. Kass; the photographs were taken by Carolin Dick and Rosanne Beatrice Howard.
R. R. Donnelley & Sons Company was printer and binder.

The endpaper photographs were taken by Rosanne Beatrice Howard.

Library of Congress Cataloging in Publication Data
Main entry under title:

Nutrition in clinical care.

Includes index.
1. Diet therapy. 2. Nutrition. 3. Food—Composition. 4. Nursing. I. Howard, Rosanne Beatrice.
II. Herbold, Nancie Harvey. [DNLM: 1. Diet therapy.
2. Nutrition. QU 145 H851n]
RM216.N84   1982   613.2   81-11803
ISBN 0-07-030514-5   AACR2

CONTENTS

List of Contributors   xi

Foreword   xiii

Preface   xv

PART ONE
FOOD: ITS NUTRITIVE SUBSTANCES AND PHYSIOLOGICAL EFFECTS

1. Nutrition: An Applied Science   3
   Rosanne Beatrice Howard

2. The Adequate Diet–The Prudent Diet   13
   Roberta Larson Duyff

3. Protein   39
   Ruth Palombo

4. Carbohydrate   57
   Carol Stollar

5. Lipids   72
   Rosanne Beatrice Howard and Nancie Harvey Herbold

6. Vitamins   90
   Patricia A. Kreutler

7. Minerals   126
   Jean Hine

8. Water and Electrolytes   153
   Grace Shen

9. The Body's Use of Food and Nutrients   168
   Christine Adamow Murray

PART TWO
FOOD, THE HUMAN ENVIRONMENT, AND HEALTH

10. Nutrition, Physical Fitness, and Athletic Performance   191
    Marilyn D. Schorin

11. The Psychology of Diet and Behavior Modification   211
    Rosanne Beatrice Howard and Richard R. Schnell

12. Developmental Considerations in Infant Feeding   227
    Robert W. Telzrow

13. Growth and Nutrition   239
    Christine E. Cronk and Rosanne Beatrice Howard

14. The Nutritional Care of the Premature Infant   287
    James L. Sutphen

15. Nutrition in Pregnancy, Lactation, and the Middle and Later Years   311
    Nancie Harvey Herbold

16. Community Nutrition   337
    Nancie Harvey Herbold

17. Nutrition and Dental Health   361
    T. Howard Howell

18. The Evaluation of Nutritional Status   374
    Nancy S. Wellman

PART THREE
THE CONSEQUENCES OF DISEASE ON NUTRITIONAL CARE

19. Malnutrition and the Immune Response   403
    Robert M. Suskind

20. The Allergic Response and Diet   418
    Mary Alice Marino

21. The Cardiovascular System   430
    Margaret L. Mikkola

22. The Gastrointestinal System   462
Christine Adamow Murray, Nancie Harvey Herbold, and Rosanne Beatrice Howard

23. The Kidneys and Urinary Tract   502
Roberta Ruhf Henry

24. The Endocrine System and Skeletal Disorders   535
Susan K. Golovin

25. Overweight and Underweight Conditions   570
Patricia A. Kreutler, Nancie Harvey Herbold, Rosanne Beatrice Howard,
and Peggy L. Pipes

26. Nutrition in Neurological Disorders and in the Care of the Disabled   594
Rosanne Beatrice Howard, Linda Fetters, and Dorothy M. MacDonald

27. Inborn Errors of Metabolism   629
Gail Neimeth Kaplan

28. Surgery, Stress, Burns, and Nutritional Care   654
Ronni Chernoff

29. Nutrition and Cancer   691
Nancie Harvey Herbold and Janet L. Sydness

Appendix A   713
Appendix B   752
Index   757

LIST OF CONTRIBUTORS

Ronni Chernoff, M.S., Ed.M., R.D.
Clinical Oncology Research Nutritionist
Hospital of the University of Pennsylvania
  Cancer Center
Philadelphia, Pennsylvania

Christine E. Cronk, Ph.D., M.S.
Anthropologist
Fels Research Institute
Yellow Springs, Ohio

Roberta Larson Duyff, M.S., R.D.
Nutrition Education Consultant
Manchester, Missouri

Linda Fetters, M.S., R.P.T.
Physical Therapy Consultant
Boston, Massachusetts

Susan K. Golovin, M.Ed., R.D.
Nutrition Consultant
San Francisco, California

Roberta Ruhf Henry, R.D.
Dialysis-Nutrition Coordinator for
  Special Research
National Cooperative Dialysis Study
Peter Bent Brigham Hospital
Boston, Massachusetts

Nancie Harvey Herbold, M.S., R.D.
Assistant Professor of Foods and Nutrition
Department of Nutrition
Simmons College
Boston, Massachusetts

Jean Hine, M.S., R.D.
Nutrition Consultant
Madison, Wisconsin

Rosanne Beatrice Howard, M.P.H., R.D.
Director of Nutrition Training in the
  Developmental Evaluation Clinic
Children's Hospital Medical Center
Boston, Massachusetts

T. Howard Howell, D.D.S.
Dean of Students
Harvard Dental School
Boston, Massachusetts

Gail Neimeth Kaplan, M.Ed., R.D.
Nutritionist
Developmental Evaluation Clinic
Children's Hospital Medical Center
Boston, Massachusetts

Patricia A. Kreutler, Ph.D.
Associate Professor
Chairman, Department of Nutrition
Simmons College
Boston, Massachusetts

Dorothy M. MacDonald, B.S., R.N.
Senior Surgical Clinic Nurse
Children's Hospital Medical Center
Boston, Massachusetts

Mary Alice Marino, M.S., R.D.
Nutrition Consultant
Fresno, California

Margaret L. Mikkola, R.D.
Research Dietitian
Arteriosclerosis Center
Massachusetts Institute of Technology
Cambridge, Massachusetts

Christine Adamow Murray, M.S., R.D.
Dietetic Internship Director
New England Deaconess Hospital
Boston, Massachusetts

Ruth Palombo, M.S., R.D.
Unit Coordinator
Ambulatory Nutrition Services
Massachusetts General Hospital
Boston, Massachusetts

Peggy L. Pipes, M.S., M.P.H., R.D.
Assistant Chief, Nutrition Section
Clinical Training Unit
Child Development and Mental Retardation
  Center
Lecturer, School of Home Economics
University of Washington
Seattle, Washington

Richard R. Schnell, Ph.D.
Director of Psychology Training
Developmental Evaluation Clinic
Children's Hospital Medical Center
Boston, Massachusetts

Marilyn D. Schorin, M.P.H., R.D.
Nutritionist, MRFIT Clinical Center
Adjunct Assistant Professor
Rutgers Medical School
Piscataway, New Jersey

Grace Shen, Ph.D., R.D.
Nutrition Director
Clinical Research Center
Children's Hospital Medical Center
Boston, Massachusetts

Carol Stollar, M.Ed., R.D.
Assistant Director for Patient Services
Frances Stern Nutrition Center
Tufts New England Medical Center
Boston, Massachusetts

Robert M. Suskind, M.D.
Professor and Chairman
College of Medicine
Department of Pediatrics
University of South Alabama
Mobile, Alabama

James L. Sutphen, M.D., Ph.D.
Assistant Professor of Pediatrics
Chief of Gastroenterology
University of Virginia
Charlottesville, Virginia

Janet L. Sydness, M.P.H., R.D.
Education Coordinator
Nutrition Services—Dietary
Children's Hospital Medical Center
Boston, Massachusetts

Robert W. Telzrow, M.D.
Assistant Professor
Department of Pediatrics
University of Washington
School of Medicine
Seattle, Washington

Nancy S. Wellman, M.S., R.D.
Chairman, Department of Dietetics
  and Nutrition
Florida International University
Miami, Florida

FOREWORD

One of the joys of practicing applied nutrition in a large city such as Boston with an abundance of academically oriented health care institutions is that its assembly of health professionals permits a deep study of vexing nutritional problems from many different perspectives. The contributors to this book are products of such an environment.

The reward for the practitioner comes in the applications which can be developed to help patients. It is in the marshalling of the facts toward the worthy end of improving human health and happiness by nutritional means that this book excels. The scientific underpinnings of nutrition as a health science are woven into discussions of clinically relevant problems from the viewpoint of the practitioner. The usual trap of the textbook is that it is either all light (or theory) or all heat (or practice). This book strikes a happy medium, as those who wrote these chapters do in their treatment of the patient. The reader will be pleased, as we were in leafing through the book, at the real-life flavor it has.

It is with great pleasure that we recommend this book to the reader. The esteemed colleagues and good friends who have put so much of their own expertise into writing it are fine clinical nutritionists. We trust that those who master the contents of this text will follow in their competent footsteps in their own later careers.

Johanna Dwyer, D.Sc., R.D.
Associate Professor
Tufts University School of Medicine
Director, Frances Stern Nutrition Center
Tufts New England Medical Center
Boston, Massachusetts

Mary Ellen Collins, M.Ed., R.D.
Director of Dietetics
Peter Bent Brigham Hospital
Boston, Massachusetts

PREFACE

This book has been planned to provide the student with the information from which a nutrition-centered health care practice can be established. The book is divided into three major areas. The first part considers Food: Its Nutritive Substances and Physiological Effects, setting forth the biochemical principles needed to understand the complex interactions of food within the human body. These basic principles are expanded in the second section, where Nutrition, the Human Environment, and Health are considered, followed by the third study area which addresses The Consequences of Disease on Nutritional Care.

Since the science of nutrition can be abstract and impersonal, the study of scientific facts needs to be tempered with a value-level application. This then adds relevancy to the facts and increases the possibility of their application. With this in mind, each chapter has been designed to give the student the information needed to understand the relevance of each nutrient to health, followed by a clinical analysis which will involve the student in the solution of concrete problems, leading to a deeper working understanding that cannot be acquired in didactic lectures, reading, or memorizing facts.

Through this clinical study approach, the student will learn to apply theory to the practical situation—to the client, thereby integrating nutrition into the health care delivery system.

At the beginning of each chapter, certain key words have been identified to facilitate learning; and questions, along with a clinical study, are included to encourage the development of the student's own clinical expertise. Discussions of the clinical studies come at the end of the chapter. Exceptions to this format are the introductory Chapter 1, which does not contain a clinical study, and Chapter 12, which has five clinical studies, discussed in the text throughout the chapter. Chapter 22 includes two clinical studies. One half of the clinical studies concern children and the others concern adults.

The study of nutrition is an applied study. Nutrients operate within a complex organism—the human body. To be effective, nutrition educators must apply the scientific facts to the human need. This is the purpose of this book—to encourage a holistic approach in nutritional care.

Rosanne Beatrice Howard
Nancie Harvey Herbold

NUTRITION IN CLINICAL CARE

PART ONE

FOOD: ITS NUTRITIVE SUBSTANCES AND PHYSIOLOGICAL EFFECTS

This section presents the principles of nutrition, which can be overwhelming to the student who is exposed for the first time to the biochemical theory on which the study of nutrition is based. The anxiety experienced by the new student is a common feeling, often compounded by the student's failure to understand the relevance of biochemical principles to clinical care. Let us assure you that, as in all other areas of study, you will master these principles with some work, greatly enhanced by an open attitude. Let us further assure you that this study area is relevant, for it is upon these basic principles that your future practice of clinical nutrition will eventually be established.

CHAPTER 1

NUTRITION: AN APPLIED SCIENCE

Rosanne Beatrice Howard

KEY WORDS
Food Ways
Present-Day Nutritional Concerns
Nutritional Education
Behavioral Change
Preventive Nutrition

People's past experiences help define their present situations—and so knowledge of the past role of food helps our understanding of nutrition in our present society.

Food not only is basic to survival but has been pertinent to the development of the human race. The quality of life has been dependent on the quality of food. It all started a few million years ago around the middle Pleistocene epoch when our distant anthropoid cousins were constrained to become hunters under the spur of ecological change.

This adaptation from a food scavenger of roots, fruits, and other vegetable foods to a hunter made it possible for the early hominids to accommodate to environmental changes. By becoming omnivorous, humanlike apes evolved to apelike humans as they increased their capacity for survival.

It seems clear that man survived the climatic changes of the middle Pleistocene by a new behavioral adaptation that affected fundamentally and irrevocably his psychosocial character; it was his change in food finding behavior among other things that finally made man, and that . . . helps to justify our recognition of the change from Australopithecus the apeman to Homo the man.[1]

The transition from food-gathering herbivore to hunter not only produced a change in diet but automatically implied group cooperation, since hunting could be carried out only by the strongest young males. Cooperative hunting and sharing the proceeds of the hunt with females and infants became the trademark of the human condition among primates.

Herein lies the anthropological and social significance of food as part of our cultural heritage. Food sharing and cooperation brought prehistoric humans together in a very intimate way in a situation that probably even encouraged speech. Our distinctly human act of hospitality, of inviting friends to dinner, is based to an extent on those earlier advantages of sharing. Food, so essential to survival, provided the incentive for socialized behavior around which society formed.

Throughout all societies, food and eating have been looked upon as symbolizing friendliness and interpersonal acceptance, and the withholding of food as rejection or punishment. Since history has been recorded, famine and the fear of hunger have plagued humankind and the most pressing human problem has been the securing of food to satisfy this hunger. Food has been used as a means of political subjugation, and often its availability has been the determining factor in the outcome of wars. According to a retrospective study of hunger by Keys and his coworkers that included wartime observations of starvation and the reported experiences of explorers, hunger becomes completely overpower-

ing and incites baseness in human behavior. This human response to hunger is the same regardless of time and place.[2]

Before humans learned to cultivate the land, satiety was dependent on whatever plants or animals inhabited the locality, giving rise to the vast range of geographical distinction among food preferences. Whatever was edible was eaten. The extent to which primitive peoples explored their food environment can be illustrated by their discovery of the remedial properties and the narcotic effect of certain herbs, roots, and leaves. Early societies were known to chew coca leaves, smoke Indian hemp, and drink tea, cocoa, and coffee.[3] For centuries the Chinese people held the belief that the plant ginseng was a panacea for disease. Remnants of these ancient

Figure 1-1
Cultural evolution of food habits. "Food ways" are passed from one generation to another.
(Photo courtesy of Jane McCotter O'Toole. Bamako, Mali, west Africa.)

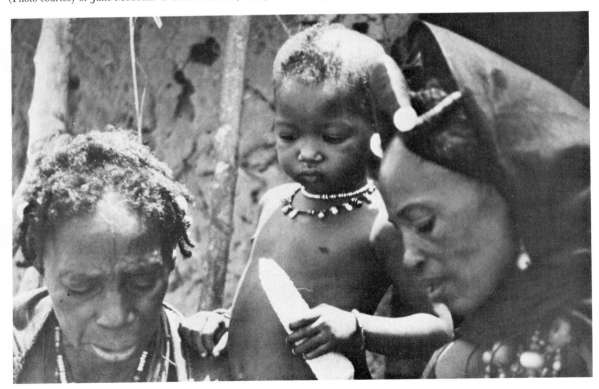

beliefs can still be found in our present culture. An appreciation of this ecological framework, a human-land interaction, helps toward an understanding of current cultural influences on food use.

From the beginning, societies developed patterns around the conduct of food activities. These standardized practices, known as *food ways,* are unique to each individual society, having evolved from different environmental factors and having been incorporated into the society to maintain the viability of the group. Food ways are part of our cultural heritage and are inculcated from birth, as the child is either placed to the breast or given a bottle.

Culture enters into the food experience, shaping and choosing the significant factors for defining the experience.[4]

Thus, culture determines *what* will be recognized as food, *when* we should have an appetite, and for *what* we should be hungry.

Because of the general American societal mixtures, there is no one cultural pattern that exists in its pure form. But whatever the potpourri, food habits develop from culturally determined values, attitudes, and beliefs. The cultural significance of food habits predates the concept of nutrition, a twentieth-century science which has helped us to define the food that humans need in order to grow and maintain health.

NUTRITION: A SCIENCE

The early knowledge of nutrition consisted of anecdotal observations that go as far back as Hippocrates, the father of medicine (460–370 B.C.), who is said to have paid strict attention to the diet of his patients as a feature of his therapeutic regimens. However, little of a scientific nature was accomplished in the development of nutrition or any science until the latter part of the eighteenth century. It was at this time that Antoine Laurent Lavoisier measured in guinea pigs and in his laboratory assistant the amount of body heat lost, oxygen consumed, and carbon dioxide expired. He concluded that respiration is a combustion process similar to the process utilized in a flame. Lavoisier's measurements taken in fasting and resting states essentially represent basal metabolism, a concept fundamental to the development of nutritional science, and are the reason that Lavoisier is known as the father of nutrition.

During the nineteenth century, considerable work was done on energy exchange and on the nature of major foodstuffs, and the energy value of a large number of foods was determined. Leiberg, Rubner, Atwater, Voit are but some of the names of researchers whose work began to bring the science of nutrition to an age. However, the progress was slow until chemical methodology had developed to the point that relatively purified foodstuffs could be isolated. Prior to 1910, vitamins and minerals had not been identified.

F. G. Hopkins (1906) in England recognized the relationship between accessory food factors, now known as *vitamins,* and the dietary deficiency syndromes known for many years and described by James Lind in his *Treatise on Scurvy* (1753). In 1912, the accessory food factors were named *vitamines* by Casimir Funk. He propounded the theory that beriberi, scurvy, pellagra, and possibly rickets were caused by *deficiency,* or the lack of special substances. He called these special substances *vitamines—vita,* the factors essential for life, and *amines,* because he thought that the antiberiberi factor he was attempting to isolate was an amine.

The vitamin hypothesis prompted new vistas of exploration and technology and by 1913 McCollum and Davis had discovered vitamin A. The continuing isolation and synthesis of vitamins and minerals is the matrix around which nutrition has developed as a field of scientific study that is closely interwoven with medicine, anatomy, physiology, chemistry, bacteriology, and agriculture.

Nutrition as we know it today is "the science that interprets the relationship of food to the functioning living organism."[5] It has been recognized as an independent field of study since

1926 with the appointment of Mary Swartz Rose as professor of nutrition at Columbia University.

NUTRITION: PRESENT-DAY CONCERNS

Advances in the science of nutrition heralded in the field of food technology, which has created improved methods of producing, preserving, and processing food. The fortification of milk with vitamins A and D, the iodization of salt, and the enrichment of flour, cornmeal, cereals, and bread are but a few illustrations. Despite these modern food processes, and despite the restoration, fortification, or enrichment of nutrients, nutrients can be lost with poor manufacturing techniques. Many questions about the continued availability of nutrients, especially the trace elements, in processed and fabricated foods are now being raised among health professionals.

In the United States the marriage of food technology and the science of nutrition, along with a great deal of capital and ingenuity, has resolved the problem of our food supply. However, these same solutions have provoked concern over the adulteration of our food supply with residues of fertilizers and additives to preserve, flavor, color, or thicken food. As far back as 1970, it was estimated that 5 lb of additives per person per year were ingested by an average citizen. Although the use of additives has guaranteed our food supply, and has probably made it safer than ever before in history, the cumulative effects are as yet unknown and their relationship to allergies, cancer, birth defects, and interactions with drugs and diets needs to be fully investigated.

Modern food technology has led to the development of many new products and convenience foods, reflected in the 12,000 items that line the shelves of the average large supermarket. The consumer is now faced with many food choices which, when carefully examined, may offer little variation. Consumer compliance and acceptance of foods, and the failure to demand from the food industry a wholesome, unadulterated food supply, are prime examples of the need for consumer education. Only after consumer education has been successful and has produced resultant changes in consumer food preferences can we expect action by the food industry toward increasing the nutritional value of the food offered to the consumer.

Fat- and sugar-rich foods, commonly known as "junk" foods or "snack" foods, have become increasingly popular. Some experts estimate that snack foods are close to comprising 30 percent of the daily caloric intake, prompting them to consider the fortification of some of these same junk foods.

The spiraling use of junk foods and the excess consumption of sugar and fat, combined with the sedentary life style, has led to the "overweight society," a product of the imbalance between essential and energy-yielding nutrients. Overweight is a problem that now affects many and knows no barriers of age, race, or income level.

The prevalance of obesity is high. However, it is difficult to determine the rate because of the different standards of obesity. In the Health and Nutrition Examination Survey conducted by the National Center for Health Statistics, 13 percent of all males 20 to 74 years of age and almost 23 percent of all females 20 to 74 years of age were obese. More black females were obese than white females, but the rates for white males and black males were similar. The prevalence of obesity for all groups increased with age.[6]

Low-fiber diets have been implicated in the growing incidence of lower bowel disease and cancer of the colon in our population. The focus on fiber relates to its role in promoting gastrointestinal motility and viscosity of the gastrointestinal contents, its interaction with bile acids, and its effects on the microbial flora, fecal bulk, and the time of passage of food through the intestine. Canned fruit juices, vegetable soups, and white bread are a few examples of the bland, low-roughage foods that permeate our food supply. The fact that foods such as these do not promote gastrointestinal motility but cause intestinal stasis is suggested as the causative factor in lower bowel disease.

The increasing use of refined carbohydrate is associated with the prevalance of dental caries, endemic to our population and found in all economic strata. It is figured that 100 lb of sugar disappears for each person per year.

According to Friend, not only has the use of refined sugars increased but the pattern of use has changed as well. While the use of sugar in households is less than what it was at the beginning of this century the use of sugar by industry in processed foods and beverages is three times greater.[7]

The problem of highly refined, sugar- and fat-rich foods is compounded by the fact that these foods are popularized in fast-food chains and restaurants across the nation.

Thirty-five percent of all food dollars is spent for meals outside the home,[8] and a quarter of this is spent in fast-food outlets.[9] Between 1963 and 1978, the sales in food stores rose 44 percent, in eating places 83 percent, and in fast-foods chains 300 percent.[10]

The fact that more people eat in restaurants is a result of the ways in which industrialization has affected our life-style and of more people living alone. Ten years ago approximately one in five households was a nonfamily household, but it is projected that by 1990 at least one-third of households will not be family households.[11] Forty-five percent of those who live alone are over 65 years of age, with another 20 percent expected during the 1980s.[12]

Another trend affecting families is the working mother, who in some instances is also becoming the sole breadwinner. In the period from 1947 to 1965 there was an increase of 131 percent in the number of mothers added to the work force, and by 1975, 39 percent of these women were mothers of preschool children.[13] Already those families which depend on women make up a disproportionate percentage of the poor. While one in three families headed by a woman is poor, only one in eighteen families headed by a man is poor, and the latest figures from 1976 to 1980 show that the trend is not slowing. The emotional stress and financial constraints of a female-headed family are changing family meals.

The working mother's family often relies on restaurants, day-care centers, and school lunch and breakfast programs. Increasingly, early food habits are influenced by forces outside the home. Also, with the emphasis on speed and efficiency, families have relied on convenience foods. With inflation, however, meal planners are becoming more judicious about how they spend their food dollars.

Another present-day concern is our per capita meat consumption of 186 pounds per year, which may reflect a belief emanating from our frontier ancestors that eating meat from strong animals conferred strength.[14] Hanes I data indicate that the mean protein intakes make up 16 percent of the total caloric intake of the American diet.[15] We appear to continue to subscribe to this notion, as meat high in saturated fat and cholesterol remains at the center of the American meal table despite its identification as a risk factor in cardiovascular disease. Furthermore, this overuse of animal protein may come to be viewed as irresponsible in the face of global food shortages and malnutrition in the third-world nations.

In the future, food scarcity may be more persistent as negative ecological trends gain momentum yearly in poor countries. The prospects are for ever-increasing dependence on North American grain stores. Since it takes approximately 5 lb of grain to produce 1 lb of meat, grain is siphoned away from human consumption.[16]

For our nation the implication is clear: we need a comprehensive nutritional policy to assure adequate food production and maintenance of quality for our global commitments as well as domestic needs. In this regard one idea has been to create a federal office that will be responsible for nutritional planning. The government's reluctance to develop a federal food and nutrition office has caused much debate within the U.S. Senate's Select Committee on Nutrition and Human Needs.[17] This committee was established in response to the discovery of malnutrition in America during the 1960s by a Senate subcommittee headed by Senator Robert Kennedy. Originally mandated to solve the problem of hunger and malnutrition in the 20 to 30 million so-identified Americans, it then broadened its scope to consider the effectiveness of federally subsidized food programs. Presently, the existing programs are tied to different special-interest groups, each oriented toward its own narrow goals, and as a consequence federal food policy has developed piecemeal.

For the most part, our nutritional problems are ones of excess or imbalance, rather than deficiency, and can be found in all socioeconomic groups, and in particular, in poverty pockets (Appalachia, the deep south, urban ghettos). Malnutrition is highest in blacks, Indians, Mexican Americans, Puerto Ricans, and the elderly. The hunger in America discovered by the Senate subcommittee and confirmed by the Ten-State Nutrition Survey conducted from 1968 to 1970 is now less severe because of the expansion of many of the federal food programs such as food stamps. However, this does not mean that Americans get the right food or enough food. It means that generally they are not starving; but with cutbacks in nutrition and social programs, this may change.

The nutritional problems of excess were examined closely by the U.S. Senate Select Committee on Nutrition and Human Needs under the leadership of Senator George McGovern. *Dietary Goals for the United States* was published in 1977.[18] While the recommended levels of consumption stimulated much controversy, they also served as the basis for a broad discussion of nutrition and its relationship to disease. During the summer of 1979, the first *Surgeon General's Report on Health Promotion and Disease Prevention* was released.[19] The guidelines in the report are compatible with the *U.S. Dietary Goals* but do not recommend specific levels of consumption. Both reports examine the relationship between overconsumption of fats, sugar, salt, and alcohol and leading causes of death (heart disease, stroke, cancer, diabetes, arteriosclerosis, and cirrhosis of the liver). In addition, they discuss the relationship of diet to the development of conditions that affect health, such as hypertension.

The allure of food cults and quackery has further compounded the nutritional status of our citizens. People look to certain combinations of food or vitamins to cure diseases such as cancer or arthritis, and conditions such as aging or mental retardation. Particularly vulnerable are those without hope, especially older adults.

Misinformation about food is often promulgated by the media, and this in turn influences children's food habits. It has been estimated that nearly 44 million children under 12 years of age who watch a moderate amount of TV see 21,300 commercials in one year. The effectiveness of this advertising can be seen in the aisles of the supermarkets, as children pressure parents for a particular product, or on the breakfast tables across the nation, each replete with several different brands of cereal, many with dubious nutritional value.

We have advanced in isolating nutrients and in applying technology to the production and processing of food, but we have progressed little in the area of adequate food distribution and the effective application of the science of nutrition to individual needs. Satisfying these latter unmet needs is necessary in order to bring about the behavioral changes and the formation of good food habits that are necessary for the improved health of the population. With the escalating cost of health care and without strong evidence to support a concomitant improvement in our nation's health, greater emphasis must be placed on preventive health services, including preventive nutrition. The goal of *preventive nutrition* is to achieve a balance between the nutrients needed for health and those which must not be eaten to excess, so as to prevent nutrition-related diseases. An example of prevention working is the decline in cardiovascular disease deaths in the last 10 years—stroke deaths are down by 32 percent, heart attacks by 22 percent. The decline shows the results that a better knowledge of risk factors involved in the disease can effect. Control of dietary risks is one aspect of preventive nutrition.[20]

Nutrition educators must broaden their scope — away from pathology and therapy, and toward normal nutrition in its positive aspects.

Efforts should focus on the establishment and protection of nutritional health rather than on crisis intervention. It is needed regardless of income, location, or cultural, social, or economic practices or level of education. Nutrition education must be a continuing process through the life cycle as new research brings new knowledge.[21]

To accomplish this goal, nutrition must be applied — a science applied to the human need.

NUTRITION: AN APPLIED SCIENCE

Nutrition education is a multidisciplinary process that involves the transfer of information, the development of motivation and the modification of food habits where needed. It must form the bridge that carries appropriate information from the research and development laboratories to the public, the ultimate user. During transport, nutrition educators and their counterparts in related professions must apply their skills and knowledge to adapt the information so it can be applied to a variety of everyday situations and then package it for distribution in a variety of ways, whether directly to the intended user or indirectly through intermediate agents.[22]

A subcommittee of the Intra-Agency Committee on Nutrition Education has proposed four basic concepts of nutritional education:

1 Nutrition is the food you eat and how the body uses it.
- We eat food to live, to grow, to keep healthy and well, and to get energy for work and play.

2 Food is made up of different nutrients needed for growth and health.

- All nutrients needed by the body are available through food.
- Eating many kinds and combinations of food can lead to a well-balanced diet.
- No food, by itself, has all the nutrients needed for full growth and health.
- Each nutrient has specific uses in the body.
- Most nutrients do their best work in the body when teamed with other nutrients.

3 All persons, throughout life, need the same nutrients, but in varying amounts.
- The amounts of nutrients needed are influenced by age, sex, body size, activity, and state of health.

4 The way that food is handled influences the amount of nutrients in the food, as well as its safety, appearance, and taste.
- Handling means everything that happens to food while it is being grown, processed, stored, and prepared for eating.

These concepts can help to launch a nutrition education program. However, any attempt to apply the science of nutrition must take into consideration that humans are part of a dynamic sociopolitical system affected by the environmental resources (climate, soil, water, energy) around them. People, whether in an affluent nation or an undeveloped country, have certain basic needs to which nutritional science must be applied, for it is from these needs that food habits develop.

Food habits of an individual are the characteristic and repetitive acts that he performs under the impetus of the need to provide himself with nourishment and simultaneously to meet an assortment of social and emotional goals. By the choices he makes, which become habit on repetition, he strives to achieve such satisfactions as security, comfort, status, pleasure, and enhancement of his ego.[23]

Since food habits are learned in response to a need and are not genetically determined, nutrition education is possible. The concern of the nutrition educator is the way in which people

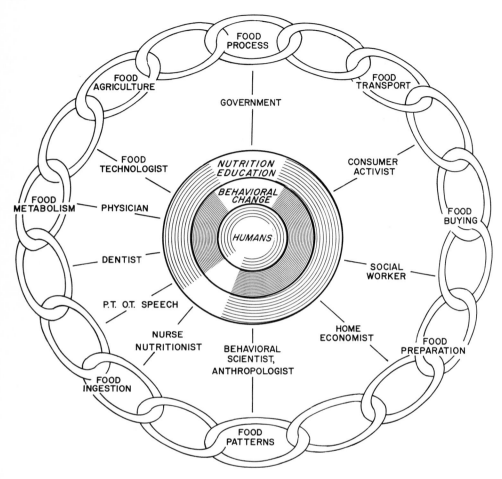

Figure 1-2
The interconnecting chain of food factors influencing nutritional education. This chain connects all factors that influence food intake and ultimately human nutritional status. Note: The term nutritionist *includes dieticians.*

learn and how this learning can bring about behavioral change.

NUTRITION: A MULTIDISCIPLINARY TEAM APPROACH

Behavioral change as an integral part of nutrition education is a complex process, and as such is best achieved through the combined efforts of a health-care team. A multidisciplinary team of physician, nurse, nutritionist, and behavioral scientist, with other members as needed (physical therapist, dentist, speech therapist, home economist, etc.), working together yet from different vantage points, formulate a plan of nutrition intervention while considering the total person, with a discipline to relate to each individual need. By focusing on the level of need, the health professional can apply the science of nutrition at that level to bring about behavioral change. There is no one way to change food behavior.

TABLE 1-1   CONSCIOUS ACTION ARISES FROM NEEDS

Basic human needs: Order of priority	Nutrition focus
Basic physiological needs (food, water, oxygen, sleep)	Food for sustenance
Safety and security	Food for growth and maintenance
Belonging and social activity	Food for social reinforcement
Esteem and status	Food for prestige
Self-realization and fulfillment	Food for optimum productivity and well-being
Need to know and understand	Nutritional education

Each program must be individually tailored to the human need.

According to Maslow, human needs are ordered in a hierarchical pattern, and as one level is reasonably satisfied the next level emerges.[24] This theoretical pattern can be a useful guide for the nutrition educator who is attempting to understand human motivation. Approaching the individual at his or her level of need may bring about the desired change (see Table 1-1).

YOUR ROLE AS A NUTRITION EDUCATOR

To be an effective nutrition educator, you must become a food therapist. You must have an understanding of food as it relates to human needs and must incorporate the role of a food expert into that of being a health professional.

By being the food experts, we should know and be interested in everything about food as it relates to people, chemically, physiologically, biochemically, economically—everything from the source to use and what happens to it in us.[25]

This is a chain which connects all the factors that influence our food intake and ultimately our nutritional status, with each link permanently and irreversibly linked to the next. A knowledge of all these links is a prerequisite to the application of the science of nutrition.

Changes in food consumption patterns de-velop within the context of cultural evolution. This evolution is responsive to human interactions and may change the food itself in some instances, as occurs with food processing. In other instances cultural changes affect the response to food as a function of lifestyle. These changes exert both positive and negative effects, they are ongoing, and it is essential that you as nutrition educator maintain credibility by being well-informed and conversant with the latest research in the field.

STUDY QUESTIONS

1   What is the cultural significance of food?

2   List all of the present-day nutritional concerns.

3   Why is nutrition education a multidisciplinary process?

4   Explain the statement "nutrition is an applied science."

5   What is your role as a nutrition educator?

REFERENCES

1   B. Campbell, *Human Evolution,* Aldine Publishing Company, Chicago, 1966, p. 235.

2   A. Keys, J. Brozek, A. Henschel, O. McIkelser, and H. L. Taylor, *The Biology of Human Starvation,* vols. 1 and 2, University of Minnesota Press, Minneapolis, 1950.

3   E. V. McCollum, *A History of Nutrition,* Riverside Press, Cambridge, Mass., 1957, p. 4.

4   D. Lee, "Cultural Factors in Dietary Choice," *American Journal of Clinical Nutrition,* **5,** March–April 1957, p. 166.

5   R. Pike and M. Brown, *Nutrition: An Integrated Approach,* 2d ed., John Wiley & Sons, Inc., New York, 1975, p. 1.

6   H. W. Miller, *Plan and Operation for the Health and Nutrition Examination Survey, United States, 1971–1973, Vital and Health Statistics,* ser. I, no. 10a, 10b, U.S. Department of Health, Education, and Welfare Publication (HRA)76–1310, Public Health Service, Health Resources Administration, National Center for Health Statistics, 1976.

7   B. Friend, L. Page, and R. Marston, "Food Consumption Patterns in the United States, 1909–1913 to 1976," in R. Levy, B. Rifkind, B. Dennis, and N. Ernst (eds.), *Nutrition, Lipids, and Coronary Heart Disease,* Raven Press, New York, 1979, pp. 489–522.

8   *U.S. Food Expenditures 1954–1978,* U.S. Department of Agriculture Agricultural Economic Report 431, 1979.

9   U.S. Bureau of the Census, "Merchandise Hire Sales, U.S. Summary," in *Census of Retail Trade,* 1972.

10 U.S. Department of Agriculture, *Farm Index,* October 1979.

11 U.S. Bureau of the Census, "Projections of the Number of Households and Families 1979–1995," in *Current Population Reports,* ser. P–20, no. 345, March 1979.

12 U.S. Bureau of the Census, "Marital Status and Living Arrangements," in *Current Population Reports,* ser. P–20, no. 338, March 1978.

13 Christian Beals, "The Case of the Vanishing Mommy," *The New York Times,* July 4, 1976, p. 28.

14 A. Berg, *The Nutrition Factor,* The Brookings Institution, Washington, D.C., 1973, p. 64.

15 S. Abraham, M. D. Carroll, C. M. Dresser, and C. L. Johnson, *Dietary Intake Findings, United States, 1971–1974,* Vital and Health Statistics, ser. 11, no 202, U.S. Department of Health, Education, and Welfare Publication (HRA)77–1647, Public Health Service, Health Resources Administration, National Center for Health Statistics, July 1977.

16 A. Berg, op. cit.

17 U.S. Select Committee on Nutrition and Human Needs, *Towards a National Nutrition Policy,* Washington, D.C., 1975.

18 U.S. Select Committee on Nutrition and Human Needs, *Dietary Goals for the United States,* staff report, 2d ed., Washington, D.C., December 1977b.

19 *Healthy People: The Surgeon General's Report of Health Promotion and Disease Prevention,* U.S. Department of Health, Education, and Welfare Publication (PHS) 79–55071, 1979.

20 National Center for Health Statistics, "Annual Summary for the United States, 1978," *Monthly Vital Statistics Reports,* **27**(13), 1979.

21 "American Dietetic Association Position Paper on Nutrition Education for the Public," *Journal of American Dietetic Association,* **62**:429, 1973.

22 R. Leverton, "Commentary: What Is Nutrition Education?" *Journal of American Dietetic Association,* **64**:17, 1974.

23 Helen H. Gifft, Marjorie B. Washbon, Gail G. Harrison, *Nutrition, Behavior and Change,* Prentice-Hall, Inc., Englewood Cliffs, N.J., 1972, p. 29.

24 A. H. Maslow, "A Theory of Human Motivation," *Psychological Review,* **50**:370–396, 1943.

25 Madge L. Meyers, "Fact and Fantasy in the Practice of Clinical Dietetics: Ninth Martha F. Trulson Memorial Lecture," *Abstracts of the 58th American Dietetic Annual Meeting,* October 1975, p. 123.

CHAPTER 2
THE ADEQUATE DIET—THE PRUDENT DIET

Roberta Larson Duyff

KEY WORDS
Food Additive
Nutrification
Restoration
Enrichment
Fortification
Nutrient Density
Empty Calorie Foods
Nutrient Labeling
Recommended Dietary Allowances
Daily Food Guide
Food Composition Tables

INTRODUCTION

An adequate diet is one that provides all the necessary nutrients in amounts needed by the body for optimum health. While specific eating practices may range widely from individual to individual, the nutrient needs of most Americans can be met by following the guidelines of two standards: the Recommended Dietary Allowances (RDA) and the food groups. Health professionals must interpret these guidelines for clients, and in doing so must consider the numerous factors that may affect the nutrient quality of the food selected. These influences include:

Food processing
Food consumption patterns
Food purchasing
Food handling and preparation

This chapter will consider these influences and their effect on the nutrient content of food and diet, to better enable the health professional to determine the effect of these influences on dietary standards.

FOOD PROCESSING

Technological advances in food processing methods have increased the number of available food products. In the early 1900s approximately 800 items were supplied to retail stores while today over 12,000 products are stocked on grocery shelves. Although the modern supermarket carries many nonfood items, a large percentage of the consumer's spending options are for edible goods. Consumers must discern which processing methods and food products will meet physical, psychological, and social needs.

The term *processing* covers a wide variety of physical steps to which food is subjected prior to consumption. Washing produce, cooking a garden vegetable at home, or refining wheat at a mill are all forms of processing; however, the term commonly refers to industrial processing before purchase. Processing foods through *preservation* techniques, the use of *additives,* and

13

nutrification has both advantages and disadvantages.

Advantages:
Storage time increased
Preparation time and effort decreased
Food safety improved
Overall product appeal improved for some people
Nutritional value improved
Food changed into edible form
More foods available

Disadvantages:
Nutrients destroyed
Cost increased
Quality changed, decreasing the overall product appeal for some people
Individuals subjected to unknown risk factors

From a nutritional standpoint, three aspects of processing must be considered: (1) the trade-off between increased availability of food and the loss of nutrients, (2) the degree of nutrient loss (e.g., home preparation often results in greater losses than commercial processing does), and (3) the relative importance of the loss (e.g., ascorbic acid is destroyed in pasteurization of milk, but milk does not contain significant quantities of the nutrient).[1]

Preservation Methods

Since most foods do not have a long storage life, processing methods have been developed to retain the nutrient value, aesthetic qualities, and functional properties of foods while reducing the possibility of microbial spoilage. There are five commonly used methods of preservation: *canning, freezing, freeze-drying, drying,* and *dehydrating.* Another, *irradiation,* is now undergoing research.

Preserved foods aid the consumer by providing a varied diet throughout the year. With the use of processed foods, seasonal changes in the food supply need not impose a major shift in one's dietary pattern. Processing allows foods to be transported over a wide geographical area as well as to be stored at home for longer periods of time. Some processing may be purely a convenience to consumers. For instance, dried and freeze-dried foods are excellent for backpacking, when refrigeration is not available.

While some nutrients are lost in the course of preservation, overall quality can remain high. In fact, canned or frozen fruits and vegetables may provide more nutrients than fresh produce that has been improperly handled during storage and preparation.

Additives

Food additives are used in food processing. They are defined as substances added to food either directly for a functional purpose *(intentional food additives)* or unintentionally during some phase of production, processing, storage, or packaging *(incidental food additives)*. Those added purposely are expected to:

Improve nutritional value
Enhance flavor
Maintain appearance, palatability, and wholesomeness
Impart and maintain a desired consistency
Control acidity or alkalinity
Impart a desired and characteristic color
Serve as maturing and bleaching agents in milling and baking
Maintain quality in processed foods, e.g., curing agents and anticaking agents

The charts in the Appendix list functions of specific additives.

While many additives are recognized as harmless components of food if eaten in moderation, the public has expressed increasing concern over the use and safety of many additives. A list has been compiled of additives that are "generally recognized as safe" (GRAS) for moderate use in food processing without serious health hazard (e.g., ascorbic acid to nutrify and to prevent browning in cut fruits and vegetables, lecithin to emulsify mayonnaise, and alum to produce crispness in pickles). Currently some commonly used additives (particularly coloring agents, nitrates, nitrites) are under debate for being potentially deleterious to health. Products that contain saccharin must carry the following warning: "Use of this product may be hazardous to your health. This product contains saccharin, which has been determined to cause cancer in laboratory animals."

The Food and Drug Administration (FDA) and businesses share the responsibility of ensuring the safe and proper use of additives by means of research and by removal of an additive from the market if necessary. The consumer's role should be to:

Keep informed about food additives, using reliable information sources.

Communicate concerns to the government and industry.

Read package labels, understanding the function of additives included.

Consume a varied diet to minimize exposure to any one additive.

Nutrification

Nutrification is both a form of processing and a type of food additive. Nutrification includes *restoration, enrichment,* and *fortification* of conventional foods and *formulation* of new foods, all methods that can increase the nutritional value of food.

Restoration is the adding of nutrients to foods to replace some of those that have been lost or removed through processing. These nutrients are usually added in amounts up to original levels. *Enrichment* is adding nutrients naturally present to levels *higher than normal.* Most enrichment is done to foods made with grain. Milling, which removes the germ and outer layers of grain, causes the loss of several nutrients, including iron, thiamin, riboflavin, and niacin. Enrichment replaces these nutrients in the product. However, it does not add back all of the trace elements that are lost in processing.

Although enrichment of bakery bread was made mandatory in 1943 for the duration of World War II, no such federal legislation currently exists. This early law, however, set a precedent for today's voluntary enrichment by some manufacturers, as well as for several state laws which mandate enrichment in some bread and cereal products. Since enrichment is not required in many states, consumers may be unaware of the added food quality it provides unless they are educated to look for an enrichment statement on a product label. In particular, foods considered as staples, such as rice and bread, should be enriched since they play such an important role in the daily diet.

Fortification is the addition of nutrients not normally present in a food. Nutrients that are used to fortify foods are those which generally are consumed in less than adequate amounts by sectors of the population. Examples include vitamin D added to milk, iodine added to table salt, vitamin C added to fruit-flavored drinks, and vitamin A added to margarine. The fact that many breakfast cereals are highly fortified may make them inappropriate for children, especially with respect to vitamin A.

Improving the quality of conventional food is done in a careful and systematic fashion. Industry is encouraged to follow guidelines which ensure the effectiveness and safety of fortification. In 1973 the Council on Food and Nutrition of the American Medical Association (AMA) and the Food and Nutrition Board of the National Research Council (NRC) recommended the nutritional improvement of conventional foods that meet the following critieria.[2]

1   The food is commonly consumed.
2   The added nutrient is:
    a   Below desirable levels of intake in diets
    b   Important to the overall diet
    c   Safe, not creating a dietary imbalance or, through excessive intake, not resulting in toxicity
    d   Stable during normal storage and usage
    e   Physiologically available from food
3   The additional cost is reasonable.

The addition of iron for enrichment and fortification has been controversial. Although pregnant and menstruating women and growing children need increased amounts of iron, the problem may not be solved by simply adding iron to foods. Both biological and technological problems must be faced. Not all iron compounds are bioavailable (i.e., in a form readily available to the body). Ferric phosphates, for instance, have limited or no bioavailability, according to research findings. Other compounds, like ferrous gluconate, ferrous sulfate, ferrous lactate, and reduced iron, have limited availability in comparison to natural iron. Addition of iron has also caused an undesirable color and flavor in foods.[3] Another consideration is that the foods to be fortified may not necessarily be consumed by the population at risk. Further research is necessary if iron deficiencies are to be prevented by simple enrichment or fortification.

Formulation

Supermarket shelves are filled with an ever-increasing number of formulated or "engineered" foods. These foods are complex mixtures of ingredients designed for a particular dietary use; both scientific and technological knowledge are employed in food processing to obtain products with predictable color, texture, odor, flavor, and nutritional quality. The products usually resemble existing, more natural products.[4] Such items include egg substitutes which have had the cholesterol and many saturated fats removed; meat substitutes, made of a soybean base, that resemble hot dogs, ground beef, or bacon; dairy substitutes made with vegetable oils, like nondairy creamers and margarine; and meal-replacement beverages and bars which have little or no resemblance to existing foods. In many developing nations where protein consumption is low, engineered foods with a soybean base have been developed to be a protein substitute (e.g., Incaparina).

The nutritional composition of engineered foods is a controversial issue. While many have been formulated to meet specific dietary needs, others have been developed purely to offer a convenience or to develop a new "taste" for the consumer. Although nutrients used to fortify the product often make a significant dietary contribution, other important nutrients, such as trace elements, may be lacking.

In order to ensure the nutritional quality of formulated foods, the AMA's Council on Food and Nutrition and the NRC's Food and Nutrition Board have established relevant guidelines.[5]

1 Formulated foods are significant to the diet if they contribute 5 percent or more of any recommended nutrient or energy requirement or if they act as substitutes for other foods.
2 Unless developed for a specific dietary reason, the substitute products should contain similar nutrients to those foods that they are formulated to resemble.
3 The quantity of protein and fat should be nutritionally appropriate to the food and its use.
4 Foods which are meal replacers should provide 25 to 50 percent of the actual or estimated RDA.
5 The energy content should be determined by the intended use.

Food processing is essential to the complex food production and marketing system in the United States. Careful selection of processed food can enhance the overall quality of the diet. Consumers need particular guidance in the appropriate use of processed food and an understanding of its nutrient value.

FOOD CONSUMPTION PATTERNS

The effect of industrialization and urbanization on family structure is reflected in the emerging food ways, or habits, of many American families, who rely heavily on fast-food chains, high-caloric snack foods, and convenience dinners. With the technological age promoting speed and efficiency, people have learned to eat quickly— standing at lunch counters and sitting behind the wheel of a car. Parents can even be seen feeding babies hastily, spooning a mouthful in before the first is swallowed. In addition, eating patterns are influenced by a host of sociological and psychological factors which transcend a conscious recognition of the health value of food. (See Chap. 10.)

Food at Home

The three-meals-a-day pattern has undergone changes in the last few years. The pattern which many people follow is that of little or no breakfast, a light lunch, and a large evening meal containing the bulk of the day's energy supply. Studies show that "gorging" at one time of the day results in single high glucose levels and continuous higher levels of free fatty acids in the serum. Smaller, more frequent meals result in lower levels.[6] The overall contribution of snacks should not be overlooked, as they can provide significant dietary components when chosen wisely. The concern over this food style is its nutritional adequacy, since foods high in calories and low in nutrients may be selected. Erratic eating patterns may also affect the utilization of nutrients. There is growing evidence of natural body rhythms that suggests better utilization of protein during the morning than at other times.[7,8] In addition, since the functions of many nutrients are interrelated a variety of foods eaten together is essential.

In the past heavy breakfasts were important for those involved in strenuous activity. However, a more sedentary life style and the many pressures on people's time have dictated changes in early morning eating patterns, for which there are several solutions. For example, for those in a hurry, meals of cheese and crackers with a piece of fresh fruit can help to supply nutritional needs.

Depending upon a person's lifestyle, a midday meal may be light or heavy. Regardless of its size, the meal should be balanced nutritionally and should fill the social and psychological needs of the individual. Bag lunches are often carried to the office and school. With careful thought these meals can fill the requirements

from all four food groups; e.g., either a peanut butter sandwich, an apple, and a carton of milk from the cafeteria or vending machine, or a ham and cheese sandwich and a can of fruit juice, can make a balanced lunch.

For most people, the evening meal is the largest of the day. Again, it should include a well-balanced selection of food. If lunch was large, this meal might be lighter. For the elderly and the bedridden, eating a larger lunch and smaller dinner is often recommended, and it may also be well advised for sedentary populations. No one pattern is recommended for dinner, as cultural patterns dictate many equally nutritious meals.

Table 2-1 provides guidelines to be considered in planning the family's daily meals and snacks.

Fast-Food Chains and Restaurants

Eating out is becoming a way of life in the United States. In 1977, 42 percent of the American food dollar went to the food service industry, and it is very likely that 50 percent of the food budget will be devoted to eating out in the 1980s.[9]

Most fast-food service has been aimed at two populations, young families and college students, although the middle-aged customer will be the target of more promotion in the 1980s. The nutritional quality of fast foods may be a problem if consumed frequently and regularly. Fast-food meals offer few choices and encourage a trend toward less variety in food intake. In general the meals are high in energy content and lack several essential nutrients (see Appendix, Nutrient Content of Typical Fast Foods). Studies indicate that the average take-out lunch consisting of a hamburger, french fried potatoes, and a milkshake provides about 800 kcal (3360 kJ). Most typical meal combinations range from 900 kcal (3690 kJ) to 1300 kcal (5330 kJ). This combination of foods may lack vitamin A, vitamin C, iron, several trace elements, and dietary fiber. Additionally, there are excessive quantities of fat, salt, and sugar. When soft drinks rather than dairy products are consumed as the bever-

TABLE 2-1   GUIDELINES FOR PLANNING MEALS AND SNACKS

1   Food patterns should be planned to provide *recommended servings from each of the four food groups* (vegetables and fruit; bread and cereal; milk and cheese; meat, poultry, fish, and beans) and should allow for sufficient calorie needs.

2   *Outside food sources* of the family, like school breakfast and lunch programs, congregate meal sites for elderly people, and restaurants should be considered as part of the food budget and total dietary program.

3   *Snacks and beverages* supplement nutrient needs. Those high in nutrients but low in calories should be readily available to members of the household.

4   *Special dietetic needs,* like fat or calorie restrictions or mechanical difficulties in eating, should be considered in overall planning in order to satisfy physical, social, and psychological needs.

5   *Aesthetic qualities* make a meal more appetizing. Variety of color, texture, flavor, temperature, and shape is important.

6   *Planning a week ahead* allows consumers to cut food costs and save time and energy.

7   The *size of the group* to be fed is an important consideration. A balanced diet cannot be eaten if there is an insufficient quantity of food. Too much food, on the other hand, may be a waste.

8   The *age of individuals* in the group is important. Young children eat less, and growing teenagers and those involved in strenuous activity may need more. Although the elderly require the same nutrients as younger adults do, their energy needs are lower.

9   *Food likes and dislikes* of family members influence the entire family's food patterns. Consideration of preferences and the provision of alternative foods when necessary helps to ensure adequate dietary consumption.

---

age, the meals are also low in calcium and riboflavin. It is important to recognize that many shakes are not made with dairy products but instead with fat-free milk solids with added thickening and sweetening agents.[9,10,11,12]

Well-balanced meals can be planned from a fast-food menu. Substitution of milk for a milkshake or soft drink will provide important nutrients without excessive calories. Including tomato and lettuce on the hamburger or adding a serving of cole slaw can help provide dietary fiber as well as vitamins A and C. Likewise, a slice of cheese will provide additional protein, B vitamins, and calcium.

Excess calories, ultimately transformed into fat, is the major dietary problem of many restaurant meals. Typical foods are fried, prepared in gravies, and buttered. Desserts are often made with large amounts of sugar and fat. Portions are generally larger than necessary. Those people who eat frequently at restaurants must learn to order those foods which balance their day's diet without adding excess calories.

The Creative Cuisine program sponsored by the American Heart Association is one way people can identify low calorie and low salt foods. In this program, some restaurants are voluntarily labeling menu items which are low in fat, sugar, and cholesterol.

Snacks

Between-meal eating is part of the American food style. Snack foods such as potato chips, pretzels, nuts, crackers, and spreads now gross $9 billion per year.[13] Coffee breaks and omnipresent vending machines are part of this pattern. Both the ubiquitousness of food and the increased purchasing power of children and adults contribute to between-meal eating. Although consumers generally do not regard snacking as an important part of the day's diet, snack foods do contribute significantly to the total diet. A study of teenagers' snacking patterns from the Ten-State Nutrition Survey showed that 23 percent of the day's total calories was consumed between meals. The average nutrient intake from snacks met or exceeded the RDA for protein, calcium, ascorbic acid, and thiamin. Intake of iron, vitamin A, and riboflavin was also significant.[14]

Since snack patterns are not only a way of life but play a significant nutritional role in the diet, nutritional educators should utilize this phenomenon and help people choose healthful snacks. Snacks which should be encouraged are those which supply nutrients, not merely calories, such as fruit, vegetables, crackers and cheese, peanut butter, nuts, whole-grain breads, milk, and milk products. Individuals who need to watch their weight should take special care to consume foods high in nutrients but low in calories, such as raw vegetables and skim milk products.

Beverages

In the day's total food pattern, beverages also play an important role. They satisfy thirst, supply nutrients, and fill psychological and social needs. While some beverages like milk and fruit and vegetable juices are excellent sources of nutrients, others provide water but few nutrients.

Like food patterns in general, the pattern of beverage consumption is changing, with the consumption of soft drinks replacing coffee and milk. Soft drinks, which are fast becoming the national beverage, provide calories but few nutrients. When consumers purchase low-caloric beverages, they do not even get calories for the money spent; moreover, such beverages use varying amounts of sugar substitutes with unknown long-term effects. The increased consumption of soft drinks is now a cause for concern. They alter the normal ratio of calcium to phosphorus in the diet because of the high phosphate content of these beverages.

Soft drinks can have a negative effect on the diet since they displace beverages which contain more nutrients. They may also pose a threat to weight and dental health because of their high sugar content. In addition, coffee, tea, cocoa, and cola beverages contain high levels of caffeine, theophylline, and theobromine. These substances are central nervous system stimulants and may also act as excessive stimulants to the cardiovascular system.

Intake of alcoholic beverages can be a problem. Nutritionally, these beverages contribute more in calories than in nutrients. Each gram of ethanol provides 7.1 kcal (29.8 kJ). Alcohol may, in fact, displace other more nutritious foods in the diet. Chronic alcohol consumption may interfere with the digestion and absorption of nutrients like thiamin, riboflavin, pyridoxine, folate, and zinc. Excessive amounts cause liver damage.

Intake of beverages should not be overlooked when one is assessing diets since it can provide many important dietary constituents. The dietary requirement of eight glasses of liquid per day is partially met by beverages. Consumers should be sure that the selection and quantity of their beverages will aid them in obtaining an adequate daily nutrient intake.

FOOD PURCHASING

Affluence, change in life-style, and the availability of a more diversified food supply have changed American patterns of food consumption. Since 1900, a notable change has occurred: sugar and fat intake have increased sharply while consumption of grain has decreased drastically. Protein intake has remained about the same, although more animal sources and fewer vegetable sources are being used, except by some more health-conscious individuals and vegetarians.

The food purchasing patterns of families are influenced by many demographic factors:

Family size. Large families and those with growing children and teenagers generally must spend more for food.

Regional differences in food costs. Traditionally costs of food are highest in the northeast while they are less in the south. Food purchased near its source of production is generally less expensive than food which must be transported. Home gardening and home preparation of food save the cost of producers' and processors' services.

Working women.   As women have entered the work force, their patterns of shopping and food preparation have changed. With less time and energy, convenience foods, simpler food preparations, and eating out are more common.

Inflation.   Inflation may negatively affect purchasing power, especially that of the poor. People who are more affluent can substitute equally nourishing but less expensive sources of food. The poor, however, are often already buying the least expensive sources of food and have few cheaper alternatives.

While food has always been a major budget item for many Americans, recent increases in food costs have made the expenditure even more significant. In 1960, food represented 16 percent of the budget, and by 1979 inflationary costs had escalated the food budget to an average of 25 percent and to over 31 percent for low-income people.[15] The rise is also reflected in the price of menu items in restaurants.

Adjustment in the expenditure for food must be based on the following factors.[16]

What foods are selected?

Where does the family buy food?

How much food is prepared at home?

Is some food produced at home?

How carefully does the family plan and make purchases?

What importance does the family place on food in relation to other family needs?

While most individuals need to be cognizant of food expenditures, those with low incomes need to be even more selective in their purchasing in order to meet basic nutrient needs. Because of their limited purchasing power, their choices are restricted.

Out of necessity, many of the poor have learned to put up with some degree of dreary monotony in eating most of the time.

An occasional feast, however, can be symbolically important. Welfare recipients who buy steaks and chops when the check is received and then eat skimpily toward the end of the month demonstrate behavior that is typical of many poor cultures around the world—the feast or famine custom of eating all you can hold when food is available and doing without when it isn't.[17]

As health professionals help families toward a more appropriate use of the food dollar, they must recognize both the limitation of resources and the psychological significance of food. Candy, potato chips, and liquor may be devices that are helping an individual to cope with life in a bleak, inner-city ghetto. Here middle-class values are inappropriate and should not interfere in counseling relationships. However, the health professional can attempt to motivate the individual toward the wise use of the food dollar, focusing on the person's own value system, what he or she feels is important, and the benefits of using a food budget.

Although federally subsidized food programs like food stamps and the special supplemental food program for women, infants, and children (see Chap. 16) have been developed to increase the purchasing power of the poor, they do not fill the gap—especially now, with federal cutbacks. More, not less, federal assistance is needed by the poor and those on fixed incomes such as the elderly and some handicapped persons.

Good nutrition begins with wise and careful purchasing behavior. With knowledge of the dynamics of the food market and skill in discerning quality products, and through nutrient labeling, unit pricing, open dating, and universal product coding, the consumer can purchase food that fits physical, social, and economic needs.

Economical Shopping

Most consumers are anxious to get the most for their food dollar. For many, careful shopping is the only way they can purchase an adequate supply of food. Supermarket psychology, however, is geared toward increasing sales. Meat counters often stretch across the ends of aisles so that customers will be attracted by meat, a high-profit item. Aisles are often long without breaks in the middle; consumers must walk the full length for a single item, passing shelves stocked with goods as they go. Cereals advertised on children's television are placed at youngsters' eye level. Store specials are also carefully placed at the ends of aisles so that they have prominence. Fresh produce is the first section that many shoppers encounter. These are items with special appeal because the consumer sees the food itself rather than a package; they are also high-profit items. A few simple suggestions can help to protect consumers from impulse shopping and allow them to cut costs and ultimately to shop wisely (see Table 2-2).

Labeling

The information provided on many food labels can help a shopper determine the contents and cost of the product, compare it to similar items on the shelf, understand how to use it, and learn

---

TABLE 2-2 GUIDELINES FOR ECONOMICAL SHOPPING

1 *Shopping lists* A consumer who plans food purchases ahead will not only eliminate unnecessary food purchases but will save time, energy, and transportation costs by not having to return to the supermarket. Also, studies indicate that shopping when hungry increases impulse buying.

2 *Store brands and generic products* Often the store brand of a specific item will cost 5 to 10 percent less than similar name-brand products. A generically labeled product with no brand name and little information on the label is even less expensive. Comparison shopping will provide the answer.

3 *Newspaper advertisements* Purchasing "specials" listed in weekly newspapers can provide savings. Although consumers were encouraged by nutrition educators in the past to take advantage of specials at many stores each week, limits on time and transportation costs may make this kind of shopping less economical.

4 *Coupons* Coupons, available through magazine and newspaper advertisements, direct mailings, and package labels, offer reduced prices on specific items, but they are useful only if the items are needed.

5 *Unit pricing* Comparison shopping is facilitated in some stores by unit pricing. This system allows consumers to compare the price on like quantities of specific products. On the shelf under each product the price per pound, serving, cup, etc., is given, rather than the price per package.

6 *Quantity purchases* If adequate storage is available and money can be tied up in food, the purchase of large quantities of food at one time can be a saving. However, buying a larger container is not a saving if the food is unused and ultimately discarded.

7 *Economy foods* By purchasing inexpensive cuts of meat, dried or evaporated milk, and less expensive produce like green beans and peas, the consumer can spend less in the supermarket for equally nutritious foods.

8 *Seasonal produce* Purchasing vegetables and fruits in season can reduce the food expenditure. If possible, it is wise to purchase large quantities for freezing or canning when they are in season, and to cook foods that are in season.

9 *Limitation of convenience foods* The consumer can generally save money by preparing food at home rather than purchasing the same item prepared. The cost of preparation is included in the price of convenience items like frozen dinners.

10 *Frequency of shopping* Research indicates that consumers spend less on food by shopping once or twice a month rather than once a week or more frequently.

11 *Food-buying cooperatives* Another way to save money on food is to become involved in a food cooperative, a nonprofit food outlet operated by its members. Consumers invest their time and energy to help the cooperative in exchange for being able to buy food at wholesale prices.

how to save money. All products must carry the following information on a package label:

Common name of the product

Name and address of the manufacturer, packer, or distributor

Variety, style, and packaging medium

Net weight or volume

Ingredients

Unless a food has a standard of identity, or a legal recipe, ingredient lists must appear on labels. All ingredients, including additives, must be listed in order by weight with those in the greatest quantity listed first. The listing is an aid to consumers who need to, or wish to, avoid certain ingredients.

Food labels must also carry a nutrient information panel if they are enriched or fortified or if an advertisement for the food makes a nutritional claim. Manufacturers may also provide this information voluntarily.

Nutrition information panels must follow a standard format. Serving size, servings per container, calories per serving, and grams of protein, carbohydrate, and fat must appear first. The amounts of eight nutrients—protein, vitamin A, vitamin C, thiamin, riboflavin, niacin, calcium, and iron—must be included in that order on the lower part of the label (see Fig. 2-1.) Other nutrients may be included at the discretion of the manufacturer. Examples of those not required but helpful for consumers to know are cholesterol, fats, sodium, and potassium.

Nutrients listed in the lower part of the label are expressed as percentages of the U.S. Recommended Daily Allowances. These are based on the Recommended Dietary Allowances (RDA) which will be discussed later in this chapter. Separate daily allowances have been defined for children under 4 and for pregnant and lactating women. The U.S. RDA should be used not to determine dietary adequacy but to compare foods. When stated on the label, cholesterol, polyunsaturated and saturated fats, and sodium and potassium are listed in milligrams and grams per serving.

Nutritional labeling can be a useful tool in

Figure 2-1
Food label with nutritional labeling and universal product coding. The food label has both mandatory information (common name of product, name and address of manufacturer, style, net weight, and ingredients) and voluntary information (nutritional labeling, storage instructions, recipe, and universal product code, which is in the lower right-hand corner). (Courtesy of National Dairy Council.)

MRS. O'LEARY'S small curd **COTTAGE CHEESE** 4% MILKFAT MINIMUM	**NUTRITION INFORMATION** (per serving)	STORE IN REFRIGERATOR

NUTRITION INFORMATION
(per serving)
Serving size = ½ cup
Servings per container = 4

| CALORIES | 120 | CARBOHYDRATE | 3 gm |
| PROTEIN | 15 gm | FAT | 5 gm |

PERCENTAGE OF U.S. RECOMMENDED DAILY ALLOWANCES (U.S. RDA)

PROTEIN	30	NIACIN	0
VITAMIN A	4	CALCIUM	6
VITAMIN C	0	IRON	0
THIAMINE (B₁)	0	VITAMIN B₁₂	10
RIBOFLAVIN (B₂)	10	PHOSPHORUS	15

INGREDIENTS: CULTURED SKIM MILK, MILK, CREAM, SALT, LOCUST BEAN GUM, GUAR GUM AND DEXTROSE

net wt. 16 oz. (1 lb.)   FRIENDLY DAIRY FOODS, INC. HOMETOWN, U.S.A. 87654

STORE IN REFRIGERATOR

COTTAGE CHEESE SALAD
Arrange lettuce on plate; top with cottage cheese, peach slices, pineapple, and fresh grapes.

12345 67890

nutrition education. A label can help consumers to identify the dietary quality of specific foods and compare them with similar items. By reading labels, persons on modified diets can decide which foods are appropriate for their daily consumption, but they must be reminded that not all nutrients are listed on all labels.

By creating a consumer awareness, nutrient labeling also pressures industry into monitoring and improving the nutritional quality of food. While this may force industry to be continually cognizant of the nutrient value of food, the food supply could become overfortified with some nutrients while those not listed on a panel could be forgotten. For this reason, a regulation was passed requiring that any food that contained added vitamins or minerals at a level of 50 percent or more of the U.S. RDA would be classified as a *dietary supplement;* supplements containing 150 percent or more of the U.S. RDA would be considered *drugs.* In the near future, other regulations may affect food labeling.

Open Dating and Universal Product Coding

Open dating is a system for informing consumers of the age and freshness of a packaged food. In the open dating system, dates have different meanings. To indicate the age of their product, manufacturers may use the packaging date or the pull date (date after which the product should be removed from the shelves).[18] Consumers can check with the store manager or the manufacturer to learn what an open date means in any particular case. It should be understood that the date indicates freshness only if the product has been properly handled and stored. A date cannot guarantee quality.[19]

Universal product coding (UPC) (see Fig. 2-1) is a new addition to many grocery labels. Its purpose is to cut costs for the retailer and ultimately for the consumer, to simplify storage, inventory, and ordering of merchandise, to speed check-out, and to reduce errors at check-out. The codes are standard ten-digit numbers with a machine-readable bar code that represents price, product, size, manufacturer, and the nature of the contents.[20] This code is read by an electronic scanning device at the check-out counter. A computerized receipt identifies the product, manufacturer, price, and weight and provides a record for consumers. Comparison shopping may be more difficult however since prices may not be marked on food packages.

FOOD HANDLING AND PREPARATION

Although the food industry influences the quality of food from the farm to the retail store, the consumer's domestic handling of the purchased food strongly affects its overall quality. Proper methods of *storage, sanitation,* and *cooking* are necessary.

Storage to Maintain Food Quality

Most food items can maintain quality in nutritional value, taste, texture, and appearance only for a finite period of time. Storage times and temperatures that are longer and higher, respectively, than optimal will result in deterioration in many foods. Other factors that may cause food spoilage include exposure to oxygen, moisture, and bacterial growth. For each product, the life and method of storage is specifically determined. All, however, must be properly covered or stored in suitable containers to protect against contamination and off-flavor.

All foods deteriorate over time. For instance, fats change through the chemical reactions of oxidation and hydrolysis. Protein molecules break down, causing textural changes and loss of functional properties like thickening and whipping qualities. Pigments change color as they oxidize, and some vitamins are lost through deterioration.[21]

The following losses, however, occur prematurely if food is not stored properly.[22]

Loss of nutrient value, such as vitamin loss and protein breakdown

Spoilage by microorganisms, enzymatic action, or insect infestation

Loss of aesthetic qualities such as color, flavor, aroma, texture, or general appearance

Loss of functional properties such as leavening activity in baking powder, thickening power in sauce mixes, or the "set" in instant puddings

Refrigeration is the preferred method for storing many fresh foods, including produce, dairy products, and all fresh meat, fish, poultry, and eggs. Food that requires refrigeration should be kept between 33°F (1°C) and 40°F (5°C); since bacteria, yeasts, and molds grow most rapidly at 50 to 120°F (10 to 49°C), an unrefrigerated product may become contaminated in as little as 3 to 4 h. Milk requires immediate refrigeration since exposure to sunlight also destroys riboflavin. Vegetables stay crisper when they are refrigerated and tightly covered. Refrigeration is also necessary for fats and oils since temperatures of 80°F (27°C) can cause rancidity. During the summer and when the refrigerator is heavily filled, the temperature should be set lower because nutrient losses are greater at these times. [23]

To maintain the quality of frozen food, the temperature inside freezers must be held at 0°F (−18°C) or lower. Most freezing compartments within refrigerators do not reach these low temperatures; therefore, storage periods in them should be short. Separate freezer units, however, generally do hold food at 0°F (−18°C) but should preferably be set even lower for long-term freezing.

Products stored at room temperature should be kept in cool, dry areas in airtight containers. This keeps moist foods like muffins from drying out and dry foods like breakfast cereals from losing their crispness. Moisture and heat are perfect conditions for bacterial growth. To protect against contamination by insects and rodents, foods should also be well sealed. Root and tuber vegetables can be stored at room temperatures not exceeding 70°F (21°C); higher temperatures cause rapid deterioration.

Sanitation in Food Handling

To minimize the incidence of food-borne illnesses (see Appendix Table A-14), food must also be handled properly. While food in the United States is among the safest in the world, many reported instances of food poisoning occur each year and many others go unreported. In 1977, 436 outbreaks of food poisoning were reported, involving 9896 individual cases. At that time bacteria caused 64 percent of these food illnesses. Chemicals caused 24 percent; parasites, 10 percent; and viruses, another 3 percent of the illnesses. In this period there were 8 resulting deaths. [24] Most of these illnesses could have been prevented if food had been handled properly.

Proper handling of food in the store is necessary for its safety. Consumers should find stores that maintain high standards of quality and cleanliness. The consumer should also follow simple rules of domestic food sanitation to eliminate the possibility of transmitting food-borne illness. Table 2-3 lists important guidelines.

Cooking Methods

Cooking enhances the palatability, digestibility, and safety of many food items. Preparation methods, however, also affect nutritional value, color, texture, taste, smell, and, ultimately, acceptability. Normal home cooking may result in high vitamin and mineral losses.

Overcooking or overheating a product can destroy its nutritive value, texture, color, and flavor. Nutrient loss primarily occurs in the water-soluble vitamins (the B complex vitamins and ascorbic acid) through leaching. Even proper cooking methods cause some nutrient loss, and overcooking may make that loss excessive.

Just as products should not be overcooked, they also should not be undercooked. Sufficiently high temperatures are necessary to destroy microorganisms. For example, meat, fish, and poultry should be cooked in order to destroy parasites, bacteria, and viruses that may be pres-

TABLE 2-3 RULES FOR SANITATION IN FOOD HANDLING

1 The refrigerator should be kept at 33 to 40°F (1° to 5°C).

2 Cooked foods should be refrigerated immediately. They should not be allowed to cool on the counter before being put in the refrigerator as this provides an ideal medium for bacterial growth.

3 Frozen foods should be thawed in the refrigerator, not on the counter.

4 Produce should be washed before it is eaten.

5 Foods that are kept at room temperature should be in airtight containers to protect them from insects, rodents, and dirt.

6 Anyone having an infectious illness (e.g., a cold) or sores on the hands should not prepare food.

7 Cans that have a leak or that bulge should be discarded *without tasting* the contents.

8 Products made with mayonnaise or cream fillings should be refrigerated immediately.

9 Hands, counter, and cooking equipment should be clean before food preparation begins.

10 A utensil should not be returned to a bowl after being licked.

11 After use, dishes, utensils, and cooking equipment should be washed in hot soapy water and carefully rinsed.

12 Hands should be washed after using the toilet or blowing the nose.

ent. Cooking destroys salmonellae. Pork in particular should be adequately cooked in order to eliminate the possibility of trichinosis. Legumes may carry toxic substances that are destroyed by cooking.

When preparing produce for cooking, the nutrient content can be retained in four ways:

1 Cut produce into larger rather than smaller pieces. The greater the exposed surface areas in cooking, the greater the loss of nutrients.

2 Scrub produce when possible rather than peel it. The outer skin of many produce items (e.g., potatoes, apples, carrots) contains abundant supplies of nutrients and fiber.

3 Use the least amount of liquid possible in cooking. Water-soluble vitamins are a particular problem since they are lost in the cooking water. The nutrient-containing liquids that remain after cooking should be saved for gravies and soups.

4 Use a shorter cooking time. Covering the pot will decrease the cooking time since the steam increases the temperature. Exceptions are vegetables like cabbage and onions that have a high sulfur content. The sulfur flavor of these vegetables becomes quite pronounced and less palatable if they are covered during cooking. Stir frying is another quick cooking method.

DETERMINATION OF DIETARY ADEQUACY

Many guides have been developed to aid consumers in making wise decisions in their food consumption patterns. With further research these guides will continue to be adjusted and updated. Ultimately, it is up to the consumers to be aware of these changes. Only then can they make informed food choices that reflect sound nutrition principles. Four guidelines have been developed to aid health professionals and consumers choose diets to meet nutrient needs:

Recommended dietary allowances
Food group systems
Nutrient density scores
Dietary guidelines for Americans

Recommended Dietary Allowances

The Recommended Dietary Allowances (RDA) represent nutritional standards for planning and

TABLE 2-4 A COMPARISON OF INTERNATIONAL NUTRIENT STANDARDS FOR SELECTED NUTRIENTS

Standard	Sex/ age	Weight, kg	kcal (kJ)	Protein, g	Fat-soluble vitamins					
					Vitamin A		Vitamin D		Vitamin E	
					μg	RE*	μg	IU	IU	mg d-α-tocopherol
Recommended intakes of nutrients, FAO/ WHO†	Male Adult	65	3000 (12,600)	37	750		2.5			
1980 Recommended Dietary Allowances, USA‡	Male 23–50	70	2700 (11,340)	56		1000		5		10
1975 Recommended daily nutrient intake, Canada§	Male 19–35	70	3000 (12,600)	56		1000		100		9

*RE: Retinol equivalents.

† H. S. Mitchell, H. J. Rynbergen, L. Anderson, and M. V. Dibble, *Nutrition in Health and Disease,* J. B. Lippincott Company, Philadephia, 1976, p. 296.

assessing dietary intake. They are defined by the Food and Nutrition Board of the National Research Council (NRC) as levels of intake of essential nutrients "designed for the maintenance of good nutrition of practically all healthy persons"[25] (see Appendix Table A-1). The guidelines are appropriately used only for normal, healthy members of the American population. Since their development in 1943, the allowances have been continually updated in accordance with the most current scientific research. Every 5 or 6 years new data are reviewed and both the RDAs and background information on nutrients and their functions are revised.

Other countries (e.g., Canada) have also developed their own standards as a means of improving nutritional status; standards have also been issued by the Food and Agriculture Organization (FAO) (see Table 2-4). Some standards give minimal nutrient needs and others list maximal nutrient needs (the latter provide a margin of safety). Most reflect nutrient needs based on differing life-styles and environments. The Canadian recommendations are similar in philosophy to those of the United States. The guidelines established by the FAO are set for minimum daily requirements and reflect the needs of a moderately active population.[26]

Determination of the RDAs Nutrient allowances are based on the most current and valid scientific evidence available. Ideally, recommendations consider (1) the *average* nutrient requirements of a representative segment of healthy people for each age group, (2) the statistical *variability* of people, and (3) the possible *increased requirement* above the average in order to meet the needs of almost all healthy Americans. A variety of research procedures are used to determine nutrient requirements. These include balance studies, biochemical measurements of nutrients, and clinical evaluations.

Scientific knowledge is well established for some nutrients, while relatively little data are available for others. Protein (see Chap. 3) is an example of a nutrient for which data are rather extensive. Establishing caloric guidelines is relatively easy since a close relationship exists between energy intake and energy expenditure. The study of vitamin A, however, has been limited.

	Water-soluble vitamins						Minerals					
Ascorbic acid, mg	Folacin, μg	Niacin, mg, NE[¶]	Riboflavin, mg	Thiamin, mg	Vitamin B_6, mg	Vitamin B_{12}, μg	Calcium, mg	Phosphorus, mg	Iodine, μg	Iron, mg	Magnesium, mg	Zinc, mg
30	200	19.8	1.8	1.2		2.0	400–500			5–9		
45	400	18.0	1.6	1.4	2.2	3.0	800	800	150	10	350	15
30	200	20.0	1.8	1.5	2.0	3.0	800	800	150	10	300	10

‡Food and Nutrition Board, *Recommended Dietary Allowances,* rev. ed. 1980, National Reserach Council Publications, National Academy of Sciences, Washington, D.C.

§Information Canada, Ottawa, KIA OS9, *Dietary Standard for Canada,* Catalog H58-26, 1975.

¶1 niacin equivalent (NE) = 1 mg niacin or 16 mg tryptophane.

Method of expression   The RDAs are grouped to apply to varying age and sex categories, and reflect the increased needs of pregnancy and lactation.

For most nutrients, the RDAs are expressed in metric measures. (The metric system is the internationally accepted standard of measure, and with the passage of the 1975 Metric Conversion Act, voluntary conversion to the metric system has been assisted through a national policy.) In the International System of Units, the *joule* is the unit of energy. Kilocalories are expressed also as kilojoules. One kilocalorie *(kcal)* equals 4.2 kilojoules *(kJ).* Historically many RDAs have been expressed in metric measure. For example, protein requirements are listed in grams while thiamin, ascorbic acid, calcium, and iron are expressed in milligrams. Several nutrients are listed in different measures. Vitamin A is given in retinol equivalents (RE); 1 RE equals 10 international units (IU) vitamin A or 1 μg retinol or 6 μg β-carotene. Niacin is listed in niacin equivalents (NE); 1 niacin equivalent equals 1 mg niacin or 60 mg of dietary tryptophan. Vitamin E is listed as α-tocopherol equivalents; 1 mg d-α-tocopherol equals alpha tocopherol equivalent (1 α-TE) 1. And last, vitamin D is listed as cholecalciferol; 10 μg cholecalciferol equals 400 international units (IU) vitamin D.

Influences on the RDA   The following factors influence the recommendations of nutrients for individuals: physiological state (growth, pregnancy, lactation), body size, sex, physical activity, environmental temperature, age, illness, and the presence of intestinal parasite.

Although *activity levels* will differ among individuals, the RDA for energy has been set to meet the needs of typically sedentary activity levels in the United States. Because of the high incidence of obesity and overweight in the United States, there is no need to include a margin of safety for energy.

Although much of the United States climate is temperate, the extreme *temperatures* found in some areas may influence nutrient needs. Prolonged exposure to cold temperatures increases requirements for energy while exposure to higher temperatures lowers these requirements due to reduced activity and energy expenditure.

As people *age* during adulthood, requirements for most nutrients do not change; however, energy need is decreased because of a lowered basal metabolic rate and reduced activity levels.

When a person is fighting *illness, surgical stress, injury, or intestinal parasites,* nutrient requirements need to be adjusted to accommodate for metabolic loss.

Interpretation and Use of the Recommended Dietary Allowances

The Recommended Dietary Allowances are grouped into three charts (See Appendix). The main chart, Recommended Daily Dietary Allowances, lists guidelines for 17 nutrients. A margin of safety has been added which allows for differences in nutrient requirements among individuals. This allowance is approximately the average requirement plus 30 to 50 percent.

The Estimated Safe and Adequate Daily Dietary Intakes of Additional Selected Vitamins and Minerals gives a suggested range of intake for 12 additional vitamins and minerals. Specific allowances have not been determined for these nutrients because there is not sufficient research yet available. Because less information is available, however, a range is given and the nutrients are not listed on the main table. The upper level should not be regularly exceeded since scientists are still determining what level is toxic.

Energy guidelines are provided in a chart entitled "Mean Heights and Weights and Recommended Energy Intake." The guideline along with a range recognizes that different people need different amounts of energy to maintain normal weight. Activity levels and age are among the factors which influence energy need. Energy allowances for children 18 and under are based on median energy intakes of children these ages who were followed in longitudinal growth studies. The values in parentheses indicate the energy intake of the 10th and 90th percentiles. Allowances for young adults are for light work. And the allowances for adults 51 and

older represent mean energy needs and allow for a 2 percent decrease in basal metabolic rate per decade and a reduction in activity of 200 kcal (840 kJ) per day between the ages of 51 and 75 and of 500 kcal (2100 kJ) and 400 kcal (1680 kJ) for men and women, respectively, over age 75. The numbers in parentheses show the range of energy intake appropriate for some adults.

As a tool for guiding nutrient intake, the RDA should be interpreted with these considerations:

1   RDAs are expressed in groupings by age, sex, and weight, with special recommendations for pregnant and lactating women.

2   RDAs do not designate a particular diet. They guide nutrient intake, not food intake.

3   RDAs are provided on the basis of daily intake. Fat-soluble vitamins are stored in the body, so that larger amounts may be consumed one day and used later; the average daily value is provided by the RDA.

4   RDAs are not designed for therapeutic needs (states of illness, stress, surgery).

5   Evidence is inadequate on which to base some allowances, such as those for adolescents, older adults, or users of contraceptives. RDAs do not completely represent the nutrient needs of these groups.

6   RDAs are appropriately used to evaluate diets of groups of people and not individual diets. When these data are coupled with clinical and biochemical evidence, dietary deficiencies can be identified. Many researchers have used *two-thirds* of the RDA as the breaking point between an adequate and an inadequate diet, which means that when the intake of a nutrient is two-thirds below the RDA, the diet may be deficient. Since the RDA is a somewhat arbitrary tool that is periodically revised on the basis of current research, *two-thirds of the RDA* must be used cautiously to express dietary adequacy.

7 RDAs do not establish the percentage of calories to be consumed from carbohydrate, fat, and protein.

8 The RDA level of protein must be exceeded in order to have adequate intakes of vitamin B_6, iron, and zinc.

9 RDAs are not established for all nutrients known to be essential to humans.

10 The RDAs are guidelines and not specific nutrient requirements for individuals. Failure of individuals to meet the RDAs does not necessarily indicate a deficiency state.

Food Group Systems

Food grouping systems are used throughout the world to translate nutritional needs such as those established by the RDAs into practical guidelines for food intake. Food groups are designed so that individuals fulfilling the specified criteria will consume necessary quantities of essential nutrients.

DAILY FOOD GUIDE

The grouping of specific foods is determined first and foremost by nutrient content, and then reflects availability of food, food patterns, and local nutrition problems (see Fig. 2-2). The system classifies foods into the following groupings according to their similarity in nutrient content: *vegetables and fruit; bread and cereal; milk and cheese; meat, poultry, fish, and beans.* Foods placed in each group have a high *nutrient density*, i.e., a high proportion of nutrients to the amount of calories (joules) supplied, whereas foods that are high in fats, oils, or sugar, and low in nutrients are classified outside the four food groups and into the *fats, sweets, and alcohol group*. These foods have a high caloric density, i.e., they have a high proportion of calories (joules) for the amount of nutrients provided (empty calories). They include sugar, potato chips, soft drinks, butter, margarine, mayonnaise, salad dressings, fats and oils, candy, jams,

Figure 2-2

Food groups. Food is classified into groups on the basis of nutrient content. By consuming recommended servings from the four groups with high nutrient density most individuals can be adequately nourished. Foods from the other groups provide calories but few nutrients. (Adapted from National Dairy Council.)

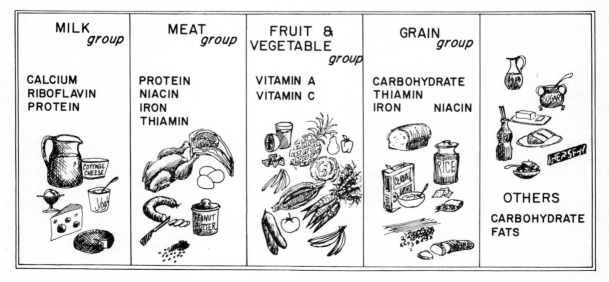

TABLE 2-5 DAILY FOOD GUIDE WITH NUTRIENT PATTERN AND RECOMMENDED QUANTITY

Group	Key nutrients	Quantity	Comments
Milk and cheese	Calcium, protein, phosphorus, riboflavin	Servings: Three for children, four for teenagers, two for adults. Add one for pregnancy and two for lactation. Serving size: 8 oz milk or yogurt 1⅛ oz cheddar or Swiss cheese 2 oz process cheese food 1½ cups ice cream or ice milk 4 tbsp or 2 oz process cheese spread or 4 tbsp Parmesan cheese 2 cups cottage cheese	Butter is not included in this group as it is a fat. Milk in foods such as pudding, sauce, and creamed soup counts toward a serving from this group. Low-fat milk products have generally the same nutrient content; however, they are lower in calories. Many milk products also contain significant amounts of vitamins A, B_6, and B_{12}.
Meat, poultry, fish, beans	Protein, B vitamins, iron	Servings: Two Serving size: 2–3 oz cooked lean meat, poultry, fish, without bones 1 egg ½ to ¾ cup cooked dry beans, dry peas, soybeans, or lentils 2 tbsp peanut butter ¼ to ½ cup nuts, sesame seeds, or sunflower seeds	Legumes, nuts, and soy extenders can be substituted for meat although the protein has a lower biological value than meat. These foods can be combined with animal or grain products to increase protein quality. Foods from this group also contribute a variety of other nutrients. Red meats are a good source of zinc. Egg yolks and liver are high in vitamin A. Dry beans, soybeans, and nuts are good sources of magnesium. Cholesterol and vitamin B_{12} are found only in animal sources. Egg yolks and organ meats contain the most cholesterol, while fish and shellfish (except shrimp) are low. Fish and poultry are also low in calories and saturated fats.
Vegetable and fruit	Vitamin A, vitamin C, carbohydrate (fiber)	Servings: Four Serving size: ½ cup vegetable or fruit 4 oz citrus juice 1 medium potato 1 medium fruit wedge of lettuce ½ medium grapefruit or cantaloupe juice of one lemon bowl of salad	One serving daily should be vitamin C–rich (e.g., citrus fruits). Vitamin A–rich foods (e.g., leafy green and yellow vegetables) should be consumed 3 or 4 times a week. Unpeeled fruits and vegetables and those with seeds such as berries contain fiber. Dark green vegetables are good sources of riboflavin, folacin, iron, and magnesium. Calcium is also found in collards, kale, mustard, turnip, and dandelion greens. Vegetables and fruits contain negligible fat.

TABLE 2-5 CONTINUED

Group	Key nutrients	Quantity	Comments

Bread and cereal (whole-grain or enriched)	Carbohydrate (fiber), B vitamins, iron	Servings: Four
		Serving size:
		  1 slice bread
		  ½ to ¾ cup cereal, cornmeal, grits, macaroni, noodles, rice, spaghetti
		  1 oz ready-to-eat cereal
			Whole-grain and enriched or fortified products are recommended grain foods. Whole-grain products also contain magnesium, folacin, and fiber. Bread and cereal products are a good source of low-quality protein. Many breakfast cereals are fortified to high levels with nutrients not normally found in cereal products; during processing, however, some essential nutrients are destroyed which are not added back. Less refined products are recommended.

Fats, sweets, alcohol	Fat, carbohydrate	Fats: In the total diet should be 35 percent of the total calories with 10 percent from polyunsaturated fat Sugar: In the total diet should not be more than 10 percent of the calorie intake Alcohol: None recommended	Unenriched, refined bakery products are included here because they provide low levels of vitamins, minerals, and protein compared to calories. The foods in this group provide mainly calories. Fats provide more than twice the calories, ounce per ounce, than carbohydrate and protein do. Alcohol contains almost twice the calories that carbohydrate and protein do. Vegetable oils are high in vitamin E and in essential fatty acids.

Source: Adapted from: *Food*, Home and Garden Bulletin No. 228, U.S. Department of Agriculture, Science and Education Administration, 1979.

jellies, syrups, sweet toppings, alcoholic beverages, refined but unenriched breads, pastries, and flour products This system also establishes the requirements for portion size and number of servings (see Table 2-5).

Daily food guide as a diet evaluation tool The food group system was designed primarily as an easy tool for the planning and evaluation of a day's meal pattern for normal, healthy individuals. A balanced diet is considered to include the recommended servings from each group. A balanced meal has one serving from each food group. The food group system was not designed to be an absolute measure of dietary quality. It is a simple, rough estimate that allows consumers and health professionals to check the intake of essential foods in order to plan a diet which offers the basic nutrient requirements for optimal health.

Certain physiological states require adjustments. For example, pregnant and lactating women require more than the usually recommended intake of foods from the meat, poultry, fish, or beans group and the milk and cheese group. A special guideline is provided for pregnancy and lactation. Infants and small children require smaller amounts of food than called for in the guideline. At the present time the daily food guide is a good system for a consumer's quick and easy dietary evaluation.

Limitations of the food group system   The following points should be considered when using food groups:

1   The high amounts of iron required by pregnant, lactating, and premenopausal women cannot be met by food group guidelines.
2   Strict adherence to the guideline without accompanying foods of high caloric density (e.g., gravies, condiments, etc.) may result in an energy intake that is lower than the needed for some individuals.
3   The guideline for protein-rich foods is high, providing excess protein in order to supply adequate quantities of vitamin B_6, iron, and zinc
4   Ready-to-eat processed and fabricated foods that are consumed in industrialized societies, like formulated fruit drinks and breakfast bars, cannot be classified into a food group because they may not follow the nutrient pattern of any one food group. In addition, they do not provide trace elements that are present in naturally occurring foods.
5   Overprocessing destroys nutrients in a given food; thus, a food may no longer represent a serving from a food group. For example, potato chips cannot be included in the vegetable and fruit group.
6   Combinations of foods like casseroles and pizzas make group classification difficult. They should often be classified into two or more groups.
7   It may be difficult to utilize the food group system when assessing the diet of particular ethnic groups (e.g., Chinese-American).

While food grouping systems have limitations, they are still an invaluable tool in nutrition counseling and education. It is essential to be flexible, understanding that a wide variety of food combinations can satisfy a person's nutrient requirements.

Food group scoring system   Food groups are simple guidelines for evaluating a patient's diet that can be used both by health professionals and by individuals themselves. This is done by recording all food intake for a 24-h period or longer and then scoring the diet using the food groups as a guideline. Generally a 3- or 7-day record provides more information about adequacy than a single-day record because an average food score can be determined (see Chapter 18).

Once the intake of food has been recorded, it should be compared with the quantity suggested by the four food groups. Table 2-6 is an example of a scoring system used to rate diets. The amount of each item consumed is recorded in one column. One point is recorded for *each full serving consumed*. Table 2-6 lists serving sizes. A score is then determined for each food group, and a grand total is assigned for the diet. The optimum scores are 12, 13, and 14 for adults, children, and teenagers, respectively. The scoring needs to be adjusted for pregnancy and lactation.

Within the milk and cheese group each age group has different requirements; as a result the total possible points to be earned will vary. The vegetable and fruit group also has special scoring requirements. In order to receive a possible 4 points in this group, one serving each of vitamin A–rich and vitamin C–rich foods must be consumed, for which a maximum of 2 points is given, with all other vegetables contributing another possible 2 points. Using this food pattern summary, data on food intake may be evaluated.

NUTRIENT DENSITY

Nutrient density, the ratio between the calorie content and the nutrient composition in a food, is a new system of indicating food quality. The resulting scores are useful in helping health professionals or consumers assess the nutritional quality of individual foods and diets. The methodology is still under investigation.

TABLE 2-6 SCORING SYSTEM FOR A FOOD RECORD

Food group	Serving size	Amount consumed	Total no. servings consumed	Total possible points	Score for food group
Milk and cheese					
Milk	1 cup			2 (adults) 3 (children) 4 (teenagers) (add 1 for pregnancy add 2 for lactation)	
Cheese	1 oz cheddar 1½ cup cottage				
Yogurt	8 oz				
Ice cream	1½ cups				
Others					
Meat, poultry, fish, and beans					
Meat, fish, poultry	3 oz				
Eggs	2			2	
Nuts	½ to 1 cup				
Legumes, beans	1 to 1½ cups				
Others					
Vegetables and fruits					
Vitamin C–rich	½ cup fruit or vegetable juice 1 medium-size fruit			1	
Vitamin A–rich	½ cup dark green or yellow fruit or vegetable			1	
Others				2	
Bread and cereal					
Bread	1 slice				
Cereal	½ cup			4	
Others					
Fats, sweets, and alcohol					
Sweets					
Fats and oils					
Soft drinks				0	
Coffee, tea					
Alcohol					
Total points					
Optimum score					
Children				13	
Teenagers				14	
Adults				12	
Pregnancy				13 (Adults) 15 (Teenagers)	
Lactation				14 (Adults) 16 (Teenagers)	

One system shows an index of nutritional quality derived using the following equation:

$$\text{Index of nutritional quality (INQ)} = \frac{\text{amount of nutrient in 1000 kcal (42 MJ) portion of food}}{\text{recommended daily allowances for that nutrient per 1000 kcal (42 MJ)}}$$

In this system, the nutrient profile of a food can be illustrated using a bar graph to show the INQ for protein, calcium, iron, vitamin A, thiamin, niacin, and vitamin C. This graphic representation gives a picture of a food's contribution to the total diet. By adding the INQ for each nutrient, a composite profile of the meal is derived.[27]

A simplified nutrient density food scoring tool has been devised to help consumers discriminate between good nutrient sources and "empty calorie" foods. The system has some limitations, however, since specific information on each nutrient is not provided. Scores are derived by adding together the INQs for the eight nutrients. Total scores for fats, sugars, soft drinks, and alcohol are zero, while those for more nutritious foods are high; for example, turnip greens score 296.[28]

Food Composition Tables as a Tool for Evaluating Diets

Food composition tables, giving the approximate nutrient content of foods, are a necessary tool for evaluating diets. Tables are expressed in either 100-g portions of a food, the edible portion of 1 lb of food, or portions commonly consumed. Energy is expressed as calories, and nutrients are generally indicated using metric measure or international units (or retinol equivalents for vitamin A). The values represent the average nutrient content of food items throughout the year and throughout the United States. An average is taken from research on a variety of weighed samples. Actual analysis is completed by government, universities, and industry.

When using composition tables for dietary evaluation, nutrient values must be considered in proper perspective. They are estimates and not the exact nutrient content of specific foods.

1   Growing conditions (e.g., sunlight, soil, climate) affect the nutrient content of the same variety of a food.

2   There is variability in a plant food, depending upon maturity, variety, season, and plant part.

3   Storage, processing, and preparation influence nutrient values.

4   The total amount of the nutrient listed may not be biologically available to an individual.

Available food composition tables include:

Composition of Foods: Raw, Processed, and Prepared, USDA Handbooks (series of handbooks for each food category), United States Department of Agriculture, Washington, D.C.

Nutritive Value of American Foods in Common Units, USDA Handbook No. 456, United States Department of Agriculture, Washington, D.C., 1975.

Food Values of Portions Commonly Used, J. A. Pennington and H. H. Church, J. B. Lippincott Co., Philadelphia, 1980, 13th ed.

DIETARY GUIDELINES FOR AMERICANS

The limitations of the food group system have resulted in other guidelines for planning healthful diets. Though controversial, the government released Dietary Guidelines for Americans

(February 1980), which can help consumers choose and prepare foods which promote overall well-being.

Because health depends on heredity, lifestyle, and attitudes, adherence to these guidelines does not necessarily guarantee health. However most health professionals agree that a diet based on moderation and variety promotes health. Disagreement about the guidelines centers on the role of the government in issuing dietary advice and the lack of conclusive evidence on the role of saturated fat and cholesterol in heart disease or sodium intake in hypertension. In addition there are concerns on the impact of the guidelines on government food programs and agriculture policy. The guidelines are summarized in Table 2-7.

The guidelines evolved from the Dietary Goals for the United States first released by the U.S. Senate Select Committee of Nutrition and Human Needs. During the summer of 1979, the first Surgeon General's Report on Health Promotion and Disease Prevention was released. It stated that Americans would probably be healthier if they followed certain dietary guidelines given what is already known or strongly suspected about the relationship between diet and disease. In the report the guidelines are compatible with the U.S. Dietary Goals but specific levels of consumption are not recommended.

TABLE 2-7 DIETARY GUIDELINES FOR AMERICANS

Eat a variety of foods.

Maintain ideal weight.

Avoid too much fat, saturated fat, and cholesterol.

Eat foods with adequate starch and fiber.

Avoid too much sugar.

Avoid too much sodium.

If you drink alcohol, do so in moderation.

Source: Ideas for Better Eating: Menus and Recipes to Make Use of the Dietary Guidelines, U.S. Department of Agriculture, Science and Education Administration, Human Nutrition, January, 1981.

THE ADEQUATE DIET— THE PRUDENT DIET

The adequate diet for our population must now become the "prudent diet" to combat many of our diet-related diseases and conditions such as coronary heart disease, obesity, and now perhaps even cancer. The prudent diet will still contain foods from the four food groups but more low-fat milk products and poultry, fish, and beans will be encouraged, with eggs kept to a maximum of three times per week. Vegetables and fruit and whole-grain breads and cereals will be emphasized for fiber, and combinations of these foods may be used to supply future protein needs and help to preserve dwindling protein reserves. The future of our health now depends on the adequate diet's becoming the prudent diet. The prudent diet contains:

Food groups	Prudent diet
Milk and cheese	Skim milk
Meat, poultry, fish, and beans	Chicken, fish, eggs 3x/wk
Vegetable and fruits	Increase
Bread and cereal	Whole-grain
Other: Fats, sweets, and alcohol	Less sugar Less fat Less salt Less alcohol Fewer additives

STUDY QUESTIONS

1 Are fortified, enriched, and engineered foods a benefit or detriment to the diet? Explain your answer.

2 What information can the label provide for the consumer?

3 What steps must be taken to reduce possibilities of food-borne illness?

4 For what purpose is the RDA used? What are its limitations?

5 In what way is the Daily Food Guide an appropriate tool for dietary evaluation?

CLINICAL STUDY 2

S., who is 32, heads a single-parent household. She works as a clerk receiving minimum wage during the day. Her 6-year-old daughter attends first grade and her 4-year-old son goes to a day-care center. Her family budget is modest. Although she receives financial assistance for her children, she does qualify for food stamps. Inflation makes grocery shopping more and more of a challenge, and often she quickly shops for the evening meal after work. Her work and family schedule also require careful budgeting of time and physical energy. This is her typical dietary pattern during a work day:

9:00 A.M.   1 cup black coffee with 1 teaspoon sugar

10:30 A.M.   1 cup black coffee with 1 teaspoon sugar, candy bar

12:30 P.M.   1 slice American cheese, lettuce leaf, and 1 tablespoon mayonnaise on 2 slices white bread, apple, 12 oz soft drink

6:00 P.M.   convenience dinner with 3 oz chopped beef, ½ cup green beans, ½ cup mashed potatoes, 2 tablespoons gravy, 1 cup black coffee with 1 teaspoon sugar

9:00 P.M.   1½ cups popcorn

Clinical study questions

1   Score this diet according to the Daily Food Guide. What is missing?

2   What recommendations would you make to improve the adequacy of this diet?

3   What suggestions would you make for economical shopping?

4   How could she prepare meals which would conserve her time and energy?

REFERENCES

1   Institute of Food Technologists' Expert Panel on Food Safety and Nutrition and the Committee on Public Information, "The Effects of Food Processing in Nutritional Values," Chicago, October 1974.

2   Food and Nutrition Board, "Improvement of the Nutritive Quality of Foods," Journal of the American Medical Association, August 27, 1973, p. 63.

3   "Problems in Iron Enrichment and Fortification of Foods," Nutrition Reviews, February 1975, p. 46.

4   Ibid., p. 65.

5   Ibid., p. 63.

6   W. M. Bortz, P. Howat, and W. L. Holmes, "The Effect of Feeding Frequency on Diurnal Plasma Free Fatty Acids and Glucose Levels," Metabolism, February 1969, p. 120.

7   R. J. Wurtmam, "Biologic Rhythms in the Body," Technical Review, March 1968, p. 3.

8   R. J. Wurtman, C. M. Rose, C. Shou, and F. F. Larin, "Daily Rhythms in the Concentrations of Various Amino Acids in Human Plasma," New England Journal of Medicine, July 25, 1968, p. 171.

9   Ross Laboratories, "Perspectives on Fast Foods," Dietetic Currents, September–October 1978, p. 25.

10   J. Goldberg, "The Fast Food Phenomenon," Family Health, April 1975, p. 39.

11   H. Appledorf, "Nutritional Analysis of Food from Fast Food Chains," Food Technology, April 1974, p. 50.

12   L. F. Chem and P. A. LaChance, "An Area of Concern: The Nutritive Profile of Fast Food Combinations," Food Product Development, October 1974, p. 40.

13   Twelfth Annual State of the Snack Food Industries Report, Snack Food Magazine, June 1980, Chicago.

14   J. A. Thomas and D. L. Call, "Eating between Meals—A Nutrition Problem Among Teenagers?" Nutrition Reviews, May 1973, p. 137.

15   U.S. Bureau of Labor Statistics, Autumn 1979 Urban Family Budgets and Comparative Indexes for Selected Urban Areas, April 30, 1980, p. 2.

16   B. Peterkin, "Food Plans and Family Budgeting," Family Economic Review, May 1975, p. 3.

17 H. H. Gift, M. B. Washbon, and G. Harrison, *Nutrition Behavior and Change,* Prentice-Hall, Inc., Englewood Cliffs, N.J., 1972, p. 104.

18 F. J. McEwen, "Consumer Problems in Relation to the Food Industries," in J. Mayer (ed.), *U.S. Nutrition Policies in the Seventies,* W. H. Freeman and Co., San Francisco, 1973, chap. 16.

19 E. F. Taylor, "Guide to Buying—Open Dating and Price per Unit," *Shopper's Guide, 1974 Yearbook of Agriculture,* U.S. Department of Agriculture, 1975.

20 Health and Consumer Product Department, "Looking Ahead to Automation in the Supermarkets," *Dow Dairy,* Fall 1975.

21 Institute of Food Technologists' Expert Panel on Food Safety and Nutrition and the Committee on Public Information, "Shelf Life of Foods," Chicago, August 1974.

22 Ibid.

23 B. C. Hobbs, *Food Poisoning and Food Hygiene,* 2d ed., Edward Arnold, Ltd., London, 1968.

24 Center for Disease Control, *Foodborne and Waterborne Disease Surveillance,* U.S. Department of Health, Education, and Welfare, Public Health Service, Atlanta, 1979.

25 Food and Nutrition Board, *Recommended Dietary Allowances,* rev. 9th ed., National Academy of Sciences, Washington, D.C., 1980.

26 J. A. Campbell, "Approaches in Revising Dietary Standards—Canadian, U.S., and International Standards Compared," *Journal of American Dietetic Association,* February 1974, p. 175.

27 R. Hansen and B. W. Wyse, "Expression of Nutrient Allowances Per 1000 Kilocalories," *Journal of American Dietetic Association,* **76:**223–227, 1980.

28 A. Dickinson and W. T. Thompson, "Nutrient Density Scores," *Journal of Nutrition Education,* July–September 1979, p. 119.

CLINICAL DISCUSSION 2

Scoring S.'s diet using the Daily Food Guide revealed a score of 6 (see Table 2-8, p. 38). The diet contained only one serving from the milk and cheese group, no vitamin A– or vitamin C–rich fruits or vegetables, only one serving from the meat, poultry, fish, and beans group, and just two servings of breads and cereals. This places her at nutritional risk for vitamins A and C, and at moderate risk for calcium, phosphorus, protein, iron, riboflavin and other B vitamins. Her diet is high in empty calories (soft drinks, candy, sugar, gravy, mayonnaise).

The following dietary changes are recommended:

1 *Morning:*
Eat breakfast instead of midmorning empty calorie snacks. Include low-cost, easy to prepare meals such as cereal, milk and fruit. Breakfast is a good time to include a vitamin C–rich fruit or juice. If possible, avoid sugar in coffee, and substitute milk for added nutrients.

2 *Lunch:*
Plan balanced meals with servings from *each* food group. Add vitamin A–rich fruits and vegetables frequently. Carried lunches could include hard-cooked eggs, tuna salad, or peanut butter. Drink milk or fruit juice instead of soft drinks. Fruit juice in cans can be frozen and used to keep a carried lunch cold.

3 *Dinner:*
Plan balanced meals. Include vitamin A–rich fruits and vegetables frequently. Drink milk as a beverage. Save money by making homemade convenience dinners. Prepare quantities of food ahead, and freeze in portions for family meals.

4 *Snacks:*
Choose snacks to balance out the day's diet. Take nutritious, less expensive snacks to work, such as a piece of fruit. Eat a balanced breakfast, so that midmorning snacks perhaps will not be necessary.

By planning ahead, S. can budget her resources—money, time, and energy—more carefully. To save time and energy, she might make shopping lists; prepare meals ahead and freeze; make quick dishes such as macaroni with cheese and tomato sauce, or omelets filled with grated cheese or chopped vegetables, or stir-fried dishes; organize her kitchen well so that she can prepare food and clean up efficiently; and do some food preparation ahead of time, such as making orange juice for breakfast the night before.

TABLE 2-8   DAILY FOOD GUIDE SCORING SYSTEM

Food group	Amount consumed	Total no. servings consumed	Total possible points	Score for food group
Milk and cheese				
Milk			2 adults (nonpregnant and nonlactating)	
Cheese	1 slice	1	3 children	1
Yogurt			4 teenagers	
Ice cream			(add 1 for pregnancy)	
Others			(add 2 for lactation)	
Meat, poultry, fish, and beans			2	
Meat, poultry, fish	3 oz chopped meat	1		1
Eggs				
Nuts or legumes				
Others				
Fruit and vegetable				
Vitamin C–rich			1	0
Vitamin A–rich			1	0
Others	1 leaf lettuce	3	2	2
	apple			
	½ cup green beans			
	½ cup mashed potatoes			
Bread and cereal			4	
Bread	2 slices white bread	2		2
Cereal				
Others				
Fats, sweets, and beverages				
Sweets	1 candy bar / 3 tsp sugar			
Fats and oils	2 tbsp gravy / 1 tbsp mayonnaise			
Beverages: e.g., coffee, tea, Coke, Kool-Aid, alcohol	12 oz soft drink / 3 cups coffee			
Others	1½ cup popcorn			
Grand total				6

Note: Optimum points: Children 13, teenagers 14, adults 12, pregnant adults 13, pregnant teenagers 15, lactating adults 14, lactating teenagers 16.

CHAPTER 3
PROTEIN

Ruth Palombo

KEY WORDS
Conjugated Proteins
Peptide Bonds
Essential Amino Acids
Nonessential Amino Acids
Transamination
DNA (Deoxyribonucleic Acid)
RNA (Ribonucleic Acid)
Deamination
Decarboxylation

INTRODUCTION

The controversy over protein requirements has sparked a lively debate in both the scientific and popular literature.[1,2] Today the subject of protein nutrition is a major political, economic, and social issue. The potential problem of world hunger cannot be taken lightly. Are we facing a protein crisis? In the mid 1970s, we were warned of a grain deficit of 85 million tons in developing countries by 1985 if food production did not increase.[3] Nutritionists, economists, and politicians speculate on ways to develop, use, and redistribute the world's agricultural resources. Still we have no national plan developed nor are we focusing our scientific and technical knowledge toward meeting the increased needs for food production around the world.

Although protein is available from many sources, each nation usually has a particular protein food or food combination which serves as its dietary staple. In the United States this food has traditionally been meat. Americans are very fond of meat, and with increasing affluence people consume more meat. Even in families with low incomes, a major part of the food budget is spent on meat, poultry, and fish, with little money left for other foods such as dairy products, fruits, and vegetables.[4] Consumers in the United States are very sensitive to meat prices. Evidence of this was the 1973 nationwide boycott of meat touched off by rising meat prices. Yet as food prices rise, many people have begun questioning whether they should change their eating practices; that is, eat less meat and more of alternative protein sources.[5]

Consumption of protein has generally been high in the United States, with patterns of inadequate intakes being a problem in only a few select age and income categories.[6,7] Sixty years ago flour and cereal products supplied 36 percent of our protein, and meat, fish, and poultry only 30 percent. Today cereal products provide 18 percent of our daily protein while meat, fish, and poultry supply 42 percent. These shifts in consumption of meat and cereal products represent major changes in the source of dietary proteins in the American diet.[8] These trends may be reversed again if the new dietary goals impact significantly on the eating patterns of Americans (see Chap. 2).

In addition to the current controversy over the use of protein, the confirmed role of protein in growth and the maintenance of body tissue, and its newly discovered role in the body's immune defense system, make the knowledge of protein essential to the student who will establish a nutrition-centered health practice.

FUNCTIONS OF PROTEINS

Proteins have a wide range of specialized functions and characteristics. They are necessary for:

1 Growth
2 Maintenance and repair of body tissues
3 Energy supply

Yet, despite the diversity of functions, proteins have some common characteristics. Proteins are large organic molecules of which simpler compounds called *amino acids* are the basic structural unit. When proteins are broken down (hydrolyzed), they split into these amino acids. All proteins contain the elements carbon, hydrogen, nitrogen, and oxygen. Many proteins contain sulfur and phosphorus and some also contain metallic components such as iron, zinc, and copper. Each gram of protein supplies 4 kcal (17 kJ) when metabolized. However, it is the presence of nitrogen that makes protein unique and differentiates it from fat and carbohydrate, the other energy-yielding nutrients in our diet.

When we eat, food proteins supply our bodies with amino acids for synthesis of body proteins and nitrogenous compounds. During normal tissue turnover some amino acids are released and are reused for synthesis of body protein. Other products of amino acid metabolism such as urea, creatinine, and uric acid are excreted in the urine. Nitrogen is also lost through many body secretions, excretions, sweat, feces, sloughed skin, hair, and nails. Therefore, in order to replace these losses, dietary proteins which supply amino acids and nitrogen are necessary throughout the life cycle, even when growth has stopped.

The human body is approximately 18 to 20 percent protein by weight. Protein provides the structural framework for our bodies. Muscles contain about 45 percent of this protein and the skeleton about 18 percent. Skin and adipose tissues contain about 10 and 4 percent respectively of the body's total protein.[9]

CLASSIFICATION OF PROTEINS

Proteins can be classified in many ways. One common method is to describe proteins as either simple or conjugated. *Simple proteins* consist of only amino acids. Upon hydrolysis, they yield only amino acids. There are no nonprotein constituents in simple proteins. *Conjugated proteins* consist of simple proteins plus a prosthetic group (nonprotein constituent). Upon hydrolysis, conjugated proteins are broken down into amino acids and other substances. Examples of conjugated proteins are nucleoproteins (protein and RNA or DNA), lipoproteins (protein and lipid), glycoproteins (protein and carbohydrate), and metaloproteins (protein and metal such as zinc, copper, or iron). Another way to group proteins is according to function (see Table 3-1).

CLASSIFICATION OF AMINO ACIDS

The general formula for the amino acids found in protein can be represented as the following:

$$NH_2 \quad \boxed{\text{Amino group}}$$
$$R - C - COOH$$
$$\boxed{\text{Side chain}} \quad H \quad \boxed{\text{Carboxyl group}}$$

As indicated, the amino acid is formulated from a carbon chain (carbon skelton), and the amino and radical groups are then added. Since the amino group is on the carbon adjacent to the carboxyl group (the alpha carbon), the amino acids having this formula are known as alpha-

TABLE 3-1 CLASSIFICATION OF PROTEIN BY FUNCTION

Classification	Body location	Example	Function
Structural proteins	Skin, cartilage, bone	Collagen	Principal substance in connective tissue
Contractile proteins	Skeletal muscle	Actin, myosin	Muscle contraction
Antibodies	Blood plasma, spleen, lymphatic cells	Alpha globulins	Disease protection
Blood proteins	Blood plasma	Albumins	Control osmotic pressure of blood
			Maintain the buffering capacity of blood pH
	Blood	Fibrinogen	Blood clotting
	Blood	Hemoglobin	Transports oxygen from lungs to all parts of the body
Hormones	Endocrine or ductless glands (thyroid, pancreas, parathyroid, adrenals, pituitary)	Insulin	Regulates carbohydrate metabolism
		Growth hormone	Stimulates overall protein synthesis and growth
Enzymes	Throughout body— nearly 2000 different enzymes known; each highly specific in function		Biological catalysts; proteins which allow chemical reactions to proceed at their proper rate
	Stomach	Pepsin	Protein digestion
	Pancreas	Trypsin and chymotrypsin	Protein digestion
Nutrient proteins		Meat, fish, chicken, milk, cheese, eggs, peanut butter, nuts, soybeans, tofu, dried peas and beans	Sources of amino acids required by humans and other animals
Viruses	Microscopic infective agents	Smallpox, measles	Cause disease
Nucleoproteins	Cell nucleus	DNA	Determines and transmits hereditary characteristics; carries genetic (hereditary) code

amino acids. All amino acids have a free carboxyl group (COOH) and a free amino group (NH$_2$) on the alpha carbon atom. Amino acids differ from each other according to their unique side chains or R groups. There are 20 different amino acids which serve as the building blocks of protein. Amino acids are usually grouped according to their chemical nature. The classification is as follows:[10]

1 Monoamino monocarboxylic: glycine, leucine, alanine, isoleucine, valine
2 Hydroxyl-containing: serine, threonine
3 Sulfur-containing: cystine, cysteine, methionine
4 Aromatic: tryosine, phenylalanine
5 Heterocyclic: proline, hydroxyproline, histidine, tryptophan
6 Diamino monocarboxylic (basic): arginine, lysine
7 Monoamino dicarboxylic (acidic): glutamic acid, aspartic acid

Amino acids are joined together in proteins by linkages called *peptide bonds:*

$$R-\underset{\underset{H}{|}}{\overset{\overset{NH_2}{|}}{C}}-COOH + H_2N-\underset{\underset{H}{|}}{\overset{\overset{R}{|}}{C}}-COOH \underset{\underset{+H_2O}{hydrolysis}}{\overset{\overset{-H_2O}{synthesis}}{\rightleftharpoons}}$$

$$R-\underset{\underset{H}{|}}{\overset{\overset{NH_2}{|}}{C}}-\boxed{\underset{\substack{Peptide\\bond}}{CO-NH}}-\underset{\underset{H}{|}}{\overset{\overset{R}{|}}{C}}-COOH$$

These linkages are formed by the attachment of the carboxylic carbon of one amino acid to the nitrogen of another amino acid. At the same time, a molecule of water is eliminated.

In protein molecules, the amino acids are linked together in long chains called *polypeptides.* (A *peptide* is two or more amino acids linked together; a *polypeptide* is many amino acids linked together.) Polypeptides are large molecules which may consist of hundreds of amino acids in the form of a helix or spiral. Some proteins consist of only one polypeptide chain; some contain two, three, or more. The specific function of each protein depends on its constituent amino acids and the arrangement of the amino acids in the polypeptide chain. The number, kind, and sequence of the amino acids (known as the *primary structure*) in each polypeptide chain of each protein is genetically determined by DNA (deoxyribonucleic acid) on the chromosomes (see "Protein Synthesis," below). Each polypeptide chain has its own unique characteristics:

1 Specific molecular weight
2 Specific chemical composition
3 Definite amino acid sequence
4 Definite three-dimensional shape

The molecular weights of proteins vary from 5000 to 1 million. Most polypeptide chains contain 100 to 300 amino acids and have a molecular weight of 12,000 to 36,000.[11]

DETERMINANTS OF PROTEIN REQUIREMENTS

Nitrogen Balance

Determining nitrogen balance provides a gross measure of protein utilization. This determination is based on the assumption that nitrogen equilibrium occurs in adults when the diet supplies adequate protein for (1) synthesis of tissues (such as hair and nails) and (2) replacement of endogenous losses in the urine, feces, sweat, and sloughed epithelial cells. Theoretically, the formula for nitrogen balance is

Nitrogen balance = dietary nitrogen intake
— nitrogen losses
(urine + feces + skin)
Balance = intake − losses

Measuring the amount of nitrogen eaten in food and comparing this to the amount excreted in the feces helps to determine nitrogen balance. A *positive nitrogen balance* indicates that the body is retaining nitrogen, while a *negative balance* signifies that more nitrogen is being catabolized than consumed. When the nitrogen in the food consumed equals what is excreted, nitrogen balance is zero and the body is in *nitrogen equilibrium*. Nitrogen balance is affected by physiological state, energy requirements, and diet.

Physiological state   Childhood growth periods, pregnancy, and lactation are characterized by a marked positive nitrogen balance. When an individual is under severe stress from infection, fever, surgical trauma, or starvation, protein is depleted from the tissues, resulting in negative nitrogen balance. There is no evidence at present to indicate that the normal stresses of daily living increase our protein needs.

Energy requirements   The body's need for energy takes priority over the body's need for nitrogen. If energy derived from fat and carbohydrate is inadequate, protein from the diet and from tissue breakdown are used for energy. Diets must be adequate in fat and carbohydrate in order to spare protein for its unique functions.

Diet   Nitrogen balance depends on the proportions of essential amino acids in the diet plus the total nitrogen intake. When an adult is in nitrogen equilibrium, this indicates that the diet is probably adequate in essential amino acids.

Essential and Nonessential Amino Acids

The proteins in the human body are made up of 20 amino acids in varying combinations. Each protein has its own unique amino acid composition. Eight of these amino acids cannot be synthesized by the body in large enough quantities to meet body needs. These amino acids, because they must be supplied by food, are known as the *essential amino acids*. They are:

Tryptophan	Valine
Leucine	Threonine
Isoleucine	Methionine
Lysine	Phenylalanine

Histidine is an essential amino acid for infants.[12] Histidine was thought to be nonessential for adults; however, a recent study suggests that this may not be the case,[13] and further studies must be done to clarify the essentiality of histidine for adults.

In order for our bodies to carry out protein synthesis, all eight essential amino acids must be present simultaneously and in the proper proportions. This means that if one essential amino acid is missing in the diet or present in a disproportionately small quantity, protein synthesis will slow down or stop completely. When a food is low in one or more of the essential amino acids, the utilization of all amino acids is reduced in the same proportion as the "limiting" amino acid.

The *nonessential* or *dispensable amino acids* can be produced by the body if there is an adequate source of nitrogen as well as carbon, hydrogen, and oxygen. The nonessential amino acids are as important as the essential amino acids in growth and body metabolism. The terms *essential* and *nonessential* refer only to how they are supplied to the body; i.e., the carbon skeleton of the essential amino acids cannot be formed in the human body and must be supplied by our diets.

After the requirement for essential amino acids has been met, the requirement for additional nitrogen can be met by any protein-containing foods in our diet, or by nitrogenous compounds such as urea or amino acids from the metabolic pool. The carbon skeletons for the nonessential amino acids can be provided from intermediary products of fat or carbohydrate metabolism. Nonessential amino acids may be formed when a carbon skeleton combines with a free amino group derived from another amino acid or from ammonia. The process by which an amino group is transferred from one amino acid to another is called *transamination*. The availability of the nonessential amino acids depends on the proper functioning of these conversion systems. In diseases in which protein formation is disturbed, such as liver disease or protein malnutrition, the failure to form nonessential amino acids may increase the severity of the illness.[14]

Our diet is the usual source of nonessential amino acids and nitrogen. When the nonessential amino acids in the diet are low, they must be formed in adequate quantities from the products of intermediary metabolism in order to allow the most efficient usage of the essential amino acids. Therefore, protein synthesis is determined by the supply of essential amino acids, as well as by the rapidity and efficiency of production of nonessential amino acids. Both the essential and nonessential amino acids must be present simultaneously and in the proper proportions for protein synthesis to proceed efficiently. For example the protein in cereal is better utilized when milk is consumed with it.

Recommended Protein Allowances

There is no universal agreement on the optimal amount of protein needed in the diet.[15] In general, the protein requirements are less than the quantities consumed by most Americans.

Adults

The Food and Nutrition Board of the National Research Council advocates a daily protein allowance of 0.8 g per kilogram of ideal body weight for adults. The 1980 recommended dietary allowance (RDA) for protein is based on the criteria listed in Table 3-2.[16]

Major changes in recommended allowances for protein were outlined in the 1974 RDAs.[17] In 1968, the RDA for a 70-kg man was 65 g protein per day and 55 g protein per day for a 58-kg woman. In 1974, the RDA for a 70-kg man was reduced to 56 g of protein per day; the RDA for a 58-kg woman was reduced to 46 g of protein per day. These changes are surrounded by controversy. The reduced RDAs for protein have been criticized as being "incompatible with sound nutritional planning."[18] The 1980 RDAs for protein are the same as the 1974 recommendations and the controversy continues.

Protein foods contain a variety of nutrients, including B_6 and some trace elements. Adequate intakes of these nutrients may be difficult to obtain within the current RDAs for protein and energy.[19] Deficiency of these nutrients is unusual since most Americans consume more protein than the current recommendations. However, problems with these nutrients might occur in certain institutionalized populations where personnel are required to keep costs down as well as meet the recommended allowances.[20]

It should be emphasized that the controversy revolves around the potentially inadequate intake of other nutrients found in protein, not the recommendation for protein per se. The current RDAs for protein more than cover the maintenance requirement for nitrogen equilibrium, in-

TABLE 3-2   CRITERIA ON WHICH RDA FOR PROTEIN IS BASED

0.47 g protein per kg body weight per day—average maintenance requirement for nitrogen, estimated from nitrogen balance studies; not for growth
+
0.14 g protein per kg body weight per day—30% over maintenance requirement to account for individual variability
0.6 g protein per kg body weight per day—allowance for high-quality protein; to cover needs of almost all healthy individuals in the U.S. (95% population)
+
0.2 g protein per kg body weight per day—additional allowance for U.S. diet, which contains a combination of high-quality and lower-nutrient-quality proteins; 75% efficiency of utilization assumed
Total 0.8 g protein per kg body weight per day—RDA for protein for adults

dividual variation, and variable utilization of mixed proteins in the American diet. However, since our knowledge of the availability, essentiality, and balance of trace elements and other less-studied nutrients is uncertain, it seems wise to plan diets around protein levels which we know are compatible with health from epidemiological studies, even though they may contain more protein than necessary to maintain nitrogen equilibrium.[21] When protein intake is limited because of poor food selection or inadequate income, the additional calories often come from low-nutrient fats, sugars, and alcohol, components which already comprise a large proportion of the American diet and contribute to our major health problems of obesity, heart disease, and dental caries.

Infants

Protein allowances for infants are based on normal growth rates, changes in body composition, and the amount of milk protein that will result in satisfactory growth. We know from clinical experience that the protein in human milk is adequate for a breast-fed infant who feeds completely at the breast of a well-nourished woman. During the first year of life, the protein content of the body increases from 11 to 14.6 percent. This increase in body protein is approximately 3.5 g per day during the first 4 months and 3.1 g per day during the next 8 months.[22] The recommended protein allowance (RDA) is 2.2 g per kilogram body weight per day for infants up to age 6 months and 2.0 g per kilogram body weight for infants age 6 months to 1 year.[23]

During early infancy, the most rapid postnatal growth period, an unusually high proportion of protein intake is used for growth. Beyond infancy, as the growth rate decreases, children and adults use an increasing proportion of their protein intake for maintenance (nongrowth) needs.

The low birth weight (LBW) infant, that is, the infant who weighs 2500 g or less at birth, has extraordinary requirements for both energy and protein during the first weeks of life. A protein intake over 2 g and less than 6 g per kilo-

gram per day is recommended for LBW infants to meet growth needs and prevent the complications of excess intake (elevated BUN, acidosis, hyperpyrexia, lethargy, diarrhea, edema). Although most commonly an intake of 3 to 4 g per kilogram per day is advised,[24,25] protein intake for the LBW infant must be individualized. When recommendations are made, consumption of an adequate calorie intake is assumed. If protein is provided intravenously, requirements may be less (see Chap. 14).[26]

Foman [27] is cautious about recommending a diet consisting solely of breast milk for infants weighing less than 1500 g. Premature LBW infants who are growing rapidly have estimated needs which may exceed the quantity of nutrients in milk.

Children and Adolescents

Studies on the nitrogen and protein requirements of children and adolescents are limited. The allowances for individuals aged 1 to 18 years are calculated from data on growth rates[28] and body composition.[29,30] The RDAs for children and adolescents are found in the Appendix.[23]

Pregnancy

During pregnancy, 30 g of protein per day beyond the normal requirement is now recommended. In 1974, the Food and Nutrition Board increased the protein allowances per day because of (1) nitrogen balance data suggesting that efficiency of protein utilization during pregnancy is lower than was previously thought, and (2) epidemiological evidence that protein intakes of healthy pregnant women tend to be higher than estimated needs.[31] These recommendations were retained in the 1980 RDA revisions.

The additional protein allowance during gestation provides for the needs of the developing fetus and surrounding tissue, maintenance protein requirements of the mother, and an adjustment for efficiency of dietary protein utilization. It is widely accepted that 925 g of protein is deposited in the fetus and surrounding tissue during pregnancy, at the rate of 0.6, 1.8, 4.8, and 6.1 g per day during the successive quarters of gestation.[32]

There are potential risks to mother and infant from low protein and inadequate food intakes. However, it is difficult to isolate the separate effects of protein and energy, since low protein intakes are often associated with low caloric intakes. When calories (joules) are inadequate, protein is used for energy needs and not for its unique functions of growth, repair, and body maintenance.

Lactation

During lactation, the RDA for protein is 64 g per day, an increase of 20 g per day for the average woman.[33] The additional dietary protein requirement during lactation can be better understood if we look at the amount of breast milk secreted and its protein content.

Average daily milk secretion is approximately 850 mL with an upper range of about 1200 mL. Human milk contains about 1.2 percent protein.[34] Therefore, 850 mL of human milk contains 10 g of protein; 1200 mL contains 15g. On the basis of this argument, the RDA for protein during lactation should be adequate for nearly all women.

The Elderly

The protein requirements of the elderly are not well documented. The evidence to date does not suggest that the protein requirements of the elderly are quantitatively different from those of other adults. However, impaired digestion and recurring episodes of chronic diseases which require repletion of body protein during convalescence may increase nutrient requirements.

DIETARY SIGNIFICANCE OF PROTEIN

Evaluation of Protein Quality

The quality of a protein is determined by its amino acid composition, which in turn determines a protein's ability to sustain growth and maintain body tissue. Therefore, biological evaluation, based on nitrogen retention in the body, is the usual method of assessing protein quality. For human studies, procedures have been developed which use nitrogen balance or growth as indices of nitrogen retention. Nitrogen retention may also be measured by direct analysis of the animal body. Procedures used to describe biological evaluation are summarized in Table 3-3. Common terms associated with the quality of protein are *protein efficiency ratio* (PER), *biological value* (BV),[35] and *net protein utilization* (NPU). For example, an egg has a PER of 3.92,[36] a BV of 93.7,[37] and an NPU of 93.5,[38] which indicates that it is a high-quality protein.

Evaluation of Protein Availability

Both the quality and quantity of protein determine the amount available for utilization. The protein content of the diet is influenced by both the quantity of the food eaten and by the protein concentration in the food. The concentration of protein in food can be calculated by multiplying the nitrogen content of the food by the factor 6.25. The nitrogen content in most protein foods is approximately 16 percent of the total grams of protein present in the food (or 6.25 × nitrogen content of the food). For example, an egg contains approximately 7 g of protein[39] and approximately 1.12 g of nitrogen (1.12 × 6.25 = 7). This value is for crude protein because a small quantity of nonprotein nitrogen is present as well as the nitrogen from protein and amino acids.[40]

Energy intake also influences protein available for body utilization. When the body's energy needs are not met by carbohydrate and fat, protein will be used for energy. Therefore, rehabilitation of a malnourished individual requires increasing the intake of both protein and calories.

The availability of amino acids is also affected by incomplete digestion and absorption. This seems to be a problem only with proteins of vegetable origin. Possible explanations are the higher fiber content of the diet and the inhibitors of digestive enzymes present in some foods which must be inactivated by heating. The ex-

TABLE 3-3 METHODS OF BIOLOGICAL EVALUATION

Procedure	Calculation formula	Experimental conditions	Study design	Comments — Advantages	Comments — Disadvantages
1 Protein efficiency ratio (PER)	$\dfrac{\text{Weight gain, g}}{\text{Protein intake}}$	Standardized dietary conditions: adequate energy intake; adequate protein intake—not excess	Small animals (laboratory rats), human infants	Simplest method; requires measure of protein intake and weight gain, inexpensive, quick	Weight gain may not be proportional to gain in body protein
2 Biological value (BV)	$\dfrac{\text{Nitrogen retained}}{\text{Nitrogen absorbed}}$ $\text{(Dietary N} = \text{urinary N} + \text{fecal N)}$ $\text{(Dietary N} - \text{fecal N)}$	Protein must be fed at or below maintenance level for maximum efficiency of utilization; BV is determined by nitrogen balance	Laboratory animals, humans	Represents proportion of absorbed nitrogen retained; this is amount of nitrogen body actually uses	No allowance for incomplete nitrogen absorption; i.e., that proportion of nitrogen absorbed by digestive tract
3 Net protein utilization (NPU)	$\dfrac{\text{Nitrogen retained}}{\text{Nitrogen intake}}$ or $\text{BV} \times \text{digestibility}$	Standardized dietary conditions: adequate energy intake; adequate protein intake—not excess; NPU is determined by amino acid pattern	Humans— NPU obtained by nitrogen balance Animals— NPU measured by nitrogen balance or by direct body analysis	Measures both biological value of absorbed amino acid mixture and digestibility of food protein; represents proportion of food nitrogen absorbed; is directly related to dietary intake of nitrogen	

cessive heat treatment that is sometimes used in the manufacture of dry milk powder, fish protein concentrates, and oil seed meals may also decrease the availability of amino acids, particularly lysine and the sulfur amino acids. Home cooking and commercial canning procedures have little or no effect on the availability of amino acids.[41]

Sources and Nutritional Value of Dietary Protein; Complete and Incomplete Proteins

Dietary protein may be derived from both animal and vegetable sources. The protein content of foods varies widely, as seen in Table 3-4.

Complete proteins contain all eight essential amino acids in approximately the correct proportions. Complete proteins—meat, fish, poultry, eggs, and dairy products (milk, cheese, yogurt)—are derived from animal sources. They have a high biological value, which enables small quantities of these foods to meet our daily protein requirements. For example 6 oz of meat, fish, or poultry plus 8 oz of milk will generously cover the protein recommended for the adult woman.

Incomplete proteins—vegetables, grains, and legumes—also contain all eight essential amino acids but are low in one or more of them. The terminology *incomplete* may be misleading since proteins of plant origin are not lacking in types of amino acids but rather are deficient in quantity and proportion. Vegetable proteins are less complete than animal proteins—not incom-

TABLE 3-4   PROTEIN AND CHOLESTEROL CONTENT OF SOME COMMON FOODS

Food	Household measure	Protein content, g*	Cholesterol content, mg†	Biological value‡ (BV)	Net protein utilization§ (NPU)
Human milk, U.S. samples	8 fl oz	2.4	35 mg▲	¶	¶
Whole milk	8 oz	9	34	84.5	81.6
Cheddar cheese	1 oz	7	28	70.6	69.8
Rice	1 cup	4.1	0	64	62.7
Lentils, cooked	1 cup	15.5	0	44.6	29.7
Lima beans, cooked	1 cup	13	0	66.5	51.5
Soybeans, cooked	1 cup	19.8	0	72.8	61.4
Sunflower seeds (hulled)	⅓ cup	11	0	69.6	58.1
Beef, lamb, pork	3 oz	23	80–90	74.3	66.9
Chicken	3 oz	20	63	74.3	72.9
Fish	3 oz	22	50–70	76	79.5
Egg	1 large	7	252	93.7	93.5

*Nutritive Value of Foods, U.S. Science and Education Administration Home and Garden Bulletin 72, U.S. Department of Agriculture, 1978.

†R. M. Feeley, P. E. Criner, and B. K. Watts. "Cholesterol Content of Foods," *Journal of American Dietetic Association*, **61**:134, August 1972.

‡*Amino-Acid Content of Foods and Biological Data on Proteins*, FAO Nutritional Studies, no. 24, Food and Agriculture Organization of the United Nations, Food Policy and Food Service, Nutrition Division, Rome, 1972.

§Ibid.

▲S. K. Kon and A. J. Cowie, *Milk: The Mammary Gland and Its Secretion*, vol. 2, Academic Press, New York, 1961, pp. 265–305.

¶No figures available.

plete. They are not as well used in the body as animal proteins are and cannot support satisfactory growth unless combined with other foods. In diets composed primarily of plant foods, the amino acids most frequently low are lysine, isoleucine, tryptophan, cysteine, and methionine.[42]

Protein Complementarity

The correction of amino acid deficiencies in plant proteins is made through a process called protein complementarity. By combining two different proteins, the essential amino acids which are low (limiting) in one food are present or complemented in the other food eaten with it, thereby improving the biological value of the protein. By eating a variety of plant proteins with complementary amino acid patterns, individuals can consume the correct quantity and proportion of amino acids without depending on animal proteins. Some good plant protein combinations are beans and rice, beans and wheat, or legumes and rice.[43]

Individuals who consume no animal foods are known as *vegans*. These vegetarians must plan their diets very carefully to include plant proteins that mutually supplement each other. Vegan parents must be particularly judicious in selecting foods for their infants and small children. Vegetable proteins have a lower biological value, are less readily digested, and are more difficult to chew than animal proteins. These problems, coupled with rapid growth, which causes an increased need for protein in infants and young children, may result in protein-calorie deficiencies.[44] For infants, soy formulas must be well processed to inactivate the enzyme inhibitors present in raw soybeans and must be supplemented with small amounts of L-methionine for improved protein quality.[45] Individuals on vegan diets must also be careful to get an adequate intake of vitamin B_{12}, a vitamin found almost exclusively in animal protein and important in the prevention of pernicious anemia (see Chap. 6).

An alternative way of improving the biological value of plant protein is to include small quantities of animal foods such as fish, eggs, or dairy products along with the vegetable proteins. Good protein mixtures would be cereal with milk, bread with cheese, or a bean and cheese casserole. Vegetarians who include eggs and dairy products are known as *lacto-ovo vegetarians*; those who include only dairy products are known as *lacto-vegetarians*. When small amounts of animal foods are eaten, vegetarians can be better assured of getting the correct supply of amino acids. Children consuming vegan or poorly planned vegetarian diets are at risk of adverse health effects from malnutrition. Also, in a few cases rickets have been reported. Deficits in length, weight, hemoglobin, and hematocrit are being observed.[46,47,48]

THE BODY'S USE OF PROTEIN

Protein Digestion

Amino acids are the end products of protein digestion as well as being the basic structural units of protein. Protein digestion begins in the stomach. The acid environment of the stomach (which is due to the secretion of hydrochloric acid by the stomach mucosa) activates the enzyme pepsin. Pepsin begins to break down the protein into large protein derivatives called proteoses and peptones. There is another special enzyme in the stomach, called rennin, which coagulates milk and begins to digest casein, the protein in milk. Rennin slows down the passage of milk from the stomach and changes the casein to a form that can be acted on by pepsin. Rennin is a particularly important enzyme for infants whose main source of dietary protein is milk. When this enzyme is deficient, milk then passes too quickly through the stomach, causing the infant to be milk-intolerant.

The next modification of protein occurs in the small intestine. Pancreatic juices containing the protein-splitting enzymes trypsin and chymotrypsin are secreted from the pancreas into the small intestine. Polypeptides and dipeptides are formed in the small intestine due to the action of these powerful enzymes on the protein from the stomach. The polypeptides are then broken down into their constituent amino acids in the small intestine by the peptidases, a mixture of carboxypeptidase (an enzyme from the pancreatic juice) and aminopeptidase and dipeptidase (enzymes found in the intestinal juices). The carboxypeptidases split the terminal peptide bond at the carboxyl end of the polypeptide chain; the aminopeptidase splits the terminal peptide bond at the free amino end of the chain. Once food proteins are converted into their constituent amino acids by the enzymatic cleavage of the peptide linkages and the mechanical action of the digestive organs, they are ready for absorption by the intestinal mucosa. This absorptive process is an active one and requires energy, provided by adenosine triphosphate (ATP). After the amino acids are absorbed, they are carried to the liver via the portal vein and are utilized through various metabolic processes.

Protein Metabolism

Protein Synthesis (Anabolism)

Amino acids from the amino acid pool leave the liver and are transported throughout the body to be used for growth, repair, and maintenance of body tissues, and formation of special compounds (enzymes, hormones, plasma proteins). An adequate supply of both essential and nonessential amino acids is needed for protein synthesis. If essential amino acids are not supplied via the diet to the cell, synthesis cannot take place. However, when the supply of nonessential amino acids is inadequate they can be synthesized in the cell through a process called *transamination*. Once the essential and nonessential amino acids are present in the cell, synthesis of specific body proteins will be genetically controlled by DNA (deoxyribonucleic acid) located in the cell nucleus (see Figure 3-1). The genetic information for the amino acid sequence (the primary structure of the protein) is stored in DNA. This information is carried by messenger RNA (ribonucleic acid) to the site of protein synthesis, the cell cytoplasm, where specific protein is produced. (See "Genes," in Chap. 13.)

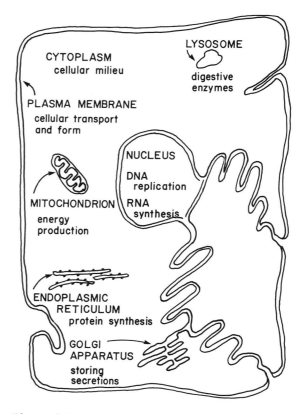

Figure 3-1
The function of cell components as related to protein metabolism.

Catabolism

Catabolism (metabolic breakdown) of amino acids involves the processes of deamination and decarboxylation. *Deamination*, the removal of the nitrogen portion ($-NH_2$) of the amino acid to form alpha-keto amino acids, occurs for the most part in the liver, although it can occur in the kidney and other organs of the body. Ultimately the nitrogen portion of the amino acid is converted to ammonia and finally to urea, which is excreted in the urine. The deaminated keto acids may be converted to nonessential amino acids by transamination or oxidized for needed energy through the Krebs cycle. According to the nature of the carbon skeleton, the oxidized ketoacids become either ketogenic amino acids or glycogenic amino acids. If energy is not required, the amino acids are converted to fat and stored in the body.

Decarboxylation, a reaction that involves the splitting off of CO_2 from the carboxyl group of the amino acid to form amines, occurs in tissues such as the kidney, liver, or intestinal flora. An example of this reaction is the decarboxylation of hydroxytryptophan to form 5-hydroxytryptamine or serotonin, the neuro-transmitter necessary for central nervous system function. (See Chap. 26.)

Figure 3-2 summarizes the sites of protein utilization.

CLINICAL APPLICATIONS

Protein Requirements and Disease

States of protein deficiency can be differentiated into clinical entities: kwashiorkor (protein malnutrition) and marasmus (protein-calorie malnutrition). (See Chap. 19.) These states of malnutrition decrease resistance to disease and also retard growth. In developing countries, the combined effects of infection and protein deficiency contribute to the high mortality rates. Diarrhea, measles, and respiratory infections are more severe and often fatal in children with protein malnutrition. In hospitalized patients, therapy is poorly tolerated and recovery from surgery or trauma is complicated when the patient is malnourished.

In certain disease states, and with extreme environmental or physiological stress or surgical trauma, protein requirements are increased because the body is catabolizing protein and nitrogen is being lost. A state of negative nitrogen balance results, lean body mass decreases, and body weight declines. Initially, when protein is withdrawn from the cells, a normal concentration of plasma proteins is maintained. However, with increasing protein depletion, plasma proteins are reduced. During convalescence from an

Figure 3-2
Sites of protein metabolism. (1) Deamination; (2) transamination; (3) decarboxylation.

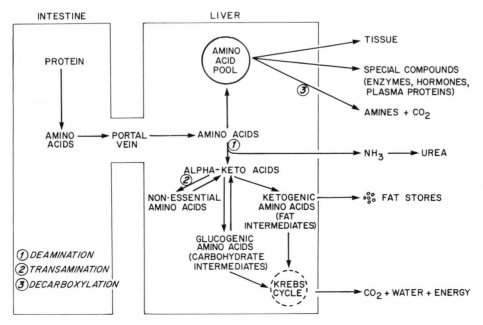

illness where protein depletion has occurred, protein and energy requirements are higher in order to replace wasted tissue

The most common biochemical tests for determination of protein nutriture, and their normal values, are total serum protein (6.0 to 8.0 g per 100 mL) and serum albumin (3.5 to 5.5 g per 100 mL).[49] Another biochemical measure being used to assess protein status is the creatinine-height index. The excretion of creatinine is reduced during states of malnutrition.[50] (See Chap. 19.)

Clinical treatment for protein-depleted patients involves the provision of extra dietary protein along with sufficient energy. It has been estimated that as much as 2 to 3 g of protein per kilogram of body weight may be necessary in severe pathological states when nitrogen losses are extensive.[51] In other milder states and during convalescence, a protein intake of 0.6 to 1.2 g per kg of body weight has been found to be adequate.[52]

In disease states involving the kidney or liver, protein intake may need to be curtailed because of the body's inability to handle the waste products of protein metabolism.

Table 3-5 lists some common conditions that alter protein requirements.

TABLE 3-5 PATHOLOGICAL CONDITIONS ALTERING PROTEIN REQUIREMENTS

Condition	Increased	Decreased
Sepsis	x	
Fever	x	
Trauma—injury	x	
Fractures	x	
Burns	x	
Gastrointestinal disorders (ileostomy, colostomy, diarrhea and other malabsorption states, ulcerative colitis)	x	
Respiratory infections	x	
Parasitic infections	x	
Bacterial infections	x	
Viral infections	x	
Hepatic coma		x
Liver disease	x	
Massive hepatic necrosis		x
Proteinuria	x	
Renal disease (glomerulonephrosis)	x	
Renal failure, acute and chronic		x
Cancer	x	
Marasmus (protein-calorie malnutrition)	x	
Kwashiorkor (protein malnutrition)	x	
Pain	x	
Anxiety or other psychological stress	x	
Profuse sweating	x	

Protein Requirements and Exercise

Exercise or heavy work does not significantly increase one's need for protein.[53] Athletes are often attracted to expensive high-protein diets and concentrated protein supplements such as high-protein drinks or powders in order to increase their body size and strength.[54] Buying these foods is an unnecessary expense since performance is not improved. In addition, excess protein can cause dehydration unless large amounts of water are consumed to help the body excrete the metabolic by-products of protein metabolism. Also, large quantities of animal protein increase the quantitiy of saturated fat and cholesterol ingested. (See Table 3-3; see also Chap. 10.)

Protein Requirements and Weight Reduction

Weight reduction does not change one's need for protein. The key factor in a weight-reduction regimen is controlling the energy intake. The diet is individualized according to nutrient needs and lifestyle. (See Chap. 25.)

Low-calorie protein diets, especially liquid-protein diets, can be hazardous. Liquid protein is hydrolyzed collagen. It is a protein source of poor biologic value, low in vitamins, minerals, and essential amino acids. It is sold in drug and grocery stores. Because of the many risks associated with low-calorie protein weight-reduction diets, particularly liquid protein, this type of diet is not recommended for infants, children, or pregnant or lactating women under any circumstances,[55] or anyone else for that matter.

The major complication of the liquid-protein diet is sudden death.[56] Although frequency is unknown, cases have been reported by the Center for Disease Control and the Food and Drug Administration.[57] The exact cause of death is unknown.

Certain clinical symptoms are noted with liquid-protein diets:[58]

1 Tachycardia in females is increased.

2 Syncope, which is a warning signal for arrhythmias, can occur.

3 Hypokalemia is present in some people.

4 Loss of lean body mass (starvation) occurs.

Even with close medical supervision, there is the risk of sudden death. Physicians cannot precisely determine when fatal heart arrhythmias may develop.

The use of liquid protein is not to be confused with the protein-sparing modified fast (PSMF). (See Chap. 25.)

FUTURE AVAILABILITY OF PROTEIN

We are living at a time when people are questioning how to best meet our nutrient needs. World population continues to rise and food production becomes more sophisticated. However, there still seems to be a lag in applying technology to solving food problems in developing countries. Further research is needed in order to define protein requirements more precisely and to advance solutions for meeting world protein needs.

In affluent countries of the world, such as the United States, substantial quantities of animal protein will continue to be eaten, even though there seems to be a growing awareness of the ecological wastefulness and potential health risks of eating large quantities of meat. As developing countries improve their living standards and enlarge their populations, the demand for animal protein will probably increase. However, because of the limits of the earth's agricultural capacity and animal resources and the high cost of animal foods, animal protein will probably never make significant nutritional contributions to the diets of most of the world's people.

In the future, we can look forward to many changes in the types of protein foods available. There will probably be an increased utilization of fish and fish protein concentrates, algae and microorganisms, oilseed meals, and textured soy proteins, and use of synthetic amino acids, especially lysine and methionine, to improve the quality of legume and cereal protein mixtures. These new foods will add greater variety to our diets and help conserve the earth's limited food resources.

STUDY QUESTIONS

1 Identify three factors that affect nitrogen balance. When does positive nitrogen balance occur? When does negative nitrogen balance occur?

2 Explain the importance of essential and nonessential amino acids in protein synthesis.

3 Why are protein requirements increased during pregnancy and lactation?

4 Describe two methods for improving the biological value of plant protein. Identify appropriate food combinations for each. What problems might a child encounter if no animal foods are consumed?

5 Describe the interrelationship between protein nutrition and disease. Identify two pathological states where (a) protein requirements are increased and (b) protein requirements are decreased.

CLINICAL STUDY 3

Past history

S. G. is a 15-month old boy who is brought to the community health center by his parents for a routine check-up. Until age 10 months, the time of the child's last clinic visit, S. G. was in good health and growing along the 10th percentile for both height and weight (height = 70 cm; weight = 8.25 kg). His parents had reported at that time that S. G. was feeding well at the breast and taking solids, consisting primarily of grains and vegetables. At approximately 10 months, S. G. began to teethe, and Mrs. G. decided to wean the child from the breast to a cup. The Gs are strict vegetarians who eat no animal foods. S. G. is being raised on a diet similar to his parents'.

Present

S. G.'s current weight and height are 7.5 kg and 70 cm. Since the 10-month visit, he has lost weight and has not grown. Currently, S. G. is eating grains, vegetables, nuts, and seeds; no animal foods or soy products are included in the diet. The nurse is concerned that the child is not eating enough and is failing to thrive as a result.

Clinical study questions

1 What would you tell the parents about protein requirements of infants and young children?

2 What practical dietary recommendations would you suggest to assure a more adequate protein intake for the child?

3 What would you tell the parents about the relationship between intake and protein utilization?

REFERENCES

1 N. S. Scrimshaw, "Shattuck Lecture—Strengths and Weaknesses of the Committee Approach: An Analysis of Past and Present Recommended Dietary Allowances for Protein in Health and Disease (Part One)," *New England Journal of Medicine*, **294** (3): 136–142, January 1976.

2 N. S. Scrimshaw, "Shattuck Lecture—Strengths and Weaknesses of the Committee Approach: An Analysis of Past and Present Recommended Dietary Allowances for Protein in Health and Disease (Part Two)," *New England Journal of Medicine*, **294** (4): 198–203, January 1976.

3   D. Morgan, "UN Reports Warn of Global Food Crisis By '85," *Boston Sunday Globe*, June 20, 1976.

4   "Dietary Levels of Households in the United States, Seasons of Year 1965–66," *Household Food Consumption Survey*, 1965–66, rep. 18, U.S. Department of Agriculture, Consumer and Food Economics Institute, Agricultural Research Service, 1974.

5   M. Pines, "Breaking the Meat Habit," in C. Lerza and M. Jacobson (eds.), *Food for People Not Profit*, Ballantine Books, New York, 1975.

6   Center for Disease Control, *10 State Nutrition Survey, 1968–1970*, V *Dietary*, U.S. Department of Health, Education, and Welfare Publication (HSM) 72-8133, Atlanta, 1972.

7   "Caloric and Selected Nutrient Values for Persons. 1–74 Years of Age, "*First Health and Nutrition Examination Survey, United States, 1971–1974*, U.S. Department of Health, Education, and Welfare Publication (PHS) 79-1657, June 1979.

8   L. Brewster and M. Jacobson, *The Changing American Diet*, Center For Science in the Public Interest, Washington, D.C., 1978, p. 65.

9   A. A. Albanese and L. A. Orto, "The Proteins and Amino Acids," in R. S. Goodhart and M. E. Shils (eds.), *Modern Nutrition in Health and Disease*, 5th ed., Lea and Febiger, Philadelphia, 1973, p. 28.

10 R. L. Pike and M. L. Brown, *Nutrition: An Integrated Approach*, 2d ed., John Wiley & Sons, Inc., New York, 1975, pp. 49–52.

11 A. L. Lehninger, *Biochemistry*, 2d ed., The Johns Hopkins University School of Medicine, Worth Publishers, Inc., New York, 1975, chap. 3.

12 S. E. Snyderman, A. Boyer, E. Roitman, L. E. Holt, Jr., and P. H. Prose, " The Histidine Requirement of the Infant," *Pediatrics*, **31**:786–801, May 1963.

13 R. L. Pike and M. L. Brown, op. cit., 860.

14 H. N. Munro and M. C. Crim, "The Proteins and Amino Acids," R. S. Goodhart and M. E. Shils (eds.), *Modern Nutrition in Health and Disease,* 6th ed., Lea nd Febigee, Phildelphia, 1980, pp. 84–86.

15 A. E. Harper, P. R. Payne, and J. C. Waterlow, "Human Protein Needs," *Lancet,* **1**:1518, June 1973.

16 Food and Nutrition Board, *Recommended Dietary Allowances*, 9th ed., National Academy of Sciences National Research Council, Washington, D.C., 1980, p. 46.

17 Food and Nutrition Board, *Recommended Dietary Allowances*, 9th ed., National Academy of Sciences, National Research Council, Washington, 1974, pp. 37–48.

18 D. H. Calloway, "Recommended Dietary Allowances for Protein and Energy," *Journal of American Dietetic Association*, **64**:161, February 1974.

19 Ibid.

20 Ibid.

21 Ibid.

22 S. Fomon, *Infant Nutrition*, 2d ed., W. B. Saunders Company, Philadelphia, 1974, chap. 6.

23 1980, op. cit., Food and Nutrition Board, pp. 39–51.

24 M. Davidson, S. Z. Levine, C. H. Bauer, and M. Dann, "Feeding Studies in Low Birthweight Infants," *Journal of Pediatrics*, May 1967, pp. 695–713.

25 L. E. Holt and S. E. Snyderman, "The Feeding of Premature and Newborn Infants," *Pediatric Clinics of North America*, **13**(4):1103–1115, November 1966.

26 S. E. Snyderman, "Amino Acid Requirements," *Intravenous Nutrition in the High Risk Infant,* John Wiley & Sons, Inc., New York, 1975, p. 210.

27 S. J. Foman, E. E. Ziegler, and H. D. Vazquez, "Human Milk and the Small Premature," unpublished address, Department of Pediatrics, University of Iowa.

28 M. L. Hathaway, "Heights and Weights of Children in the United States," *USDA Home Economics Research Report No. 2,* U.S. Government Printing Office, Washington, D.C. 1957, p. 131.

29 E. M. Widdowson and J. W. T. Dickerson, "Chemical Composition of the Body," in C. L. Comar and F. Bronner (eds.), *Mineral Metabolism,* vol. II, pt A. Academic Press, New York, 1963, pp. 1–247.

30 S. Fomon, op. cit, pp. 118–151.

31 1980, op. cit., Food and Nutrition Board, pp. 39–51.

32 F. E. Hytten and I. Leitch, *The Physiology of Human Pregnancy,* 2d ed., F. A. Davis Co., Philadelphia, Blackwell Scientific Publications, Oxford, 1971.

33 1980, op. cit., Food and Nutrition Board, pp. 39–51.

34 *Nutrition in Pregnancy and Lactation*, WHO Technical Report, ser. 302, World Health Organization, Geneva, 1965, p. 54.

35 H. H. Mitchell, "A Method of Determining the Biological Value of Protein," *Journal of Biological Chemistry*, **58**:873–922, January 1924.

36 *Amino-Acid Content of Foods and Biological Data on Proteins,* FAO Nutritional Studies, no. 24, Food and Agriculture Organization of the United Nations, Food Policy and Food Science Service, Nutrition Division, Rome, 1972, p. 180.

37 Ibid.

38 Ibid.

39 USDA Science and Education Administration, "Nutritive Value of Foods," *Home and Garden Bulletin No. 72,* Washington, D.C., 1978.

40 *Protein Requirements,* FAO Nutrition Meetings Report, ser. 37, Food and Agriculture Organization/World Health Organization, 1965, p. 41.

41 Ibid., p. 24.

42 F. M. Lappe, *Diet for a Small Planet,* Ballantine Books, New York, 1975, pp. 80, 81.

43 Ibid., p. 81.

44 *Protein Requirements*, op. cit., p. 24.

45 S. Foman, op. cit., pp. 387–390.

46 J. T. Dwyer, R. Palombo, H. Thorne, I. Valadian, and R. B. Reed, "Preschoolers on Alternate Life-Style Diets," *Journal of American Dietetic Association*, **72**:264–270, 1978. (March).

47 J. R. K. Robson, J. E. Konlande, F. A. Larkin, P. H. O'Connor, and H. Y. Liu, "Zen Macrobiotic Dietary Problems in Infancy," *Pediatrics*, **53**:326–329, 1974.

48 P. T. Brown and J. G. Bergan, "Dietary Status of 'New' Vegetarians," *Journal of American Dietetic Association*, **67**:455–459, 1975.

49 J. Wallach, *Interpretation of Diagnostic Tests*, Little, Brown and Co., Boston, 1970, p. 9.

50 Committee Report, "Assessment of Protein Nutritional Status," *American Journal of Clinical Nutrition*, **23**(6):807–819, June 1970.

51 *Protein Requirements*, op. cit., p. 30.

52 H. S. Soroff, E. Pearson, and C. P. Artz, "An Estimation of the Nitrogen Requirements for Equilibrium in Burned Patients," *Surgery, Gynecology, and Obstetrics*, **112**:159–172, February 1961.

53 N. J. Smith, *Food for Sport*, Bull Publishing Co., Palo Alto, Calif., 1976, chap. 1, pp. 16–20.

54 Ibid., chap. 3, p. 48.

55 D. Kennedy, *H.E.W. News*, November 9, 1977.

56 R. R. Michiel, J. S. Sneider, R. A. Dickstein, J. Hayman, and R. H. Eich, "Sudden Death in a Patient on a Liquid Protein Diet," *New England Journal of Medicine*, **298**:1005–1007, May 1978.

57 R. R. Michiel, ibid.

58 B. R. Bistrian, "Recent Developments in the Treatment of Obesity with Particular Reference to Semistarvation Ketogenic Regimens," *Diabetes Care*, **1**(6):379–384, November–December, 1978.

CLINICAL DISCUSSION 3

Treatment

While breast feeding, S. G. seemed to be receiving an adequate intake of protein and calories from breast milk, supplemented by vegetables and grains. Evidence of this is S. G.'s consistent growth along the 10th percentile for both height and weight for his first 10 months of life, which was consistent with his familial pattern. When S. G. stopped breast feeding, his growth problems began. On a diet consisting of only grains, vegetables, nuts, and seeds, S. G. was unable to consume an intake of protein and energy adequate to sustain growth. His weight loss is evidence of an inadequate energy intake. This would suggest that the protein consumed was used primarily to meet energy needs.

Children who follow vegan diets are consuming proteins which have lower biological value, are less readily digested, and are more difficult to chew. These problems, coupled with rapid growth, which causes an increased need for protein in young children, may result in protein-calorie deficiences.

Treatment involves increasing both protein and energy in the diet. The G.'s were referred to the nutritionist at the health center for careful dietary evaluation and nutritional counseling.

Nutritional education

The parents were counseled on the nutritional value of animal and vegetable proteins. Since the G.'s are strict vegetarians, they were not amenable to including animal foods in the child's diet. Careful instruction in the mechanics of protein complementarity was the primary focus of nutritional education. The parents were also encouraged to include some soy products and a well-processed commercial soy formula.

Follow-up plans

The patient was seen weekly by the nurse and nutritionist for weight checks, growth monitoring, and supportive nutritional care to ensure adequate protein and caloric intakes and developmental feeding progress.

CHAPTER 4

CARBOHYDRATE

Carol Stollar

KEY WORDS
Monosaccharides
Disaccharides
Polysaccharides
Glycogen
Fiber
Gluconeogenesis
Glycogenolysis
Glycolysis

INTRODUCTION

Changing patterns in carbohydrate consumption—an increase in the use of highly refined carbohydrate (milled, bleached flour) and an excessive sugar intake—are products of our technological age that are provoking nutritional concern. Now being examined are cause-effect relationships between the lack of fiber in the American diet and the incidence of lower bowel disease, atherosclerosis, obesity, and cancer; and between excessive sugar intake and dental caries. A knowledge of carbohydrate, its food sources, and its metabolism is essential for health professionals who are working toward preventing the above disorders and treating other disease states such as diabetes mellitus, malabsorption, allergies, and inborn errors of metabolism such as galactosemia. Even to counteract the food misinformation of the low-carbohydrate, quick-weight-loss reduction diet a knowledge of carbohydrate is necessary. This chapter will provide the student with the information to be a competent, well-informed nutrition educator in all areas requiring a basic knowledge of carbohydrate.

DEFINITION OF CARBOHYDRATE

Carbohydrate is the term used to describe any of various neutral compounds of carbon, hydrogen, and oxygen, most of which are formed by green plants. As sugars, starches, and cellulose, carbohydrate is the major energy source in the human diet, comprising 45 to 55 percent of the energy in the American diet and up to 80 to 90 percent in the diets of those in the developing nations where vegetation is lush and livestock production and refrigeration are limited.

Carbohydrate and its potential energy originate in chlorophyll-containing plants, which synthesize carbohydrate from carbon dioxide and water, using energy from the sun in a process known as photosynthesis:

$$6H_2O + 6CO_2 \xrightarrow{\text{light}} C_6H_{12}O_6 + 6O_2$$

Water   Carbon dioxide   Sugar   Oxygen

The carbohydrate formed consists of carbon, hydrogen, and water, and so the term *carbohydrate* indicates somewhat the basic chemical composition. However, the term gives no real indication of the chemical structure, and the implied formula excludes many members of this class. The term *saccharide* is more appropriate since it allows for classification into monosaccharides, disaccharides, and polysaccharides.

CLASSIFICATION OF CARBOHYDRATES

Carbohydrates are divided into three main groups according to the number of *saccharides,* or *sugar units,* comprising the basic structure. They are:

> *Monosaccharides* The simplest form of carbohydrate, consisting of a single sugar. (Single)
>
> *Disaccharides* A more complex form of carbohydrate, consisting of two sugars or two monosaccharides. (Double)
>
> *Polysaccharides* The most complex carbohydrate, consisting of many units of one or more monosaccharides. (Many)

Monosaccharides

The structure of a simple sugar of monosaccharide is a carbon chain:

$$-\overset{|}{\underset{|}{C}}-\overset{|}{\underset{|}{C}}-\overset{|}{\underset{|}{C}}-\overset{|}{\underset{|}{C}}\ -\overset{|}{\underset{|}{C}}-\overset{|}{\underset{|}{C}}-\overset{|}{\underset{|}{C}}-\overset{|}{\underset{|}{C}}-$$

with hydrogen and oxygen atoms attached singly or in groups known as *aldehydes* (an alcohol that has been oxidized and contains a $C-H$ group) or *ketones* (a compound containing a $C=O$ group):

Glucose (an aldose)

Fructose (a ketose)

According to the number of carbons present in the basic structure, the monosaccharides are grouped as follows:

Trioses	3 Carbons
Tetroses	4 Carbons
Pentoses	5 Carbons
Hexoses	6 Carbons
Heptoses	7 Carbons

The hexoses are nutritionally the most important of the monosaccharides.

Hexoses (6-Carbon Sugars)

The four monosaccharides in the hexose group are glucose, fructose, galactose, and mannose.

Glucose The most abundant monosaccharide, glucose is found in a natural state in many fruits, such as ripe grapes (known therefore as grape sugar), plums, dates, and figs. It is also a constituent of disaccharides (sucrose, lactose, maltose), of the polysaccharides, and of glycogen, starch, and cellulose. Glucose is the form in which carbohydrate is used by the body—the form that is transported in the bloodstream and oxidized in the cell for energy. Glucose is present in the systemic venous blood, when a person is resting after a meal, in the following concentrations:

Whole blood 60 to 100 mg per 100 mL
Plasma 65 to 110 mg per 100 mL

There are no clinically significant sex or age differences in blood glucose concentrations except that values are low (30 mg per 100 mL) in the newborn and tend to be somewhat higher than average in the elderly.

Glucose is also known as *dextrose* because it is the dextrorotatory form of the molecule (which means that in a chemical reaction this compound rotates a plane of polarized light toward the right). Dextrose is produced commercially by the hydrolysis of starch (hydrolysis is a chemical process of decomposition involving the splitting of a chemical bond and the addition of the elements of water). The product formed is dextrose (corn syrup), which is often added to cow's milk in order to modify it for infant feeding. Dextrose is also used in intravenous therapy along with water and electrolytes.

Fructose Fructose, known also as *fruit sugar,* is found in its natural state in many fruits, including apples and pears, and in honey, and is a constituent of sucrose and the polysaccharide inulin. It is the sweetest of the monosaccharides. When ingested orally, fructose does not need insulin for metabolism and does not appear to significantly stimulate the release of glucagon and growth hormone. Large amounts of fructose may cause flatulence and osmotic diarrhea.[1] Fructose in food can be used directly for energy or can be converted to glucose derivatives.

Fructose is also called *levulose* as it is the levorotatory form of the molecule (which means that as an optically active molecule it rotates a plane of light to the left).

Galactose Galactose is found in nature only in a combined form. In the human body it is a constituent of lactose (milk sugar), certain glucopro-

teins, and the complex glycosides of nervous tissue. Galactose is converted to glucose in the liver. During lactation, the human body converts glucose to galactose in the mammary tissue for the synthesis of the lactose component of breast milk.

Milk is the primary source of this sugar. Legumes also contain galactose which, after digestion, may be available to the human body. (These food sources are of note in planning a diet for a child with galactosemia, an inborn error of metabolism that necessitates the removal of all food sources of galactose. See Chap. 27.)

Pentoses (5-Carbon Sugars)

Among the important pentoses are arabinose, xylose, ribose, 2-deoxy-D-ribose, and xylulose. Arabinose and xylose are examples of naturally occurring pentoses found in foods; nuts are a good source. Ribose and deoxyribose are synthesized in the body and are integral components of the nucleic acids ribonucleic acid (RNA) and deoxyribonucleic acid (DNA). Ribose is also a part of coenzymes derived from the vitamins niacin and riboflavin.

The body is capable of synthesizing its own supply of pentose from glucose by way of the pentose shunt (pentose phosphate pathway) and from glucuronic acid. Normally the body produces glucuronic acid (a monosaccharide derivative) from glucose.

The pentose phosphate pathway is important as an alternative pathway for glucose oxidation. This route does not require adenosine triphosphate, and about 30 percent of glucose metabolism in liver cells takes place by this mechanism.

Xyloses may appear in the urine after the ingestion of large amounts of certain fruits such as cherries and plums, causing a condition known as alimentary pentosuria. As a result of a benign inborn error of metabolism (a familial type of pentosuria), xylulose is excreted in the urine independently of the nature of the diet.

Xylose can be used as an indicator of carbohydrate malabsorption. A known amount (25

g) is ingested and its appearance in the urine is then monitored. When less than 4.5 g is excreted in 5 h (if the patient has normal renal function), impaired carbohydrate absorptive capacity is indicated.

Disaccharides

A disaccharide is composed of two monosaccharides which are joined together by a glycosidic linkage with the release of one molecule of water. For example:

Monosaccharide + monosaccharide →
disaccharide + water

$$C_6H_{12}O_6 + C_6H_{12}O_6 \rightarrow C_{12}H_{22}O_{11} + H_2O$$
Glucose   Glucose   Maltose   Water

The disaccharides include sucrose (glucose and fructose), maltose (glucose and glucose), and lactose (glucose and galactose).

Sucrose Sucrose (glucose and fructose) is the common granulated *table sugar,* obtained from sugar cane, sugar beets, and the sap of maple trees. Many fruits and vegetables such as bananas, dates, ripe pineapple, green peas, and sweet potatoes contain sucrose in its natural state. Many food products are now processed with large amounts of sugar; consequently, sucrose now comprises about 15 to 20 percent of our total calories in our daily food intake. It has been estimated that slightly over 100 lb of sugar is used per person per year in the United States.

Lactose Lactose (glucose and galactose) or *milk sugar,* is the sugar found in milk and is unique to mammals. Lactose comprises about 7½ percent of the total content of human milk and 4¼ percent of cow's milk. When milk products are fermented, or milk sours, much of the lactose is converted to lactic acid, which gives sour milk and yogurt their characteristic flavor. In cheesemaking, the whey (the fluid part of soured milk) is removed and, since lactose is soluble in the whey, the hard, ripened cheeses

(cheddar, Swiss, mozzarella) that are made from the curds contain only trace amounts of lactose.

Lactose is hydrolyzed to glucose and galactose in the cells of the intestinal mucosa. When the enzyme lactase is absent or deficient, symptoms of cramping and flatulence may occur (see Chap. 22).

Maltose Maltose (glucose and glucose), or *malt sugar,* is not present in a natural state but is produced by the action of the amylase enzymes on polysaccharides like starch and glycogen. It is of little dietary significance except for its contribution to the process of beer making, in which the action of the enzyme diastase on grain (starch) produces the first step in alcohol production. Cereals, corn syrup, and baby foods produced by hydrolysis of cereal grains contain some maltose.

Sweetness of Sugar
The sweetness of sugar is perceived on the tip of the tongue. Taste is a highly individualized response influenced by many factors, including genetic predisposition and environmental conditioning, and so the degree of sweetness perceived by different individuals is variable.

The sweetness of various sugars is measured by a subjective sensory test, in which individuals are asked to judge the relative sweetness of the sugars at differing concentrations. Sucrose is usually used as the standard of comparison and is given a value of 100 (see Table 4-1).

Polysaccharides

Polysaccharides are complex carbohydrates composed of large numbers of monosaccharide units linked together. Polysaccharides can be divided into two groups—those that have a function in energy storage and those that have structural roles.

Storage function: starch (plants)
glycogen (animals)
dextran
inulin

TABLE 4-1 COMPARISON OF SWEETNESS OF SUGARS AND OTHER SWEETENERS

Sugar or sweetener	Degree of sweetness
Sucrose	100
Lactose	39
Maltose	46
Sorbitol	50
D-Mannose	59
Galactose	63
D-Glucose	69
D-Fructose	114
Xylitol	120
Sodium cyclamate*	1500–3100
Saccharin*	24,000–35,000

Scale: Compared with sucrose = 100

*These are artificial sweeteners.

Source: Adapted from L. W. Aurand and A. E. Woods, *Food Chemistry,* Avi Publishing Company, Westport, Conn., 1973.

Structural function: cellulose

hemicelluloses

pectin

agar, alginates, and

carageen

lignin

Storage Forms

Starch Starch is a storage form of carbohydrate in plants where it acts as a food reserve, freeing monosaccharides as they are needed. It is the most significant source of carbohydrate in the human diet. The basic structure of the starch molecule is composed of glucose units, which range in number from 250 to 1000 units per molecule. These monosaccharide units are arranged in a straight chain such as is found in amylose or in a branched-chain configuration as in amylopectin. Starch from most sources is a mixture of amylose and amylopectin.

Starch granules differ in size and shape and are completely insoluble in cold water. However, with moist heat the starch grains swell, breaking the cell wall and making it more digestible. As starch cooks, it thickens because of the gel-like quality of amylopectin.

Starch is found in plant seeds, particularly cereal grains, and in tubers, fruits, and roots. Legumes and nuts also contain significant amounts of starch. The use of starch differs around the world according to local sources. In the United States, wheat, oats, rye, barley, corn, potatoes, and rice are important. In other countries, millet, sweet potato, taro, breadfruit, cassava, and plantain are staples.

The digestion of starch to maltose is accomplished in the body by the digestive enzyme α-amylase, found in the saliva (where starch digestion begins) and in the pancreatic juice present in the small intestine (where starch digestion is completed). *Dextrins* are the intermediate products of starch digestion.

Starch → dextrins → maltose → glucose

Dextrins are utilized in baby foods, breakfast cereals, and malt mixtures.

Glycogen The animal equivalent of starch, glycogen, consists of branched-chain polysaccharides of great and varying length. The human body stores glycogen in small amounts in the liver and muscle tissue where it serves as a source of glucose when needed for energy and helps to maintain blood glucose levels. Glycogen is of little importance as a dietary source of carbohydrate.

Dextrans Dextrans are substances produced when certain bacteria grow on a sugar substrate. They are branched-chain polysaccharides but differ from glycogen and starch in the nature of their linkages. Dextrans form the substrate for the plaque on the surface of teeth that is implicated in the formation of dental caries (see Chap. 17).

Dextran is used intravenously in solution as a plasma expander after blood loss to increase blood volume through osmotic pressure. It is slowly utilized, remaining in the blood for 24 h or more.

Inulin   Inulin is a fructose-containing polysaccharide found in the Jerusalem artichoke. It can be utilized for energy. Inulin is filtered by the kidney but not reabsorbed and is therefore used to determine kidney function. This test is known as the *inulin clearance test.*

Structural Forms

These are polysaccharides such as cellulose, hemicellulose, and pectin that give rigidity and structure to plant cell walls.

Cellulose   Cellulose is the most plentiful organic compound in the world. It is found in the stems, roots, leaves, hulls, and seed coverings of plants. It has been estimated that only 15 percent of cellulose undergoes bacterial breakdown in the large intestine. Thus, for the most part, cellulose stays whole in the digestive tract, lending bulk to the diet, stimulating peristalsis, moving food along through the intestine, and holding water in the fecal mass, all of which aids in elimination.

Hemicellulose   Hemicellulose was a term originally applied to a mixture of nondigestible polysaccharides extracted from plants, since they were thought to be related to cellulose. More recently, chemical analysis has shown that these substances are not related to cellulose but are composed of polysaccharides of various sugars, including xylose, glucose, and mannose, and are sometimes called *noncellulosic polysaccharides.*

Hemicelluloses are present in whole wheat; carrots, cabbage, and other leafy vegetables; and common fruits, such as peaches, pears, apples, and melons. Hemicelluloses are considered to be the factor in dietary fiber that is associated with increasing stool bulk. About 96 percent of hemicellulose may undergo bacterial breakdown in the small intestine, with end products of gases (carbon dioxide, methane) and volatile fatty acids.

Pectins   Pectins are nondigestible polysaccharides with a colloidal property. They are often classified with hemicellulose. They are soluble in hot water, forming a gel. This property is utilized in preparing fruit jams and jellies and also makes them useful in certain drugs. For example, pectin is used with an absorbent, kaolin, in the treatment of diarrhea. Pectin is found in the rind of citrus fruits and in the skin of apples.

Agar, alginates, and carageen   These are nondigestible polysaccharides found in seaweed and having properties that allow gel formation. Agar is used to make kosher gelatin since it contains no animal products and it can be used under the Jewish dietary laws. Agar is also used as a culture medium on which bacterial growth can be studied (agar plate). Carageen and alginates are additives used to emulsify, stabilize, and thicken, especially in milk products such as ice cream and evaporated milk.

Lignin   Lignin is a woody substance closely bound to cellulose in plants and therefore is grouped with the polysaccharides. It lends fiber to the diet and is now being used in special high-fiber products such as bread.

Derivatives of Polysaccharides: Mucopolysaccharides

Mucopolysaccharides are heteropolysaccharides that are found in combination with protein in body structures and secretions. They tend to be viscous in nature and are usually found in the substance surrounding connective tissues.

Hyaluronic acid is a mucopolysaccharide that assists in lubricating joints and is present as a gel-like substance filling the space between capillaries and cells in connective tissue. *Chondroitin* and *chondroitin sulfate* are mucopolysaccharides that form the matrix of cartilage and the intercellular substance of other connective tissues. *Heparin,* another derivative of polysaccharides, is the anticoagulant that helps to prevent fibrin clots. It also plays a role with lipoprotein lipase in clearing chylomicrons from plasma. It occurs in most cells as part of the granules in which histamine is stored.

THE FIBER CONTENT OF THE DIET

Crude fiber consists of the residue remaining after plant material is treated with acid, alkali, ether, alcohol and water. This is mainly cellulose and lignin. Dietary fiber is usually characterized as the structural components of the plant cell wall (cellulose, lignin, noncellulosic polysaccharides)and nonstructural polysaccharides (gum, mucilage, waxes, cutins, and algal polysaccharides) left after digestions by animal enzymes. Dietary fiber may be three to five times greater than crude fiber.

It has been shown that fiber has the capacity to take up water and form a gel; diminish absorption of fat and nitrogen; bind metal ions such as calcium, zinc, and iron; and bind bile salts. Guar gum and pectin have been reported to be hypercholesterolemic and alter the pattern of glucose absorption in humans.[2] A major role for fiber known since the time of Hippocrates has been the "normalization" of transit time of laxation and the increasing of stool bulk. Addition of large amounts of fiber to one's diet may cause diarrhea, gas, and other signs of intestinal distress.[3]

The composition of plant fiber differs with the age and source of the plant and the amount of processing it has undergone. For example, the dietary fiber content of cereals depends on the degree to which it has been refined. It can range from 3.5 g per 100 g for white flour to 13.5 g per 100 g for whole grain flour. Bran, the coat of the grain seed, can be from 30 g per 100 g for fine-sieved to 48 g per 100 g for coarse-cut, showing that surface area may play a role in its properties (see Table 4-2). The usual mixed diet eaten in the United States contains about 20 g per day.[4]

THE BODY'S USE OF CARBOHYDRATE

Functions

The functions of carbohydrate in the human body are important and varied:

1   It is a source of energy and potential energy.

TABLE 4-2   CONTENT OF DIETARY FIBER

Product	Dietary fiber, g/100g
Cereals and vegetables	
White flour	3.45
Whole grain flour	13.51
Rice, long grain	2.74
Rice, not milled	12.7
All-Bran	26.7
Grape Nuts	7.0
Rice Krispies	4.5
Peas, frozen	7.8
Baked beans, canned	7.3
Corn, canned	5.7
Broccoli, cooked	4.1
Carrot, cooked	3.7
Potato, raw	3.5
Cabbage, cooked	2.8
Lettuce, raw	1.5
Tomato, raw	1.4
Fruit	
Raisins	4.4
Apple (skin only)	3.7
Apple (flesh only)	1.4
Peaches (flesh and skin)	2.3
Grapefruit (canned)	0.44

Source: Adapted from Southgate et al., *Journal of Human Nutrition*, **30**:303, 1976.

2   It is a starting material for the synthesis of other types of compounds in the body, such as fatty acids and certain amino acids.

3   It plays a role in the structure of many compounds that are biologically important: glycolipids, glycoproteins, heparin, nucleic acids.

As a source of energy, 1 g of carbohydrate equals 4.1 kcal (or approximately 17.2 kJ).

Glucose is the form of carbohydrate utilized by the body. The brain is especially dependent on a continuous supply of glucose, as are the red blood cells. After digestion and absorption, glucose is either oxidized or converted to glycogen and stored in the muscles, heart, and liver, while excess is converted to fat and stored as adipose tissues.

It is necessary to ingest carbohydrate in sufficient amounts at regular intervals because it is not stored in large amounts in the body. In persons weighing 70 kg, the following distribution is seen:

Sites of concentration	Amount, g	
Muscle	245	
Liver	108	
Blood and extracellular fluid	17	
Total	370	[× 4 kcal/g (17.2 kJ/g) = 1480 kcal (6216 kJ)]

The amount of energy in this stored glycogen provides only enough calories (joules) for half a day for such a person if engaged in a sedentary occupation. The infant, whose liver is one-tenth the size of the adult liver, has much smaller glycogen reserves and is dependent on frequent feedings for an adequate glycogen supply.

When there is a limited supply of carbohydrate, adipose tissue is utilized and then protein stores, as the nonnitrogenous fraction of the protein is converted to energy. This is why carbohydrate has what is termed a *protein-sparing action.* An ample supply of carbohydrate allows the body to conserve protein for tissue maintenance and growth.

Digestion and Absorption

Digestion of carbohydrate is primarily a function of the small intestine, although some breakdown begins in the mouth. The final products of digestion of carbohydrate are glucose, fructose, and galactose (see Fig. 4-1).

The comparative rates of absorption of monosaccharides through the cells of the intestinal mucosa and into the portal bloodstream, in decreasing order of absorption, are as follows: galactose, glucose, fructose, mannose, and the

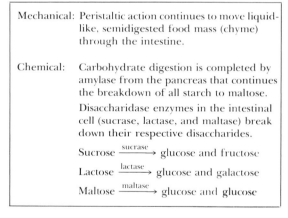

Figure 4-1
The digestion of carbohydrate.

pentoses. Very small amounts of glucose may be absorbed from the stomach. The main site of absorption is in the small intestine, particularly in the duodenum.

Sugars are absorbed in the following mechanisms:

1　*Diffusion*—the process whereby particles in solution randomly move from areas of high concentration to low, thus equalizing the concentration. This is dependent on the sugar concentration between the intestinal lumen, mucosal cells, and blood plasma. Mannose and the pentoses utilize this method.

2 *Active transport*—a process which requires energy to carry particles in solution from an area of lesser to an area of greater concentration. This process requires the use of an energy-dependent carrier system involving sodium to transport sugars through the mucosal cell. Glucose and galactose use this mode of transport.

There is a limiting rate of absorption of about 1 g per kilogram of body weight per hour. Approximately ½ to 1 h after a meal, the blood glucose reaches a maximum of 130 mg per 100 ml, then decreases in 2 to 2½ h to approximately 70 to 90 mg per 100 mL. (This blood glucose curve provides the basis of the glucose tolerance test that is used to diagnose underlying pathology of carbohydrate metabolism; see Chap. 24.) *Hypoglycemia* is the term used to indicate blood sugar levels below the normal range, while hyperglycemia indicates ranges above, and normoglycemia indicates levels within the normal range.

At blood levels about 160 to 190 mg per 100 mL, glucose cannot be reabsorbed by the kidney tubules and is therefore excreted in the urine; this level is called the *renal threshold.*

If blood glucose levels fall markedly, central nervous system signs and symptoms such as dizziness, convulsions, and loss of consciousness may occur. Sustained and profound hypoglycemia may cause irreversible brain damage since the brain has no stored glucose and is dependent on a constant supply.

Metabolism

The prime site of carbohydrate metabolism is the liver. Here glucose is carried after absorption and is stored as glycogen. Fructose and galactose are converted here to glucose, which in turn is stored as glycogen or used for energy.

Other tissues of the body, including adipose, muscle, and renal tissue, are active sites of glucose metabolism. However, for the most part energy metabolism goes on in all cells of the body.

The first stage of glucose metabolism occurs in the cell cytoplasm. In this state, called *glycolysis,* or glucose breakdown, the glucose molecule is split into smaller fragments and phosphorylated (i.e., phosphorus is added to glucose), yielding some energy and glucose 6-phosphate. This glycolytic pathway is known as the *Embden-Myerhof pathway.* The glucose 6-phosphate is then either converted to glycogen (a process known as *gluconeogenesis*) and stored (in the liver or muscle), or proceeds in the presence of oxygen to be converted to pyruvic acid (in the absence of oxygen, to lactic acid). Pyruvic acid then enters the mitochondria of the cell where the oxidative steps of the tricarboxylic acid cycle *(Krebs cycle)* take place, and carbon dioxide, water, and energy are formed (see Fig. 9-7). Ninety percent of the energy derived from carbohydrate is metabolized in this manner.

Another pathway for glucose metabolism is the *pentose phosphate shunt* of the Embden-Myerhof pathway, in which the glucose 6-phosphate is side-channeled to produce pentoses for nucleic acid synthesis and an important enzyme factor called *reduced niacin adenine dinucleotide phosphate* (NADPH), which is needed for the synthesis of fatty acids and steroids.

When energy demands for glucose have been satisfied, and the demand as an intermediate for other types of compounds (e.g., synthesis of nonessential amino acids) has been fulfilled, along with repletion of the storage reserves in tissues and in circulation, excess glucose is then converted to fat through the process of *lipogenesis,* and the fat is stored in various tissues throughout the body.

When there is a need for glucose, glycogen stores in the liver are converted to glucose in the process of *glycogenolysis* and then released into the bloodstream. Glycogen stored in muscle can be used only for immediate local energy and is not available for circulation. If the work or exercise imposed on the body is greater than the

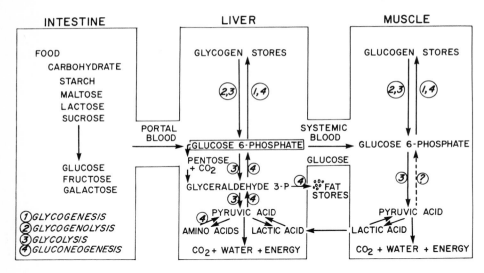

Figure 4-2

The sources and routes of carbohydrate utilization. (1) Glycogenesis; (2) glycogenolysis; (3) glycolysis; (4) gluconeogenesis. (Adapted from A. Cantarow and M. Trumperer, *Clinical Biochemistry*, W. B. Saunders Co., Philadelphia, 1975.)

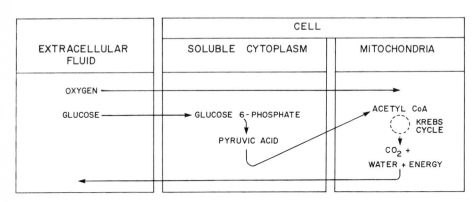

Figure 4-3

The metabolism of glucose within the cell.

oxygen available, the anaerobic process of the Embden-Meyerhof pathway takes place and the glucose is then converted to lactic acid instead of pyruvic acid. The lactic acid is then transported to the liver and converted to glucose and returned to the exercising muscle.

Both proteins and fat are noncarbohydrate sources of glucose. They are converted to glucose by the process of *gluconeogenesis* when energy is needed. Several hormones are crucial to the regulation and integration of the mechanisms for supplying glucose to the blood from the liver and its utilization by the tissues. Insulin, glucagon, epinephrine, thyroxine, and the pituitary hormones are the major influences on glucose metabolism (see Table 4-3).

TABLE 4-3 HORMONAL CONTROL OF CARBOHYDRATE METABOLISM

Hormone	Effect on carbohydrate metabolism	Effect on blood glucose levels
Insulin	Promotes glucose uptake by the cell	Decreases
	Increases glycogen formation from glucose in the muscle	
	Stimulates conversion of glucose to fat	
Glucagon	Stimulates glycogen breakdown and glyconeogenesis in the liver	Increases
Epinephrine	Accelerates glycogenolysis in the liver and muscles, causing a decrease in the glycogen content of these structures	Increases (and blood lactic acid increases)
Thyroxine	Accelerates liver glycogenolysis	Increases
	May increase glucose absorption from the small intestine	
Hydrocortisone	Promotes gluconeogenesis in the liver	Increases
Growth hormone	Acts as an insulin antagonist, thereby depressing glucose utilization by the cell	Increases

DIETARY REQUIREMENTS AND SOURCE OF CARBOHYDRATES

Requirements

The daily requirement for carbohydrate in the diet has not been established by the National Research Council, although there is evidence that humans require at least 100 g per day to provide energy for the nervous system. When carbohydrate is the only source of energy in the diet, the fasting individual requires closer to 150 g per day to prevent tissue (muscle) breakdown. Most adult Americans consume diets that provide 200 to 300 g of carbohydrate per day, which constitutes somewhere between 40 and 50 percent of the calories in our diet. Grain products contribute 40 percent of the carbohydrate in our diet; fruits and vegetables contribute 23 percent. Milk and beverages such as soft drinks or fruit drinks were both about 11 percent. Sugar and sweets constitute approximately 6 percent, but this does not include sweetener as ingredients in other beverages and food products (e.g., ketchup, peanut butter).[5]

Dietary Sources

Both the nature and the amount of carbohydrate in the American diet has changed over the past 40 years. The total carbohydrate content of the diet has declined because of a decreased intake of flour and cereal products. Also, milk, fruit, and vegetable consumption has decreased, causing net losses in dietary carbohydrate. This in part reflects the change from the temporary increase in the use of carbohydrate during the depression years when cereals and potatoes were the more affordable entities. Since that time, increasing prosperity has led to the greater use of meat and dairy products, which are also carriers of saturated fat.

While the amount of carbohydrate has decreased, the type of carbohydrate consumed has changed markedly, with a precipitous rise in sugar consumption. Sugar now contributes 53 percent of the carbohydrate in our national food supply. This large proportion of sugar is related to the greater use of processed foods and soft drinks.

Ripening and processing causes changes in the nature of carbohydrate. In the ripening process in some plants, such as bananas, starch is changed to sugar; in others, such as corn, sugar may be changed to starch as the seed matures. Drying foods such as fruit and vegetables causes a relative increase in their carbohydrate content. Food processors have even modified starch to improve the functionality of a variety of food products. The starch is treated by adding small amounts of chemicals to a suspension of starch granules in water and then all the chemicals that have not reacted with the starch are removed during processing. This processing alters the properties of the starch; however, it does not alter its energy value or digestibility.[6] However, the use of modified food starch in baby foods has caused some concern over the inability of some infants to absorb the modified starch, with consequent diarrhea. It is estimated that over 150 million lb of modified starches are used yearly in salad dressings, fruit pie fillings, canned soups, gravies, frozen dinners, and baby foods.[7] In these products, the modified food starches serve as thickeners, fillers, moisture adsorbents, and carriers for fats, oils, and flavors.

It is apparent that the trend in carbohydrate consumption favors the consumption of carbohydrate in processed foods over that from fresh foods. For the most part, natural food sources of carbohydrate are cereal grains, fruits, vegetables, milk, and concentrated sweets (see Table 4-4).

In food composition tables, carbohydrate is usually listed as total carbohydrate with no differentiation between crude (unavailable) and dietary (available) carbohydrate, and no identification of whether the carbohydrate content is composed of monosaccharides, disaccharides, or polysaccharides. The carbohydrate content of fruit consists mainly of the monosaccharides glucose and fructose, with some disaccharides in the form of sugar, and the polysaccharides cellulose, hemicellulose, dextrins, and pectin. Vegetables have varying amounts of sucrose and starch, with small amounts of glucose and fructose. The root tuber and seed variety of vegetable (potatoes, sweet potatoes, beans, beets, carrots,

TABLE 4-4 THE PERCENTAGE OF CARBOHYDRATE IN FOODS (AVERAGE)

Food	Percentage of carbohydrate
Sugar	99–96
Honey	82
Corn syrup	75
Flour (wheat)	72
Bread	50
Rice	80
Oatmeal	68
Dry corn, cold	85
Dry corn, sugar-coated	91
Bran	
Nuts	7–30
Vegetables	
Legumes, cooked	20
Potatoes, cooked	15
Others	2.5–18
Fruits	
Fresh	6–15
Canned in syrup	20–27
Dried	60–70
Milk	5

squash) have a higher starch and sucrose content, while the leafy vegetables contribute appreciable amounts of cellulose and hemicellulose.

CLINICAL APPLICATIONS

There are many normal (physiologic) conditions and abnormal conditions (disease states) which affect carbohydrate metabolism, as reflected in altered levels of blood glucose (see Tables 4-5 and 4-6), the most common condition being diabetes mellitus (see Chap. 24). There is also some controversy at present about the role of carbohydrate in the causation of coronary heart disease[9] (see Chap. 21). Some of these conditions will require the dietary regulation of the type of carbohydrate, the amount of carbohydrate, or both. It is therefore important for the student to be able to differentiate between the various types of carbohydrate and their food sources.

ADER

TABLE 4-5 DISEASE STATES ALTERING BLOOD GLUCOSE LEVELS

Condition	Increase	Decrease	Condition	Increase	Decrease
Stress (shock, burns, anaesthesia)	X		Extrapancreatic tumors—stomach, adrenal		X
Increased circulating adrenalin from injection or adrenalin-producing tumors	X		Hepatic disease		X
Diabetes mellitus—insulin-dependent or resistant	X		Leucine sensitivity		
ACTH or adrenal steroid therapy	X		Any severe liver disease—cirrhosis, hepatitis, tumors, enzyme deficiencies, Von Gierke's galactosemia		
Acute pancreatitis	X		Poisons		
Wernicke's encephalopathy—thiamine deficiency	X		Endocrine disorders		X
Some central nervous system lesions—subarachnoid hemorrhage	X		Addison's disease and hypopituitarism		
Insulin excess		X	Hypothyroidism		
Insulin overdose or overeffectiveness			Absorptive disturbances		X
Oral antidiabetic agent overdose			Gastroenterostomy, postgastrectomy		X
Pancreatic disorders		X	Malnutrition		X
Islet cell tumor			Ethanol-induced hypoglycemia		X
Pancreatitis			"Reactive" hypoglycemia		X
Glucagon deficiency			After alimentary hyperglycemia		
			Latent diabetes		
			Nervous, high-strung individuals		
			Hypothalamic lesions		X

Source: Adapted from J. Wallach, *Interpretation of Diagnostic Tests*, 3d ed., Little, Brown and Company, Boston, 1978.

TABLE 4-6 PHYSIOLOGICAL CONDITIONS ALTERING BLOOD GLUCOSE LEVELS

Condition	Increase	Decrease
Pain	X (transitory)	
Intense emotion	X (transitory)	
Brief strenuous exercise	X (transitory)	
Protracted strenuous exercise		X
Prematurity in infants		X

Carbohydrate and Dental Caries

Glucose and, to lesser degrees, other disaccharides and monosaccharides play a role in dental caries. Bacteria in the mouth utilize the sugar to produce an acid that invades the enamel of the teeth, causing cavities (see Chap. 17).

Carbohydrate and Exercise

Research has shown that carbohydrate is the preferred energy source for the working muscles of a person in training. Carbohydrate loading is practiced by some athletes. The muscles must be worked to exhaustion 1 week prior to the athletic competition. A diet high in protein and fat is eaten for 3 days; thereafter a high carbohydrate diet is consumed until the day of the athletic event.[10] This promotes maximum glycogen stores, which enhances physical endurance. Weight gain up to 2.5–3.5 kg can occur because of water held with stored glycogen.[11] The use of this regime is controversial. (See Chap. 10.)

Carbohydrate and Weight Reduction

Weight-reduction diets which are low in carbohydrate become popular every few years. Some stress foods high in protein and fat (Dr. Atkins) while others emphasize lean protein as the predominating nutrient with very small amounts of fat and carbohydrate included (Scarsdale diet). The high-fat, low-calorie diet may lead to hyperketonemia and hyperuricemia.[12] A diet which lacks any carbohydrate can lead to ketosis, excessive breakdown of tissue protein, and fluid loss as well as loss of cations, especially sodium.[13] Minimum amounts, 50 to 100 g of digestible carbohydrate, can prevent these undesirable effects. Therefore, vegetables, fruits, and whole-grain breads and cereals should be included in weight-reduction programs.

Carbohydrate and Malabsorption Syndrome

Individuals who have an enzyme lack (disaccharidase deficiency) are unable to digest disaccharides. This causes a state of malabsorption that results in diarrhea, abdominal cramps, flatulence, and failure to thrive. Treatment involves the removal of disaccharides from the diet and supplementation to replace the missing foods. For example, the lactose-intolerant individual, who lacks the enzyme lactase, must avoid milk and milk products, and a milk-free formula or supplement must be provided to replace the missing nutrients (see Chap. 22).

STUDY QUESTIONS

1 Differentiate between a monosaccharide, a disaccharide, and a polysaccharide and give an example of each.
2 What are the main sources of carbohydrate in the American diet?
3 Describe the functions of dietary fiber and list important sources.
4 Trace the route of carbohydrate from ingestion to metabolism.
5 What is the recommended level of carbohydrate in the diet?

CLINICAL STUDY 4

Susan, a 26-year-old active professional, arrives at the company health service with the chief complaint of general lethargy, abdominal pain, and constipation.

A physical examination revealed a normal healthy woman with a height of 5 ft 4 in and weight of 115 lb. Laboratory analysis and gastrointestinal x-ray series were normal. Present diet includes the following meal pattern:

Breakfast	*4 oz orange juice*
	1 English muffin with margarine
	coffee with milk and sugar
Midmorning	*coffee with milk and sugar*
	jelly doughnut
Lunch	*tuna fish sandwich*
	12 oz Coke
	1 candy bar
Dinner	*chicken breast*
	french fried potatoes
	squash
	chocolate cake
	coffee with milk and sugar

On the basis of the normal clinical and laboratory findings, the diagnosis of constipation was made and Susan was referred to the nutritionist for counseling.

Clinical study questions

1 *What types of carbohydrate are excessive in the diet? What types are negligible?*
2 *Outline a diet plan incorporating the type of carbohydrate sources that are lacking.*
3 *How does fiber promote intestinal function?*

REFERENCES

1 V. Marks and E. Samols, "Intestinal Factors and the Regulation of Insulin Secretion," *Advances in Metabolic Disorders* 4:1–38, 1970.

2 J. H. Cummings, Nutritional Implications of Dietary Fiber, *American Journal of Clinical Nutrition,* 31:521–529, 1978.

3 M. Eastwood, "Volvulus of the Colon," in G. A. Spiller and R. J. Amen (eds.), *Fiber in Human Nutrition,* New York, Plenum Publishing Company, 1978.

4 D. A. T. Southgate, "Dietary Fiber: Analysis and Food Sources," *American Journal of Clinical Nutrition,* 31:S107–S110, 1978.

5 *Food and Nutrient Intakes of Individuals in One Day in the United States, Spring 1977,* U.S. Department of Agriculture, Science and Education Administration, September 1980.

6 *Toxicological Evaluation of Some Enzymes, Modified Starches and Certain Other Substances,* WHO Publication 1, Food Additives Series, World Health Organization, Geneva, 1972.

7 *Sugar Report,* U.S. Department of Agriculture, Agricultural Stabilization and Conservation Service, no. 241, 1972.

8 M. G. Hardinge, J. B. Swarner, and H. Crooks, "Carbohydrate in Foods," *Journal of the American Dietetic Association,* 46:197–204, 1965.

9 E. L. Bierman, "Carbohydrates, Sucrose and Human Disease," *American Journal of Clinical Nutrition,* 32:2712–2722, 1979.

10 P. O. Astrand, "Nutrition and Work Performance," *Federation Proceedings,* 26:1772–1777, 1967.

11 K. Ollson and B. Saltin, Diet and Fluids in Training and Competition, *Scandanavian Journal of Rehabilitation Medicine,* 3:31, 1971.

12 S. B. Lewis, J. P. Wallin, S. Kane, and J. E. Gerich, "Effect of Diet Composition on Metabolic Adaptations to Hypocaloric Nutrition: Comparison of High Carbohydrate and High Fat Isocaloric Diets," *American Journal of Clinical Nutrition,* 30:160, 1977.

13 D. H. Calloway, Dietary Components that Yield Energy, *Environmental Biology and Medicine,* 1:175–186, 1971.

CLINICAL DISCUSSION 4

Review of the diet shows the excessive use of refined carbohydrate in the form of baked goods, candy bars, and soft drinks. The lack of fruits, vegetables, whole-grain breads and cereals, and nuts makes the diet low in polysaccharides (cellulose, hemicellulose, lignin, and pectin) and thus low in dietary fiber.

Dietary fiber promotes intestinal function by its ability to take up water and swell, to absorb organic molecules such as bile salts, to exchange cations, and to form a gel. Therefore, Susan was encouraged to increase dietary fiber by including more fresh fruits, vegetables, whole grains (especially bran), and nuts in meals and snacks. In addition, foods with special laxative effect (prunes, apricots, and raisins) were encouraged, along with water and fruit juices. She was also encouraged to increase her activity and incorporate a daily exercise program into her life-style. The following plan was devised.

Breakfast	prune juice
	½ grapefruit
	raisin bran or granola with milk
Midmorning	bran muffin and coffee
Lunch	tuna fish sandwich on whole-wheat bread with lettuce and tomato
	apple
	milk
Midafternoon	juice
	soy nuts
Dinner	meat, fish, or poultry
	2 vegetables (peas and carrots)
	salad
	fruit
	seltzer water

CHAPTER 5

LIPIDS

Rosanne Beatrice Howard
and
Nancie Harvey Herbold

KEY WORDS
Saturated Fats
Unsaturated Fats
Essential Fatty Acids
Medium-Chain Triglycerides
Cholesterol
Phospholipid

INTRODUCTION

The incidence of coronary heart disease has prompted epidemiological surveys of risk factors among populations. Lower average serum cholesterol levels and fewer heart attacks are found in countries where consumption of saturated fat and cholesterol is low.[1] Since increased levels of serum cholesterol and triglycerides have been identified as associated risk factors, much attention has been focused on dietary lipids and their role in the causation, treatment, and prevention of coronary heart disease.

This concern over the type and amount of fat in the diet necessitates a knowledge of lipid function in the human body. In addition there are many conditions, such as biliary obstruction, hypothyroidism, nephrosis, and pancreatic disease, that have associated abnormalities in plasma lipid transport. Also, certain genetic diseases (Tay-Sachs, Gaucher's, Niemann-Pick disease), although not amenable to dietary treatment, have an inherent lipid storage disorder, which further demonstrates the need for health professionals to have an acquaintance with lipid metabolism.

In the human body, lipid has many important roles. Probably the most important quantitatively is that of fuel, since lipid provides twice the energy of carbohydrate and protein. One gram of fat supplies 9.3 kcal (39.06 kJ), while 1 g of either protein or carbohydrate provides 4.1 kcal (17.22 kJ). Lipid is not only an effective fuel source but is the body's storage form of energy, for, unlike carbohydrate and protein, it can be stored in almost unlimited quantity. All cells of the body, except for those of the central nervous system and the erythrocytes, are able to use fatty acids as a source of energy.

Besides providing a storehouse of energy, fat depots exert an insulating effect in the body and cushion the internal organs. Another important function of lipid is that of supplying compounds that cannot be synthesized by the human body, and the fat-soluble vitamins (A, D, E, and K), which are classified as lipids. Some compounds derived from lipids are important building blocks of biologically active materials, for example, the prostaglandins, substances with hormone-like activity that cause many effects in the body. Other lipids that are compounded with proteins, namely lipoproteins, function as structural components of the cell membrane. In the diet, fats have a satiety effect, since fats are digested and absorbed more slowly than carbohydrate and protein.

This chapter considers these functions of lipids within the body and those lipids involved in clinically significant abnormalities.

DEFINITION OF LIPIDS

When lipids are liquid at room temperature, they are called *oils,* and when they are solid at

room temperature, they are called *fats.* Fats and oils can be either visible or invisible to the human eye. The so-called *invisible fats* are those dispersed within a food, such as that within nuts and egg yolks, whereas the visible fats such as butter or vegetable oil are readily apparent to the consumer.

As a group, lipids comprise a heterogeneous collection (fats, oils, waxes, and related organic substances) that are related by the fact that they are poorly soluble in water but are soluble in organic solvents such as ethanol or ether. (This solubility property is utilized in extraction of lipids from tissues.) Lipids are also related by the fact that in their molecular structure there is usually a fatty acid or a fatty acid derivative.

TABLE 5-1 CHEMICAL REACTIONS OF LIPIDS

Property	Reaction	Comments
Hydrogenation	Liquid oils become solid fats by the introduction of hydrogen. This hardening process is used commercially to produce solid cooking fats and margarine from liquid vegetable oils. In processing, the unsaturated bonds of the fatty acids become saturated by the hydrogen gas, in the presence of a catalyst (nickel, palladium, or platinum).	Since this processing affects the degree of saturation, this has significance in determining the vegetable-oil margarine appropriate for diets high in polyunsaturates. The harder the margarine, the less polyunsaturated, which inhibits the ability to alter serum cholesterol.
Iodine number	The iodine number is the amount of iodine that can be retained by 100 g of fat. It reflects the average number of double bonds or the degree of unsaturation of a lipid.	Vegetable oils have a high iodine number and animal fats have a low iodine number. Individuals on a diet lowering blood cholesterol would want to consume fats with a high iodine number, as they would be unsaturated fats.
Saponification (hydrolysis)	Occurs when a fat is hydrolyzed by alkali. Salts are formed (soaps) from the liberation of free fatty acids and glycerol.	Formation of insoluble soaps in the GI tract, whereby fat combines with calcium to form a soap which is excreted in the feces (steatorrhea).
Rancidity	Caused by hydrolysis or oxidation. Oxidation occurs when the double bonds are broken and form peroxides, aldehydes, ketones, and acids, which have an unpleasant odor and flavor. Oxidation requires oxygen and is accelerated by heat, light, moisture, and acids.	Rancidity may be slowed down by storing food in air-tight containers, and in green or brown containers which are light-proof. Vitamin E is a natural antioxidant which may be present in vegetable fat but not animal fat. Vitamin A can become inactivated in rancid fats.

These fatty acids are similar to carbohydrate and contain the same elements—carbon, hydrogen, and oxygen—but there is less oxygen relative to the amounts of carbon and hydrogen in fatty acids than in carbohydrate. Table 5-1 summarizes the chemical reactions of lipids.

CLASSIFICATION OF LIPIDS

Since lipids are such a heterogeneous group, classification is best conceptualized by considering only those lipids that are significant to human nutrition, and then grouping these lipids into two categories, major constituents and minor constituents, based on the amount of lipid present in body tissue (Table 5-2). The minor constituents, fat-soluble vitamins and prostaglandins, are present in minute amounts, milligrams or less. Those in the major category, fatty acids, fatty acid derivatives, and sterols, are present in somewhat larger amounts (e.g., the average amount of cholesterol in serum ranges from 140 to 310 mg per 100 mL in individuals between the ages of 30 and 50; see Chap. 21).[2]

TABLE 5-2 CLASSIFICATION OF LIPIDS ACCORDING TO PRESENCE IN THE BODY

I   Major constituents
   A   Fatty acids
   B   Fatty-acid derivatives
      1   Fatty acids with glycerol: glycerides
      2   Cholesterol esters
      3   Phospholipids: phosphatides (lecithin, cephalin), plasmalogens, sphingomyelins
      4   Glycolipids: cerebrosides, gangliosides
   C   Sterol alcohols
      1   Free cholesterol
      2   Bile acids
      3   Steroids
II Minor constituents
   A   Fat-soluble vitamins: carotene, vitamins A, D, E, K
   B   Prostaglandins

Source: Adapted from Montgomery et al., *Biochemistry: A Case Oriented Approach*, C. V. Mosby Company, St. Louis, 1974, chap. 8.

MAJOR CONSTITUENTS OF LIPIDS IN BODY TISSUE

Fatty Acids

Saturated and Unsaturated Fatty Acids

Fatty acids are the basic structural units of lipids. Fatty acids vary in the number of carbon atoms in the molecule and therefore vary considerably in chain length, with most having an even number of carbon atoms and a straight chain. Fatty acids can be grouped according to chain length into short, medium, and long:

> Short-chain fatty acids: 2 to 4 carbon atoms
> Medium-chain fatty acids: 6 to 10 carbon atoms
> Long-chain fatty acids: 12 to 26 carbon atoms

Fatty acids also vary in another important chemical characteristic, the degree of *saturation* or *unsaturation* (see Fig. 5-1). These terms describe the basic carbon chain and the degree to which it is filled with hydrogen. This is an important concept: the degree of saturation of the lipid determines the effect within the body, namely, the effect on the serum cholesterol, since the position of unsaturation influences the breakup point of the chain in metabolism, affecting the body's ability to modify the molecule and to metabolize the remaining fragments. Saturated fats raise the serum cholesterol, monounsaturated fats have no effect, and polyunsaturated fats lower the serum cholesterol.

An important characteristic of polyunsaturated fatty acids is the shape of the molecule. In unprocessed foods, polyunsaturated fatty acids normally occur in what is known as a *cis* configuration, which means that the fatty acid is folded back upon itself at each of the double bonds. During processing, the cis form may be converted to the unfolded or *trans* form and thereby acquires different nutritional properties. An example would be linoleic acid, which loses its effectiveness as an essential fatty acid during processing when converted from the cis to the trans form.

1 Carbon has a valence of four, which means that in a chemical reaction four atoms may attach to the carbon atom to form a compound.

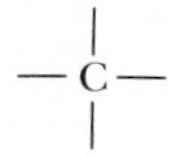

$$-\overset{|}{\underset{|}{C}}-$$

2 During a chemical reaction in which all the valence bonds of a fatty acid become filled with hydrogen, the compound formed is referred to as *saturated*, that is, *"saturated with hydrogen."*

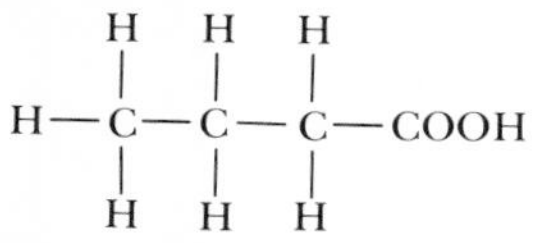

```
      H   H   H
      |   |   |
  H — C — C — C — COOH
      |   |   |
      H   H   H
```

Saturated fat, butyric acid (C$_4$: O)
(4 carbon atoms, no double bond,
found in butter)

3 In the carbon chain of the fatty acid, when there are two less hydrogen atoms attached to the carbon atom, the carbon atoms join their two available valence bonds and make a *mutual bond*. Adding this new mutual bond to an existing bond forms a *double bond*, thereby creating a state of *unsaturation*, which provides room for more hydrogen. It is the number of double bonds present along the carbon chain of the fatty acid that determines the degree of saturation. When there are many double bonds present in a fatty acid, there is more space available to combine hydrogen, and the fatty acid is known as *polyunsaturated*. When there is only one double bond in the fatty acid, it is known as *monounsaturated*.

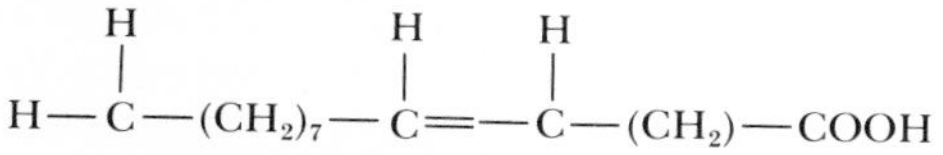

```
      H                H   H
      |                |   |
  H — C —(CH₂)₇— C ═ C —(CH₂)— COOH
      |
      H
```

Monounsaturated, oleic acid (C$_{18}$: 1)
(18 carbon atoms, 1 double bond
found in olive oil)

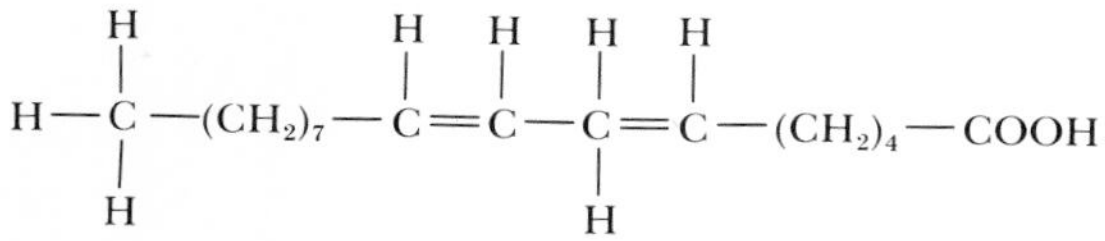

```
      H              H   H   H   H
      |              |   |   |   |
  H — C —(CH₂)₇— C ═ C — C ═ C —(CH₂)₄— COOH
      |                  |
      H                  H
```

Polyunsaturated, linoleic acid (C$_{18}$: 2)
(18 carbon atoms, 2 double bonds
found in vegetable oils)

Figure 5-1
The process of saturation of a fatty acid.

Tables 5-3 and 5-4 (p. 76) list the saturated and unsaturated fatty acids occurring in nature, along with their chemical formulas.

Saturated fatty acids which have carbon chains with fewer than 10 even-numbered carbon atoms are liquid at room temperature, and the melting and boiling points rise as the chains get longer. Those fatty acids with more than 10 carbon atoms are solid at room temperature. Saturated fatty acids with 10 carbons or fewer are usually not present in animal fats. The most abundant saturated fatty acids in animal fats are myristic (C$_{14}$), palmitic (C$_{16}$), and stearic (C$_{18}$). Those saturated fatty acids with fewer than 12 carbons and those with more than 18 have little effect on serum cholesterol, while those in between, lauric (C$_{12}$), myristic (C$_{14}$), and palmitic (C$_{16}$), have the strongest effect of the saturated fatty acids in raising the serum cholesterol in the human body.[3] Animal fat (dairy products, meat) is the abundant source of saturated fatty acids.

All of the common unsaturated fatty acids are liquid at room temperature. Oleic, palmitoleic, linoleic, and linolenic acids are the most unsaturated fatty acids found in nature. They occur in the oils of vegetable and cereal products, such as soy, corn, cottonseed, and safflower oils.

Certain unsaturated fatty acids have been identified as essential to the body because of the fact that:

1 The body is unable to synthesize these fatty acids.

2 The absence of this fatty acid will cause a deficiency state.

Essential Fatty Acids (EFA)

There are two polyunsaturated fatty acids that cannot be synthesized in the human body and must be supplied by the diet. These *essential fatty acids* (EFA) are linoleic and arachidonic. However, arachidonic acid can be formed in the body from linoleic acid and therefore only linoleic acid is actually essential to humans.

Essential fatty acids are necessary to maintain the function and integrity of the cellular and subcellular membranes in tissue metabolism.

TABLE 5-3   SOME NATURALLY OCCURRING SATURATED FATTY ACIDS

Molecular formula	Common name	Systematic name	Number of C atoms
$C_2H_4O_2$	Acetic		2
$C_3H_6O_2$	Propionic		3
$C_4H_8O_2$	n-Butyric		4
$C_6H_{12}O_2$	Caproic	n-Hexanoic	6
$C_8H_{16}O_2$	Caprylic	n-Octanoic	8
$C_9H_{18}O_2$	Pelargonic	n-Nonanoic	9
$C_{10}H_{20}O_2$	Capric	n-Decanoic	10
$C_{12}H_{24}O_2$	Lauric	n-Dodecanoic	12
$C_{14}H_{28}O_2$	Myristic	n-Tetradecanoic	14
$C_{16}H_{32}O_2$	Palmitic*	n-Hexadecanoic	16
$C_{18}H_{36}O_2$	Stearic*	n-Octadecanoic	18
$C_{20}H_{40}O_2$	Arachidic	n-Eicosanoic	20
$C_{22}H_{44}O_2$	Behenic	n-Docosanoic	22
$C_{24}H_{48}O_2$	Lignoceric	n-Tetracosanoic	24
$C_{26}H_{52}O_2$	Cerotic	n-Hexacosanoic	26
$C_{28}H_{56}O_2$	Montanic	n-Octacosanoic	28

*The most common saturated fatty acids in animal fats.

TABLE 5-4   SOME NATURALLY OCCURRING UNSATURATED FATTY ACIDS

Molecular formula	Common name	Systematic name	Number of C atoms	Number of double bonds
$C_{16}H_{30}O_2$	Palmitoleic*	9-Hexadecenoic	16	1
$C_{18}H_{34}O_2$	Oleic*	cis-9-Octadecenoic	18	1
$C_{18}H_{34}O_2$	Elaidic	trans-9-Octadecenoic	18	1
$C_{18}H_{34}O_2$	Vaccenic	11-Octadecenoic	18	1
$C_{18}H_{32}O_2$	Linoleic*	cis,cis-9,12-Octadecadienoic	18	2
$C_{18}H_{30}O_2$	Linolenic*	9,12,15-Octadecatrienoic	18	3
$C_{18}H_{30}O_2$	Eleostearic	9,11,13-Octadecatrienoic	18	3
$C_{20}H_{32}O_2$	Arachidonic	5,8,11,14-Eicosatetraenoic	20	4

*The most common unsaturated fatty acids in animal fats.

Linoleic acid derivatives are also necessary for prostaglandin synthesis. Prostaglandins are hormonelike compounds which have many and varied functions in the human body. They are known to stimulate smooth-muscle contractions, to reduce blood pressure, to inhibit gastric secretions, and to activate or antagonize other hormones.

When linoleic acid is not present in the diet, symptoms of deficiency appear:

Scaly skin

Sparse hair growth

Poor wound healing

Thrombocytopenia (decrease in blood platelets)

The developmental and behavioral changes in progeny of rats fed an EFA-deficient diet during pregnancy and lactation were less pronounced than those resulting from deficiencies of a number of other nutrients. Nevertheless, a brief exposure of the developing fetus to dietary EFA deficiency did impair the development of reflexes; in particular, the startle reaction to sound was most severely affected.[4]

The analysis of blood serum, plasma, or erythrocytes for certain unsaturated fatty acids is used as a diagnostic means of recognizing a dietary deficiency of linoleic acid. Biochemical evidence of EFA deficiency includes a decrease in plasma lipids, arachidonic acid, and linoleic acid, and an increase in 5,8,11-eicosatrienoic, palmitoleic, and oleic acids.[5,6,7] With depletion eicosatrienoic acid becomes detectable in serum. An earlier diagnostic tool of EFA deficiency was an increase in the ratio of trienoic to tetraenoic fatty acids (triene/tetraene ratio) of more than 0.4.[8]

Essential fatty acid deficiency has been reported in hospitalized infants and adults who have been kept on fat-free total parenteral nutrition for several weeks.[9] Infants fed skim milk formulas for extended periods of time without fatty acid supplementation can also become fatty acid-deficient.[10] Once linoleic acid is added to the diet, symptoms of EFA deficiency disappear. To prevent fatty acid deficiency the National Research Council recommends an intake of 1 to 2 percent of the total calories as essential fatty acids.[11] Good sources of linoleic acid are corn, cottonseed, peanut, soybean, and safflower oils.

For infants, particular attention should be given to providing 1 to 3 percent of the energy as linoleic acid, because of the rapid growth period and limited body stores. The American Academy of Pediatrics recommends that infant formula contain 3 percent of its caloric value as essential fatty acids.[12] It has been found that the average linoleic acid content of breast milk from United States mothers amounts to 4 to 5 percent of the total breast milk calories. But variations are found in other populations and are related to the mother's nutritional status and diet.[13]

Essential fatty acids appear to play a role in the regulation of cholesterol metabolism, especially cholesterol transport, its transformation into metabolic products, and the excretion of some of these products. It has been shown that a diet high in essential fatty acids reduces high levels of serum cholesterol in experimental animals and in humans.[14]

Fatty Acid Derivatives

Fatty acids are rarely found free in nature but are combined to other moieties by an ester linkage or an amide linkage, and the complex lipids thus formed can be considered fatty acid derivatives. [An *ester linkage* is a chemical bond that connects an alcohol and an acid of an ester, as in the formation of glycerides (see below). An *amide linkage* connects the alpha-carboxyl group of one amino acid to the alpha-amino group of another amino acid; this linkage becomes operative when fat and protein combine to form a lipoprotein.]

Fatty Acids with Glycerol (Glycerides)
Upon hydrolysis, simple lipids yield fatty acids and glycerol. Glycerol is a sweet viscous liquid that is closely allied to carbohydrate, which it can be converted to within the body. Glycerol contains three hydroxyl (OH) groups, which makes it an alcohol. When the acidic (COOH) groups of the fatty acids react with the alcoholic OH of glycerol, a neutral fat or glyceride results. This process, whereby a compound is formed from an alcohol and a fatty acid by the removal of water, is known as *esterification,* and the product formed is known as an *ester.*

These fatty acid esters of glycerol are known as *acylglycerol* (*acyl group* is the name for the fatty acid moiety in lipid esters) and are commonly called *glycerides* (see Fig. 5-2). There are three general types of glycerides, mono-, di-, and triglycerides. The distinction between them depends on the number of glycerol alcohol groups esterified.

In the human body, monoglycerides are important in digestion and as metabolic intermediates, which is almost the exclusive role of diglycerides. Triglycerides are the major transport and storage form of fatty acids. The average triglyceride content of blood plasma is 140 to 225 mg per 100 mL. These triglycerides for the most part contain long-chain fatty acids.

Medium-chain triglycerides (MCT)—those triglycerides containing medium-chain fatty acids— have been used effectively in the treatment of patients with impaired absorption or digestion of fat (e.g., from biliary obstruction, pancreatic insufficiency, chronic pancreatitis, or cystic fibrosis). These triglycerides contain fatty acids with 8 and 10 carbon atoms and are a mixture of octanoic (C_8) and decanoic (C_{10}) fatty acids. Data gathered from rat studies suggest that MCT may have a depressive effect on fat stores and a reductive effect on lipogenesis. This information, if supported by human studies, may have clinical significance for obesity control.[15] A commercially prepared MCT product is made from coconut oil, which contains octanoic and decanoic acids. When the coconut oil is hydrolyzed, the octanoic and decanoic acids are esterified with glycerol and the resulting product, MCT oil, contains 75 percent octanoic acid and 25 percent decanoic acid.

MCT derives its special effect from the fact that it is digested and metabolized differently from long-chain triglycerides. These medium-chain triglycerides are rapidly hydrolyzed and absorbed directly into the intestinal mucosa where intramucosal lipolysis occurs. They do not require bile salts, chylomicron formation, nor lymphatic transport, and they travel directly to the liver. For example, in the condition known as *a-beta-lipoproteinemia*, absorption of long-chain fatty acids is impaired because of an inherited defect which interferes with the synthesis of low-density lipoproteins. MCT can be used as a dietary supplement to provide a source of dietary fat and energy. Also, MCT is being used to induce ketosis in patients with intractable seizure disorders. Inducing a ketotic state has been shown to be somewhat effective in controlling certain types of seizures in patients who have not responded to drug therapy (Chap. 26).

MCT now provides the fat component of several infant formulas used for children with defects in fat assimilation (Portagen and Pregestimil; Mead Johnson). It is used as a source of readily absorbable energy providing 8.3 kcal (34.8 kJ) per mL for individuals suffering from malabsorptive states.

MCT does not provide a source of essential fatty acid. It is a light yellow oil with a slightly acrid taste that is somewhat apparent only when

Figure 5-2
The formation of a triglyceride. R_1, R_2, and R_3 represent different or identical fatty acids.

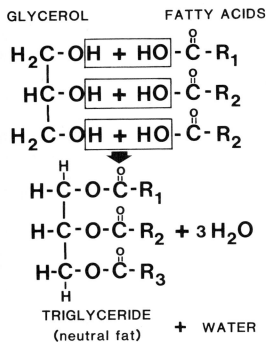

it is added to foods during cooking or preparation.

Cholesterol Esters and Free Cholesterol

Although these compounds should be differentiated by strict classification we will consider them together because of their interrelating role within the body.

Cholesterol is an alcohol and is therefore capable of forming esters with fatty acids. Cholesterol esters contain fatty acids esterified to a 3-beta-hydroxyl group of a steroid ring. The fatty acid component of the ester usually has a long carbon chain and is frequently unsaturated. These cholesterol esters are the storage form of cholesterol and are found in the plasma, constituting two-thirds of the total cholesterol there. In fact, most of the cholesterol that accumulates in the walls of atherosclerotic arteries is esterified. Free or unesterified cholesterol exists in smaller amounts, for the most part in plasma lipoproteins and cell membranes.

Most cholesterol contained in the diet is present as the free sterol and is readily absorbable. It is only present in foods of animal origin, especially meats, glandular organs, egg yolk, whole milk, cheese, and fats. Plants do not have cholesterol but contain other sterols, known as phytosterols, which are poorly absorbed by the human body. These sterols, such as β-sitosterol, if fed in large quantities, are known to inhibit cholesterol absorption. This property is utilized clinically in patients with elevated serum cholesterol levels in an attempt to reduce cholesterol absorption.

In addition to the exogenous supply of cholesterol from food sources, the human body synthesizes cholesterol and thus provides an endogenous supply. Cholesterol is synthesized in most tissues of the body (with the possible exception of the human brain), but primarily in the liver, which regulates cholesterol synthesis.[16] According to Hanes I, the mean per capita intake of cholesterol is 366 mg per day, of which between 40 and 50 percent is absorbed (see Chap. 21).[17]

The fact that the body can synthesize cholesterol has led to some confusion with respect to the effectiveness of low-cholesterol diets in reducing serum cholesterol. It should be noted that although synthesis continues in a normal person on a low-cholesterol and low-saturated-fat diet, the synthesis does not replace that which is taken away from the diet, so that the blood cholesterol level does become somewhat lower. Also, there are certain factors that influence the amount of cholesterol absorbed. They are as follows:[18,19]

The total amount of cholesterol per feeding

The frequency of ingestion

The type of dietary fat fed with cholesterol

Age

Past dietary intake

The body's efficiency in synthesizing cholesterol relates to its important functions within the human body. Cholesterol is a structural component of cell membranes and plasma lipoproteins and is converted in the liver to bile acids. Another important role is that it is a precursor to steroid and sex hormones. In the adrenals, cholesterol, perhaps as a sulfate, is the precursor for pregnenolone, which is the precursor for progesterone, testosterone, and the estrogens, and is also the precursor of the adrenocortical steroids such as aldosterone and cortisol. In the skin, cholesterol serves as the precursor of vitamin D when, on exposure to sunlight or ultraviolet irradiation, 7-dehydrocholesterol is converted to active vitamin D.

Phospholipids

Phospholipids are another class of compound lipids. They are composed of fatty acids, phosphoric acid, and a nitrogenous base. The functions of phospholipids in the body are:

1 Formation of structural elements within the cell

2 Synthesis of cholesterol

3 Carrier in the transport of fatty acids and protein

Phospholipids can be subdivided into three groups:

Phosphatides (lecithin, cephalin)
Plasmalogens
Sphingomyelins

We will focus our attention on the phosphatides and sphingomyelins, as they have the most dietary significance.

Phosphatides (lecithin, cephalin) Phosphatides are derivatives of glycerol phosphate. Upon hydrolysis (the splitting of a compound by the addition of water) phosphatides yield one molecule of phosphoric acid and two molecules of fatty acid. Usually the phosphoric acid is bound to a nitrogenous compound such as choline, in which case it is called phosphatidyl choline. Choline, a vitamin, must be supplied in the diet or synthesized in the body in order to form lecithin. *Lecithin* is composed of glycerol, fatty acid, and the nitrogenous base choline. It is a component of the erythrocyte plasma membrane and is distributed in the cells of the body. Egg yolks and soybeans are excellent sources of lecithin. Lecithin is produced commercially from soybeans for use as an emulsifying agent in such foods as mayonnaise and salad dressings. *Cephalins* are another group of phosphatides that are found in egg yolks and animal tissues, especially brain. Cephalin is present in thromboplastin, which is needed in the blood clotting process.[20]

Sphingomyelins The sphingomyelins are found in the nerves and brain tissue and are components of the myelin sheath which acts as an insulator around the nerve fibers. Sphingomyelins are composed of:

Fatty acids
Phosphoric acid
Choline
Sphingosine

Niemann-Pick disease is a lipid-storage disorder of childhood that is due to the lack of sphingomyelinase, the enzyme needed for the breakdown of spingomyelin. Because of the lack of this enzyme, sphingomyelin is not broken down, and hence is deposited in all organs and tissues of the body. This disease is fatal and many stricken children do not live beyond the age of three.[21]

Glycolipids

Glycolipids are composed of fatty acids, carbohydrate, and nitrogen. Included in this classification of glycolipids are cerebrosides and gangliosides.

Cerebrosides are found in high concentrations in the white matter of the brain and are a component of myelin. They are also found in lesser amounts in the blood serum, erythrocytes, spleen, and kidney. Cerebrosides are composed of:

Sphingosine
Fatty acids (22 to 24 carbon atoms)
Galactose

Gangliosides are also found in the brain and nerve tissue and are typical constituents of synaptic membranes. Gangliosides are composed of:

Sphingosine
Fatty acids (22 to 24 carbon atoms)
Glucose and galactose
Complex compounds containing an amino acid sugar

A number of diseases are caused by a deficiency of the ganglioside enzyme. In Tay-Sachs disease, one such disorder, a large amount of gangliosides is deposited in the gray matter of the brain. It is a disease of infancy and is generally fatal.

THE BODY'S USE OF FAT

Fats play many important roles in human nutrition. Fats contained in foods are sources of energy, of essential fatty acids, and of fat-soluble vitamins. Food fats give flavor to our foods and help to delay the onset of hunger, as fat remains in the stomach longer than carbohydrate or protein. Fat deposits in the adipose tissue insulate the body and cushion the body's organs.

Fats provide twice as much energy as carbohydrate or protein does and therefore are the most concentrated source of energy available to the body. One gram of fat provides 9.3 kcal (39.06 kJ), compared with 4.1 kcal (17.22 kJ) from 1 g of either carbohydrate or protein. Fatty acids can be utilized as a source of energy by all the cells in the body except for the erythrocytes and cells of the central nervous system. Fat can be stored in the adipose tissue and therefore becomes a form of stored energy.

Digestion and Absorption of Fat

Glycerides

Fat digestion does not actually begin until the fat reaches the first section of the small intestine, the duodenum. The secretions which aid in the enzymatic breakdown of fats are:

1   The bile salts, produced by the liver and secreted by the gallbladder
2   Pancreatic lipases, produced and secreted by the pancreas
3   Enteric lipase, secreted by the walls of the intestine

With the aid of the bile salts emulsification takes place. The lipids are divided into small globules which increase the surface area and thereby facilitate enzyme penetration. Aggregation of the bile salts into micelles and the formation of mixed micelles with the products of fat digestion then take place.

Then pancreatic and enteric lipases break the mixed micelles into monoglycerides, diglycerides, fatty acids, and glycerol. Glycerol, monoglycerides, diglycerides, and medium-chain fatty acids (10 carbon atoms or less) are absorbed directly into the portal blood system from the intestine and are transported to the liver. Long-chain fatty acids (over 14 carbon atoms) are first esterified to form neutral fat within the mucosal wall of the intestine and then combine with cholesterol, phospholipids, and protein to form chylomicrons. The chylomicrons are absorbed from the intestine into the lymphatic system and are transported from the thoracic duct to the left subclavian vein, where they enter the venous blood and are carried to the liver. Sixty to seventy percent of dietary fat is absorbed via this route (see Fig. 5-3, p. 82). The remainder, cholesterol and phospholipids, is absorbed by a different route.

Cholesterol

Once dietary cholesterol reaches the small intestine, most of it is esterified with fatty acids by pancreatic cholesterol esterase. This esterified cholesterol is absorbed via the lymphatic system and converted to bile acids in the liver. When bile acids are needed for digestion they are excreted into the small intestine and reabsorbed with the digested fat. This process, which is known as the *enterohepatic cycle,* regulates cholesterol synthesis by negative feedback. It is this endogenous synthesis that makes dietary restriction of cholesterol not totally effective in regulating serum cholesterol (see Fig. 5-3).

Phospholipids

Phospholipids are ingested in food in the form of lecithin. They may also by synthesized by the small intestine. Dietary phospholipids can be absorbed directly into the portal system, while synthesized phospholipids are incorporated into chylomicrons and absorbed via the lymphatics (see Fig. 5-3).

Fat Absorption Test

Some fat is not absorbed but is excreted via the stool. An excretion of fecal fat about 6 g per day is a condition known as *steatorrhea.* Steatorrhea is caused by a malabsorption of fat due to defective breakdown and absorption.

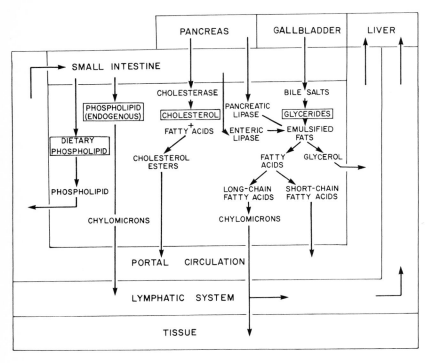

Figure 5-3
The various mechanisms of fat absorption.

Normal adults can absorb up to 300 g of fat daily. A fecal fat test is used in the diagnosis of many gastrointestinal disorders. The test involves the use of a high-fat diet: patients must consume a diet of 100 g of fat daily for 3 days prior to a stool collection. If the amount of fat in the collected stool exceeds 6 g (6 percent of the ingested fat), steatorrhea exists and various disorders must be ruled out.[22] In the child, a loss of fecal fat greater than 5 percent of the ingested fat constitutes steatorrhea.[23]

Metabolism of Fat

Once chylomicrons reach the liver they are metabolized or are converted to alpha- and beta-lipoproteins which are used for energy, if needed, or stored in adipose tissue.

Fat storage is an active process. *Lipogenesis* (synthesis and deposition of fat) and *lipolysis* (mobilization and oxidation of fat) are ongoing processes. Fatty acids and glycerol are the end products of these reactions. The hydrolysis of triglycerides to glycerol and fatty acid is one of the first steps in fat synthesis and deposition. Fatty acids are further broken down during oxidation into two carbon units and acetyl CoA. Thereafter, fat follows the same oxidative pathway as carbohydrate (the Krebs cycle; see Chap. 9). See Fig. 5-4.

Incomplete oxidation of fat, such as occurs during states of fasting or uncontrolled diabetes mellitus, leads to the formation of ketone bodies (acetoacetic acid, beta-hydroxybutyric acid, and acetone) and accumulation in the blood (ketonemia) with subsequent excretion in the urine (ketonuria). This state is known as *ketosis*. Under this condition, the brain, which normally uses glucose for energy, utilizes ketone bodies. To a limited extent, other tissues of the body also utilize ketones in lieu of glucose.

Since glycerol cannot be oxidized by most

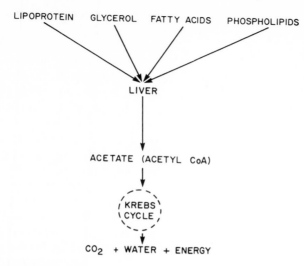

Figure 5-4
The metabolism of fat.

tissues of the body, it is transported to the liver where it combines with fatty acids to form triglycerides and is then transported to the cells. The liver plays an important role in fat metabolism; its functions are summarized as follows:

1 Synthesis of triglycerides from carbohydrate
2 Synthesis of cholesterol from triglycerides
3 Synthesis of phospholipid and lipoprotein from protein
4 Clearance of phospholipid, cholesterol, and lipoprotein from the plasma

In addition to the liver, hormones also affect fat metabolism, causing fat to be mobilized, synthesized, utilized, or released from tissue stores. Table 5-5 summarizes the effect of the body's hormones on fat metabolism.

Deposition of Fat

When fat has been metabolized and energy requirements have been met, excess fat is stored or deposited in certain anatomical sites, which include subcutaneous tissue, the peritoneal cavity, and intramuscular tissue.

The storage or deposition of excessive fat results in obesity. Normally fat comprises approximately 30 percent of body weight in the female and 16 percent of body weight in the male.[24] During these periods fat is transported from the storage depots to the actively metabolizing tissue requiring energy. Those depots found under the skin respond first to dietary deprivation.

Types of Fat Deposition

Both age and diet affect the deposition and the composition of body fat. For example, the composition of adipose tissue of a newborn differs markedly from that of an elderly individual. In the newborn period, only 40 percent of adipose tissue is composed of lipid (the other 60 percent is mostly water with some nitrogen); however, in the elderly, adipose tissue contains approximately 75 percent lipid. Also, with age there is a tendency for more fat to be deposited since activity patterns usually decrease, and there may not be a concomitant decrease in food intake.

The fact that diet affects the type of body fat deposition has been demonstrated by animal studies. In animals fed on diets high in saturated

TABLE 5-5   HORMONES AFFECTING FAT METABOLISM

Hormone	Effect on fat
↓ *Insulin*	↓ Fat synthesis ↑ Fat mobilization
↑ *Insulin*	↑ Fat synthesis ↓ Fat mobilization
↑ *Growth hormone*	↑ Release of FFA (free fatty acids) from adipose tissue
↑ *Thyroxine*	↑ Mobilization of fat by energy metabolism
↑ *ACTH (adrenocorticotropic hormone)*	↑ Mobilization of fat by energy metabolism
↑ *Glucocorticoids*	↑ Fat mobilization
↑ *Epinephrine*	↑ Fat mobilization
↑ *Glucagon*	↑ Fat mobilization ↓ Fat synthesis

fatty acids, the depot of animal fat was also high in saturated fatty acids. A comparable phenomenon was observed with diets high in unsaturated fatty acid. Humans consuming a high polyunsaturated diet have lower serum cholesterol levels and adipose tissue that is higher in unsaturated fatty acids than are found in individuals maintained on high saturated fatty acid diet.

The extrapolation of this information to animal husbandry may provide a new therapeutic tool in the prevention of heart disease, whereby a change in animal feeds that alters the adipose tissue of animals might produce an effect on the type of fat in the human diet. A reduction in the amount of fat produced in animals is already quite evident from the difference between corn-fed and grass-fed animals, with the latter having fewer fat stores.

DIETARY SIGNIFICANCE AND REQUIREMENTS OF FAT

In the United States, evidence of the effect of dietary fat composition on blood lipid levels has changed the research, production, and sales of fats and fatty acids. Since the early 1960s, there has been a profound increase in the consumption of salad and cooking oils. In the Hanes Survey, 38 percent of energy intake was contributed by fat. Forty percent of that intake came from saturated fat sources.[25]

With the introduction of tub-type margarines and more stick-type margarines with higher levels of unsaturation, there has been a marked increase in the polyunsaturates/saturates ratio (P/S ratio) of the visible fat portion of the diet. The P/S ratio indicates the quantitative relationship between the polyunsaturated and the saturated fatty acids in the diet. Of interest is the increase in the P/S ratio, which was 0.5 to 1 in 1959 and grew to 1 to 1 in 1971.[26] Some questions have been raised as to whether the amounts of highly unsaturated fatty acids should be increased much above present levels and whether or not polyunsaturated fatty acids are benign compounds imposing risk with large consumption. The committee on Dietary Allowances rec-

ommends an upper limit of 10 percent of caloric intake as polyunsaturated fatty acids.[27]

The issues surrounding the P/S ratio of the diet remain unresolved, but current clinical practice is to limit the total amount of fat and within the fat limitations to use polyunsaturates in the diet. An increase in the P/S ratio is achieved by placing dietary emphasis on vegetable oils (safflower, corn, soybean, sunflower, sesame) and margarines, and reducing the saturated fat intake by limiting animal meats and dairy products, with fish and fowl used as substitutes.

The total fat content of the diet has no specific requirement other than to provide enough to supply the essential fatty acids and the fat-soluble vitamins. It is estimated that a diet containing between 15 and 25 g of appropriate food fat should provide the dietary requirement for fat (see Table 5-6).[28] The American Heart Association has recommended that 35 percent of the total calories in the diet be derived from fat (see Chap. 21).[29]

During infancy, clinical experience indicates that 30 to 55 percent of the energy should be provided from fat. Diets deviating from this range upwardly tax the infant's digestive and

TABLE 5-6   THE FAT COMPOSITION OF SELECTED FOODS

Food	Household measure	Fat, g
Milk (whole)	8 oz	12.0
Milk (skim)	8 oz	0.2
Beef (ground lean)	3 oz	9.1
Chicken (breast)	3 oz	5.1
Fish (halibut)	3 oz	6.0
Margarine (stick type)	1 tsp	3.8
Butter (stick type)	1 tsp	3.8
Corn oil	1 tbsp	13.6
Peanut butter	1 tbsp	8.1
Salad dressing	1 tbsp	11.2

Source: Nutritive Value of American Foods, U.S. Department of Agriculture Handbook 456, Agriculture Research Service, 1975.

excretory capabilities.[30] With lower fat intakes, the carbohydrate and protein content of the diet increases. An increase in carbohydrate causes an increase in disaccharides in the intestinal lumen which may exceed the existing disaccharidase activity and cause diarrhea. An increase in protein may present an excessive renal solute load to the immature kidney. It is interesting to note that 50 percent of the calories in human milk are derived from fat, and therefore most commercial formulas which are produced to simulate human milk provide between 35 and 50 percent of the calories as fat.

Clinical Application

There are many conditions which affect lipid metabolism, as reflected in altered levels of lipid in blood plasma (see Tables 5-7 and 5-8). Some of these conditions will require regulation of dietary fat. For the most part, those conditions requiring fat modification or reduction are malabsorption syndromes, gallbladder disease, coronary heart disease, diabetes mellitus, fatty liver, cystic fibrosis, and obesity. Other conditions require fat additions, for example, the underweight individual or the use of fat to induce ketosis in seizure patients (see Chap. 26).

Dietary fat is regulated by changing the total amount of fat in the diet, by changing the type of fat in the diet, or by changing both. In order to be effective in helping the patient to modify the dietary intake, the student will need to understand the differences between saturated fatty acids, polyunsaturated fatty acids, cholesterol, and medium-chain triglycerides and to know their functions in the human body.

Dietary fat is becoming a significant risk factor in coronary heart disease and a possible risk factor in cancer of the colon and breast. In epidemiological surveys high-fat diets (also high in animal protein) have been identified as risk factors in countries with a high incidence of bowel cancer.[31] Therefore, the control of fat is an important tenet of preventive nutrition. In addition, our population, for the most part sedentary, does not require the extra energy from fat.

TABLE 5-7 AVERAGE VALUES OF LIPID CONTENT OF BLOOD PLASMA*

Type	Age, yr	Value, mg per 100 mL
Cholesterol† (total)	Birth	40–90
	1–19	120–230
	20–29	120–240
	30–39	140–270
	40–49	150–310
	50–59	160–330
Cholesterol esters		Determined by 60–75% of the total cholesterol values
Triglycerides	1–19	10–140
	20–29	10–140
	30–39	10–150
	40–49	10–160
	50–59	10–190
Phospholipids		60–350
Vitamin A		65–275 IU
		20 µg per 100 mL
Vitamin E (tocopherol)		>0.5 mg per 100 mL
Carotene		100–300 IU
Vitamin D		0.7–3.3 IU per mL (Procedure not generally available.) Indirect estimate by serum alkaline phosphatase, calcium, and phosphorus

*Normal values vary depending on the individual laboratory and the method used.

†Total serum cholesterol as measured in the laboratory represents the sum total of cholesterol contained in high-density lipoprotein (HDL), low-density lipoprotein (LDL), very-low-density lipoprotein (VLDL), and the chylomicrons.

A prudent, fat-controlled diet should be initiated during the early years of life. There are many risk factors to our health in our environment, such as noise and pollution, that cannot be easily controlled; however, fat can be controlled, and you as a future health professional, through nutrition education, can help our population to adopt the prudent diet and elicit the control of fat necessary to foster health (see Chap. 2).

TABLE 5-8   CONDITIONS ALTERING LIPID CONTENT OF BLOOD PLASMA

Blood lipid	Condition	Increased in	Decreased in
Triglycerides	Familial hyperlipidemia	X	
	Liver diseases	X	
	Nephrotic syndrome	X	
	Diabetes mellitus (higher values correlate with hyperglycemia and poorer control of diabetes; reduced by insulin therapy)	X	
	Pancreatitis	X	
	Von Gierke's disease	X	
	Acute myocardial infarction (rise to peak in 3 wk; increase may persist for 1 yr)	X	
	Malnutrition		X
	Congenital a-beta-lipoproteinemia (rare disease characterized by acanthocytes, absence of serum low-density lipoproteins, very low serum triglyceride values—i.e., less than 6 mg per 100 mL)		X
Cholesterol	Idiopathic hypercholesterolemia	X	
	Biliary obstruction (stone, carcinoma, etc., of duct; cholangiolitic cirrhosis)	X	
	Von Gierke's disease	X	
	Hypothyroidism	X	
	Nephrosis (due to chronic nephritis, renal vein thrombosis, amyloidosis, systemic lupus erythematosus, periarteritis, diabetic glomerulosclerosis)	X	
	Pancreatic disease	X	
	Diabetes mellitus	X	
	Total pancreatectomy	X	
	Chronic pancreatitis (some cases)	X	
	Pregnancy	X	
	Severe liver damage (due to chemicals, drugs, hepatitis)		X
	Hyperthyroidism		X
	Malnutrition (e.g., starvation, terminal neoplasm, uremia, malabsorption in steatorrhea)		X
	Chronic anemia		X
	Pernicious anemia (in relapse)		X
	Hemolytic anemias		X
	Marked hypochromic anemia		X
	Cortisone and ACTH therapy		X
	A-beta-lipoproteinemia Tangier disease		X
Carotenoids	Excessive intake (especially carrots)	X	
	Postprandial hyperlipemia	X	
	Hyperlipemia (e.g., essential hyperlipemia)	X	
	Diabetes mellitus	X	
	Hypothyroidism	X	

TABLE 5-8   CONTINUED

Blood lipid	Condition	Increased in	Decreased in
Carotenoids (*continued*)	Carotenoid-poor diet (blood level falls within 1 week, while vitamin A level is unaffected by dietary change for 6 mo because of much larger body stores)		×
	Malabsorption syndrome (a very useful screening test for malabsorption)		×
	Liver disease		×
	High fever		×
Lipoproteins	Alterations in familial lipoprotein abnormalities	*	*
	Tangier disease [marked decrease (heterozygous) or absence (homozygous) of high-density lipoprotein; pre-beta-lipoprotein is absent]		
	A-beta-lipoproteinemia (low-density beta-lipoproteins are absent; high-density lipoproteins are normal; patients also have acanthotic RBCs and low serum carotene levels)		

*See Chap. 17.

Source: Jacques Wallach, *Interpretation of Diagnostic Tests: A Handbook Synopsis of Laboratory Medicine,* 3d ed., Little, Brown Company, Boston, 1978.

STUDY QUESTIONS

1 Explain the difference between a polyunsaturated fat and a saturated fat.

2 What unsaturated fatty acids have been identified as essential to the body and why are they called "essential"?

3 What is the role of cholesterol in the body?

4 The mode of absorption of fat differs according to chain length. What is the clinical significance?

5 Excessive storage of fat results in obesity. What is the mechanism of fat deposition and in what areas of the body is fat stored?

CLINICAL STUDY 5

A 3-month-old girl was brought to the clinic because of irritability and marked failure to thrive. The past history revealed that at 3 weeks of age, the infant had been changed to a skim milk formula in attempts to control diarrhea.

On physical examination, the infant was found to be growing 2 standard deviations from the mean,

with a height of 56.3 cm and a weight of 5.2 kg. Noted were scaly dermatitis on the forehead, the medial ends of the eyebrows, the points of the shoulders, and the scalp; multiple subcutaneous hemorrhages; and sparse hair. Present diet includes eight 6-oz bottles of skim milk, 3 oz of orange juice, and 4 teaspoons of rice cereal, providing a total of 537 kcal (2255 kJ) or

100 kcal (420 kJ) per kilogram per day. The infant was receiving supplemental vitamins A, C, and D.

Laboratory analysis revealed eicosatrienoic acid of 0.85 mg per dL, a serum cholesterol level of 115 mg per 100 mL, a total serum lipid level of 200 mg per 100 mL, a hemoglobin level of 9.8 g per 100 mL, a hematocrit of 31 percent, and a platelet count of 4.5 × 10⁻⁵ mm³.

Clinical questions

1 From the biochemical profile and clinical state, what deficiency state would you identify?

2 Based on your diagnosis, what recommendations would you make?

3 How would you relate the symptoms exhibited in this patient to the role of the missing nutrient?

REFERENCES

1 *Healthy People: The Surgeon General's Report on Health Promotion and Disease Prevention, DHEW (PHS) Publication*, U.S. Department of Health, Education and Welfare Publication (PHS) 79-550 71, 1979.

2 J. Wallach, *Interpretation of Diagnostic Tests: A Handbook Synopsis of Laboratory Medicine*, 3d ed., Little, Brown and Company, Boston, 1978.

3 H. B. Brown, "Food Patterns That Lower Blood Lipids in Man," *Journal of American Dietetic Association*, **58**:303, 1971.

4 M. S. Lamptey and B. L. Walker, "Physical and Neurological Development of Female Rats Fed an Essential Fatty Acid Deficient Diet During Pregnancy and/or Lactation," *Journal of Nutrition*, **108**:351-357, 1978.

5 J. F. Mead, "The Metabolism of Polyunsaturated Fatty Acids," in R. T. Folman (ed.), *Progress in Chemistry of Fats and Other Lipids*, vol. 9, Pergamon Press, Inc., New York, 1968, pp. 159-192.

6 B. Samuelson, "Biosynthesis of Prostaglandins," *Federation Proceedings*, **31**:1442, 1972.

7 Z. Friedman, A. Daron, M. Stahlman, and J. Oates, "Rapid Onset of EFA Deficiency in the Newborn," *Pediatrics*, **58**(5):640-648, November 1976.

8 W. F. Cuthbertson, "Essential Fatty Acid Requirements in Infancy," *American Journal of Clinical Nutrition*, **29**:559-568, May 1976.

9 M. Caldwell, H. Jonsson, and H. B. Othersen, Jr., "Essential Fatty Acid Deficiency in an Infant Receiving Prolonged Parental Alimentation," *Journal of Pediatrics*, **81**:894, 1972.

10 J. R. Paulsrud, L. Pensler, C. F. Whitten, S. Stewart, and R. T. Holman, "Essential Fatty Acid Deficiency in Infants Induced by Fat Free Intravenous Feedings," *American Journal of Clinical Nutrition*, **25**:897, 1972.

11 Food and Nutrition Board, *Recommended Dietary Allowances*, 9th ed., 1980, p. 34.

12 American Academy of Pediatrics, "Commentary on Breast Feeding and Infant Formulas Including Standards for Formulas," *Pediatrics*, **57**:278-285, 1976.

13 Cuthbertson, op. cit., p. 565.

14 Brown, op. cit., p. 303.

15 M. M. Lavau and S. A. Hashim, "Effects of Medium Chain Triglycerides on Lipogenesis and Fat in the Rat," *Journal of Nutrition*, **108**:613-620, 1978.

16 R. Goodhart and M. Shils, *Modern Nutrition in Health and Disease*, Lea & Febiger, Philadelphia, 1980, p. 131.

17 S. Abraham, M. D. Carroll, C. M. Dresser, and C. L. Johnson, "Dietary Intake Findings, United States, 1971-1974," *Vital and Health Statistics*, ser. 11, no. 202, DHEW Publication no. (HRA) 77-1647, Health Resources Administration, Washington, D.C., July 1977, p. 38.

18 D. S. Goodman, "Cholesterol Ester Metabolism," *Physiological Reviews*, **45**:747-839, 1965.

19 L. Swell, E. C. Trout, J. R. Hooper, H. Field, and C. R. Treadwell, "The Mechanism of Cholesterol Absorption," *Annals of New York Academy of Science*, **72**:813, 1959.

20 A. C. Guyton, *Textbook of Medical Physiology*, 5th ed., W. B. Saunders Company, Philadelphia, 1976, p. 924.

21 R. Pike and M. Brown, *Nutrition: An Integrated Approach*, 2d ed., John Wiley & Sons, New York, 1975, p. 46.

22 J. Wallach, *Interpretation of Diagnostic Tests*, 3d ed., Little, Brown, Boston, 1978, p. 141.

23 Nelson, op. cit., p. 1078.

24 Pike and Brown, op. cit., p. 805.

25 Abraham et al., op. cit., p. 44.

26 American Medical Association, *Nutrients in Processed Foods*, vol. 3, *Fats and Carbohydrates*, Publishing Sciences Group, Inc., Acton, Mass., 1975, p. 8.

27 Food and Nutrition Board, op. cit., p. 35.

28 Ibid., p. 33.
29 American Heart Association Committee on Nutrition, Diet, and Coronary Heart Disease, A Statement for Physicians and Other Health Professionals, 1978.
30 S. J. Foman, *Infant Nutrition,* W. B. Saunders Company, Philadelphia, 1974, p. 164.
31 J. Berg, "Nutrition and Cancer," *Seminars in Oncology,* 3(1):17ff.

CLINICAL DISCUSSION 5

This infant shows the classic signs of essential fatty acid deficiency. Since essential fatty acids are necessary to maintain the function and integrity of the cellular and subcellular membranes, changes in the skin manifest the deficiency state. It is speculated that the change in the fatty acid composition of the phospholipid of the membranes is the primary lesion of the EFA deficiency.*

All of these symptoms were reversed within a 2-week period by the administration of linoleic acid. The infant was gaining steadily and thriving on iron-fortified Similac, in which linoleic acid constitutes 15 percent of the total calories, providing more than the 1 to 3 percent of the total calories recommended to be fed as linoleic acid. The parents were counseled regarding baby-food additions and the hazards of using skim milk during the first year of life.

*E. F. Sinclair, in R. Paoletti (ed.), *Lipid Pharmacology,* Academic Press, New York, 1964, p. 237.

CHAPTER 6
VITAMINS

Patricia A. Kreutler

KEY WORDS
Fat-Soluble Vitamins
Water-Soluble Vitamins
Vitamin Deficiency
Vitamin Toxicity
Retinol Equivalents
Cholecalciferol
Tocopherol
Niacin Equivalents
Megavitamin Therapy
Vitamin Supplements

INTRODUCTION

The vitamin story has had many exciting chapters. The current popular and scientific interest in nutrition, coupled with concerns about vitamin deficiencies and possible excesses caused by supplementation, promises to maintain the momentum in the efforts to unravel their mechanism of action. In addition, new discoveries about the interactions of the vitamins with drugs and other nutrients have generated another focus for research.

The word *vitamine* was proposed by Casimir Funk in 1911 to describe a new "food factor" found to be necessary for health and life, but chemically different from the essential nutrients known at that time, namely, carbohydrates, fats, and proteins. As more and more of these factors were discovered, it was found that they were not all amines, but a variety of chemical compounds: and the general name was changed to *vitamin*.

By definition, vitamins are organic compounds that are required by the body in trace amounts to perform specific cellular functions. They are considered essential because they cannot be synthesized in sufficient amounts by the body, and an exogenous source is therefore required. Although a single nutrient class, vitamins are a heterogeneous group, because they differ in their chemistry, function, and distribution in foods.

Much of what we know about vitamins has resulted from the so-called deficiency diseases. Recognition of what happens when an essential substance is missing very often leads to definition of its particular and important function, and this has certainly been true in the study of vitamins. These compounds act as cofactors in biochemical reactions involving the transport and metabolism of other nutrients, and may perform structural functions as well.

Vitamins are generally divided into groups on the basis of their solubility. Vitamins A, D, E, and K are soluble in fat and fat solvents. This property is reflected in their distribution in foods, storage in the body, and mechanism of excretion. Because our bodies can store them, they do not have to be consumed every day, and there is also the danger of toxicity, particularly for vitamins A and D.

Vitamin C and the B complex vitamins are water-soluble, and because amounts in excess of what our bodies need are readily excreted, they must be provided in the diet regularly.

Because no one food contains all the vitamins our body needs, it is important to consume a variety of foods to ensure an adequate intake.

A vitamin deficiency can be classified as either primary or secondary. Primary deficiency is caused by consuming an inadequate intake; in secondary deficiency, the recommended allowance may be ingested, but because of disease, medication, or physiological states such as pregnancy, lactation, and growth, the actual individual requirement is increased. Regardless of the etiology of the deficiency, insufficient vitamin intake for a prolonged period of time will be reflected in a decrease in the serum and tissue levels of the vitamin, followed by or coincident with a decrease in the biochemical function for which it is required, and finally the manifestations of a clinical deficiency disease will appear.

FAT-SOLUBLE VITAMINS

Vitamin A

History and Discovery

Shortly after Funk proposed the vitamin theory, two independent groups of researchers reported the existence of a fat-soluble substance that affected growth and reproduction in rats, and might be a candidate for the newly designated vitamin category. In 1912 Osborne and Mendel, working at Yale, noted that rats demonstrated growth failure when milk fat was removed from their diet, and eye lesions also were apparent. Reintroduction of milk fat abated the symptoms. At about the same time, McCollum and Davis from the University of Wisconsin fed rats purified diets with the fat provided by lard. These rats failed to grow after several months, and also developed eye disease. If the rats were then provided with butterfat or egg yolk, the symptoms were reversed. The unidentified fat-soluble substance was named *vitamin A*. The next step in the understanding of this new growth factor was the work of Steenbock, who identified a yellow pigment, carotene, from yellow vegetables; this pigment also demonstrated growth-promoting properties, and was further identified as a precursor of the vitamin found in animal products.

In 1937 a fat-soluble substance with the physiological properties of vitamin A was isolated from cod liver oil, and in 1946 the vitamin was synthesized. It is colorless and heat-stable, but labile to oxygen and ultraviolet light.

Chemistry

Preformed vitamin A exists in three forms, retinol (an alcohol), retinal (an aldehyde), and retinoic acid. All of these are biologically active, although there is some specificity of function among various forms. Figure 6-1 demonstrates the chemical relationship between the three forms. Most of the vitamin A we ingest from food exists in the alcohol form, which can be reversibly oxidized to the aldehyde form. It is the latter which is functional in the response of vision in dim light. Further oxidation produces the acid form, which is no longer useful in the visual cycle, but which retains the growth-promoting properties of the vitamin.

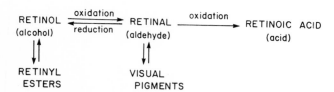

Figure 6-1
Chemical relationship between the three forms of preformed vitamin A—retinol, retinal, and retinoic acid.

Metabolism

Preformed vitamin A usually occurs in foods as a retinol ester. After ingestion, the vitamin is hydrolyzed by pancreatic or intestinal enzymes to retinol and the fatty acid. Because vitamin A is a fat-soluble substance, those factors which enhance fat absorption also increase the absorption of the vitamin. After uptake of retinol into the mucosal cell, it is rapidly reesterified, primarily with palmitate, and is packaged into chylomicrons for transport via the lymph to the general circulation.

Provitamin A (α-, γ-, and especially β-carotene) is converted to vitamin A, primarily in the intestinal mucosa. Theoretically, one molecule of β-carotene will produce two molecules of retinol, but the cleavage enzyme is only about 50 percent effective; in addition, only one-third of the β-carotene which exists in food is absorbed. The net result is that β-carotene is approximately one-sixth as effective as the same amount of preformed vitamin A. This fact is reflected in the recommended dietary allowance (RDA) for vitamin A, which is expressed as retinol equivalents (RE).

After absorption, vitamin A is transported to the liver, where it is stored as the alcohol ester. When vitamin A is needed by the body, it is mobilized from the liver and transported to the tissues by a special transport protein, retinol-binding protein (RBP). The protein forms a complex with prealbumin, which serves to protect against excessive loss of the vitamin and RBP from the kidney and therefore in the urine. The release of the binding protein appears to be dependent on the presence of vitamin A in the liver. Also, protein deficiency affects vitamin A status, probably by decreasing the synthesis of RBP. After dietary rehabilitation of malnourished patients, serum levels of both RBP and vitamin A increase.[1]

The role of zinc in vitamin A metabolism is unclear. Smith et al.[2] reported that zinc deficiency in animals is associated with decreased mobilization of vitamin A, and linked this finding to a decrease in RBP synthesis.[3] Other researchers have demonstrated that zinc deficiency can cause abnormal dark adaptation in humans.[4] However, zinc supplementation to people who are not zinc-deficient has no elevating effect on plasma vitamin A levels.[5,6] A review of the interaction of vitamin A and zinc has been published.[7]

Several other clinical conditions have been implicated in vitamin A metabolism. Liver disease decreases serum levels of the vitamin and its binding protein, whereas in renal disease an increase is observed.[8] Several drugs have been shown to influence vitamin A status as well. Oral contraceptives increase serum vitamin A and RBP levels; cholestyramine (a drug used to lower blood cholesterol) and mineral oil interfere with its absorption.

Function

The only physiological function of vitamin A that has been clearly defined in biochemical terms is its role in the so-called visual cycle. In 1967 George Wald earned a Nobel Prize for this discovery. Night blindness results from vitamin A deficiency, because the vitamin is required to regenerate the chemical which allows us to see in dim light. Rhodopsin is the complex of opsin (a protein present in the rods of the eye) and the retinal form of vitamin A. A simplified scheme of the process is shown in Fig. 6-2. Because some retinal is degraded in the process of rhodopsin degradation caused by bright light, additional vitamin A is necessary to regenerate the

Figure 6-2
Function of vitamin A in the visual cycle.

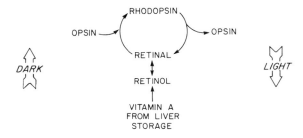

complex. Thus, normal vision cannot be attained quickly after rhodopsin bleaching by bright light, such as that from an oncoming car, unless there is an ample supply of stored vitamin A.

While only retinol and retinal can be used for maintenance of the visual cycle, all three forms function in maintaining growth. Rats fed retinoic acid will maintain their growth rate, but will soon develop eye lesions. Some research suggests that vitamin A allows the maturation of osteoblasts to osteoclasts, a conversion necessary for the remodeling and therefore continued growth of bone.[9]

Vitamin A is also required for the maintenance of epithelial tissue; that is, of the cells which are found in the outer layers of the skin as well as lining the gastrointestinal, respiratory, and urogenital tracts. Likewise, in tooth development vitamin A is necessary for the normal differentiation and function of the ameloblasts, cells of ectodermal origin which are responsible for the formation of dental enamel.

Vitamin A deficiency results in a transformation of epithelial cells from soft, moist tissue to cells which are hard and dry or keratinized. This effect has been related to the protective effect of vitamin A in maintaining the integrity of epithelial tissue against infective organisms, particularly of the respiratory tract. The biochemical effect of vitamin A in this function is not clear; it may exert a direct effect on the synthesis of mucopolysaccharides and glycoproteins.

Dietary Allowances and Sources

Allowances for vitamin A are expressed as retinol equivalents (RE).[10] This term, which replaces international units (IU), was introduced to take into account the presence of both preformed vitamin A and its pro-vitamin carotene in foodstuffs, and the relative efficiency of carotene utilization. Allowances related to age and sex can be found in the RDA table (see Appendix, Table A-1).

Retinol equivalents can be calculated by using the following information:

$$1 \text{ RE} = 1 \ \mu\text{g retinol}$$
$$= 6 \ \mu\text{g } \beta\text{-carotene}$$
$$= 12 \ \mu\text{g other carotenes}$$
$$= 3.33 \text{ IU activity from retinol}$$
$$= 10.0 \text{ IU activity from } \beta\text{-carotene}$$

Food sources of preformed vitamin A are liver, kidney, whole milk, eggs, and butter. Skim milk and margarine are frequently fortified with vitamin A. Major sources of provitamin A are yellow and green leafy vegetables, such as carrots, squash, kale, spinach, pumpkin, and red or green peppers. The deeper the green or yellow color, the higher the carotene content will be.

Processing and cooking cause little loss of vitamin A. Because the vitamin is insoluble in water, there is no loss in cooking. Some processing, in fact, such as mashing, cutting, or pureeing, may increase the availability of carotenes in plant products by rupturing cell walls and making the provitamin more available.[11]

Clinical Deficiency

Less than an optimal supply of vitamin A results in some classic deficiency symptoms, which are night blindness, growth retardation, reproductive failure (in laboratory animals), and an increased susceptibility to infections, particularly those affecting the respiratory tract. The most serious public health problem associated with vitamin A deficiency is blindness due to changes in the eye tissue, leading to irreversible corneal damage. In xerophthalmia, keratinization of epithelial cells leads to a decrease in the protective secretions of the eye. The eye becomes dry and the cornea eventually loses its sensitivity. Continuation of the deficiency results in a lesion known as a Bitot's spot, and if unchecked, causes keratomalacia, when severe visual impairment and even blindness may result. These severe signs of deficiency are widespread in India, South and East Asia, Africa, and Latin America. It is no coincidence that these areas are also those which have a high prevalence of protein-energy malnutrition. Preventive programs of vitamin A administration are effective in reducing the incidence and prevalence of xerophthalmia and keratomalacia.[12]

Toxicity Symptoms

Because vitamin A is fat-soluble, it is capable of being stored in the body, and the potential for toxicity exists. Hypervitaminosis A is a condition that includes symptoms of nausea, headache, peeling and flaking of skin, dizziness, and pain in the long bones. Progression to a chronic state may lead to growth failure and hair loss. Vitamin A toxicity symptoms have been reported on intakes of 10,000 to 75,000 IU per day. Toxicity in children usually can be traced to overzealous vitamin supplementation with commercial vitamin preparations. Less commonly, it is caused by prolonged ingestion of foods which are rich in vitamin A.[13] Symptoms generally disappear when the vitamin is discontinued, although some residual effects have been noted in children. Increased intake of provitamin A results in a reversible skin pigmentation as a result of carotenemia.

The experimental use of retinoids for the chemoprevention of cancer[14-16] and severe acne[17,18] is being currently investigated. These compounds are not available for general use, and because of the potential for vitamin A toxicity, the public should be cautioned that the vitamin A supplements presently on the market are not known to have any cancer-preventing effects. Large intakes may produce a toxicity state.

Vitamin D

History and Discovery

Vitamin D has been known as the "sunshine vitamin" or the "rickets-preventive factor," names which are related to the confusing history of the vitamin and to its role in preventing a debilitating bone disease. Cod liver oil had been used for centuries as a cure for rickets, a disease in which bone calcification is hampered, leading to bowed legs and knock-knees. It was not until the early part of this century that Mellanby presented evidence of a fat-soluble substance in the oil that could cure rickets in dogs. In 1924

Steenbock and Hess discovered independently that ultraviolet light would give antirachitic properties to certain foods. These findings began to resolve the long debate that involved the etiology of rickets. Because the disease existed in children living in crowded, smoky industrial cities, many thought that it was an infectious disease. It was also noted that dark-skinned people who moved to England from the tropics were more susceptible to the bone deformity. We now know, from much research, that both food and sunlight have antirachitic properties. A new period of vitamin D research unfolded within the past two decades. It is recognized that the vitamin is converted in the body to an active form which exerts a physiological effect on calcium metabolism.

Chemistry and Properties

As with vitamin A, there is a provitamin-vitamin relationship with vitamin D. Plant substances contain a sterol called ergosterol which is activated by ultraviolet light and converted to ergocalciferol, or vitamin D_2. In animal tissues, including the human body, 7-dehydrocholesterol in skin is converted by ultraviolet light (sunshine) to cholecalciferol, or vitamin D_3. These fat-soluble substances are stable to heat and light.

Measurement

Vitamin D activity has been expressed as International Units, but the preferred unit is micrograms of cholecalciferol (1 IU = 0.025 μg cholecalciferol). Only recently have techniques been developed to measure cholecalciferol directly. For many years, the standardized line test was used to quantitate vitamin D activity. In this time-consuming and expensive bioassay method, rats are treated with graded doses of vitamin D after rickets has been produced. Histological examination of the rats' long bones demonstrates areas of calcification (noted by a line that becomes visible after the bone is stained with silver nitrate) which are proportional to the amount of vitamin D administered.

Metabolism

Dietary vitamin D is absorbed from the small intestine in the presence of bile and is transported into the circulation via the lymph in chylomicrons, in much the same way as vitamin A. Again, factors which increase or interfere with fat absorption will influence the rate at which dietary vitamin D is absorbed. The vitamin is removed from the circulation into the liver, where it is stored, although not to as great an extent as is vitamin A. Cholecalciferol produced in skin by ultraviolet light is absorbed into the blood.

An exciting chapter in the history of vitamin D unfolded when it was discovered that the liver contains an enzyme which can hydroxylate cholecalciferol, forming 25-hydroxycholecalciferol [25(OH)D_3]. A specific transport protein carries 25(OH)D_3 from the liver to the kidney, where another hydroxylation takes place to produce 1,25-dihydroxycholecalciferol [1,25(OH)$_2$$D_3$], thus far identified as the most active form of the vitamin. Renal hydroxylation of 25(OH)D_3 appears to be at least partially regulated by parathyroid hormone; in turn, low serum calcium and phosphate levels stimulate the release of parathyroid hormone. Growth hormone may also increase the synthesis of 1,25(OH)$_2$$D_3$.[19]

Reserves of vitamin D are found in liver, bone, brain, and skin; some vitamin D metabolites are excreted in the bile.

Function

A primary role of vitamin D is to increase the absorption of dietary calcium in a manner which strongly suggests an endocrine function of 1,25(OH)$_2$$D_3$.[20] Interaction of the vitamin (hormone) with DNA in intestinal cells ultimately induces the synthesis of a specific calcium-binding protein, which binds dietary calcium and promotes its absorption. Phosphorus absorption is also increased, perhaps by a similar mechanism.

Vitamin D also exerts a specific effect on bone. Bone acts as a reserve to maintain the tightly controlled level of calcium in the blood.

When serum calcium falls, vitamin D increases the release of calcium from bone to increase serum levels of the mineral. While there is indirect evidence that 1,25(OH)$_2$$D_3$ acts on bone in a manner analagous to its action in the intestine, no specific receptors or functional proteins have yet been identified. Vitamin D also has an effect on bone mineralization, although the mechanism is not clear. In vitamin D deficiency, bone mineralization is impaired, resulting in osteomalacia in adults and rickets in children.

Other tissues are also responsive to 1,25(OH)$_2$$D_3$. Phosphate reabsorption by kidney tubules is increased by the vitamin, and the release of insulin and other hormones may be mediated by this hormonelike compound.[21]

Clinical Implications

With the recognition that vitamin D is converted to active forms within the body, the use of synthetic analogues [1α(OH)D_3 or 1,25(OH)$_2$$D_3$] to correct bone diseases associated with vitamin D–resistant rickets is being investigated. In kidney and liver disease, bone disease sometimes occurs, and this is understandable if we consider that reduced hydroxylation of cholecalciferol may result from the primary disease. The possibility also exists that an inborn error of metabolism, resulting from a genetic defect in production of the kidney enzyme hydroxylase, can cause vitamin D–resistant rickets as well. Patients often do not respond to massive doses of either vitamin D_2 or D_3, whereas high doses of 25(OH)D_3 and much smaller doses of 1α(OH)D_3 or 1,25(OH)$_2$$D_3$ appear to correct the situation. Another interesting approach to the treatment of vitamin–D resistant syndromes has recently been proposed. Exposure to ultraviolet light after application of 1α,25(OH)$_2$-7-dehydrocholesterol to the skin resulted in an increase in the level of 1,25(OH)$_2$$D_3$ in the blood.[22]

Certain drugs are known to antagonize the effects of vitamin D. Corticosteroids have a negative effect on vitamin D and calcium metabolism; patients with Cushing's disease (overproduction of hydrocortisone) and those undergoing cortisone therapy may develop osteoporosis. Thus, the requirement for D_3 increases in these conditions. The use of anticonvulsant drugs has been associated with the development of rickets or osteomalacia. Many patients taking these medications have decreased levels of serum $25(OH)D_3$ but normal or elevated levels of $1,25(OH)_2D_3$.[23] The drugs may have a direct effect on the responsiveness of bone or the intestine to the actions of vitamin D. Cholestyramine, a drug used in cardiovascular disease, decreases the amount of bile, which is necessary for the absorption of the vitamin.

Dietary Allowances and Sources

Naturally occurring vitamin D is found only in small and insignificant amounts in common foods, such as cream, butter, eggs, and liver. Therefore, we rely on fortified foods or fish liver oil for our vitamin D requirements. Because children are highly susceptible to rickets, milk has been chosen as the vehicle for vitamin D fortification at a level of 400 IU per qt, equivalent to 10 μg of cholecalciferol.

Sunlight is the major nonfood source of the vitamin. For many of us, our requirement for the vitamin can be suitably obtained by this means. However, geography and climate modify the amount of sunlight, cultural customs and city living may diminish the amount of exposure, and infants and elderly people often do not get enought sunlight. Ultraviolet light cannot penetrate ordinary window glass, smog, or clouds; in addition, dark-skinned people living in temperate zones may not get enough exposure. Thus, certain population groups need an exogenous source of vitamin D,[24] and this is generally provided by fortified milk.

The dietary requirement for vitamin D has been difficult to determine, since a part of the necessary amount is supplied by regular exposure to sunlight. The Food and Nutrition Board recommends a daily intake of 10 μg cholecalciferol from birth through 18 years, 7.5 μg from 19 to 22 years, and 5 μg for adults. Pregnant and lactating women should receive an additional 5 μg per day.

Clinical Deficiency

Rickets, formerly quite prevalent in infants and children, and identified as early as 1645, is characterized by bone malformation caused by insufficient deposition of calcium and phosphorus. Long bones are affected, so that bowed legs and knock-knees are generally found; ribs, skull, and pelvic bones exhibit changes as well. Because mineralization is diminished, a tendency toward a thickening of wrists and ankles also exists. Poorly calcified and late-erupting teeth are often found in children with rickets. While the incidence of rickets in the United States is rare today, children who consume strict vegetarian diets are at risk of developing the deficiency disease,[25] unless regular sunlight exposure is assured. Occasional cases of rickets in breast-fed infants have been reported, leading to recommendations for vitamin D supplementation.[26] However, current guidelines for infant feeding do not include routine supplementation with vitamin D (see Table 13-5).

The counterpart of rickets in adults is osteomalacia, characterized by decalcification of bone shafts, increasing the tendency for fractures. Osteomalacia is especially prevalent in women, particularly among the elderly and following repeated pregnancies. Vitamin D and occasional calcium supplements may be beneficial.

Toxicity

Hypervitaminosis D can occur when excess vitamin D is provided in the diet, generally as supplements of cod liver oil. Symptoms produced by the condition are generally related to those produced by hypercalcemia, which results from increased intestinal absorption and bone mobilization; they include nausea, weight loss, anorexia, calcification of bones and soft tissues, head pain, and in children a reduction in growth rate. Certain infants may develop hypercalcemia on vitamin D intakes of 45 to 50 μg cholecalciferol per day, and symptoms have been documented in adults receiving more than 2500 μg per day. However, much lower levels of vitamin D may result in hypercalcemia. As with vitamin A, total intake must be monitored: pediatricians and parents should be aware of the importance of vitamin D, but also that overuse of the vitamin may produce pathological changes.

Vitamin E

History and Discovery

The presence of a dietary factor necessary for reproduction in the rat was recognized in 1922 by Evans and Bishop; 2 years later, Sure named it the "antisterility vitamin" or vitamin E. In the 1930s the substance was isolated from wheat germ oil and named *tocopherol,* from the Greek "to bear offspring."

Since that time, many investigators have sought to define its role in human nutrition. Many of the clinical signs apparent in vitamin E-deficient animals have not been documented in humans, and the role of the vitamin is not completely understood at the present time.

Chemistry and Properties

Compounds with vitamin E activity (tocopherols and tocotrienols) are oily yellow liquids; they are heat-stable, but deteriorate upon exposure to air and light and on contact with iron and lead. Because they are readily oxidized, they prevent the oxidative breakdown of other substances, notably vitamin A and polyunsaturated fatty acids (PUFA). Vitamin E, then, can be described as a chemical antioxidant, and the α-tocopherol form exhibits the greatest biological activity.

Measurement

Biological activity has been expressed in terms of International Units, with 1 mg of commercially available dl-α-tocopherol acetate designated as 1 IU. Other forms have higher activities per unit weight. In order to estimate the total vitamin E activity of foods and diets, the term α-tocopherol equivalent has been introduced. One milligram of α-tocopherol equivalent is equal to 1 mg α-tocopherol, 2 mg of β-tocopherol, 10 mg of γ-tocopherol, or 3.3 mg of α-tocotrienol. Thus the total vitamin E activity can be calculated as milligram α-tocopherol equivalents. If only the amount of α-tocopherol is provided, that figure is multiplied by 1.2 to correct for the presence of other tocopherols.

Metabolism

Vitamin E is absorbed as are other fats and fat-soluble substances: it requires the presence of bile, and once absorbed into the mucosal cell, the vitamin is carried with chylomicrons to the general circulation via the lymph. The efficiency of absorption is relatively low and is further decreased by mineral oil and by conditions which affect fat absorption in general. Vitamin E is stored in liver and muscle, with significant amounts present in adipose tissue. Fat mobilization also releases vitamin E into the circulation. Metabolites of the vitamin are excreted in urine and feces.

Function

For many years, the vitamin has been "in search of a disease." Since the function of most nutrients has not been elucidated until deficiency symptoms have been produced, the lack of definite disease states has hampered the search for a physiological function of the tocopherols. However, several roles have been postulated. There is some evidence that the vitamin acts as a cofactor in the cytochrome system of the electron transport chain. A few studies have suggested a role for the vitamin in erythropoiesis (through an effect on heme synthesis); however, a recent report indicates that vitamin E is not normally required for this function, except perhaps for patients with protein-energy malnutrition or anemia of unknown etiology.[27]

By far the most attractive and best-understood role of vitamin E relates to its antioxidant properties. Through its effect in trapping free radicals (highly reactive compounds produced in biological systems which induce lipid peroxidation and subsequent cellular damage), vitamin E protects cellular and intracellular structures. Accumulating evidence shows that the vitamin spares polyunsaturated fatty acids, vitamin A, sulfur-containing enzymes, and cell membranes from peroxidation. In this regard, some research suggests that the aging process is accelerated by the effects of free radicals; these observations have led some extremists to advocate large doses of vitamin E to prevent aging. But the evidence is not yet strong enough to establish a cause-effect relationship, and the research surrounding the aging process itself is controversial. Therefore, widespread use of large vitamin E intakes is not warranted, particularly since scientists do not yet know precisely how it functions in the body.

An interesting relationship between the mineral selenium and vitamin E has been observed. Selenium is a cofactor necessary for the activity of glutathione peroxidase, whose function is to prevent cellular peroxidation. Selenium can replace some of the vitamin E needed for certain functions, thus reinforcing the idea that the primary role of the vitamin is as an antioxidant.

Indeed, some clinical uses of vitamin E are predicated on its antioxidant effect. Neonates with bronchopulmonary dysplasia,[28] low-birth-weight infants with hemolytic anemia[29] and persons with sickle cell anemia[30] or glucose-6-phosphate dehydrogenase deficiency[31] have benefited from vitamin E therapy. Horwitt has reviewed the therapeutic uses of vitamin E.[32]

The antioxidant functions of vitamin E have been those most extensively studied, but other roles may be important. As one scientist has said, "There is the nagging suspicion that there is a very important use for the vitamin and we are just not smart enough to see it."[33]

Dietary Allowances and Sources

The Food and Nutrition Board first set a recommended dietary allowance for vitamin E in 1968. The figures have been revised and the current recommendations are considered to be adequate for persons consuming balanced diets, with usual amounts of polyunsaturated fatty acids. The minimum requirement for adults is probably not more than 3 to 4 mg α-tocopherol equivalents per day; the RDA for men and women are 10 and 8 mg α-tocopherol equivalents, respectively. Most investigators agree that the requirement for vitamin E increases with the content of polyunsaturated fat in the diet. Although a precise ratio cannot be defined, diets as consumed in the United States [with a mg α-tocopherol equivalent: grams PUFA (polyunsaturated fatty acid) ratio of 0.4] are apparently satisfactory.

The major sources of vitamin E in the American diet are fats and oils, particularly the vegetable oils, which are also rich sources of polyunsaturated fatty acids. Animal foods are generally poor sources of the vitamin, although liver and egg contain moderate amounts. Cereals and legumes are also moderate sources.[34]

Clinical Deficiency

Clinical evidence of deficiency is almost entirely restricted to premature infants. Newborn infants in general tend to have low plasma levels of vitamin E, and the levels normally rise (particularly in breast-fed infants) by about 1 month of age. Several reports have cited cases in which premature infants showed signs of irritability and edema,[35,36] accompanied by a hemolytic anemia. The deficiency was traced to their drinking an iron-fortifed commercial formula which was low in vitamin E. Iron can exacerbate vitamin E deficiency in premature infants because it increases the rate of free radical formation.

Normally, vitamin E deficiency is difficult to produce. In the most extensive study thus far, adult men who consumed diets low in the vitamin for 3 years showed no symptoms, even though their plasma tocopherol fell to low levels. A slight decrease in red blood cell stability was apparent, but there were no clinical signs of anemia.[37]

Groups at risk of developing a vitamin E deficiency include premature infants and individuals who have a defect in the ability to absorb dietary fat, including patients with cystic fibrosis.

There is no substantial experimental evidence to suggest that vitamin E will prevent or cure muscular dystrophy, the aging process, cancer, ulcers, infertility, or sexual impotence, or that it will increase athletic performance, for which the use of vitamin E in pharmacological amounts has been advocated.

Clinical Toxicity

Although symptoms of toxicity have been produced in chicks, the risk of toxicity in humans is apparently less than that caused by excess consumption of vitamins A and D. Nevertheless, the potential for hypervitaminosis E exists; large doses of vitamin E interfere with the blood clotting mechanism and may increase the risk of hemorrhage coincident with a vitamin K deficiency.[38]

Vitamin K

History and Discovery

In 1935 Henrik Dam, a Danish scientist, identified a severe hemorrhagic disease in newly hatched chicks fed a ration adequate in all known essential nutrients. Analysis of blood showed a decrease in the amount of prothrombin, a factor involved in the normal blood clotting mechanism. Addition of hog liver fat or alfalfa to the ration improved and prevented the condition. The antihemorrhagic factor was named *vitamin K* for *k*oagulation vitamin.

Chemistry and Properties

Vitamin K is a fat-soluble yellowish crystalline compound that is stable to heat, air, and moisture. It is destroyed upon exposure to strong acids, alkalis, and light. There are several forms of the vitamin, all belonging to a family of chemical compounds called quinones. Vitamin K_1 (phylloquinone) occurs naturally in green plants; vitamin K_2 (menaquinone) is a product of bacterial synthesis in the intestine. In addition, several compounds with vitamin K activity have been synthesized.

Measurement

No present system of standardization exists. The vitamin can be measured in micrograms of a pure synthetic compound, and a bioassay based on coagulation time in chicks has been used to quantify the vitamin.

Metabolism

Vitamin K is absorbed, with the aid of bile, in the upper part of the small intestine. Since it follows the same absorptive pattern as dietary fat, any interference with fat absorption will affect the absorption of vitamin K. Effective water-soluble preparations exist for patients with fat malabsorption syndromes.

After absorption, chylomicrons carry the vitamin to the liver, where much of the vitamin is transferred to β-lipoproteins. Liver concentrates the vitamin for a short period of time, and small amounts appear in heart, skin, muscle, and kidney. Storage of the vitamin in the human body is not extensive. Metabolites of vitamin K are excreted in bile and urine.

Function

The best-known function of vitamin K is in the blood clotting mechanism, a process which depends on the presence of many protein factors. Prothrombin (factor II) is essential for the mechanism, and is directly affected by vitamin K. It is also known that the synthesis or activation of three other blood clotting factors (factors VII, IX, and X) are responsive to the vitamin. (It should be noted that vitamin K offers no therapeutic value to patients with hemophilia.) Knowledge of the molecular role of vitamin K in the blood clotting process has been studied largely during the last 10 years. Vitamin K undergoes reduction, and in its active form catalyzes the carboxylation of specific glutamic acid residues in the four blood clotting proteins.[39,40] This carboxylation facilitates the binding of calcium and phospholipids necessary for blood clotting. Similar carboxylated calcium-binding proteins whose synthesis is responsive to vitamin K have been identified in bone and kidney.[41]

Dietary Allowances and Sources

There is no RDA for vitamin K, but in 1980 the Food and Nutrition Board established a "safe and adequate daily dietary intake" of 70 to 140 μg for adults. It has been estimated that the total requirement for vitamin K is 2 μg per kilogram body weight. The lower end of the suggested range of intake assumes that one-half of the requirement is supplied by bacterial synthesis; the upper figure, that diet provides the entire requirement. In any case, deficiency is uncommon.

Newborn infants present a special circumstance, however, because placental transport of the vitamin is limited, and because the normal intestinal flora does not establish itself until some time after birth. Thus, it has been standard practice to administer 1 mg of vitamin K to newborn infants to prevent hemorrhagic disease.

In addition to the extensive bacterial synthesis of the vitamin, vitamin K is found in cabbage, cauliflower, spinach, alfalfa, and other leafy vegetables. Egg yolk and liver also provide moderate amounts. Human milk contains little of the vitamin.

Clinical Deficiency

Under normal conditions, vitamin K deficiency is unlikely. Interference with fat absorption, the presence of liver disease, the use of sulfonamides and tetracycline (which will depress bacterial synthesis), and the administration of anticoagulants, which antagonize the effects of vitamin K, and of some anticonvulsants, which increase its turnover, may precipitate deficiency symptoms, the only one of which thus far identified is a defect in blood coagulation.

Toxicity

If given in large doses over a prolonged period of time, vitamin K may produce hemolytic anemia and jaundice in the infant. Vitamin K_3, a synthetic form of the vitamin also known as menadione, has been removed from the list of over-the-counter drug preparations because of its toxic effect on membranes of red blood cells.

WATER-SOLUBLE VITAMINS

Ascorbic Acid

History and Discovery

Scurvy is one of the oldest deficiency diseases recognized by science, having been reported as early as 1500 B.C. It was a seasonal disease, and ruined many sailing and exploring expeditions, causing widespread morbidity and mortality. In a now classic nutrition experiment, James Lind in 1735 demonstrated that sailors provided with two oranges and lemons daily were cured of their disease; as citrus fruits were added to the rations of British sailors, the men were known as "limeys."

In 1907, Holst and Frölich produced scurvy in guinea pigs, one of the few species which cannot synthesize the vitamin. Humans, monkeys, and other more obscure animal species also are unable to synthesize the compound; it must be provided in the diet.

In the 1930s, crystalline vitamin C had been isolated, and it was officially named *ascorbic acid*.

Chemistry and Properties

Ascorbic acid is a white, crystalline material that is water-soluble and stable in dry form. In solution it is easily oxidized, particularly when heated, exposed to alkali, light, copper, or iron. It is the most unstable of all the vitamins, and precautions must be taken to prevent its loss during the storage and preparation of food.

Ascorbic acid has a structure closely related to monosaccharides, and exists in two biologically active forms. L-ascorbic acid can be oxidized to L-dehydroascorbic acid, which has approximately 80 percent of the activity of the reduced form. Dehydroascorbic acid is readily and irreversibly converted to diketogulonic acid, a form which has no antiscorbutic activity.

Metabolism

Ascorbic acid is readily absorbed from the small intestine; the mode of transport is controversial and may depend upon whether vitamin C is a required vitamin for the particular species studied. The efficiency of absorption decreases as the amount ingested increases. It is transported to the liver via the portal vein, and from the liver it is distributed to all tissues. There is a moderate amount of storage in liver and spleen, with a high concentration found in the adrenal gland, an observation which has led to much speculation on its relationship to steroid synthesis. Body stores generally amount to about 1500 mg.[42] Tissue levels in kidney, liver, spleen, and adrenal gland appear to be in equilibrium with serum, and there is a limited amount of storage in the leukocytes, or white blood cells. Leukocytes take up the vitamin when tissue demands have been met, and white blood cell levels have been used to evaluate vitamin C status in humans.

Metabolites of vitamin C are excreted primarily in the urine, as ascorbic acid and oxalic acid; some is expired as carbon dioxide. Approximately 3 percent of the body pool is catabolized daily.

Several drugs have been shown to affect the metabolism of vitamin C. Among those which increase the urinary excretion of the vitamin are adrenal steroids, sulfonamides, tetracycline, and salicylates. Leukocyte and plasma levels are decreased by salicylates, tetracycline, and indomethacin. The effect of oral contraceptives on vitamin C metabolism is ambiguous, with some investigators reporting a decrease in plasma and leukocyte levels of the vitamin, and others showing no effect.[43] Cigarette smokers generally have lower plasma vitamin C levels than do nonsmokers, although results to the contrary have appeared in the literature.[44]

Function

Unlike the other water-soluble vitamins, ascorbic acid has not been positively identified as a catalyst or coenzyme in any metabolic system. Its biochemical mode of action has not been determined; some investigators feel that its reducing powers may account for its function, but this is a relatively nonspecific effect. However, some specific roles of the vitamin, again based on studies of deficiency states, have been identified.

The most basic function of vitamin C thus far identified is its role in collagen formation. Collagen is a protein which makes up connective tissue found in skin, bones, teeth, and muscle. Ascorbic acid appears to exert a posttranslational effect on the hydroxylation of proline and lysine to form hydroxyproline and hydroxylysine, substances present exclusively in collagen.[45]

The function of vitamin C in wound healing was recognized years ago. Ascorbic acid migrates to the site of the wound and presumably plays a role in the collagen formation required for such healing. It is for this reason that many physicians recommend vitamin C treatment in postsurgical and burn patients. Vitamin C also has a positive effect on bone and dentin formation. Other sites of vitamin C action are related to neurotransmitter synthesis. Tyrosine and tryptophan hydroxylation require ascorbic acid, as does the conversion of dopa (3,4-dihydroxyphenylalanine) to norepinephrine.

Ascorbic acid enhances iron absorption by reducing the ferric form generally found in foods to the more readily absorbed ferrous form. Ingestion of 25 to 75 mg of vitamin C with an iron-containing meal will significantly improve the absorption of the mineral.[46] Iron supplements frequently contain ascorbic acid to promote absorption of the mineral. Ascorbic acid also influences the distribution of iron stores.

An interesting role for ascorbic acid in cholesterol metabolism, and thus its role in atherosclerosis, is a subject of controversy. Spittle[47] reported that daily doses of 1 g of ascorbic acid reduced the serum cholesterol level in young adults, but had no effect on older adults. However, Peterson et al. gave nine hypercholesterolemic patients 4 g of ascorbic acid per day for 2 months and noted no change in serum cholesterol levels.[48] It has been postulated that any cholesterol-lowering effect of the vitamin is mediated by a metabolite, ascorbic acid sulfate. More research needs to be done in this area.

The much-heralded use of vitamin C for the prevention and cure of the common cold has not been strongly supported by scientific evidence. Linus Pauling recommended that 0.5 to 5 g per day would prevent and reduce the symptoms of a cold. One of the best controlled studies to test this hypothesis was done by Anderson et al. in Canada. Using 800 subjects in a double-blind study, they reported a beneficial effect of ascorbic acid on the frequency and severity of colds, but cautioned that it was a pharmacological rather than a nutritional effect.[49] Large doses of vitamin C may have an antihistaminelike effect, and thus ameliorate some of the symptoms of a cold. A study by Coulehan et al. involving 868 schoolchildren showed no effect of vitamin C supplementation. Of the children receiving ascorbic acid, 133 were ill with 166 cold episodes, and the mean duration of illness was 5.5 days. Among the control children who received placebos, 129 suffered 159 colds, with a mean duration of 5.8 days. The differences between these figures are not statistically significant.[50] Worthington-Roberts has presented a concise summary of work in this controversial area.[51]

Undoubtedly, the controversy will remain unresolved until more definite criteria for "colds" and their symptoms can be determined. Meanwhile, most of the available evidence suggests that the beneficial effects of vitamin C in preventing colds or reducing their symptoms is minimal and highly subjective. Moreover, concern about potential unwanted side effects of massive doses of the vitamin further suggest that individuals should not embark on a Pauling-type regimen of ascorbic acid supplementation.

One of the newest proposed functions of vitamin C is its relationship to the prevention and cure of cancer. Cameron and Pauling reported that the general well-being of patients was improved and survival times were prolonged by daily administration of 10 g of ascorbic acid,[52] but a controlled study did not support their conclusions.[53] Additional research is being done to determine the possible interaction.

Dietary Allowances and Sources

Although 10 mg of ascorbic acid per day will prevent scurvy, the level required for maintenance of health is considerably higher. The Food and Nutrition Board has currently set 60 mg as the recommended allowance for adults, with increases to 80 and 100 mg for pregnant and lactating women, respectively. Because of the body's limited storage capacity, a daily intake of the vitamin is recommended.

Commonly available fruits and vegetables are the richest sources of the vitamin. Fruits and vegetables provide 94 percent of our vitamin C intake, with broccoli, cantaloupe, and strawberries being excellent sources, in addition to the citrus fruits. The amount of vitamin C in products varies according to the variety, time of harvesting, processing procedures, and even the part of the plant. Because vitamin C is so easily destroyed, care must be taken to preserve its content. Frozen vegetables should be plunged into already boiling water, baking soda should never be added to cooking water, and there should be a minimum of chopping and cutting of foods before cooking. Vitamin C will leach out into the cooking water and is also destroyed by the heat and exposure to air.

Less well known sources of vitamin C are the acerola (or West Indian cherry), rose hips, papaya, guava, and black currants. While potatoes do not have a high concentration of the vitamin, the quantity in which they are eaten in some population groups makes them a valuable source of the vitamin.

Clinical Deficiency

Scurvy is characterized by general weakness and lassitude, swollen joints, spongy and bleeding gums and loose teeth, and delayed wound healing. Muscle cramps, aching bones, anemia, and dry, rough skin are also symptoms. Infantile scurvy, because of the effect of vitamin C on bone formation, is manifested by a characteristic "frog's leg" position, and the child shows anorexia, lip tenderness, and extremely sensitive arms and legs—a generally irritable child. Scurvy is rare in breast-fed infants, unless of course their mothers are deficient in the vitamin. Bottle-fed infants may require supplementation, depending on the formula used (see Table 13-5). Scurvy is relatively rare in this country, though occasional epidemics are found. These are generally related to custom, ignorance, and poverty, but in two cases were due to technology. Blacks in the South were accustomed to consuming "pot likker," the liquid in which vegetables were cooked. When social changes led them to abandon this practice, children developed scurvy. Early in this century, pasteurization of milk, which destroyed the ascorbic acid, led to a scurvy outbreak. Fortunately, scurvy has been all but eradicated as a nutritional disease.

Toxicity

Because vitamin C is a water-soluble vitamin and little is stored, toxicity symptoms are unexpected. However, with many advocating the ingestion of very large doses to prevent the common cold, several effects have been noted. Large doses cause abdominal cramps and diarrhea in some people, and several investigators have reported the induction of kidney stones. Because excess amounts of ascorbic acid are excreted in the urine and the vitamin is structurally similar to glucose, false results have been obtained when monitoring patients for urinary glucose excretion.

Other findings relate to vitamin B_{12} status: decreased levels of serum vitamin B_{12} have been reported in some persons taking large amounts of vitamin C,[54] but this may be due to problems in the assay method rather than an effect on absorption of vitamin B_{12}. Hogenkamp presented the view that the interaction may be significant only in people who have a disorder of cobalamin metabolism.[55] Some physicians have warned that large ascorbic acid intakes during pregnancy may create a "vitamin C-dependent" fetus whose requirements after birth may exceed the normal level. Clearly, further study is required to assess the risk-benefit ratio in prescribing high doses of ascorbic acid.

Thiamin (Vitamin B_1)

History and Discovery

Beriberi is a nutritional deficiency disease which was recognized as early as 2600 B.C. by the Chinese. It takes its name from the Sinhalese words which mean "I cannot," which appropriately describes the clinical state. In 1855 a Japanese naval officer named Takaki cured the disease by feeding milk and meat to his men. In 1897 a Dutch physician, Eijkman, who was working in Java, noted that the chickens in the yard of the prison hospital had symptoms similar to those of his patients with beriberi. Replacement of polished rice by brown rice in the poultry rations reversed their condition. Studies in later years demonstrated that an "accessory food factor" was present in the outer husk of rice. It was named vitamin B; subsequent investigators showed that there was more than one accessory food factor, and the antiberiberi factor was renamed vitamin B_1. Thiamin was isolated in 1926, and in 1936 R. R. Williams succeeded in synthesizing the vitamin.

Chemistry and Properties

The name *thiamine* was given to this substance because it contains a sulfur molecule (a thio group) and an amine. The vitamin is available commercially as thiamin hydrochloride. It is a crystalline yellowish-white compound that is water-soluble and has a nutlike taste and odor. In the dry form, it is heat- and oxygen-stable. In solution, it becomes heat-labile, particularly in alkali. For these reasons, baking soda should not be added to vegetables as a color preservative, and minimal amounts of water should be used when cooking. In addition, the sulfur dioxide used in processing dried fruits destroys their thiamin content.

Metabolism

Dietary thiamin is absorbed from the upper part of the small intestine. In large amounts, it is passively absorbed. In smaller amounts, the absorptive process is an active one, requiring energy and sodium. Evidence suggests that thiamin is phosphorylated within the mucosal cell and is transported via the portal vein and then into the general circulation. Although bacteria in the gastrointestinal tract do synthesize thiamin, the product of their metabolism is thiamin pyrophosphate, which cannot be absorbed and is therefore unavailable. Alcohol and barbiturates decrease thiamin absorption.

Limited reserves of thiamin are found in the human body; of the 30 mg stored, 50 percent is found in muscle tissue. Amounts in excess of what the cells can use are excreted in the urine, either as intact thiamin or as the pyrimidine and thiazole moieties. Mercurial diuretics increase urinary loss of the vitamin.

Function

Thiamin, as thiamin pyrophosphate (TPP), functions as an important coenzyme in energy metabolism. Thiamin pyrophosphate is required for the oxidative decarboxylation of alpha-keto acids such as pyruvate and alpha-keto-glutarate, and the keto analogues of the branched-chain amino acids. It is also required for the transketolase reactions of the hexose monophosphate shunt (pentose phosphate pathway), and therefore plays an indirect role in nucleic acid, fatty acid, and steroid metabolism. Thaimin is needed for the metabolism of carbohydrates, proteins, and fats, and for the conversion of tryptophan to niacin.

In addition to its coenzyme role, thiamin pyrophosphate may have a specific role in neurophysiology, which may explain the devasting effects of thiamin deficiency on the nervous system. Itokawa and Cooper[56] have suggested that thiamin pyrophosphate (or thiamin triphosphate) is a component of the nerve cell membrane, and is part of the mechanism required for propagation of an electrical potential along the axon. However, other research does not support this hypothesis,[57] and the mechanism of thiamin deficiency in the production of neurological symptoms remains unresolved.

Biochemical Assessment

Several tests were developed to evaluate thiamin status in humans. Measurement of the vitamin in blood and urine, and blood levels of pyruvate and alpha-ketoglutarate, have been used to estimate the adequacy of thiamin stores. A load test has also been used. In this test, a standardized dose of thiamin (5 mg) is administered, and the urinary content of thiamin 4 h later is measured. An acceptable concentration, indicating adequate status, is more than 80 μg; a deficient subject will have less than 20 μg in a 4-h urine sample.

In recent years, a functional test to evaluate thiamin status has been developed.[58,59] Erythro-cyte transketolase activity is measured; this may be a more reliable index of a subclinical deficiency state than blood or urine levels of the vitamin.[60] The activity of this thiamin-dependent enzyme decreases in times of vitamin deficiency and is stimulated in vitro by addition of thiamin pyrophosphate. When thiamin status is adequate, stimulation does not occur or is only slight, while in marginally and severely deficient subjects there is at least a 16 percent increase in enzyme activity following addition of the cofactor.

Dietary Allowances and Sources

Because of thiamin's importance in the metabolism of the energy-yielding nutrients, the daily requirement is based on the energy content of the diet. Sauberlich et al. have recently confirmed that the minimum requirement for thiamin is 0.3 mg per 1000 kcal (0.3 mg per 4200 kJ).[61] The present recommended dietary allowance, based on excretion of thiamin and its metabolites, the effects of graded doses on signs of clinical deficiency, and the effect on the level of erythrocyte transketolase activity, is 0.5 mg per 1000 kcal per day (0.5 mg per 4200 kJ per day). A minimum of 1 mg per day is recommended for adults and the elderly, even when energy intake is less than 2000 kcal (8400 kJ).

Thiamin is found in a wide variety of animal and plant foods, but occurs in large amounts in only a few. Pork and wheat germ are excellent sources. Whole grains and enriched grain products are the best daily sources, because of the quantity in which they are eaten. Milk and milk products are generally not good sources of the vitamin, but do make a contribution to the daily intake. In general, fruits and vegetables should not be relied upon to provide a significant source of thiamin.[62]

Clinical Deficiency

The classic symptoms of beriberi affect the nervous, cardiovascular, and gastrointestinal systems. Infantile beriberi is a disease of rapid onset, striking infants whose mothers are in poor thiamin status. Cyanosis, tachycardia, vomiting, convulsions, and death follow if treatment is not instituted promptly.

In adults, the disease manifests itself in one of two ways, each, however, characterized by irritability, disorderly thinking, and nausea. "Dry" beriberi is a wasting disease, with nervous manifestations and paralysis of the lower extremities. In "wet" beriberi the edema associated with heart failure is the predominant sign, with noticeable swelling of the limbs, feet, and heart.

In addition to deficiency symptoms produced by inadequate intake of the vitamin, antivitamins can alter thiamin status. Thiaminase, a heat-labile enzyme present in uncooked shellfish and some types of freshwater fish, causes hydrolysis of the vitamin. A heat-stable factor found in certain plants is related to caffein and tannic acids, both components of tea; this also has antithiamin effects.

Chronic alcoholics may also become thiamin deficient, for several reasons. Low thiamin intake, impaired intestinal absorption, a phosphorylating defect, and apotransketolase deficiency have been implicated in their condition.

Patients with primary deficiency can be treated with physiological doses of thiamin. Thiamin has been used in pharmacological doses to treat patients with several inborn errors of metabolism, such as lactic acidosis due to low activity of liver pyruvate carboxylase, and branched-chain ketoaciduria due to decreased activity of keto acid dehydrogenase.[63]

Beriberi has been eradicated in the United States, largely because of the enrichment of grain products. In areas of the world where enrichment is not a standard processing procedure, and people subsist on a diet of polished rice, beriberi remains a public health problem.

Riboflavin (Vitamin B₂)

History and Discovery

In the 1920s it was recognized that there was more than one B vitamin, since some growth-promoting properties were retained after heat treatment had destroyed the antiberiberi properties of certain foods. In 1933 a yellow-green pigment was isolated from milk, and was found also in liver and eggs. The compound was identified as part of "Warburg's yellow enzyme," and in 1935 vitamin B_2 was synthesized.

Chemistry and Properties

Vitamin B_2 is a member of the chemical family called *flavins*, which are fluorescent compounds. Attached to the flavin moiety is a five-carbon sugar, ribose; the newly identified vitamin was therefore christened *riboflavin*. It is stable to heat, acid, and oxygen, but is unstable in alkaline solution and is readily destroyed by light. The relatively high riboflavin content in milk requires that milk be packaged in an opaque container to prevent decomposition by light.

Metabolism

Riboflavin is absorbed from the small intestine; it must be phosphorylated, and there appears to be a specific transport system required for its absorption. It is transported to the liver by albumin, where it is further phosphorylated. Absorption of the vitamin increases with age, and riboflavin is apparently better absorbed when eaten with a meal than when ingested separately. Although the liver and kidney have moderate amounts of riboflavin, little of the vitamin is stored and it must therefore be supplied regularly. When dietary intake is low, however, the body's capacity for maintaining riboflavin stores is greater than that for storing thiamin. Excess riboflavin is excreted in the urine.

Several drugs affect the metabolism of this vitamin. Tetracycline and the thiazide diuretics increase urinary excretion, as does probenecid (used in the treatment of gout). The latter drug also causes a decrease in absorption. Sulfonamides depress bacterial synthesis of the vitamin, but to what extent bacteria normally serve as a source of riboflavin is questionable. Some oral contraceptive preparations have been associated with a reduction in serum levels of the vitamin, although no deficiency symptoms have been noted.

Function

Riboflavin functions in conjunction with phosphoric acid as two coenzymes which are necessary for the release of energy from carbohydrates, fats, and proteins. Flavin mononucleotide (FMN) and flavin adenine dinucleotide (FAD) are important coenzymes which catalyze oxidation-reduction reactions, notably in the electron transport system, where adenosine triphosphate (ATP) and water are produced. The coenzymes also function in the tricarboxylic acid cycle in dehydrogenase reactions and in fatty acid oxidation. Oxidative deamination of amino acids requires the vitamin as FMN. The vitamin may also play a role in corticosteroid synthesis and in the production of red blood cells in the bone marrow.

Biochemical Assessment

Urinary levels of riboflavin have been used to evaluate vitamin status, but these primarily reflect immediate past intake and are easily influenced by temperature, stress, and exercise. Therefore, other methods have been sought. A functional test similar to that described for thiamin has been developed and shows promise as an indicator. Riboflavin is bound to the enzyme glutathione reductase, an erythrocyte enzyme required to maintain the levels of reduced glutathione, necessary for the maintenance of red blood cell membranes. Results are usually expressed in terms of *activity coefficients,* determined by the in vitro addition of FAD to the assay mixture. The coefficient is 1.0 to 1.2 if adequate riboflavin is present, and increases to greater than 1.4 if the subject is at high risk of developing a riboflavin deficiency.[64]

Dietary Allowances and Sources

The 1980 recommendations for riboflavin are based on energy intake, being set at 0.6 mg per 1000 kcal (0.6 mg per 4200 kJ). Thus, for adult men and women, daily intakes should be 1.6 and 1.2 mg, respectively. A minimum intake of 1.2 mg per day is recommended for adults and the elderly.

Riboflavin is widely distributed in food, but, like thiamin, only in small amounts in most commonly eaten foods. Milk and milk products, organ meats, and green leafy vegetables provide a substantial part of our daily intake. Although cereals and breads enriched with the vitamin do not contain large amounts, they too contribute significant amounts of riboflavin to our food supply. Strict vegetarians may have a marginal intake of the vitamin, since riboflavin consumption is apt to be low if milk is not part of the diet.[65] A recent study of an adolescent population has also demonstrated that riboflavin status is correlated with milk intake.[66]

Clinical Deficiency

Riboflavin deficiency generally occurs in concert with other B vitamin deficiencies, and the specific clinical signs associated with riboflavin are less dramatic than those seen in beriberi and pellagra (niacin deficiency). Vitamin deficiency results in growth retardation and several abnormalities of the mouth and eyes. Cracks at the corners of the mouth (cheilosis) appear, and the tongue becomes smooth and purplish (glossitis). Dry and scaly skin is also apparent. The eyes may itch, become sensitive to light, and be susceptible to strain and fatigue.

There is no known toxicity from the vitamin.

Pyridoxine (Vitamin B₆)

History and Discovery

Another of the water-soluble vitamins, sought after because none of the known B vitamins could cure a specific type of dermatitis in rats, was isolated in 1938, synthesized in 1939, and named *pyridoxine.*

Chemistry and Properties

Vitamin B_6 is a complex of closely related compounds, all of which are interconvertible and biologically active. The parent compound is a pyridine with either an alcohol (pyridoxine), aldehyde (pyridoxal), or amine (pyridoxamine) group attached to the pyridine nucleus. The complex is a white, crystalline, and odorless compound which is both water- and alcohol-soluble. It is heat-stable in acid solution, and is relatively heat-labile in an alkaline medium and upon exposure to light.

Metabolism
The absorption of pyridoxine from the upper segment of the small intestine is unremarkable, except perhaps in children with acute celiac disease, chronic alcoholics (synthetic pyridoxine preparations appear to be better absorbed by the latter group), and persons who have had a jejunoileal bypass for the treatment of obesity. After absorption, all three forms are converted to pyridoxal phosphate or pyridoxamine phosphate. There is only limited storage of the vitamin in human tissue, occurring mostly in muscle. The primary metabolite is pyridoxic acid, which is excreted in the urine.

Function
Pyridoxine functions as a coenzyme, pyridoxal phosphate, in protein, carbohydrate, and perhaps fatty acid metabolism. By far the most extensive function of the vitamin is its role in protein and amino acid metabolism. It functions as a coenzyme in several types of reactions: transamination and deamination (gluconeogenesis and the synthesis of nonessential amino acids), decarboxylation (serotonin, norepinephrine, and histamine synthesis), and desulfuration (conversion of serine to cysteine). Pyridoxal phosphate is required for the formation of a heme precursor, delta-amino-levulinic acid. It appears to stabilize phosphorylase, which functions to release glucose-1-phosphate from liver and muscle glycogen. It may also be involved in the conversion of linoleic to arachidonic acid. Evidence has accumulated that vitamin B_6 is also important in cell-mediated immunity.[67]

An important function of the vitamin is its role in the conversion of tryptophan to niacin, and the deficiency therefore may be manifested to some extent as niacin deficiency. In fact, a limited intake of pyridoxine may play a contributory role in the pathogenesis of pellagra.

Biochemical Assessment
The traditional method of evaluating pyridoxine status has been the tryptophan load test. In a B_6-deficiency state, administration of a large dose of tryptophan results in an abnormally high urinary excretion of xanthurenic acid, an intermediary product in the conversion of the amino acid to niacin. Urinary excretion of the vitamin or of pyridoxic acid has also been used to determine adequacy. More recently, a functional test has been developed, in which erythrocyte levels of glutamic acid–oxaloacetate transaminase activity (EGOT) or glutamic acid–pyruvate transaminase activity (EGPT) are measured. In vitro simulation with pyridoxal phosphate is used as a measure of in vivo pyridoxine deficiency.

Dietary Allowances and Sources
As a result of the close association between protein metabolism and vitamin B_6, is it not surprising that the requirement for pyridoxine is increased with increasing intakes of protein. Although vitamin B_6 is present in a wide variety of foodstuffs, concern about its availability has been raised. The Food and Nutrition Board has set the daily recommended allowance at 2.2 mg for adult men, and 2.0 mg for adult women. These recommendations are based on a ratio of 0.02 mg of the vitamin per gram of dietary protein,[68] with average protein intakes of 110 and 100 g for men and women respectively. The allowance during pregnancy is 2.6 mg per day. This corresponds to the increase in protein allowance. While some research has suggested that the allowance should be even higher,[69] the Food and Nutrition Board concluded that no such recommendation is justified on the basis of available evidence.

Of concern also is the fact that many women taking oral contraceptive agents demonstrate abnormal tryptophan metabolism which can be normalized by large doses of pyridoxine. Many investigations have been carried out to determine the clinical significance of this finding. Most researchers now feel that pharmacological pyridoxine supplementation is probably unnecessary for most women, although some benefit has been seen in women who show signs of depression. This finding has been related to the role of pyridoxine in serotonin synthesis.

Requirements for infants (0.3 to 0.6 mg per day) are largely based on studies which followed an incident about 20 years ago, in which vitamin B_6 was accidentally destroyed in a commercial infant formula. The resulting deficiency produced irritability and convulsions in the infants.

Very little is known about nutritional requirements in general for the elderly. Since this age group is becoming a proportionally larger segment of our population, it behooves nutritional researchers to look into this important question. Some evidence suggests that vitamin B_6 requirements may increase with age.[70,71]

Several medical conditions requiring drug therapy have been shown to affect pyridoxine status, and therefore to affect the requirement for the vitamin. Antitubercular drugs, such as cycloserine and isoniazid (INH), bind with the vitamin and if used without adjuvant B_6 therapy result in serious neurological symptoms. Therefore, pyridoxine supplementation accompanies administration of these drugs. The use of the antibiotic chloramphenicol also produces neuritis, and this untoward effect can be prevented by simultaneous administration of large amounts of pyridoxine. Hydralazine (an antihypertensive agent) and certain diuretics also cause increased urinary loss of vitamin B_6. Penicillamine, which is used in the treatment of Wilson's disease and rheumatoid arthritis, also increases the requirement for pyridoxine. Finally, levodopa (L-dopa), used in the treatment of Parkinson's disease, can cause a polyneuropathy related to pyridoxine depletion. Unfortunately, increasing the intake of pyridoxine decreases the effectiveness of L-dopa; the use of carbidopa (which enhances the effects of L-dopa) and B_6 with L-dopa therapy is recommended.

The best dietary sources of pyridoxine are pork, wheat germ, organ and muscle meats, whole grain cereals, and bananas. Milk and eggs provide only limited amounts.[72]

Clinical Deficiency

Rats deficient in pyridoxine develop a characteristic dermatitis and growth failure, weakness, and mental changes, which cannot be counteracted with niacin. Adults given a pyridoxine antagonist (deoxypyridoxine) develop nausea, depression, neuritis, dermatitis, and microcytic anemia. The most extreme symptom of severe pyridoxine deficiency involves the central nervous system, as demonstrated by the incident with the overprocessed infant formula and by the effects of certain medications. The incidence of vitamin B_6 deficiency in alcoholic populations has been estimated at 20 to 30 percent.[73]

Vitamin B_6 has been used therapeutically in certain inborn errors of amino acid metabolism, such as homocystinuria. Pharmacologic doses of the vitamin enhance the activity of the defective enzyme in some cases. (See Chap. 27.)

Toxicity

While vitamin B_6 is relatively nontoxic, therapeutic doses of 150 mg per day may induce sleepiness. Daily supplements of 200 mg per day have produced a vitamin B_6–dependency state after withdrawal of the vitamin.

Niacin (Nicotinic Acid)

History and Discovery

In the early part of this century, thousands of Americans, mostly poor southerners, were suffering from a debilitating disease that resulted in many of them being confined to mental institutions. It was a disease that had been described by Casal of Spain in 1735 and also was rampant in Italy, where it received its name, pellagra (rough skin). Although many theories were proposed for its existence, Goldberger clearly and gallantly determined that it was a dietary deficiency disease, although he was unable to identify the pellagra-preventive factor. Diets based on cornmeal appeared to precipitate the symptoms, and high-quality protein diets prevented or cured them. It was not until 1937, when El-vehjem demonstrated that nicotinic acid cured blacktongue in dogs, the counterpart of human pellagra, that nicotinic acid, or niacin, was recognized as a dietary essential. Further research elucidated the reason why high-protein diets abated the symptoms, when it was recognized that tryptophan is a precursor from which the body can synthesize niacin.

Chemistry and Properties

Niacin (nicotinic acid) is a white crystalline powder that is remarkably stable to light, heat, acid, and alkali, but because it is water-soluble, may be lost in cooking water.

Metabolism

Niacin is rapidly absorbed in the upper part of the small intestine, probably by passive diffusion. It is readily converted to nicotinamide, the metabolically active form of the vitamin. Limited storage exists in the body and the vitamin is excreted in the urine as N-methylnicotin-amide or 2-pyridone.

Niacin can be synthesized from tryptophan. Many studies have indicated that when 60 mg of the amino acid are ingested, enough is oxidized to produce 1 mg of niacin, although this approximation may not apply in certain conditions such as pregnancy. The synthesis of niacin requires pyridoxine, riboflavin, and thiamin; deficiencies of these vitamins may also be implicated in the etiology of pellagra.

Function

Niacin and its active form nicotinamide are intimately related to energy release from fat, carbohydrate, and protein. The vitamin functions as a part of two important coenzymes, NAD (nicotinamide adenine dinucleotide) and NADP (nicotinamide adenine dinucleotide phosphate), which are involved with hydrogen transfer in metabolic reactions, in both their oxidized and reduced forms (NADH and NADPH). The coenzymes are utilized in the glycolytic and tricarboxylic acid pathways, and in the synthesis and breakdown of fatty acids. Transfer of hy-drogen from NADH to the riboflavin-containing coenzymes occurs in the electron transport system, by which ATP and water are formed. NADP is utilized in the pentose phosphate pathway, in which ribose is synthesized. Thus, a variety of important metabolic pathways are influenced by the availability of niacin.

Biochemical Assessment

Dietary surveys do not provide a good index of niacin status, as there is a question about the availability of niacin in foods. Biochemical methods of estimation are more meaningful, although present methods are not particularly suitable or accurate. Measurement of niacin metabolites in urine, and recently the ratio of 2-pyridone to N-methylnicotinamide, have been used. Measurement of NAD levels in blood has been disappointing; there are no satisfactory and reliable differences between pellagrins and normals. Clearly, more research is needed, particularly to identify subclinical cases of pellagra.

Dietary Allowances and Sources

The allowance for niacin is based on niacin equivalents, to take into account its in vivo synthesis from tryptophan. One niacin equivalent (NE) is defined as 1 mg niacin or 60 mg tryptophan. Allowances for niacin are based on caloric intake, 6.6 NE per 1000 kcal (6.6 NE per 4200 kJ), with the recommendation that a minimum of 13 NE per day be ingested, even at energy intakes of less than 2000 kcal (8400 kJ). Note that the requirement for this vitamin is considerably higher than that recommended for any of the other water-soluble vitamins. Pregnancy increases the daily recommended allowance by 2 NE, and lactation by 4 NE. Patients with Hartnup's disease (a rare familial disorder in which there is decreased intestinal absorption and renal reabsorption of the neutral amino acids, including tryptophan) often develop pellagralike symptoms which are responsive to niacin treatment.

Meat, poultry, and fish are better sources of niacin than are plant products, on the basis not only of preformed niacin content, but also of their tryptophan content. Enrichment procedures have also made enriched bread and bread products good sources of the vitamin, primarily because of the quantity in which they are eaten, although our weight-conscious society often shuns these products. Peanut butter can be an important source of the vitamin. Fruits and vegetables are generally poor sources; milk and eggs have little preformed niacin, but are good sources of tryptophan.

Clinical Deficiency

Pellagra is the classic disease associated with niacin deficiency and is characterized by the "three D's": *dermatitis, diarrhea,* and *dementia* (a fourth "D," *death,* is often added). The observed dermatitis is interesting in that the rash generally shows a symmetrical pattern and is accentuated by exposure to sun or heat. *Casal's necklace* describes the rash apparent in the neck area of affected persons. Mouth, tongue, and intestinal tissues become inflamed in niacin deficiency. Mental confusion, anxiety, and depression are manifestations of the effects of the disease on the central nervous system. Many of the symptoms are reminiscent of riboflavin and thiamin deficiencies; recent work suggests that pellagra is a mixed deficiency and that riboflavin and thiamin (and perhaps also pyridoxine) nutriture are important factors in its development. In addition, millet (sorghum)-based diets may be responsible for the onset of pellagra in some cases. This grain contains high concentrations of available niacin and is not low in tryptophan, but it is high in leucine content; this branched-chain amino acid may interfere with the conversion of tryptophan to niacin.

Fortunately, most pellagra has disappeared in the United States. It is still found, however, in the corn-eating countries of Europe. Of interest is the fact that the people of Latin and Central America have not been prone to pellagra, even though their dietary staple is corn. This is probably related to the fact that the corn is treated with lime salts, which may release bound forms of niacin and make the vitamin available for absorption.

Toxicity and Pharmacological Effects

Large doses of nicotinic acid (but not nicotinamide) have a vasodilating effect, causing transient tingling and flushing of the skin.

Pharmacological doses of niacin (3 g or more daily) have been used to lower serum cholesterol and lipoprotein levels. The Coronary Drug Project Research Group recently released a statement concerning the safety and efficacy of this form of treatment:

> [*There is*] no evidence that niacin influences mortality of survivors of myocardial infarction; this medication may be slightly beneficial in protecting persons to some degree against recurrent nonfatal myocardial infarctions. However, because of the excess incidence of arrhythmias, gastrointestinal problems, and abnormal chemistry findings in the niacin group, great care and caution must be exercised if this drug is to be used for treatment of persons with coronary heart disease.[74]

Another highly publicized use of nicotinic acid has been in the treatment of schizophrenia. In addition to questionable effects on the mental disorder, massive doses of the vitamin may cause liver injury. Diabetes and activation of peptic ulcers may also be long-term consequences of nicotinic acid therapy. Niacin is not, therefore, a totally harmless water-soluble vitamin.

Pantothenic Acid

History and Discovery

This B vitamin gets its name from the Greek *pantos,* meaning "everywhere"; its ubiquitous presence in all plants and animals led to its nomenclature. The vitamin was recognized as essential for several species, including humans, and was isolated in 1938 and synthesized in 1940.

Chemistry and Properties

Pantothenic acid is a yellow oily liquid, but is crystalline in its commercially available form, calcium pantothenate. It is soluble in water and alcohol, and is easily decomposed by alkali, acid, and heat.

Metabolism

Little is known about the absorption of pantothenic acid, although it is probably absorbed by diffusion from the upper part of the small intestine. The vitamin is converted to its active forms, and there is limited storage in liver, adrenal gland, brain, kidney, and heart. It is excreted primarily in urine.

Function

The essentiality of pantothenic acid was recognized when it was determined that it was part of the coenzyme A molecule, a very important compound in intermediary metabolism. Coenzyme A forms thioesters with carboxylic acids, and is intimately involved in the metabolism of carbohydrate, protein, and fat. Acetyl CoA, the entry point for many compounds into the tricarboxylic acid cycle, is also involved in fatty acid and sterol synthesis. It provides acetyl groups for acetylcholine, a neurotransmitter, and is also required for the synthesis of porphyrin, the pigment portion of the hemoglobin molecule.

Another function of pantothenic acid is its role in the structure of acyl carrier protein (ACP), necessary for the transport of acetyl CoA from mitochondria to cytoplasm for use in fatty acid synthesis. ACP is required in all subsequent steps of fatty acid synthesis.

Dietary Allowances and Sources

Lack of adequate evidence about the actual requirement for pantothenic acid has led the Food and Nutrition Board to suggest a daily intake of 4 to 7 mg of the vitamin. A higher intake may be needed by pregnant and lactating women. It has been estimated that the average American diet contains 7 mg per day,[75] with variations between 5 and 20 mg per day.

Although pantothenic acid is present in all foods, eggs, liver, yeast, salmon, and heart are the best-known sources. Mushrooms, cauliflower, molasses, and peanuts are also good sources. In general, fruits are relatively poor sources of the vitamin. Grains are an important source of pantothenic acid; however, approximately 50 percent is lost in the milling process.

Clinical Deficiency

One of the reasons that the Food and Nutrition Board has not been able to set a recommended dietary allowance is that no spontaneous deficiencies of pantothenic acid have been shown to occur in humans. In fact, experimentally induced deficiencies, by use of either purified diets or pantothenic acid antagonists, have not been "successful" either, in that they, too, are difficult to produce. In one study, subjects on a deficient diet experienced insomnia, leg cramps, and paresthesias of hands and feet. Addition of an antagonist produced burning feet, insulin sensitivity, and mental depression.

Lower species do show specific signs of deficiency: chicks develop ocular dermatitis and spinal cord degeneration, and rats develop red whiskers, growth failure, alopecia, and graying of hair. Contrary to the claims of vitamin advocates, pantothenic acid will not prevent the appearance of gray hair in humans.

In some patients treated with streptomycin, a polyneuropathy may develop which is responsive to pantothenic acid. One report suggests that in patients with chronic ulcerative and granulomatous colitis a block in the conversion of pantothenic acid to coenzyme A occurs within the intestine.[76]

The vitamin has been used clinically after surgery to stimulate gastrointestinal motility, but large doses will cause diarrhea and should be avoided.

Biotin

History and Discovery

Variably known as vitamin H and coenzyme R, biotin was recognized as a growth factor for microorganisms in 1924. It was synthesized in 1943 and recognized as a compound which protected rats against "egg white injury," caused by the feeding of raw egg whites. Symptoms which appeared included dermatitis, paralysis of the hind legs, and a characteristic alopecia around the eye, appropriately called "spectacle eye." Cooked egg white did not produce these signs. It is now known that raw egg white contains a heat-labile protein, avidin, which binds dietary biotin and makes it unavailable for absorption.

Chemistry and Properties
Biotin is a sulfur-containing monocarboxylic acid which is water- and alcohol-soluble. It is stable to heat but destroyed by oxidation, alkali, and strong acids.

Metabolism
Except for its being made unavailable for absorption by avidin, the absorption of biotin from the gastrointestinal tract is unremarkable. In addition, synthesis of the vitamin by intestinal bacteria is extensive and probably largely available to humans. Little is known about its storage, and most of it appears to be excreted intact in the urine.

Function
Biotin is a component of several important enzyme systems, particularly those involved in carbohydrate and fat metabolism. The vitamin acts as a carbon dioxide carrier in carboxylation reactions whereby carbon chains are lengthened. Examples are the conversion of pyruvate to oxaloacetate and the production of malonyl coenzyme A for fatty acid synthesis.[77]

Dietary Allowances and Sources
No allowance has been set by the Food and Nutrition Board for biotin, although a safe and adequate estimated intake of 100 to 200 μg per day has been proposed. Most American diets contain at least this much, and intestinal production by the microflora seems to provide a substantial amount.

Although few foods have been analyzed for biotin content, it is present in milk, liver, egg yolk, mushrooms, and legumes.

Clinical Deficiency
Biotin deficiency has been produced in animals by dietary means. Until recently, however, human deficiency could only be produced by feeding large amounts of raw egg white. Symptoms include dermatitis, anorexia, lassitude, muscle pain, and nausea. Evidence suggests that seborrheic dermatitis seen in infants less than 6 months of age is due to nutritional biotin deficiency. The condition responds rapidly to biotin therapy.

Consumption of an occasional raw egg, as in an eggnog, will not precipitate deficiency symptoms. It is only large amounts, estimated to be more than 20 eggs per day, that cause biotin deficiency. This equivalent is highly unlikely in the typical American diet.

Folic Acid

History and Discovery
In 1931 Wills reported an often fatal macrocytic anemia among the pregnant women of India, and suggested that it might be a symptom of a dietary deficiency disease. Further investigation with animals led to the conclusion that the substance was identical to a bacterial growth factor isolated from spinach leaves. Folic acid (from the Latin *folium,* meaning "leaf") was subsequently isolated and synthesized in 1948.

Chemistry and Properties
The folacin group of water-soluble crystalline yellow compounds contains several forms of the vitamin which are biologically active. The parent compound is known as *folic acid* or *pteroylglutamic acid* (PGA), the latter describing its chemical nature: pteroic acid (of which para-aminobenzoic acid, once thought to be an essential vitamin, is a part) and one or more molecules of glutamic acid. Folacin is a heat-labile compound in acid solution, and it is unstable to sunlight in the dry form. Considerable loss of the vitamin occurs in high temperature processing and during storage, with various forms of the vitamin exhibiting different degrees of thermal stability.

Metabolism
The primary site of folate absorption is the upper part of the small intestine, where both active and passive transport contribute to its entry into mucosal cells. Before dietary folate, which

is present primarily as polyglutamates, can be absorbed, excess glutamates must be enzymatically removed by conjugase, a hydrolytic enzyme present in intestinal cells. The rate of absorption of dietary folate may be inversely related to the length of the polyglutamate chain, and current research is attempting to determine the availability of the various forms of folate.[78] The monoglutamate form is transported to the liver, where it is converted to one of its metabolically active compounds.

Liver stores contain about half of the vitamin found in the body, although folate is found in all cells. It is bound to a protein for transport and storage. Small amounts are found in the urine, as a folate metabolite.

The metabolism of folate may be influenced at several points by interactions with pharmaceutical agents. Among those which cause a decrease in its absorption are alcohol, the antitubercular drugs, aminosalicylic acid cycloserine, and some anticonvulsants. The antimalarial drugs trimethoprim and pyrimethamine inactive folate; methotrexate is a powerful folate antagonist used in antitumor treatment. The use of oral contraceptives has been associated with decreased levels of serum folate.

Function

A discussion of the function of folic acid requires discussion of its own metabolism. Folic acid is reduced to tetrahydrofolic acid (THFA) in the presence of NADPH (a niacin coenzyme). Addition of a one-carbon fragment to one or two of the nitrogen molecules in pteroic acid completes the synthesis of the active coenzyme form of folic acid. As the coenzyme, folate participates in the transfer of single carbon units (formyl, methyl) to intermediates in the biosynthesis of purine and pyrimidine (precursors for the nucleic acids), and in several amino acid interconversions. The latter reactions include the methylation of homocysteine to methionine, and the conversion of histidine to glutamic acid.

Folacin is required for heme synthesis, and is necessary for the formation of blood cells in the bone marrow, and for their maturation.

Generally speaking, folic acid needs are highest in tissues with a rapid turnover rate, because of their increased rate of nucleic acid and protein synthesis.

Biochemical Assessment

Serum folate levels of less than 3 ng per mL are indicative of a folic acid deficiency. Another widely used assessment method is the histidine load. Histidine requires folate for its metabolism and when the vitamin is not available, an intermediary metabolite, formiminoglutamic acid (FIGLU), accumulates and is excreted in the urine. After a 20-g histidine load, more than 50 mg of FIGLU in a 12-h urine sample is considered abnormal and suggestive of a folic acid deficiency.

Dietary Allowances and Sources

The recommended dietary allowance for adults is 100 μg per day. Because requirements are substantially increased during periods of extensive cell multiplication (owing to the role of folic acid in nucleic acid synthesis), the allowances for pregnancy and lactation are 800 and 500 μg per day, respectively. Rodriguez has published an extensive review of human requirements for folacin.[79]

Folic acid is found in green leafy vegetables, liver, fish, meat and poultry, legumes, and whole grains.[80] Chemical determinations of folate vary widely; newer and more accurate analyses are being developed.

Clinical Deficiency

In humans, folate deficiency results in megaloblastic anemia, gastrointestinal disturbances, glossitis, and growth retardation. Folacin deficiency symptoms in the elderly have been linked to both inadequate intake and inefficient absorption.[81,82] A deficiency of the vitamin itself will cause structural changes in the small intestine,[83,84] further interfering with the absorption of the folate that is present in the diet, as well as other nutrients.

Because of the close relationship between folic acid and vitamin B_{12} metabolism, several of the same clinical signs appear when either of these is deficient. It should be stressed that folate will cure the anemia due to B_{12} deficiency, but will not alleviate the more serious neurological symptoms that accompany the anemia in B_{12} deficiency.

Vitamin B_{12}

History and Discovery
In 1926 pernicious anemia was a fatal disease of unknown origin, characterized by neurological damage and megaloblastic anemia. Castle postulated the existence of an *intrinsic factor,* which he believed to be present in gastric secretions, and an *extrinsic factor,* both at the time unidentified, which were involved in the etiology of the disease. When physicians in Boston demonstrated that liver cured patients with pernicious anemia,[85] the search for the so-called extrinsic factor began. In 1948, the isolation of vitamin B_{12} from liver proved to be a turning point in the understanding of the disease.

Chemistry and Properties
Vitamin B_{12} is a complex molecule which was not synthesized in the laboratory until 1973. It contains the mineral cobalt and is an extremely potent compound. It is a water-soluble reddish molecule and is sensitive to acid, alkali, and oxidizing agents.

Metabolism
The unfolding of the B_{12} mystery was a challenge to biochemists. The vitamin, presumably because of its large size, is poorly absorbed without the presence of intrinsic factor, a large glycoprotein secreted by gastric cells. Vitamin B_{12} is released from food and combines with intrinsic factor in the stomach. The complex is bound to a receptor in the intestinal wall; this attachment is calcium-dependent. The vitamin is released from its carrier and transported through intestinal cells into the bloodstream, where it is carried by transcobalamin, a transport protein, to the tissues. Storage occurs in the liver, and in contrast to other water-soluble vitamins, the ex-

tent to which this vitamin is conserved is substantial. An efficient enterohepatic circulation of the vitamin contributes to its relatively long storage time. Excess vitamin B_{12} is excreted in the urine.

Absorption of vitamin B_{12} appears to decrease with age, and in iron and pyridoxine deficiency. Diminished absorption occurs in patients with gastritis and those with congenital intrinsic factor deficiency.

Function
Vitamin B_{12} functions as a coenzyme in cellular reactions. The synthesis of nucleic acids is dependent upon vitamin B_{12}, and this is related to its interactions with folate metabolism. Vitamin B_{12} is necessary for the regeneration of tetrahydrofolate from 5-methyltetrahydrofolate; without the return of THFA, DNA synthesis is impaired. The metabolism of odd-chain fatty acids is also B_{12}-dependent, as is the conversion of homocysteine to methionine.

Biochemical Assessment
Evaluation of nutritional status can be done by measuring serum levels of B_{12}, and, less frequently, by determining the amount of methylmalonic acid (MMA) in the urine. MMA requires B_{12} for its conversion to succinic acid, and in the absence of the vitamin, urinary excretion is increased, which is diagnostic of a vitamin B_{12} deficiency. A newer method of assessment relies upon the degree of vitamin B_{12} stimulation of in vitro DNA synthesis. This test is analogous to the stimulation tests described for thiamin, riboflavin, and vitamin B_6.

Dietary Allowances and Sources
The present recommendation for vitamin B_{12} intake is 3 μg per day for adults, increasing to 4 μg during pregnancy and lactation. In patients whose liver stores have been depleted, 15 μg per day is recommended.

Neither plants nor animals can synthesize vitamin B_{12}. Consequently, the vitamin is available only from foods of animal origin, because the animals have accumulated it from their resident population of microorganisms, which are capable of the biosynthesis of vitamin B_{12}. The only reliable sources, then, are meats, eggs, fish, poultry, and dairy products. Plant foods contain no vitamin B_{12} unless they are specifically fortified or contaminated with microorganisms.

The distribution of vitamin B_{12} in our food supply raises some interesting questions about the vitamin B_{12} status of strict vegetarians. While it has been proposed that intestinal bacterial synthesis in humans provides enough vitamin B_{12} to prevent deficiency symptoms, it is generally agreed that absorption of the vitamin from that source is minimal. Fermented foods, such as tempeh, may contain some of the vitamin, but should not be relied upon to meet vitamin B_{12} needs.

Clinical Deficiency

Signs of vitamin B_{12} deficiency are manifested by both blood and nervous system disorders. The megaloblastic anemia is presumably due to the effect that the vitamin has on maturation of immature red blood cells; nervous system disorders may be due to defective myelin synthesis and fatty acid metabolism. Pernicious anemia is classically due to the congenital absence of intrinsic factor, in which case milligram doses of vitamin B_{12} must be administered parenterally on a daily basis. Iatrogenic (physician-induced) deficiency is produced by gastrectomy or surgical removal of the ileum. Malabsorptive states may induce a deficiency. In some populations, infestation of the gastrointestinal tract with a particular fish tapeworm, which dissociates the B_{12}-intrinsic factor complex, may precipitate a deficiency state.

Of increasing concern to nutritionists is the effect of a strict vegetarian diet on vitamin B_{12} status. Adults who choose this type of diet generally have enough of the vitamin stored in their liver to last for 5 or 6 years before deficiency symptoms set in. However, breast-fed infants of vegetarian mothers[86] and children consuming a vegetarian diet have not accumulated stores of the vitamin and are at higher risk of developing a deficiency. Parents are urged to include at least some animal products (milk and eggs) in their children's diets. If that is unacceptable, fortified soy milk or a vitamin preparation containing vitamin B_{12} is necessary.

VITAMINLIKE FACTORS

There are several compounds which at one time or another have been considered as vitamins. As we learn more about their metabolism and function, a decision will be made as to their inclusion in the vitamin category.

Choline

Choline is a bitter-tasting, water-soluble compound that is widely distributed in plant and animal tissues. It can be synthesized by the human body in the presence of sufficient serine, methionine, folate, and vitamin B_{12}, but probably not in amounts adequate for the maintenance of health. Choline is used as a source of labile methyl groups needed for synthetic processes, and is a structural component of phospholipids (lecithin and sphingomyelin) in addition to being a precursor of acetylcholine. Along with methionine, choline is known as a *lipotropic factor* that is "fat-attracting," and is necessary for the prevention of fatty liver. Fatty liver is observed in kwashiorkor and alcoholism; choline has been used to treat the condition. Under normal circumstances, choline deficiency does not occur in humans; sources of this compound include egg yolk, organ meats, legumes, and wheat germ. Dietary requirements are not known; the average American diet provides 400 to 900 mg per day, and this appears to be sufficient.

Inositol

Inositol is a colorless water-soluble compound and is structurally related to glucose. In animal tissues it occurs as a component of phospholipids in muscle, and this is its primary function in man; phytic acid, an inositol-phosphate com-

TABLE 6-1   SUMMARY OF THE VITAMINS

Vitamin	RDA for adults	Food sources	Biological functions	Signs of deficiency	Signs of toxicity
A (retinol, carotenes)	W:* 800 RE 4000 IU M: 1000 RE 5000 IU	Liver, whole milk, butter, fortified milk and margarine, dark green leafy vegetables, yellow-orange vegetables and fruits	Maintains vision in dim light, maintains integrity of epithelial tissue, promotes skeletal growth	Night blindness, xerophthalmia, impaired tooth and bone development, keratinization of epithelial tissues	Loss of hair, pain in bones and joints, hepatomegaly, dry skin, bulging of fontanelles and growth failure in children
D (calciferol)	5 μg = 200 IU	Fortified milk, some in liver, sardines and salmon, fish liver oils (sunlight)	Promotes absorption of dietary calcium and phosphorus, promotes tooth and skeletal development	Rickets in children, and osteomalacia in adults	Soft tissue calcification, bone demineralization
E (tocopherol)	W: 8 mg α-TE M: 10 mg α-TE	Vegetable oils, wheat germ, legumes, green leafy vegetables	Chemical antioxidant: protects vitamin A and PUFA from oxidation, stabilizes cell membranes	Deficiency unlikely; hemolysis of red blood cells	Toxicity unlikely; may decrease blood clotting time
K (phyllo- and mena-quinones)	70–140 μg†	Dark green leafy vegetables, liver (intestinal bacterial synthesis)	Necessary for blood clotting; formation of prothrombin and osteocalcin	Prolonged clotting time	Hemolytic anemia and jaundice in infants
Thiamin (B₁)	W: 1.0 mg M: 1.4 mg	Brewer's yeast, pork, liver, legumes, nuts, whole grain and enriched bread and cereals	Necessary for energy production from carbohydrate, fat, and protein; transmission of nerve impulses?	Beriberi; edema, cardiac failure, changes in nerve functioning, anorexia	None reported
Riboflavin (B₂)	W: 1.2 mg M: 1.6 mg	Dairy products, organ meats, whole grain and enriched breads and cereals, green leafy vegetables	As coenzymes FAD and FMN, participates in hydrogen transfer reactions	Cheilosis, glossitis, dry scaly skin, itchy eyes	None reported
Niacin (nicotinic acid, nicotinamide)	W: 13 mg NE M: 18 mg NE	Meats, liver, whole grain breads and cereals, legumes (tryptophan is precursor)	As coenzymes NAD and NADP, participates in carbohydrate, fat, and protein metabolism; hydrogen transfer reactions	Pellagra; diarrhea, dermatitis, change in nerve function	Nicotinic acid: skin flush, liver injury, activation of peptic ulcer

*W = women; M = men.
†Estimated safe and adequate daily dietary intake.

TABLE 6-1   CONTINUED

Vitamin	RDA for adults	Food sources	Biological functions	Signs of deficiency	Signs of toxicity
Pyridoxine (B$_6$)	W:* 2.0 mg M: 2.2 mg	Liver, bananas, beef, pork, corn, brussels sprouts, wheat germ	As coenzyme PLP for transamination and decarboxylation reactions; essential for conversion of tryptophan to niacin	Microcytic anemia, mental depression, muscle weakness	Sleepiness; B$_6$ dependence
Biotin	100–200 µg†	Liver, meats, oatmeal, legumes, mushrooms, milk (intestinal bacterial synthesis)	Participates in CO_2–transfer reactions	Not likely; seborrheic dermatitis in infants	None reported
Pantothenic acid	4–7 mg†	Eggs, liver, salmon, mushrooms; present in all foods	As part of coenzyme A, participates in synthesis and catabolism of many nutrients; necessary for metabolism of carbohydrate, protein, and fat	Not likely; Induced deficiency produces insomnia, fatigue and irritability	Large doses may cause diarrhea
Folacin (folic acid)	400 µg	Green leafy vegetables, organ meats, legumes, broccoli, beets	As coenzyme THFA, transfers single carbon units in amino acid and nucleic acid metabolism; maturation of red blood cells	Megaloblastic anemia	None reported
Vitamin B$_{12}$	3 µg	Animal products (dairy, meats); fortified cereal products and fortified soy milk	Transfers single carbon units in nucleic acid metabolism; related to folate metabolism; maturation of red blood cells; nerve conduction?	Megaloblastic and pernicious anemia	None reported
Ascorbic acid (vitamin C)	60 mg	Citrus fruits, strawberries, green peppers, melons, broccoli, potato	Enhances iron absorption, promotes collagen synthesis	Scurvy, bleeding gums, swollen joints, muscle cramps; fights infection	Diarrhea, rebound scurvy, kidney stones

*W = women; M = men.

†Estimated safe and adequate daily dietary intake.

plex, is found in plants and is known to decrease the absorption of calcium and iron. Besides its occurrence in large amounts in common foods, the body appears to be able to synthesize adequate amounts; most researchers no longer include it as a vitamin.

Ubiquinone

Ubiquinone or coenzyme Q, chemically related to vitamin K, is present in mitochondria and plays a major role in the operation of the electron transport system. Adequate in vivo synthesis takes place in humans, and its inclusion as a vitamin is not warranted.

Lipoic Acid

Another substance that serves as a coenzyme in intermediary metabolism is also synthesized in sufficient amounts by the human body. Lipoic acid is a sulfur-containing fat-soluble compound that functions in conjunction with thiamin pyrophosphate in decarboxylation reactions, particularly the conversion of pyruvate to acetyl CoA.

NONVITAMINS

Despite popular claims, which are unsupported thus far by reliable scientific evidence, there is no essential nutrient function for laetrile (erroneously named vitamin B_{17}) or pangamic acid (misnamed vitamin B_{15}).[87,88]

Laetrile, in particular, has aroused popular curiosity because of its postulated benefits in the cure and prevention of cancer. However, there is no scientific evidence at this time that it is either safe or effective in cancer therapy.[89] In any case, it is not a vitamin, because it fails to meet two of the criteria for defining a vitamin: it does not perform an essential biochemical function in the body, and its absence from the diet produces no deficiency symptoms.

VITAMIN SUPPLEMENTATION

We have become a vitamin-conscious society. A misunderstanding of the biochemical role of the vitamins has led to suggestions that people will enjoy better health, be less tired, and possibly live longer if they increase their vitamin intake.

Vitamin supplementation may be appropriate when prescribed for people recovering from illnesses, to facilitate their return to health and adequate nutritional status. Also, supplementation is sometimes necessary for people who are regularly taking medications which are known to influence vitamin metabolism. But self-medication with high-level multivitamin supplements should only be undertaken under the supervision of a physician.

Today, the increasing use of highly processed foods in our society has generated concern that some of the water-soluble vitamins (vitamin B_6 and folic acid, for example) are being systematically removed from our food supply. Generally speaking, consumption of a diverse and balanced diet (with a minimum of highly processed foods) will ensure adequate vitamin intake, unless the calorie intake falls below 1000 to 1200 kcal (4.2 to 5.0 mJ) daily. Then the use of a supplement containing 100 percent of the U.S. RDA may be reasonable.

In most cases, when people eat regular, balanced, and varied meals containing all essential nutrients, the extra vitamins are not needed, and the water-soluble nutrients are excreted. A vitamin supplement does not ensure adequate nutrient intake in the absence of food. So they should not be relied on as a replacement for food! (See Table 6-2).

On the other hand, the widespread availability and consumption of vitamin-fortified foods has raised a different issue. Cereals, baby foods, candy bars, beverages, and dessert items have been increasingly fortified with vitamins (and some minerals). Two major issues are apparent. Many of the fortified foods are high-calorie, high-sugar, and high-fat snack-type foods which frequently replace more nutrient-dense foods in

TABLE 6-2 COMPOSITION OF MULTIVITAMIN SUPPLEMENTS

Supplement	Recommended dose	Vitamin A, IU	Vitamin D, IU	Vitamin E, IU	Vitamin C, mg	Thiamin, mg	Riboflavin, mg	Niacin, mg	Pyridoxine, mg	Vitamin B$_{12}$, µg	Folic acid, µg	Pantothenic acid, mg	Fluoride, mg	Biotin, µg
Ce-Vi-Sol Drops[a]	0.6 mL	...	...	...	35	...	...	...	...	...	...	...	...	...
Poly-Vi-Flor Infant Drops[a]	1 mL	1500	400	5	35	0.5	0.6	8	0.4	2	...	...	0.5	...
Poly-Vi-Sol Multivitamin Drops[a]	1 mL	1500	400	5	35	0.5	0.6	8	0.4	2	...	...	...	...
Tri-Vi-Flor Infant Drops[a]	1 mL	1500	400	...	35	...	...	...	...	...	...	...	0.5	...
Tri-Vi-Sol Infant Drops[a]	1 mL	1500	400	...	35	...	...	...	...	...	...	...	...	...
Vi-Penta Multi-Vitamin Drops[b]	0.6 mL	5000	400	2	50	1.0	1.0	10	1.0	...	...	10	...	30
Chocks-Bugs Bunny Multivitamin Supplement[c]	1 tablet	2500	400	15	60	1.05	1.2	13.5	1.05	4.5	300	...	...	...
Pals Multivitamins[d]	1 tablet	3500	400	...	60	0.8	1.3	14	1.0	2.5	50	5	...	...
One-A-Day Vitamins[c]	1 tablet	5000	400	15	60	1.5	1.7	20	2.0	6	400	...	...	...
Stresstabs 600[e]	1 tablet	...	...	30	600	15	15	100	5.0	12	...	20	...	...
Unicap[f]	1 tablet	5000	400	15	60	1.5	1.7	20	2.0	6	400	...	...	...

[a]Mead Johnson, Evansville, Ind.
[b]Roche Laboratories, Nutley, N.J.
[c]Miles Laboratories, Inc., Elkhart, Ind.
[d]Bristol-Myers Products, New York, N.Y.
[e]Lederle Laboratories, Wayne, N.J.
[f]Upjohn Company, Kalamazoo, Mich.

Sources: Physicians Desk Reference for Non-Prescription Drugs, Medical Economics Company, Oradell, N.J., 1980. Physicians Desk Reference, 35th ed., Medical Economics Company, Oradell, N.J., 1981.

the total diet. Secondly, overconsumption of these highly fortified products, especially consumption of adult cereals by children, often results in the intake of several times the RDA for many nutrients. Considering the natural availability of vitamins in our food supply, and the potential toxic effects of some of the vitamins, the indiscriminate addition of vitamins to foods is unnecessary.

MEGAVITAMINS

The use of vitamins in doses of at least ten times the RDA is popularly known as megavitamin therapy. The term *orthomolecular therapy* was introduced by Linus Pauling in 1968 to describe treatment based on substances that are found in or are used by the body, such as hormones and vitamins. Massive doses of niacin, for example, have been used in an attempt to lower blood lipid levels; niacin, ascorbic acid, and other water-soluble vitamins have been used in the treatment of schizophrenia. In recent years, advocates of megavitamin therapy have claimed that this approach is useful in the treatment of autism, hyperactivity in children, arthritis, learning disabilities, cancer, and a number of other conditions. To date, most of the evidence to support its efficacy is anecdotal in nature, and data from well-controlled scientific studies do not substantiate the claims.

Although the postulated benefits of megavitamin therapy cannot be ascribed to correction of a documented biochemical abnormality in most cases, there are some clinical conditions in which large doses of a *specific* vitamin are effective. Several vitamin-dependency disorders have been identified; in these inborn errors of metabolism a pharmacologic amount of a particular vitamin will stimulate a poorly functioning enzyme. There is a predictable, known, and rapid response in the absence of other treatment which is not found in schizophrenic patients.

Large doses of vitamins can also compensate for the effects of prescribed medications that are known to interfere with the absorption, func-

tion, or excretion of that vitamin. An example is the use of the antituberculous drug isoniazid, which increases the need for vitamin B_6.

But aside from these relatively few and specifically defined disorders, the use of megavitamin therapy is not warranted; there is little evidence of benefit and the potential for undesirable and toxic side effects. And individuals certainly should not take it upon themselves to consume massive amounts of vitamins; the assumption that "if some is good, more is better" is not scientifically valid.

CONCLUSION

Although the classic signs of vitamin deficiency are seldom manifest in our population, certain altered physiological states and diseases can place individuals at nutritional risk. Since these deficiencies evolve in a gradual continuum and in clusters, the diagnosis must be based on medical and diet histories, and on physical, laboratory, and anthropometric data. Medical and surgical patients, by virtue of their conditions, are at particular risk and should be monitored accordingly. However, given the wrong circumstances, anyone can be at risk of developing vitamin deficiencies, especially the poor, the ignorant, and the elderly. It is the astute health professional who looks for the obscure signs of vitamin deficiencies rather than the classic manifestations, and who counsels against the indiscriminate use of vitamin supplements and large amounts of vitamin-fortified foods.

In terms of basic research in the vitamin field, several priorities have been identified: standardization of existing methods and development of new methods of assessing vitamin status, better definition of marginal and optimal intakes, identification of the withdrawal effects following supplementation with therapeutic dosages, the interaction of other nutrients and drugs with vitamins, and the impact of a marginal vitamin supply on health.[90] Such questions promise to make the field of vitamin research an exciting one for years to come.

STUDY QUESTIONS

1   What are the similarities and differences between the fat-soluble and water-soluble vitamins?

2   What are the chief symptoms of vitamin A deficiency? Vitamin D? Vitamin E? Vitamin K?

3   Explain three specific types of information you might use to determine nutritional status with regard to the vitamins. Of what value is this information in nutrition education?

4   How would you describe the general function of vitamins in the body?

5   What are the potential dangers of "super-fortification" of foods?

6   Name three vitamins to which strict vegetarians must pay particular attention. Identify acceptable food sources of these vitamins.

CLINICAL STUDY 6

Cathy is a 26-year-old woman who went to her university health service complaining of leg, ankle, and back pain; fatigue; insomnia; and hair loss. She also reported that she had chronic headaches which were interfering with her preparation for her doctoral examinations in chemistry.

A medical examination and history revealed the following: height, 165 cm (66 in); weight, 50 kg (110 lb); no previous hospitalizations or severe illness, regular menstrual cycles, a 20-lb weight loss (3 years prior to her clinic visit) after she adopted a lacto-vegetarian plan of eating. Her change in diet was prompted by health considerations and a limited income as a graduate student. She was concerned about her vitamin intake, and routinely took two low-level multivitamin supplements containing 5000 IU of vitamin A per day. Approximately 1 year before her visit to the health service she read an article about some research that "vitamin A prevented cancer." Since there was a family history of cancer, she decided to increase her intake of vitamin A and began taking capsules containing 25,000 IU four times a day in addition to her regular multivitamin supplements. Suspecting hypervitaminosis A, her physician ordered a serum vitamin A determination in addition to the usual laboratory tests. All the lab tests were within the normal range, except for vitamin A, which was 150 μg per dL (normal 30 to 60 μg per dL).

A diet history revealed that Cathy consumed an average of 2 cups of vitamin A–fortified skim milk, 2 oz of cheddar cheese, and 4 teaspoons of fortified margarine per day. The rest of her diet included a variety of whole grain breads, brown rice, fruits, vegetables, and legumes, providing about 1500 kcal (6.3 mJ) per day.

On the basis of the clinical, biochemical and dietary findings, a diagnosis of hypervitaminosis A was made.

Clinical study questions

1   *What was Cathy's daily minimum intake of vitamin A?*

2   *How would additional foods contribute to her total intake of the vitamin?*

3   *What is the treatment for hypervitaminosis A?*

4   *How would you explain to Cathy, an obviously intelligent woman, that she doesn't need vitamin A supplements?*

5   *She asks you how she can ensure an adequate intake of nutrients without using supplements, since she plans to continue her lacto-vegetarian pattern of eating. What would you tell her?*

REFERENCES

1   F. R. Smith et al., "Plasma Vitamin A, Retinol-binding Protein and Prealbumin Concentrations in Protein-Calorie Malnutrition. III. Response to Varying Dietary Treatments," *American Journal of Clinical Nutrition,* **28**:732, 1975.

2   J. Smith, Jr., et al., "Zinc: A Trace Element Essential in Vitamin A Metabolism," *Science,* **181**:954, 1973.

3   J. E. Smith et al., "The Effect of Zinc Deficiency on the Metabolism of Retinol-binding in the Rat," *Journal of Laboratory and Clinical Medicine,* **84**:692, 1974.

4   S. A. Morrison et al., "Zinc Deficiency: A Cause of Abnormal Dark Adaptation in Cirrhotics," *American Journal of Clinical Nutrition,* **31**:276, 1978.

5   H. D. Palin et al., "The Effect of Oral Zinc Supplementation on Plasma Levels of Vitamin A and Retinol-binding Protein," *American Journal of Clinical Nutrition,* **32**:1253, 1979.

6   P. L. Hooper et al., "Zinc and Vitamin A," *American Journal of Clinical Nutrition,* **33**:2395, 1980.

7   N. W. Solomons and R. M. Russell, "The Interaction of Vitamin A and Zinc: Implications for Human Nutrition," *American Journal of Clinical Nutrition,* **33**:2031, 1980.

8   F. R. Smith and D. S. Goodman, "The Effects of Diseases of the Liver, Thyroid and Kidneys on the Transport of Vitamin A in Human Plasma," *Journal of Clinical Investigation,* **50**:2426, 1971.

9   S. S. Harris et al., "Vitamin A Deficiency and New Bone Growth: Histologic Changes," *Journal of Oral Pathology,* **7**:85, 1978.

10 Food and Nutrition Board, *Recommended Dietary Allowances,* rev. 9th ed., National Academy of Sciences, Washington, D.C., 1980.

11 Institute of Food Technologists, "The Effects of Food Processing on Nutritional Values," *Nutrition Reviews,* **33**:123, 1975.

12 D. P. Sinha and F. B. Bang, "The Effect of Massive Doses of Vitamin A on the Signs of Vitamin A Deficiency in Preschool Children," *American Journal of Clinical Nutrition,* **29**:110, 1976.

13 C. P. Mahoney et al., "Chronic Vitamin A Intoxication in Infants Fed Chicken Liver," *Pediatrics,* **65**:893, 1980.

14 A. E. Rogers et al., "Induction by Dimethylhydrazine of Intestinal Carcinoma in Normal Rats and Rats Fed High or Low Levels of Vitamin A," *Cancer Research,* **33**:1003, 1973.

15 U. Saffiotti et al., "Experimental Cancer of the Lung. Inhibition by Vitamin A of the Induction of Tracheobronchial Squamous Metaplasia and Squamous Cell Tumors," *Cancer,* **20**:857, 1967.

16 M. B. Sporn and D. L. Newton, "Chemoprevention of Cancer with Retinoids," *Federation Proceedings,* **38**:2528, 1979.

17 G. L. Peck et al., "Prolonged Remission of Cystic and Conglobate Acne with 13-*cis*-Retinoic Acid," *New England Journal of Medicine,* **300**:329, 1979.

18 Medical News, "Experimental Retinoid Effective in Treatment of Severe Acne," *Journal of the American Medical Association,* **243**:11, 1980.

19 E. Spanos et al., "Effect of Growth Hormone on Vitamin D Metabolism," *Nature,* **273**:246, 1978.

20 M. R. Haussler and T. A. McCain, "Basic and Clinical Concepts Related to Vitamin D Metabolism and Action," *New England Journal of Medicine,* **297**:974, 1977.

21 A. W. Norman et al., "Vitamin D Deficiency Inhibits Pancreatic Secretion of Insulin," *Science,* **209**:823, 1980.

22 M. F. Holick et al., "The Photoproduction of $1\alpha,25$-Dihydroxy-vitamin D_3 in Skin. An Approach to the Therapy of Vitamin D-resistant Syndromes," *New England Journal of Medicine,* **303**:349, 1980.

23 W. Jubiz et al., "Plasma 1,25-Dihydroxyvitamin D Levels in Patients Receiving Anticonvulsant Drugs," *Journal of Clinical and Endocrinological Metabolism,* **44**:617, 1977.

24 F. Konishi and S. L. Harrison, "Vitamin D for Adults," *Journal of Nutrition Education,* **11**:120, 1980.

25 J. T. Dwyer et al., "Risk of Nutritional Rickets among Vegetarian Children," *American Journal of Diseases of Children,* **133**:134, 1979.

26 S. J. Fomon and F. G. Strauss, "Nutrient Deficiencies in Breast-fed Infants," *New England Journal of Medicine,* **299**:355, 1978.

27 J. R. Drake and C. O. Fitch, "Status of Vitamin E as an Erythropoietic Factor," *American Journal of Clinical Nutrition,* **33**:2386, 1980.

28 R. A. Ehrenkranz et al., "Amelioration of Bronchopulmonary Dysplasia after Vitamin E Administration," *New England Journal of Medicine,* **299**:564, 1978.

29 F. A. Oski, "Metabolism and Physiological Roles of Vitamin E," *Hospital Practice,* **12**:79, 1977.

30 C. L. Natta et al., "A Decrease in Irreversibly Sickled Erythrocytes in Sickle Cell Anemia Patients Given Vitamin E," *American Journal of Clinical Nutrition,* **33**:968, 1980.

31 L. Corash et al., "Reduced Chronic Hemolysis during High Dose Vitamin E Administration in Mediterranean-type Glucose-6-Phosphate Dehydrogenase Deficiency," *New England Journal of Medicine,* **303**:416, 1980.

32 M. K. Horwitt, "Therapeutic Uses of Vitamin E in Medicine," *Nutrition Reviews*, 38:105, 1980.

33 A. L. Tappel, "Vitamin E," *Nutrition Today*, 8(4):4, 1973.

34 P. J. McLaughlin and J. L. Weihrauch, "Vitamin E Content of Foods," *Journal of the American Dietetic Association*, 75:647, 1979.

35 J. H. Ritchie et al., "Edema and Hemolytic Anemia in Premature Infants. A Vitamin E Deficiency Syndrome," *New England Journal of Medicine*, 279:1185, 1968.

36 F. A. Oski and L. A. Barness, "Vitamin E Deficiency: A Previously Unrecognized Cause of Hemolytic Anemia in Premature Infants," *Journal of Pediatrics*, 70:211, 1967.

37 M. K. Horwitt, "Vitamin E and Lipid Metabolism in Man," *American Journal of Clinical Nutrition*, 8:451, 1960.

38 J. J. Corrigan and F. I. Marcuss, "Coagulopathy Associated with Vitamin E Ingestion," *Journal of the American Medical Association*, 230:1300, 1974.

39 G. L. Nelsestuen et al., "The Mode of Action of Vitamin K. Identification of Gamma-Carboxylglutamic Acid as a Component of Prothrombin," *Journal of Biological Chemistry*, 249:6347, 1974.

40 C. T. Esmon et al., "A New Carboxylation Reaction. The Vitamin K-dependent Incorporation of $H^{14}CO_3$ into Prothrombin," *Journal of Biological Chemistry*, 250:4744, 1975.

41 P. M. Gallop et al., "Carboxylated Calcium-binding Proteins and Vitamin K," *New England Journal of Medicine*, 302:1460, 1980.

42 A. Kallner et al., "Steady-state Turnover and Body Pool of Ascorbic Acid in Man," *American Journal of Clinical Nutrition*, 32:530, 1979.

43 V. J. Thorp, "Effect of Oral Contraceptive Agents on Vitamin and Mineral Requirements," *Journal of the American Dietetic Association*, 76:581, 1980.

44 D. L. Yeung, "Relationships between Cigarette Smoking, Oral Contraceptives, and Plasma Vitamins A, E, C, and Plasma Triglyceride and Cholesterol," *American Journal of Clinical Nutrition*, 29:1216, 1976.

45 "The Function of Ascorbic Acid in Collagen Formation," *Nutrition Reviews*, 36:118, 1978.

46 E. R. Monsen et al., "Estimation of Available Dietary Iron," *American Journal of Clinical Nutrition*, 31:134, 1978.

47 C. R. Spittle, "Atherosclerosis and Vitamin C," *Lancet*, 2:1280, 1971.

48 V. E. Peterson et al., "Quantification of Plasma Cholesterol and Triglyceride Levels in Hypercholesterolemic Subjects Receiving Ascorbic Acid Supplements," *American Journal of Clinical Nutrition*, 28:584, 1975.

49 T. W. Anderson et al., "Vitamin C and the Common Cold: A Double Blind Trial," *Canadian Medical Association Journal*, 107:503, 1972.

50 J. L. Coulehan et al., "Vitamin C and Acute Illness in Navajo Schoolchildren," *New England Journal of Medicine*, 295:973, 1976.

51 B. S. Worthington-Roberts, "The Water-soluble Vitamins," *Contemporary Developments in Nutrition*, The C. V. Mosby Company, St. Louis, 1981, pp. 201–205.

52 E. Cameron and L. Pauling, "Supplemental Ascorbate in the Supportive Treatment of Cancer. I. Prolongation of Survival Times in Terminal Human Cancer," *Proceedings of the National Academy of Science*, 73:3685, 1976.

53 E. T. Creagan et al., "Failure of High-dose Vitamin C (Ascorbic Acid) Therapy to Benefit Patients with Advanced Cancer. A Controlled Trial," *New England Journal of Medicine*, 301:687, 1979.

54 E. Jacob et al., "Low Serum Vitamin B_{12} Levels in Patients Receiving Ascorbic Acid in Megadoses: Studies Concerning the Effect of Ascorbate on Radioisotope Vitamin B_{12} Assay," *American Journal of Clinical Nutrition*, 31:253, 1978.

55 H. P. C. Hogenkamp, "The Interactions between Vitamin B_{12} and Vitamin C," *American Journal of Clinical Nutrition*, 33:1, 1980.

56 Y. Itokawa and J. R. Cooper, "Ion Movements and Thiamin. II. The Release of the Vitamin from Membrane Fragments," *Biochimica et Biophysica Acta*, 196:274, 1970.

57 K. Berman and R. A. Fishman, "Thiamin Phosphate Metabolism and Possible Independent Functions of Thiamin in Brain," *Journal of Neurochemistry*, 24:457, 1975.

58 M. Brin, "Erythrocyte Transketolase Activity in Early Thiamine Deficiency," *Annals of the New York Academy of Sciences*, 98:528, 1962.

59 Y. H. Chong and G. S. Ho, "Erythrocyte Transketolase Activity," *American Journal of Clinical Nutrition*, 23:261, 1970.

60 B. Wood et al., "A Study of Partial Thiamin Restriction in Human Volunteers," *American Journal of Clinical Nutrition*, 33:848, 1980.

61 H. E. Sauberlich et al., "Thiamin Requirement of the Adult Human," *American Journal of Clinical Nutrition*, 32:2237, 1979.

62 M. H. Dong et al., "Thiamin, Riboflavin and Vitamin B_6 Contents of Selected Foods as Served," *Journal of the American Dietetic Association*, 76:156, 1980.

63 C. R. Scriver, "Vitamin-responsive Inborn Errors of Metabolism," *Metabolism*, 22:1319, 1973.

64 H. E. Sauberlich et al., "Application of the Erythrocyte Glutathione Reductase Assay in Evaluating

Riboflavin Status in a High School Student Population," *American Journal of Clinical Nutrition,* **25**:756, 1972.

65 J. G. Bergan and P. T. Brown, "Nutritional Status of 'New' Vegetarians," *Journal of the American Dietetic Association,* **76**:151, 1980.

66 R. Lopez et al., "Riboflavin Deficiency in an Adolescent Population in New York City," *American Journal of Clinical Nutrition,* **33**:1283, 1980.

67 L. C. Robson et al., "Vitamin B$_6$ and Immunity," in National Research Council, *Human Vitamin B$_6$ Requirements,* National Academy of Science, Washington, D.C., 1978, pp. 162–179.

68 Bureau of Nutritional Sciences, *Dietary Standards for Canada,* Department of National Health and Welfare, Ottawa, Canada, 1975.

69 L. Lumeng et al., "Adequacy of Vitamin B$_6$ Supplementation during Pregnancy: A Prospective Study," *American Journal of Clinical Nutrition,* **29**:1376, 1976.

70 C. S. Rose et al., "Age Differences in Vitamin B$_6$ Status of 617 Men," *American Journal of Clinical Nutrition,* **29**:847, 1976.

71 S. C. Vir and A. H. G. Love, "Vitamin B$_6$ Status of the Hospitalized Aged," *American Journal of Clinical Nutrition,* **31**:1383, 1978.

72 M. H. Dong et al., op. cit.

73 T.-K. Li, "Factors Influencing Vitamin B$_6$ Requirement in Alcoholism," in National Research Council, *Human Vitamin B$_6$ Requirements,* National Academy of Science, Washington, D.C., 1978, pp. 210–225.

74 The Coronary Drug Project Research Group, "Clofibrate and Niacin in Coronary Heart Disease," *Journal of the American Medical Association,* **321**:360, 1975.

75 P. C. Fry et al., "Metabolic Response to a Pantothenic Acid Deficient Diet in Humans," *Journal of Nutritional Science and Vitaminology,* **22**:339, 1976.

76 J. J. Ellestad-Sayed et al., "Pantothenic Acid, Coenzyme A, and Human Chronic Ulcerative and Granulomatous Colitis," *American Journal of Clinical Nutrition,* **29**:1333, 1976.

77 J. P.Bonjour, "Biotin in Man's Nutrition and Therapy-A Review," *International Journal of Vitamin and Nutritional Research,* **47**:107, 1977.

78 C. H. Halsted, "The Intestinal Absorption of Folates," *American Journal of Clinical Nutrition,* **32**:846, 1979.

79 M. S. Rodriguez, "A Conspectus of Research on Folacin Requirements of Man," *Journal of Nutrition,* **108**:1983, 1978.

80 B. P. Perloff and P. R. Butrum, "Folacin in Selected Foods," *Journal of the American Dietetic Association,* **70**:161, 1977.

81 L. B. Bailey et al., "Folacin and Iron Status and Hematological Findings in Predominately Black Elderly Persons from Urban Low-income Households," *American Journal of Clinical Nutrition,* **32**:2346, 1979.

82 H. Baker et al., "Severe Impairment of Dietary Folate Utilization in the Elderly," *Journal of the American Geriatrics Society,* **26**:218, 1978.

83 L. Elsborg, "Reversible Malabsorption of Folic Acid in the Elderly with Nutritional Folate Deficiency," *Acta Haematologica,* **55**:140, 1976.

84 G. P. Davidson and R. R. W. Townley, "Structural and Functional Abnormalities of the Small Intestine Due to Nutritional Folic Acid Deficiency in Infancy," *Pediatrics,* **90**:590, 1977.

85 G. R. Minot and W. P. Murphy, "Treatment of Pernicious Anemia by a Special Diet," *Journal of the American Medical Association,* **87**:470, 1926.

86 M. C. Higginbottom et al., "A Syndrome of Methylmalonic Aciduria, Homocystinuria, Megaloblastic Anemia, and Neurologic Abnormalities in a Vitamin B$_{12}$-deficient Infant of a Strict Vegetarian," *New England Journal of Medicine,* **299**:317, 1978.

87 V. Herbert, "The Nutritionally and Metabolically Destructive 'Nutritional and Metabolic Antineoplastid Diet' of Laetrile Proponents," *American Journal of Clinical Nutrition,* **32**:96, 1979.

88 V. Herbert, "Pangamic Acid ('Vitamin B$_{15}$')," *American Journal of Clinical Nutrition,* **32**:1534, 1979.

89 V. Herbert, "Laetrile: The Cult of Cyanide. Promoting Poison for Profit," in *Nutrition Cultism: Facts and Fictions,* G. F. Stickley Company, Philadelphia, 1980, pp. 15–106.

90 M. S. Bamji et al., "Research Priorities in the Field of Vitamin Deficiency in Man," *American Journal of Clinical Nutrition,* **32**:1982, 1979.

CLINICAL DISCUSSION 6

On the basis of her daily supplements and the dairy foods in her usual diet, Cathy ingested a minimum of 112,200 IU of vitamin A per day. This intake is more than 25 times the RDA. If the additional foods in her diet included carrots, dark green leafy vegetables, apricots, tomatoes, and cantaloupe, for example, significantly higher amounts of vitamin A (as carotene) would be consumed.

The response of adults to large oral doses of vitamin A is highly variable, but Cathy clearly demonstrated a toxic response, primarily due to the inclusion of the high-potency vitamin A capsules during the previous year. She was told to discontinue the vitamin supplements, and could expect that within a few days her symptoms would subside.

While Cathy is probably aware of the commonly known functions of vitamin A that most children learn in school, she may be unaware of its potential for toxicity. Since she is a graduate student in chemistry, however, you should be able to easily explain the effect of its fat-soluble nature in terms of storage in the body. It would also be helpful to explain to her the basis for the RDAs: that they are set to meet the nutritional needs of practically all healthy people in the United States. It is especially important to point out that the results of the research linking cancer prevention and vitamin A are primarily based on work with animals using synthetic analogues of the vitamin which are different from retinol.

Help her identify food items which she likes, which are inexpensive, and which are in keeping with her abstinence from meat, fish, poultry, and eggs. She will discover that she can easily meet the RDA by continuing her intake of vitamin-A fortified dairy products, and by including vitamin-A rich vegetables and fruits in her diet. Her other nutrient needs should also be met by her usual diet, especially if the milk she drinks is fortified with vitamin D. She should include whole grains and bananas in her diet occasionally to increase her intake of vitamin B_6, which may be limited in a nonmeat diet.

On Cathy's return visit, which took place 3 months later, her symptoms were gone, her serum levels of vitamin A were found to be in the normal range, she was pleased with her meal pattern, and she had passed her doctoral examination!

CHAPTER 7

MINERALS

Jean Hine

KEY WORDS
Macrominerals
Microminerals
Calcium/Phosphorus Ratio
Tetany
Osteoporosis
Iron Deficiency Anemia
Ferritin
Goiter

INTRODUCTION

Foods we eat supply us with the inorganic elements, or minerals, which are essential to the body's metabolic processes. The mineral content of food varies with local soil and water conditions. The total mineral content of a food is determined by burning a specific amount of the food and weighing the remaining ash, which is then analyzed for the individual mineral content.

Of the 103 known elements 11 constitute the bulk of living matter, while the remainder are present in much smaller or trace amounts. Essentiality is not related to abundance of a mineral in nature. For example, lead is abundant, but not essential to animal life. Minerals can be viewed as falling into two categories: those required in amounts at or above 100 mg per day (*macrominerals* or *trace elements*) and those needed in amounts no higher than a few milligrams per day (*microminerals* or *trace elements*) (Table 7-1). Calcium, chloride, magnesium, phosphorus, potassium, sodium, and sulfur are classified as macrominerals and have well-documented roles in human nutrition. Essential trace elements are cobalt, copper, iodine, iron, magnesium, manganese, molybdenum, and zinc. Chromium, fluorine, and selenium appear to be essential for most species, including humans.[1] Roles for nickel, silicon, tin, vanadium and arsenic have been identified in some laboratory animals and they may have some essential functions in humans as well. (See Table 7-2, p. 128.)

Within the body, minerals serve a variety of functions: as essential activators for a number of enzyme-catalyzed reactions (namely, zinc, molybdenum, and manganese), as components of skeletal structure (calcium and phosphorus), in hemoglobin synthesis and red blood cell formation (iron, cobalt, copper), and as part of thyroid hormone (iodine). In addition, they control the water and electrolyte balance (sodium, potassium, calcium, phosphorus, chlorine) and are

Note: Supported by UAF federal grant Project MCT-3000-915-080.

TABLE 7-1 MACROMINERALS AND
MICROMINERALS OR TRACE ELEMENTS

Macrominerals	Microminerals or trace elements
Calcium	Arsenic*
Chloride	Cadmium*
Magnesium	Chromium
Phosphorus	Cobalt*
Potassium	Copper
Sodium	Fluorine
Sulfur	Iodine
	Iron
	Manganese
	Molybdenum
	Nickel*
	Selenium
	Silicon*
	Tin*
	Vanadium*
	Zinc

*Trace elements known to be essential for some animal species but no data available on human requirement.

necessary for nerve cell function (calcium, magnesium).

The Food and Nutrition Board of the National Academy of Sciences has established recommended dietary allowances for calcium, phosphorus, iron, iodine, magnesium, and zinc. In the 9th edition of the *Recommended Dietary Allowances* estimated safe and adequate daily dietary intakes have been designated for copper, manganese, fluoride, chromium, selenium, and molybdenum. That publication also states that although requirements for cobalt, nickel, vanadium, silicon, tin, arsenic, and cadmium have been determined for some animal species, there are no data from which an estimate of human requirements can be derived;[2] consequently, much research on the need for these elements is under way. Investigations have been stimulated by the increasing concern over the pollution of our environment and its possible effect on the mineral content of food. The inclusion of a wide variety of foods in the diet formerly assured an adequate intake of most minerals: however, due to negative ecological trends, modern food processing, and changing food habits, this assertion may be questionable. However, it is still a generally accepted notion that when a diet provides sufficient amounts of calcium, iron, and iodine, the intake of other minerals will be adequate to meet body needs.

Mineral absorption is influenced by both endogenous and exogenous factors. Once in the blood, the minerals are bound to protein, act as free ions, or are assigned to a specific transport carrier. They are then utilized, stored in the liver, skin, skeleton and possibly in adipose tissue, or excreted in the urine, feces, sweat, and bile.

In human physiology, the minerals are interrelated; they do not function with circumscribed roles but work in concert. However, for the sake of discussion, this chapter will examine each mineral separately: calcium, phosphorus, sulfur, magnesium, iron, iodine, fluorine, chromium, manganese, cobalt, zinc, selenium, molybdenum, and copper. (Sodium, potassium, and chloride will be discussed in Chap. 8.) This chapter will elucidate the importance of these minerals in human nutrition and emphasize the effects of illness on mineral metabolism.

MACROMINERALS

Calcium

A 70-kg adult's body contains approximately 1200 g of calcium, 99 percent of which is found in the skeleton. In the bones, calcium is present in the form of deposits of calcium phosphates in a soft, fibrous, organic matrix.[3] The unique structure of the matrix is required for normal calcification. The principal inorganic compound of bone is a form of calcium phosphate which is similar to the mineral hydroxyapatite:

$$Ca_{10}(PO_4)_6(OH)_2$$

TABLE 7-2   SUMMARY OF BODY CONTENT, HOMEOSTASIS AND DIETARY RECOMMENDATIONS FOR TRACE ELEMENTS

| Name | Body content | Dietary recommendations | | % Absorption | Plasma levels | Excretion (primary route) |
		Safe	Adequate			
Chromium	<6 mg		0.01–0.2 mg	1–25	0.2–2 mgdL	Urine
Copper	80 mg			40–60		
Fluoride	2.6–4 g		0.05–0.30 mg	Very high	97–164 mgdL	Feces (bile)
			0.1–4.0 mg	Very high	3.5 mgdL	Urine
Iodine	10–25 mg	40–190 µg		Very high	4.5–10 mgdL	Urine
Iron	4–5 g	10–18 mg		15–35 heme 2–20 nonheme	87–187 mgdL	Feces, menstrual blood
Manganese	12–20 mg		0.5–5 mg	6	0.054–6.1 mgdL	Feces (bile)
Molybdenum	<5 mg		0.03–0.5 mg	>50	0.6–2.7 mgdL	Urine
Selenium	6–10 mg		0.01–0.2 mg	75	9.8–32.7 mgdL	Urine
Zinc	1.6–2.3 mg	3–25 mg		20–40	67–183 mgdL	Feces (bile)

Sources:

1. K. M. Stika and G. H. Morrison, "Analytical Methods for the Mineral Content of Human Tissues," *Federation Proceedings*, **40**:2115, 1981.

2. Food and Nutrition Board, *Recommended Dietary Allowances*, rev. 9th ed., National Academy of Sciences.

3. I. H. Tipton and M. J. Cook, *Trace Elements in Human Tissues*, Part II, *Adult Subjects From the United States, Health Physics*, **9**:103, 1963.

4. E. J. Underwood, *Trace Elements in Human and Animal Nutrition*, 4th ed., Academic Press, New York, 1977.

The precise chemical nature of bone is unknown because of transitional forms which are present as the bone matures and because of ion exchange and substitution that can take place in the crystalline structure. It is known that calcium in the bone is precipitated initially as an amorphous material which is changed to a crystalline precipitate and subsequently converted to the final crystal.[4] In adult bone, approximately 40 percent of the total calcium is present in the form of a non-apatite material; in younger persons, the amorphous material predominates. Sodium and small amounts of carbonate and magnesium are also present in bone.

Function

Bone formation Bone is constantly being formed and resorbed. In adults, the skeleton is completely replaced every 10 to 12 years. However, in children the renewal process takes only 1 to 2 years.[5] The formation of bone and the control mechanisms which influence formation and dissolution are incompletely understood. Bone is formed by *osteoblasts,* which form new bone crystals in the matrix by the deposition of calcium phosphate. *Osteoclasts* balance this process by resorbing or phagocytizing and digesting the minute bone crystals. Physical stress stimulates osteoblastic deposition of bone and bone is deposited in proportion to the load that the bone must carry. For example, bones are heavier in athletes than in nonathletes; and when an individual is in a cast and continues to walk on one leg, the bone of the disabled leg becomes thin and decalcified while the bone in the opposite leg remains thick and calcified.

Calcium in the skeletal framework is in a dynamic state of equilibrium with body tissues and fluids, and balance mechanisms work to maintain the level of calcium in the plasma within its narrow normal range. In fact, the rate of exchange between the plasma and bone calcium is greater than the rate of original deposition of new bone. The calcium stored in the trabeculae at the ends of bones is most readily mobilized and responds to the increasing demands during pregnancy, lactation, and periods of malnutrition. The calcium contained in the dentin and enamel of teeth is more stable. This fact negates the old wives' tale that for every baby, the mother loses a tooth.

In teeth, the crystalline salts are similar to those of bone and are composed basically of the hydroxyapatite with absorbed carbonates and varying cations bound together as a hard crystalline substance. As in bone, new salts are constantly being deposited, while old salts are being resorbed from the teeth. This deposition and resorption occurs mainly in the cementum with some activity in the dentin and minimal occurrence in the enamel (see Chap. 17).

Circulating calcium The small but significant quantity of circulating calcium operates under strict homeostatic regulation and plays a crucial role in maintenance of normal body function. Levels of calcium range from 8.5 to 10.5 mg per 100 mL (somewhat higher in children) with no more than a 10 percent variation.[6] The level of circulating calcium is independent of the dietary calcium intake and tightly regulated by the parathyroid hormone and calcitonin.

Calcium is present in the serum mostly in a soluble ionized form; the remainder occurs in a protein-bound form (mainly bound to albumin and globulins), with very small quantities complexed with organic acids. Blood calcium functions in the following roles:

1 *Transmission of nerve impulses.* Calcium is necessary for the release of neurotransmitters such as acetylcholine, serotonin, and norepinephrine from nerve endings.

2 *Muscle contraction.* Muscle is composed of many long cells or fibers, formed by many longitudinally arranged fibrils containing hundreds of protein myofilaments composed of myosin and actin. Beside the myofilaments is the sarcoplasmic reticulum, a system of fine tubes which contain sacs in which calcium ions are stored. These calcium ions are essential for the actin, myosin, and adenosine triphosphate (ATP, a high-

energy phosphate compound) to function in muscle contraction. The contraction of muscle or the sliding of filaments involves cross-linking between actin and myosin. Contraction is initiated when the nerve signal reaches the muscle fiber, calcium is released from the reticulum sacs into the fluid surrounding the filaments where it is bound to the calcium-receptive protein of muscle (troponin), ATP is cleared into ADP and inorganic phosphate, and contraction occurs. The calcium immediately returns to the storage vesicles in the sarcoplasmic reticulum and the muscle relaxes. Magnesium is also essential to this process, since it is required for the release of energy from the cell. Without a source of energy or a loss of ATP, necessary to cause a separation of the actin and myosin filaments, muscles remain stiff, accounting for the rigor mortis that develops in muscle after death.

With low levels of circulating calcium, *tetany* occurs. Tetany is a symptom complex characterized by increased neuromuscular excitability. It is a state in which the nerve fibers become so excitable that they discharge spontaneously, initiating nerve impulses that pass to peripheral skeletal muscles, where they elicit tetanic contractions which may lead to cardiac and respiratory failure. Usually, tetany occurs when the blood concentration of the calcium falls below 8 mg per 100 ml, which is 30 percent below the normal calcium concentration.

3   *Blood coagulation.* Calcium is required for the conversion of prothrombin to thrombin during formation of the fibrin clot (see Chap. 6). Since blood clotting is normal in hypocalcemic tetany, it can be inferred that only minute quantities of calcium are required for prothrombin activation.

4   *Enzyme activation.* Calcium is necessary for the activation of certain enzymes, including pancreatic lipase, plasma lipoprotein lipase, phospholipase, and phosphorylase kinase.

5   *Cell membrane permeability.* Calcium regulates the transport of ions across cell membranes.

6   *Maintenance of the integrity of the intracellular cement substances and of various membranes.*

7   *Enhancement of normal cardiac function.* Fluctuations in calcium blood levels affect cardiac function.

Absorption and Utilization

Calcium is principally absorbed in the duodenum by means of an active process.[7] Only 20 to 30 percent of dietary calcium is absorbed and the remainder is excreted in the feces, urine, and sweat. The amount of calcium absorbed is controlled by the following factors:

1   *Body need.* With a small dietary supply or an increased need, the body becomes more efficient in absorption. A state of increased need is found during growth, pregnancy, stress, and calcium depletion. Under usual conditions, calcium absorption is not increased proportionately with an increased intake.

2   *Intestinal pH.* An acid pH enhances calcium absorption, since calcium salts, namely phosphates and carbonates, are soluble in acid solutions and relatively insoluble in an alkaline medium; thus, the normal gastric hydrochloric acid is necessary to facilitate efficient absorption.

3   *Food components.* Substances in food that exert an influence over calcium absorption can be grouped into three categories: those exerting a positive, a negative, or a questionable effect.

- *Vitamin D.* The major regulator of calcium absorption is 1,25-dihydroxycholecalciferol, an active metabolite of vitamin D produced by the kidney. When the plasma calcium level goes down, production of the metabolite is stimulated; when the plasma calcium goes up, lesser amounts of the metabolite are produced.

- *Calcium/phosphorus ratio.* Although some animal studies suggest an optimum dietary calcium/phosphorus intake ratio to be 2 to 1, the most recent edition of the Recommended Dietary Allowances has established a 1 to 1 relationship, or a ratio of unity.[8] There have been recent concerns regarding changes in the calcium/phosphorus ratio in the United States as a result of increased use of phosphates as food additives. Most recent estimates suggest a ratio of about 1 to 1.5 or 1 to 1.6. This appears to be acceptable, but this topic needs more research.

- *Lactose.* Lactose, the disaccharide found in milk, may promote calcium absorption. Two mechanisms have been suggested to explain this effect. Lactose is absorbed slowly and it is possible that a free sugar in the ileum could change the flora, thereby lowering the pH. An acid pH enhances calcium absorption. Others have suggested that lactose may combine with calcium to form a chelate which could protect it from precipitation and consequently promote absorption.

- *Protein.* A diet adequate in protein, particularly the amino acids lysine, arginine, and serine, has been viewed as exerting a positive effect on calcium absorption.

- *Oxalic acid and phytic acid.* High levels of oxalic acid (found in spinach, chocolate, greens, rhubarb) and phytic acid (found in the outer husk of cereal grain) form insoluble salts which lower the concentration of ionizable calcium in the gut, with the net result of increasing the level of fecal calcium. This is not considered to be a problem when the dietary level of calcium is sufficiently liberal. Also, in research studies, subjects who were fed high-phytate diets adapted to the diets and, after a short period of negative balance, absorbed normal amounts of calcium.

4 *Quantity of bile salts present.* Fats must be properly digested and absorbed or calcium absorption can be inhibited. When fats are not absorbed either because they are not hydrolyzed by lipases or because the absorption of fatty acids is impaired, fatty acids combine with free calcium and form insoluble calcium soaps, which are excreted. Also, the fat-soluble vitamin D is not absorbed, promoting a deficiency state (calcium deficiency can occur in prolonged obstructive jaundice, pancreative insufficiency, celiac disease, and sprue).

5 *Serum level of inorganic phosphorus.* The metabolism of calcium is closely related to that of phosphorus, and a serum calcium/phosphorus ratio must be maintained (serum calcium level, 8.5 to 10.5 mg per 100 mL; serum phosphorus level, 2.0 to 4.5 mg per 100 mL).[9] A change in the serum calcium/phosphorus ratio, such as is seen in kidney disease, interferes with calcium absorption.

6 *Hormonal influences.* Both the parathyroid and thyroid glands are active in influencing calcium homeostasis. When circulating plasma calcium drops, the parathyroid gland releases parathyroid hormone, which acts to (*a*) liberate calcium from the bone and (*b*) increase calcium reabsorption from the renal tubules. At the same time, the parathyroid hormone causes phosphorus excretion, via the urine, thus maintaining the calcium-phosphorus ratio. Calcitonin, a hormone formed by the thyroid gland, is secreted when plasma calcium levels are elevated. Calcitonin acts at the bone site to block removal of calcium from the bone fluid compartment.

Excretion

Of the calcium ingested, 70 to 80 percent is excreted. When serum calcium is depressed or dietary intake is low, calcium absorption is more efficient, and vitamin D works in concert with parathyroid hormone to promote conservation of calcium by the kidney tubules. High levels of serum calcium initiate secretion of calcitonin which results in loss of calcium via the urine. Calcium excreted in the stool is mostly unabsorbed calcium from food. In persons with steatorrhea, substantial amounts of calcium can be lost in the stool. Calcium is also lost via bile and digestive secretions, and in sweat:

Calcium losses	Amount
Fecal	100 to 200 mg per day
Urine	150 mg per day
Bile and digestive secretions	500 mg per day
Sweat	Depends on temperature; may be as high as 1 mg per day

Dietary Allowances

Evidence regarding human calcium needs has been derived from balance studies, in which calcium intake and excretion are measured. In a normal adult, it is assumed that the requirement for calcium will be equal to the excretion and that individuals can adapt to different levels of calcium intake. Since it is difficult to establish a base line of need, there has been much discussion concerning the levels of calcium requirements.

The 1980 edition of the National Academy of Sciences *Recommended Dietary Allowances* advises 60 mg per kilogram body weight for infants, an amount of calcium typically received by breast-fed infants.[10] A dietary intake of 800 mg per day has been recommended for adults and children except those 11 to 18 years of age for whom an intake of 1200 mg per day is suggested. Pregnant and lactating women are encouraged to increase their intake by 400 mg daily, i.e., a pregnant teenager should be ingesting more than 1.5 g.

The committee does acknowledge the growth needs of children and the fact that adults are capable of maintaining a positive balance on lower intakes. The WHO Food and Agriculture Organization suggests an adult intake of 400 to 500 mg per day. The recommended intake for calcium is therefore probably somewhere between 500 and 800 mg per day. However, for several reasons it seems inadvisable to recommend low intakes.

1 The yet undefined role of calcium intake in the pathogenesis of osteoporosis

2 The mounting evidence that calcium excretion is promoted by diets high in protein[11]

3 The possibility that high phosphorus intake also promotes calcium excretion

4 A likely decreased ability to absorb calcium with increasing age

Dietary Sources

Milk and milk products are the richest food sources of calcium. Without the use of milk products, which provide 60 percent of the dietary calcium, it is very difficult to meet the recommended levels of intake. Foods containing smaller amounts of calcium are grains, fruits, nuts, vegetables, shellfish such as clams and oysters, fish (sardines and salmon), eggs, and molasses. In certain areas of the country, the drinking water may contain absorbable calcium. Table 7-3 compares the calcium content of selected foods.

Supplementation

When calcium supplements are necessary, calcium lactate and calcium gluconate are the therapeutic agents of choice. Approximately 30 to 50 percent of the available calcium is absorbed. Calcium lactate is often prescribed because it is less expensive than calcium gluconate. Calcium gluconate, however, may be preferred because of its better taste.

Children who are allergic to cow's milk or who have another condition that precludes its use in the diet will need a milk substitute, such as a soy formula, or a calcium supplement to meet their needs. Other individuals, under no therapeutic restriction but eating diets that are

TABLE 7-3 CALCIUM CONTENT OF SELECTED FOODS

Type	Household measure	Weight, g	Calcium content, mg
Milk, whole*	1 cup	244	288
Milk, skim*	1 cup	244	296
Yogurt (made from whole milk)	8 oz	226	251
Cheddar cheese	1 oz	28	213
Cottage cheese (creamed)	1 oz	28	27
Ice cream (10% fat)	1 cup	133	194
Vanilla pudding (made with milk)	1 cup	255	298
Blackstrap molasses	1 tbsp	20	137

*Cow's milk contains approximately 4 times the amount of calcium in an equal volume of human milk.
Source: *Nutritive Value of American Foods,* U.S. Department of Agricultural Handbook 456, Agriculture Research Service, 1975.

minimal in calcium, can increase their dietary intake by adding fluid milk or milk solids to soups, gravies, casseroles, or baked goods. Very high protein regimens should be avoided.

Clinical Application

There are many disease conditions that cause clinical disturbances of calcium metabolism which are reflected in abnormalities of serum calcium or of the skeletal framework. Tables 7-4, 7-5, and 7-6 (pp. 134–135) summarize those conditions that alter calcium metabolism as reflected in serum levels, urinary excretion, and fecal excretion. Although the conditions causing these alterations will be discussed in detail in later chapters, it is important to acknowledge the interrelationship between calcium and the disease state.

Osteoporosis is a metabolic disorder that causes a decrease in the amount of bone (deossification) without any change in its chemical composition or histological structure. Osteoporosis is most prevalent in postmenopausal women and in men over the age of 50. It is more common in females than in males. Some investigation had suggested that decreased estrogen levels has been observed among females with osteoporosis; however, recent studies have shown differences only in progesterone levels. Other factors associated with deossification are malnutrition, especially protein malnutrition, conditions associated with protein breakdown (e.g., Cushing's syndrome), acromegaly, hyperthyroidism, lack of exercise, and prolonged immobilization. Bone demineralization can also occur following a prolonged course of corticosteroid therapy.

Osteoporosis per se causes no disability, except that it increases the likelihood of fractures. However, there are several clinical symptoms of osteoporosis. Hypercalciuria may develop initially, especially when prolonged immobilization is a factor and renal calculi form. Besides bone fractures, other symptoms of osteoporosis include weakness, anorexia, hip and back pain, muscle tenderness, and cramping. Stooped posture and a loss of height result from a shrinking vertebral column.

The best prophylaxis for middle-aged persons is to remain physically active. Cyclic administration of estrogen has been used in the treatment of osteoporosis. It frequently relieves pain and has been suggested to be the only long-term treatment which prevents additional fractures. Results of such hormonal therapy and calcium and fluoride supplements have been highly variable.

TABLE 7-4   CONDITIONS ALTERING SERUM CALCIUM LEVELS

Condition	Serum calcium level	
	Increase	Decreased
Hyperparathyroidism (primary and secondary)	×	
Hematological malignances	×	
Vitamin D intoxication	×	
Milk alkali syndrome	×	
Acute osteoporosis	×	
Idiopathic hypercalciuria in infants	×	
Hypoparathyroidism		×
Calcium or vitamin D malabsorption		×
Cachexia		×
Nephrotic syndrome and chronic renal disease		×
Celiac disease		×
Cystic fibrosis		×
Acute pancreatitis		×
Late pregnancy		×

Source: Adapted from J. Wallach, *Interpretation of Diagnostic Tests,* 3d ed., Little, Brown and Company, Boston, 1978.

TABLE 7-5   CONDITIONS ALTERING URINARY CALCIUM LEVELS

Condition	Urinary calcium	
	Increased	Decreased
High calcium diet (excessive milk intake)	×	
Hyperparathyroidism	×	
Hyperthyroidism	×	
Idiopathic hypercalciuria	×	
Immobilization (especially in children)	×	
Osteoporosis	×	
Vitamin D intoxication	×	
Renal tubular acidosis	×	
Hypoparathyroidism		×
Rickets, osteomalacia		×
Steatorrhea		×
Renal failure		×

Source: Adapted from J. Wallach, *Interpretation of Diagnostic Tests,* 3d ed., Little, Brown and Company, Boston, 1978.

TABLE 7-6 CONDITIONS ALTERING FECAL CALCIUM LEVELS

	Fecal calcium level	
Condition	Increased	Decreased
Rickets	X	
Osteomalacia	X	
Sprue	X	
Celiac disease	X	
Chronic nephrosis	X	

Source: Adapted from J. Wallach, Interpretation of Diagnostic Tests, 3d ed., Little, Brown and Company, Boston, 1978.

Because osteoporotic bones have already lost both calcium and phosphate it would seem reasonable to conclude that diets low in these minerals might accelerate the process. However, there is no firm evidence to support this contention. A 1972 investigation found no significant correlation between the calcium intake and the bone density of middle-aged subjects.[12]

Phosphorus

After calcium, phosphorus is the most abundant mineral in the body. There are approximately 12 g of phosphorus per kilogram of fat-free body tissue. Although most phosphorus (85 percent) is present in the skeleton, smaller amounts are found in the red blood cells and plasma. The plasma inorganic phosphate level in adults is usually 3.0 to 4.5 mg per 100 mL. Infants may have levels up to 6.0 mg per 100 mL up to 1 year of age.[13]

Function

All body cells contain organic phosphates, which play a vital role in cellular functioning:

1 *Component of ribonucleic acid (RNA) and deoxyribonucleic acid (DNA).* The nucleic proteins involved in reproduction, cell division, and transmission of hereditary traits.

2 *Component of cellular membranes.* Phospholipids which are present in cell membranes are major determinants of cell permeability.

3 *Phosphorylation in metabolic pathways.* For example, the oxidation of carbohydrate, culminating in the formation of adenosine triphosphate (ATP), requires phosphorus because phosphorylation is a required step in the metabolism of monosaccharides.

4 *Component of high-energy phosphate compounds.* Phosphorus is a part of the structure of adenosine diphosphate (ADP) and ATP, which are compounds involved in processes related to the storage and release of energy.

5 *Component of B vitamin coenzymes.* Several B vitamins (e.g., thiamin) are effective only in the coenzyme form, which contains phosphorus (thiamin pyrophosphate).

Absorption and Utilization

Approximately 70 percent of the phosphorus that is ingested is absorbed. There is minimal control over the absorption of phosphorus and body content is principally regulated by urinary excretion. Provided that vitamin D intake is adequate, wide variations in the intake ratio of calcium to phosphorus are tolerated. An acid pH in the upper intestine and normal motility of the gastrointestinal tract promote absorption of phosphorus.

Dietary Allowances

There is little direct information concerning the human requirement for phosphorus. Phosphorus is present in nearly all foods and, consequently, dietary deficiency in humans is unlikely. In adults, the intake of phosphorus often exceeds that of calcium because meat is rich in phosphorus and phosphates are common food additives. Page and Friend estimated the average daily adult intake of phosphorus of U.S. adults to be 1500 to 1600 mg.[14] The intake recommended by the National Academy of Sciences is the same as that for calcium, except in the infant. Current evidence supports a calcium/phosphorus ratio of 1.5 to 1 in early infancy decreasing to 1 to 1 by 1 year of age. The calcium/phosphorus ratio of cow milk is 1.2 to 1 while in human milk it is 2 to 1. Infants on formulas derived from soybeans or other vegetable sources may not get sufficient phosphorus because some of it is in the form of phytate and consequently not readily available for absorption.[15]

Dietary Sources

Because phosphorus is present in nearly all foods, there is no indication that human intake of the mineral is ever low enough to interfere with vital body processes. Diets which provide adequate levels of protein and calcium can be inferred to contain a sufficient amount of phosphorus as well. Foods rich in phosphorus include milk and milk products, nuts, legumes, cereals, meat, fish, poultry, and eggs. Cow milk has a greater phosphorus content than human milk.

Clinical Application

Depletion of body phosphorus can result from prolonged intake of high doses of nonabsorbable antacids. Clinical signs of depletion are weakness, anorexia, malaise, bone pain, and bone demineralization, coupled with a marked increase in urinary calcium excretion. Treatment involves discontinuing the use of antacids and ingestion of a diet high in phosphorus. Metabolism of phosphorus can be disturbed in many disease states, especially in kidney and bone disorders (see Chaps. 23 and 24).

Sulfur

Sulfur is found in all body cells and is essential to life. It is principally found as a part of the protein structure of the living cell. Sulfur-containing compounds play several important roles in the body. Sulfur and nitrogen metabolism are closely related.

Function

1 *Part of the structure of amino acids.*   Sulfur is a component of the chemical structure of methionine, cysteine, and cystine (the double form of cysteine). Keratin, the protein of hair, is rich in sulfur.

2 *Component of two known vitamins.* Thiamin and biotin contain sulfur.

3 *Required for many oxidation-reduction reactions and coenzymes.*   Enzyme systems containing coenzyme A and glutathione depend on free sulfhydryl (SH) groups for their activity. SH groups are important in tissue respiration. Other organic compounds of sulfur include heparin, lipoic acid, ergothioneine, taurocholic acid, and chondroitin sulfate.

4 *Contained in blood and other tissues.*   Small amounts of inorganic sulfates, along with sodium and potassium, are present in blood and other tissues.

5 *Active in detoxification mechanisms.* Sulfur-containing compounds such as sulfuric acid combine with other components to detoxify compounds which would otherwise be harmful to the body.

6 *Contained in polysaccharides.* Sulfur is a part of polysaccharides found in cartilage, tendons, bones, and skin.

No conclusive studies of sulfur intake and output have been reported in the literature. This can probably be attributed to the difficulty in estimating small amounts of sulfur. An adult normally excretes between 1 and 2 g of sulfur daily, of which 75 to 80 percent is in the form of sulfate. Some effects of protein deficiency may be due to inadequate synthesis of sulfur-containing enzymes or polysaccharides.

Dietary Allowances and Dietary Sources

No specific recommendation for sulfur intake has been established. The primary sources of sulfur in the diet are the sulfur-containing amino acids. A mixed diet providing 100 g of protein will provide a range of 0.6 to 1.6 g of sulfur.[16]

Magnesium

A 70-kg human contains 20 to 28 g of magnesium.[17] Magnesium is found principally in bone and muscle tissue. Magnesium plays a central role in intermediary metabolism. The normal range of magnesium in the serum is 1.5 to 2.5 meq per L.[18] Unlike calcium, there is no hormonal control of blood magnesium levels.

Function

1 *Is essential for the mobilization of calcium from bone.*

2 *Ranks after potassium as having the most important intracellular action.*

3 *Is a part of many enzyme systems.* It is essential for cellular respiration; specifically, in the oxidative phosphorylation process leading to the formation of ATP. It is critical to all phosphate transfer systems. It functions as an activator for many of the enzymes of the glycolytic systems.

4 *Plays a role in protein synthesis.* Magnesium binds messenger RNA. It is also important in the synthesis and degradation of DNA.

5 *Is important in neuromuscular transmission.*

6 *Plays a possible role in the prevention of cardiovascular disease.*[19]

Absorption and Excretion

There is great variability in the levels of magnesium intake. Approximately 30 to 40 percent of the magnesium that is ingested is absorbed and utilized by the body. Magnesium is absorbed from the entire small bowel and to a small extent in the colon, particulary in infants.[20] Several factors influence the absorption of magnesium; among these are the amounts of calcium, phosphate, and lactose in the diet; intestinal transit time; and the rate of water absorption from the gastrointestinal tract. Maintenance of a normal range of magnesium in the blood depends on a balance between absorption and renal excretion.

Magnesium is lost via both urine and feces. In contrast to most other minerals, the major excretory route of magnesium is the urine. Consequently, magnesium homeostasis can be disturbed as a result of kidney disease. Gastric juice is relatively high in magnesium content, so that significant amounts can be lost during prolonged episodes of vomiting or diarrhea.

Dietary Allowances

A magnesium intake of 350 mg for men and 300 mg for women has been suggested. Human milk contains 4 mg per 100 mL, and recommendations for infants have been formulated in relation to that level. Recommendations for childhood and adolescence are estimates, designed to allow for rapid bone growth.[21] To date, there is little information concerning needs during pregnancy and lactation.

Dietary Sources

The mineral is widely distributed in foods, particularly in vegetables, which contain chlorophyll, a magnesium porphyrin. The typical diet in Western countries provides about 5 mg of magnesium per kilogram of body weight per day. Oriental persons typically ingest a diet rich in magnesium and their intake has been found to be approximately 6 to 10 mg per kilogram of body weight per day.

Clinical Application

Acute deficiency in humans is manifested by tremors, tetany, repetitive involuntary movements, seizures, mental disorientation, and tachycardia. Magnesium deficiency affects calcium, phosphorus, and sodium metabolism.

Several clinical conditions can predispose the individual to magnesium deficiency. Among these are malabsorption syndromes, loss of gastrointestinal fluids, chronic diarrhea, and ulcerative colitis. Severe protein depletion such as that which occurs in protein-calorie malnutrition can increase the risk of magnesium depletion. Increased renal excretion of magnesium can result from the use of diuretics and can occur in severe alcoholism. Prolonged parenteral feed-

TABLE 7-7   CONDITIONS ALTERING SERUM MAGNESIUM LEVELS

Condition	Serum magnesium level	
	Increased	Decreased
Renal failure	X	
Diabetic coma	X	
Hypothyroidism	X	
Addison's disease and after adrenalectomy	X	
Controlled diabetes mellitus in older age groups	X	
Administration of magnesium-containing antacids	X	
Malabsorption and abnormal loss of gastrointestinal fluids*		X
Acute alcoholism or alcoholic cirrhosis		X
Insulin treatment of diabetic coma		X
Hyperthyroidism		X
Aldosteronism		X
Hyperparathyroidism		X
Hypoparathyroidism		X
Lytic tumors of bone		X
Renal disease		X
Excessive lactation		X
Acute pancreatitis		X

*E.g., nontropical sprue, small bowel resection, biliary and intestinal fistulas, abdominal irradiation, prolonged aspiration of intestinal contents; celiac disease and other causes of steatorrhea.

Source: Adapted from J. Wallach, *Interpretation of Diagnostic Tests,* 3d ed., Little, Brown and Company, Boston, 1978.

ing using solutions which contain little or no magnesium can lead to deficiency. Patients on hemodialysis should be carefully observed for signs of hypomagnesemia. Conditions that elevate or decrease serum magnesium levels are summarized in Table 7-7.

MICROMINERALS/TRACE ELEMENTS

Iron

Function

The body of a 70 kg adult contains between 4 and 5 g of iron. Of this, 70 percent may be clas-sified as functional or essential iron and 30 percent as storage iron. Because of its presence in the hemoprotein enzymes and in the cytochromes, iron is vitally involved in the oxidative mechanisms of all living cells. It is complexed with a variety of protein molecules which determine its function. When the iron-containing pigment heme combines with the colorless protein globin, the resultant molecule is hemoglobin. Iron is also combined in other enzymes such as catalase, peroxidase, and Warburg's respiratory enzyme which perform their electron transport in tissue respiration by virtue of their iron content.

As part of hemoglobin, four atoms of iron are combined with two alpha- and two beta-polypeptide chains and four protoporphyrin molecules. The hemoglobin molecule is 4 percent heme and 96 percent globin. The ability of hemoglobin to carry oxygen from the lungs to the tissues and to carry carbon dioxide back relates to the presence of iron in the heme molecule. Without iron, the oxygen supply to tissues is diminished and hypoxia of blood and tissues results.

Absorption

Newer evidence suggests that the amount of iron potentially available from foods is dependent on the amount of iron supplied, the form of iron consumed, and the composition of the meal in which the iron source is consumed. The availability of food iron is best considered separately from heme iron and nonheme iron.[22] Heme iron comes from hemoglobin and myoglobin and is absorbed as the intact iron porphyrin complex, with its iron being freed in the intestinal mucosal cell. The percent of heme iron usually absorbed from the diet is high in contrast to the amount of nonheme iron. Additionally, iron stores influence the efficiency of absorption. For example, an individual with no iron stores may absorb 35 percent of heme iron when ingested as meat, while another person with iron stores in the range of 500 mg would absorb only 25 percent of the iron from an identical amount ingested.

The primary absorption site for iron is in the upper small intestine (duodenum and jejunum), although a limited amount is absorbed in the stomach. The iron status of the individual and the composition of the meal exert an effect on the absorption of nonheme iron. Unique to nonheme iron is the fact that the amount absorbed can be altered by components of foods eaten concomitantly. Dietary factors which can increase the absorption of nonheme iron as much as fourfold are ascorbic acid and the so-called meat factor.[23] The term *meat factor* is used by Cook et al. to underscore the importance of meat, fish, and poultry in iron nutriture.

These foods contribute heme iron which is absorbed efficiently and promotes the absorption of nonheme iron. Although neither protein nor animal protein per se increases iron absorption, as the amounts of ascorbic acid and the meat factor in a meal increase, so does iron absorption. On the other hand, milk, cheese, and eggs do not increase and may even depress the uptake of nonheme iron.

There are great differences in the availability of different forms of iron for absorption.[24] Most available is ferrous sulfate; other organic complexes or chelates of iron are also easily absorbed. The availability of reduced metallic iron is moderate and is probably related to the particle size of the preparation. Iron phosphates and carbonates are poorly absorbed.

Absorption is sometimes impaired in persons who have had total or subtotal gastrectomies and in those who have had portions of the small intestine removed.

Absorption of iron is an active process. Mucosal cells of the duodenum and jejunum send part of the iron directly to the bloodstream where most of it is bound as *apoferritin*. This protein combines with iron to form *ferritin*. Ferritin is the major storage form of iron in the tissues and the serum ferritin concentration is in direct equilibrium with the total body iron content. Radioimmunoassays of serum ferritin are used to identify minor deficiencies of iron before a frank clinical deficiency state develops. *Hemosiderin* is another storage form of iron.

Excretion

Under usual circumstances, little iron is absorbed and the amounts excreted in the urine are small. Iron is also lost in feces and sweat and, in women, as a result of blood losses during menstruation and pregnancy. Menstrual losses of iron can vary widely.[25] The average amount of iron lost during each menstrual period is 30 mg. Because of the small percentage of iron absorbed, and the amount lost monthly, females have a higher iron requirement than males.

There is no physiological mechanism which allows the body to excrete excess iron effectively.

Therefore, control of absorption is the first line of defense in preventing the accumulation of iron in toxic amounts in body tissues. Acute iron toxicity has been observed in children who have ingested large numbers of oral iron supplements (often as a result of obtaining iron pills used by other family members). Ingestion of 3 to 18 g of iron can be fatal to young children.

A genetically transmitted condition known as idiopathic hemochromatosis results in a large accumulation of iron stores over time. Clinical manifestations of the disorder occur between 40 and 60 years of age. It is more prevalent in males. The principle organs involved are the liver, pancreas, heart, and gonads.[26]

Dietary Allowances
During the life cycle, there appear to be three periods when iron intake may be inadequate: (1) infancy, especially for infants born of women with low stores; (2) adolescence, due to the growth spurt and onset of menstruation in girls; and (3) pregnancy and childbirth. The increased need during pregnancy is due to increased blood volume, necessitating an increased production of red blood cells to maintain a near-normal hematocrit. Also, an average of 270 mg of iron is transferred to the fetus and another 240 mg is lost at delivery. Iron stores in the normal infant born at term are exhausted in 3 to 6 months if not replaced.

Consequently, recommendations for infants and women are generous. The recommended allowance in infancy is 10 mg per day.[27] Recently, there have been data published which suggest that breast-fed infants absorb iron from breast milk with greater efficiency than those on a cow milk–based formula.[28] Recommended daily allowances are 10 mg for infants and 15 mg for children. The allowance for women of childbearing age is 18 mg per day, which allows for the needs imposed by menstruation, pregnancy, and lactation. A woman on an adequate diet, ingesting energy at the recommended levels, will only derive 9 to 12 mg of iron per day from dietary sources. It can be particularly difficult to ingest adequate amounts if the woman is a vegetarian. During pregnancy, a supplementary intake of 30 to 60 mg of iron per day is recommended. For postmenopausal women and for men, an intake of 10 mg per day is recommended.

Dietary Sources of Iron
There is some variation in the amount of heme iron in different kinds of meats. In beef, lamb, and chicken 50 to 60 percent of the iron is heme iron while 30 to 40 percent of the iron in pork, liver, and fish is present in the heme form. Nonheme iron sources include grains, fruits, eggs, and dairy products in addition to nonheme iron from poultry, meat, and fish and from soluble iron supplements.

Table 7-8 demonstrates how to calculate the absorbable iron from different types of meals. Table 7-9 shows sources of heme and nonheme iron.

Clinical Application
The primary consequence of iron deficiency is anemia. The causes of iron-deficiency anemia are given in Table 7-10. They can be summarized under four categories:

1 Iron-poor diet
2 Increased iron losses
3 Malabsorption of iron
4 Increased iron requirements

Iron-deficiency anemia is characterized as microcytic hypochromic anemia because the red cells are small (microcytic) and pale (hypochromic). As anemia develops, there is a natural sequence of compensatory mechanisms. Initially, as iron stores become depleted, the body becomes more efficient in iron absorption. Then the serum level of iron decreases and the iron-binding capacity of serum transferrin increases.[29] The percent of transferrin saturation is indicative of the amount of iron available to the erythroid marrow for red blood cell formation (average values: serum iron, 80 to 160 μg per 100 mL in males, 50 to 150 μg per 100 mL in females;

TABLE 7-8 FACTORS FOR ESTIMATING PERCENT OF DIETARY IRON ABSORPTION

Iron stores	Percentage of iron absorbed in relationship to stores			
	0 mg	250 mg	500 mg*	1000 mg
Heme iron	35	28	23	15
Nonheme iron				
A. *Low availability meal*				
1. < 30 g meat, fish or poultry	5	4	3	2
or				
2. < 25 mg ascorbic acid				
B *Medium availability meal*				
1. 30–90 g meat, poultry, or fish	10	7	5	3
or				
2. 25–75 mg ascorbic acid				
C. *High availability meal*				
1. > 90 g meat, poultry, or fish				
or	20	12	8	4
2. > 75 mg ascorbic acid				
or				
3. 30–90 g meat, fish, or poultry, plus 35–75 mg ascorbic acid				

Source: Adapted from E. R. Monsen et al., "Estimation of Available Dietary Iron," *American Journal of Clinical Nutrition*, **31**:133, 1978.

*Authors recommend using 500-mg stores for most dietary calculations.

TABLE 7-9 SOURCES OF HEME AND NONHEME IRON

Heme iron sources*	Nonheme iron sources
Beef	Whole or enriched grains
Chicken	Dairy products
Fish	Eggs
Lamb	Fruits
Liver	Nonheme iron from poultry, liver, meat, and fish
Pork	Soluble iron supplements

*Assume a 40% heme iron content for animal tissues including poultry, liver, meat, and fish.

TABLE 7-10 CAUSES OF IRON DEFICIENCY

I Iron-poor diet
II Increased iron loss
  A Excessive menstrual flow
  B Chronic blood loss
    1 Peptic ulcer
    2 Lesions of gastrointestinal tract
    3 Lesions of genitourinary tract
  C Chronic hemoglobinuria
  D Parasitic infections (e.g., hookworm)
  E Blood loss from other causes (surgery, trauma)
III Malabsorption of iron
  A Postgastrectomy
  B Small-bowel disease
IV Increased iron requirements
  A Pregnancy
  B Infancy

Source: J. A. Koepke, "Iron Deficiency Anemia," *Postgraduate Medicine*, **163**:163, 1972.

iron-binding capacity, 250 to 410 μg per 100 mL; percent saturation, 20 to 55 percent; transferrin, 205 to 374 mg per 100 mL).[30]

As time progresses, the red cell pattern emerges. If the anemia is untreated, characteristic tissue changes may appear, including spoon nails, cheilosis, glossitis, and, on rare occasions, a membranous obstruction of the upper esophagus (see Fig. 7.1, which shows the progression of iron-deficiency anemia).

Clinical signs of mild iron-deficiency anemia are weakness, lassitude, and fatigue. Pagophagia (ice eating) has been observed in some iron-deficient persons. Some investigators have suggested that in utero or during the first 2 years of life an infant may sustain permanent damage through effects on the cerebral oxidative metabolism, neurotransmitter synthesis, or brain cell mitosis.[31] Others have documented disruptive behavior in anemic adolescents. There have also been observations of apathetic and irritable behavior, along with short attention span, in anemic preschool youngsters.[32] These behaviors were observed in children with hemoglobins in the 8.5 to 10 g range.

The incidence of iron deficiency may be as high as 20 percent among children in certain populations.

The hematocrit and the hemoglobin level are used as routine screening measures of populations. These measures must be interpreted according to the individual's age and physiological state, since variations in total blood volume affect the definition of anemia (see Table 7-11, p. 144).

In the treatment of iron-deficiency anemia, nutrition education should be teamed with the use of oral supplements. The nutritional counseling should emphasize selection of foods that are adequate in iron and ascorbic acid. Parents of young children may need additional help introducing new foods and weaning from the breast or bottle.

Oral administration of ferrous salts (sulfate, gluconate, or fumarate) is the usual treatment recommended for uncomplicated iron-deficiency anemia. The therapeutic dose is calculated in terms of elemental iron present, and varies with the type of iron used. Ferrous sulfate yields 20 percent elemental iron. A total daily dose of 4.5 to 6 mg per kilogram of body weight is divided into three doses, which is considered optimal for bone marrow utilization. Iron should be given between meals to avoid interference with absorption from chelating agents contained in foods. Ingestion of milk interferes with absorption, and medication should not be administered with milk.

Within 7 days following the initiation of oral iron therapy, the hemoglobin level should begin to rise. Within 1 week to 2 months, the hemoglobin values approach normal levels; however, oral iron therapy should be continued for 6 months to 12 months if stores are to be repleted.

An excessive intake or accumulation of iron can also cause problems. Hemocromatosis, as mentioned earlier, is a genetic disorder of iron metabolism which is characterized by a large accumulation of iron, as hemosiderin, in the tissues. Hepatic, pancreatic, and cardiac problems are commonly observed in persons with hemocromatosis. A slate-gray skin color, diabetes mellitus, and hepatic cirrhosis are classic signs of the disorder. The excessive accumulation of iron is the result of long-term elevated absorption of iron.[33]

In the treatment of hemochromatosis, the objective is to remove excess iron from the body. Usually, phlebotomy (incision of a vein and removal of blood) is the method used to achieve mobilization of parenchymal iron stores. The diabetes mellitus is generally treated with insulin.

Besides hemocromatosis, there are several other conditions which may result in markedly increased levels of iron. Among these are repeated transfusions, excessive administration of intravenous iron, and excessive intake of dietary or supplementary iron, causing an increased storage of iron or hemosiderosis. Acute iron toxicity has caused death in some young children

HOW IRON DEFICIENCY EVOLVES:

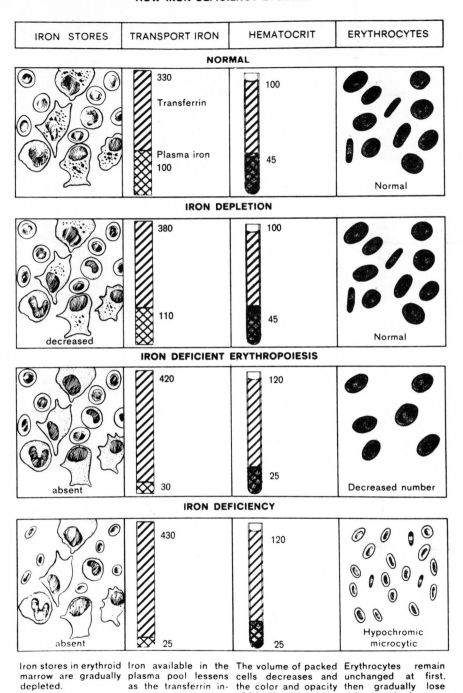

IRON STORES	TRANSPORT IRON	HEMATOCRIT	ERYTHROCYTES

NORMAL

Iron stores in erythroid marrow are gradually depleted.

Iron available in the plasma pool lessens as the transferrin increases.

The volume of packed cells decreases and the color and opacity of blood plasma fade.

Erythrocytes remain unchanged at first, then gradually lose color and become smaller.

Figure 7-1
The progression of iron-deficiency anemia. (From Clement Finch, "Iron Metabolism," *Nutrition Today,* Summer 1969, p. 6.)

143

TABLE 7-11   NORMAL VALUES BY AGES

Age	Hemoglobin, g	Hematocrit, %
6–23 months	10	31
2–5 years	11	34
6–14 years	12	37
15 years + (male)	13	40
15 years + (female)	12	37
15 years + (pregnant female)	11	34

Source: Center for Disease Control, U.S. Department of Health, Education, and Welfare.

who have inadvertently ingested several iron tablets. Ingestion of 3 to 18 g can cause vomiting, diarrhea, acidosis, hyperventilation, and lowered blood pressure, which can lead to death from shock.

Iodine

The adult body contains approximately 10 to 20 mg of iodine. Most iodine is concentrated in the thyroid gland and deficiency states cause an enlargement of the gland, producing a swelling in the front part of the neck (goiter). (See Chap. 24.)

Function

The sole function of iodine is to serve as a component of the thyroid hormones thyroxine and triiodothyronine, and of other compounds produced by the thyroid gland.

Absorption and Excretion

Dietary intake is converted to iodide in the gastrointestinal tract; iodide is efficiently absorbed. The thyroid gland is the only tissue that has a capability for utilizing iodide, which it does in the synthesis of the two thyroid hormones, thyroxine and triiodothyronine. The activity of the thyroid gland is regulated by thyroid stimulating hormone (TSH), which is secreted by the pituitary gland. There is no mechanism which allows for the conservation of iodine in the face of dietary deficiency. Iodine is excreted via the urine.

Dietary Allowances

Because of the variation in soil content of iodine, the dietary need for the mineral is probably different in different regions of the country. In general, it is recommended that an intake of 100 μg daily will provide a sufficient amount of iodine, providing that intake of goitrogens (substances that have antithyroid activity) is limited. Goitrin is a goitrogen and is found in turnips, rutabagas, and other members of the cabbage family. It is unlikely that goiter will develop solely as the result of ingesting large amounts of these foods. Some medicines, such as the thiocarbamides, are also known for their antithyroid activity.

Dietary Sources

Seafood is the only naturally occurring major source of iodine. The iodine content of a particular agricultural food can vary greatly depending on local variations in soil and fertilizers. Generally, land nearer the sea has a better natural iodine content than the midwest. Iodized salt provides a primary source of iodine for many persons. Also, milk and bread made with iodate dough conditioners can be considered as contributors to dietary iodine. The practice of using iodate in bread making is on the decline. In spite of a recent increase in dietary iodine to levels well in excess of those recommended, there has been no evidence of adverse reactions to this excess.[34]

Clinical Application

Iodine deficiency, manifested as simple goiter, can occur in areas where the soil is low in iodine and dietary intake of iodine-rich substances such as seafoods and iodized salt is inadequate to meet body needs. Endemic goiter (see Chap. 24) occurs principally in two areas of the United States: the Great Lakes and the Rocky Mountain regions. Treatment involves administration of iodine-containing preparations, ingestion of a diet rich in iodine, and use of iodized salt. Originally, iodine deficiency was considered to be the cause of all cases of goiter. However, iodine replacement therapy alone has not always been effective in eliminating goiter. Consequently, those treating goiter have carefully monitored the efficacy of iodine replacement therapy.

During fetal or neonatal periods, thyroid deficiency results in cretinism, a syndrome of infancy and early childhood (see Chap. 24). The etiology can be identified as an abnormal development of the thyroid gland, an inborn error of thyroid hormone metabolism, or, in endemic goiter regions, a maternal dietary iodine deficiency.

Clinical signs of cretinism are thick, dry skin, thick lips, and a broad face. Infants with cretinism usually are lethargic and show mild to severe mental retardation; hypotonia, hypothermia, and constipation are also noted.

Treatment involves administration of dessicated thyroid until a euthyroid (normal) state is achieved. Adequate dietary intake of iodine is stressed and use of iodized salt is recommended.

Fluoride

Fluoride is widely distributed in soils and water as well as in plant and animal life. Traces of this mineral are present in teeth, bones, skin, and the thyroid gland.

Function

Fluoride provides protection against dental caries (see Chap. 17). It has been suggested that fluoride may strengthen the structure of the tooth and limit the solubility of tooth minerals.[35] Although its anticariogenic action is especially important during the growth years, it persists throughout adult life.

Fluoride is an inhibitor of some enzyme systems, such as enolase, the enzyme in the process that converts glyceric to pyruvic acid during glycolysis. Inhibition of the Krebs (citric acid) cycle has also been described. Excess intake of fluoride can affect metabolism. Ingestion within a short period of time of 3 to 5 g of fluoride can be lethal.

Dietary Allowances and Sources

There are no specific dietary recommendations relating to fluoride intake. Dietary intake has been observed to range from 0.3 mg per day in low-fluoride areas to 3.1 mg per day in high-fluoride areas.[36]

Drinking water can provide a major source of fluoride. Many areas have fluoridated their water supplies to a standard level of 1 ppm (part per million), which equals 1 mg of fluoride per liter of water. Seafood and tea are considered to be good dietary sources of the mineral.

Clinical Application

Poor fluoride status appears to result in an increased incidence of dental caries (see Chap. 17). Some researchers have studied the use of fluoride in the treatment of osteoporosis and Paget's disease of bone. To date, results are inconclusive, although some patients with osteoporosis have been reported to be improved through administration of sodium fluoride.

Fluoride can be poisonous if consumed in large amounts. Toxicity has been identified in industrial workers handling fluoride-containing substances such as cryolite. One of the initial signs of fluoride excess (fluorosis) is mottling of tooth enamel. Toxic signs include anorexia and sclerosis of the spine.

Copper

Copper is an essential mineral for most animal species. The highest concentrations of copper in the body are found in the liver, kidney, and blood. The normal plasma level ranges from 100 to 200 μg per 100 mL.[37] Copper is also present in muscle, liver, brain, heart, and kidney tissues.

Function

The mineral is a constituent of several enzymes or is essential in their activity; these include superoxide dismutase, tyrosinase, lysyl oxidase, dopamine B–hydroxylase, and cytochrome C–oxidase. Together with iron, copper is required for the synthesis of hemoglobin. The copper-binding protein in plasma is ceruloplasmin, which may play an important role in the release and transport of iron from storage cells to plasma transferrin. In order for normal hemoglobin synthesis to occur, iron must be transported by transferrin from storage sites in the liver and intestine to the bone marrow. Cerebrocuprein is a copper protein which has been isolated from brain tissue.

The role of copper in human nutrition is incompletely understood; it is suggested that it may be involved in collagen and bone formation, in maintenance of myelin in the nervous system, and in gastrointestinal function.

Absorption and Excretion

In the human, absorption of copper occurs mainly in the stomach and duodenum. Approximately 40 to 60 percent of dietary copper is absorbed. Copper absorption is regulated at the intestinal mucosa. There may be competition with zinc, molybdenum, sulfates, phytates, and ascorbic acid for absorption. In contrast to the enhancing effect ascorbic acid has on nonheme iron very high levels of ascorbic acid intake may inhibit copper absorption. The major excretory route of copper is via the bile.[38] Lesser amounts are excreted in the saliva, urine, sweat, and menstrual blood.

Dietary Allowances and Sources

Copper intakes ranging from 1.3 to 2 mg per day seem to be adequate for adolescents and adults. The typical American diet probably supplies 3 to 5 mg of copper per day. Recently, it has been observed that institutional diets may contain less than 1 mg per day. For children, an intake of 0.08 mg per kilogram of body weight per day appears adequate. The amount of copper recommended for full-term infants may not be sufficient for premature infants because of the infants' low copper reserves. Infant formulas used to the exclusion of other foods should furnish 100 mg per kilogram of body weight.[39] The richest food sources of copper are liver (calf, lamb, and beef), crustaceans, and shellfish, especially Atlantic oysters. Other good sources are nuts and seeds, high-protein cereals, dried fruits, poultry, fish, meats, legumes, and root and leafy vegetables. The copper content of water may be significant where copper piping is used.

Clinical Application

Copper deficiency, as manifested in hypocupremia, has been observed in individuals with protein-calorie malnutrition, sprue, cystic fibrosis, or kidney disease, and in those undergoing prolonged parenteral nutrition. Infants who were maintained for extended periods of time on diets consisting only of milk manifested symptoms similar to those seen in copper-deficient animals.[40,41,42] These symptoms include hyperproteinemia, hypocupremia, anemia, poor growth, neutropenia (a decrease in neutrophilic leukocytes in the blood), and low ceruloplasmin levels. These symptoms are reversed by the administration of iron and copper.[43]

Menkes' steely hair syndrome is an X-linked recessive inborn error of copper metabolism which causes steel wool–like texture of the hair (due to lack of keratinization), mental retardation, hypothermia, low plasma copper, skeletal changes, and degenerative changes in heart tissue. Those affected are severely deficient in copper because of their inability to absorb it from the gastrointestinal tract. The profound copper deficiency can be partially corrected by parenteral administration of copper.[44]

Wilson's disease is a rare autosomal recessive disease which is characterized by degeneration of brain tissue and cirrhosis of the liver. It seems a paradox that while serum copper and copper content of ceruloplasmin are low, concomitantly large amounts of copper are deposited in the liver, brain, cornea, and kidney.

Therapy for this disorder involves use of a chelating agent which promotes copper excretion. This agent must be used with care as it also drastically increases urinary zinc and can thereby cause zinc deficiency. A low-copper diet has been viewed as an effective therapeutic adjunct. Dietary intake of copper is typically reduced to 1.0 to 1.5 mg per day. More stringent dietary restriction has been viewed as impractical.[45] If diagnosed early and treated throughout life, prognosis is fairly good for those who have the disorder.

Table 7-12 presents a summary of disorders which can affect serum copper.

It has been postulated that a metabolic zinc-copper imbalance may be a major factor in the etiology of coronary heart disease.[46] This imbalance, a relative or absolute deficiency of copper with a high ratio of zinc to copper, may result in hypercholesterolemia and an increased mortality due to coronary heart disease.

Zinc

The human body contains 2 to 3 g of zinc. Although the need for zinc in animals has been recognized for several decades, clinical signs of human zinc deficiency were initially described in 1961 in males living in the middle east. Ten years later, similar symptoms were documented in females. Conditioned zinc deficiency has been described in persons with regional gastroenteritis, cirrhosis, infectious disease, cystic fibrosis, nephrotic syndrome, and pancreatic insufficiency.

Function

Zinc is an essential constituent for the activity of a number of metalloenzymes such as carbonic anhydrase, carboxypeptidase, alkaline phosphatase, aspartate transcarbamylase, mannosidase, aminopeptidase, dehydrogenases, dipeptidase, superoxide dismutase, and DNA polymerase. Zinc is a component of insulin and has a role in taste and olfactory acuity. It is required for protein synthesis and hence for growth and sexual

TABLE 7-12 CONDITIONS CAUSING AN INCREASE OR DECREASE IN SERUM COPPER

Increased in
  Anemia
    Pernicious anemia
    Megaloblastic anemia of pregnancy
    Iron-deficiency anemia
    Aplastic anemia
  Leukemia, acute and chronic
  Infection, acute and chronic
  Malignant lymphoma
  Hemochromatosis
  Collagen diseases
  Hyperthyroidism, hypothroidism
Decreased in
  Nephrosis
  Wilson's disease
  Acute leukemia in remission
  Some iron-deficiency anemias of childhood requiring both copper and iron therapy
  Protein-calorie malnutrition

Source: Adapted from J. Wallach, *Interpretation of Diagnostic Tests,* 3d ed., Little, Brown and Company, Boston, 1978, p. 112.

maturation. Zinc has been identified as important in the wound-healing process.[47]

Absorption and Excretion

Approximately 20 to 40 percent of dietary zinc is absorbed.[48] The pancreas secretes a zinc-binding ligand into the intestinal lumen. It appears that zinc of animal origin is more readily available than zinc of plant origin. Presence of phytates in the diet can compromise the absorption of zinc. These phytates tend to form insoluble zinc-phytate complexes. High levels of calcium can further decrease zinc availability by forming a zinc-calcium-phytate complex. Geophagia (clay eating) has also been noted to interfere with absorption of zinc.

Excretion of the mineral is via gastrointestinal and pancreatic secretions. Zinc is also excreted in urine, sweat, and menstrual blood. Body reserves of zinc are not easily mobilized, and consequently there is a need for a regular intake of the mineral, particularly during periods of growth and stress.

Dietary Allowances and Sources

The 1980 edition of the National Academy of Sciences *Recommended Dietary Allowances* suggests a zinc intake of 15 mg per day for the adult, with an additional 5 mg per day during pregnancy and 10 mg during lactation. Recommendations for infants and children range from 3 mg for infants up to 6 months of age, to 10 mg for early childhood. In general, the body requirement for zinc is related to body size and rate of growth.

Though zinc is widely distributed in foods, perhaps the best source is red meats. Seafood, particularly Atlantic oysters, are also high in zinc content. The zinc content of foods is subject to wide variation, related to a net loss of zinc in the soil due to natural leaching, erosion, and constant removal of crops without repletion.

Clinical Application

One study of 35 persons with zinc deficiency noted hypogeusia (diminished taste sensation), anorexia, weight loss, and psychological problems.[49] Another noted poor growth and impaired taste acuity in school-aged children.[50] Growth retardation, sexual immaturity, and skin lesions have been observed in other zinc-deficient subjects. The results of an investigation of pregnant Turkish women suggests a need for additional study of zinc nutritional status during pregnancy.[51] Various teratogenic effects of zinc deficiency have been noted in the offspring of zinc-deficient rats and chicks. Some have suggested that zinc deficiency impedes wound healing through allowing lipid peroxidation of cellular membranes. Administration of supplementary zinc allows stabilization of the cell membranes through decreasing lipid preoxidation of these structures.

Zinc toxicity can occur as a result of eating foods stored in galvanized containers. Toxic signs are gastrointestinal distress, vomiting, diarrhea, and fever.

Several conditions known to lower serum zinc levels are pregnancy, upper respiratory infections, kidney disease, sickle cell anemia, myocardial infarction, and malignant neoplasms. Oral contraceptives may also lower serum zinc. Zinc levels are decreased in pernicious anemia; however, this is reversed by vitamin B_{12} therapy. The metabolism of zinc is significantly altered in persons with alcoholic cirrhosis of the liver, since a key step in the metabolism of alcohol requires an enzyme containing zinc (liver alcohol dehydrogenase).

Although plasma, red cell content, and hair zinc levels are often reported, there is no single acceptable index of zinc nutritional status. Moreover, contamination of samples poses an analytical problem.

Manganese

The role of manganese in human nutrition has received little attention. Analysis of biological samples requires sophisticated techniques. One investigator inadvertently produced manganese deficiency in human subjects while attempting to restrict vitamin K and hence concluded that both vitamin K and manganese may be necessary for production of normal prothrombin. In animals, manganese is required for proper collagen and bone formation. The largest concentrations of manganese are found in the bone, liver, kidney, pancreas, and pituitary. The adult human body contains approximately 12 to 20 mg of manganese.[52]

Function, Absorption, and Excretion

Manganese is important in bone formation, brain function, growth, and reproduction. It is a component of several enzyme systems.

Manganese is absorbed rather poorly from the gastrointestinal tract. About 4–6 percent of the 2.5 to 7 mg typically ingested by adults is absorbed from the small intestine. High levels of calcium and phosphorus in the diet are known to diminish absorption. Excretion of manganese is through the bile and pancreatic juice.

Dietary Allowances and Sources

No formal recommendations for manganese intake have been established. Since no cases of overt deficiency have been described in humans, it seems reasonable to assume that the average daily intake of 2.5 to 7 mg meets the requirement.

Nuts, seeds, and whole grains are good sources of manganese; fruits and vegetables provide moderate amounts. Tea is exceptionally rich in manganese content.

Cobalt

Cobalt is a component of vitamin B_{12} (see Chap. 6). The bacterial synthesis of vitamin B_{12} requires the mineral. Nonruminant species meet this requirement for cobalt through ingestion of vitamin B_{12}. Cobalt is well absorbed by animals and humans, and absorption is increased in iron deficiency. In fact, there is mutual antagonism between iron and cobalt at the absorptive level. Cobalt is excreted in the urine.

Selenium

Selenium is found in body tissues in concentrations that vary with the level and chemical form of selenium in the diet. The kidney and liver generally carry the highest concentrations of selenium. Selenium is an essential component of the enzyme glutathione peroxidase. It is known that glutathione protects red blood cells through destruction of hydrogen peroxide and fatty acid hydroperoxides through reactions catalyzed by glutathione peroxidase. This role for selenium clarifies the relationship between vitamin E and selenium in the prevention of lipid peroxidation.

Although suboptimal selenium nutriture has been observed in severely malnourished persons, neither overt deficiency nor excess has been reported. To date, no recommended dietary allowance has been set. The average American diet provides about 50 to 150 μg per day. High-protein foods such as meats and seafoods have been found to be the best sources of selenium. Although grains can provide a reasonable source, their content varies depending on the soil in which they are grown.

It has been suggested that cystic fibrosis is a disease possibly caused by nutritional deficiency of selenium; however, there is no direct evidence to support the contention that a lack of the element plays either a role in the etiology of the disorder or in its treatment.[53] There is a danger of developing signs of selenium toxicity when the mineral is administered in large amounts.

Chromium

Chromium is involved in glucose metabolism through promoting the action of insulin. The form of chromium present in brewer's yeast is highly utilizable. In some individuals with diabetes an improvement of glucose tolerance has been observed following the administration of chromium. Also, research has demonstrated improvement in glucose tolerance of malnourished children as a result of chromium administration.

The mean daily chromium intake of subjects consuming institutional diets has been reported as 52 to 78 μg daily.[54] Approximately 10 to 25 percent of chromium from foods is absorbed. Sources of chromium include most animal proteins (except fish), whole grains, and brewer's yeast. Refinements of cereal products can markedly lower the chromium content and this loss is not replaced by current fortification. In the United States the organ content of chromium declines with increasing age. This phenomenon has not been observed in all parts of the world. Low chromium status may play a role in adult-onset diabetes, rendering insulin less effective. Several investigators have suggested that marginal chromium deficiencies may occur among elderly persons, pregnant women, and those suffering from protein-calorie malnutrition. There is no basis upon which to establish a firm recommendation for chromium intake.

Molybdenum

Molybdenum is an essential component of xanthine oxidase, the enzyme responsible for the conversion of xanthine to uric acid. Xanthine arises from the degradation of nucleic acids. The estimated average intake of the mineral in the United States is approximately 100 μg. Molybdenum content of foods varies with the content of the soil. Major sources of molybdenum are meat, grains, and legumes. Intakes of moderate amounts of molybdenum can lead to increased excretion of copper.[55]

Other Minerals

Signs of nickel, vanadium, and silicon deficiency have been produced in animal species, and it is possible that a human requirement exists. To date, however, there are no data to confirm such needs.

Arsenic, cadmium, and tin may also be essential elements, but further investigations are warranted. Deficiency of these minerals has been documented to impede growth and reproduction in animals.

INTERACTIONS

Researchers have proposed a mechanism for predicting and demonstrating interactions among minerals which are important in nutrition and metabolism. Their existence prevents the tabulation of precise requirements for humans. In some cases, two minerals are chemically similar to one another and can compete for binding sites on a transport protein (e.g., zinc and copper). In others, insoluble complexes are precipitated (e.g., calcium, phytate, and zinc can form an unavailable complex). To add to the confusion, we have insufficient knowledge concerning action to take when a nutrient can enhance the absorption of one element while depressing the uptake of another. For example, ascorbic acid promotes the absorption of iron; however, large amounts of ascorbic acid are known to impede the uptake of copper. Medications can interfere with mineral utilization. Within the realm of interactions, many important questions remain unanswered. Investigators with well-designed research will assist in unraveling the metabolic mysteries which complicate our understanding of human nutrition.

STUDY QUESTIONS

1   Differentiate between macrominerals and trace elements.
2   Describe the interrelating role of calcium and phosphorus in the human body.
3   Cite the factors which influence calcium absorption.
4   Describe the progression of iron-deficiency anemia in the human body. What clinical and laboratory symptoms would you expect to find?
5   What predisposing factors lead to magnesium deficiency?

CLINICAL STUDY 7

Past history

Jeremy, aged 19 months, was brought by his parents to the clinic pediatrician with the chief complaints of listlessness, irritability, and constipation. The past history was unremarkable. Initially, he fed well on a standard infant formula (not fortified with iron) and accepted all baby foods well. At 6 months of age, when junior foods were introduced, food refusals became pronounced, and Jeremy developed very specific preferences which excluded meat and vegetables.

Present history

Physical examination revealed a pale child whose height was at the 25th percentile for his age and whose weight was between the 50th and 75th percen-

tiles. Laboratory analysis revealed the following: hemoglobin 9.6 g per 100 mL, hematocrit 31 percent, serum iron 59 μg per 100 mL, iron-binding capacity 365 μg per 100 mL, and saturation of transferrin less than 16 percent.

Present food intake consists of 40 oz of milk, 8 oz of fruit juice, presweetened cereal, white toast, canned vegetable soup, ice cream and canned spaghetti. Although drinking from a cup, Jeremy continues to take a bottle at nap and bedtime. Intake of iron was esti- *mated to be 4.5 mg, protein intake 45 g, and ascorbic acid 15 mg.*

Clinical study questions

1 *Based on laboratory and clinical findings and dietary intake, what condition would you diagnose?*

2 *Why is the serum iron-binding capacity value high when the hemoglobin value is low?*

3 *What are your recommendations for treatment?*

REFERENCES

1 E. Underwood, *Trace Elements in Human and Animal Nutrition,* 4th ed., Academic Press, New York, 1977, p. 1.

2 Food and Nutrition Board, *Recommended Dietary Allowances,* 9th ed., National Academy of Sciences, National Research Council, Washington, 1980, pp. 181–182.

3 Food and Nutrition Board, op. cit., p. 125.

4 A. S. Posner, "Crystal Chemistry of Bone Mineral," *Physiology Review,* **49**:766, 1969.

5 S. Davidson, R. Passmore, J. Brock, and A. Truswell, *Human Nutrition and Dietetics,* 7th ed., Churchill and Livingston, London, 1979, p. 91.

6 J. Wallach, *Interpretation of Diagnostic Tests: A Handbook Synopsis of Laboratory Medicine,* 3d ed., Little, Brown and Company, Boston, 1978, p. 8.

7 W. F. Ganong (ed.), *Medical Physiology,* 9th ed., Lange Medical Publications, Los Altos, Calif., 1979, p. 370.

8 Food and Nutrition Board, op. cit., p. 126.

9 Wallach, op. cit., pp. 8, 10.

10 Food and Nutrition Board, op. cit., pp. 129–130.

11 S. Schuette, M. Zemel, and H. Linkswiler, "Studies on the Mechanism of Protein-induced Hypercalciuria in Older Men and Women," *Journal of Nutrition,* **110**:305, 1980.

12 S. Garn, "The Course of Bone Gain and Phases of Bone Loss," *Orthopedic Clinics of North America,* **3**:503, 1972.

13 Wallach, op. cit., p. 10.

14 L. Page and B. Friend, "The Changing United States Diet," *Bioscience,* **28**:192, 1978.

15 S. J. Fomon, *Infant Nutrition,* 2d ed., W. B. Saunders Company, Philadelphia, 1974, p. 271.

16 Davidson, op. cit., p. 121.

17 R. Goodhart and M. Shils, *Modern Nutrition in Health and Disease,* 6th ed., Lea and Febiger, Philadelphia, 1979, p. 310.

18 Wallach, op. cit., p. 9.

19 R. Misironi, *Trace Elements in the Etiology of Cardiovascular Disease,* WHO Technical Report 5, World Health Organization, Geneva, 1974, p. 628.

20 A. Prasad and D. Oberleas (eds.), *Trace Elements in Human Health and Disease,* vol. 2, Academic Press, New York, 1976, p. 1.

21 Food and Nutrition Board, op. cit., p. 135.

22 E. Monsen, L. Hallberg, M. Layrisse, D. Hegsted, J. Cook, W. Mertz, and C. Finch, "Estimation of Available Dietary Iron," *American Journal of Clinical Nutrition,* **31**:134, 1978.

23 J. Cook and E. Monsen, "Food Iron, 1: Use of a Semi-Sythetic Diet to Study Absorption of Nonheme Iron," *American Journal of Clinical Nutrition,* **28**:1289, 1975.

24 J. Fritz, *Measures to Increase Iron in Foods and Diets,* Food and Nutrition Board, National Academy of Sciences, National Research Council, Washington, 1970, p. 633.

25 A. Jacobs and E. Butler, "Menstrual Blood Loss in Iron Deficiency Anemia," *Lancet,* **2**:407, 1965.

26 A. Harvey, R. Johns, A. Owens, and R. Ross, *The Principles and Practice of Medicine,* 19th ed., Appleton, Century, Crofts, New York, 1976, p. 909.

27 Food and Nutrition Board, op. cit., pp. 138–139.

28 J. McMillan, A. Landaw, and S. Oski, "Iron Sufficiency in Breast-fed Infants and the Availability of Iron From Human Milk," *Pediatrics,* **58**:686, 1976.

29 Committee on Nutrition of the American Academy of Pediatrics, "Iron Balance and Requirements in Infancy," *Pediatrics,* **43**:134, 1969.

30 Wallach, op. cit., pp. 9, 10.

31 Pollet and Leibel, "Iron Deficiency and Behavior," *Journal of Pediatrics,* **88**:372, 1976.

32 M. S. Read, "Anemia and Behavior," *Moderne Problems des Paediatri,* **14**:189, 1975.

33 J. Stanbury, J. Wyngaarden, and D. Frederickson, *The Metabolic Basis of Inherited Disease,* 4th ed., McGraw-Hill, New York, 1978, pp. 1126–1164.

34 Food and Nutrition Board, op. cit., p. 149.

35 Goodhart and Shils, op. cit., p. 871.

36 J. C. Muhler, "The Supply of Fluorine to Man," sec. 11, in *Fluorine and Human Health*, World Health Organization, Geneva, 1970, pp. 32–40.

37 Wallach, op. cit., p. 9.

38 K. Mason, "A Conspectus of Copper Metabolism and Requirements of Man," *Journal of Nutrition*, **109**:1979, 1979.

39 Food and Nutrition Board, op. cit., p. 152.

40 Underwood, op. cit., pp. 91, 92.

41 K. Mason, op. cit., p. 1985.

42 R. S. Goodhart and M. Shils, op. cit., p. 418.

43 Stanbury, op. cit., pp. 1098–1126.

44 Stanbury, op. cit., p. 1116.

45 Stanbury, op. cit., p. 1103.

46 L. M. Klevay, "Coronary Heart Disease: The Zinc/Copper Hypothesis." *American Journal of Clinical Nutrition*, **28**:764, 1975.

47 Underwood, op. cit., p. 218.

48 *Trace Elements in Human Nutrition, Technical Report 532*, World Health Organization, Geneva, 1973, pp. 9–14.

49 R. Henkin, P. Schecter, R. Hoye and C. Mattern, "Idiopathic Hypogeusia with Dysgeusia, Hyposonia, and Dysosmia: A New Syndrome," *Journal of the American Medical Association*, **217**:434, 1971.

50 K. Hambridge, P. Walravens, R. Brown, J. Webster, S. White, M. Anthony, and M. Roth, "Zinc Nutrition of Preschool Children in the Denver Head Start Program," *American Journal of Clinical Nutrition*, **29**:734, 1976.

51 A. O. Cavdar, E. Babacon, A. Arcasoy, and W. Ertem, "Effect of Nutrition on Serum Zinc Concentration during Pregnancy in Turkish Women," *American Journal of Clinical Nutrition*, **33**:542, 1980.

52 Goodhart and Shils, op. cit., 418.

53 Editor's Column, "Selenium and Cystic Fibrosis," *Journal of Pediatrics*, **96**:421, 1980.

54 O. Levander, "Selenium and Chromium in Human Nutrition," *Journal of the American Dietetic Association*, **66**:338, 1975.

55 T. A. Tsongas, R.R. Meglen, P.A. Walravens, and W.R. Schappel, "Molybdenum in the Diet: An Estimate of Average Daily Intake in the United States," *American Journal of Clinical Nutrition* **33**:1103, 1980.

CLINICAL DISCUSSION 7

On the basis of clinical and laboratory findings, the diagnosis of iron-deficiency anemia was made. An oral supplement of ferrous sulfate was prescribed with specific instructions regarding administration. The recommended dose was 3 mL per day (the daily dose should give 4.5 to 6 mg of elemental iron per kilogram of body weight), given between meals in fruit juice or water (never milk).

Within 7 days, the hemoglobin began to rise, and after 8 weeks values had returned to normal. Therapy was continued for 8 months. (A common error is to discontinue iron after 2 or 3 months, but therapy should be continued for 6 to 12 months to replete stores.) Since food intake was providing only 4.5 mg of iron (the recommended dietary allowance is 15 mg), iron-containing foods, especially "heme sources" including lean red meat, liver, and iron-fortified cereals, and whole-grain breads were encouraged. Citrus juices and vitamin C–rich foods were recommended to enhance iron absorption.

Since Jeremy had very definite food preferences, his parents were counseled about normal developmental feeding issues (i.e., toddler feeding behavior; see Chap. 13) and weaning was suggested. With respect to Jeremy's constipation, his parents were advised that since iron medication can also cause constipation, it was important to include prunes, juices, water, and bran in Jeremy's diet on a daily basis. Milk was curtailed to 24 oz per day, enough to provide requirements without interfering with appetite for solid foods. Also, the parents were counseled against the hazards of leaving the iron medication within easy reach of the child. Follow-up well-child care with laboratory analysis occurred at 3-month intervals over the next year.

CHAPTER 8

WATER AND ELECTROLYTES

Grace Shen

KEY WORDS
Electrolyte
Ions
Osmotic Pressure
Sodium
Potassium
Chloride
Dehydration
Acidosis
Alkalosis

INTRODUCTION

The fundamental unit of life in all living organisms is the cell. Each cell of the human body is bathed in a tissue fluid of water and certain electrolytes (sodium, potassium, calcium, magnesium, chloride, phosphate, and sulfate) and is regulated by the integration of many physiological processes.

Illness, trauma, or surgery can cause an alteration in the amount and composition of tissue fluids, which may have profound effects (dehydration, shock, death) if not corrected by the administration of suitable replacement fluids. Successful fluid and electrolyte therapy is based on the fundamental concepts governing water and electrolytes, which this chapter presents.

BODY WATER

Function

All biological functions require a suitable concentration of water as the solvent for inorganic electrolytes and other substances. Thus, water is an essential nutrient. As the most important body solvent, it provides a normal constant internal environment for body function. It serves as the vehicle to deliver oxygen and nutrients to tissue and cells. It excretes wastes from the body. It is essential for metabolism. In periods of growth, it also expands different fluid compartments. Water is the largest single component of the body, and a loss of even 10 percent can cause metabolic disorders.

Body Water Distribution

Two-thirds of the total body weight consists of water. It is distributed throughout the body in all cells, in the extracellular fluids, and in the solid supporting structures of the body. However, there are three designated functional fluid compartments: the intracellular compartment (the cellular fluid), which contains the largest percentage of water; the extracellular (intravas-

TABLE 8-1 BODY FLUID COMPARTMENTS IN THE ADULT MALE

Compartment	Volume in males, mL	Percentage of body weight
Plasma	3,500	5
Interstitial fluid	10,500	15
Total extracellular fluid	14,000	20
Intracellular compartment	28,000	40
Total	42,000	60

Source: Adapted from J. H. Bland, Clinical Metabolism of Body Water and Electrolytes, W. B. Saunders Company, Philadelpha, 1963, p. 36.

cular) compartment (the plasma); and the extravascular compartment (the interstitial fluid) (see Table 8-1).

Total body water as a percentage of body weight changes with age from 78 percent of body weight at birth to 60 percent by adulthood. This is related to a changing body surface area and metabolic activity, both of which are high in infancy. Also, body water tends to decrease as body fat increases, since fat is essentially water-free; the leaner and more muscular a person is, the higher the body content of water. Thus, total body water is 60 percent of body weight for a normal person, 50 percent for an obese person, and 70 percent for a lean person.

Water Balance

Normally there is a maintenance or balance between the *intake* and *output* of water, and an osmotic equilibrium between the diferent body fluid compartments.

Water intake is controlled by the thirst center in the hypothalamus, which is stimulated by a rise in the tonicity of the extracellular fluid, or by the generalized dehydration of all tissues. Water output is controlled by the antidiuretic hormone of the posterior pituitary gland. This hormone is secreted in response to an increase in the osmotic pressure of the blood plasma.

Water intake has two routes, *ingestion* and *metabolism*. The chief sources of fluid intake in health are (1) liquids and (2) water derived from solid foods, which can contain considerable amounts of water. For example, bread contains 38 percent moisture; potato 60 percent, and cooked meat 50 percent. In a normal diet, 350 mL of the daily water intake may be derived from solid food.

Metabolic water is water obtained from chemical oxidation of foodstuffs; carbohydrate, protein, and fat in the body must therefore be considered as part of the fluid intake. Thus, 1 g of food protein provides 0.41 g of water; 1 g of food carbohydrate provides 0.61 g of water; and 1 g of food fat provides 1.07 g of water. Under abnormal conditions imposed by disease states or starvation, the catabolism of body tissue also yields water. One kilogram (2.2 lb) of oxidized body fat will yield 1 L or 1000 mL of water.

Water output or elimination is largely through secretion of urine by the kidneys. Part of the urine is obligatory water, obligated to excrete the end products of metabolism, and the rest is facultative water, varying with conditions (diet, temperature). Normally an adult has to excrete a minimum of 500 mL of urine as obligatory water in order to eliminate approximately 25 g of urea produced in the average daily metabolism of protein and other metabolic waste products. Total urine output, including facultative losses, for an adult male is between 1000 and 1500 mL per day.

TABLE 8-2 WATER INTAKE AND OUTPUT IN ADULTS

Mode of intake	Amount, mL	Mode of output	Amount, mL
Water and other beverage	1250	Insensible perspiration	
Water of solid foods	1000	Skin	600
Metabolically produced	350	Lungs	400
		Sweat	50
		Feces	100
		Urine	1450
Total	2600	Total	2600

Source: Adapted from Emanuel Goldberger, *A Primer of Water, Electrolyte and Acid-Base Syndromes,* 5th ed., Lea and Febiger, Philadelphia, 1975, p. 48.

Other water losses are:

100 mL in feces

600 to 700 mL as insensible perspiration or evaporation through the skin

400 to 500 mL in air expired through breathing

Both expiration and insensible perspiration (not sweating) are electrolyte-free water. The amount of water lost by sweating under conditions of moderate temperature and humidity is small and fairly constant. Under these conditions, the electrolyte losses are also small. However, with elevated temperature or vigorous exercise, water and electrolyte losses can be excessive (e.g., an athlete can lose up to 5 lb during a marathon run or a tennis match). In lactating women, water is also lost in the breast milk.

For the most part, the amount of water taken in each day approximates the amount of water lost (see Table 8-2 above).

The daily minimum fluid intake should cover the total amount lost per day through the lungs, skin, feces, and urine. Water requirements are based on body size and determined per kilogram of body weight (see Table 8-3). If based on recommended energy intake, it is suggested that the daily intake be 1 mL of fluid per kcal (4.2 mL per kJ) for adults and 1.5 mL of fluid per kcal (4.2 mL per kJ) for infants.

TABLE 8-3 WATER REQUIREMENT
Milliliters per kilogram body weight*

	Age, years	Water, mL per kilogram body weight
Infants	Birth–1	120–100
Children	1–10	60–80
Adolescents	11–18	41–55
Adults	19–51+	20–30

*The daily maintenance requirement is based on body surface area, at 1500 to 2000 mL per m² of surface area per 24 h.
Source: Adapted from G. H. Bell, *Textbook of Physiology and Biochemistry,* 6th ed., Williams and Wilkins Company, Baltimore, 1965, p. 166; and W. Waring and L. Jeansonne, *Practical Manual of Pediatrics,* The C. V. Mosby Company, St. Louis, 1975, p. 217.

INFLUENCES ON THE DISTRIBUTION OF BODY WATER

The influences that control the body water distribution are (1) the solutes present in the body water and (2) membrane pressure or osmotic pressure.

Solutes are substances that can be dissolved in a solvent to make a solution. There are three types of solutes governing changes in the body fluids—*electrolytes* (e.g., sodium chloride), *nonelectrolytes* (e.g., glucose, urea, creatinine), and *large molecules* (e.g., plasma protein).

Solutes

Electrolytes are electrically charged particles when they are dissociated in aqueous solutions. *Ions* are the dissociated particles of electrolytes in solution which carry the electric charges. A positively charged ion is a *cation,* while a negatively charged ion is an *anion.*

The main cations in the body fluids are sodium (Na^+), potassium (K^+), calcium (Ca^{2+}), and magnesium (Mg^{2+}). The main anions in the body fluids are chloride (Cl^-), bicarbonate (HCO_3^-), phosphate (HPO_4^{2-}), and ions of organic acids such as lactate, pyruvate acetoacetate, and many proteinates.

Electrolytes are essential for forming and retaining water in the extracellular and intracellular compartments and are evenly distributed between the compartments (see Table 8-4).

The even distribution of such positive and negative charges is known as electroneutrality. This ionic equilibrium within the body fluid compartments maintains the homeostasis within the body. Homeostasis is affected by both electrolyte concentration—the number of particles per unit volume, expressed as *millimoles* (mmol); and the electrolyte activity—the number of charges present, expressed as *milliequivalents* (meq).

The conversion formulas are:

$$mmol \text{ per } L = \frac{mg/100 \text{ mL} \times 10}{molecular \text{ wt}}$$

$$meq = \frac{mg/100 \text{ mL} \times valence}{atomic \text{ wt}}$$

In case of ions containing one electric charge (such as sodium, potassium, and chloride), the numerical values for millimoles and milliequivalents are the same. However, with ions carrying two charges or having a valence of two, such as calcium or magnesium, the values for milliequivalents and millimoles are different in the

TABLE 8-4   IONIC CONCENTRATION IN EXTRACELLULAR FLUID (ECF) AND INTRACELLULAR FLUID (ICF)

		Extracellular fluid		Intracellular fluid	
Cation	Anion	Cation, meq/L	Anion, meq/L	Cation, meq/L	Anion, meq/L
Na^+		142		11	
K^+		5		164	
Ca^{2+}		5		2	
Mg^{2+}		3		28	
	Cl^-		103		
	HCO_3^-		27		10
	HPO_4^{2-}		2		105
	SO_4^{2-}		1		20
	Protein		16		65
	Organic acids		6		5
Total		155	155	205	205

Source: Adapted from D. Black, *Essentials of Fluid Balance,* 4th ed., Blackwell Scientific Publications, Oxford, 1969, p. 9.

solution, since there are more charges present in the solution once the compound with the higher valence is dissolved.

For example, 1 L in which 24 mg of magnesium is dissolved contains only 1 mmol of magnesium but 2 meq of magnesium.

Role of Membranes in Fluid and Electrolyte Distribution

Since all biological membranes which separate extracellular and intracellular fluids are completely permeable to water, the total solute concentrations in both extracellular fluid and intracellular fluid are approximately equal. Water molecules will move from the extracellular fluid to the intracellular fluid when the latter has a higher solute concentration. The reverse process occurs when the solute concentration of the extracellular fluid is higher—water then moves to it.

Membrane pressure exerts a significant influence on body water distribution. A living cell membrane is the site of continuous activity; molecules of solute and water are constantly being transported to and fro across the cell membrane, which is semipermeable, producing a membrane barrier. Each molecule of solute added to a solution occupies an element of volume formerly occupied by water molecules. The more solute added, the greater the number of water molecules displaced and the greater the pressure against the membrane.

Osmotic pressure can be defined as the pressure exerted by a solute on a semipermeable membrane in order to attract water. Since the amount of pressure is proportional to the concentration of the solute or numbers of molecules or ions present, the measure of osmotic pressure is the number of particles present in a unit of volume. The unit of measurement of the osmotic activity is the *milliosmol* (mosmol), representing the amount of work that dissolved particles must do in order to draw fluid through a semipermeable membrane. It is a measure of the osmotic contribution of a solute to a solution. Since a solute ionizes in water, the osmotic pressure depends on the number of ions or particles present in solution rather than on the amount of solute present. For example, 1 mmol of calcium chloride produces 3 mosmol, while 1 mmol of sodium chloride produces 2 mosmol and 1 mmol of a nonelectrolyte such as glucose produces 1 mosmol.

There are several mechanisms by which water and solutes move across a semipermeable membrane; among these are osmosis, diffusion, filtration, active transport, and pinocytosis.

Osmosis   The net diffusion of water between two compartments separated by a semipermeable membrane is known as osmosis. This process occurs in the simple movement of water through a semipermeable membrane.

Diffusion   When the pressure on the two sides of a membrane is *equal,* the solute molecules move across the separating membrane from a region of higher concentration to a region of lower concentration. This process is known as diffusion.

Filtration   Water molecules are filtered through membranes when there is a difference in pressure on the two sides of the membrane.

Active transport (energy-dependent)   When the solute molecules must cross a membrane against significant pressure, both energy (which comes from cell metabolism) and some vehicle of transport is required. This process is called active transport. For example, glucose is absorbed from the intestinal lumen and is actively transported across the intestinal wall by the *sodium pump.* Amino acids and fatty acids also enter and leave the cell by active transport (see Chap. 9).

Pinocytosis   Through the mechanism of pinocytosis, the cell membrane forms a pocket *(vesicle)* on the cell surface, engulfing molecules which are eventually released into the cell cytoplasm. Pinocytosis provides a major route for the entry of molecules into the cell. Proteins, fats, and various ions appear to increase the rate of vesicle formation in certain cells and use this mechanism as the mode of cell entry.

Role of the Kidneys in Regulation of Fluid and Electrolytes

In regulating the fluid and electrolyte balance, the kidneys, more than any other organ, control the volume, the osmolality, and the composition of the extracellular fluid compartment in accordance with the body's constantly changing needs.

Whenever there is a change in the extracellular fluid volume, the kidneys can vary the urinary volume to handle the water load (see Fig. 8-1). In response to hypovolemia (a decrease in the blood plasma volume) the renin-angiotensin system of the kidneys is activated, which stimulates the adrenal gland to release aldosterone and facilitates the reabsorption of sodium and water by the kidneys (see also "Sodium: Balance Mechanisms," below). This interaction between aldosterone and the kidneys can maintain the normal ratio of water to solute in the body at 3.3 mL of water to 1 mosmol of electrolyte.

Whenever there is a change in tonicity of the extracellular fluid, the kidneys can change the urine osmolarity from 50 mosmol per kg of water [giving urine a specific gravity (sp gr) of 1.001] to 1300 mosmol per kg of water (urine sp gr 1.040). The kidneys regulate the concentration of solutes in this way through interaction with the hypothalamus and the pituitary gland. The hypothalamus secretes an antidiuretic hormone (ADH) which is stored in the pituitary (see Fig. 8-2). The function of ADH is to promote an increase in water reabsorption by the kidneys. When the osmotic pressure of the blood plasma increases, that is, in response to hypertonicity of the extracellular fluid, the pituitary gland releases ADH, which stimulates the kidneys to reabsorb more water. In this way, the release of ADH helps in the production of concentrated urine and the restoration of a normal extracellular fluid volume. With hypotonicity of

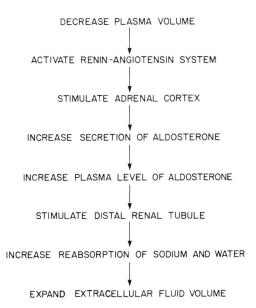

DECREASE PLASMA VOLUME

↓

ACTIVATE RENIN-ANGIOTENSIN SYSTEM

↓

STIMULATE ADRENAL CORTEX

↓

INCREASE SECRETION OF ALDOSTERONE

↓

INCREASE PLASMA LEVEL OF ALDOSTERONE

↓

STIMULATE DISTAL RENAL TUBULE

↓

INCREASE REABSORPTION OF SODIUM AND WATER

↓

EXPAND EXTRACELLULAR FLUID VOLUME

Figure 8-1

Interaction between the renin-angiotensin system of the kidney and the adrenal cortex, serving to stabilize the volume of body fluids.

Figure 8-2

Interactions between the release of antidiuretic hormone by the hypothalamus and water reabsorption by the kidneys, serving to stabilize the osmotic pressure of the body fluids.

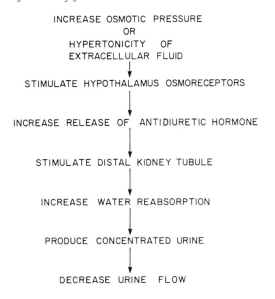

INCREASE OSMOTIC PRESSURE
OR
HYPERTONICITY OF
EXTRACELLULAR FLUID

↓

STIMULATE HYPOTHALAMUS OSMORECEPTORS

↓

INCREASE RELEASE OF ANTIDIURETIC HORMONE

↓

STIMULATE DISTAL KIDNEY TUBULE

↓

INCREASE WATER REABSORPTION

↓

PRODUCE CONCENTRATED URINE

↓

DECREASE URINE FLOW

the extracellular fluid, no ADH is released and a diluted urine is excreted.

Role of the Gastrointestinal Tract in Regulation of Fluid and Electrolytes

Besides the kidneys, the gastrointestinal tract, the lungs, and the skin also play a role in regulating the fluid and electrolyte balance.

The exchange of water and electrolytes between the extracellular compartment and the gastrointestinal tract is considerable, with a negligible loss of gastrointestinal secretions. However, persistent vomiting, diarrhea, or drainage from an intestinal fistula may quickly cause a serious contraction in volume of the extracellular fluid compartment, and a serious deficiency of potassium, chloride, and bicarbonates. In determining replacement needs, both the volume and the electrolyte composition of vomitus, diarrhea fluids, and drainage fluids must be considered. The approximate electrolyte content of these fluids is summarized in Table 8-5.

Role of Lungs and Skin in Regulation of Fluid and Electrolytes

Normal insensible water loss from the lungs and the skin is mainly electrolyte-free water, ranging in volume from 250 mL to 750 mL per day. It increases in cases of fever, hyperventilation, dyspnea, and burns, as well as in some trauma to the body, including surgery.

ELECTROLYTES

Sodium

Distribution in the Body

Sodium is the principal cation of the extracellular fluid, found in concentrations between 136 and 145 meq per L while only approximately 10 meq per L is found in the extracellular fluid. Of the exchangeable sodium, 90 percent is in the extracellular compartment; the remainder is in the intracellular fluid and in bone. The chief function of sodium is to maintain osmotic pressure in the extracellular fluid compartment.

Sodium in the body is in the form of sodium chloride—that is, the same as common table salt. Under normal conditions an individual consumes about 85 to 100 meq of salt per day (5 to 10 g per day). Ninety percent of the sodium intake is then excreted in the urine. Stool and sweat losses are less than 10 meq per day. In the adult, sodium intake and excretion are in equilibrium. For children, a positive sodium balance is necessary to expand the extracellular fluid compartment during growth.

The kidneys are the principal sodium excretory organ and regulate excretion closely. The body is very efficient in sodium conservation. In case of zero intake of sodium, the kidneys and sweat glands reduce the sodium output to zero. The body can maintain sodium balance with an intake of as little as 12 to 15 meq (0.2 to 0.3 g) of sodium per day and can tolerate an acute load of 400 meq (9.2 g) per day.

Balance Mechanisms

Sodium balance is controlled by the reninangiotensin-aldosterone system. Angiotensinogen is a liver plasma protein, circulating in the blood. Renin is an enzyme secreted by the kidneys which catalyzes angiotensinogen to angiotensin. The angiotensin in turn stimulates the secretion of aldosterone by the adrenals. With sodium de-

TABLE 8-5 ELECTROLYTE COMPOSITION OF FLUID LOSSES FROM VOMITING, DIARRHEA, AND FISTULA DRAINAGE

Type of fluid	Sodium, meq per L	Potassium, meq per L
Gastric (suction, vomiting)	75	15
Small bowel (suction, vomiting)	135	15
Diarrhea	50	40

Source: Adapted from W. Waring and L. Jeansonne, *Practical Manual of Pediatrics*, The C. V. Mosby Company, St. Louis, 1975, p. 220.

pletion, the secretion of renin by the kidneys is in inverse proportion to the amount of sodium present in the tubules of the kidneys. This increased production of renin by the kidneys is followed by the formation of angiotensin in the plasma. Angiotensin then stimulates the release of aldosterone from the adrenal cortex, which causes the kidneys to reabsorb sodium. In the complete absence of aldosterone, as occurs in Addison's disease, the patient may excrete 25 g of salt per day, whereas excretion may be negligible when aldosterone is present in large quantities.

Daily Sodium Intake

Daily intake of sodium is regulated more by taste, custom, and habit than by need. The normal intake ranges from 100 to 300 meq, or 6 to 18 g of sodium chloride per day. The quantity of sodium in most infant formulas is around 3.3 meq per 100 kcal (420 kJ) which means that a 3-month-old infant consuming 600 kcal (2520 kJ) per day would take 20 meq of sodium daily. Certain commercially prepared strained and junior foods (e.g., dinners, vegetables) provide 12 meq of sodium per 100 kcal (420 kJ). Earlier, salt was added to certain infant foods primarily to cater to the taste of the parents rather than to meet nutritional needs. This caused concern regarding the long-term effect on the incidence of cardiovascular disease, raising the question whether early introduction of salt into infants' food creates a "taste" for salt that leads to overuse later in life. Since 1970, the amount of sodium chloride added to baby foods has been decreased. The Recommended Dietary Allowances (1980) give the requirements of sodium for different ages (see Table 8-6).

Clinical Application

Disorders arise when sodium intake or losses exceed the adaptive balance mechanisms. This can occur in conditions resulting from kidney or heart failure. In renal disease problems are due to the inability of the kidneys to excrete sodium normally, whereas in heart failure the problem is caused by increased levels of aldosterone, which promotes the retention of sodium. In such cases sodium intake may be restricted. In other conditions, such as the nephrotic salt-losing syndrome or adrenal insufficiency, there is sodium loss because of renal or adrenal cortical damage. Vomiting, diarrhea, drainage from an intestinal fistula, and other extrarenal losses of sodium may also cause a problem of excess losses. Without replacement therapy, the volume of water in the extracellular space or the sodium concentration in all extracellular water (including plasma) or both may fall, leading to dehydration, shock, and death.

TABLE 8-6   ESTIMATED SAFE AND ADEQUATE DAILY DIETARY INTAKES OF SODIUM, POTASSIUM, AND CHLORIDE

		Sodium		Potassium		Chloride	
	Age, years	mg	meq	mg	meq	mg	meq
Infants	0 –0.5	115– 350	5–15.2	350– 925	8.9– 23.7	275– 700	7.8– 19.7
	0.5– 1	250– 750	10.9– 32.6	425–1275	10.9– 32.7	400–1200	11.3– 33.8
Children	1 – 3	325– 975	14.1– 42.4	550–1650	14.1– 34.6	500–1500	14.1– 42.3
	4 – 6	450–1350	19.6– 58.7	775–2325	19.9– 59.6	700–2100	19.7– 59.2
Adolescents	7 – 10	600–1800	26.1– 78.3	1000–3000	25.6– 76.9	925–2775	26.1– 78.2
	11 +	900–2700	39.1–117.4	1525–4575	39.1–117.3	1400–4575	42.0–118.3
Adults		1100–3300	47.8–143.5	1875–5625	48.1–144.2	1700–5100	47.9–143.7

Source: **Food and Nutrition Board,** Recommended Dietary Allowances, rev. 9th ed., National Academy of Sciences, Washington, D. C., 1980.

Potassium

Distribution in the Body

Potassium is the chief cation in the intracellular compartment. There is approximately 164 meq of potassium per L of intracellular fluid. In the extracellular compartment, potassium is present in small amounts, 5 meq per L; however, the cation is very significant for maintenance of body process and survival. The body contains a total of 3200 meq of cellular potassium, and only 70 meq of potassium in the extracellular fluid. Since potassium is the predominant cation of cells, its distribution among the organs of the body is related to their cell number. Retention of this potassium is associated with an increase in the lean body mass, and the total-body counting of the naturally occurring radioactive isotope of potassium, ^{40}K, is an indirect measure of the total body potassium.

Balance Mechanism

The minimum amount of potassium that the body can function with is approximately 30 meq, while the maximum load is approximately 400 meq per day. Normally, 90 percent of the potassium intake is excreted in the urine; stool and sweat losses are less than 10 meq per day. In the adult body, the potassium intake and output are in equilibrium. However, a positive balance is necessary for children, to increase their cellular growth and expand the intracellular fluid compartment. There is always an obligatory potassium loss even with negligible intake. In contrast to sodium ions, which are completely reabsorbed when the plasma sodium level is low, the reabsorption of potassium ions from renal tubules does not increase when the plasma potassium level is low. Normally, reabsorption of potassium from the glomerular filtrate takes place in the proximal tubules and some potassium is secreted into the urine in the distal part of the tubules. The average serum potassium levels are maintained between 3.5 and 5.5 meq per L.

The chief function of extracellular potassium is to control cardiac function and muscle and nerve irritability. The heart muscle is subject to injury if the serum potassium is outside the range of 3 to 7 meq per L. Intracellular potassium is essential in many cellular enzymatic functions, such as glycogen synthesis and glucose degradation, and in amino acid uptake. In homeostasis, the total-body potassium and the extracellular potassium remain relatively constant. Since potassium can enter cells easily, the potassium of the liver, kidneys, lungs, gastrointestinal tract, and muscle is exchanged rapidly.

Potassium Intake and Dietary Sources

The dietary intake of potassium must be adequate to maintain electrolyte balance in the body. Potassium is widely distributed in milk, meats, fruits, and vegetables, and the usual intake is somewhere between 50 and 150 meq (1.9 to 5.8 g) per day. It is estimated that adults need approximately 64.1 meq (2.5 g) per day of potassium and children, according to their age, need between 25 and 100 meq (0.98 to 3.9 g) per day. The Recommended Dietary Allowances (1980) give the requirements for different ages (see Table 8-6).

Potassium supplementation must be administered with care when potassium deficiency occurs. This can result from low potassium intake or from excessive losses due to diarrhea, diabetic acidosis, other disease states, or use of drugs such as diuretics, steroids, and purgatives.

Clinical Application

Potassium deficiency can cause structural and functional changes in the intestines, myocardium, kidney, tubules, pancreas, and liver. Under abnormal conditions, causing cellular breakdown, such as hemolysis, acidosis, and starvation, potassium moves from the intracellular fluid compartment to the extracellular fluid compartment, and potassium losses can result from renal as well as extrarenal origin. Renal losses can be exaggerated by diuresis, acidosis, renal tubular damage, or excessive secretion of adrenocortical hormone, as occurs in

Cushing's syndrome. Extrarenal losses usually take the form of vomiting, diarrhea, and intestinal fistula drainage. Usually the loss of potassium from the upper gastrointestinal tract is insignificant. However, losses from the lower gastrointestinal tract may be considerable in abnormal conditions.

Chloride

Distribution in the Body

Chloride is the predominant anion in the extracellular fluid compartment, providing two-thirds of the anions in the plasma. It is almost entirely absent within cells and occurs mainly in combination with sodium. The extracellular fluid compartment normally contains about 80 percent of the body chloride. The plasma normally contains 100 to 110 meq per L and the red blood cells about 58 meq per L. The principal role of chloride is to regulate the osmotic pressure and water content of the body. It is also the predominant component in the gastric juice. The chloride anion acts as a coenzyme for digestive amylases. It helps to buffer the acid-base balance of blood by exchange of chloride from the plasma for bicarbonate from the red blood cells.

Balance Mechanism

The plasma chloride level is affected only slightly by the ingestion of chloride; it decreases about 2 meq per L at the height of gastric secretion because of the need to produce hydrochloric acid. Approximately twice the quanity of chloride present in the plasma is secreted daily in the gastric juice and is reabsorbed again.

In healthy adults the chloride intake and output are in equilibrium. Normally more than 90 percent of the body chloride is excreted in the urine, the remainder mostly in the feces and sweat. But a positive balance is necessary for children in order to expand the extracellular fluid compartment. The rate of urinary chloride excretion depends on the chloride intake and the water balance. The retention of chloride occurs readily during periods of fluid retention (edema).

Chloride Intake and Dietary Sources

Most dietary chloride is derived from dairy products and meat with some from vegetables and fruit. The chloride content of foods is roughly proportional to the sodium content and inversely proportional to the potassium content. The daily intake is about 60 to 100 meq (3.5 to 5.9 g).

Human milk provides about 11 meq per L and infant formulas must be formulated to provide this amount. Reports of adverse effects of a chloride-deficient formula with failure to thrive and hypochloremic metabolic alkalosis led to the August 1979 recall of two infant formulas (Neo-Mull-Soy and Cho-Free) by Syntex laboratories, Palo Alto, California. Most infants who developed metabolic alkalosis were using these formulas as their sole source of nutrition for at least 2 months. When chloride was replaced and another formula was used, the infants recovered and did not show signs of severe developmental disability. The Center for Disease Control is collaborating with the National Institutes of Health in a follow-up study of infants who developed metabolic alkalosis after consuming the chloride-deficient formulas. During the 1978–1979 period when the chloride-deficient formulas were produced approximately 120 infants were identified with metabolic alkalosis. (See below.)

Clinical Application

Starvation, fever, vomiting, diarrhea, and excessive sweating will lower the urinary chloride output. When the plasma chloride is low, the urinary excretion of chloride is markedly decreased except in adrenal cortical insufficiency. Deficit of adrenocortical hormone increases the chloride output by interfering with tubular reabsorption of chloride. In abnormal conditions such as starvation, fever, diarrhea, excessive vomiting, and excessive sweating there is a decrease in the plasma chloride. As with the marked loss of potassium, the marked loss of chloride can result in hypokalemic alkalosis for the following reasons: If there is a decrease in the chloride concentration in the extracellular fluid, there is a concomitant increase in the bicarbonate concentration, which leads to the state of alkalosis. Since the availability of chloride ions as anions to accompany sodium is limited, the reabsorption of sodium is diminished. However, there is a mechanism for the reabsorption of sodium without chloride, known as the *exchange mechanism*, whereby there is an accelerated excretion of potassium in the urine in exchange for sodium reabsorption without chloride ions. Therefore, in replacement therapy, if potassium is supplied without chloride, hypokalemic alkalosis may persist. Chloride supplementation in addition to the potassium is needed to correct hypokalemic alkalosis (see below).

Acid-Base Balance

Water and electrolytes act together within the body to maintain the acid-base balance.

The acidity or alkalinity of a substance or a solution is determined by the concentration of hydrogen ions. The more hydrogen ions present, the more a solution is acid; a decrease in hydrogen ions makes the solution more alkaline or basic. The degree of acidity is expressed by the symbol *pH*. The pH of a solution is defined as the negative logarithm of the hydrogen ion concentration. The definition is based on the fact that the quantity of hydrogen ions present in a solution is best expressed mathematically as a negative logarithm, since the weight of hydrogen in water is about one ten millionth of a gram per liter (0.0000001 or 10^{-7} g). Therefore, a hydrogen ion concentration of 0.0000001 g per L equals 10^{-7} g per L or a pH of 7.

A solution with a *pH of 7* is at the neutral point between an acid and a base because at that concentration the number of hydrogen ions (H^+) is in equilibrium with the number of basic or hydroxyl ions (OH^-). Because of the use of a negative "log," an acid solution has a pH below 7 and a basic solution has a pH greater than 7.

Buffer Systems

The body, through a buffer system (see Figure 8-3), maintains the extracellular fluid within a narrow pH range of 7.35 to 7.45. The buffer system involves certain combinations of chemicals in the extracellular fluid which can act as buffers or protectors against changes in the hydrogen ion concentration. The importance of this system lies in the fact that the chemical processes of living cells are exceedingly sensitive to changes in pH.

A *buffer* is a substance capable of maintaining the relative concentration of hydrogen and hydroxyl ions in a solution by neutralizing within limits and offsetting rapid changes. It is a mixture of acidic and alkaline components which are protective against either added acid or base. When a strong acid is added to a buffered solution, the base component of the acid-base buffer combines with the added acid to form a weaker acid. Similarly, when a strong base is added to the buffered solution, the acid compo-

Figure 8-3

The buffer system of the body, which maintains a ratio of 1 part carbonic acid to 20 parts bicarbonate (1:20). (Adapted from *Fluid and Electrolytes; Some Practical Guides to Clinical Use,* Abbott Laboratories, North Chicago, May 1969, p. 23.)

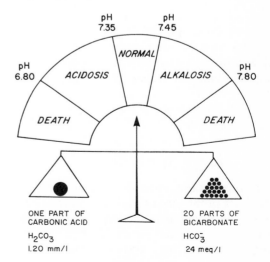

nent of the acid-base buffer donates ionized hydrogen to form a weaker base and restore the pH.

Although there are several buffer systems in the human body, the most important one in the extracellular fluid is the *carbonic acid–sodium bicarbonate system* (H_2CO_3-$NaHCO_3$). Under normal conditions a ratio of 1 part carbonic acid to 20 parts bicarbonate is present (1:20).

When the extracellular environment becomes more acid, the buffer system activates. The bicarbonate ions alkalize, since they have an affinity for hydrogen ions, binding them, removing them from solution, and thereby neutralizing or buffering the effect of the acid. This is observed in the following reaction:

$$H^+Cl^- + Na^+HCO_3^- \rightarrow Na^+Cl^- + H_2CO_3$$

Hydro-   Sodium   Salt   Carbonic
chloric   bicarbonate   acid
acid

These events cause the bicarbonate/carbonic acid ratio to become altered, giving an acid pH. The carbonic acid formed is excreted via the lungs as carbon dioxide—the depth and rate of breathing increase to exhale more carbon dioxide and control the level of carbonic acid in the blood:

$$H_2CO_3 \xrightarrow{\text{carbonic anhydrase}} CO_2 + H_2O$$

This increased exhalation of carbon dioxide decreases the raw material for carbonic acid production, while the decreased level of sodium bicarbonate signals the renal tubules to reabsorb sodium. Both of these mechanisms serve to restore the 1:20 ratio of the buffer system; i.e., 1 part carbonic acid to 20 parts bicarbonate.

Disturbances in Acid-Base Balance

Disturbances of the acid-base balance consist of major shifts in the electrolyte patterns related to failure of the compensatory responses of the buffer system, the lungs, or the kidneys. The resulting conditions are referred to clinically as *acidosis,* in which an increase in hydrogen ion concentration causes a shift in pH to an acidic medium, or *alkalosis,* the opposite state, in which the hydrogen ion concentration is below normal, causing a shift in pH to a basic medium.

The disturbances of the acid-base balance of the body are characterized according to their origin: imbalances caused by failure of the lungs are either respiratory acidosis or respiratory alkalosis; imbalances caused by failure of the renal system are either metabolic acidosis or metabolic alkalosis.

Acid-base disturbances are differentiated by determining three components of the blood: (1) the respiratory component, plasma carbon dioxide pressure or P_{CO_2} (normal range 35 to 45 mmHg); (2) the metabolic component, plasma bicarbonate or HCO_3 (normal range 22 to 26 meq per L); and (3) the blood pH (normal 7.40; normal range 7.35 to 7.45).

Acidosis and Alkalosis

Respiratory Acidosis
Respiratory acidosis is due to disturbances in regulatory mechanisms in the respiratory center, or to disorders of muscles involved in respiration, or to diseases of the lungs such as emphysema. These conditions cause a retention of carbon dioxide (CO_2), with an increase in the partial pressure of CO_2 (P_{CO_2}) and carbonic acid (H_2CO_3) and a decrease in pH.

Respiratory Alkalosis
Respiratory alkalosis is due to hyperventilation, which causes a decreased arterial P_{CO_2} and an elevated pH. It is associated with many stressful conditions. Hyperventilation also results from many hypermetabolic states. It is common in gram-negative sepsis and peritonitis, salicylate poisoning, and encephalitis.

Metabolic Acidosis
Metabolic acidosis is due to a loss of base resulting from disorders of either the kidney or the gastrointestinal tract. Causes include the accumulation of acidic compounds in the extracellu-

lar fluid, such as occurs in lactic acid acidosis of diabetes, and renal failure involving retention of phosphates, sulfates, and organic acid anions as a result of the kidney's inability to regenerate bicarbonate. Metabolic acidosis also occurs with improper use of parenteral hyperalimentation solutions, in other diseases causing loss of bicarbonates from extracellular fluids and in renal tubular acidosis, which causes abnormal loss of bicarbonate from renal tubules. Loss of small intestinal secretions from fistulas, vomiting, and diarrhea may also induce metabolic acidosis.

Metabolic Alkalosis

Metabolic alkalosis is due to a loss of acid by either the renal or the gastrointestinal route. Examples of diseases due to gastrointestinal loss are pyloric obstruction and loss of hydrochloric acid from the stomach via a gastric tube. Metabolic alkalosis of renal origin is usually caused by loss of potassium from the kidney. Diuretics, which are used in many different diseases, are likely to cause this problem.

CLINICAL APPLICATIONS

Principles of Electrolyte Therapy

When the normal oral route is insufficient to replace fluid and electrolyte substances as a result of surgery, dehydration, or severe burns, parenteral fluid therapy must be instituted. This therapy is based on the principles of providing the body with optimal amounts of water and a suitable mixture of electrolytes in order to either maintain water and electrolyte balance or replace frank losses. The principles discussed above under the sections on body water distribution, electrolyte composition of fluid compartments, and acid-base balance become operational in considering replacement therapy.

Each patient requires a special therapeutic formulation to meet specific needs, which must be closely monitored and reevaluated on a daily basis. The average daily maintenance requirements of sodium, water, potassium, and glucose per square meter of body surface area must be

TABLE 8-7 AVERAGE DAILY MAINTENANCE REQUIREMENT FOR ELECTROLYTE THERAPY

Nutrient	Amount required per m^2 in 24 h*
Water	200 mL
Sodium	40 meq
Potassium	30 meq
Glucose	100 g

*m^2 = square meter of body surface area.
Source: Adapted from W. Waring and L. Jeansonne, *Practical Manual of Pediatrics*, The C. V. Mosby Company, St. Louis, 1975, p. 218.

considered for parenteral therapy (see Table 8-7, above).

The normally functioning kidney is selectively able to retain or excrete ions as needed and thereby maintain water and electrolyte balance. However, in illness states requiring replacement therapy, the osmolarity of the patient's serum, the urine volume, and the fluid and electrolyte intake must be carefully monitored. A 24-h flow sheet (input-output) is recommended for this purpose.

Dehydration

Dehydration is a consequence of deficits of either water or electrolytes or both water and electrolytes. Two conditions may result: *hypotonic dehydration* or *hypertonic dehydration*. When there is a loss of electrolytes in excess of water, the result is hypotonic dehydration. It is seen in patients with diarrhea whose fluid losses have been replaced with excessive amounts of carbohydrates in water solutions without added electrolytes. When there is a loss of water in excess of electrolytes, the result is hypertonic dehydration.

Infants are particularly sensitive to shifts in fluid and electrolyte balance and are prone to hypertonic dehydration because of their large body surface area and relatively greater evaporative losses. For example, a 1-year-old child weighing 10 kg has a body surface area of 0.50 m², whereas an adult weighing 68 kg has a body surface area of 1.8 m², which is not proportionately higher. (See Appendix for nomogram to determine body surface area.)

Another factor making the infant particularly vulnerable to hypertonic dehydration is that the infant kidney is immature in its ability to concentrate urine. (Infants can concentrate urine only to 553 mosmol per L whereas adults concentrate urine to 1200 mosmol per L.) Also, the fact that infants are totally dependent on others for their fluid intake places them at further risk. This dependency for water is also true for debilitated, elderly, or handicapped patients, all of whom should be closely monitored for signs of dehydration (dry parched lips, scant and thick saliva, reduced urine output), especially during states of fever or illness.

STUDY QUESTIONS

1 What is the role of water within the human body?

2 How is water distributed within the body and what are the influences on the pattern of distribution?

3 Does water intake equal water losses on a daily basis? Describe.

4 What are the rules of the kidney, lungs, skin, and gastrointestinal tract in regulating the body's fluid and electrolyte balance?

5 How does the body maintain the extracellular fluid within a narrow pH range of 7.35 to 7.45?

CLINICAL STUDY 8

A 7-month-old male infant with moderate dehydration and lethargy was brought to the emergency ward for therapy. The parents reported that on the advice of their physician, they had been treating a 7-day bout of infantile diarrhea with boiled skim milk, which they had been giving the infant for 2 days.

On physical examination the infant was found to be lethargic and semicomatose, with dry mouth and parched lips. Admission weight was 6.3 kg, which represented a weight loss of 0.7 kg, or 10 percent of body weight. Laboratory analysis revealed the following:

blood urea nitrogen	*40 mg per 100 mL (average, 8 to 18 mg per 100 mL)*
serum sodium	*159 meq per L (average, 134 to 145 meq per L)*
serum potassium	*5.5 meq per L (average, 3.5 to 5 meq per L)*
serum chloride	*110 meq per L (average, 98 to 100 meq per L)*
serum bicarbonate	*15 meq per L (average, 25 meq per L)*
urinary specific gravity, with collection by catheter	*1.027 (average, 1.018)*

Clinical study questions

1 *List those factors involved in precipitating hypertonic dehydration.*

2 *How does the body respond to hypertonic dehydration?*

3 *How would you monitor the effectiveness of the fluid and electrolyte therapy?*

BIBLIOGRAPHY

Black, D. A. K.: *Essentials of Fluid Balance,* 4th ed., Blackwell Scientific Publication, Oxford, 1969.

Bland, John, H. (ed.): *Clinical Metabolism of Body Water and Electrolytes,* W. B. Saunders Company, Philadelphia, 1963.

Christensen, Halvor, N.: *Diagnostic Biochemistry,* Oxford University Press, New York, 1959.

Gamble, James L.: *Chemical Anatomy, Physiology and Pathology of Extracellular Fluid,* 6th ed., Harvard University Press, Cambridge, Mass., 1967.

Goldberger, Emanuel: *A Primer of Water, Electrolyte and Acid-Base Syndromes,* 5th ed., Lea & Febiger, Philadelphia, 1975.

Linshaw, M. A. et al.: "Hypochloremic Alkalosis in Infants Associated with Soy Protein Formula," 635–640, **96**:*Journal of Pediatrics,* April 1980.

Loeb, John N.: "Current Concepts: The Hyperosmolar State," *New England Journal of Medicine,* **290**: 1184, 1974.

Snively, William D., and Michael J. Sweeney: *Fluid Balance Handbook for Practitioners,* Charles C Thomas Publisher, Springfield, Ill., 1956.

Talbot, Nathan B., Richie H. Robert, and Crawford D. John: *Metabolic Homeostatis,* Harvard University Press, Cambridge, Mass., 1959.

Waring, William W., and Louis Jeansonne: *Practical Manual of Pediatrics,* The C. V. Mosby Company, St. Louis, 1975.

Welt, Louis G.: *Clinical Disorders of Hydration and Acid-Base Equilibrium,* Little, Brown and Company, Boston, 1959.

Wolfsdorf, J., and B. Senior: "Failure to Thrive and Metabolic Alkalosis: Adverse Effects of a Chloride-Deficient Formula in Two Infants," *Journal of American Medical Association,* **243**:1068–1070, March 14, 1980.

CLINICAL DISCUSSION 8

The child was diagnosed as having hypertonic dehydration and metabolic acidosis resulting from losses of water, sodium, potassium, and bicarbonate caused by the diarrhea and further complicated by the use of a concentrated high "renal solute load" formula of boiled skim milk. The serum levels of potassium, sodium, and bicarbonate reflect the electrolyte imbalance. The increase in urine specific gravity shows the decrease in extracellular fluid which prompted the hypothalamus to stimulate pituitary secretion of antidiuretic hormone (ADH). In turn, the ADH signaled the kidneys to facilitate the reabsorption of water. However, the extreme losses of electrolytes from the diarrhea were worsened by the use of the concentrated boiled skim milk formula, which has a renal solute load of 308 mosmol per L (whole cow's milk has a renal solute load of 221 mosmol per L). Adequate fluid intake is needed in order to excrete the solute load. Since the infant's body was unable to maintain homeostasis, the infant became dehydrated and developed metabolic acidosis, because of an accumulation of strong acid in the extracellular fluid.

The infant was admitted to the hospital and rehydrated with intravenous therapy. Since 150 mL per kilogram of body weight per day is an infant's normal fluid requirement, fluid replacement of sodium involved giving 15 to 30 meq of sodium per liter of fluid each day, in a 5 percent dextrose solution. Potassium was withheld until adequate fluid volume was assured, and was then added to the intravenous fluid. Replacement therapy was monitored by serum electrolyte levels. The patient was discharged after 4 days, by which time the laboratory findings had returned to normal and the diarrhea had subsided. The parents were advised against the hazards of using a boiled milk formula.

CHAPTER 9

THE BODY'S USE OF FOOD AND NUTRIENTS

Christine Adamow Murray

KEY WORDS
Absorption
Anabolism
Basal Metabolic Rate
Calorie
Catabolism
Digestion
Krebs Cycle
Embden-Meyerhof Glycolytic Pathway
Glycolysis
Gluconeogenesis
Glycogenolysis
Joule
Metabolism

INTRODUCTION

The body's utilization of food is one of the most impressive and important human functions. The nutrients, when allowed to follow an uninterrupted course through the 10 ft of the small intestine and onward to the colon, provide for the building, unkeep, and operation of the body.

Having previously considered the nutrients on an individual basis, we will now examine their interrelationships within the gastrointestinal system. In this chapter the process of nutrient utilization will be considered on the basis of the specific contribution made by each of the various gastrointestinal organs in successive order, so as to help the student follow the common pathway of food from digestion to excretion (see Fig. 9-1). It is important for the student who will become a health professional to recognize the significant contributions of each gastrointestinal organ to the biochemical breakdown and final utilization of food.

This chapter will enable the health professional to understand the processes of digestion, absorption, and metabolism as a whole, as the consequences of food digestion and energy metabolism are discussed and related to body composition. It is with the understanding of an integrated gastrointestinal system that the health professional can conceptually integrate nutrients into the human system and forward the practice of nutrition-centered health care.

INGESTION

The process of digestion begins with the intake of food into the alimentary tract. There are many factors contributing to the individual's selection of foods that ultimately affect the body's nutritional status. Food availability, eye appeal, cultural preferences, and taste—all influence the daily nutrient intake.

Four primary groups of taste buds, located on the papillae of the tongue (Fig. 9-2), enable an individual to perceive the tastes of sweet, sour, salty, and bitter. With these four basic

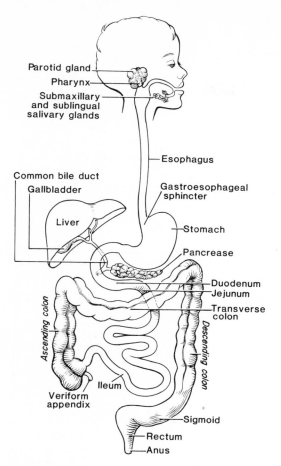

Figure 9-1
The gastrointestinal system.

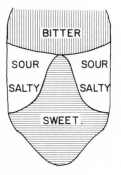

Figure 9-2
Primary sets of taste buds.

tastes an individual is able to perceive hundreds of taste combinations. The number of taste buds increases slightly during childhood to become representative of a variety of tastes, and declines after the age of 45. During the adult years there are over 10,000 taste receptors located along the entire surface of the tongue.

Mouth

The primary mechanical action occurring in the oral cavity is the mastication of ingested food. Through the grinding bilateral motion of the teeth, food particles are broken into smaller units and mixed with saliva. The process of digestion begins at this point because saliva contains the starch-splitting enzyme, salivary amylase. This enzyme is secreted in response to the presence of food as an unconditioned reflex. It has been shown that the conscious act of thinking about food can also trigger its secretions as a conditioned response. Salivary amylase acts on starch molecules to produce units of maltose, a simple sugar, in the presence of the optimal oral pH of 6.9. However, as with all enzyme-catalyzed reactions, the length of time that the enzyme is in contact with the substrate will significantly affect the degree of starch breakdown that occurs in the oral cavity. Therefore, the longer the mastication time, the greater the degree of starch degradation taking place in the mouth.

However, the amount of time that food is actually chewed depends on a multitude of variables. The nature of the food, the amount of conversation, individual habit, and early training all contribute to the mastication time and eventually to the extent of starch breakdown in the oral cavity.

Following mastication, involuntary reflex actions close the passages going from the pharynx to the nose and trachea, allowing the swallowing reflex to initiate the passage of food to the esophagus.

Swallowing can be started at will or by the stimulation of a number of areas in the mouth and pharynx.

The preformed food mixture is now able to proceed towards the antrum of the stomach via the esophagus. The esophagus utilizes strong muscular contractions to propel the food mass through its length to the stomach. At the lower end of the esophagus the muscle is slightly hypertrophied to form the gastroesophageal constriction. This muscle allows for passage of the swallowed food into the stomach and prevents reflux of the stomach contents into the upper esophagus where the acid gastric secretions could damage the esophageal mucosa.

DIGESTION

Stomach

The gastric mucosa resembles the foothills of a large mountain range. The stomach's interior is heaped in folds and ridges which contribute significantly to the process of digestion. Closer examination of the mucosa reveals column-shaped cells, called *columnar epithelial cells*. A microscopic view of these cells reveals the presence of tiny pores leading to the gastric glands from which the gastric secretions that are responsible for aiding digestion arise. These secretions are the products of the parietal, chief, and mucous gastric cells (see Fig. 9-3). Each of these cells is specific for its contribution to digestion.

Figure 9-3
Gastric gland showing cells responsible for gastric secretions. (Adapted from A. C. Guyton, *Textbook of Medical Physiology*, W. B. Saunders, Philadelphia, 1976.)

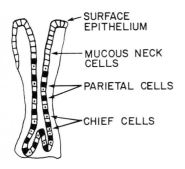

SURFACE EPITHELIUM

MUCOUS NECK CELLS

PARIETAL CELLS

CHIEF CELLS

Parietal cells   The parietal cells rising from the glandular mucosal lining of the stomach are the production sites of hydrochloric acid. The normal stomach contains sufficient hydrochloric acid to produce a pH of 1 or an acid medium many times more acidic than lemon juice. The production of this acid, a complicated process, is stimulated by the gastrointestinal hormone, gastrin, upon distention of the stomach by food. Davenport reported that the body uses 324 kcal (1360.8 kJ) to produce the normal hydrochloric acid content found in the stomach at 1 h after a meal.[1] Hydrochloric acid is fundamental in the digestive process by acting to:

1   Partially split some glucose molecules from starch
2   Slightly alter the condition of fats and proteins in preparation for further action by other digestive enzymes
3   Activate the transformation of pepsinogen to active pepsin, a protein-digesting enzyme

Chief cells   The gastric mucosa also produces enzymes that digest protein and certain fats. Pepsin is the major protein-digesting (proteolytic) enzyme and is manufactured in the chief cells of the gastric mucosa. Pepsin breaks down large protein molecules to form peptides (see Chap. 3). This enzyme relies on the acid medium of the stomach for its proteolytic action. In the absence of the hydrochloric acid, pepsin is relatively inactive and very little protein digestion will occur.[2]

Besides producing pepsin, the lining of the stomach secretes gastric lipase. This enzyme acts principally on fats containing short- and medium-chain fatty acids (see Chap. 5), yielding smaller units of short-chain or free fatty acids. The stomach contains no enzymes specific for carbohydrate digestion. However, a negligible amount of starch digestion can occur in the stomach from swallowed salivary amylase or regurgitated pancreatic amylase.

Mucous cells   The mucous cells of the stomach produce another important gastric product, mucus. Mucus creates the slimy, slippery appearance of the gastric lining and seems to be a protective element. It is believed to lubricate the mucosal surface of the stomach and to protect the stomach from harmful irritants.

Gastric digestion relies not only on biochemical reactions, but also on various mechanical actions of the stomach wall. Immediately upon entry of food particles into the stomach cavity, tonus or mixing waves move along the stomach wall to help the gastric secretions combine with the stomach's contents. Besides these mixing waves, strong peristaltic movements occur in the gastric musculature which squeeze the partially digested food particles toward the body of the stomach. Once the food has become mixed with the gastric secretions it is called *chyme*. Chyme has a murky, milky color and a semifluid consistency.

Stomach emptying is aided by peristaltic waves moving from the stomach to the duodenum. Opposition to passage of the food is created by the pylorus. However, the creation of a pressure gradient and certain tonic contractions allow for emptying of the chyme from the stomach cavity into the duodenum.

Gastric emptying is regulated by neural and hormonal controls as well as by the physical properties of the chyme. Additional factors affecting the rate of emptying are:

Particle size
Viscosity of the chyme
Osmotic pressure
Gastric acidity
Gastric volume

Monosaccharides tend to pass through the stomach quickly in proportion to their duodenal osmolarity, while complex carbohydrates such as cellulose (a polysaccharide providing bulk in the normal diet) pass through the gut most rapidly because of the body's inability to break down the molecule's organic bond. (See Chap. 3.) In contrast, protein molecules increase the release of the hormones gastrin and cholecystokinin, which tends to inhibit gastric motility. However, fatty meals tend to empty from the stomach most slowly because they stimulate mucosal production of enterogastrone. This hormone is absorbed into the blood and within minutes inhibits gastric motility, thereby slowing the stomach's emptying time and prolonging the digestion time of fats in the small intestine. It is for this reason that meals high in fat are said to have a high satiety value.

Pancreas, Liver, Gallbladder, and Small Intestine

The digestive process proceeds toward the small intestine, where the pancreatic duct supplies the duodenum with enzymes for protein, fat, and carbohydrate breakdown. The pancreas is stimulated by the hormones secretin, cholecystokinin, and pancreozymin to produce several important digestive enzymes. These enzymes act on the partially digested nutrients to prepare them for the absorption process in the small bowel.

Two pancreatic enzymes, hydrolase and cholesterol esterase, which act on the esters of glycerol and cholesterol respectively, depend on bile salts for their action. The liver is weakly stimulated by the hormone secretin to secrete bile. Cholecystokinin stimulates the gallbladder to contract and allow the flow of bile to mix with the contents of the duodenum. These hormones are synthesized by the intestine and are released when the contents of the stomach pass to the duodenum. In the duodenum, bile acts as an emulsifying agent, improving the solubility of fat molecules and thus aiding the process of fat absorption. The major components of bile are conjugated bile acids, bile salts, pigments, and cholesterol. Bile salts act as detergents that contain both fat- and water-attracting regions. Their action in fat and cholesterol digestion is to allow these nutrients to form a complex called a *micelle*. This micellar complex allows the otherwise insoluble fat and cholesterol molecules to enter into aqueous solution, thereby facilitating their uptake by cells of the intestinal wall (see Table 9-1, p. 172).

TABLE 9-1 DIGESTIVE ENZYMES AND SECRETIONS RESPONSIBLE FOR THE BIOCHEMICAL DEGRADATION OF PROTEIN, FAT, AND CARBOHYDRATE

Site	Secretion	Substrate	Product
Oral cavity	Salivary amalyse (ptylin)	Starch	Maltose
Stomach	Hydrochloric acid	Pepsinogen	Pepsin
	Pepsin	Protein	Peptides
	Gastric lipase	Fat	Medium-chain triglycerides and short-chain fatty acids
Pancreas	Trypsin	Protein, polypeptides	Smaller polypeptides
	Chymotrypsin	Protein, polypeptides	Smaller polypeptides
	Carboxypeptidases	Polypeptides	Lower peptides and amino acids
	Amylase	Starch	Dextrins
	Lipase	Fats	Monoacylglycerols, fatty acids, and glycerols
	Cholesterase	Cholesterol	Cholesterol esters with fatty acids
Gallbladder, liver	Bile	Unemulsified fats	Micelle

Gastrointestinal Flora

Normally, there are approximately 10^{14} living bacterial cells in the gut.[3] The effect of the gastrointestinal flora in the digestion-absorption process is often overlooked.

The most commonly found enteric bacteria are anaerobic streptococci, gram-positive bacilli, gram-negative cocci, and gram-negative bacilli. These bacteria inhabit the lower small intestine of humans and are found embedded in the mucus attached to the intestinal mucosa. However, they are found in significant numbers only in the large intestine.

The gastrointestinal tract is sterile at birth but becomes inhabited by bacteria via the oral route within the first few days of life. The diet is the principal determinant of the type of bacteria that will inhabit the gastrointestinal tract. All surfaces of the human body are covered with a normal flora population which has been shown to be stable in composition. Relatively lit-

tle is known concerning the control of this population on the body's surface, including the gastrointestinal colonies.

Moore and Holdeman have reported the presence of 400 to 500 different kinds of bacteria in the feces of the population studied.[4] Their study indicated the existence of a strong interaction between the microenvironment and mechanisms by which one bacterial population controls the growth of others.

Intestinal bacteria are responsible for the production of several enzymes involved in the digestive and absorptive process. Many members of the body's normal bacterial flora produce fatty acids and carbon dioxide and are responsible for the formation of flatus in the gut and lower gastrointestinal tract. The gastrointestinal flora also serves as a catalyst in the production of bile acids and in the intermediate stages of carbohydrate and fat digestion.

Colonic bacteria are capable of producing

vitamin K and several of the B complex vitamins. *Staphylococcus aureus,* a common gastrointestinal inhabitant, is responsible for the synthesis of vitamin K. Vitamin K injections are necessary for newborn infants because they lack an intestinal flora at birth and therefore lack vitamin K, which is needed to prevent hemorrhages.

The presence of bacteria has also been shown to alter the mucosal structure of the intestinal wall. In animals raised in a sterile environment, the intestinal wall appears thinner and lighter in composition when compared to the thicker mucosal structure of the bacteria-inhabited gastrointestinal tract of ordinary animals. Nutritional and environmental factors affect the normal intestinal flora and can affect the resulting function of the inhabited gastrointestinal structure. One of the frequent side effects of antibiotic therapy is sterilization of the bowel. Research is underway to determine the level of antibiotic ingestion that is necessary to effect a change in the gastrointestinal population resulting from the action of these drugs on the gastrointestinal flora. At present, there are few data citing the limits of antibiotic usage that will result in decreasing the bacterial colonization of the lower gastrointestinal tract.

Shapiro showed that a yogurt supplement containing *Lactobacillus bulgarius* and *Staphylococcus thermophilus* can aid in restoring the physiological balance and bacterial colonization of the small bowel after extensive antibiotic therapy in some disease states.[5] The implications of extensive antibiotic use and its effect on the intestinal bacterial flora remain of concern in long-term antibiotic therapy.

Currently, the extensive use of enteral nutrition support raises many questions on the effect of liquid formula diets on the bacterial colonization of the gut.[6] Early studies using a glucose-based defined formula diet demonstrated a significant decrease in the quantity and nature of the intestinal bacterial flora. However, subsequent studies have not had similar outcomes. It seems that the decrease in number of intestinal microorganisms is probably related to the decrease in stool volume and frequency resulting from extended use of liquid diets. The significance of the alterations in gut flora as well as the change in stool properties is not clearly determined.

Neurohormonal Control of Digestion

Until now, digestion has been viewed in this chapter as a chemical and mechanical process utilizing the secretions and muscular actions of the pancreas, liver, gallbladder, and stomach. Four hormones have been identified as the initiators of enzyme secretions—gastrin, cholecystokinin, pancreozymin, and secretin. It is also important to understand the significant neurohormonal control that is exerted on the digestive process.

The complex interconnections between the cerebral cortex, hypothalamus, and vagus nerve have been explored by Go and Summerskill.[7] The homeostasis of the digestive process is shown to be coordinated by both local and central mechanisms while being modified by neural, hormonal, and metabolic relationships.

The process of digestion becomes an integrated process by virtue of impulses transmitted via the vagus nerve which regulate the gastrointestinal secretions that are ultimately responsible for the digestive process. These impulses arise from the ventral medial center of the hypothalamus (believed to be the center of satiety) in response to blood sugar levels, initiating a feeling of hunger when the blood sugar level is below normal. In response to the hypoglycemia, secretion of insulin and glucagon are regulated by the pancreas, and gastrointestinal secretions begin urging the initiation of eating.

The presence of food in the gut as well as vagal stimulation initiates the secretion of the hormones gastrin from the gastric mucosa and secretin, cholecystokinin, and pancreozymin from the intestinal mucosa. The central nervous system and gastrointestinal system influence each other by vagal efferent and afferent pathways, resulting in the secretion of these gastrointestinal hormones.

These hormones in turn are responsible for stimulation of the stomach, intestine, liver, gallbladder, and pancreas to produce the specific enzymes that are necessary to further the breakdown of nutrients in the gut. Thus the integrated mechanisms of hunger, ingestion, and digestion are regulated.

Bearing in mind the relationship between the neural cortical centers and hormone secretions, it becomes clear that digestion can be significantly affected by a disturbance in the delicate neural biochemistry. Stress, anxiety, fatigue, and illness can alter vagal control of the

gastrointestinal secretion and may thereby interrupt the dynamics of the digestive process. Therefore, in order to understand how the digestive process contributes to a homeostatic milieu, the role of the brain in relation to the process of food utilization must not be overlooked (see Fig. 9-4).

ABSORPTION

Stomach

Very little absorption takes place in the stomach. It functions rather as an organ of preparation for the digestion and absorption that are carried out in the gut.

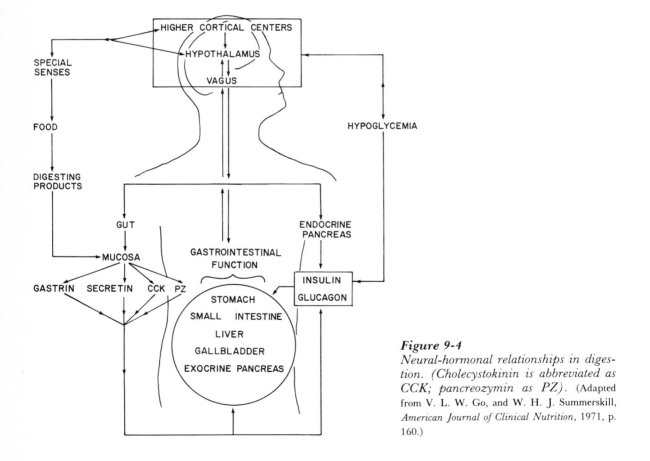

Figure 9-4

Neural-hormonal relationships in digestion. (Cholecystokinin is abbreviated as CCK; pancreozymin as PZ). (Adapted from V. L. W. Go, and W. H. J. Summerskill, *American Journal of Clinical Nutrition,* 1971, p. 160.)

Small Intestine
(Small Bowel)

The small bowel is the primary site of nutrient absorption. It is approximately 300 cm (10 ft) long; however, its absorbing surface is larger than one-third of a football field. The large absorptive surface of the small bowel is due mainly to its mucosal structure. The exterior, or serosal, surface of the small intestine appears smooth. However, the inside luminal or mucosal surface is heaped in folds. On microscopic examination of this irregular mucosal surface, fingerlike projections known as *villi* are evident. When these villi are examined more closely with high-power electron microscopy, the epithelial cells covering these villi are seen to be covered themselves with bristlelike projections known as the *microvilli.* This luminal surface housing the microvilli is known as the *brush border.* The presence of the villi and the microvilli enlarges the potential absorptive surface of the small intestine to an area as much as 600 times greater than the outside serosal area.

The mucosal lining of the small intestine consists of a single layer of columnar epithelial cells that rests on a layer of supporting connective tissue, the *lamina propria.* Figure 9-5 (p. 176) illustrates the structure of the jejunal mucosa, showing the columnar epithelial cells, nuclei, and villi. Note the contribution of the villi to the increased absorptive capacity of the small bowel.

Mucosal Function

The primary function of the small intestine is to absorb the end products of digestion. Once inside the mucosal cell, the nutrients traverse the membrane and are carried through the serosal layer and eventually enter the intestinal fluid. From here, the nutrients are able to pass through the vascular network or lymphatic capillary network for transport to the sites of metabolism.

Mucosal Transport

A knowledge of the various means of molecular transport is important in understanding the passage of nutrient molecules to their sites of absorption and metabolism (see Fig. 9-6). The mucosal cells require special transport systems to accommodate the cellular absorption of nutrient molecules. These transport systems are known as:

Passive diffusion
Bulk flow
Solvent drag
Carrier-mediated diffusion
Active transport
Sodium pump

The six transport systems are discussed in turn in the following paragraphs.

Passive diffusion   Absorption from the duodenum usually occurs by *passive diffusion.* Passive diffusion, or osmotic pressure, allows substances that are small enough in size to pass from one side of a membrane to the other, from an area of greater concentration to one of lesser concentration. Monosaccharides, fat-soluble vitamins, and several water-soluble vitamins pass across the intestinal mucosa via passive diffusion.

Bulk flow   In bulk flow negatively charged ions such as chloride move from an area of higher concentration to an area of lesser concentration in an attempt to equalize the osmotic pressure.

Solvent drag   Some molecules may be small enough to pass through the intestinal mucosal pores, thus utilizing the transport process known as *solvent drag.*

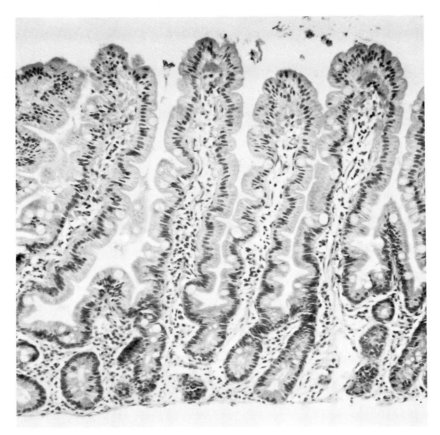

Figure 9-5
Photomicrograph of human jejunal mucosa. Note the tall, fingerlike villi and short crypts (ratio, approximately 4 : 1). The cells lining the villi are columnar, with basally oriented nuclei and an even surface layer. Lamina propria and supporting elements show normal cellularity. (Original magnification × 125. Photo courtesy of Dr. Richard J. Grand.)

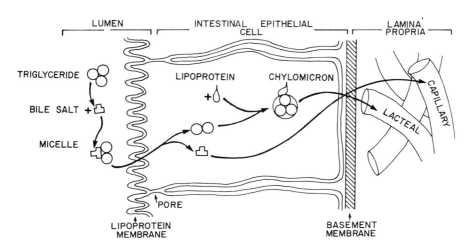

Figure 9-6
Intestinal epithelial absorption.
(Adapted from F. J. Ingelfinger, *Nutrition Today*, 2:3, 1967.)

Carrier-mediated diffusion   Following a meal, when the contents of the intestinal lumen are high in digested carbohydrates and proteins, a means for ferrying these molecules into the blood from the gut is needed. The intestinal epithelium contains a large quantity of carriers that act as ferries to transport these water-soluble complexes through the lipoprotein membrane. Passive diffusion of this type is known as *carrier-mediated diffusion*.

Active transport   Transporting a substance against an electrochemical gradient or other forces is known as *active transport*. It differs from passive transport in that more energy is required to transport materials against a gradient to permit a homeostatic equilibrium of concentration. Although there is much disagreement over which substances rely on active transport, the major nutrients believed to enlist this mechanism include sodium, calcium, iron, glucose, galactose, many amino acids, and vitamin B_{12}.

Sodium pump   The final transport phenomenon to be considered here is the *sodium pump*. Possibly this mechanism is the most crucial of all.

This system has the ability to extract sodium ions from isotonic or even hypotonic salt solutions in the intestinal lumen, in order to move sodium into, through, and out of the intestinal epithelial cell and into the vessels draining the area. The movement of this positively charged ion produces an electrical gradient which allows negatively charged ions to follow. Thus, an osmotic pressure is created, and water molecules move in response to the pressure gradient.

Large Intestine

Most of the ingested water and electrolytes are absorbed in the colon. Sodium and chloride ions are actively absorbed in the proximal half of the colon, creating an osmotic gradient. This osmotic gradient between the intestinal lumen and the plasma is the major determinant of water absorption. The normal colon absorbs approximately 1400 mL of water daily, with the movement of the water molecules closely paralleling movement of the sodium ions that are present.

A few bacteria in the colon are capable of digesting small amounts of cellulose. However, the major portion of ingested cellulose, of hemicellulose, and of other roughage is excreted from the body as the principal component of the feces.

The rectum plays a small part in water and sodium absorption, and is most involved with the process of elimination.

Protein Absorption

(See also Chap. 3.) The intestinal mucosa allows for a small, nutritionally insignificant, amount of large, intact protein molecules to pass into the epithelial cells. Gastric, pancreatic, and intestinal enzymes break large protein molecules into the smaller amino acids. Through active transport, amino acids are absorbed into the intestinal mucosa.

Several factors affect macromolecular transport, as follows:

1   *Presence of localized antibodies.*   Local antibody deficiency may increase the number of large protein molecules that are absorbed. An example can be found in the fish-protein–sensitive individual. When fish protein is ingested by an individual who has developed an antibody to the protein, an allergic reaction to the protein molecule occurs at the site of the antibody, thus blocking the protein molecule and ultimately affecting its absorption.

2 *Anatomy of the intestinal mucosa.* Alterations in the mucosal barrier, such as ulceration, inflammation, or mucosal surface changes, will affect the receptor sites for nutrient absorption and hinder the transport of the large protein molecule.

3 *Physiology of lysosomes.* Lysosomes are composed of hydrolytic enzymes. Normal lysosomal function permits acid hydrolysis of proteins to amino acids and glycogen to glucose. Therefore, lysosomal dysfunction can interefere with the intracellular digestion process and affect the transport of large protein molecules.

4 *Gastric acidity.* Finally, low gastric acidity, pancreatic insufficiency, and other factors can alter the ability of the gut to absorb large nutrient molecules and thus can interfere with the absorption of proteins.

Lipid Absorption

(See also Chap. 5.) Fat absorption is a process involving several interdependent steps. Fat is most often ingested as triglycerides. In the upper small bowel, pancreatic enzymes and secretions split the larger fat molecules into smaller fatty acid units. Bile salts help to emulsify these fatty acids and put them into solution, forming a unit known as a *micelle* for continuation in the absorption process. Once in solution, the fat molecules which are traveling as a micellar complex are able to reach the microvilli of the small intestine. Here the complex splits, the bile salts travel down to be reabsorbed in the distal ileum, and the free fatty acids and monoglycerides are reassembled to form a new triglyceride. To enable the passage of this newly formed triglyceride through the intestinal lumen, a small droplet of a protein called a *beta-lipoprotein* surrounds the fat molecule. The new compound, called a *chylomicron,* is the form that can penetrate the epithelium of the lamina propria, or basement membrane, of the small intestine. The chylomicron enters the lymphatic system via the lamina propria and travels through the portal blood system, completing the process of fat absorption.

Cholesterol absorption (see also Chap. 5) is poorly understood. Cholesterol is usually ingested with fat and requires the pancreatic enzyme cholesterol esterase to emulsify the compound and make it available for absorption via the intestinal lumen. Cholesterol is also synthesized in the intestinal mucosa, which makes absorption studies difficult to execute. There is evidence that cholesterol absorption occurs at a steady rate when dietary intake is moderate but seems to increase with the ingestion of a diet high in fats.

Carbohydrate Absorption

(See also Chap. 4.) Carbohydrate is most often ingested as a disaccharide or polysaccharide. Salivary and pancreatic enzymes break the complex molecules into disaccharides which are then passed on to the intestinal lumen. Because of their still large molecular structure, the partially digested disaccharides are acted on by a variety of disaccharidases found in the microvilli of the intestinal lumen. These enzymes split the molecules into their constituent simple sugars, or monosaccharides—glucose, fructose, and galactose.

Glucose is water-soluble and, despite its large molecular size, is readily transported across the lipoprotein membrane. Other six-carbon sugars can also be absorbed readily because of their ability to pass through the narrow passages of the luminal pore system. Glucose can be absorbed actively or passively, depending on the degree of concentration in the gut. Because of the nature of this transport, glucose is capable of being absorbed even when the concentration of sugar in the blood is relatively high, as in diabetes mellitus.

Once absorbed, the monosaccharides enter the capillary network and circulate throughout the blood system.

Vitamin and Mineral Absorption

It is important to remember that ingestion of a meal will result in the intake of a variety of vitamins and minerals along with the basic nutrients. The small intestine is the site of absorption for these vitamins and minerals, the most active absorptive area being the lower part of the duodenum and the first part of the jejunum (see Table 9-2; also see Chaps. 6, 7, and 8).

METABOLISM

The process of food ingestion, breakdown, and utilization involves a number of biochemical processes aided by enzyme-catalyzed reactions.

TABLE 9-2 SITE OF ABSORPTION OF NUTRIENTS FROM THE GASTROINTESTINAL TRACT

Nutrient	Site of absorption
Glucose	Lower duodenum, upper jejunum
Sucrose	Lower jejunum, ileum
Lactose	Jejunum, upper ileum
Maltose	Jejunum, upper ileum
Amino acids	Lower duodenum, jejunum
Fats	Lower duodenum, upper jejunum
Cholesterol	Lumen of small intestine
Iron	Duodenum (limited absorption), jejunum
Calcium	Duodenum
Vitamin D	Ileum (disputed)
Vitamin A	Duodenum, jejunum
Vitamin E	Duodenum
Vitamin K	Duodenum
Folic acid	Upper duodenum
Pyridoxine	Jejunum
Riboflavin	Duodenum
Thiamin	Duodenum
Ascorbic acid	Jejunum
Water	Colon

It is important to understand that the major outcome of the digestion and absorption process is the production of energy.

In the living cell the nutrients work synergistically in cellular metabolism. Through this metabolic process energy is released and utilized for the synthesis of the cell's own biochemical composition and by-products.

Metabolism is the sum total of all the chemical processes occurring in the body that result in the utilization of ingested food. Energy production is a result of the body's ability to digest, absorb, and finally metabolize nutrients.

The Measurement of Energy

The body's ability to do work and operate its biochemical system is dependent on the production of energy. Energy can be measured in units of heat equivalents. A *calorie* is a unit of heat measurement. In nutritional and physiological studies the traditional unit of heat measurement has been the large calorie or *kilocalorie* (equal to 1000 small calories), which is defined as the amount of heat required to raise 1 kg of water 1°C. In practice, the terms calorie and kilocalorie are used interchangeably as a measure of food energy content.

In the International System of Measurements the *joule* is the unit of energy; 1 calorie (1 kcal) equals 4.184 joules (4.184 kJ). Caloric values of food may be converted to the metric equivalent (joules) by multiplying the number of calories by 4.184. For example: 1 g of carbohydrate contains 4 kcal or approximately 17 kJ.

Through the use of an instrument known as a bomb calorimeter, energy values have been determined for a large variety of foodstuffs. A specific amount of food is placed in the inner center of the calorimeter and the instrument is submerged in water. In the presence of oxygen, the food is ignited and burned. The water surrounding the food chamber increases in temperature during the combustion process, signifying the number of calories obtained through the oxidation of the food.

With this process, the *fuel factor,* or average number of calories per gram of nutrient, has been established for each of the three energy-producing nutrients and for alcohol:

1 g of carbohydrate	= 4 calories (kcal)
	= 17 joules (kJ)
1 g of protein	= 4 kcal
	= 17 kJ

1 g of fat	= 9 kcal
	= 37.6 kJ
1 g of alcohol	= 7 kcal
	= 29.3 kJ

CATABOLISM

Catabolism is the metabolic process involving the breakdown of molecules, resulting in the release of energy. Figure 9-7 shows the interrela-

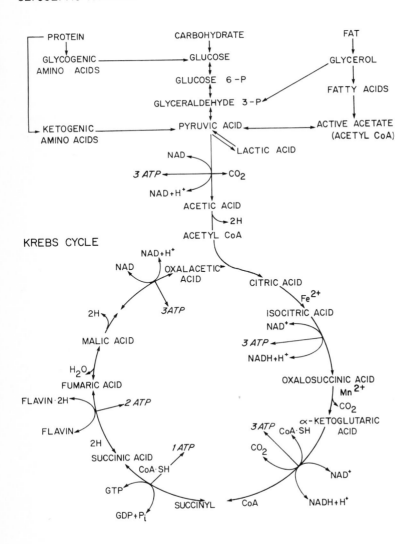

EMBDEN-MEYERHOF GLYCOLYTIC PATHWAY

KREBS CYCLE

Figure 9-7

Interrelationships between the two energy-producing cycles—the Embden-Meyerhof glycolytic pathway and the Krebs cycle. A total of 38 molecules of ATP (adenosine triphosphate) is produced from the combination of these cycles for every 1 molecule of glucose.

tionships between carbohydrate, protein, and fat during the catabolic process.

These compounds are all processed eventually in the same cycle for the production of energy. This cycle, known as the *Krebs cycle* (or *tricarboxylic acid cycle* or *citric acid cycle*), produces about 90 percent of the body's energy requirements of adenosine triphosphate (ATP). ATP is a high-energy compound which provides the body with an easy source of energy in a stored form.

Several vitamins are needed to catalyze certain reactions within the Krebs cycle:

Pantothenic acid

Niacin

Lipoic acid

Thiamin

Riboflavin

Nutrient catabolism yields 2 molecules of ATP from the Embden-Meyerhof glycolytic pathway and 36 ATP molecules from the electron transport chain for every glucose molecule catabolized. Thus, the body receives a constant supply of chemical energy to maintain its physiological and biochemical functions.

ATP is stored in a small metabolic pool for use as needed. However, because of the body's constant need for energy, there is a rapid turnover in this pool.

All products of endogenous or exogenous metabolism have been shown to be in a state of active turnover. The concept of a metabolic pool has been elaborated in relation to protein metabolism and synthesis.[8] The steady state of flux of all living matter clearly demonstrates the process of the rapid state of turnover of free-circulating amino acids available for anabolism and protein synthesis. Thus, the metabolic pool is the quantity of a substance that is in a state of rapid turnover.

Carbohydrate Catabolism

(See also Chap. 4.) Glucose is converted through a series of biochemical reactions from a 6-carbon sugar to pyruvic acid, allowing entry of this molecule into the energy-producing Krebs cycle. This sequence of catabolic reactions, referred to as *glycolysis,* results in the release of energy and the production of pyruvic acid. In this process of glycolysis, two molecules of the high-energy compound ATP are used and four are produced, with the net gain of two molecules available for immediate use. The pyruvic acid, under aerobic conditions (available oxygen), then enters the Krebs cycle. However, when there is insufficient oxygen or under anaerobic conditions such as during heavy exercise, the pyruvic acid is converted to lactic acid and does not enter the Krebs cycle. The lactic acid accumulates in the blood and can be converted back to glucose, mostly in the liver.

Protein Catabolism

(See also Chap. 3.) Early studies have led to the classification of amino acids into two categories according to the type of end products after degradation: those amino acids with glucose as an end product are known as *glycogenic,* whereas those amino acids producing ketone bodies are known as *ketogenic* amino acids (see Table 9-3).

TABLE 9-3 CLASSIFICATION OF AMINO ACIDS FORMED BY CATABOLISM OF PROTEIN

Glycogenic	Ketogenic	Glycogenic and ketogenic
Alanine	Leucine	Isoleucine
Arginine		Lysine
Aspartic acid		Phenylalanine
Cystine		Tyrosine
Glutamic acid		
Glycine		
Histidine		
Hydroxyproline		
Proline		
Serine		
Threonine		
Tryptophan		
Valine		

Glycogenic amino acids are deaminated by coenzyme vitamin B_6 to form pyruvic acid in the Embden-Meyerhof pathway. They may undergo decarboxylation to form acetic acid or they may go through the process of gluconeogenesis to form glucose and glycogen. Gluconeogenesis is the formation of glucose from noncarbohydrate sources. Ketogenic amino acids are processed as fatty acids and are eventually converted to acetyl coenzyme A (acetyl CoA).

Fat Catabolism

Fatty acids undergo a degradation process resulting in the formation of acetyl coenzyme A, allowing entry into the same pathway as carbohydrate.

ANABOLISM

Anabolism is the biochemical process of synthesizing large molecules from small molecules. This process is responsible for the maintenance of body tissue and ultimately for the synthesis of body components. Nutrients in excess of the energy needs of the cells are used for growth, development, and body maintenance.

Glucose is converted to glycogen by the liver and is stored in that organ when there is more glucose in the circulation than can be used by the cells for energy. Glycogen is also stored in muscle tissue and can be used for muscle function during periods of increased exercise or muscular stress that will require increased energy needs. Liver stores of glycogen can be mobilized and converted back to glucose by the process known as glycogenolysis. *Glycogenolysis* is the process resulting in the conversion of glycogen to glucose for eventual entry into the Krebs cycle. In starvation or with energy-deficient diets, liver and muscle stores are mobilized to provide glucose for energy and cellular functioning (see also Chap. 4). Fat stores are also mobilized for energy through the breakdown of lipid molecules. Resynthesis of these molecules to glucose supplies the body with energy when the exogenous supplies of energy are limited.

Glycerol, an intermediate metabolic product of lipid digestion, can enter the Krebs cycle or can be reconverted to glucose or glycogen. Glycogenic amino acids can provide energy through entry into the Krebs cycle or can be converted to glucose for either conversion to glycogen or the production of energy.

The process of *gluconeogensis* (glucose production from a noncarbohydrate source) provides a source of glucose for circulation or for storage or glycogen. However, since glucose production results from the degradation of protein, fats, and carbohydrates, it must be noted that ingesting these nutrients in amounts beyond normal energy demands can result in the increase of glucose in the system. Since all amino acids, carbohydrates, fatty acids, glycerol, and glucose eventually enter the Krebs cycle, the potential for increased lipid synthesis in response to increased nutrient intake is real. The energy that is produced as a result of these nutrients' entering the Krebs cycle will be converted to storage forms of glycogen or fat. Thus, the response to a nutrient intake that is greater than the energy need is the production of adipose tissue as a source of stored energy.

Besides carbon dioxide and water, energy is one of the major metabolic products derived from the utilization of ingested food (Table 9-4). A metabolic homeostasis, with energy input (nutrient intake) equaling energy output (catabolism), results in the maintenance of essential body functions.

BASAL METABOLIC RATE

Energy expenditure can be defined as the metabolic cost of a period of work. This cost can be calculated as gross kilocalories (kilojoules) or net kilocalories (kilojoules). However, the net kilocalories used by the body include two other factors that must be deducted from the net caloric expenditure during a period of work: (1) the basal metabolic rate and (2) the specific dynamic action of food.

The *basal metabolic rate* (BMR) is the energy expended by an awake individual at rest.

TABLE 9-4   FINAL PRODUCTS OF NUTRIENT DIGESTION, ANABOLISM, AND
CATABOLISM

Nutrient	Digestion	Anabolism	Catabolism
Protein	Amino acids	Tissue, enzymes, hormones, fat	CO_2, energy, H_2O urea
Fat	Fatty acids and glycerol	Fat	CO_2, energy, H_2O
Carbohydrate	Monosaccharides	Glycogen and fat	CO_2, energy, H_2O

The BMR requires the individual to be at physical, digestive, and emotional rest. The rate of oxygen consumption can be used as a measure of energy expenditure. Energy costs are most often expressed in kilocalories per minute but can be readily converted to kilocalories per 24 h.

The BMR can be measured by direct or indirect methods or determining oxygen consumption and carbon dioxide expiration per unit of specified time. The individual is required to observe a 12-h fast to ensure that the energy costs of digestion are excluded. With the individual awake and in a reclining position, the oxygen and carbon dioxide status are recorded.

The BMR is influenced by many factors:

Age
Body size
Temperature
Physical exercise
Fever
Specific dynamic action of food

Because of these variables it is difficult to predict the basal metabolic requirements of an individual. However, the BMR is commonly calculated by allowing 24 kcal per kilogram body weight (101 kJ per kilogram body weight) per day:

$$BMR = 24 \text{ kcal} \times \text{weight (kg)/day}$$
$$= 101 \text{ kJ} \times \text{weight (kg)/day}$$

Any condition that increases or decreases the body's expenditure of energy will inevitably reflect a proportionate change in the BMR. Some conditions that alter the BMR are listed in Table 9-5 (p. 184).

Age   Infants' and children's energy requirements increase with growth in size. BMR can be calculated using standardized tables or equations based on body surface area.[9] Energy requirements increase during the first 12 months of life from approximately 30 cal per m^2 per h to approximately 50 cal per m^2 per h by year 2. Basal energy requirements gradually decline to the level of approximately 30 to 40 cal per m^2 per h in adult years. Measurement of body surface which corresponds to approximate heights and weights can be derived through the use of nomograms (Appendix, Fig. A-1).

The basal oxygen consumption per kilogram of body weight decreases approximately 5 to 10 percent every 10 years after age 14. This decrease reflects a general decrease in cellular growth and activity and seems to be at the lowest levels in the elderly population over 65 years of age.

Body size   The relationship between body size and metabolism is an inverse proportion. The smaller the animal the larger the BMR. In early studies done with animals of various sizes, it was found that an indirect relationship existed between metabolism and body weight. However, there seems to be a direct relationship between body surface area and BMR. That is, the larger the organism's surface area the greater the metabolic rate. This seems to be due to the processes

TABLE 9-5   CONDITIONS ALTERING BASAL METABOLIC RATE

Condition	Increase	Possible increase	Decrease	Possible decrease
Increased physical activity	X			
Pregnancy	X			
Fever	X			
Endocrine disorders				
Hyperthyroidism	X			
Hypersecretion of pituitary gland		X		
Cushing's syndrome		X		
Tumors of adrenal glands		X		
Blood diseases				
Leukemia (most often)	X			
Pernicious anemia		X		
Essential hypertension		X		
Myocardial stress	X			
Diabetes insipidus		X		
Shock			X	
Malnutrition			X	
Anemia (severe)				X
Chronic arthritis				X
Peptic Ulcer				X
Nephrotic syndrome (lipid nephrosis)			X	
Endocrine disorders				
Hypothyroidism			X	
Addison's disease				X
Hypopituitarism				X
Nervous system diseases				
Schizophrenia				X
Psychoneurosis				X
Autonomic imbalance (vagotonia)				X

Source: Adapted from A. Cantarow and M. Trumperer, *Clinical Biochemistry,* W. B. Saunders Company, Philadelphia, 1975.

of temperature regulation and heat loss, which are both related to surface area. Therefore, as surface area increases, the BMR increases to compensate for heat loss and to help control body temperature.

Environmental temperature   Exposure to cold increases energy needs in response to the increased need for maintenance of body heat. Studies have shown that the metabolic rates of people living in the arctic are 10 to 20 percent higher than those of people living in tropical areas. This increase reflects an adaptation of the thyroid gland, resulting in increased thyroid secretion in cold climates and decreased secretion in warm climates.

Physical exercise Physical activity increases the BMR in proportion to the type of exercise and the manner in which the activity is undertaken.

Fever Disease and physiological stress increase the BMR 7 percent for every 1°F above the norm. This is because every chemical reaction in vitro or in vivo increases its reaction 130 percent for every rise in temperature of 50°F (10°C). Therefore a body temperature of 105°F (40.5°C) represents a 49 percent increase in the metabolic rate.

Specific dynamic action of food net energy expenditure is a result of the energy required to maintain metabolic processes when the body is at rest, plus the energy produced after the ingestion of food. Energy is measured in units of heat, as previously mentioned. It has been reported that heat production increases during food ingestion. This effect of food on the production of heat is referred to as the *specific dynamic action* (SDA) of food. The SDA accounts for approximately 10 percent of the total energy intake but represents the energy value of the nutrient that is not available to the body for metabolism. Some of the ingested food is not absorbed by the body and is excreted as feces. These losses are due to the SDA and the excretion of the metabolic by-products creatinine, urea, and other organic components of the urine. The caloric values of foods as listed in diet tables are energy values for the food items after the SDA and other losses have been deducted.

ENERGY REQUIREMENTS

An individual's caloric or energy requirements are a function of the whole psychosocial-physiological state. Muscular activity influences the body's total energy needs perhaps more than any other environmental factor. In determining the average energy need of an individual, it is necessary to assess activity level as related to lifestyle and add this increased need to the BMR. In very broad terms, a sedentary life-style will require additional calories equal to 30 percent of the BMR. Moderate activity will increase the energy needs by 40 percent of the BMR, and a very active life-style will increase the caloric needs by 50 percent of the BMR. For example, 1 60-kg woman who leads a very active and full day would require 2160 kcal (9072 kJ) to accommodate her BMR and daily activity needs, as illustrated below:

BMR = 60 kg × 24 kcal per day
    = 1440 kcal per day = 6048 kJ per day
Heavy activity = 50% BMR = 50% × 1440
    = 720 kcal per day = 3024 kJ per day
Total energy needs
    = BMR + calculated activity requirement
Total energy needs per day = 1440 + 720
    = 2160 kcal per day = 9072 kJ per day

This method for determining an individual's energy needs can be made more specific by determining exact energy expenditure per day by activity (see Chap. 10).

Emotional stress, growth, muscle activity, health, and body size are key factors in determining the body's energy needs for energy balance. The Food and Nutrition Board of the National Academy of Sciences–National Research Council has established energy allowances for adults on the basis of age and sex (see Appendix). These figures are to be used as a guideline in determining energy needs. It must be remembered that any deviation from the individual's normal psychosocial-physiological status will reflect an increase or decrease in these estimated energy needs, depending upon the nature of the change.

BODY COMPOSITION

Body composition can be defined as the chemical composition of the body's stores of:

    Bone tissue
    Connective tissue
    Soft tissue
    Adipose tissue

In vitro and in vivo studies have been utilized to determine the exact chemical composition of the body's tissues. Via chemical analysis there seems to be general agreement on body composition of vitamins, minerals, and other nutrients. Friis-Hansen has quantitated the percentage of mineral, protein, and fat composition for the water-free body area as 6, 16, and 18 percent respectively.[10] In determining exact proportions of body nutrients, it has been estimated through chemical analysis that 25 to 50 percent of the body is water-free tissue.

The difficulties of studying the human body by direct chemical analysis plus the desirability of studying in vitro measurements has led to the development of indirect methods of determining body composition, namely:

Bone density
Fat fold measurements
Radiography
Anthropometric measurements

Anthropometric Measurements

Body measurements provide a good estimation of fat stores and thus give an indication of body composition. Traditionally, height and weight measurements have been utilized to relate physical size to an estimated set of standards established by the National Research Council. However, bone and muscle, as well as adipose tissue, cannot be quantitated accurately by these gross measurements.[11] The use of skinfold calipers can aid in the estimation of body fat stores via measurement of skinfold thickness (see Chap. 13). Skinfold thickness standards have been established for measurement of the triceps muscle and abdominal and midthigh regions.

Body density, as demonstrated by Ingalls and by Baker and Newman, can provide an accurate measurement of lean body mass, defined as the whole body less the excess fat.[12,13] Submersion of the entire body in a tankful of water, and then recording the air volume in the lungs and measuring the rise in water volume, can provide statistics that yield the body density of the subject through mathematical equations.

Body density is related to the physical activity of the individual, which increases metabolism and places extra stress on muscles and bones, thus affecting lean body mass.

Factors Affecting Body Composition

The study of body composition must take into account the functional, physiological, genetic, and nutritional factors that are significant determinants of body tissue structure.

Diet has an effect on body composition, perhaps most evident in the bone density and extent of adipose tissue. Bone density has been shown to vary up to 50 percent among individuals with similar stature. The amount of bone mineral seems to be greater in males than in females, greater in adults than in adolescents, and greater in individuals with higher calcium and phosphorus intakes.

According to Garn, subcutaneous fat deposits are greater in females than in males.[14] This may be due to the role of adipose tissue as insulation during childbearing.

Weight loss can significantly affect total body composition by decreasing adipose tissue stores. When increased exercise is coupled with an energy deficient diet, fat stores will be mobilized and converted to energy in order to accommodate for the increased energy expenditure caused by increased activity.

Body composition has been studied in relation to onset of menarche and sexual development. During puberty, the development of secondary sex characteristics is accompanied by a rapid linear growth spurt, changes in the quantity and distribution of adipose tissue, and other physiological changes. Marshall suggests that despite the apparent increase in total body water and fat in pubescent girls, *age of onset of menarche is not determined by attaining a critical weight or percent of lean body mass as fat.*[15] As the body approaches maturity, the electrolytes in the diet and the ratio of these electrolytes to dietary protein seem to influence body composition, reflected in an increase of these nutrients per kilogram of body weight.

STUDY QUESTIONS

1 Starting with the "port of entry," follow a meal progressively through the gastrointestinal system.

2 What are the neurohormonal control mechanisms that are operative in the process of digestion?

3 Describe the interrelationships between carbohydrate, protein, and fat metabolism in the body.

4 List those factors influencing the basal metabolic rate.

5 How would you go about calculating your own daily energy needs? Proceed to do so.

CLINICAL STUDY 9

S. J. is a 14-year-old girl who has come to the clinic for weight reduction. She is 63 in (160 cm) tall and weighs 145 lb (65.9 kg). Nutrition history reveals an energy intake of 2400 kcal (protein 90 g; fat 105 g, carbohydrate 274 g.) She spends her free time sewing, cooking, babysitting, and listening to music.

Clinical study questions

1 What factors effect energy requirements for S. J.?
2 What is an ideal weight for S. J.? Why?
3 Calculate the energy requirements for S. J.
4 Calculate a balanced calorie deficit diet for this young girl.

REFERENCES

1 H. W. Davenport, *Physiology of the Digestive Tract,* Year Book Medical Publishers, Inc., Chicago, 1961.
2 M. H. Sleisenger, Protein Digestion and Absorption. *New England Journal of Medicine,* **300**(12):659–663, March 1979.
3 Williams, "Benefit and Mischief from Commensal Bacteria," *Journal of Clinical Pathology,* **26**:811–818, 1973.
4 W. E. C. Moore and L. V. Holdeman, "Human Fecal Flora: The Normal Flora of 20 Japanese-Hawaiians," *Applied Microbiology,* **27**:961, 1974.
5 S. Shapiro, "Control of Antibiotic Induced Gastrointestinal Symptoms with Yogurt," *Clinical Medicines,* **7**(2):295–301, 1960.
6 N. S. LeLeiko, C. A. Murray, and H. N. Munro, *Enteral Support of the Hospitalized Child,* in R. Suskind (ed.), *Textbook of Pediatric Nutrition,* Raven Press, New York, 1981.
7 V. L. W. Go and W. H. J. Summerskill, "Digestion, Maldigestion, and the G.I. Hormones," *American Journal of Clinical Nutrition,* **24**:160–167, 1971.
8 H. N. Munro, "Free Amino Acid Pools and Their Role in Regulation," in H. N. Munro (ed.), *Mammalian Protein Metabolism,* vol. IV, Academic Press, New York, 1970.
9 W. E. Nelson (ed.), *Textbook of Pediatrics,* W. B. Saunders Company, Philadelphia, 1979, chaps. 2, 5.
10 B. Friis-Hansen, "Body Composition during Growth," *Pediatrics,* **47**(ii), January 1971.
11 G. E. Kandell, "Evaluating Body Composition," *Aerospace Medicine,* **40**:486, 1969.
12 A. Ward, M. Pollock, A. Jackson, J. Ayres, G. Pape, "A Comparison of Body Fat Determined by Underwater Weighing and Volume Displacement," *American Journal of Physiology,* **234**(1):E 94-6, January 1978.
13 J. Brozek, G. Grande, J. Anderson, A. Keys, "Densitometric Analysis of Body Composition: Revision of Some Quantitative Assumptions," *Annals of the New York Academy of Sciences,* **110**:113–140, 1963.
14 R. Steen et al., "Body Composition in 70-Year-Old Females and Males in Goth, Sweden: A Population Study," *Acta Medica Scandinavica, Supplementum,* **611**:87–112, 1977.

15 W. A. Marshall, "The Relationship of Puberty to Other Maturity Indicators and Body Composition in Man," *Journal of Reproduction and Fertility*, **52**: 437–443, 1978.

CLINICAL DISCUSSION 9

S. J. is an adolescent girl. Her energy requirements are directly affected by her (1) age, (2) sex, (3) level of activity, (4) present weight for height, and (5) her immediate need to lose weight.

Basal caloric requirements for maintenence are calculated on the basis of current weight for height. Thus in order to achieve weight loss, caloric intake must be based on ideal body weight.

Activity level is an important factor in the determination of energy requirements. S. J. has a fairly sendentary life-style. Therefore an allowance of 30 percent of estimated BMR caloric requirements will accommodate her activity level.

To determine an ideal weight for height, standardized growth charts are used. A height of 63 in (160 cm) places S. J. at the 50th percentile for height for age based on the National Center for Health Statistics (NCHS) Growth Charts. Her weight of 145 lb (65.9 kg) places her at the 90th percentile. An ideal weight for S. J. should be determined by her height. A weight of 118 lb (53.6 kg) is considered to be ideal for a 14-year-old girl growing at the 50th percentile for height using NCHS standards.

On the basis of this ideal weight as derived from NCHS growth standards, S. J.'s basal energy requirements are 1286 kcal per day (5381 KJ per day):

$$\begin{aligned} BMR &= 53.6 \text{ kg} \times 24 \text{ kcal per day} \\ &= 1286 \text{ kcal per day} \\ &= 5381 \text{ kJ per day} \end{aligned}$$

To determine caloric needs for a sedentary life-style, an allowance of 30 percent of the BMR caloric requirements is added to the BMR needs:

$$\begin{aligned} \text{Sedentary activity} &= 30\% \text{ BMR} \\ &= 30\% \times 1286 \\ &= 386 \text{ kcal per day} \\ &= 1615 \text{ kJ per day} \end{aligned}$$

Total energy requirement is the sum of the basal metabolic requirement plus energy requirements for activity. Therefore, S. J. will require approximately 1672 kcal per day (6996 kJ) to maintain an ideal weight of 118 lb (53.6 kg). This energy level includes the energy cost of growth which is included in the BMR calculation of 24 kcal per day. A 1600 kcal (6996 kJ) diet represents a daily calorie deficit which should mean a weight loss of at least 1 lb per week.

PART TWO

FOOD, THE HUMAN ENVIRONMENT, AND HEALTH

The principles of nutrition operate not in a vacuum but in a human environment, an environment that is dynamic and impinged on by both internal and external forces. This section examines the forces operative within the individual—growth, development, pregnancy, lactation, and aging—and those outside the individual within the community. The final two chapters examine health as indicated by good oral hygiene and nutritional status.

CHAPTER 10

NUTRITION, PHYSICAL FITNESS, AND ATHLETIC PERFORMANCE

Marilyn D. Schorin

KEY WORDS
Aerobic Exercise
Anaerobic Exercise
Isotonic Exercise
Carbohydrate Loading
Fluid Replacement
Sports Anemia
Preevent Meals

INTRODUCTION

The difference between the superstar athlete and the average man and woman will probably never be satisfactorily explained in physiological, biochemical, or even genetic terms. The aspects of training, genetic endowment, and nutrition that can be scientifically studied allow the competitor to meet realistic expectations of control and performance. Other traits that are poorly understood and appear to vary widely from one individual to another lend themselves to myths and faddish practices among the naive and uninformed.

For generations, athletes have consumed red meat in the pursuit of power and strength. The origin of this symbolic relationship comes from the early years of Western civilization, when meat was prized but rarely eaten. Athletes are continually searching for the superdiet or the miracle food that will provide them with an edge over their opponents. These attitudes make them vulnerable to mercenary promoters. A review of dietary practices of the Olympic athletes at the 1972 games in Munich[1] revealed many American contenders consuming megadoses of vitamins C, E, B_6, and B_{12}, wheat germ, and liver protein supplements. Some athletes questioned were using the supplements more for psychological assurance than from belief in a nutritional advantage.

This chapter examines the nutritional aspects of sports. Effective counseling of the athlete or physically active person requires an understanding of how activity changes nutritional requirements.

Competitive and recreational athletes may find it beneficial to keep a log of the type and duration of their activities. This sports log helps the athlete to note improvement over time. As an adjunct to activity monitoring, sports enthusiasts should be encouraged to record periodically their food and beverage intake. With the help of this sports log, nutritionists can teach people to monitor a variety of dietary influences on performance. Factors such as fluid replacement needs, the effects of caffeine and ethanol, nutritional balance of the overall diet, and the positive and negative reactions to specific foods can all be evaluated. Each of these is discussed in greater detail later in this chapter.

TYPES OF EXERCISES

The perspective of Americans toward participatory sports has undergone an enormous change in recent years. Fitness clubs have sprung up nationwide, cycling and ski touring have found new recruits, and city streets are filled with joggers. The goal is to become physically fit. Some exercises are clearly better adapted to promoting fitness than others. The following categories describe the various types of exercises.

Isometric exercises strengthen muscles by pushing one set of muscles against another. The force of each muscle grouping is equal, so no movement is evident; for example, push the

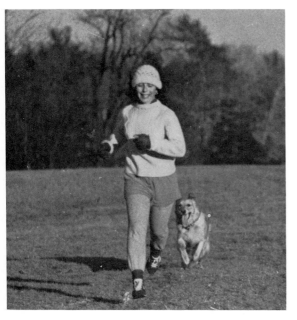

Figure 10-1
You don't have to be a super athlete to be physically fit. (Photo courtesy of John E. Howard, Jr.)

palms of your hands together as hard as possible. The activity has a low oxygen demand and does not lead to greater efficiency of the vascular and respiratory systems.

Isotonic exercises strengthen muscles as they push against an object to produce movement. Examples of isotonic exercises are calisthenics, weight lifting, and bowling. Like isometrics, isotonic exercises do not provide any cardiovascular benefits. They may, in fact, be detrimental to persons at high risk of cardiovascular disease because of the intense requirement for blood by muscles close to the heart. In limited amounts, they are useful when incorporated into warming-up and cooling-down routines.

Anaerobic, meaning "without oxygen," identifies exercises that are very short in duration, although the overall movement of the body may be similar to that in the beneficial aerobic activities. Activities such as the 100-yd dash, shot put, and football are primarily anaerobic.

Aerobic exercises utilize oxygen. The oxygen supply to the muscles will be enhanced and the efficiency of the heart will be improved during a training program designed to increase aerobic capacity. The term *aerobics* was coined by Dr. Kenneth Cooper of Dallas for a series of aerobic exercises to develop fitness which could be self-monitored. Any activities which can be carried on continuously for more than a few minutes are aerobic exercises, but they must be longer and of a certain intensity to promote fitness. (See Appendix B: American College of Sports Medicine position statements.)

ENERGY PRODUCTION

Human beings derive energy to perform activities from stored fuels (see Table 10-1). That energy can theoretically be provided by protein, carbohydrate, or fat. In reality, however, most protein in the body exists either in essential cell structures or as vital compounds such as hormones and enzymes. The body attempts to spare utilization of its protein for energy. Studies of nitrogen excretion in the well-nourished individual reveal no significant differences during pe-

TABLE 10-1   ENERGY EXPENDITURE IN VARIOUS ACTIVITIES

(The figures are based upon the caloric expenditure of a 150-lb individual)

Activity	kcal expended per 10 min
Sedentary	
Canoeing, leisurely	30
Carpet sweeping	33
Cooking	33
Dancing, ballroom	35
Eating	16
Standing quietly	18
Typing, electric	18
Typing, manual	21
Moderate	
Badminton	66
Calisthenics	49
Climbing hills, with no load	82
Cycling, 5.5 mi/h	44
Dancing, vigorous, disco	56
Gardening, mowing	76
Golf—without golf cart	58
Tennis	74
Walking, 3 mi/h	40
Mopping floors	39
Vigorous	
Circuit Training	126
Football	90
Gardening, digging	86
Racquetball	88
Running, 9-min miles	131
Running, 7-min miles	153
Skiing, cross-country	108
Skiing, downhill	81
Squash	102
Swimming, slow crawl	87
Swimming, fast crawl	106

Source: Adapted from A. Garth Fisher and R. K. Conlee, *The Complete Book of Physical Fitness,* Brigham Young University Press, Provo, Utah, 1979; and F. I. Katch and W. D. McArdle, *Nutrition, Weight Control and Exercise,* Houghton Mifflin Company, Bostom, 1977.

riods of exercise over the resting state, thus indicating that proteins are not being broken down to meet the increased energy needs associated with exercise. Only in cases of starvation will the protein be mobilized. Therefore, the predominantly available fuels are really limited to fat and carbohydrate.

Humans are able to store a limited amount of carbohydrate in the form of glycogen. A nonobese adult male weighing about 70 kg stores roughly 450 g of glycogen, equivalent to less than 2000 kcal (8368 kJ). Yet the human body is able to store unlimited quantities of fat. In that same 70-kg man, fat accounts for over 16 kg, or more than 140,000 kcal (586 MJ), roughly 85 percent of body fuel stores.

Researchers can determine the type of fuel utilized in a particular activity by measuring the nonprotein respiratory quotient. Respiratory quotient (RQ) is defined as the volume of CO_2 produced per volume of O_2 utilized:

$$RQ = \frac{CO_2 \text{ produced}}{O_2 \text{ inspired}}$$

A value of 1.00 indicates that carbohydrate is being metabolized; fat metabolism has an RQ of 0.7. In the resting state, the RQ is about 0.8, indicating the almost total reliance upon fat as a metabolic fuel. The RQ of the brain remains 1.00 except during starvation, because glucose is that organ's preferred fuel.

With activity, the RQ will change depending upon the intensity and duration of exercise. The intensity of activity is measured in terms of aerobic power, which is the maximal volume of oxygen consumed per unit of time [it may also be called *maximal oxygen uptake* or *maximal oxygen consumption* (abbreviated V_{O_2} max)]. If an activity is very intense and requires the player to perform at nearly 100 percent capacity, the RQ will be close to 1.00. Leisurely walking may require less than 50 percent V_{O_2} max and burn more fat. The body also changes from metabolizing carbohydrate to metabolizing fat during long endurance contests, as the carbohydrate stores become depleted over time.

Humans have two systems available for energy production. The choice depends upon the intensity and duration of the activity. The systems are anaerobic metabolism, which requires no oxygen, and aerobic metabolism. Usually, a combination of both systems is used. The shift from anaerobic to aerobic metabolism is gradual. The durations presented here are approximations.

Adenosine triphosphate (ATP) is the energy compound of the body. It is present in limited amounts, so that the supply of ATP must continually be replenished. Phosphocreatine (PC) exists in equilibrium with ATP and, for very short periods, will replace ATP as it is expended. This anaerobic breakdown of phosphate compound is critical in events to a maximum duration of about 8 s, such as the 100-m dash, the javelin throw, and the shot put.[2]

As that immediate supply of energy abates, the body switches to lactic acid production, reflecting the breakdown of glycogen. Only a limited amount of energy can be produced by this anaerobic metabolism as compared to complete oxidation. However, this system of energy production is important in sports such as gymnastic routines, speed skating, runs of up to about 440 yd, and the beginning yards of longer-distance runs. After 1 min of maximal effort, anaerobic metabolism will be providing 67 to 70 percent of the energy; after 2 min, this declines to 50 percent.

If the body were not able to shift to energy derived primarily from oxidative breakdown of fuels after that time, exhaustion would quickly set in. Oxidative metabolism involves the breakdown of 2-carbon fragments through the tricarboxylic acid (Krebs) cycle and electron transport system. (See Chap. 9.) The amount of energy produced through aerobic metabolism is substantially greater than that available via lactic acid production. Theoretically, as long as fuel is available to be metabolized and oxygen can be provided, exhaustion may be delayed.

From a practical standpoint, however, one will become exhausted after 2 to 4 h of intense activity. That is because the body shows a preference for energy derived from carbohydrate over that from fat. Even with plenty of fat still remaining after several hours of hard work, when the carbohydrate stores in the muscle are depleted, it is difficult to continue the activity. The fastest and most direct route to making ATP via oxidative metabolism is the glycolytic pathway. Therefore, carbohydrate produces more energy during activity than fat does.

Site of Energy Production

Within the muscle cell are specialized centers for aerobic and anaerobic glycolysis. The sarcoplasm contains the enzymes for anaerobic energy production, from the phosphorylation of glycogen to glucose 6-phosphate (after intermediary steps) to pyruvic acid and thence to lactic acid.

If carbohydrate breakdown is to proceed, the pathways used are the Krebs cycle and electron transport, which take place within the mitochondria. So much more energy can be produced aerobically that the mitochondria have been called the "powerhouse" of the cell (see Chap. 9).

One would anticipate that given the specialization for metabolism, the cells of elite short- and long-distance athletes would look very different. In fact, elite marathon runners show both increased number of, and increased enzyme activity in, mitochondria. That is, through endurance training, they have been able to expand their capability for oxidative metabolism, and run both with greater intensity and for longer duration.

Types of Muscle Fibers

Not only are the individual cells so differentiated, but the muscle cells are organized into muscle fibers, which are also notable for their distinct enzyme activities. *Fast twitch* (FT) *fibers* play an important role in short, intense bursts of activity. *Slow twitch* (ST) *fibers* are better adapted to repeated contractions over a prolonged period of time. Slow twitch fibers have more mitochondria and more enzyme activity for the Krebs cycle, the electron transport system, and fatty acid breakdown. Fast twitch fibers have more enzyme activity for anaerobic glycolysis.[3]

Again an examination of elite runners revealed significant differences in the number of FT and ST fibers. Marathon runners had a preponderance of ST fibers, while more FT fibers were found in world-class sprinters. The type and distribution of fibers are apparently genetically determined. Some coaches and exercise physiologists are advocating that young runners undergo muscle fiber analysis so that if they have more FT fibers, they will not be coached in distance events for which they are unsuited.

Glycogen Utilization and Storage

The brief discussion of cellular physiology and muscle fiber types provides a basis for grasping how the body utilizes fuels during exercise. In very short bursts of activity, the ATP-phosphocreatine system plays the major role, as stated earlier. The utilization of PC has little impact on glycogen and none at all on fatty acids or blood glucose. The glycogen that is used is broken down to lactic acid. If frequent, intense bursts of activity are punctuated with rest, the phosphocreatine could continue to provide the high-energy phosphates necessary to make ATP. Glycogen content would decline, but not substantially.

An athlete doing maximal work for about 1 h will utilize glycogen aerobically to produce energy. Most likely, after 1 h, the glycogen storage will be significantly depleted, but not empty.

Liver Glycogen

The body stores glycogen in both the liver and muscle. The liver has the capacity to store relatively large amounts of this high-molecular-weight substance, up to 8 percent of its weight. The function of liver glycogen is to maintain blood glucose, although during long endurance events such as marathon runs, it can be used to supplement muscle glycogen.[4,5]

Blood glucose levels are little altered during short-term, moderate-intensity exercise. During short-term, severe exercise, they may rise 20 to 30 mg per 100 mL. This is due to an increase in splanchnic glucose output from two to five times normal, proportional to the severity of the exercise. After 90 min or more of exercise, the blood glucose levels will have fallen from 10 to 40 mg per 100 mL.[6]

Muscle Glycogen

All skeletal muscles store some glycogen. Fatigue or exhaustion after long periods of exercise (60 to 180 min) correlates well with the depletion of muscle glycogen.[7,8] Subjects report a heavy feeling in their muscles and are unable to continue exercising, even though plenty of substrate is potentially available in the form of triglycerides.

Muscle glycogen utilization must be localized to the site where it is stored, for the principal enzyme releasing glucose from glucose 6-phosphate, glucose 6-phosphatase, is absent from human muscle. But glycogen from liver may be used to supplement the immediate energy needs of a carbohydrate-depleted muscle, for the liver contains this enzyme. However, the reciprocal cannot occur; i.e., muscle glycogen cannot eliminate hypoglycemia which results from a glycogen-depleted liver.

A second consequence of the absence of this enzyme in muscle is that one glycogen-bulging muscle cannot be tapped to aid a depleted one. For example, if the calf, or gastrocnemius, muscle becomes exhausted by running, a renewed supply of complex carbohydrate cannot be supplied by the biceps. When even one muscle's glycogen stores are depleted, the individual must stop exercising that muscle shortly thereafter, until that particular glycogen depot can be replenished.

The body responds to exercise of 40 min or more by making efforts to spare its muscle glycogen. Triglycerides are increasingly mobilized from adipose tissue, and fatty acids are oxidized for energy.[9] The fatty acids will be broken down to 2-carbon fragments that will enter the TCA (tricarboxylic acid) cycle as acetyl CoA. Acetyl CoA is metabolized aerobically. The shift to a reliance upon fatty acids is gradual, providing about 10 percent of the energy after 1 h of work, but about 50 percent after 4 h.[10] Yet, as stated earlier, if carbohydrate stores in the muscle are depleted, a person will become exhausted even when there is ostensibly a great deal of energy still available in the form of fat.

The situation is not substantially different during light exercise. Light exercise would be defined as exercise at less than 50 percent Vo_2 max. The lower intensity of this activity allows the body to use aerobic metabolism almost exclusively. The energy will be provided by a combination of glucose, glycogen, and fatty acids. As the duration of this activity increases, fatty acids will be called out to provide more and more of the energy.

There is some controversy over how much of an exercising muscle's energy supply derives from muscle glycogen vs. circulating blood glucose. Some studies indicate that muscle stores of glycogen will provide nearly all the carbohydrate substrate at 60 to 80 percent Vo_2 max; others indicate that heavy exercise leads to a greater uptake of glucose by the muscle to provide as much as 80 percent of the energy.[11-13]

The proponents of the theory of glucose as the primary metabolic substrate for the muscle are in the minority. However, one report did show that leg uptake of glucose was decidedly less when subjects consumed a high-fat–high-protein diet as compared to a mixed or a high-carbohydrate diet.[14] A good deal more evidence points to the role of muscle glycogen as the most significant determinant of energy available to perform work.

Training alone enables the muscle to store more glycogen. In experiments exercising one leg and resting the other in the course of 1 month, investigators were able to show almost a doubling of muscle glycogen levels in the trained leg vs. the control.[15] Any activity designed to increase the level of muscle glycogen stored or to spare the stores should thus expand exercise time and delay exhaustion.

It has been found that training is not the only factor influencing the level of glycogen stored in skeletal muscle. Diet can profoundly affect the size of these stores.[16] In the exemplary study in this field, subjects performed exhaustive exercise at 75 percent of their maximal oxygen uptake, leading to a depletion of the initial glycogen stores. They were then fed either a carbohydrate-free, mixed, or high-carbohydrate regimen for three days. Low glycogen levels prevailed after the carbohydrate-free diet, while glycogen levels two to three times normal were present after the carbohydrate-rich diet.[17] The researchers also noted that blood glucose was markedly depressed during the exercise test administered after the carbohydrate-free diet.

A significant aspect of this depletion-resynthesis phenomenon is that it is localized to the specific muscle group exercised. The one-leg-exercise–one-leg-rest experimental design gives clear evidence of the specificity of depletion and loading.

NUTRIENTS FOR EXERCISE

Carbohydrate

The preceding information on muscle glycogen has been formulated into a dietary and exercise regime for endurance athletes. It is called *carbohydrate loading* or *glycogen loading*. The procedure is to begin 1 week before a competition and to exercise the leg muscles to exhaustion. For runners, this may mean a 17 to 20 mi run. To ensure depletion, the athlete should exercise the following day, again to exhaustion. During this time, the athlete should consume a high-fat–high-protein diet, low in carbohydrates, for 3 days. These 3 days are called the *depletion phase.*

The supersaturation phase, followed for 3 days prior to the competition, consists of little or no exercise in order to allow the glycogen reserves to refill. The diet is a high-carbohydrate regime. It should also be high in calories so that the carbohydrate calories do not replace protein.

There is no special diet prescribed for the

day of competition. The general guidelines for preevent meals should be considered.

Pros and Cons of Carbohydrate Loading

The depletion of muscle glycogen reserves has been noted to occur in many runners at about the 20th mile in a marathon race. This point has been called "the wall." Runners report that it is very difficult to keep moving once this state has been reached. Yet a marathon race lasts 26.2 mi. That is why marathoners are constantly striving to discover ways to make more fuel available or to make what they have last longer. The singular advantage of carbohydrate loading is that it offers the opportunity to increase the most readily available fuel and prolong endurance.

Yet many runners experience some aggravating side effects that cause them to eschew the potential benefits of this regime. The major concern is an inability to train during the crucial 3 days before competition. There is a great psychological letdown for some athletes in merely resting and letting the glycogen stores fill, knowing that their opponents may be out working in the last bit of training.

If, during the loading or supersaturation phase, the athlete consumes large amounts of fruit or concentrated sugars, diarrhea may be an uncomfortable side effect. The competitor may also experience a heavy or stiff feeling in the muscles during this second phase, since the storage of glycogen takes with it additional water. For each gram of glycogen stored, 2.7 g of water will be added.[18] Runners may, in fact, use weight changes as a guide to how successful the carbohydrate loading is. Costill says that the glycogen-loaded runner will weigh between 1 and 3 lb more than normal.[19]

Another factor in carbohydrate loading is that there is a great deal of individual variability in the length of time necessary to saturate the glycogen stores. Whereas some people may need 3 days, as recommended in the standard regime, others may require 5 or even 6 days, in which case, if they follow the standard model, they will be competing in a semidepleted state. [The test used in research and one that runners may

undergo to find out just how long it takes them to supersaturate is a needle biopsy of their quadriceps femoris (thigh) muscle. A small sample of muscle, 10 to 20 mg, can be removed by means of a large needle and then examined for glycogen content.]

Given that trained distance runners have as a baseline a higher muscle glycogen content than untrained subjects, and considering the severity of some of these concerns about the full glycogen loading plan, it seems safer to recommend the supersaturation phase alone. Some increase in stores is achieved, although not as great as that accompanying depletion. Costill asserts that most endurance athletes have resting muscle glycogen levels of 150 to 250 mmol per kilogram of muscle, roughly two or three times the 80 to 100 mmol per kilogram in untrained athletes, and equal to the values usually reported for carbohydrate-loaded muscle.[20]

Many researchers have expressed concern about the frequency of using this regimen. If the body becomes accustomed to having very high levels of muscle glycogen, it becomes more difficult to deplete. Then one is not able to supersaturate a habitually supersaturated muscle. Clearly, more research must be done on the value and methodology of this controversial dietary practice.

It is currently very faddish to claim to use carbohydrate loading. However, in a survey of runners done at Rutgers Medical School, the sports nutritionists found that the term was being used to define everything from a pasta meal the night before a race to the 7-day program. Respondents claimed that they were carbohydrate loading for every event from a 30-mi ultramarathon to a 2-mi race. This showed not only that athletes need more knowledge about just what carbohydrate loading is but that they need to know for which events it will be useful.

Carbohydrate loading will only be beneficial for events in which one is in danger of becoming depleted of glycogen. These are events of 1 hour or more continuous activity in which the individual is performing at greater than 75 or 80 percent of aerobic capacity. Most intermittent activities are not appropriate vehicles for carbohydrate loading, even if the total game or event time is 1 h or more. Examples of activities for which carbohydrate loading is inappropriate include basketball, football, downhill skiing, and middle-distance running. Appropriate activities for carbohydrate loading include long-distance running, cross-country skiing, distance cycling. If the workload is at an intensity less than 75 percent Vo_2 max but continues for several hours, it is likely that the drop in blood sugar will be larger than the decrease in glycogen. The competitor in that instance should be aware of the symptoms of hypoglycemia, such as dizziness and confusion, and take steps to alleviate the situation.

In summary, carbohydrates are the most important fuel for activity of more than a few seconds' duration. Methods exist to increase its availability and to spare it, but they need further refinement. The exercising public must be educated on how to use these techniques properly.

Fluid/Dehydration

Dehydration can be a serious problem for both recreational and competitive athletes. Each year there are scores of cases of heatstroke resulting from inadequate consumption and improper timing of fluid intake. Prevention of dehydration depends not only upon achieving and maintaining normohydration during and after an athletic event but also upon attaining a state of optimal hydration before competition. Many studies have been done to investigate various formulations of sports beverages, examining how rapidly they are absorbed and utilized as well as any side effects that may accompany their ingestion.[21-24]

Sweat is hypotonic relative to body fluids. It is less concentrated in electrolytes than blood. The secretion of sweat is the body's principal cooling mechanism. As the body's internal temperature rises, sweat glands begin to produce perspiration, which, when evaporated, will cool the individual. Internal temperatures may go up in response to increased environmental temperatures or increased metabolic activity of skeletal muscle. Physical activity in a hot environment places the athlete in double jeopardy.

Even though sweaty bodies conjure up negative societal responses, recreational athletes should not attempt to restrict the production of sweat. Golfers, tennis and racquetball players, and joggers should be advised not to wear antiperspirants during activity, for they may hinder the cooling apparatus from working effectively. Deodorants and showers can be used after the event to control undesirable odors that may accompany sweat. The sweat itself is a necessary body secretion.

A number of investigators have found that losses of body weight of 3 percent or more from dehydration can impair physical performance.[25-29] The fluid and electrolyte losses do not vary substantially whether the dehydration occurs by thermal means (sauna or hot environmental temperature) or by activity. Heart rates increase in response to submaximal workload.[30] In the dehydrated athlete, cardiac output and stroke volume decline at 6.8 percent weight loss.[31] Others noted a significant decrease in plasma in dehydrated subjects that could not be completely restored after a 4-h period of rehydration.[32] The dehydration also causes an increase in plasma sodium concentration,[33,34] which raises concern for athletes' unwise use of salt tablets (see below).

Two separate and distinct groups of athletes suffer the effects of dehydration: athletes for whom the dehydration is a consequence of the sport and those for whom the dehydration is an intentional adjunct to training. Athletes involved in sports lasting more than a few minutes lose water in proportion to the amount of calories they burn. In marathon runners, the total fluid loss may be from 8 to 13 lb. If these runners were not allowed to replace any of that fluid during the race, they would lose even more weight and would be vulnerable to cardiovascular injury. These athletes must strive to maintain normal hydration and to replace as rapidly as possible all of the fluid lost during the athletic event.

Wrestlers constitute most of the second group of athletes. They practice intentional dehydration as a form of weight control. Weight classes for high school and college wrestlers are listed in Table 10-2. More than 50 percent of wrestlers normally (i.e., preseason) weigh in the middle classes,[35] but only a limited number of wrestlers may be assigned to each class. A student wishing to compete, then, will frequently be advised to lose weight but will be given little professional guidance. So common in the past were dehydrating facilities in high schools and colleges that the *Wrestling Rule Book* (1979–80) of the National Federation of State High School Associations states specifically that "the use of a sweat box, hot showers, whirlpools or similar 'artificial' heat devices for weight reduction purposes is prohibited. The use of diuretics and/or drugs for weight reduction is prohibited."[36] What is not ruled out and is widely abused today are food and fluid restriction, vomiting, laxatives, and intense sweat-producing exercise just prior to weigh-in. These put athletes in an impaired state before competition.

TABLE 10-2   WEIGHT CLASSES FOR HIGH SCHOOL AND COLLEGE WRESTLERS

High school	College
98 lb (44.5 kg)	....
105 lb (47.6 kg)	....
112 lb (50.8 kg)	118 lb (53.5 kg)
119 lb (54.0 kg)	126 lb (57.2 kg)
126 lb (57.2 kg)	134 lb (60.8 kg)
132 lb (59.9 kg)	142 lb (64.4 kg)
138 lb (62.6 kg)	150 lb (68.0 kg)
145 lb (65.8 kg)	158 lb (71.7 kg)
155 lb (70.3 kg)	167 lb (75.8 kg)
167 lb (75.7 kg)	177 lb (80.3 kg)
185 lb (83.9 kg)	190 lb (86.2 kg)
Unlimited	Unlimited

Source: From National Collegiate Wrestling Association, *1980 NCAA Wrestling*, Shaunee Mission, Kansas City, Mo., 1979, p. W-5.

Since there is a 5-h period between official weigh-in and the start of a match, many wrestlers use this time to attempt to rehydrate. Hematocrits and plasma protein concentrations measured after weighing in and just prior to competition reveal that partial rehydration occurs, but the wrestlers are nonetheless competing in a state of semidehydration.[37]

The urinary profiles of champion high school wrestlers in Iowa confirm the theory.[38] The level of dehydration of the athletes observed might not be normalized during the 5 h between weighing in and competing. Further, the high levels of urinary potassium could be associated with renal ischemia.[39]

The dehydration, of course, is an unfortunate consequence of the weight loss, not the rationale for it. There is concern not only for the precompetition weight loss but for the seasonal pattern of keeping weight down, in that it might interrupt normal growth.[40] In examining the amount of weight actually lost, 747 Iowa high school wrestlers were weighed 17 days before certification and again at certification.[41] The average weight loss was 6.8 lb (3.1 kg), or 4.9 percent of inital body weight, while a considerable number of them lost 10 percent or more of their body weight. With the exception of the three heavier classes, most wrestlers lost 5 to 6 percent of their initial body weight. After the end of the season, the wrestlers gained an average of 13.6 lb (6.2 kg), or approximately 11 percent, compared with the 7.2 lb that would be predicted on the basis of growth changes. The large postseason weight gain was an unconscious attempt to "catch up" to their predicted place in the growth curve.

Few would complain if these wrestlers were obese or averaged more than 15 percent body fat and if the weight loss had been conducted in a manner to lose primarily fat. But it has been shown that wrestlers in the lower weight divisions average about 4.2 percent body fat.[42] When they embark on weight reduction programs, the majority of their loss comes from lean body tissue and fluids. The dehydration compromises their entire physiological functioning.

Several solutions have been suggested, ranging from increasing the number of people that may compete in the middleweight divisions, to increasing the size of those divisions, to granting a longer time period between weighing in and actual competition to allow for more complete rehydration. The American College of Sports Medicine[43] states that "the potential health hazards created by the procedures used to 'make weight' by wrestlers can be eliminated if state and national organizations will:

1. *Assess the body composition of each wrestler several weeks in advance of the competitive season. Individuals with a fat content less than five percent of their certified body weight should receive medical clearance before being allowed to compete.*
2. *Emphasize the fact that the daily caloric requirements of wrestlers should be obtained from a balanced diet and determined on the basis of age, body surface area, growth and physical activity levels. The minimal caloric needs of wrestlers in high schools and colleges will range from 1200 to 2400 kcal/day (5020–10,040 kJ/day); therefore, it is the responsibility of coaches, school officials, physicians and parents to discourage wrestlers from securing less than their minimal needs without prior medical approval.*
3. *Discourage the practice of fluid deprivation and dehydration. This can be accomplished by:*
   a. *Educating the coaches and wrestlers on the physiological consequences and medical complications that can occur as a result of these practices.*
   b. *Prohibiting the single or combined use of rubber suits, steam rooms, hot boxes, saunas, laxatives, and diuretics to "make weight."*
   c. *Scheduling weigh-ins just prior to competition.*
   d. *Scheduling more official weigh-ins between team matches.*
4. *Permit more participants/teams to compete in those weight classes (119–145 pounds) which have the highest percentages of wrestlers certified for competition.*
5. *Standardize regulations concerning the eligibility rules at championship tournaments so that individuals can only participate in those weight classes*

in which they had the highest frequencies of matches throughout the season.
6. *Encourage local and county organizations to systematically collect data on the hydration state of wrestlers and its relation to growth and development.*

So far the situation remains the same. Health professionals must continue to try to reach both coaches and wrestlers with education and to encourage weight management programs to begin long before the seasonal training.

Most of the work on intentional weight loss by athletes has been performed on high school and college wrestlers, but a new class of athletic dieters is emerging, the gymnasts. A group with small body size to begin with, these athletes strive to weigh as little as possible and use all of the techniques established over the years by wrestlers. More studies need to be done on weight changes and competitive performance for these athletes.

Rapid Fluid Replacement

For most active individuals, dehydration is an unintentional consequence of their involvement in sports. They would like to find ways to prevent, blunt, or delay its effects so that it does not interfere with their performance. This involves being optimally or even "hyperhydrated" before competition. Depending upon whether the activity is intermittent or continuous, it entails consumption of an appropriate beverage during breaks or during the workout. Hyperthermia and circulatory stress resulting from endurance activities can be prevented by fluid replacement during the exercise. Additional weight loss during the activity should be replaced with rapidly absorbed beverages as soon as possible after the activity.

Hyperhydration is loading up with water just prior to a competition.[44] Previously, it held particular attraction for marathon runners since international rules governing the 26.2-mi race used to prohibit water stations before the 10-km mark. Fortunately, this official policy was amended in 1975 (see Appendix: ACSM "Position Statement on Heat Injuries"). Some water will be released by metabolism of glycogen, but if the body has a supply of extra fluid to draw upon, the effects of hyperthermia may be delayed. Athletes engaging in short-term events are unlikely to benefit from last-minute drinks, but those participating in endurance contests should consider consuming large amounts of fluid in the hour prior to the competition or, in any case, about 0.5 L immediately before the start.[45] Costill advocates drinking 400 to 500 mL of water or very dilute sugar beverages 15 to 30 min before competition.[46]

The composition, timing, and temperature of beverages taken during competition have been studied at length. Plain water is absorbed fastest, and even small amounts of carbohydrate slow gastric emptying. Of course an individual's tolerance to endurance exercise is limited by the energy available to do work and by the amount of water lost as sweat. Fluid replacement may counteract both of these fatiguing factors by providing rapidly absorbable liquids that can cool the body and by providing readily usable carbohydrate.

Content of Fluid Replacement Solutions

Carbohydrate content of fluid The more carbohydrate a beverage contains, the more slowly it will empty from the stomach. However, variations among individuals exist with regard to gastric emptying time and even within the same individual at different times. One study compared gastric emptying rates of Gatorade, Body Punch, Brake Time (no longer manufactured), and water.[47] Gatorade, with 4.6 g carbohydrate per 100 mL, was emptied 35 to 40 percent less rapidly than any of the other beverages. Potassium has also been shown to slow gastric emptying time. Sodium will increase gastric emptying up to a point, beyond which the opposite effect will occur. Chloride ions appear to have no effect upon emptying rates. Although both carbohydrate and water should be present to prolong endurance, it is usually better to look for the beverage that can deliver the most water to the body in the fastest possible time. During long bouts of low-intensity exercise in cool weather, carbohydrate content may be the most important factor, but in warm climates, high humidity, or intense exercise, water balance will be compromised first, and the body's need for water outweighs other nutritional considerations. Therefore, either plain water or dilute sugar beverages would be superior in most cases.

Electrolyte content of fluid The issue of timing of electrolyte replacement is still very controversial. Electrolytes—potassium, sodium, chloride, and magnesium—are lost in sweat. These electrolytes need to be replaced. However, it is debated whether these electrolytes should be replaced during exercise, along with the glucose or water, or whether replacement can be delayed until subsequent meals.[48]

The American College of Sports Medicine has issued guidelines for the composition of beverages to be consumed during competition.[49] "It is the responsibility of the race sponsors to provide fluids which contain small amounts of sugar (less than 2.5 g. glucose per 100 ml of water) and electrolytes (less than 10 meq sodium and 5 meq potassium per liter of solution)." See Table 10-3 (p. 202) for common beverages of rapid fluid replacement and their dilutions.

Temperature of Fluids

Temperature of the beverages also influences gastric emptying. One report noted that 50 percent of the cold ($5°C$) test solution was emptied from the stomach within 15 min after ingestion, while only 27 percent of the warmer ($35°C$) solution was emptied during the same time period.[50] It has been shown that cold water reduces the gastric temperature and that this thermal change may increase gastric motility and rapid flow through the jejunum. For this reason, cold beverages are recommended for rapid fluid replacement.

The volume of beverage consumed has an effect as well. An increase in volume up to a maximum of 600 mL causes a progressively greater rate of emptying. Therefore, quantities

TABLE 10-3 DRINKS FOR RAPID FLUID REPLACEMENT

Water	Use as is
Seltzer water	Use as is
Club soda	Use as is
ERG Punch*	Use as is
Body Punch*	Use as is
Gatorade	Mix 1 part Gatorade and 2 parts water
Bike Half Time Punch*	Mix 1 part B.H.T.P. and 2 parts water
Sportade*	Mix 1 part Sportade and 3 parts water
Fruit juices and fruit drinks	Mix 1 part juice and 7 parts water
Cola and other carbonated beverages, sugar-sweetened	Mix 1 part soda and 3 parts water
Cola and other carbonated beverages, artificially sweetened	Use as is

*Made according to manufacturer's directions.

Source: Best, Fisher, Galandak and M. Schorin, "Guide fo Rapid Fluid Replacement in Exercise." Adapted from D. L. Costill, "A Scientific Approach to Distance Running," *Track and Field News,* Los Altos, Calif., 1979; and American College of Sports Medicine, "Position Statement on Heat Injuries," Medicine and Science in Sports, 7:vii, 1975.

as large as up to 600 mL can be tolerated and should be consumed to direct the fluid into the circulation quickly.

Fluid Replacement after Exercise

Weight loss can be used as a guide to the amount of fluid to be replaced. The guideline is based on the fact that 1 pt of water weighs 1 lb and the weight lost during athletic activity is principally water. Since the goal of fluid replacement is to return rapidly to normohydration, one indication of recovery is body weight equal to precompetition weight. Thirst is not an adequate guide to fluid replacement needs. Therefore, it is important that athletes be taught the simple guideline to replace each pound of weight lost with 1 pt of water or appropriately diluted beverage.

Unfortunately, many high school and college teams do not keep scales in the gym or on the playing field. It is strongly recommended that one be purchased so that the athletes can learn to monitor their own fluid replacement needs. The scale should be available during practice sessions and regular games.

It is better not to return to full-strength sugary drinks until sufficient beverages needed for fluid replacement have been consumed. This is important because a sugary beverage is not absorbed as quickly as a dilute drink and rehydration will be delayed. Also, the athlete is likely to become satiated more quickly with a high-sugar drink and not to consume enough water for replacement.

It is very fashionable in some circles to drink beer or other alcoholic beverages after playing tennis, racquetball, or "working out." Although the social pleasures cannot be denied, the solutes in alcoholic beverages, including beer, slow down the rate of gastric emptying and delay rehydration. Adults should be counseled to consume ethanol only after their initial fluid replacement needs have been met.

Salt Tablets

Each salt tablet contains about 0.5 g of sodium chloride. Typically, salt tablets are taken by those who have been sweating profusely. Their primary need is for water. Four 8-oz glasses of water must be consumed along with every salt tablet to ensure dilution of the salt. In the absence of the additional water, fluids will be drawn into the extracellular fluid from the cells in order to equalize the osmolarity of the fluid compartments.[51] The intracellular fluid may become severely depleted (see Chap. 8). Thus, salt tablets may promote the cellular dehydration that the sports enthusiast intended to offset.

Protein

Protein provides virtually none of the energy for physical activity. Almost all of that energy comes from carbohydrate and fat. If protein intake exceeds the body's requirement, the amino acids will be deaminated and the carbon skeletons re-synthesized into glycogen or fat. Then, the protein may indirectly contribute to the energy needs of the active person, but, of course, the means is rather inefficient from the perspective of energy production.

The most difficult notion to dispel is the belief that building large muscles requires massive inputs of protein, the stuff of which muscles are made. The literature contains references recommending anywhere from 0.5 to 3 g protein per kilogram body weight daily.[53-55] The best evidence indicates that, although there may be some additional protein requirement during intensive conditioning, that extra amount is quite small compared to the total protein requirement.[56-58] The following example may help to elucidate this confusing problem.

A vigorous training program may lead to the biosynthesis of ⅕ lb (approximately 90 g) of new muscle per week; the total weight gain will be substantially larger due to the concomitant formation of necessary vascular, neural, and interstitial components. Since muscle is about 60 percent protein, ⅕ lb of muscle corresponds to an increased need of about 54 g of protein (60 percent of 90 g) per week. The daily extra requirement from this very intensive muscle-building program is less than 8 g protein. The recommended dietary allowance (RDA) for protein for a 70-kg male is 56 g.[59] The muscle-building programs would increase his requirement to 64 g protein (56 + 8 = 64).

If this seems like a large increase in protein requirement, perhaps it would be useful to compare it to what Americans are typically consuming. The latest Hanes data reveal that the average American male consumes 103 g protein daily; the teenage male takes in even more.[60] Thus, regardless of the increased protein requirement engendered by a strenuous training program, athletes are probably already eating far in excess of their true need for this nutrient.

The additional protein requirement exists only during a period of intensive muscle building. To maintain fitness, the RDA values are sufficient.

Age Differences

The guidelines described in this section apply to all ages, since the RDA for protein does not vary significantly, ranging from about 0.9 g per kilogram per day in the adolescent to 0.8 g per kilogram per day in the adult. An intake of 1 g protein per kilogram per day should be sufficient for trained athletes of any age.

Sex Differences

Male and female athletes have equivalent protein requirements, based upon their body weight. Males, as a rule, have larger muscle mass; a male hormone, testosterone, promotes protein synthesis, which is, in part, responsible for men's increased musculature. Testosterone-like compounds have been developed for use by athletes to imitate this muscle-building (anabolic) effect. In addition to enhancing muscular development, these anabolic steroids have a number of undesirable side effects. Of particular concern, from both a physiological and psychological perspective, is their masculinizing effect upon females. They are not currently used in the United States.

Protein Supplements

It is evident that protein is not in short supply in the American diet. This dismantles the primary argument for protein supplementation. The high cost of many of these products relative to milk is another strong reason *against* recommending them.

In summary, a great deal of folklore persists about the protein needs of athletes. Few studies have documented adequately the rationale for large protein intakes, but most researchers agree that up to 3 g per kilogram per day of protein is not harmful.

Sports Anemia

The term *sports anemia* was coined in 1954 to describe a transient anemia that occurs during the initial phase of any intensive conditioning program.[61,62] Serum protein, red blood cells, hemoglobin, and hematocrit all decline at the start of an exercise program, although in time they return to normal levels.[63] The suggestion was made that if protein intake were inadequate, developing muscles would have to rob from available protein sources such as blood proteins. Subsequent studies have found the anemia to persist despite very high protein intakes. Therefore, sports anemia does not per se indicate a protein deficiency. Yet this condition is still used as a rationale for enormous portions of meat for many athletes.

Vitamins and Minerals

Athletes are caught in the same dilemma as the general public with regard to the issue of vitamins. They understand that it is unlikely for them to look for a frank deficiency of individual vitamins, but the symptoms of subacute deficiencies are vague enough that any deviation in training capabilities may be attributed to "vitamin deficiency." Active people often believe that vitamins not only prevent illness but can also promote "health." A number of athletes have even attributed to some vitamins the effect of improving performance, or *ergogenic effects.*

The need for extra energy for highly active individuals puts a stress on requirements for two B vitamins, thiamin and niacin. Both of these are essential to oxidative metabolism of carbohydrates. The RDA has accounted for the variable demands by presenting allowances per 1000 cal. (See Chap. 6 for the specific requirements of these vitamins.)

There is no evidence of any increased need for, or ergogenic effect of, vitamin B_{12} or vitamin E. The evidence for an enhanced effect of ascorbic acid does point to the possibility of improved performance with megadoses of the vitamin, but the results are not clear enough to recommend this strategy routinely.[64] On the other hand, vitamin C intakes in pharmacologic doses cause diarrhea and reportedly have led to the formation of calcium oxalate kidney stones.

Age Differences
The variations in vitamin and mineral requirements for different age groups are not changed by activity.

Sex Differences
The major sex difference in nutritional requirements is the high female need for iron in the adult as compared to that of the male. Since anemia affects the oxygen-carrying mechanism of the blood, a low iron intake may impair the body's ability to maintain optimum oxygenation of the muscles, thus diminishing performance.

Vitamin Supplements
No strong case can be made for boosting vitamin or mineral intakes beyond the RDA. It is unlikely that supplements of single vitamins will be useful to the athlete. Large amounts of fat-soluble vitamins can cause harm. Active people who are eating balanced diets do not require additional vitamins and minerals to perform physical activity. However, there are generally no detrimental effects associated with consuming a multivitamin pill. The multivitamin supplement is useful for athletes not adhering to a balanced diet.

To summarize the athlete's vitamin needs, a well-balanced diet providing adequate energy is also likely to fulfill the athlete's vitamin and mineral requirements. No competitive advantage is gained by taking large doses of any vitamins, although no harm will be caused by taking a multivitamin tablet that provides the RDA levels.

PREEVENT MEALS

Few areas in sports are fraught with as much misinformation and faddish practices as are preevent meals. It is difficult to carry out controlled studies of the effect of the pregame meal on performance because of the complex web of psychological and physiological factors determining the outcome of the competition. The following general guidelines reflect the current thinking about preevent meals, but are subject to individual variation (see Table 10-4).

Timing

If the pregame meal will be solid food, it is best to finish eating 2½ to 3 h before game time. This

TABLE 10-4 SAMPLE PREEVENT MEALS

Breakfast—500 kcal	Breakfast—700 kcal
6 oz orange juice	8 oz apple juice
1 cup cooked cereal	2 slices French toast
1 tsp sugar	3 tsp margarine
1 slice toast	2 tbsp syrup
1 tsp margarine	8 oz skim milk*
12 oz skim milk*	

Lunch—500 kcal	Lunch—700 kcal
8 oz low-fat milk*	8 oz low-fat milk*
8 oz water or diet soda	8 oz water or diet soda
Peanut butter sandwich:	Ham sandwich:
2 slices bread	2 slices bread
2 tbsp peanut butter	2 oz boiled ham
2 tsp jelly	1 tsp mayonnaise
1 banana	½ cup canned peaches
	1 plain cookie

*Low-fat and skim milk are used for two reasons: (1) Excess fat slows gastric emptying, and this meal should be out of the GI tract by game time. (2) More of the energy will come from carbohydrates, the preferred energy source.

will allow sufficient time for food to leave the stomach and upper bowel. Once the competition has begun, the athlete does not want to divert blood from muscles to the stomach. Liquid meals, because of their rapid digestion, may be taken as late as 1 h before the game. Marathon runners generally prefer not to eat for 4 to 6 h before a race, but again are able to tolerate liquid meals. The meal should be light to moderate in size; athletes should avoid overeating. It is not harmful to allow more than 3 h between a meal and the game, but many teenage athletes, accustomed to very high energy intakes, will become hungry and fatigued if the interval between meals forces a substantial reduction in caloric intake. Energy for the competition, for the most part, is not provided by the pregame meal. All individuals in training should be advised to eat nutritious and calorically adequate meals during their entire training period. Meals eaten the day before the game or race will contribute most of the energy for the event.

Fluids

The preevent meal should encourage maximum hydration. The amount of fluid to be taken depends upon such factors as duration of competition, ambient temperature and humidity, ability to rehydrate during competition, and the psychological state of the sportsperson.

In humid or hot settings, whether indoors or outdoors, the preevent meal should provide at least two 8-oz glasses of fluid. (Guidelines for hydration are detailed in the section on fluids earlier in this chapter.)

Familiarity and Acceptance

Only those foods that are familiar to the athlete and have not caused digestive problems in the past should be included in the pregame meal. This is one of the most important guidelines. In fact, psychological factors exert such power that if an athlete believes a certain food or beverage provides a competitive edge, he or she is very likely to perform better than usual after consuming it. When counseling athletes, it is best, for this same reason, not to disabuse them of their current practices; a positive attitude toward their diets may be far more important in winning than the composition of the pregame meal.

As a rule, dry beans and gas-producing vegetables should be eliminated from preevent meals; they may cause diarrhea or intestinal discomfort during the competition. Some athletes also react adversely to highly spiced foods and to salads. Keeping a record of food intake during training and over the course of a competitive season will enable athletes to tailor meals to their own individual preferences and tolerances.

Composition

Carbohydrates offer the most expeditious choice for the pregame meal. They are easily digested, pass directly to the liver to supplement the liver glycogen, and help maintain blood glucose levels. Complex carbohydrates are preferable to simple sugars; highly concentrated sugary foods may cause dehydration and diarrhea. Fats tend to slow the rate of gastric emptying; a high-fat meal will still be in the stomach 3 h later. Fats should be incorporated into the pregame meal for taste and satiety value but should be limited in quantity. Fried foods, fatty meats, whole milk, and ice cream should be avoided.

Protein, too, tends to slow the rate of gastric emptying. Performance may be compromised by a high-protein meal because the body must consume energy in converting protein to carbohydrate. If energy is diverted to metabolizing protein rather than to providing fuel for the muscles, the individual may not be able to rally energy when and where it is most needed.

Liquid Meals

In some cases, liquid meals offer an advantage over solid food. They can be well-balanced and come in a wide variety of flavors. These meals pass readily through the digestive tract, rarely causing any gastrointestinal discomfort. Thus, they may be consumed up to 1 h before game time. They are economical and do not require any preparation, ideal features for the traveling team.

Although a number of products on the market are milk-based, choosing a lactose-free or low-lactose beverage will ensure the absence of any adverse reaction in lactose-intolerant athletes. Two commercially available products in this category are Ensure® (Ross Laboratories, lactose-free) and Sustacal® (Mead Johnson, 6 g lactose per 12 fl oz).

Many athletes are initially skeptical about the benefits and satisfaction afforded by a liquid meal. It may take a season or more to convince the players and their coaches that under certain circumstances, liquid meals offer a promising alternative to restaurant food. However, they should be cautioned that all liquid meals are not equally appropriate.

Alcohol

Ethanol should not be incorporated in preevent meals on the basis of its nutritional properties.

Some athletes do claim that their performance is enhanced by its inclusion. Excessive consumption of ethanol causes impaired coordination, which makes it contraindicated for any serious athlete. On the other hand, depression of central nervous system anxiety centers may actually relax the athlete, and procedures that have become well established during training may proceed without tension interfering. Tolerance will vary from one individual to another; competition day is not the time to experiment.

Caffeine

Caffeine has no untoward effect upon performance when taken during the preevent meal. Several investigators have been searching for its role in performance. Researchers looking at female performance to exhaustion on a bicycle ergometer in response to a small, medium, or large dose of caffeine or a placebo found no significant effect upon time to exhaustion, maximal heart rate, or rating of perceived exhaustion.[65] They conclude that while caffeine may be helpful in performing sustained mental tasks, it cannot serve as an ergogenic aid to improve energy or delay exhaustion in physical activity.

Taking a different tack, one group of researchers observed that since exhaustion during endurance activity seems to coincide with depletion of muscle glycogen, if the muscle glycogen could be spared, a racer would be less concerned with running out of energy. They noted that although there is still plenty of fat available in adipose tissue at the end of a race, if it could be mobilized in greater quantity, this would be one method of sparing muscle glycogen. In two different papers, they reported that caffeine increases the rate of lipolysis, thus sparing glycogen depletion from the liver and skeletal muscles.[66,67] They noted a significant increase in the amount of work that could be performed during a given amount of time after ingesting caffeine.

This is still a controversial issue for which across-the-board recommendations cannot be made. Yet for the serious competitor in long-distance events, caffeine ingestion offers one more possibility for improving endurance. If one is going to try this approach, Costill recommends a double-strength cup of coffee about 60 min before a 10-mi training run to get a feel for one's reactions.[68]

It is important to note that, particularly on a hot day, coffee can be dehydrating by stimulating the production of urine. If caffeine is taken in cola drinks, the high sugar concentration will also have a dehydrating effect.

CONCLUSION

The nutritional requirements of athletes vary in proportion to certain physical parameters of the individuals, such as body weight and leanness, environmental temperature and humidity, and the duration and intensity of the activity. Conditioning places demands on athletes for enhanced muscle development, which may require an increase in protein intake, but by far the most significant need is for additional energy. Vitamin requirements should be determined by total energy intake rather than by adhering to the RDA standard for the "reference" woman or man. The digestion and absorption of a meal will depend not only upon the timing of food and beverage relative to competition but also upon the athlete's emotional state. (See Appendix B for American College of Sports Medicine position statements.)

STUDY QUESTIONS

1 For which events would the glycogen supercompensation regime be recommended, and why?

2 Why is it important not to eat 1½ to 2 h before an athletic contest?

3 What are the differences between male and female athletes' nutritional requirements?

4 What would the protein requirement be for a 15-year-old 55-kg boy who wanted to gain weight for the football team?

5 Explain why a golfer going out to play 18 holes on an 85°F day would not benefit by first consuming 8 oz of orange juice with a salt tablet.

CLINICAL STUDY 10

J. F. is a 14-year-old female athlete on the junior high school track team. She reported experiencing a "funny" quivering feeling in her stomach and dizzy spells following either an intensive workout or a track meet. The meets and workouts usually took place after school.

Her physician ordered electrocardiographic and glucose tolerance tests, both of which were within normal limits. A physical examination revealed no unusual findings.

A 3-day food anaylsis showed that J. F. was consuming a wide variety of foods, totaling roughly 2500 to 2800 cal per day. Her meal pattern consisted of lunch, dinner, an after-school snack, and an after-dinner snack. Typical snacks included hamburgers, milk shakes, pie, or cookies.

Clinical study questions

1 From the information presented, do you think J. F. may have a nutrition-related problem?

2 Could she have a problem of inadequate fluid replacement?

3 How would you assess whether the timing and composition of her meals and snacks are appropriate?

REFERENCES

1 E. Darden, "Olympic Athletes View Vitamins and Victories," *Journal of Home Economics,* **65**:8, 1973.

2 M. H. Williams, *Nutritional Aspects of Human Physical and Athletic Performance,* Charles C Thomas, Springfield, Illinois, 1976.

3 J. O. Holloszy, L. B. Oscai, P. A. Mole, and I. J. Don, "Biochemical Adaptations to Endurance Exercise in Skeletal Muscle," in B. Pernow and B. Saltin (eds.), *Muscle Metabolism during Exercise,* Plenum Press, New York, 1971.

4 E. Hultman and L. H. Nillson, "Liver Glycogen in Man. Effect of Different Diets and Muscular Exercise," in B. Pernow and B. Saltin (eds.), *Muscle Metabolism During Exercise,* Plenum Press, New York, 1971.

5 J. Wahren, G. Ahlborg, P. Felig, and L. Jorfeldt, "Glucose Metabolism During Exercise in Man," in B. Pernow and B. Saltin (eds.), *Muscle Metabolism During Exercise,* Plenum Press, New York, 1971.

6 P. Felig, J. Wahren, and R. Hendler, "Influence of Oral Glucose Ingestion on Splanchnic Glucose and Gluconeogenic Substrate Metabolism in Man," *Diabetes,* **24**:468, 1975.

7 L. Hermansen, E. Hultman, and B. Saltin, "Muscle Glycogen during Prolonged Severe Exercise," *Acta Physiologica Scandinavica,* **71**:129, 1967.

8 E. Hultman, "Studies on Muscle Metabolism of Glycogen and Active Phosphate in Man with Special Reference to Exercise and Diet," *Scandinavian Journal of Clinical and Laboratory Investigation,* **19**: (Suppl. 94), 1967.

9 P. Paul and W. L. Holmes, "Free Fatty Acid and Glucose Metabolism during Increased Energy Expenditure and After Training," *Medicine and Science in Sports,* **7**:176, 1975.

10 P. Felig and J. Wahren, "Fuel Homeostasis in Exercise," *New England Journal of Medicine,* **293**:1078, 1975.

11 C. K. Chapler and W. N. Stainsby, "Carbohydrate Metabolism in Contracting Dog Skeletal Muscle in Situ," *American Journal of Physiology,* **215**:995, 1968.

12 B. Martin, S. Robinson, and D. Robertshaw, "Influence of Diet on Leg Uptake of Glucose during Heavy Exercise," *American Journal of Clinical Nutrition,* **31**:62, 1978.

13 B. Saltin and J. Karlsson, "Muscle Glycogen Utilization during Work of Different Intensities," in B. Pernow and B. Saltin (eds.), *Muscle Metabolism during Exercise,* Plenum Press, New York, 1971.

14 B. Martin et al., op. cit.

15 J. Bergstrom and E. Hultman, "Muscle Glycogen Synthesis after Exercise: An Enhancing Factor Localized to the Muscle Cells in Man," *Nature,* **210**:309, 1966.

16 J. Karlssonand B. Saltin, "Diet, Muscle Glycogen and Endurance Performance," *Journal of Applied Physiology: Respiratory, Environmental and Exercise Physiology,* **31**:203, 1971.

17 J. Bergstrom, L. Hermansen, E. Hultman, and B. Saltin, "Diet, Muscle Glycogen and Physical Performance," *Acta Physiologica Scandinavica,* **71**:140, 1976.

18 P. O. Astrand and K. Rodahl, *Textbook of Work Physiology,* 2d ed., McGraw-Hill Book Company, New York, 1977.

19 D. L. Costill, *A Scientific Approach to Distance Running, Track and Field News,* Los Altos, Calif., 1979, p. 121.

20 Ibid., p. 120.

21 Ibid., pp. 90–93.

22 D. L. Costill, W. F. Kammer, and A. Fisher, "Fluid Ingestion During Distance Running," *Archives of Environmental Health,* **21**:520, 1970.

23 E. F. Coyle, D. L. Costill, W. J. Fink, and D. G. Hoopes, "Gastric Emptying Rates for Selected Athletic Drinks," *Research Quarterly,* **49**:119, 1978.

24 J. S. Fordtran and B. Saltin, "Gastric Emptying and Intestinal Absorption during Prolonged Severe Exercise," *Journal of Applied Physiology: Respiratory, Environmental and Exercise Physiology,* **23**:331, 1967.

25 E. Buskirk, P. F. Iampetro, and D. E. Bass, "Work Performance after Dehydration: Effects of Physical Conditioning and Heat Acclimatization," *Journal of Applied Physiology: Respiratory, Environmental and Exercise Physiology,* **12**:189, 1958.

26 J. Mayer and B. Bullen, "Nutrition and Athletic Performance," *Physiological Reviews,* **40**:369, 1960.

27 P. M. Ribisl, "Rapid Weight Reduction in Wrestling," *Journal of Sports Medicine and Physical Fitness,* **3**:55, 1975.

28 C. B. Sproles, D. P. Smith, R. J. Byrd, and T. E. Allen, "Circulatory Responses to Submaximal Exercise after Dehydration and Rehydration," *Journal of Sports Medicine and Physical Fitness,* **16**:98, 1976.

29 P. Vaccaro, D. W. Zausner, and J. R. Cade, "Changes in Body Weight, Hematocrit and Plasma Protein Concentration Due to Dehydration and Rehydration in Wrestlers," *Journal of Sports Medicine and Physical Fitness,* **16**:45, 1976.

30 W. K. Palmer, "Selected Physiological Responses of Normal Young Men Following Dehydration and Rehydration," *Research Quarterly,* **39**:1054, 1968.

31 C. B. Sproles et al., op. cit.

32 D. L. Costill and K. E. Sparks, "Rapid Fluid Replacement Following Thermal Dehydration," *Journal of Applied Physiology: Respiratory, Environmental and Exercise Physiology,* **34**:299, 1973.

33 J. R. Cade, H. J. Free, A. M. De Quesada, D. L. Shires, and L. Roby, "Changes in Body Fluid Composition and Volume during Vigorous Exercise by Athletes," *Journal of Sports Medicine and Physical Fitness,* **11**:1972, 1971.

34 P. Vaccaro et al., op. cit.

35 F. I. Katch and E. D. Michal, "Body Composition of High School Wrestlers According to Age and Wrestling Weight Category," *Medicine and Science in Sports,* **3**:190, 1971.

36 *1979–1980 Wrestling Rule Book,* National Federation of State High School Associations, Kansas City, Mo., 1980, p. 15.

37 P. M. Ribisl and W. G. Herbert, "Effects of Rapid Weight Reduction and Subsequent Rehydration upon the Physical Working Capacity of Wrestlers," *Research Quarterly,* **41**:536, 1970.

38 F. I. Katch and W. D. McArdle, *Nutrition, Weight Control and Exercise,* Houghton Mifflin Co., Boston, 1977.

39 E. J. Zambraski, C. M. Tipton, H. R. Jordon, W. K. Palmer, and T. K. Tcheng, "Iowa Wrestling Study: Urinary Profiles of State Finalists Prior to Competition," *Medicine and Science in Sports,* **6**:129, 1974.

40 N. Smith, *Food for Sport,* Bull Publishing Co., Palo Alto, Calif., 1976, p. 138.

41 T. Tcheng and C. Tipton, "Iowa Wrestling Study: Anthropometric Measurement and the Prediction of a 'Minimal' Body Weight for High School Wrestlers," *Medicine and Science in Sports,* **5**:1, 1973.

42 F. I. Katch and E. D. Michal, op. cit.

43 American College of Sports Medicine, "Position Stand on Weight Loss in Wrestlers," *Medicine and Science in Sports,* **8**:xi, 1976.

44 M. H. Williams, op. cit.

45 Ibid.

46 D. L. Costill, 1979, op. cit.

47 D. L. Costill and B. Saltin, "Factors Limiting Gastric Emptying during Rest and Exercise," *Journal of Applied Physiology: Respiratory, Environmental and Exercise Physiology,* **37**:679, 1974.

48 D. L. Costill, R. Cote, E. Miller, and S. Wynder, "Water and Electrolyte Replacement during Repeated Days of Work in the Heat," *Aviation Space and Environmental Medicine,* **46**:795, 1975.

49 American College of Sports Medicine, "Position Statement on Heat Injuries," *Medicine and Science in Sports,* **7**:vii, 1975.

50 D. L. Costill and B. Saltin, op. cit.

51 W. S. Ladell, "Effects of Water and Salt Intake Upon Performance of Men Working in Hot and Humid Environments," *Journal of Physiology,* **127**:11, 1955.

52 M. L. Best, F. T. Fisher, D. Galandak, and M. D. Schorin, *Guide for Rapid Fluid Replacement in Exercise,* pamphlet, 1979.

53 P. O. Astrand and K. Rodahl, op. cit.

54 R. C. Darling, R. E. Johnson, G. C. Pitts, C. F. Consolazio, and P. F. Robinson, "Effects of Variations in Dietary Protein on the Physical Well-being of Men Doing Manual Work," *Journal of Nutrition,* **28**:273, 1944.

55 M. H. Williams, op. cit.

56 C. F. Consolazio, H. L. Johnson, R. A. Nelson, J. G. Dramise, and J. H. Skala, "Protein Metabolism during Intensive Physical Training in the Young Adult," *American Journal of Clinical Nutrition,* **28**:29, 1975.

57 B. Torun, N. S. Scrimshaw, and V. R. Young, "Effect of Isometric Exercises on Body Potassium and Dietary Protein Requirements of Young Men," *American Journal of Clinical Nutrition,* **30**:1983, 1977.

58 P. Rasch, "Protein Dietary Supplementation and Physical Performance," *Medicine and Science in Sports,* **1**:195, 1969.

59 *Recommended Dietary Allowances,* 9th rev. ed., National Academy of Sciences, Food and Nutrition Board, Washington, 1980.

60 *Dietary Intake Source Data, United States, 1971–1974,* U.S. Department of Health, Education, and Welfare, 1979. National Center for Health Statistics: *Dietary Intake Findings, United States, 1971–1974,* by S. Abraham, M. D. Carroll, C. M. Dresser, C. L. Johnson. Vitaland Health Statistic Series II—No. 202 D.H.E.W. Pub. No. (HRA) 77–1647. Health Resources Administration, Washington, U.S. Gov. Printing Office. 1979.

61 R. Yamaji, "Studies on Protein Metabolism in Muscular Exercise. II. Changes of Blood Properties in Training of Hard Muscular Exercise," *Journal of the Physiological Society of Japan,* **13**:483, 1951.

62 H. Yoshimura, "Anemia during Physical Training (Sports Anemia)," *Nutrition Reviews,* **28**:251, 1970.

63 C. F. Consolazio et al., op. cit.

64 M. H. Williams, op. cit.

65 R. Perkins and M. H. Williams, "Effect of Caffeine Upon Maximal Muscular Endurance of Females," *Medicine and Science in Sports,* **7**:221, 1975.

66 D. L. Costill, G. P. Dalsky, and W. J. Fink, "Effects of Caffeine Ingestion on Metabolism and Exercise Performance," *Medicine and Science in Sports,* **10**:155, 1978.

67 J. L. Ivy, D. L. Costill, W. J. Fink, and R. W. Lower, "Influence of Caffeine and Carbohydrate Feedings on Endurance Performance," *Medicine and Science in Sports,* **11**:6, 1979.

68 D. L. Costill, 1979, op. cit.

CLINICAL DISCUSSION 10

Yes, J. F. may have a nutrition-related problem in that she is eating energy-dense foods for her after-school snack at about the time she works out or competes.

Fluid replacement may be a problem, but there is no indication of her fluid consumption in the case presented. However, if the after-school snack is taken with fluid, the high sugar content may prevent rapid absorption.

The dizziness may be due to a hypoglycemic condition precipitated by sugary foods before practice. The sugar will cause an outpouring of insulin, which helps the glucose enter cells. Exercise, too, makes the cells more receptive to glucose. The combined effect of exercise and insulin may lead to a depressed blood sugar. You should check for glucose consumption 15 min to 1 h before activity. If present, a hypoglycemic response is likely. Similarly, the ingestion of concentrated carbohydrates up to 2 h before intensive exercise demands that some of the energy required for activity be diverted to absorption of the food.

CHAPTER 11

THE PSYCHOLOGY OF DIET AND BEHAVIOR MODIFICATION

*Rosanne Beatrice Howard
and Richard R. Schnell*

KEY WORDS
Food Symbol
Feeding Problem
Helping Relationship
Diet Counseling
Observational Learning
Stimulus-Response Learning
Operant Learning
Reinforcement
Extinction
Guiding Behavior
Self-Management

THE PSYCHOLOGY OF DIET

Rosanne Beatrice Howard

INTRODUCTION

Success in diet counseling depends on directives being followed. This can only be accomplished when health professionals involved in diet counseling look beyond the food that is eaten and consider all those factors influencing food behavior, a process implied in the word *psychodietetics.*[1] Psychodietetics describes the complex interaction between diet and behavior and the need to look beyond the diet to the emotional aspects of eating—the need to consider all that is going on "in between the food and the mouth." This means considering all the determinants of food intake—sensory, personal, social. It involves taking an interest in clients—in their feelings and attitudes about food—and giving them careful consideration in the planning of a diet. To do so, the nutrition educator must establish a counseling relationship that is a helping relationship. This section on psychology of diet focuses on the determinants of food intake and the approach needed to influence the formation of positive food habits. We begin by reflecting on the meaning of food: the diversity of meanings and how food meanings are acquired.

THE MEANING OF FOOD

Food choices are influenced by a whole host of factors that include:

Cultural background

Religious beliefs

Psychological acceptance (pleasing to see, taste, smell, feel)

General economic situation (inflation, depression, recession)

Family finances

Susceptibility to advertising media

Level of education

Emotions

Society

Both consciously and unconsciously, all individuals are influenced by these factors as they make their food choices. However, these factors impinge differently on each individual causing each individual to evolve his or her own unique food meanings or symbols.

Food is essential for both the body and spirit. It not only calls forth much of thinking and emotion, but food can also be endowed readily with meaning and attitudes that are indeed "the body and the soul" of the person who partakes or rejects the food available to him. The ability of the body and spirit to utilize food may change within any given person in the face of any stress (be it physical, societal, or emotional) that is of sufficient duration and of such timing as to influence the balance within which the organism was operating in the immediate past. . . .[2]

Symbolic Meanings of Food

A categorization of food symbolisms is a somewhat arbitrary task; however, it does provide a framework around which to organize those meanings that are primarily operative in any individual (see Table 11-1). For the most part, food meanings of consequence relate to security. These food meanings emanate from the residual emotions of infancy and make the individual secure, whether biologically, socially, or emotionally secure. It is through food and feeding that an individual learns trust in the environment. As a child is held, cuddled, and fed, biological as well as emotional needs are met. Thereafter, a full stomach is identified with the person who provides the satisfaction, and food becomes "love." Developmentally, many food problems may emanate from this basic perception, as the toddler and the adolescent refuse food in their struggle to establish their own ego identity (see Chap. 13).

Food Symbolism and Illness

Feelings regarding food are difficult to intellectualize. During stress and illness, distortions of food behavior and a poor or fluctuating appetite

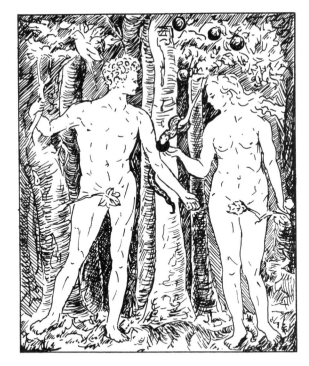

Figure 11-1
The apple—a universal food symbol of human weakness.

are often the first signs of underlying pathology. In these periods, food can be used as an emotional crutch to gain security. For example, individuals may sublimate anxiety by eating continually or may seek attention in the same way. Hospitalized patients may manipulate the staff by rejecting food or making impossible requests (e.g., wanting the breakfast egg cooked exactly 2½ min—no more, no less).

Food also can be used as a vehicle by which stressed, handicapped, or debilitated individuals seek to exert control over their environment. In fact, one's relationship to food may be the last vestige of personal control as all else fails—eyes, motor ability, bladder and bowel control.

With illness and hospitalization, regression in feeding behavior and food preferences may occur. For example, an adult patient might show a preference for baby foods despite having

TABLE 11-1   SYMBOLIC MEANINGS OF FOOD

Food symbol	Symbol formation
Love Security Trust Gratification Sensory pleasure	Food from early feeding experiences imparts feelings of security, trust, love; the infant that suckles from breast or bottle is cuddled closely, is filled with warm milk, feels sensory pleasure.
Reward Punishment	Food can be used as a method of discipline, withheld to enforce behavior (a tool to provoke fear or hunger) or given as a reward for good behavior.
Self-fulfillment	Food, so paramount to the infant's development, can become the focus of the parent-child relationship and, as such, the means through which parents achieve self-fulfillment. For example, the act of feeding becomes the act of nurturing, and the fulfillment of parental esteem is heavily at stake in feeding the family.
Religion: Foods that derive a separate meaning only from religious rites on feast days, e.g., matzo *Prestige:* Foods whose major value is to demonstrate an ability to pay, e.g., gourmet or exotic foods such as caviar or quality foods such as brand-name products *Taboo:* Foods proscribed for irrational and nonscientific reasons, e.g., Hindu prohibition of beef *Socialization:* Food and eating that carry the perceptible symbolic undertone of sociability, e.g., a wedding banquet, testimonial dinner, holiday feast, coffee klatch, cocktail party *Health:* Foods purported to have magical properties, e.g., used to cure ailments, ward off old age, or function as aphrodisiacs	Food customs are part of our cultural heritage. From the beginning, societies developed patterns around the conduct of food activities. These standardized practices are unique to each society, having evolved from different environmental factors and having been incorporated into the society to maintain the viability of the group.
"Language": Meat, steak, potatoes — Masculinity, aggression Vegetables, fruits — Feminity Fruits ("bearing fruit," fruition) — Love, affection, sexuality Olives — Sophistication or adult taste Peanut butter — Childhood	Foods communicate meanings that justify the simile of a language.

Source: Adapted from H. B. Moore, "The Meaning of Food," *The American Journal of Clinical Nutrition,* 77–82, 1957.

the ability to masticate table food. The stress of hospitalization may cause a weaned child to seek his or her bottle and refuse food. The ability of the child to accommodate to stress and separation from parents depends on the child's age and stage of development. For the newborn to 6-month-old child, there is little separation anxiety. However, anxiety may be observed as the child approaches the 6th month and begins to develop a strong attachment to the parent, so that adequate substitute mothering becomes difficult to provide. For all children under 4 years old, sudden prolonged separation can be overwhelming, and food often becomes the vehicle through which the children vent their frustrations as they initiate the separation process, a process described by Robertson as a progression from protest to despair to denial.[3]

In the protest phase, children cry a great deal and look for sights and sounds indicative of their parents. Next, children withdraw, as crying diminishes and apathy sets in. They make little attempt to alter their environment. With the onset of the denial phase, children demonstrate interest in their surroundings and acceptance of separation. They may appear to have forgotten their parents, even ignoring a parent's presence and allowing departure without complaint. An awareness of this process is important for health professionals who are working in a pediatric setting, when they attempt to interpret the cause of indifferent appetite or a regression in food behavior.

Feeding Problems

There are three main ways in which the function of eating is open to disturbance.[4]

1   *Organic feeding disturbances.* Feeding problems related to severe physical illness, weakness, exhaustion, strain, or certain states of convalescence affecting the individual's drive to survive or the need for food
2   *Nonorganic feeding disturbances.* Feeding problems related to an interference with the pleasurable character of eating such as occurs when a feeding schedule is imposed on a child with no allowance for individualization of frequency, quantity, or method of feeding (feeding situations that lack a sense of synchrony between the food provider and the child, with little or no attention paid by the provider to the cues emanating from the child)
3   *Neurotic feeding disturbances.* Feeding problems occurring when the function of

eating is drawn deeply into the circle of the individual's emotional life (and is used as an outlet for libidinal or aggressive tendencies), causing extremes of appetite and aberrant food behavior, which can be seen in the following conditions:

- *Pica.* The persistent ingestion of substances commonly considered unfit as food. Investigations support the concept that the interaction between the child and the mother is a critical factor in the development of pica, which in part represents oral fixation serving as a relief of the child's anxiety in response to an absent or inadequately functioning mother.[5,6]
- *Rumination.* The regurgitation of previously swallowed food and the rechewing and reswallowing of the food. Findings suggest that the syndrome develops in response to a disordered relationship between parents and infant.[7]
- *Anorexia nervosa.* A psychophysiologic disorder in which the ascetic pursuit of thinness is used as a tool in an individual's struggle for control—for a sense of identity and effectiveness.[8]

These major types of feeding disturbances are separated for the purpose of theoretical consideration; however, when observed clinically they are invariably intermixed and interrelated.

Organic feeding problems can lay the groundwork for the nonorganic type, as observed in the child with a tracheoesophageal fistula who, after the period of surgical repair, refuses food by mouth when it is first introduced, since the child's only knowledge of food and of the pleasure of feeling full has been by way of a gastrostomy tube.

Neurotic disturbances arise after the loss of pleasure in the function of eating. The child just described is at risk of developing a neurotic superstructure around feeding. Anticipatory guidance for the parents and the staff working with this child, along with the considerate handling that allows some self-determination, can help the child reacquire pleasure in the function of eating. Before intervention is made, a determination of the organic vs. the functional components of the feeding problem must be completed. This is aided by an interdisciplinary feeding evaluation in which a pediatrician, nutritionist, psychologist, and physical or occupational therapist take part.

Examples of neurotic or functional feeding disturbances include those related to weight gain following some traumatic emotional experience. Although no doubt with some genetic component, feeding is learned from birth. Learning is necessary for its organization into patterns.

Feeding patterns can be changed. This change is a challenge to the nutrition educator. Sometimes the nutrition educator can become overly concerned with giving information and does not help the client to understand his or her food behavior, which is the goal of diet counseling.

DIET COUNSELING: AN INSTRUMENT OF CHANGE

Diet counseling is defined as "providing individualized professional guidance to assist a person in adjusting his daily food consumption to meet his health needs."[9] The definition does not imply how this is effectively done.

To be effective, information must be presented in such a way that the individual will discover personal meaning in it. The problem of helping people to learn is the problem of creating a closer meaningful relationship between the information and the self. This is the *basic principle of learning:* the closer the events are perceived to the self, the more likely it is that behavior will be affected.[10] This is vastly different from *knowing* the information, which comes from acquiring information, a task at which most nutrition educators are proficient. Until clients do something with the information, it is unlikely to affect them in any important way. When clients are confronted with a prohibited food, they do not have time to decide what to do

about it. They will naturally do those things that are most closely related to self and their past experiences. The importance of moving information into a closer and meaningful relationship to the self is thus evident, and that movement can be facilitated by establishing a helping relationship with the patient.

A Helping Relationship in Diet Counseling

Diet counseling begins with a patient interview, which all too often approximates an interrogation for the purposes of filling in a nutritional history form. This is unfortunate because it is during this initial interview that a rapport is developed between the patient and the nutrition educator which determines the success or failure in diet counseling. The ability to *engender trust* and *understanding* of the problem during this time may determine the patient's progress, and is essentially the basis of a helping relationship.

Carl Rogers, the noted psychologist, identified three characteristics necessary for effective helping: the counselor's *empathy, genuineness,* and *unconditional positive regard for his or her client.* He also once observed, in an article on the nature of the helping relationship, that it didn't seem to make much difference how helpers behaved so long as their intent was to be helpful.[11] There is no control implied. Since diet means food control, patients often tend to regard the nutrition educator as the controlling, rather than the helping, agent. Consequently, the walls are built between patient and nutrition educator before the process begins. The nutrition educator may also have walls already built, but of another variety—namely, those emanating from preconceived attitudes about certain cultural or economic backgrounds. Professional objectivity does not allow for any one value system to interfere with patient management. It is important for nutrition educators as helpers to understand themselves as they begin to interface with other human beings in a counseling relationship and to hold in respect the personal and society values of patients.

A changing diet can be perceived as a detriment or a benefit, depending on one's value system. For example, an individual with the cultural tenets of poverty and a present-oriented, fatalistic outlook may find the concept of food planning completely alien. The same response may also be encountered with the directive to ghetto parents to remove candy from their children's diet (since candy may be the only attainable pleasure in a bleak inner-city environment). Another negative response may be encountered when cultural practices endorse a prolonged period of bottle feeding or breast feeding and instructions are given to wean a child.

An important factor affecting the discovery of meaning and susceptibility to change is the threat to predetermined perceptions. Resistance to change is normal. The nutrition educator must help people to change perceptions, not cause them to defend those they already have. For example, some vegetarians may reject nutrition information that does not fit into their frame of reference on the premise that their practices are ecologically sound in terms of health and environment. The greater the degree of threat, the more tenaciously a person will hold to perceptions, ideals, or practices.

The Nutritional Interview

To understand the consequences of the diet prescription, a considerable knowledge of the patient is necessary. This can be gathered through the nutritional interview. Once the approach is decided upon, the objectives are to obtain reliable information in a manner that is both efficient and considerate of the patient. Helfer and Hess have identified 11 behaviors, 9 of them desirable and 2 undesirable, for evaluating the interviewing skills of medical students and physicians.[12] These can be applied to nutrition educators as well. They are as follows:

1 Observes social amenities
2 Invites expression of concern
3 Reassures, shows sympathy and warmth
4 Explains rationale
5 Inquires about the effect of illness
6 Clarifies prior statement or question
7 Makes nonleading inquiries
8 Makes leading inquiries
9 Uses common words
10 Ignores or shows misunderstanding; cuts off communication
11 Is impatient; shows lack of empathy

There are many different nutritional interview forms used to obtain information (see Appendix). However, there is no place on the forms to measure *feeling tones, incidental remarks,* and *body language* that give meaningful clues to the patient's attitudes and experiences, yet these are important in gathering knowledge which will aid the nutritional educator in helping patients to learn how to incorporate nutritional information into their way of life.

The Process of Learning as Part of Diet Counseling

During the course of the nutritional interview the nutrition educator must determine what change is needed in the diet, the individual's food habits, the feasibility of change, how best to go about making the necessary change, and how to plan for change. The key to planned change is motivation, which involves helping the individual to discover a *personal meaning* in the change. In every individual, self-concern is pervasive in deciding how to act.

To a healthy person, health does not serve as a motivational force to change eating patterns. Usually only when well-being is threatened will diet action be taken voluntarily, but even in these circumstances a person's perception of health is affected by age, and by biological and emotional factors. An example is the adolescent diabetic who is in poor control of his illness. Concerned with the here and now and with peer relations, this teenager will not be motivated by the threat of secondary diabetic complications. Other avenues, such as social or academic incentives, must be sought to motivate diet change.

Besides considering the motivational forces that are operative within the individual, the nutrition educator must establish a receptive framework for learning. Conditions must allow flexibility and the freedom for verbal exchange. Responses from the patient could be encouraged. Tension can be reduced by incorporating phrases like "let's think this through together."

The learning environment can be further enhanced by incorporating illustrative tools (food models, flip charts, videotapes, learning machines). Also, the techniques of behavior modification can be utilized to help focus the attention of the patient on his or her own observable food behavior; these techniques will help to define the problem and to specify behaviors that must be increased, decreased, eliminated, or instituted in order to alleviate or solve the problem (see "Behavior Modification").

Food habits are practiced and maintained by selective perception in which new nutritional information is evaluted. Nutrition education must be presented within the individual's framework of selective perceptions, the framework of self-needs and values. Krech et al. state that "the

foods an individual chooses must not only satisfy his hunger but also be congruent with himself as a certain kind of person."[13] It is with this in mind, and with the attitude of developing a helping relationship, that the nutrition educator should commence counseling.

Nutrition Education

Since nutrition is one of the cornerstones in preventing illness, in maintaining health, it is essential to convey to the public the current state of knowledge and the potential benefits of modifying dietary habits. Nutrition education is part of many federal food programs. It is taking place in schools, clinics, and even supermarkets and food cooperatives around the country. In face-to-face counseling sessions, in group situations, and through television, radio, and the print media, a variety of tools are used to help each individual discover the personal meaning in dietary change. Table 11-2 summarizes some of the learning activities that can be used to get both children and adults involved in learning about nutrition. Because food habits are so ingrained, behavioral techniques may be needed to bring about change. The next section will explain the principles of behavior modification.

TABLE 11-2 NUTRITIONAL LEARNING ACTIVITIES THAT ENCOURAGE PARTICIPANT INVOLVEMENT

In school

Games (charades, puzzles, worksheets)
Snacking workshop emphasizing nutritious snacks
Food fairs
Menu planning for the cafeteria
Gardening/growing plants in the classroom or watching beans sprout
Writing poems, plays, or puppet shows about nutrition
Using dance and music
Peer teaching (where older schoolchildren help younger ones learn about food)

In the community

Newsletter
Consumer hot line
Nutritious recipe contest

BEHAVIOR MODIFICATION*

Richard R. Schnell

INTRODUCTION

How can socially important maladaptive eating behaviors be changed? The procedures employed in changing or modifying any behavior often hinge upon the theoretical conceptions of personality and behavior that one holds. Traditionally, personality and subsequent behavior have been viewed as a consequence of psychic forces within the person, such as drives, needs, and motives. Problem behavior is seen as a symptom of dysfunction within the personality. To alter behavior requires that underlying aspects of the personality be uncovered. Another major position on ways of changing behavior, which has mushroomed in popularity during the past few years, is the so-called behavioral approach. This position has its roots in the psychology of learning. The behavioral approach explains behavior as the product of external environmental, situational, and social determinants. Behaviors, in the main, are seen as learned and therefore as something that can be changed or modified through appropriate learning procedures. Problem behaviors are not seen as signs of a problem, but as the problem itself.

In day-to-day situations these two major approaches can, and often do, overlap to a great extent. Also, despite allegiance to either one of the positions, it is obvious that aspects of the other approach might be useful in a particular circumstance to change behavior in a desired direction. There is no need to see the two viewpoints as incompatible or antagonistic to each other.

This section on behavior modification focuses on some of the basic issues in employing a behavioral approach and presents a case study

*Research upon which this section is based was supported in part through the U.S. Department of Health, Education, and Welfare: Maternal and Child Health Service (Project 928).

to demonstrate the utility of the approach in clinical nutrition.

LEARNING AND BEHAVIOR

Current learning research has focused on three major approaches: observational learning, stimulus-response learning, and operant learning. In applying these different ways of changing behavior, the distinctions between them become blurred, and different aspects of each approach may often be used within the same situation. The operant approach receives the most attention here because it appears to have the most flexibility for use in applied situations.

Observational Learning

Observational learning requires observation of the behavior of another person (model) to cause learning to take place. The observer need not overtly respond at the time but will later imitate the behavior. Parents can often be heard commenting on how the behavior of their child was close to perfect before the child went to school and was exposed to the behavior of many other children; with other children for models the child's behavior has taken a turn for the worse in the eyes of the parents. The qualities of the model exert an influence on the learning that takes place. When there are several models, when they are similar to the observer, and when they have high prestige and status, the observer is more likely to imitate the model.[14,15] The consequences associated with certain behaviors also influence whether the behaviors will be imitated. The importance of consequences is discussed further in the operant learning section.

Stimulus-Response Learning

Stimulus-response learning, or *conditioning* (also known as classic conditioning), was originally studied by Pavlov. In this type of learning, stimuli that produce a strong reflexive (unlearned) action, such as salivating to the taste of food, are paired with a neutral stimulus which does not elicit the response, such as the sound of a bell. This pairing of stimuli eventually results in the neutral stimulus's (e.g., the bell alone) being able to elicit the response (e.g., salivating). In this type of learning, an event can take on new powers in producing a behavior. The event must be paired with a stimulus that already elicits the behavior of interest and must precede the behavior to be able to produce the behavior without the original stimulus being present.

Desensitization is one of the widely used techniques of behavior modification which has evolved from the stimulus-response approach.[16] The technique has enjoyed success when applied to specific anxieties and phobias. In using desensitization, stimuli that appear to elicit fear or anxiety are paired with an alternative and incompatible response to the fear such as relaxation. Desensitization breaks the stimulus-response association by developing an incompatible response to the same stimulus. Typically the person is exposed to the fear-eliciting stimuli in the order of their ability to arouse anxiety. Thus, the least anxiety-producing stimulus is used first and is coupled with the relaxation response. As the person is able to relax in its presence, the next level of anxiety-producing stimulus is introduced until the ability of this stimulus to produce anxiety is eliminated. Some researchers have claimed that desensitization is an effective technique in increasing food intake in people who have anorexia nervosa.[17]

Operant Learning

The history of operant learning, or *operant conditioning,* as it is most commonly called, begins with B. F. Skinner. Operant approaches focus on the learning that takes place as a result of the consequences of behavior. Positive consequences are systematically used to shape desired behaviors. In the case of operant learning, the consequences determine how a stimulus influences the probability of a response's occurring and, potentially, the intensity, speed, and magnitude of the response.[18] It can easily be seen that much of our behavior might be affected by this approach, as most of us feel that the consequences of behavior have a direct influence on whether or not we perform certain behaviors. Operant learning, however, implies more, in that systematic procedures must be applied to gain control over the behavior. The following section is an exposition of some of the most important components of operant learning.

PRINCIPLES OF OPERANT LEARNING

As in most theories of learning, the operant paradigm depends upon certain basic principles. The most basic, of course, is that behavior is controlled by the events or consequences that immediately follow it. Below are some of the essential ingredients necessary to an understanding of the operant approach.

Reinforcement

The behavior to be influenced is usually referred to as the *target behavior*. An event which immediately follows a target behavior and alters that behavior is called a *reinforcer*. Those reinforcers which follow a target behavior and which increase its frequency of occurrence are known as *positive reinforcers* or *rewards*. Those reinforcers which increase its frequency when *removed* after a target behavior are known as *negative reinforcers* or *aversive stimuli*.

When a behavior is followed immediately by positive reinforcing consequences, it will increase in strength. It should be noted that consequences that are rewarding for some people may not be for others, so that the best way to determine whether a consequence is reinforcing is to observe its effects upon behavior. If praising a child for eating a certain vegetable increases consumption of that vegetable, then the praise is reinforcing the behavior of eating that vegetable. Positive reinforcers can be divided into two categories, those which do not depend upon prior learning for their reinforcement value, e.g., water to a thirsty individual; and others, which have become reinforcing by being paired with an unlearned reinforcer, e.g., money. Essentially unlearned reinforcers are called *primary reinforcers,* while learned reinforcers are referred to as *secondary reinforcers.*

An increase in target behavior is a sign of reinforcement, whether the reinforcing is positive or negative. A stimulus can only be negatively reinforcing if its removal causes the target behavior to increase. In negative reinforcement an aversive stimulus is presented to an individual before a response begins. The aversive stimulus is removed or moderated immediately after the appropriate response occurs. Negative reinforcement is not the same thing as punishment. Punishment is defined in operant terms as something that decreases the frequency of a response. Typically, in punishment an aversive stimulus is presented after a behavior is performed, which tends to decrease that behavior.

Punishment is often less effective than reinforcement and therefore is not as widely used in operant learning. Negative reinforcement is also used less often than positive reinforcement because positive reinforcement is usually as effective or more so, as well as being more socially acceptable. Negative reinforcement, however, can be useful in extreme situations in which positive reinforcement is difficult. Lovaas and his colleagues[19] have used it to develop more socially appropriate behavior in autistic children. Because other approaches had failed, an electric shock was used as the negative reinforcer. When the autistic child began engaging in more socially acceptable behaviors such as moving toward or touching an adult, the mild shock was terminated. Although the method is repugnant, it did result in behavior change which could not be accomplished in any other known way. Whether that is adequate justification for its use remains a matter of dispute.

The frequency of the reinforcement that follows a desired behavior is an important variable. If reinforcement follows each occurrence of a desired behavior, it is called *continuous reinforcement.* Continuous reinforcement is most effective in the acquisition of new behavior. Reinforcement that does not occur every time a target response is made is called *intermittent reinforcement.* Intermittent reinforcement is most effective in maintaining a behavior once it is established. Behavior is much more resistant to change if it is intermittently reinforced.

Extinction

Behaviors will decrease in frequency of occurrence if they are no longer reinforced. The process of stopping reinforcement of a behavior is called *extinction.* When a behavior is not reinforced, the behavior is reduced or eliminated. Extinction should be clearly distinguished from punishment, in which an aversive stimulus follows a behavior and thus decreases its frequency. Extinction requires the total absence of reinforcement. Extinction can contribute to problem behavior, as well as help to change it. Positive behavior can be inadvertently extinguished by ignoring it. The child who always behaves well during mealtime may never be given any attention (extinction), while the disruptive child may be given a good deal of parental attention (reinforcement) for misbehavior. Absence of reinforcement tends to weaken any behavior.

Guiding Behavior

If a desired behavior does not occur frequently or at all, it is difficult to reinforce it so that the behavior will increase in frequency. In this case a process called *shaping* can be used which reinforces closer and closer approximations to the desired behavior. Shaping uses behaviors which resemble the desired behavior and which the individual already frequently produces. These behaviors are initially reinforced, and then reinforcement is altered so that the behavior must become more and more like that of the target behavior if it is to be reinforced. If one were trying to get an individual to eat half as much at mealtimes, it might prove difficult to reinforce that behavior because it might not readily occur. Systematically rewarding the person's eating somewhat less over a period of time until the person finally reached the appropriate amount would probably give better results.

Another procedure which facilitates the occurrence of a behavior which can be reinforced is called *prompting*. By helping someone begin the behavior, faster approximations to the final behavior can be made. This can be accomplished by simple maneuvers like instructing or even physically guiding the person. For example, you might explain how to hold a knife to cut meat to an older child, while with a younger child you might help to guide the spoon from plate to mouth.

Self-Management

The principles already elaborated are most often used by someone to change the behavior of another. Usually the person who systematically attempts to alter the behavior of another is a professional in a discipline such as psychology, but others can be trained to apply behavioral techniques. Parents can serve as behavioral change agents for their children.[20] The greatest efficiency could be gained by educating individuals to exert control over their own behavior in problem situations according to the principles discussed previously. This would allow individuals to help themselves rather than become dependent upon others. Self-management techniques are being actively evaluated.[21,22]

In self-management procedures people are trained to control their own behavior by use of shaping and prompting, and by delivering reinforcement or punishment to themselves. They are required to monitor their own behavior. The most obvious merit of self-management techniques is also a potential problem. Since the individuals exert the control over the consequences of their behavior, they may not choose to follow through on a behavioral program.

APPLICATION

Research

Over the years a great deal of research using both humans and animals has been devoted to developing behavior modification techniques. One of the results has been the application of these techniques to problems related to eating.

Problems in eating behavior have become relatively important to our affluent society. Attention has been directed to those who eat too little or too much. In the case of those who significantly lose their appetite for food *(anorexia nervosa)* behavioral techniques have appeared to be helpful although they have not yet been widely used.[23,24]

In the area of weight control for obesity, behavioral techniques have been used widely. Differing behavioral approaches have proved useful, but a number of issues remain. It has been demonstrated that weight reduction can usually be accomplished with behavioral techniques, but the reduction is often difficult to maintain.[25] Some investigators have approached the problem by examining how everyday eating habits are influenced by eating-related environmental cues, while others have examined the influence of emotional states on eating habits.[26] Self-management techniques for weight loss have gained popularity, with self-reward strategies appearing to be more effective than other strategies.[27] Behavioral treatment of obesity has produced weight losses as good as, or better than, most forms of outpatient treatment, with clear maintenance of the results. Nevertheless, permanent losses still tend to be small.[28] In general, which techniques will be most useful for initiating and maintaining weight loss still depend upon the individual situation.

Common Concerns

In describing behavior modification it becomes evident that the principles are not necessarily new, and in fact many of the techniques are practiced by, and on, all of us in a variety of situations. The principles and techniques of behavior modification are deeply woven into the fabric of major social institutions and human existence, in general, as evidenced by child rearing, education, business, government and law, and religion.[29] Although we can see aspects of behavior modification at work in components of our everyday life, the important ingredient for the use of such techniques in changing behavior is that they be *systematically* and *consistently* applied. If they are not so used, their impact on behavior is not likely to be as great. Often these conditions cannot be obtained in our daily lives. It takes concern over a significant problem to mount a specific, systematic, and consistent program. With powerful enough consequences and systematic reinforcement, behavior change in most situations is possible.

Although the techniques of behavior modification are relatively simple, their effects can be quite striking. It should be kept in mind that the techniques employed in modifying behavior are double-edged in that they can be used to promote socially relevant goals or they can be used in the service of less than ethical ends. In addition, the techniques themselves can lead into problematic territory, as in choosing negative reinforcers or punishments. The use of aversive stimuli or consequences must be employed with great caution. Because the techniques are potentially so powerful, a great deal of responsibility is placed on those who would use them. Careful consideration should always be given to ethical issues before behavior modification techniques are employed.

CONCLUSION

As you have seen, a knowledge of some of the principles of operant learning can help in structuring the environment so that desirable behaviors can be learned; or, more precisely, the environment changes behavior, which in turn changes the environment.[30] There are certain procedures that need to be followed if a learning program is to be instituted. The behavior to be changed must be clearly described and observed. A base line of present behavior is recorded for later use in ascertaining whether learning has taken place. Then the learning procedures are determined and begun. Typically an attempt is made to modify the behavior by rearranging the consequences that follow the behavior. The behavior is continuously recorded, often with the use of graphs, to give feedback on the effectiveness of the procedures. Often the procedures will be adjusted to promote maximum learning. If they are not working, they can be rapidly disregarded. The behaviors at the end of the procedures can be compared with the initial base line data to demonstrate behavior changes.

STUDY QUESTIONS

1 List those factors that influence food choices.
2 What is the significance of food symbols?
3 What are the three ways in which the function of eating is open to disturbance?
4 How can a helping relationship be incorporated into diet counseling?
5 What is the goal of diet counseling?
6 Differentiate between observational learning, stimulus-response learning, and operant learning.
7 What is meant by *reinforcement?*
8 "Extinction should be clearly distinguished from punishment, in which an aversive stimulus follows a behavior and thus decreases its frequency." Explain this statement.
9 How can the techniques of behavior modification be used in nutrition practice?

CLINICAL STUDY 11

This case is devoted to a demonstration of how behavioral techniques were applied in a specific and complex situation to help Teddy, a child, modify his feeding behavior. The case will convey some of the complexities and problems in using a behavioral approach as well as demonstrating some of its advantages.

Past history

When we first met Teddy he was a 22-month-old boy with profound failure to thrive, cerebral palsy with generalized hypotonia, and phenotypic anomalies. Teddy had a striking physical appearance because of his small size, his hypotonia, and his unusual head, which had fine, dry hair, frontal bossing of the skull,

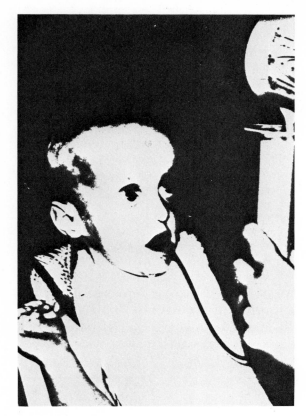

Figure 11-2
The negative rather than the positive print of Teddy was used to protect his identity. It shows him being fed by tube, which was passed into his mouth at each meal.

and shallow ocular orbits which made his eyes prominent. Teddy lived at home with only his mother, who had lived in several cities during his 22 months.

Because he was unable to suck and swallow at birth, he was begun on gavage feeding. Tube feeding continued because of persistent regurgitation, poor sucking and swallowing reflexes, and choking. Instead of passing the tube through his nasopharynx, his mother gave him the tube to swallow. However, all attempts at oral feeding had failed. With the progression of time he became conditioned to his feeding tube, and his response to oral feeding became further complicated by his lack of taste experience and his oral defensiveness. No physical abnormalities appeared to be present that required the use of the tube. He

had no major illnesses except for a brief bout of pneumonia for which he was hospitalized at 1 year of age. There was a history of recurrent urinary tract infections. His medical care had been erratic, with his mother receiving little help or encouragement. Developmentally, he had smiled at 2 to 3 months and rolled over at 1 year. He had only a few bubbling sounds at 22 months of age, and was not yet walking.

Present history
At age 22 months he was admitted to Children's Hospital Medical Center for failure to thrive. He had a bone age of 9 months, with multiple growth-arrest lines, consistent with erratic food intake and malnutrition. His tube feeding had consisted of soy formula with an estimated caloric intake of 640 kcal (2688 kJ) per day. In the hospital, his tube feeding mixture was expanded to include all the basic food groups and was supplemented with multivitamins, vitamin K, B complex, folic acid, and iron. Upon discharge from the hospital, he was enrolled in a physical therapy program and followed as an outpatient.

An outpatient program was introduced with the following goals:

1   Observation and documentation of Teddy's feeding behavior and his interaction with his mother
2   Weekly physical therapy sessions to develop better gross motor skills
3   Reduction of Teddy's oral sensitivity and introduction of foods orally
4   Monitoring of Teddy's growth, and of his nutrient intake

Weekly sessions were held for Teddy and his mother with the nutritionist. At these times, Teddy and his mother could be observed in a feeding situation and his feeding problems discussed. Teddy was encouraged to bring his hand to his mouth and to suck on his fingers. The nutritionist and mother would gently rub his gums with their fingers prior to feedings to decrease heightened oral sensitivity. A bottle and finger foods were presented along with the tube so that he would come to associate these with mealtime. This routine continued over a 6-month period, but he gained little in the way of actual food acceptance. He did, however, come to explore objects with his mouth, and he became less orally defensive.

Teddy's mother tried oral feeding with him both at home and on her weekly visits to the hospital by attempting to get him to accept many different kinds of food. Many new foods with different shapes, colors, and tastes were presented, but without success. Teddy would not try any food orally, and his mother found it difficult to persevere with any food once he had rejected it. After each refusal to eat orally, he was always tube-fed, a practice that further conditioned him to the tube.

Because of the lack of success in getting him to eat orally, a barium-swallow x-ray examination was performed. The result was a report of no coordinated muscle activity and no visible normal swallowing motions. However, we had observed how well Teddy swallowed his tube, and his ability to handle secretions was improving. Also, he had been known to drink water from a cup during episodes of throat inflammation. It was concluded that much of Teddy's inability to swallow was related to learned behavior and not due to physiological problems.

The physical therapy program had helped him to make some gains in motor development. During the 8 months since his discharge from the hospital, he had acquired sitting balance at the 5- to 6-month level, crawled with an alternate pattern at the 8-month level, and was cruising alone to tables at the 11- to 12-month level. Cognitively, he was functioning at the 15-month level on nonverbal tasks, and his expressive language skills were at the 11-month level.

Teddy was still not showing significant catch-up growth on his tube feeding regimen. It was then decided that there would have to be a more concerted effort at oral feeding.

Clinical study questions

1 Apply behavioral techniques to the case presented, identifying the target behavior and possible primary reinforcers.

2 Designate team members from the medical staff needed to implement Teddy's feeding program.

3 Explain the terms positive, negative, *and* continuous reinforcement *in relationship to this case.*

REFERENCES

1 M. D. Manning, "The Psychodynamics of Dietetics," *Nursing Outlook,* April 1965, p. 57.

2 C. G. Babcock, "Attitudes and the Use of Food," *Journal of the American Dietetic Association,* **38**:547, 1961.

3 J. Robertson, *Young Children in Hospitals,* Tavistock Publications, London, 1958, pp. 20–23.

4 Anna Freud, "The Psychoanalytic Study of Infantile Feeding Disturbances," in *The Psychoanalytic Study of the Child,* New York, 1947, pp. 119–132.

5 S. M. Pueschel, S. Cullen, R. Howard, and M. Cullinane, "Pica and Lead Poisoning," a study conducted in the Developmental Evaluation Clinic, Children's Hospital Medical Center, Boston, Mass. (to be published).

6 R. Lourie, E. Layman, and F. Millican, "Why Children Eat Things That Are Not Food," *Children,* **10**:143–146, 1963.

7 J. B. Richmond, D. Eddy, and M. Green, "Rumination: A Psychosomatic Syndrome of Infancy," *Pediatrics,* **22**:49–55, 1958.

8 H. Bruch, *Eating Disorders, Obesity, Anorexia Nervosa and the Person Within,* Basic Books, Inc., Publishers, New York, 1973.

9 American Dietetic Association Position Paper on Diet Counseling, *Journal of the American Dietetic Association,* **66**:571, 1975.

10 A. Combs, D. Avila, and W. Purkey, *Helping Relationships,* Allyn and Bacon, Inc., Boston, 1976, p. 93.

11 C. R. Rogers, "The Characteristics of a Helping Relationship," *Personnel and Guidance Journal,* **37**:6–16, 1958.

12 R. D. Helfer and J. Hess, "An Experimental Model for Making Objective Measurements of Interviewing Skills," *Journal of Clinical Psychology,* **26**:327, 1970.

13 D. Krech, R. S. Crutchfield, and E. L. Ballachecy, *Individual in Society,* McGraw-Hill Book Company, New York, 1963, p. 83.

14 A. Bandura, "Psychotherapy Based upon Modeling Principles," in A. E. Bergin and S. L. Garfield (eds.), *Handbook of Psychotherapy and Behavior Change: An Empirical Analysis,* John Wiley & Sons, Inc., New York, 1971.

15 S. Rachman, "Clinical Application of Observational Learning, Imitation, and Modeling," *Behavior Therapy,* **3**:379–397, 1972.

16 J. Wolpe, *Psychotherapy by Reciprocal Inhibition,* Stanford University Press, Stanford, Calif., 1958.

17 A. T. Schnurer, R. R. Rubin, and A. Roy, "Systematic Desensitization of Anorexia Nervosa Seen as a Weight Problem," *Journal of Behavior Therapy and Experimental Psychiatry,* **4**:149–153, 1973.

18 A. E. Kazdin, *Behavior Modification in Applied Settings,* The Dorsey Press, Homewood, Ill., 1975.

19 O. I. Lovaas, B. Schoeffer, and J. Q. Simmons, "Building Social Behavior in Autistic Children by Use of Electric Shock," *Journal of Experimental Research in Personality,* **1**:99–109, 1965.

20 B. P. Berkowitz and A. M. Graziana, "Training Parents as Behavior Therapists: A Review," *Behavioral Research and Therapy,* **10**:297–317, 1972.

21 M. R. Goddfried and M. Merbaum, *Behavior Change Through Self Control,* Holt, Rinehart and Winston, Inc., New York, 1973.

22 M. J. Mahoney, "Research Issues in Behavior Management," *Behavior Therapy,* **3**:45–63, 1972.

23 F. J. Bianco, "Rapid Treatment of Two Cases of Anorexia Nervosa," *Journal of Behavior Therapy and Experimental Psychiatry,* **3**:223–224, 1972.

24 A. Stunkard, "New Therapies for the Eating Disorders: Behavior Modification of Obesity and Anorexia Nervosa," *Archives of General Psychiatry,* **26**:391–398, 1972.

25 R. B. Stuart and B. Davis, *Slim Chance in a Fat World,* Research Press, 2621 North Mattis Avenue, Champaign, Ill., 1972.

26 G. R. Leon and K. Chamberlain, "Comparison of Daily Eating Habits and Emotional Status of Overweight Persons Successful or Unsuccessful in Maintaining a Weight Loss," *Journal of Consulting and Clinical Psychology,* **61**:108–115, 1973.

27 M. J. Mahoney, N. G. Moura, and T. E. Wade, "Relative Efficiency of Self Reward, Self Punishment, and Self Monitoring Techniques for Weight Loss," *Journal of Consulting and Clinical Psychology,* **40**:404–407, 1973.

28 S. C. Wooley, O. W. Wooley, and S. R. Dyrenforth, "Theoretical, Practical, and Social Issues in Behavioral Treatments of Obesity," *Journal of Applied Behavior Analysis,* **12**(1):3–25, 1979.

29 A. Bandura, *Principles of Behavior Modification,* Holt, Rinehart and Winston, Inc., New York, 1969.

30 Ibid.

CLINICAL DISCUSSION 11

A team comprising a physical therapist, psychologist, pediatrician, nurse, speech patholo-gist, and nutritionist met and devised a program to begin oral feeding that might be best accomplished in a very structured environment. The goal was to wean Teddy from his tube and to provide food by the oral route. It was decided to admit Teddy to the hospital since the attempt at gradual weaning on an outpatient basis had not been successful.

Changing Teddy's behavior toward food required very careful planning. Before his hospitalization the program for Teddy was discussed with the nurses and physicians who would be in contact with Teddy so that their behavior would be in concert with the program. It was decided that the most effective way to make oral food reinforcing for him was to have him be hungry before oral feeding was attempted. Heretofore he had always been tube-fed when he refused food presented orally. He had become quite adept at handling anyone, especially his mother, who tried to get him to sample food orally. He had no need to try food, for his tube feeding would always occur regardless of his behavior. In order to facilitate his learning to eat orally the tube was entirely discarded and no one in the hospital was to feed him this way. A very important concern was that without the tube feeding he could become dehydrated and begin to lose weight if he did not start eating. We decided the risk was worth taking since no other approach had shown any sign of working. Everyone connected with Teddy had to be reassured that we would not let him starve to death and within the hospital environment fluid balance could be reestablished intravenously if the need arose.

Initially we wished to involve his mother in getting him to eat in the hospital; but she felt that the situation would be very stressful for her, although she agreed with the intent of the program. She therefore left town for the first week of the program. Because of Teddy's difficulties she tended to be overprotective toward him and could not bear to see him unhappy or distressed. For about the first 3 years of his life she alone could feed Teddy. They were inseparable and literally tied by the tube.

To get him eating as quickly as possible a program with the highest amount of consistency was implemented. One person, the physical therapist, was selected to feed him at the same times each day and in the same place. The physical therapist already had had positive experiences with Teddy, as she had been the one encouraging and promoting the development of his motor skills. Teddy was given baby food with Isomil. At first he refused to try the food but after several sessions when he obviously was becoming hungrier he began to try it. Because he was no longer being tube-fed the food he received orally served as a primary reinforcement as it assuaged his hunger. The physical therapist also responded with praise and attention each time he ate a spoonful or drank a mouthful of food. He did, however, present a great deal of negative behavior such as crying and fussing when the food was offered. This behavior was extinguished by removal of the physical therapist's attention. The therapist would turn away from Teddy until the negative behavior stopped. Within 1 week, Teddy was drinking Isomil from a cup and had begun to accept baby food on a spoon with a notable decrease in negative behavior.

After an initial weight loss, Teddy's weight stabilized and he began to regain weight. When his mother returned she was trained in the feeding procedures that the physical therapist had used and was instructed never to return to tube feeding. Teddy was then discharged from the hospital and followed at biweekly intervals. Although he was now eating orally at home he demonstrated many negative, manipulative, and controlling food behaviors with his mother to the extent that he would only eat foods he preferred and not try any others. His mother found it difficult to be consistent in her attempts to get him to try new foods.

The behavior modification program had demonstrated success in helping Teddy to learn to eat orally and his growth began to improve. However, the development of completely appropriate eating habits was not accomplished at that time because that part of the program depended upon his mother, who found it difficult to maintain the program at home despite supportive counseling.

With his new feeding pattern Teddy also showed general developmental gains in many areas, and the degree of his developmental retardation was significantly reduced.

CHAPTER 12

DEVELOPMENTAL CONSIDERATIONS IN INFANT FEEDING

Robert W. Telzrow

KEY WORDS
Interaction
Synchrony
Autonomy
Temperament

INTRODUCTION

Some of the most attractive and nutritionally balanced meals prepared for infants by both parents and dietitians go untouched. The solutions to this dilemma rarely lie in the foods themselves but in the fact that "eating does not occur as an isolated phenomenon but as part of a complex of interlocking social and biological conditions."[1] Nowhere, perhaps, is the old adage "You can lead a horse to water, but you can't make him drink" truer than in a consideration of infant feeding. While this is obvious to most, it is surprising how often some need to be reminded of it.

Some studies have been concerned with the effects of nutrition on growth and development while frequently showing little interest in other environmental effects. By contrast, other studies devoted to enhancing the cognitive and social environment of infants (stimulation programs) have given little consideration to food as a major factor in the infant's experience. Obviously, an awareness of the interaction between food and environment is necessary but often absent.

In this chapter, the postnatal environmental influences on feeding development are presented, with citation of those periods in the child's early development when the interaction between feeding and important developmental variables can result in either excellent opportunities for both the parent and child or, as a consequence of these influences, feeding problems. Throughout this chapter the discussion is supported with clinical studies which give the health care professional the background needed to identify stages of child development around which anticipatory guidance can be given.

The nutritional status of the mother prior to conception and during pregnancy influences the

Note: The reader should note that this chapter has a somewhat different format: there are five "clinical studies," and—as is explained in the Introduction—these are placed not at the end of the chapter but rather at appropriate points within the text. The "clinical discussions" are omitted, as these studies are discussed in the chapter text.

outcome of the pregnancy and, ultimately, how infants are able to react to their environments and to feed. The effect of malnutrition on brain growth and subsequent development and the specialized feeding techniques needed for the "small for gestational age" (SGA) infant are topics covered in later chapters. (See Chapters 13 and 14.) Although not covered in this chapter, these factors are important influences on infant feeding.

POSTNATAL ENVIRONMENTAL INFLUENCES ON FEEDING BEHAVIOR

Age 0 to 2 Months

Infant Sucking Patterns

In a series of studies reported by Kaye,[1] newborn infants have been shown to have a natural, regular, rhythmic sucking pattern consisting of bursts of sucking followed by pauses. The length of the bursts appears to be dependent on milk flow (longer if the flow is rapid, shorter if flow is insufficient), whereas the length of the pauses appears to be related to interactions between the infant and its mother.

Contrary to popular belief, stimulation (jiggling the bottle, etc.) during the pauses reduces the likelihood of the infant's immediately returning to a burst pattern of sucking. In fact, pauses during which the infant is stimulated are longer than pauses during which the infant is not stimulated. Stopping the stimulation, on the other hand, does increase somewhat the infant's return to sucking. Kaye has shown that over the first 2 weeks, mothers changed the way in which they stimulated their infants during these pause periods. Instead of stimulating until the child began to suck again, as they had done, the mothers would stimulate briefly and then wait for the infant to respond before stimulating again.

This resulted in shortening both the duration of the stimulation and the duration of the pauses, and suggests that the mothers, in responding to the tendency of the infant to resume feeding when the stimulation stopped, had changed their responses during the pauses. This

indicates early evidence of a synchrony (mutual awareness) between the partners.

An additional aspect of infant sucking is the role of maternal parity. Studies by Thoman et al.[2,3] suggest that the feeding behavior of the infant differs as a function of parity independent of the contribution of the mother. They observed that infants born to multiparous mothers had more feeding intervals (pauses in feeding) than those of primiparous mothers. This was shown by recording the feeding behavior of these newborns while they were being fed by an experienced nurse for their first feeding. In contrast, however, when given their babies, it was the primiparous mothers who used a greater number of feeding intervals and spent more time in nonfeeding activities. It appeared that multiparous mothers were more sensitive to the infant's cues

in the observation that infants of multiparous mothers sucked more during breast feeding and consumed more during bottle feedings, even though the primiparous mothers spent more time feeding their infants and stimulated them more to get them to suck.[4]

Thoman[5] suggested that the primiparous mothers, because of their relative inexperience and increased eagerness, might be more likely to miss the types of cues or observations that Kaye is describing and to go on stimulating their infants, thus prolonging the feeding. The length of time that these differences persist is unknown. Kaye, in his report, makes no reference to differences in parity. Brody,[6] however, showed in an earlier report that for infants up to 7 months of age there still were more feeding intervals among primiparous mothers.

This is not a question of the primiparous mother's underfeeding her infant, and thus is not a pattern which demands intervention. Certainly, the known higher expectations of primiparous mothers, both of themselves and of their infants, raise the likelihood of dissynchrony and subsequent feeding problems. If, however, as Kaye suggests, the changing burst-and-pause pattern shows evidence of synchrony and contains the elements of learning to give and take turns and learning how to anticipate one an- other's behavior, then the apparent inefficiency in feeding suggested in the frequent "interven- tions" of the parent may in fact be serving a dif- ferent purpose for the parent and child, namely, providing an opportunity for social exchange be- tween the parent and the infant.

It would be wrong to place undue emphasis on efficiency in a feeding interaction at a time when a parent, especially a primiparous parent, is in the process of trying to find regularity in an interaction. That it might take a primiparous parent longer should not surprise anyone. There is no suggestion at this time that this relative inefficiency is in any way disorganizing to the infant, or that it in any way renders the infant incapable of good social interactions during those prolonged pause periods.

Attachment

One of the most important tasks awaiting new- borns is the development of ties between them- selves and their parents, referred to as the *at- tachment process*. An important component of this attachment is the establishment of a com- munication system between the infant and the caregiver within the first few months. When functional, this system shows a high degree of synchrony between the participants. When it fails, a lack of synchrony is evident.

Because feeding and feeding-related inter- actions occupy much of the infant's awake time during the first months, it is not surprising that major opportunities for further development of this synchrony occur during feeding times (see Fig. 12-1). These episodes can be very inform- ative windows through which to view the attach- ment process. In fact, a correlation has been shown between events occurring around feed- ings in the first 3 months of life and the success- ful subsequent development of attachment be- tween the infant and the mother.[7,8]

Since feeding problems often occur between some of the most apparently attached parents and their infants, it is necessary to differentiate between securely attached parent-infant pairs and anxiously attached pairs. The securely at-

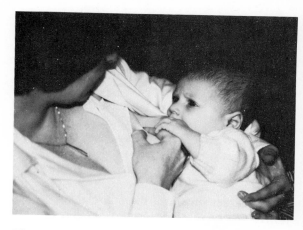

Figure 12-1
Hand-to-hand, mouth-to-breast synchrony in feeding.

tached child at 1 year of age is able, to use the parent as a secure base and shows a balance be- tween exploring the environment from that base and staying close to it when stressed or needy. Following separation (e.g., having a baby-sitter for the afternoon) the infant shows positive be- havior toward the parent when reunited (e.g., brightening, smiling, or cuddling). An anxiously attached child, on the other hand, at a similar age shows an imbalance between staying close and exploring. Following separation this child frequently shows a mixture of positive behavior and negative behavior (avoiding proximity, striking the parent, or even ignoring the parent).

Ainsworth and Bell[9] have shown that where synchrony has been achieved to a high degree in the first 3 months, as seen in the feeding inter- action, subsequent attachment is strong. There are four points which they use to assess the de- gree of synchrony in a feeding situation. All have excellent applicability.

1 The timing of the feeding—is it in response to a signal by the infant or determined pri- marily for the parent's convenience?

2 Who determines the amount of food ingested and the end of the feeding? Is it the infant or does the parent insist on a predetermined amount?

3 Is there tact in handling the infant's preferences when solid foods are introduced?

4 Who sets the pace or rate of intake? Is it in accordance with the baby's own rate or the caregiver's?

Securely attached infants had mothers who scored higher on these items and were felt to be more attuned to the infant's rhythm, signals, preferences, and pacing. This suggests a heightened awareness of the individuality of these infants and demonstrates the interaction between nutrition and other aspects of development (in this case, affective growth). Implications for counseling should center on promoting this awareness. This might best be done during the newborn period by fostering in parents an awareness of the unique qualities and individuality that newborns possess. Fostering this awareness becomes especially important in infants who are premature or have congenital anomalies, because these conditions impose stress on the attachment process. Also helpful in some cases would be encouraging the parent and child to be alone for some of the feeding episodes where they will not be distracted by ongoing events in their household.

Disorganization of Normal Rhythms Secondary to Organic Illness

There are a number of events that can occur to both parents and infants alike which have an effect on each one's ability to be attuned to these signals and rhythms and which thus affect infant feeding. (See Clinical Study 12-1.)

Here is a case where an infant has become disorganized in areas of state control (a loss of control over normal rhythms like sleeping and waking cycles) following the stress of hyperbilirubinemia and the use of phototherapy. (Phototherapy is a process which takes advantage of the fact that bilirubin concentration can be reduced by exposure to visible light, primarily in the blue spectral range, which minimizes the need for exchange transfusion. Therapy is necessary when bilirubin concentration becomes elevated to levels which can cause brain damage.) Behavioral effects of jaundice and phototherapy have been shown to be manifested as altered state control and poor interactive qualities (responsiveness to social stimuli such as faces and

---

CLINICAL STUDY 12-1
DISORGANIZATION SECONDARY TO ORGANIC ILLNESS

Timothy A. was a 2.95-kg infant born following a 38-week gestation. Pregnancy, labor, and delivery were benign. He was a slow eater during the first few days, but his mother persisted and he took up to 2 oz at most feedings. On the third day he was noticeably jaundiced and appeared sleepier than usual. His serum bilirubin level rose to 18.0 mg/dL, and fluorescent phototherapy was begun. He remained blindfolded and under the fluorescent lights for 3 days except for brief feeding periods. His mother had been discharged but was able to visit once a day to feed him.

Timothy's bilirubin responded to light treatment

and he was discharged. However, when he arrived home he appeared to be overly sleepy, and to have many brief episodes of being irritable. If left alone, he would sleep 6 or 7 hours at a time. He would then become very hungry and have difficulty taking his bottle while so irritable. When his parents tried to wake him up sooner, he often fell asleep after taking only an ounce. This meant he was getting no more than 10 to 12 oz of formula in a day. His mother became more and more concerned and began to question her own ability to care for her child. In addition she also began to wonder whether Timothy was ill or abnormal.

voices).[10] These effects appear to persist for at least 1 week following phototherapy.

Jaundice and phototherapy are by no means the only disorganizing influences on the newborn. Medication during delivery, for example, can also have such effects if not used sparingly.[11] Other infants have poor state control for reasons we do not understand.

This information is important because we know that the infant's level of participation in the parent-child interaction is of such significance that it becomes a major determinant of parental care-giving responses. It is not uncommon for a disorganized child to elicit confusion and concern in parents. This brings into play the uncertainties and fears that all parents have, leading some to respond to their unpredictable child by being unpredictable themselves. Support by health care personnel during these episodes is necessary. Proper information about the child's transient disorganization and suggestions for intervention which might minimize this disorganization would be appropriate, including, where applicable, a feeding schedule.

For example, in Timothy's case, a suggestion on how to arouse a sleepy baby would be appropriate. If we were to arouse him indiscriminately, we might undermine any attempts on his part to organize his own sleep cycles. Waking him when he is in a light sleep state minimizes this disruption. Light sleep is easy to recognize: eye movements are noticeable under the eyelids, respiration is irregular, and body movements are frequent. Following arousal from light sleep the infant is more prone to respond to a feeding. Seeing this as the infant's problem, and recognizing that the parents can help resolve it with proper information, will minimize the kinds of responses noted in the case example. Since there is some evidence of dehydration following phototherapy, which can certainly contribute to these observed behaviors, appropriate fluid intake can then be maintained.

Environmental and Emotional Stimulation

One of the more striking examples of the interaction between environment and nutrition is seen in the infant with failure to thrive. (See Clinical Study 12-2.) Powell et al.[12,13] described children of varying ages with signs of possible hypopituitarism (decreased ACTH reserve and diminished release of growth hormone) who were also noted to have very bizarre behaviors, ravenous appetites, failure to grow, and very stressed home lives. Restoration of their depressed growth hormone levels occurred following their removal from the stressed environment. Following this, growth was rapid unless they returned home, in which case they stopped growing and growth hormone levels diminished. Administration of growth hormone without altering their environment was less successful than changing their environment alone, suggesting an altered psychological response to growth hormone.[14,15]

These reports, along with others, have increased physicians' awareness of environmental (nonorganic) failure to thrive to the point where the presence of an infant on a pediatric ward with a diagnosis of nonorganic failure to thrive has become almost routine. Such infants have a variety of histories, and only a few show the picture of possible hypopituitarism.

When first encountered, these infants have weights below the 3d percentile. Some also show a falloff in length and head circumference. They are pathetic, unhappy-looking babies with sunken, wary eyes. They frequently show very little motor activity. One striking observation is that if hospitalized and put on an optimal caloric intake, they often do not begin to gain weight for up to 2 weeks. Some (about one-third) actually lose weight while in the hospital.

A study by Rosenn et al.[16] has defined the failure-to-thrive infant behaviorally and has chronicled the infant's behavior during the recovery period. It showed that the infant with nonorganic failure to thrive, when compared to those with organic failure to thrive or to controls, preferred distal to proximal social interactions. The child would show eye contact from a distance but would look away when approached. Such infants preferred objects to people. If handed a toy, they would use it to keep

CLINICAL STUDY 12-2
ENVIRONMENTAL AND EMOTIONAL STIMULATION

Amanda C. was a 2½-month-old baby admitted to the hospital because of failure to thrive. Her perinatal history was unremarkable. She had been born weighing 3.32 kg to a gravida 4, para 4, 24-year-old mother. While in the nursery she was an alert baby with no feeding difficulties. When seen at her 6-week follow-up visit she was still at just above her birth weight but overall appeared healthy. Her mother expressed minimal concern over this and felt that Amanda ate well. She described her as an easy baby. One month later, on follow-up, she was still not gaining weight (3.75 kg) and was admitted to the hospital.

Her physical examination showed her to be somewhat hypotonic, with poor head control and possibly some spasticity in her lower limbs. Neurological consultation raised the question of cerebral palsy. Behaviorally she showed evidence of neglect. She showed initial interest but no excitement when interacting with the nursing staff. There was no quick smile or the rhythmic churning of her arms and legs that one

expects from a 2- to 3-month-old. Instead she averted her gaze, her respirations became irregular, and her arms remained flexed with her hands held back on either side of her head. At times she showed mottling of her skin. Her behavior suggested that she was incapable of interacting without being easily overstimulated, as evidenced by changes in respiration and the vascular instability of mottling.

Mrs. C. was very depressed, and her history revealed that she had been so from the time she first learned she was pregnant with Amanda. Her marriage had been a disappointment. She lost many of her friends following the birth of her oldest son because she had to quit her job. She had been planning to return to work when she realized she was pregnant with Amanda. The sight of Mrs. C. sitting with Amanda lying on her lap in a limp, almost rag doll, posture yet still staring at her mother's expressionless face, with Mrs. C. unable to look back at her daughter, told the whole story.

---

the observer away rather than to draw the observer into an interaction (social exchange) as the controls did. These and other behaviors were scored using an approach-withdrawal scale which places infant behaviors on a continuum ranging from extremely negative to extremely positive.

The study suggests that when weight gain begins to occur, it follows by 24 to 48 h a change in the infant's behavior profile from the preceding negative description seen in Amanda to a positive one similar to that of the controls.

Animal studies have also shown the interactive effect of nutrition and environment. Levitsky and Barnes[17] found that the adverse behavioral effects of early malnutrition in rats were exaggerated in a deprived environment and significantly reduced in an enriched environment.

They suggested two possible mechanisms, as follows:

Malnutrition may change the experience or perception of the environment during the period of early development by physiologically rendering the animal less capable of receiving, or integrating, or both, information about the environment. Another mechanism may be purely behavioral. Malnutrition may produce behaviors which themselves are incompatible with the incorporation of environmental information necessary for optimal cognitive growth.[18]

The converse would also appear to be true, in that environmental events such as neglect may alter children emotionally and physiologically to the extent that they make poor use of the nutrients they have been given.

When these data are applied to our clinical experience, we can easily see the child, apathetic and withdrawn because of malnutrition or the lack of appropriate social stimulation or frequently both, incapable of either processing information from the environment or interacting with it.

It is remarkable how, in the light of this affront, children are able to recover when they are given an appropriate environment, including good nutrition.

In Amanda's case an intervention program was designed to provide her with a more appropriate social experience. This had to be done gradually because it was so easy to give her more stimulation than she could tolerate. Using a primary nursing approach that allowed the nurse to develop a relationship with Amanda, at Amanda's own pace, was the first step. Often such children can only tolerate being stimulated for brief periods of time and through a single sensory modality. Amanda was cuddled when fed and only spoken to softly. She was not bounced or played with in any way which elicited too much response from her. Following the first week she began to have eye contact with the nurse while being fed. This was the first sign of a trusting relationship. Continued efforts paid off and she soon began to gain weight; with that,

her abnormal muscle tone and questionable neurological signs resolved.

Age 2 to 4 Months

Most feeding problems which arise in healthy children from this point on center on two issues. The first is the parent's concern (often unfounded) over inadequate intake; the second is concern over allowing the child to become the master of what he or she eats. In this section we discuss a number of developmental milestones, infants' differences in temperament, and parental concerns which have a bearing on how children eat and how much they eat. (See Clinical Study 12-3.)

Quantity of Intake

Concern about whether a child is getting enough to eat is universal. The particular problems encountered by Jason's parents are common manifestations of this concern. Jason's fussiness always seemed to be less when he was sucking. This was interpreted to mean that he was hungry. We know now that a lot of sucking by infants is not related to hunger. Nonnutritive sucking appears to be a way in which infants quiet themselves. It helps them contain themselves in much the same way that adults do

---

CLINICAL STUDY 12-3
QUANTITY OF INTAKE

Jason Q. was an excellent eater. He was born weighing 3.868 kg following an uneventful pregnancy, labor, and delivery. His mother, age 28, planned to nurse him as she had her two older children. Jason, however, never appeared to be satisfied. Unlike his two older siblings, Jason was a very intense, fussy baby. His parents found themselves supplementing his feedings with a bottle by the time he was 2 or 3 weeks of age. This satisfied him for a while but soon

he was fussing again. Cereal was added to his milk for a few weeks, and by 7 weeks of age he had been introduced to a number of solid foods. Most of it came back out as soon as it was in Jason's mouth. He occasionally gagged and even vomited. At other times when fed he would suck on his fingers. When he did this, he did not have as much difficulty with eating. It seemed that the harder Jason's parents tried, the more he would gag and spit up.

when they swaddle or hold a crying, fussy baby. The difference is that sucking is the baby's own attempt to accomplish this. Since offering the breast or bottle does quiet the baby, it reinforces the notion of hunger as the cause. In addition, it fails to allow the child an opportunity to begin to achieve competence in controlling some of his or her own frustration.

Suckle-Swallow Reflex

The second problem in this case grew out of the first. Solid foods were introduced in response to Jason's apparent hunger. Newborns do not have the ability to swallow voluntarily much before 10 or 12 weeks of age. They can swallow only if their sucking reflex is stimulated first. Even when voluntary swallowing does occur, the infant will still suck on its fingers while attempting to swallow. Although it did not happen in Jason's case, this hand-to-mouth behavior is frequently discouraged by parents who see it as interfering with their attempts to feed their child.

Age 4 to 9 Months

As a child develops, new skills and a broader awareness of the environment change the ways in which the child approaches a feeding.

Response to Breast Feeding

Sharon is an excellent example of three common feeding problems. (See Clinical Study 12-4.) The first is seen in her response to nursing. She would appear to be uninterested, and in fact Mrs. E. felt Sharon had begun to wean herself. What we are seeing is how individual temperament influences behavior. Sharon, while showing herself to be highly adaptable when she began to nurse and with the introduction of solids, is also showing that she is very easily distracted. Extraneous stimuli, such as another adult in the room or minor noises, are now capable of attracting her attention, making her curious, and interfering with her ongoing behavior.

This seems to be more common among breast-fed infants, perhaps because the nursing child's field of vision is more confined by this position. It can usually be handled by firmly coaxing the child back and by nursing in a quiet room with dim light at least once or twice a day (preferably morning and evening), when distractions are at a minimum. With minimal distractions the child is able to focus on the ongoing feeding process and is usually reinforced by the parent's more relaxed and focused response.

Acquisition of Reaching

The second development of significance is Sharon's acquisition of reaching. As with any new skill, it is immediately put to use to explore her environment. In Sharon's case, she becomes interested in her mother's face, in combination with her distractibility and reaches out in gross sweeping movements. As her reach develops, she gets great pleasure in going after almost anything and putting it into her mouth. Almost simultaneous with this acquisitiion of reaching is the first evidence of autonomy.

Autonomy

We see in Sharon's case real evidence of preference and independence. Food preferences are not necessarily part of a child's genetic endowment but are acquired and thus individualized. Every household has a number a common foods missing from the dinner table because of the preferences of the adult members. Why then are parents unaware or intolerant of food preferences in their children?

To a large extent it has to do with control, and represents the starting point for most of the feeding problems encountered in the infant and preschooler. The development of autonomy and independence is every bit as important as the development of attachment. The participants in this process are the very people with whom the infant has just set up a dependent relationship. Most parents find the dependency needs of infants quite gratifying, so that when the child begins to separate from the parents and to become autonomous, they often feel a sense of loss. This is compounded by the child's vacillations between dependency and autonomy. Here is where

CLINICAL STUDY 12-4
INFANT'S RESPONSE TO BREAST FEEDING; ACQUISITION OF REACHING; AUTONOMY

Sharon E. is a 6-month-old infant brought to the clinic because of a feeding problem. She had been a healthy infant whose only medical contact had been for well-child visits. Mrs. E. had been successful in nursing Sharon. At 4 months of age solid foods were introduced, with Sharon taking to them in her usual eager way.

Now, however, when her mother attempts to nurse her, Sharon is continuously pushing away from the nipple after a few sucks. She will look around the room, return briefly to the breast, and look around again. If her mother is speaking to another person or

if there is any activity or noise in the room, the pushing away is more frequent. At other times she looks up at her mother and becomes interested in reaching for her mother's face and hair.

In addition, both parents report difficulties in giving her solids. She frequently turns away as the spoon approaches, waving her arms wildly and occasionally sending the spoon flying. There are certain foods which she repeatedly spits out. Because of this her parents became concerned about her food intake and sought help. Her physical examination was entirely normal.

---

allowing the child to be a more active participant in feeding should begin (see Fig. 12-2).

With the acquisition of an evolving pincer grasp using thumb and forefinger, children's reach will soon be developed to the point where

Figure 12-2
Sarah, age 7 months. The first evidence of autonomy is almost simultaneous with the acquisition of reaching.

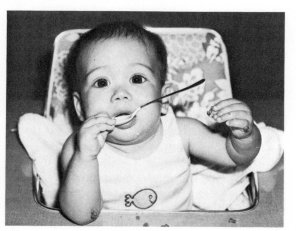

they will happily be picking up pieces of food and stuffing themselves. They will also use these skills to explore their food. Finger foods allow this to happen. Usually parents still need to be actively involved in feeding at this point and frequently need ways to deal with the reaching and grabbing of the infant while the reach and pincer grasp are still inefficient. Giving babies something to hold in each hand, like a breadstick or a spoon, eliminates the grabbing and provides something for them to feed themselves. The spoon will in time facilitate imitative behavior when the child is ready to use it competently at about 15 or 16 months of age.

Spitting Up
Spitting up in infancy is common. There are a number of infants, however, who spit up regularly, sometimes 1 or 2 times per meal. An evaluation should be done on any infant who spits up this frequently. Some of these babies have chalasia (relaxation of a bodily opening such as a cardiac sphincter, a cause of vomiting in infants)[19] and are helped by being fed and kept upright in a chalasia chair for a period of time following their feeding. On occasion surgery is

CLINICAL STUDY 12-5
SPITTING UP

Daniel R. was hospitalized at 7 months of age because of failure to thrive. Mrs. R., aged 24, described a normal pregnancy, labor, and delivery. She reported that Daniel had been spitting up since birth. At age 2½ weeks, after he had been seen by his pediatrician, his milk was changed to a soy-based formula. This seemed to work for a few weeks, following which he began to spit up again. Subsequent formula changes also proved to be unsuccessful. At about 3 months of age cereals and fruits had been introduced with no change in his symptoms. Gradually he showed evidence of a decline in his growth curve. At birth he had weighed 3.26 kg and was 51 cm long. By his sixth month he was in the 3d percentile for weight and was falling off in his length. A complete evaluation including a search for occult infection, malabsorption, chronic disease such as cystic fibrosis, evidence of central nervous system damage, and evidence of deprivation proved negative.

Daniel was described by his parents as a very intense child. When he cried, it was long and loud; when he was happy, he was beside himself. His response to a new toy or new food was very positive. He always smiled at everyone he saw. He frequently was excited just prior to spitting up. These would often be times when he was playing with his mother or father.

indicated. Other concerns, such as pyloric stenosis, also need to be considered during the newborn period.

A few of these infants, such as Daniel, who have no physical explanation for their failure to grow, end up being hospitalized. (See Clinical Study 12-5.) An understanding of the infant's temperament should be part of any evaluation. Among the children who make up "spitters" are a group like Daniel. They do not show the behaviors, described previously, of children with environmental failure to thrive. Almost in complete contrast, they are intense, easily excited infants who show good qualities of interaction and evidence of appropriate interpersonal experience. They frequently spit up when excited or in any way stressed.

This spitting up is often interpreted as overfeeding, and parents frequently try to deal with it by feeding the child less. At times this is done gradually and unknowingly, so that when such children are hospitalized, they are being given less than adequate nutrition. The feeding experience usually becomes so negative and unrewarding that it affects the way in which the parents view their child. Almost universally the parents feel like failures.

When fed an adequate diet, while the parents receive support and reassurance, these infants gain weight even while continuing to spit up. Thus the notion that they fail to grow because of the food lost from spitting up is untrue. It is because they are underfed by their parents in response to their spitting up. This problem becomes much less frequent between 12 and 16 months of age. Interestingly, these infants remain intense children who in later years when stressed or excited (by birthdays, first day of school, etc.) often respond by vomiting.

Age 9 to 16 Months

Independence
The list of milestones during this period is significant—the infant will pull to stand, will cruise, and probably will walk; he or she will have developed a reach and pincer grasp and will be able to manipulate and explore the environment; meaningful words will be uttered; a sense of spatial awareness, of the permanency of

objects, of employing means to achieve ends, and of making causal connections will have developed. Throughout all these accomplishments is a rapidly growing sense of competence and independence. By the end of this period children are quite capable of feeding themselves and will in fact insist on it (see Fig. 12-3).

By not encouraging independence, parents frequently find themselves with a feeding problem. The two parental concerns (about enough to eat and about allowing autonomy) remain at the base of most feeding problems in healthy children at this age. An example of concern over the child's getting enough to eat is seen in the amount of food that children in this age group

Figure 12-3

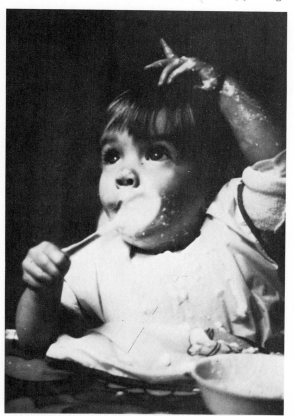

"I'd rather do it myself." Seana, age 12 months, is becoming more independent, insisting on self-feeding.

are given. Until the child is 8 or 9 months of age some parents use commercially prepared baby foods which come in standardized volumes. These parents mistakenly assume that the baby-food jar represents a desired, scientifically determined volume of food. This standard offers comfort and reassurance to parents. Once table foods are introduced, however, the parents' standard becomes whatever they determine it to be—usually a subjective percentage of an adult portion.

Once a standard has been set, an expectation has also been set. The child's own physiological response to food—an awareness of hunger or satiety—and attempts at autonomy have become challenged. The result is often food on the floor, an angry and frustrated parent, and a crying child. How much simpler it would be to put small amounts of food (chopped and cut table food) in front of children and to let them set their own pace and determine their own volume. It is wise to put out only small amounts at a time since children's temptation to play with and throw food seems to increase with the amount in front of them.

CONCLUSION

At this point it is important to consider the adage cited at the beginning of this chapter in light of what has been said in the preceding discussion about parental concerns over adequate volumes and the encouragement of autonomy in feeding. It is important to remember when bringing the horse to the trough that the objective is to satisfy the horse's thirst and not to drain the trough. Likewise, the goal in feeding children should be to satisfy their hunger and caloric needs and not to get them to clean their plates. Further, optimal nutrition, a legitimate long-range goal, can be accomplished only by being aware of a child's total growth process. There clearly are times when meeting minimal daily requirements will appear as a challenge. An approach which appreciates the value of promoting the inherent sense of competence and mastery already present in children will minimize areas of conflict such as those described in this chapter. The end result will be a child who is not only well nourished physically but also well nourished cognitively and emotionally.

STUDY QUESTIONS

1 What are the prenatal influences that can affect infant feeding behavior?

2 Describe the postnatal influences on feeding behavior in the infant between the ages of birth and 2 months, 2 and 4 months, 4 and 9 months, 9 and 16 months.

3 How would you assess the degree of synchrony between a parent and child in a feeding situation?

4 Describe the behavioral characteristics of a child with nonorganic failure to thrive.

5 What are the major issues that surround feeding problems in the second year of life?

REFERENCS

1 K. Kaye, "Toward the Origin of Dialogue," paper prepared for the Loch Lomond Symposium, University of Strathelyde, September 1975.

2 E. B. Thoman, "Development of Synchrony in Mother-Infant Interaction in Feeding and Other Situations," paper presented at symposium of the American Institute of Nutrition, Federation of American Societies of Experimental Biology: Effects of Nutrition on Maternal-Infant Interaction, Atlantic City, N.J., April 9, 1974.

3 E. G. Thoman, C. R. Barnett, and P. H. Leiderman, "Feeding Behaviors of Newborn Infants as a Function of Parity of the Mother," *Child Development* **42**:1471–1483, 1971.

4 E. G. Thoman, op. cit.

5 Ibid.

6 S. Brody, *Patterns of Mothering*, International Universities Press, Inc., New York, 1966.

7 M. D. S. Ainsworth and S. M. Bell, "Some Contemporary Patterns of Mother-Infant Interaction in the Feeding Situation," in A. Ambrose (ed.), *Stimulation in Early Infancy,* Academic Press, New York, 1969, pp. 133–170.

8 M. D. S. Ainsworth, S. M. Bell, and D. J. Stayton, "Individual Differences in Strange-Situation Behavior of One-Year-Olds," in H. R. Schaffer (ed.), *The Origins of Human Social Relations,* Academic Press, New York, 1971, pp. 17–52.

9 M. D. S. Ainsworth and S. M. Bell, op. cit, pp. 133–170.

10 D. M.Snyder, R. W. Telzrow, E. Tronick, H. Als, and T. B. Brazelton, "The Effects of Phototherapy on Neonatal Behavior," *Proceedings of the Society of Pediatric Research,* April 1976.

11 E. Tronick, S. Wise, H. Als, L. Adamson, J. Scanlon, and T. B. Brazelton, "Regional Obstetric Anesthesia and Newborn Behavior: Effect over the First Ten Days of Life," *Pediatrics* **58**:94–100, 1976.

12 G. F. Powell, J. A. Brasel, and R. M. Blizzard, "Functional Deprivation and Growth Retardation Simulating Idiopathic Hypopituitarism. I. Clinical Evaluation of the Syndrome," *New England Journal of Medicine* **276**:1271–1278, 1967.

13 G. F. Powell, J. A. Brasel, S. Raiti, and R. M. Blizzard, "Emotional Deprivation and Growth Retardation Simulating Idiopathic Hypopituitarism. II. Endocrinologic Evaluation of the Syndrome," *New England Journal of Medicine,* **276**:1279, 1967.

14 Ibid.

15 S. D. Frasier and M. L. Rallison, "Growth Retardation and Emotional Deprivation: Relative Resistance to Treatment with Human Growth Hormone," *Journal of Pediatrics* **80**:603–609, 1972.

16 D. Rosenn, L. Stein, and M. Bates, "The Differentiation of Organic from Environmental Failure to Thrive," paper presented at the meetings of the American Pediatric Society and Society for Pediatric Research, April 1975.

17 D. A. Levitsky and R. H. Barnes, "Nutritional and Environmental Interactions in the Behavioral Development of the Rat: Long-Term Effects," *Science,* **176**:68–71, 1972.

18 Ibid.

19 *Dorland's Illustrated Medical Dictionary,* 24th ed., W. B. Saunders Company, Philadelphia, 1965.

CHAPTER 13

GROWTH AND NUTRITION

Christine E. Cronk
Rosanne Beatrice Howard

KEY WORDS
Growth
Critical Periods
Growth Velocity
Cumulative Growth
Growth Assessment
Age Needs
Stage Needs

INTRODUCTION

Growth is the outward sign of a positive interaction between nutrition, genetics, and time. Nutrition operates within the confines of one's genetic background and environment to maximize growth potential. With a greater understanding of growth as presented in the first part of this chapter, the student will better understand nutritional needs through the life cycle.

Although chronological age is used as a point of demarcation to describe nutrient needs, it should be remembered that it is physiological age which is the true determinant. The spectrum of human variability is broad, and because a child is chronologically 13, he or she is not necessarily an adolescent; nor is a person at 65 always elderly. Within a single family, all ages and stages may be represented, and the nutrient needs of everybody must be considered. The influences of nutrition on the human body are continuous, with one generation passing the effect on to the next. It is a circular process, as portrayed in the Wheel of Life (Fig. 13-1, p. 240).

GROWTH

Christine E. Cronk

DEFINITION

Growth, which is one measure of nutrient effectiveness in early life, is the increase in size attendant upon development of the organism from embryo to adult. It implies the physiological accretion of tissue, which in turn reflects the acquisition of protein and water.[1]

PROCESSES AND MECHANISMS UNDERLYING GROWTH

Growth takes place by way of three processes: (1) an increase in cell number, known as *hyperplasia;* (2) growth in cell size, or *hypertrophy;* and (3) an increase in the size of the intercellular matrix (material between cells). Newer studies indicate that the first two processes are not separated in time. Once cell division is under

239

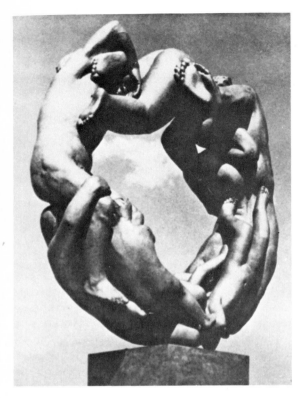

Figure 13-1
The wheel of life. (Gustav Vigeland, The Vigeland Sculpture Park, Oslo, Norway.)

way, cell size increases as cells divide; and cells continue dividing even after cell size has stabilized.[2,3] While most tissues enlarge by way of a combination of hyperplasia and hypertrophy, some tissues grow mainly by way of increases in cell size (muscle and fat, for example) and others, most importantly bone, get larger by way of an enlarging intercellular matrix.

Tissues are most vulnerable during early development. Consequently, nutritional deficiencies occurring during this period are significant and may be irremediable. This fact underlies the concept of *critical phases* of growth. In contrast to this, disruptions or deficiencies that take place during the later phases of growth when cell enlargement predominates are more easily corrected.

The three growth processes are controlled by a number of internal and external factors, including genes, hormones (and related central nervous system factors), and environmental or extrinsic influences.

Genes

Understanding the genetics of growth requires two different kinds of information: that concerning the relationship of genes to cell division and enlargement, and that concerning the inheritance of size. Within the nucleus of every cell are long strands of genetic material, deoxyribonucleic acid (DNA), which is organized in the shape of a double helix. During cell division, these long strands are coiled up into structures called *chromosomes*. The *genes* are segments of these long DNA strands, each gene being defined by a particular sequence of chemical bases. This sequence is a code or blueprint for how the cell should construct a particular protein from the raw materials (amino acids) that are available in the cell cytoplasm.

The code is carried from the nucleus into the cytoplasm by messenger ribonucleic acid (mRNA), which is single-stranded and is constructed at certain spots on the DNA strand. The mRNA moves into the cytoplasm and attaches itself to a spot called a *ribosome*. A second RNA, transfer RNA, also formed within the cell nucleus, collects the appropriate amino acids, brings them to the ribosomes to which their corresponding mRNA is attached, and hooks them onto the mRNA in the appropriate coded order. When the protein is completed, it is released into the cytoplasm. This then is the link between the genes and their expression in the structure of the body.

Growth is one aspect of the realization of the genetic plan. In general, body size, weight, and head circumference are polygenically inherited; i.e., each involves more than one set of genes, in contrast to such traits as eye color or blood group (ABO), which depend on a single genic locus. This is not surprising since the combination of tissues and physiological processes on which growth depends are so various. From the standpoint of population genetics, an individual will tend to grow in the fashion and attain a size characteristic of his or her racial or ethnic group. This population variation simply reflects the "gene pool" created by restrictions of mating, whether determined geographically, socially, or otherwise. In turn, an individual's size will closely resemble that of his or her parents and siblings, the similarity arising from the even more restricted gene pool involved. Understanding this similarity is useful in growth assessment because it allows for a more accurate idea of how big an individual child "should" be.

Hormones

The hormones most important to growth are pituitary growth hormone, thyroxine, and insulin (see Chap. 24). At adolescence the sex hormones, including testosterone, estrogen, and the adrenal androgens, play a part in both the pubertal growth spurt and the subsequent completion of bone maturation.

Extrinsic Factors Influencing Growth

Nutrition

Several environmental factors are important in maintaining growth. First is adequate *nutrition*. At least a minimum intake of nutrients, vitamins, and minerals appropriate to body size is essential for support of normal growth. Severe and chronic malnutrition will lead to profound growth failure and wasting (as in kwashiorkor and marasmus) (see Chap. 19). Less severe deficiencies, however, may also affect growth.

Secular Trend, Immigration, and Socioeconomic Status

Three phenomena that are observable in growth differences among groups of people (rather than differences between individuals within a group) are related in part or in total to a decline in the incidence of nutritional deficiency. *Secular trend* is a temporal phenomenon that has been evident in at least the last century, whereby European

populations (and other populations where documentation has been provided) have appeared to mature earlier (i.e., reach final height sooner and grow bigger than earlier generations). This size increase is due to a differential increase in the size of long bones (as opposed to other tissues) and was most clearly demonstrated in Bowles's 1932 study of Harvard University fathers and sons.[4] Secular trend is partially due to improvements in diet, but may also be related to a host of other factors (e.g., improved health). The most recent United States growth data available[5] have demonstrated that the secular trend in this country has essentially ceased since 1955.

A phenomenon related to secular trend is the larger stature of second-generation immigrants to the United States. Again, nutritional and health factors account for this difference.

Larger average size characterizes higher *socioeconomic status*. This is clearest in third-world nations where differences in diet among the various socioeconomic classes are marked. Many studies of Guatemalan child growth, for example, establish the size advantage of the privileged Ladinos over the rural Guatemalan children.[6]

Health and Emotions

The *relative state of health* of the child influences growth. Ordinary illnesses like upper respiratory tract infections or chicken pox are usually not severe or prolonged enough to interfere with growth. Chronic, repeated, or severe illnesses, however, may conserve the body's resources for maintenance purposes, with few resources left for growth, so that growth arrest occurs. However, the arrested growth is often followed by a period of *catch-up growth*.[7] Catch-up growth is a phenomenon related to the fact that each individual is genetically programmed to be a certain size by the time growth ceases. If growth deficiency occurs, the body somehow recognizes this and makes up the deficit by growing faster than normal. In addition to recovery after illness, catch-up growth characterizes recovery from malnutrition, recovery from growth failure due to emotional deprivation, and recovery from some intrauterine growth retardation syndromes.

When the condition is ameliorated (as in surgical repair of a congenital heart defect), there is potential for catch-up growth. In general, enhanced velocity is most marked at the beginning of the catch-up period and then slower as children reach their appropriate growth channel. There appear to be two different patterns of catch-up growth. The first, or that pattern which is termed *true catch-up*, is characterized by very rapid velocity immediately after the end of an illness or with the introduction of therapy, and continuing until the appropriate growth channel is achieved. The second pattern involves only slightly increased or average growth velocity, but with the total growing period extended. With this pattern children continue growing later than peers. Also, both patterns of catch-up growth may occur during the recovery period.

The potential and completeness of catch-up growth depend upon a number of factors. The period of growth during which the insult occurred is important. Growth interruption during prenatal life and infancy are least well compensated by catch-up growth because of the interruption of a critical phase of growth. (See above, "Processes and Mechanisms Underlying Growth.") During childhood and adolescence, growth failure is more recoverable. It is frequently noted that girls are more resistant to being diverted from their growth channels and better able to regain growth than boys. Finally, the completeness of catch-up will depend on individual qualities (e.g., genetic endowment) and the quality of those variables usually affecting growth (e.g., nutrition).

The mechanism for catch-up growth is not well understood. Tanner suggested that there is a tally somewhere in the central nervous system representing the ideal genetically programmed growth curve. When a mismatch between this representation and actual size is detected, a signal is sent to peripheral cells. The actual cause

of the increased velocity is also not known. Tanner suggests that increased somatomedin or greater receptivity of cartilage and other cells to growth promotion may underlie this phenomenon.[8] For a more complete discussion, the reader is referred to Tanner[9] and to Prader et al.[10].

Emotions may also affect growth. While the mechanism for the growth failure observed in some neglected children is not understood in detail, it is presumed to be related to the close connection between neural centers for emotion and those controlling many other important physiological functions.

PERIODS OF BODY GROWTH

There are several distinct periods of growth, characterized by relatively accelerated periods and intervening steady periods of increase. While height and weight are closely interrelated, their individual schedules exhibit differences. Periods of accelerated growth are evident at *mid* and *later gestation, early infancy,* and *adolescence.* These periods are interspersed with times of slower growth that occur immediately postconceptionally and during mid and late childhood. A less dramatic mid-childhood spurt of growth occurs in some children between 8 and 10 years of age (see Fig. 13-2).

Prenatal Growth

The very first part of growth, occurring from conception until 12 weeks after conception, is known as the *embryonic phase.* After fertilization of the ovum, division of the first several generations of cells occurs simultaneously, with a consequent geometric increase in cell number. Soon the dividing times become staggered, and the cells differentiate into those that will give rise to all the important tissues and organs, in a process known as *morphogenesis.* At this point the cells are also increasing in size.

During the embryonic period the placenta transports and stores nutrients and synthesizes proteins and hormones. Important insults to the

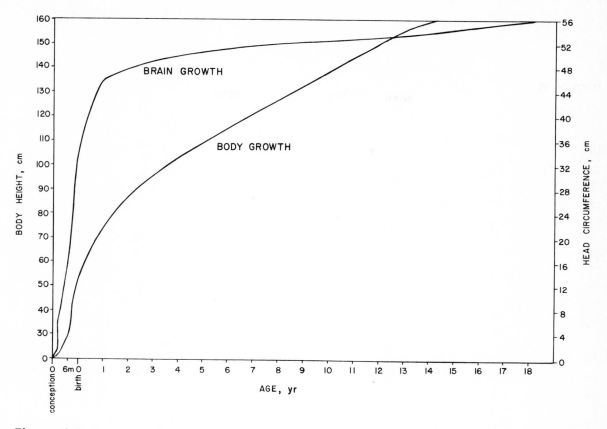

Figure 13-2
Growth of the head and body from conception to 18 years. Head growth is most rapid prenatally and in the early postnatal months. It is nearly complete by age 1 year. Body growth is rapid in the late prenatal period and early postnatal years. However, final body size depends on a continued, steady rate of growth throughout childhood.

embryo such as infections, the introduction of harmful drugs or chemicals, or severe trauma may result in spontaneous abortion or in important anomalies. While the embryo is well protected during this time, inadequate nutrition may influence the integrity of its growth.

Beginning between 8 and 12 weeks after conception, the embryo becomes a *fetus,* a relatively more independent organism with primitive reflexes, a beating heart, and a functioning renal system. The fetal period is characterized by the most rapid increase in length (during the

second trimester) and weight (during the final trimester) of the entire life cycle. In addition, the organ systems continue to differentiate and improve in function. Rapid growth occurs in all tissues and organ systems by expanding cell numbers. An increase in cell size occurs simultaneously in some tissues.

The integrity of fetal growth can be affected by smoking, high altitude, infection, toxemia of pregnancy, and the introduction of teratogenic agents. Although debate continues, some investigations demonstrate that pathophysiologic changes and compromise of growth occur in the fetus in the presence of maternal malnutrition.[11]

Birth Size

At birth, a child's size will reflect two factors: limitations imposed by the mechanics of birth (i.e., the size of the birth canal as it relates to the head size of the child) and those imposed by variations in the intrauterine environment. Birth size will be related more closely to these maternal factors than to a child's own genetic predisposition. Preterm babies will be smaller than those born at term (40 weeks). Because conceptional dates are often difficult to determine, distinguishing a child who is preterm from one who is small for reasons of inadequate intrauterine nutrient supply is often difficult. Charts are available as aids for such determinations.[12,13]

Postnatal Growth

Growth after birth can be roughly divided into three periods:

> *Infancy:* birth to 2 years
> *Childhood:* 2 to 10 or 11 years
> *Adolescence:* 10 or 11 to maturity (16 to 21 years)

Reference to Fig. 13-2 provides a general idea of the shape of the cumulative curve for postnatal growth. (See "Growth Terminology," below, for a discussion of the cumulative curve.)

Growth in *length* is most rapid in early life. A child has increased from birth length by 20 percent at 3 months, by 50 percent at 1 year, and by 75 percent at 2 years. Size at 2 to 2½ years is generally 50 percent of adult size. In the first 6 to 12 months of life children destined to be big grow faster and climb to higher percentile levels while smaller children grow more slowly, thus moving on to lower percentile levels. The percentile level established during this early infant growth is usually maintained at least until adolescence. Growth velocity decelerates steadily between birth and 4 to 5 years of age. Between age 5 years and just prior to adolescence, annual increments in length are about the same, although there may be seasonal variations in these gains (with peaks occurring between mid-April and mid-June).

Gains in length primarily reflect bone growth in three components: head, trunk (i.e., the spinal column), and legs. Since head height is 95 percent complete by 10 years of age, it comprises a greater percentage of the total length earlier in life than it does later. Growth in the first year of life occurs largely in the trunk, which gains 60 percent of its final adult size in this interval. Between 1 year and adolescence the most impressive relative growth takes place in the bones of the legs (about 66 percent of their total growth). The adolescent growth spurt is mainly due to increases in trunk length. Because of the differential growth rates of the components of stature, the body has a characteristic appearance at different ages.

Weight at birth is 3×10^6 times the weight of the ovum. The velocity of weight gain reaches its peak for the entire life cycle just after the early neonatal weight loss. Within the first few weeks after birth, weight gain proceeds very rapidly. Birth weight is doubled by 5 months, tripled by 1 year, and quadrupled by 3 years. As with length, increases in weight after the third or fourth year are steady, showing an unchanging annual velocity. Seasonal peaks also occur in weight, the winter months being characterized by the most rapid weight gains.

Weight gain is a composite of growth in all body tissues (muscle, bone, fat, and the organs). Its relation to length may be expressed in the formula called the *ponderal index:* $100 \times$ weight/length. The ponderal index is highest in infancy and early childhood (when weight is greatest relative to body surface area and length). It gradually falls toward the end of the adolescent growth spurt, after which it rises to the level it had attained at about age 8 or 9 years. The relation of bone weight to body weight is fairly constant throughout life. Skeletal muscle weight rises from 25 percent of body weight in infancy to 40 percent by adulthood. Changes in fat composition are discussed below.

Adolescence is the second postnatal period of rapid growth, and a number of its features are important:

1   Changes at adolescence include:
    a Rapid growth in height and weight
    b Changes in body composition (primarily in proportions of fat, muscle, and bone) that are more marked in boys than in girls
    c Development of secondary sex characteristics
       (1) In girls these include breast development; appearance and elaboration of pubic and axillary hair; menarche; differential deposition of adipose tissue on hips, thighs, and buttocks; and characteristic changes of facial architecture.
       (2) In boys these include growth in the size of penis and testes; appearance and elaboration of pubic, axillary, body, and facial hair; increase in size of the larynx; broadening of the shoulder girdle; and increase in skeletal musculature.

2   In general, adolescent changes occur earlier in girls (between 9 and 16 years) than in boys (between 12 and 18 years).

3   Onset of pubertal development is controlled largely by circulating hormones. The mechanisms timing the release of these hormones are not well understood.

4   There is a wide variation in the times of onset and completion of the events of puberty, but the sequence of events is usually the same. Because of this variation, the use of growth charts and percentile levels is not reliable during adolescence.

Brain Growth

The schedule for brain growth differs from that for the body (see Fig. 13-2). In general the brain grows more rapidly and completes growth ear-

lier than the rest of the body. Its growth is most rapid during the last trimester of gestation and the first postnatal months. By 1½ years of age its growth is 90 percent completed, and by 10 years of age it is 95 percent complete. No real adolescent growth spurt is evident in head circumference.

The growth schedule of different parts of the brain is important to the understanding of the potential effects of pre- and postnatal nutritional inadequacies. During the first 10 weeks of gestation the brain differentiates into its main parts. The cerebrum, which accounts for 85 percent of brain weight, increases in volume by means of an increase in the numbers of sulci (convolutions), which develop rapidly beginning at about 15 weeks of gestation. The rapid increase in volume of the cerebrum accounts for the largest part of the *first* growth spurt of the brain (occurring between 18 and 20 weeks postconception) and is largely due to neuronal hyperplasia. The number of cells established at this time will characterize the brain for life. During both the periods of differentiation and the periods of neuronal multiplication, the fetus is well protected by the intrauterine environment; as a consequence, maternal malnutrition at these times may have less impact on the growing brain than at later times. A second spurt in growth is evident at 32 weeks of gestation. This second period of rapid development and much of the subsequent growth of the brain are attributable to the tremendous increase in dendritic complexity and synaptic interconnectivity of the neurons rather than to an actual increase in cell number. The cerebellum, a part of the brain located below the cerebrum and at the posterior end of the head, exhibits a different growth schedule. Its rapid cell multiplication begins during the last month of gestation and proceeds very rapidly during the first year of life. A particularly rapid phase in the cycle of cerebellar growth occurs at 5 months postnatally. The velocity of cerebellar growth is greater than that of the cerebrum. It begins later and is nearly completed by 18 months, at which time the cerebrum and other parts of the brain are only 60 percent of their final weight. Cerebellar growth takes place at a time when the growing fetus and then the infant is much more susceptible to the effects of malnutrition. Some investigators[14,15] have suggested that because of both the rate and the timing of its rapid increase, the cerebellum, which controls integration of motor activities, is most susceptible to the effects of malnutrition, particularly protein deprivation, during this period. The strongest evidence of this comes from animal research which demonstrates important limitations in cognitive functioning in all species subjected to nutritional deprivation during critical periods of postnatal brain growth.

In human research studies, malnourished children have demonstrated smaller head circumferences and, on postmortem analysis, reduced brain weight and protein content.[16] However, the distinction between the effects on intellectual functioning produced by nutritional limitation and effects which are due to other elements of environmental deprivation is difficult to disentangle.[17]

Adipose Tissue Growth

The dynamics of the growth of adipose tissue are of special interest because fat composition (as measured by skinfold thickness) is a useful means of assessing nutritional status. Table 13-1 shows body fat composition at various ages.

Girls are approximately 25 percent fatter than boys from birth onward. During the first part of intrauterine growth there is almost no adipose tissue. Fat begins to accumulate in the second trimester, but it increases most rapidly between the second fetal month and 6 months postnatally. During this time, fat acts to ensure energy stores for the rapidly growing body and to provide extra insulation for immature thermal regulation. Weight gain by the average infant is approximately 38 percent fat between birth and age 6 months but is only about 11 percent of the weight gained between 6 months and 1 year. A reverse relationship is evident between fat and protein composition of weight gain in that age interval. Between 1 year and 6 to 8 years of age there is a relatively lower percentage of body fat. The relative fat composition increases again at 9 years as part of the adolescent growth phase. At the end of the adolescent growth spurt the ratio of fat to body size again recedes to about that observed at birth. The prepubescent growth spurt in adipose tissue precedes that of muscle and bone. Consequently,

TABLE 13-1 BODY FAT COMPOSITION AT VARIOUS STAGES OF DEVELOPMENT

Age	Body fat, % of total body weight
End of second trimester	0.5*
Birth (accrued in last 2 prenatal months)	12*
4 months	16*
6 months	26.3†
1 year	24†
4–6 years	22*
7–9 years	24*
10–12 years	28*
Adulthood	18*

*Source: Icie G. Macy and Harriet J. Kelly, *Chemical Anthropology: A New Approach to Growth in Children*, University of Chicago Press, Chicago, 1957, pp. 78–79.

†Source: Samuel Fomon, *Infant Nutrition*, 2d ed., W. B. Saunders Company, Philadelphia, 1974, p. 74.

excess weight for height may be manifest at the onset of adolescence. It should be noted that this "fat phase" is transient and not predictive of adulthood obesity.

Like other body tissues, adipose tissue increases by proliferation in cell number and increase in cell size. During the past two decades a large literature supported the idea that adipose cell proliferation occurred only during infancy and that an accumulation of a large number of fat cells (adipocytes) at that period of development possibly predisposed an individual to overweight or obesity at later ages (see, for example, references 18 and 19). Reexaminations of the evidence [20] and new studies of human adipose tissue from individuals of various ages [21,22] show that cell proliferation probably continues into adolescence and adulthood, although difficulties with accurate assessment of adipocyte number inhibit firm statements concerning the exact nature of adipose tissue growth. Reliable studies of the natural history of body fatness are few. However, the literature generally indicates that adult fatness levels have only a weak relationship to levels apparent in infancy.[23] Status during later childhood and adolescence is more predictive of status in adulthood.

Measurement of fat composition can be accomplished fairly simply in a clinical setting by use of skinfold measurements or indices of body fatness based on height and weight. Recommendations for the most appropriate clinical indicators for total body fat and percent body fat are available.[24] Such measures are useful in assessment of obesity or malnutrition.

Growth Terminology

Three terms are essential in growth assessment: cumulative growth, growth velocity, and percentile levels. *Cumulative growth* is absolute growth, an individual's size at any point in time. Height and weight charts (see Fig. 13-5 on p. 253) provide a graph of cumulative growth. *Growth velocity* or incremental growth is the rate of growth during some interval of time (e.g., 1 year or 6 months). It is obtained by subtracting an earlier measure from one taken later. Charts for increments for height, weight, and head circumference are also available. Detection of abnormally fast or slow growth is accomplished by use of *percentile levels*. The National Center for Health Statistics (NCHS) charts (Fig. 13-5) show curves for the 5th through the 95th percentiles. Children at the 50th percentile will be average for their age while those at the 5th or 95th percentiles will be respectively smaller and larger than their agemates. Because of the regular and predictable course of growth, a particular child will tend to stay within the same percentile level (beginning at about 6 to 12 months of age) throughout life. Maintenance of this percentile level depends on normal growth velocity. Deviations from the established percentile level will often indicate abnormal growth. These concepts are important to the discussion of growth assessment below.

THE ASSESSMENT OF GROWTH

The assessment of growth has three components: information gathering, anthropometric measurement, and data analysis.

Information Gathering

The health professional, in looking at a child with a growth problem, is concerned with identifying both those problems directly attributable to dietary factors and those in which diet is a secondary but contributory factor. Because feeding difficulties and other aspects of diet are often synergistic with other phenomena related to poor growth, such determinations can be difficult. It is therefore essential to make a thorough documentation of all relevant information.

1 *Longitudinal data on growth.* As many serial measurements as possible of height (or length), weight, and head circumference should be taken. These may be available in the child's hospital record, through the pediatrician or family physician, or in the baby book kept by the mother. In the case of very

young children birth records (which will most often document birth length, weight, head circumference, and chest circumference) should be obtained. These data will be important in identifying whether the current measurements represent the beginning, continuation, or intensification of an abnormal growth pattern. It should also be clear that without some idea of when growth abnormalities began, the isolation of the cause is more difficult. Finally, when more data are available, a better documentation of growth pattern is possible. Growth patterns, rather than single data points, are of the greatest use.

While these sources of data may provide a rough idea of a child's growth, it is important to remember that an inaccurate measurement may be misleading in the assessment of serial growth. A mistake of 2 cm in length at a young age may, for example, shift a child from the 25th to the 5th percentile on the NCHS growth charts. Thus, it is important to evaluate the quality of the measurements drawn from records in order to avoid mistakes. (See Table 13-2.)

2 *Health history.* Besides obtaining a diet history (see Appendix), a careful documentation of health status through life should be made.

   a Certain major disease entities have a known association with growth problems. These include diseases of the major organs, and inborn metabolic and endocrine disorders. Prenatally acquired infections (e.g., rubella) can seriously limit postnatal growth. Finally, surgery or prolonged hospitalization may slow growth. Some of these disease processes permanently impair growth. Others, including prenatal infections, may be followed by recovery (i.e., catch-up growth).

   b Sporadic or chronic minor illnesses, such as upper respiratory infections, may temporarily cause weight loss and slow the velocity of linear growth. Because ground lost during episodes of surgery, hospitalization, or illness will be regained, it is essential not to confuse these temporary setbacks with growth failure that requires intervention.

3 *Relevant background data.* A child's growth pattern and size at any point in time will be related to the height and build of other family members, to racial or ethnic background, and to environmental circumstances. Data on each of these are necessary for accurate assessment. Documentation of the size of as many other immediate and extended family members as is feasible will give some idea about the propriety of a child's size in the family context. Data on socioeconomic background and the family's country of origin are important because of the clearly different expectations for growth often associated with these factors (see preceding discussion). It may be necessary to obtain standards appropriate for these variables, such as those presented by Knott on Puerto Rican children.[25]

Measurement

Several measurements may be used for the assessment of growth. Each is a very general measure of the integrity of the biological operations of the individual being assessed. A complete definition of these and other useful measurements is available.[26]

Recumbent length is the measure used for assessing size in young children. Some standards are based on recumbent length till age 2 years (NCHS charts, for example) while others carry these standards to age 6. Because the recumbent length for a given child is about 2 cm greater than the child's standing height, the standards available will dictate which measurement is to be used.

Recumbent length is measured on a table with an immovable head piece and a movable foot piece. A measuring tape (preferably graduated in millimeters) runs along the table's

TABLE 13-2 COMMON MEASUREMENT ERRORS

All measurements	Inadequate instrument
	Restless child (procedure should be postponed)
	Reading part of instrument not fixed when value taken
	Reading
	Recording errors
Length	Incorrect age for instrument
	Footwear or headwear not removed
	Head not in correct plane
	Head not firmly against fixed end of board
	Child not straight along board
	Body arched
	Knees bent
	Feet not vertical to movable board
	Board not firmly against heels
Height	Incorrect age for instrument
	Footwear or headwear not removed
	Feet not straight nor flat on vertical platform or wall
	Knees bent
	Body arched or buttocks forward (body not straight)
	Shoulders not straight on board
	Head not in correct plane
	Headboard not firmly on crown of child's head
Weight	Room cold, no privacy
	Scale not calibrated to zero
	Child wearing unreasonable amount of clothing
	Child moving or anxious due to prior misregard
Head circumference	Occipital protuberance/supraorbital landmarks poorly defined
	Hair crushed inadequately, ears under tape
	Tape tension and position poorly maintained by time of reading
	Headwear not removed
Triceps fatfold	Wrong arm (should be left arm)
	Mid-arm point or posterior plane incorrectly measured or marked
	Arm not loose by side during measurement
	Examiner not comfortable nor level with child
	Finger-thumb pinch or caliper placement too deep (muscle) or too superficial (skin)
	Caliper jaws not at marked site
	Reading done too early or too late (should be 2 to 3 seconds)
	At time of reading, pinch not maintained, caliper handle not fully released
Arm circumference	Tape too thick, stretched or creased
	Wrong arm (should be left arm)
	Mid-arm point incorrectly measured or marked
	Arm not loosely hanging by side during measurement
	Examiner not comfortable nor level with child
	Tape around arm, not at midpoint; too tight (causing skin contour indentation), too loose (inadequately opposed)

Source: A. J. Zerfas, I. J. Shorr, and C. G. Newman, "Office Assessment of Nutritional Status," *Pediatric Clinics of North America,* **24**:253–272, 1977.

length. The child is placed on his or her back with the head brought against the head piece and is held there with gentle pressure. The head, shoulders, hips, and feet are oriented in a single line as they would be for a standing measurement. The knees are held flattened against the table, and the toes point upward. The movable board is brought against the bottom of the feet with gentle pressure. Each measure should be repeated at least three times with any necessary adjustments in body orientation. Immediate accurate recording of each of the three measures is essential. The three measures should then be averaged.

Standing height is best measured with a fixed, rather than a free-standing, measuring device (see Fig. 13-3). The child is positioned with the back snugly against the measuring device. The feet should be close together and touching the device, and the back should show as little curvature as possible. The whole body should be carefully centered, the head held erect with the gaze straight ahead. The movable board should contact the top of the head midsagittally. Three repeated measurements should be taken and averaged.

Weight is best measured using a beam balance scales with nondetachable weights. As little clothing as possible should be worn. However, with serial measures the same amount of clothing should be worn at each measurment. For infants, scales weighing to the nearest gram are desirable. The balance of the scale should be checked before each weighing. An infant should either be laid on the scale (if body size permits) or seated with the center of gravity at the exact center of the scale. On such sensitive scales, several different values should be tried to see which offers the best balance. An average of the best-balanced values should be taken.

Head circumference is taken with a measuring tape that is preferably made of fiberglass or steel rather than cloth. The tape is applied above the bony eminence slightly above the eyebrows and around the widest part of the back of the head. The largest point is sought, again with three averaged measurements.

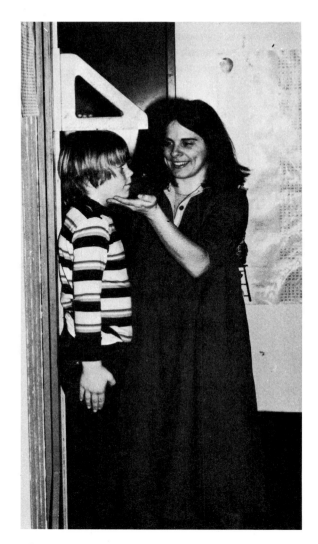

Figure 13-3
Standing height is best measured with a fixed, rather than a free-standing, measuring device.

Body fat is measured by skinfold thickness, arm circumference, and thigh circumference, as follows.

1 *Skinfold thickness:* Skinfolds comprise the skin and a layer of subcutaneous fat pulled away from the underlying muscle (see Fig. 13-4). While there are a number of body

sites where subcutaneous fat might be measured, two are easily used and have a reasonably high correlation with whole body fat composition. These are the triceps and subscapular skinfolds.

a   *Triceps skinfolds* are measured on one of the arms. The one measured should be that on which available standards are based. There are two instruments, the Lange and the Holtain calipers, that may be used for the procedure. With a tape measure, the midpoint of the upper arm between the bony eminence at the shoulder (the acromion) and the olecranon (the lateral eminence at the elbow) is located. This midpoint is best marked with a felt-tip pen. The arm is held relaxed. The skinfold is grasped between the examiner's index finger and thumb at the back of the arm 1 cm above the marked midpoint, and the calipers applied at the mark. The left hand maintains the pinch throughout the measurement.

b   *Subscapular folds* are taken at a point just below the lowest most lateral point of the shoulder blade in the line of the natural skin cleavage. Both triceps and subscapular readings are made to the nearest 0.5

Figure 13-4
Measurement of triceps skinfold thickness: (a) location of the midpoint of the upper arm; (b) application of the Lange calipers for measurement of triceps skinfold; (c) representation of the tissues of the arm (bone, fat, and skin) and measurement of skinfold thickness.

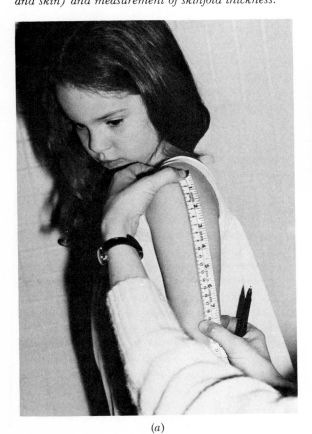

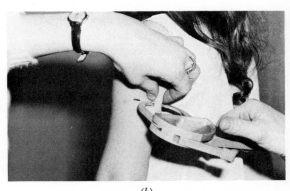

(b)

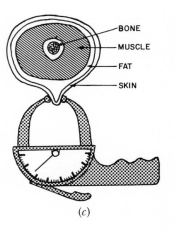

(a)

(c)

mm at about 3 seconds after the application of the calipers. Again three readings with averaging are essential. (See Appendix for skinfold standards.)

2 *Arm circumference* (the circumference of the upper arm taken at the point midway between the acromion and the olecranon process) and maximum thigh circumference (the broadest circumference located on the thigh) are sometimes substituted for skinfold thickness in the assessment of malnutrition in field or survey situations when measurement accuracy is not well controlled. From the *United States Ten-State Nutrition Survey of 1968-1970,* Frisancho derived percentiles for right upper arm circumference and triceps skinfold. From these measurements for each individual, the arm muscle diameter and arm muscle circumference may be calculated.[27] Arm circumference is not recommended as an index of obesity.

Trowbridge and Staehling assessed the use of arm circumference for age and arm circumference for height in identifying various levels of malnutrition in a third-world population.[28] They found that arm circumference for age had the greatest sensitivity and specificity in identifying severe malnutrition (those at 60 percent or less of median weight for age). Arm circumference alone had the best sensitivity and specificity in identifying less severe malnutrition.

3 *Thigh circumference* (the broadest circumference located on the thigh), like arm circumference, is not recommended as an index of obesity. Zeitlin found that maximum thigh circumference was slightly more sensitive in identifying malnutrition than upper arm circumference in her sample of American children from birth to 5 years old. Reference data for maximum thigh circumference can be found here.[29]

Data Analysis: Use of Growth Charts

The most commonly used tools for assessment of growth data are charts that plot the size of chil-

dren by percentile level at consecutive ages (Fig. 13-5). The particular charts included here are selected for their high quality (in terms of sample size used and statistical rendering). Serial measurements should be plotted. Increments in size between serial measurement can be calculated and plotted on available charts.[30] A number of observations should then be made concerning these data points and the following questions asked:

1 What is the child's current percentile level? If this is the only measurement available for this child, measures below the 3d percentile or above the 97th percentile should arouse particular concern.

2 How does the current measure relate to the child's past measurement? Has the percentile level remained stable, or has the child fallen or risen to a different percentile level? Are increments in size since the last examination within the normal range?

3 How do the various measures interrelate?
   a Height/weight relations are best plotted on the newly generated height/weight grid. When these standards are unavailable, separate graphs with height/weight plots more than two percentile levels apart are worthy of note.
   b Skinfold measures are best plotted by weight and age,[31,32] although age plots alone[33] are useful initially. Plots should be in line with percentile levels for weight.
   c The relation of head circumference to body size is not straightforward. In general a 0.25 correlation coefficient exists between stature and head circumference, indicating that it is not necessarily the case that big bodies and big heads (and vice versa) go together. There are certain characteristic relationships between head and body size during growth. At birth head circumference is larger than chest circumference, but by age 1 year the opposite is true. Deviation from this relationship usually indicates deficits in body growth. One example of a cause for such a devia-

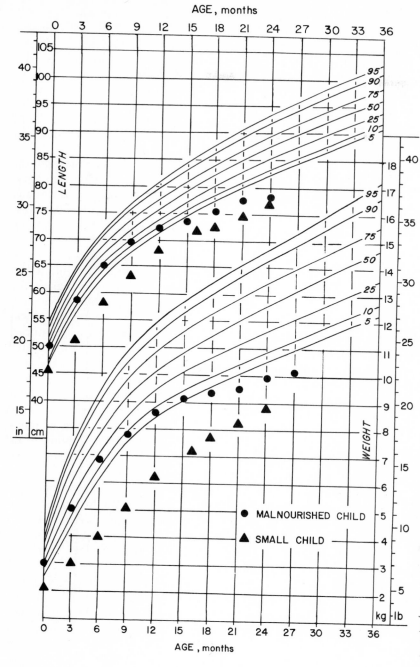

AGE, months

Figure 13-5
Serial measurements of length and weight of two children with abnormal growth patterns (see text for discussion). (Adapted from National Center for Health Statistics charts.) *The NCHS charts plot 5th through 95th percentiles. Normal children will generally fall within the upper and lower percentile limits and will maintain a particular percentile level throughout childhood.*

● MALNOURISHED CHILD

▲ SMALL CHILD

tion is growth retardation due to emotional deprivation. (See "Failure to Thrive," in Chap. 26.)

4 How do plots of other family members compare with that of the child? The reliability for predicting a child's size on this basis is limited. Two percentile levels of difference between a child and all the rest of the family is significant. More exacting standards can be used.[34a]

5 At what ages have important illnesses, surgery, etc., occurred? These should be marked on the growth chart so that deviations from growth channels relative to them are evident.

CASE APPLICATION: INTERPRETATION OF DEVIANT GROWTH

Growth charts plot data for a given child on a biologically normal curve. Consequently, patterns of growth that deviate from this curve can be easily seen. Two examples of unusual patterns in height and weight growth are given here.

Pattern #1 (Fig. 13-5) is the characteristic pattern of growth in height and weight for a chronically malnourished child. Weight drops precipitously at age 6 months and continues to move further below the 3d percentile, thus showing deficient velocity throughout the period plotted. Height begins to drop in percentiles (showing deficient velocity) somewhat after the weight falloff. The curve that is estimated through the points given is unlike the shapes of those on the normal chart. Plots of increments during this age interval would be at lower percentiles as well.

Pattern #2 (Fig. 13-5) shows a child who was born at term but was small for gestational dates. At age 2 years, this child is continuing to grow at an essentially normal velocity but remains below the 3d percentile. Such a pattern indicates a child either whose nutrition in utero was so inadequate as to compromise growth re-

covery or whose own internal biology is growth limiting.

NUTRITION THROUGH THE GROWING YEARS

Rosanne Beatrice Howard

INTRODUCTION

Food is both the source of nutrients and the source of nurturance; it is the interpersonal matrix through which we learn about ourselves and our environment. In the process of nourishing, we feed more than food with its 50-odd known nutrients; we nurture and feed feelings as well.

Although the foods and techniques (breast vs. bottle) considered appropriate for infant and child feeding have varied over the centuries, the interpersonal aspects of feeding have prevailed. The Colonial mother breast-fed by the clock, sometimes utilizing the services of a wet nurse, and prepared pap (flour or bread boiled in water with or without the addition of some milk) and panada (sometimes a synonym for pap; also, a mixture of various cereals, flours, or breads with some butter or milk cooked in broth)[34b] as supplementary feedings.[35] A combination of ignorance and folklore influenced early infant feeding, and certain fruits and vegetables were forbidden for fear of infantile diarrhea.

With industrialization, urbanization, and the commercial activities of the formula industry, the bottle became a status symbol from the 1930s to the early 1970s. The mother fed her baby on demand with ready-to-feed formulas and baby foods.

Then, during the 1970s, with a back-to-nature emphasis in our culture, a suspicion about the adulteration of our food supply, and an accumulating body of research on the nutritional benifits of breast milk, there came a resurgence in breast feeding. Results of surveys of mothers conducted from 1955 to 1978 indicate that the incidence and duration of breast feeding substantially increased during the years 1971 to 1978. This trend is evident in all demographic categories of mothers.[36] The American Academy of Pediatrics,[37,38] the American Medical Association,[39] and the American Public Health Association[40] issued position papers which encourage breast feeding (see "Lactation," in Chap. 15). Human milk is considered the best source of nourishment for the young infant. However, the decision to breast feed should be made free from pressure, and the needs of both parents and infants should be considered. With changing roles in the family, mothers are returning to work, and househusbands are becoming more prevalent. Many infants are intermittently breast- and formula-fed because of schedules.

INFANT

From birth, feeding is a learned experience as the infant is placed at the breast or given a bottle, as soon as possible if in good physical condition. Usually 4 hours after birth, the normal, full-term infant is fed with 10 percent dextrose in water or plain water. Only after successful feeding is breast or formula feeding begun. There is some evidence that nutritive sucking behavior in the newborn is affected by obstetric sedation, with the infants sucking at significantly lower rates and pressures and consuming

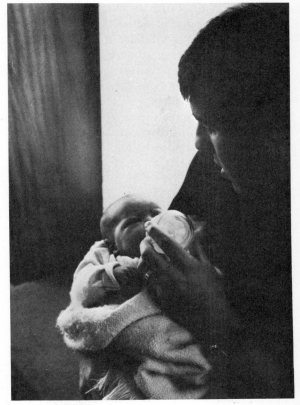

Figure 13-6
Fathers are getting more involved in feeding.

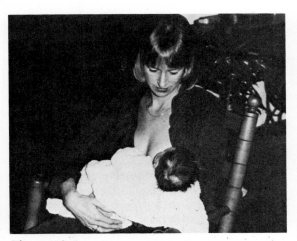

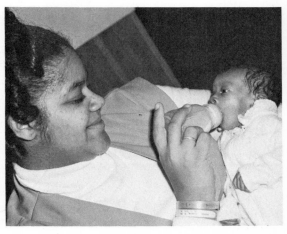

Figure 13-7
The mother and child, a "feeding couple." Because they are a "feeding couple," the needs of both must be considered in determining which mode of feeding is best. (Photo courtesy of Jane McCotter O'Toole.)

less.[41] This lack of responsiveness is important for the nurse to recognize since this can interfere with nutrient intake and the developing mother-child relationship, as anxiety, tension, or frustration on the part of the mother can negatively reinforce the infant's early feeding experience.

During the first year of life, the infant progresses from a totally dependent, somewhat passive, feeder to an active participant with a fair amount of independence. This transition follows the sequence of head, trunk, gross, and fine motor control as the infant's reflexive behavior becomes voluntary. The infant will learn to chew and swallow rather than to suck solid foods, to drink from a cup, and to acquire all the manipulative skills that are necessary for independent feeding (see Table 13-3, which summarizes the development of feeding skills).

Growth is rapid and nutrient needs closely parallel growth. (See the first part of this chapter.) Energy needs approximate 115 kcal (481.1 kJ) per kilogram of body weight during the first 6 months and 105 kcal (439.3 kJ) per kilogram during the second half of the first year.

Protein needs for the first 6 months are 2.2 g per kilogram of body weight and 2.0 g per kilogram during the second part of the first year.[42] For the most part, breast milk or a sterilized formula with supplementary vitamins and iron can provide the needed nutrients for the first 5 to 6 months. Cow's milk and skim milk are not suitable for infant feeding.

Proprietary formulas are processed to simulate human milk and are supplemented with vitamins and minerals except for fluoride. Special care is given to maintaining the ratio of calcium to phosphorus, to monitoring the renal solute load, and to replacing trace elements. Iron is added to many proprietary formulas, which is advised by the American Academy of Pediatrics. The formulas are available in ready-feed, liquid concentrate, and/or powdered form. Table 13-4 (pp. 258–261) compares the composition of breast milk with that of a number of commercially available formulas.

The infant's need for vitamin-mineral supplementation is determined by the type of feeding.[43] (See Table 13-5, p. 262, which summarizes guidelines for the use of supplements in healthy infants and children.)

Fluoride is not included on Table 13-5. The Committee on Nutrition of the American Academy favored initiating fluoride supplements shortly after birth in breast-fed infants but also recognized that fluoride could be initiated at 6 months of age.[44]

TABLE 13-3 DEVELOPMENT OF FEEDING SKILLS

Age	Oral and neuromuscular development	Feeding behavior
Birth	Rooting reflex	Turns mouth toward nipple or any object brushing cheek
	Suckle-swallow reflex	Initially sucking and swallowing are not differentiated; a stimulus introduced into the mouth elicits vigorous sucking followed by a swallow if liquid is present
		Initial swallowing involves the posterior of the tongue; by 9–12 weeks anterior portion is increasingly involved which facilitates ingestion of semisolid food
		Pushes food out when placed on tongue; strong the first 9 weeks

TABLE 13-3 CONTINUED

Age	Oral and neuromuscular development	Feeding behavior
Birth (continued)	Suckle-swallow reflex (continued)	By 6–10 weeks recognizes the position in which he or she is fed and begins mouthing and sucking when placed in this position
3–6 months	Beginning coordination between eyes and body movements	Explores world with eyes, fingers, hands, and mouth; starts reaching for objects at 4 months but overshoots; hands get in the way during feeding
	Learning to reach mouth with hands at 4 months	Finger sucking—by 6 months all objects go into the mouth
	Able to grasp objects voluntarily at 5 months	May continue to push out food placed on tongue
		Grasps objects in mittenlike fashion
	Sucking reflex becomes voluntary and lateral motions of the jaw begin	Can approximate lips to the rim of cup by 5 months; chewing action begins; by 6 months begins drinking from cup
6–12 months	Eyes and hands working together	Brings hand to mouth; at 7 months able to feed self biscuit
	Sits erect with support at 6 months	Bangs cup and objects on table at 7 months
	Sits erect without support at 9 months	
	Development of grasp (finger to thumb opposition)	Holds own bottle at 9–12 months
		Pincer approach to food
		Pokes at food with index finger at 10 months
	Reaches to objects at 10 months	Reaches for food and utensils including those beyond reach; pushes plate around with spoon; throws eating utensils; insists on holding spoon, not to put in mouth but to return to plate or cup.
1–3 years	Development of manual dexterity	Increased desire to feed self
		15 months—begins to use spoon but turns it before reaching mouth; may hold cup, likely to tilt the cup rather than head, causing spilling
		18 months—eats with spoon, spills frequently, turns spoon in mouth; holds glass with both hands
		2 years—inserts spoon correctly, occasionally with one hand; holds glass; plays with food; distinguishes between food and inedible materials
		2–3 years—self-feeding complete with occasional spilling; uses fork; pours from pitcher; obtains drink of water from faucet

Source: Getchel and Howard, "Nutrition in Development," chap. 10, in Scipien et al., Comprehensive Pediatric Nursing, McGraw-Hill Book Company, New York, 1979, p. 163.

TABLE 13-4   INFANT FORMULA PRODUCT COMPARISON WITH BREAST MILK AND COW'S MILK

Formula	Nutrient source			Energy per oz		Nutrients g/100 mL		
	Protein	Carbohydrate	Fat	kcal	kJ	Pro	Carbohydrate	Fat
Breast milk	Lactalbumin, casein	Lactose	High in olein, low in volatile fatty acids	22	92	1.1	6.8	4.5
Cow's milk	Lactalbumin, casein	Lactose	Milk fat	20	84	3.5	4.9	3.7
Well infant formulas								
Similac (Ross)	Nonfat cow's milk	Lactose	Soy oil, coconut oil	20	84	1.5	7.3	3.6
Enfamil (MJ)	Nonfat cow's milk	Lactose	Soy oil, coconut oil	20	84	1.5	7.0	3.7
Premature								
Similac Low Birth Weight (Ross)	Nonfat cow's milk	Lactose, polycose	Soy oil, coconut oil, MCT oil	24	100	2.2	8.5	4.5
Enfamil Premature (MJ)	Demineralized whey, nonfat cow's milk	Glucose polymers, lactose	Corn oil, MCT oil, coconut oil	24	100	2.4	8.9	4.1
Increased energy/oz								
Similac 24 with Iron (Ross)	Nonfat cow's milk	Lactose	Soy oil, coconut oil	24	100	2.2	8.5	4.3
Similac 27	Cow's milk	Lactose	Coconut oil, soy oil,	27	113	2.5	9.5	4.8
Enfamil 24 with Iron (MJ)	Nonfat cow's milk	Lactose	Soy oil, coconut oil	24	100	1.8	8.3	4.5
Decreased energy/oz								
Similac 13 with Iron (Ross)	Cow's milk	Lactose	Coconut oil, soy oil	13.2	55.2	1.1	4.6	2.3
Enfamil 13 (MJ)	Nonfat cow's milk	Lactose	Soy oil, coconut oil	13.2	55.2	1.0	4.5	2.4
Electrodialyzed								
SMA (Wyeth)	Nonfat cow's milk, demineralized whey	Lactose	Oleo, coconut oil	20	84	1.5	7.2	3.6
PM 60/40 (Ross)	Nonfat cow's milk, demineralized whey	Lactose	Safflower oil, soybean oil	20	84	1.6	7.6	3.5
Soy protein-lactose free								
Isomil (Ross)	Soy protein isolate	Corn syrup, sucrose	Coconut oil, soy oil	20	84	2.0	6.8	3.6
Prosobee (MJ)	Soy protein isolate, supplement with L-methionine	Corn syrup solids	Soy oil, coconut oil	20	84	2.0	6.9	3.6

Mg/100 mL	Minerals					Osmolality mosmol/kg H_2O	Renal solute load mosmol/L	Considerations
Iron	meq/L							
	Ca^{2+}	P^{2+}	Na^+	K^+	Cl^-			
0.1–0.15	17	8	7	13	11	300	75	See Chap. 15, Table 15-4.
0.05	59	60	22	35	28	288	23	Cow's milk alone is not suitable for an infant formula. Evaporated milk is diluted 1 part evaporated milk, 2 parts water, with 5% corn syrup added.
— c̄ iron 1.2	26	23	11	20	15	290	108	Formulas used for normal infant feeding. Formula with iron recommended. (Some infants do not tolerate iron-fortified formulas. With usage they may become colicky and/or constipated.)
— c̄ iron 1.2	28	27	12	18	15	290	110	
0.3	36	33	16	26	24	290	154	Formulas modified to meet the increased growth needs of the premature infant (see Chap. 14).
0.12	48	28	14	23	19	300	220	
0.15	36	33	14	27	21	360	150	Formulas used for infants with a limited intake or infants recovering from illness with increased energy needs.
Tr.	40	36	17	32	22	420	171	
1.52	33	33	15	21	18	355	130	
0.7	20	18	10	15	12	190	84	Formulas used with infants who have not been fed enterally for several days/weeks. Also, used when a conservative initial formula is needed for newborns during first 24–48-hour period.
0.10	18	18	8	12	10	182	70	
1.26	22	20	6.5	14.4	10.4	300	91	Formulas provide a lower renal solute load and lower amounts of sodium and potassium. (Whey is demineralized by electrophoresis.) Protein and mineral content is comparable to breast milk. Formulas are used with infants who have impaired renal or cardiovascular function and infants with diabetes insipidus.
0.26	20	12	7	15	7	260	92	
1.2	35	24	13	18	15	250	126	Formulas used for infants with milk sensitivity or lactose or sucrose intolerance, and for infants with galactosemia.
1.3	32	32	18.7	18	16	160	127	Other soy-based formulas are Neomulsoy and CHO-Free (Syntex).

(Continued)

TABLE 13-4 CONTINUED

Formula	Nutrient source			Energy per oz		Nutrients g/100 mL		
	Protein	Carbohydrate	Fat	kcal	kJ	Pro	Carbohydrate	Fat
Hydrolyzed protein								
Nutramigen (MJ)	Casein hydrolysate	Sucrose, modified tapioca starch	Corn oil	20	84	2.2	8.8	2.6
Pregestimil (MJ)	Casein hydrolysate, L-trytophan, L-cystine, L-tyrosine	Corn syrup solids, modified tapioca starch	Corn oil MCT	20	84	1.9	9.1	2.7
High protein-lower fat								
Probana (MJ)	Whole nonfat cow's milk, banana powder, casein hydrolysate	Dextrose, banana powder, lactose	Milk fat, corn oil	20	84	4.2	7.9	2.2
Altered fat-lactose free								
Portagen (MJ)	Sodium caseinate	Corn syrup solids, sucrose	MCT oil (88%), corn oil (12%)	20	84	2.4	7.8	3.2
Inborn errors of metabolism								
Lofenalac (MJ)	Casein hydrolysate (most phenylalanine removed), fortified with tyrosine, tryptophan, histidine, methionine	Corn syrup solids, modified tapioca starch	Corn oil	20	84	2.2	8.8	2.7
Phenyl-free (MJ)	Amino acids	Sucrose, corn syrup solids, modified tapioca starch	Corn oil	25	105	3.8	6.2	.64
Carbohydrate-free								
CHO-Free (Syntex)	Soy protein isolate		Soy oil	20	84	1.8	6.4 c̄ added CHO	3.5
Transition formula								
Advance (Ross)	Cow milk, soy protein	Corn syrup, lactose	Soy oil, corn oil	20	84	2.0	5.5	2.7

Note: List is not inclusive of all available formulas. Nutrient composition of these formulas continually changes. For up-to-date information, contact formula company.

Mg/100 mL	Minerals meq/L					Osmolality mosmol/kg H_2O	Renal solute load mosmol/L	Considerations
Iron	Ca^{2+}	P^{2+}	Na^+	K^+	Cl^-			
1.27	32	28	14	17	13	443	130	Formulas used for infants sensitive to intact protein, and infants recovering from prolonged diarrhea. These formulas avoid possible GI absorption of intact protein because the protein is hydrolyzed. The formulas contain a high percentage of free amino acids, and the remainder of the protein is in the peptide form.
1.27	32	25	14	18	16	338	125	
0.15	58	53	27	31	21	592	250	Formula high in protein (24% of calories), and lower in fat. Formula is used for infants with poor absorption (celiac disease, acute diarrhea).
1.88	32	28	14	22	16	236	150	Formula high in MCT oil which is more readily hydrolyzed and absorbed. The formula is used with infants who have a defect in the hydrolysis of fat, (C.F., pancreatic insufficiency, chronic liver disease, biliary atresia, or obstruction), a defect in absorption (sprue, idiopathic steatorrhea, resection of intestine, blind-loop syndrome), a defective lipoprotein-lipase system (hyperchylomicronemia) or faulty chylomicron formation (β-lipoproteinemia), or defects in fat transportation (intestinal lymphatic obstruction, lymphangiectasia, chylothorax, chyluria, chylous ascites exudative enteropathy).
1.3	32	28	13.9	17.4	13.3	454	130	Formula used for infants and children with phenylketonuria. Initially to meet phenylalanine needs, whole milk or formula is added (see Chap. 27).
2.3	57	55.2	20.7	34.1	26.8	920	170	Formula used for older children with phenylketonuria. The formula contains no phenylalanine (see Chap. 27).
1.04	41.6	40.3	15.8	23	14.4	480 c̄ added dextrose	125	Formula used for infants with carbohydrate intolerances. Carbohydrate of choice can be added (i.e., polycose, dextrose) slowly to provide 6.4% of total energy.
1.2	26	23	13	22	16	210	131	Formula used as a transition between infant formula and cow's milk.

TABLE 13-5 GUIDELINES FOR USE OF SUPPLEMENTS IN HEALTHY INFANTS AND CHILDREN[a]

Child	Multivitamin-multimineral	Vitamins			Minerals
		D	E	Folate	Iron
Term infants					
Breast-fed	0	±	0	0	±[b]
Formula-fed	0	0	0	0	0
Preterm infants					
Breast-fed[c]	+[c]	+	±[d]	±[c]	+
Formula-fed[c]	+[c]	+	±[d]	±[c]	+[b]
Older infants (after 6 mo)					
Normal	0	0	0	0	±[b]
High-risk[e]	+	0	0	0	±
Children					
Normal	0	0	0	0	0
High-risk	+	0	0	0	0
Pregnant teenager					
Normal	±	0	0	±	+
High-risk[f]	+	0	0	+	+

[a]Symbols indicate: +, that a supplement is usually indicated; ±, that it is possibly or sometimes indicated; 0, that it is not usually indicated. Vitamin K for newborn infants and fluoride in areas where there is insufficient fluoride in the water supply are not shown.

[b]Iron-fortified formula and/or infant cereal is a more convenient and reliable source of iron than a supplement.

[c]Multivitamin supplement (plus added folate) is needed primarily when calorie intake is below approximately 300 kcal/day or when the infant weighs 2.5 kg; vitamin D should be supplied at least until 6 months of age in breast-fed infants. Iron should be started by 2 months of age (see text).

[d]Vitamin E should be in a form that is well absorbed by small, premature infants. If this form of vitamin E is approved for use in formulas, it need not be given separately to formula-fed infants. Infants fed breast milk are less susceptible to vitamin E deficiency.

[e]Multivitamin-multimineral preparation (including iron) is preferred to use of iron alone.

[f]Multivitamin-multimineral preparation (including iron and folate) is preferred to use of iron alone or iron and folate alone.

Source: Committee on Nutrition, "Vitamin and Mineral Supplement Needs in Normal Children in the United States," *Pediatrics,* **66**:1015, 1980. Copyright American Academy of Pediatrics 1980.

With formula-fed infants, if powdered or concentrated formula is used, fluoride supplements should be administered only if the community water supply contains less than 0.3 ppm of fluoride. Ready-to-use formulas are processed with water low in fluoride, so the recommendation for infants on these formulas is the same as for the breast-fed infant.

The premature or low-birth-weight infant has special nutrient needs (see Chap. 14). Parents of these infants need counseling on possible atypical feeding behavior. The infant may have trouble sucking or have an irregular feeding schedule (see Chap. 12, Clinical Study 12-1).

During this early period most healthy infants need between 6 and 8 feedings. As the child's stomach capacity (2 tablespoons at birth) increases, feedings are spaced further apart, with a large amount of individual variation. Parents of both the breast-fed and bottle-fed infant will need the assurance that appetite is the best indicator of the amount of formula the infant should take. (A rough way to estimate the amount per feeding during the first 5 months is to take the infant's age in months and add 3 to get the total ounces per feeding.) Parents should be helped to recognize the components of infant feeding behavior (e.g., satiety; see Chap. 12). It is the failure to recognize infant cues such as satiety that has caused some pediatricians to blame the bottle for overfeeding and relate this to the cause of childhood obesity. It is postulated that since the bottle-fed infant relies on external cues emanating from the parent, the infant does not learn to rely on internal cues, thereby causing a functional deficit in hunger awareness with resultant weight gain. However, this theory of infantile obesity is highly speculative. The etiology is complex (see Chap. 25). Parents should allow the infant to stop eating at the earliest indication of satiety.

Baby Foods

Around 3½ to 4 months of age, the infant's thrusting movement of the tongue, used to extract milk from the nipple, is diminishing, along with the birth stores of iron if the infant is not on an iron-fortified formula or an iron supplement. Both these physiological processes indicate a beginning readiness for strained foods. However, there is no nutritional advantage to early introduction of baby foods.[45,46] It can be mutually frustrating to infant and parent alike as the infant pushes food out with the tongue (because of the thrusting reflex) and the parent spoons it back in. In addition, there is no evidence to support the claim that early introduction of food promotes night sleep. The achievement of an 8-h sleep interval is a developmental stage that can begin early in the second month[47] but on the average begins between 3 and 4 months of life.

Baby foods should be added one at a time (one to two foods per week), and the child with a family history of allergy should be watched closely (see Chap. 20). Parents should understand that the infant's ability to eat solid food will improve with practice and that food pushed out of the mouth is not indicative of dislike or stubbornness but, rather, of inexperience. Placing solids more to the center of the tongue with a slight downward pressure as the spoon is removed will facilitate the swallowing of the food.

The sequence of food introduction will vary with cultural practice and pediatricians' preferences, with the usual sequence being cereal, then fruit, followed by vegetables and meats.

With the introduction of solid foods recommended for breast- and formula-fed infants at 5 to 6 months, the sequence of food introductions appears to be of little consequence.[48] Foods with relatively high protein content (cereal with milk, meat, poultry) should be encouraged as the infant is introduced to vegetables and fruit. It is recommended that juices be introduced when the infant is able to drink from the cup, to avoid nursing bottle syndrome (see Chap. 17). With an allergy history, a special alert is given on feeding wheat cereal, orange juice, and whole egg, which is usually delayed to the end of the first year.

The selection of baby foods is important since replacement of formula with nutritionally inferior food can lead to a poor nutritional state; also, these foods have a high energy density which easily contributes to childhood obesity. Four categories of commercially prepared strained and junior foods—fruits, soups, dinners, desserts—account for 60 percent of baby-food sales.[49] Unfortunately, three out of these four have distinct disadvantages. Soups and dinners with high water content have less protein when compared to plain baby meat (a better protein buy) and have modified food starches added, the effect of which has never been fully tested on infants. However, with the later introduction of food, starch digestion is not a problem. Desserts contain sugar, raising concern about early conditioning to sugar. (For the same reason and for dental concerns, parents should be discouraged from adding sugar to cereal or to water bottles.) Both the sugar and salt added to

TABLE 13-6   ENERGY AND PROTEIN VALUES OF SELECTED BABY FOODS

Type	Amount, tbsp	Energy		Protein, g
		kcal	kJ	
Baby rice cereal (dry)	1	10	42	trace
Baby oatmeal cereal (dry)	1	10	42	0.33
Strained rice cereal with applesauce and bananas	1	9.8	41	0.05
Strained beef*	1	13	51	1.9
Strained chicken*	1	19	80	1.9
High-meat dinner* beef with vegetables	1	11.2	47	0.8
Strained vegetables and beef	1	9.4	39	0.4
Strained carrots	1	3.6	15	0.1
Strained applesauce	1	10	42	
Strained peaches	1	10	42	

*Compare the protein in high-meat dinner with the protein in strained beef and chicken and vegetables and beef.

Source: Nutrient Values of Gerber Baby Foods, 1979.

baby foods has provoked consumer concern, which has prompted the major baby-food companies to reduce and, in some products, to remove these additives completely (e.g., fruit is processed without sugar). Table 13-6 lists the energy and protein content of some commercial baby foods.

Baby cereals are supplemented with calcium and phosphorus, and are fortified with thiamin, riboflavin, niacin, and iron. Infants' dry cereals are processed with electrolytic iron powder of small particle size, which is of high bioavailability, according to animal studies. The use of infants' cereal is encouraged until 18 months of age since cereals not prepared specifically for infants contain a variety of types of iron of possibly poor bioavailability.[50]

Homemade versus Commercially Prepared Baby Foods

Many parents are now preparing their own baby-food mixtures with blenders or baby-food mills or grinders instead of buying commercially prepared foods. At present there is no strong opinion favoring either practice, assuming that home cooking techniques are sanitary and that cost is not the factor in decision making.

In making baby foods, parents can control and even eliminate the amount of additives such as sugar, salt, and modified starch, yet some would argue that there is greater predictability of the vitamin content in manufactured foods because of rigid production control.

Homemade baby foods may contain greater caloric density and a higher salt content than expected. Kerr et al. found that the amount of added salt of 70 samples of homemade baby foods prepared by 36 mothers was 64 percent higher than the maximum (100 mg sodium per 100 g of food) acceptable sodium level for commercially prepared foods recommended by the Food and Nutrition Board, National Academy of Sciences.[51] However, with good techniques for food buying, handling, storing, and preparation, a nutrient-concentrated baby food can be the final product, since less water is added during preparation.

With home-prepared baby food, the question of nitrite content has been raised. Plant nitrates commonly found in carrots, spinach, and beets can be converted under certain conditions to nitrites before consumption by the infant and, with consumption, can lead to methemoglobinemia. Cases have been reported from the consumption of home-prepared spinach soup, carrot soup, and carrot juice, whereas no cases of methemoglobinemia have been reported with commercially prepared foods because of the processing technique. Eliminating home-prepared beets, carrots, and spinach from the infant's diet can remove this potential health hazard.[52] Beets, whether they are prepared at home or commercially prepared, are not generally recommended for infant diets because of their high nitrate content.

Increasing Texture in the Infant's Diet

An infant does not need teeth before having texture introduced into his or her diet; the baby can begin getting accustomed to texture near the end of the fifth month, even as infant foods are introduced. Small amounts of soft mashed table foods (such as regular canned applesauce) can be mixed into baby food. With infant food introductions delayed until 5 to 6 months, the infant will not stay at the strained food stage for long. Gradually less baby food and more table food can be added to the mixture as the child develops more tongue mobility and the lateral motions of the jaw commence (6 to 7 months), usually accompanied by the first appearance of the primary teeth (5 to 7 months). Failure to observe developmental readiness for texture makes the introduction increasingly difficult with the passage of time, and the child is at risk of developing the "soft-solid syndrome."[53]

By 6 to 7 months, the child shows a readiness to begin munching (see Fig. 13-8, p. 266). As children achieve sitting balance and eye-hand coordination, finger feeding can be encouraged.

Hard toast, zwieback, and biscuits can initiate the feeding experience and help soothe gums that may be sore from teething. Thereafter, as they achieve motor control and sitting balance, foods with different textures, shapes, colors, and smells will stimulate their interest and promote food learning experiences. Cooked vegetables, meats, cheddar cheese sticks, tofu, fruit, and enriched cereals are good choices. Stringy foods, nuts, and raisins can cause choking and should not be offered. Table 13-7 (pp. 267–268) summarizes the transition of infant feeding during the first year of life.

The Transition to Whole Milk

Iron-fortified formulas may be continued well into the latter part of the first year. When the infant is over 6 months old and eating 200 g of strained foods, which is equivalent to 1.5 jars of strained food, whole milk may be introduced.[54]

With the introduction of whole milk, the infant may regurgitate a sour vomitus, because of the presence of butyric acid (a volatile fatty acid) in the butter fat. Also, constipation may occur because of a change in the curd tension of the protein.

Skim milk is not recommended during the first 12 months because the lack of the essential fatty acid, linoleic acid, and the low caloric density prompt the infant to compensate by an increased consumption of solid baby food to meet appetite needs, thereby causing a disproportionate distribution of energy from carbohydrate and protein.

The introduction of whole milk into the infant's diet has been identified as a factor in the occurrence of iron-deficiency anemia. The mechanism is associated with microscopic changes in the gastrointestinal tract, leading to impaired iron absorption.[55] However, Fomon does not consider this factor relevant to feeding older infants receiving 200 g of strained food daily and either an iron-fortified infant cereal or a medicinal iron supplement.[56]

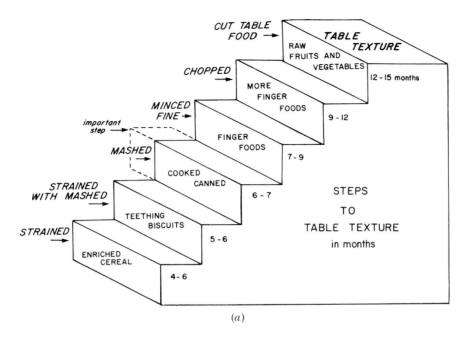

(a)

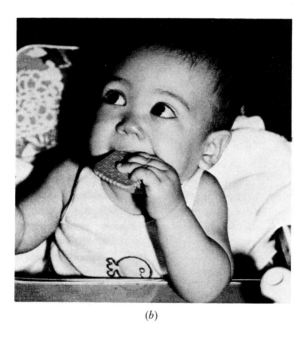

(b)

Figure 13-8
The steps to table-food texture at the 6- to 7-month level. (Adapted from Nutrition Service, Children's Hospital Medical Center, *Steps to Table Texture*, Boston, Massachusetts.)

TABLE 13-7   FEEDING GUIDELINES FOR INFANTS DURING THE FIRST 6 MONTHS*

	0–2 weeks	2 weeks–2 mo	2 mo	3 mo	4–5 mo	5–6 mo
Formula						
Per feeding	2–3 oz	3–5 oz	5 oz	6–6½ oz	7–8 oz	7–8 oz
Average total	22 oz	28 oz	30 oz	32–34 oz	32 oz	28 oz
Number of feedings	6–8	5–6	5–6	5	4–5	4–5
Food texture	Liquids	Liquids	Liquids	Liquids	Baby soft	Baby soft
Food additions						
Apple juice†						3–4 oz
Baby cereal, enriched					2–2½ tbsp, B & S	3 tbsp, B & S
Strained fruits					1½–3 tbsp, B, L, & S	2–3 tbsp, B, L, & S
Strained vegetables					1–2 tbsp, L	2–3 tbsp, L
Strained meats						1–2 tbsp, L
Egg yolk or baby egg yolk						½ med or 1 tbsp
Teething biscuit						½–1
Total calories	440	560	600	660–680	729–788	791–870
Recommended calories 117 cal/kg	410	410–608	608	667	725–784	784–878
Oral and neuromuscular development related to food intake	Rooting, sucking, swallowing	Rooting, sucking, swallowing	Rooting, sucking, swallowing	Extrusion reflex diminishes; sucking becomes voluntary	Learning to put hands to mouth; develops grasp	Munching begins; can approximate lips to rim of cup

*Calculations based on male growing at the 50th percentile for height and weight.

†Offer from the cup.

B = breakfast, L = lunch, S = supper

(Continued)

TABLE 13-7 (CONTINUED) FEEDING GUIDELINES FOR INFANTS 6 TO 12 MONTHS OLD*

	6–7 mo	7–8 mo	8–9 mo	9–10 mo	10–11 mo	11–12 mo
Whole milk						
Per feeding	8 oz†	8 oz	8 oz	8 oz	8 oz	8 oz
Average total	28 oz	28 oz	24 oz	24 oz	24 oz	24 oz
Number of feedings	3–4	3–4	3	3	3	3
Food texture	Gradual increase ⟶		Mashed table ⟶			Cut fine
Food items						
Orange juice	4 oz	4 oz	4 oz	4 oz	4 oz	4 oz
Fortified cereal	½ cup, B	½ cup, B	½ cup, B	½ cup, B	½ cup, B	½ cup, B
Fruit, canned or fresh	4 tsp, B, L, & S	4 tsp, B, L, & S	2 tbsp, L & S	2 tbsp, L & S	3 tbsp, L & S	3 tbsp, L & S
Vegetables	1½ tbsp, L & S	2 tbsp, L & S	2 tbsp, L & S	2 tbsp, L & S	3 tbsp, L & S	3 tbsp, L & S
Meat, fish, poultry	1 tbsp, L & S	2 tbsp, L & S	2 tbsp, L & S	2 tbsp, L & S	2½ tbsp, L & S	2½ tbsp, L & S
Egg yolk or baby egg yolk	1 med yolk, or 2 tbsp	1 med yolk, or 2 tbsp	1 med yolk or 2 tbsp	1 whole egg	1 whole egg	1 whole egg
Teething biscuit or bread	1 biscuit	1 biscuit	½ slice bread	½ slice bread	½ slice bread	½ slice bread
Starch—potato, rice, macaroni			2 tbsp, S	2 tbsp, S	2 tbsp, S	2 tbsp, S
Dessert—custard, pudding						2 tbsp, S
Butter			1 tsp	1 tsp	1 tsp	1 tsp
Total calories	859	876	937	974	1037	1069
Recommended calories (108 kcal/kg)	810–864	864–918	918–972	972–1015	1015–1048	1048–1083
Oral and neuromuscular development related to food intake	Begins using cup	Sits erect with support; Feeds self biscuit ⟶ Without support		Holds bottle	Picks up small food items and releases	Will hold and lick spoon after dipped into food; self-feeding

*Calculations based on male growing at the 50th percentile for height and weight.

†Offer small amounts (2–4 oz) when milk is presented from the cup.

B = breakfast, L = lunch, S = supper

Source: E. Getchel and R. B. Howard, "Nutrition in Development," in G. Scipierl et al., *Comprehensive Pediatric Nursing,* McGraw-Hill Book Company, New York, 1979, p. 161.

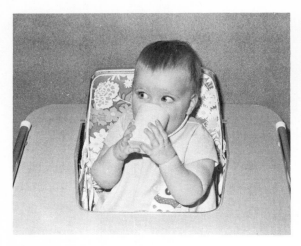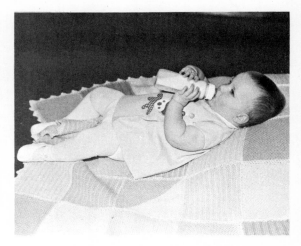

Figure 13-9
Weaning, a gradual process. As the child takes more from the cup, less will be required from the bottle.

Weaning

By definition, *to wean* is to detach affections from something long desired. Weaning a child marks that period of transition from breast or bottle feeding to a more solid food diet and cup drinking. Preparation for weaning begins in the second half of the first year. By 5 to 6 months of age, infants are beginning to be able to approximate their lips to the rim of a cup (a good time to introduce juice); and by the time they are 1 year old, they can hold and drink from a cup with assistance. As the infant can take more from the cup, less will be needed from the bottle. Somewhere between 1 and 2 years, the transition from the bottle is usually complete. While there is no specific age for weaning, it is suggested that weaning be a gradual process accomplished over a period of time, not overnight. The early practice of bottle propping, leading to empty feeding experiences, and excessive breast or bottle feeding, promoting dependency, may negatively affect the weaning process. During the weaning process, some children will refuse to drink milk from the cup, causing the concerned parent to continue with the bottle. Offering alternative milk substitutes (cheese, yogurt,

milk puddings, milk-based soups) to replace the calcium source can alleviate the concern without interfering with the weaning process.

Infant Feeding Problems

The feeding process undergoes many changes in the first year as the child progresses from six to eight breast or bottle feedings to the cup, table foods, and three meals. This process of food input and elimination is subject to an enormous range of management issues which are commonly manifested as "classic infant feeding problems" (e.g., colic), which exclude all those problems emanating from any underlying pathological conditions (i.e., congenital heart disease, Chap. 21; malabsorption, Chap. 22; failure to thrive without organic reason, Chap. 26; inborn errors of metabolism, Chap. 27). Table 13-8 (pp. 270–272) summarizes the causes and dietary treatment of nutritional failure. With the average infant, inquiries into the amount of formula or food intake, the technique of feeding or formula preparation, and the emotional climate in the home can help to identify the problem area.[57] Table 13-9 (pp. 273–274) suggests some practical approaches to infant feeding problems.

TABLE 13-8 CAUSES AND DIETARY TREATMENT OF NUTRITIONAL FAILURE

Cause	Example	Disease or condition	Therapeutic diet	Pediatric concerns
Defective food intake Quantitative	Sensory-motor deprivation (see Chap. 26)	Failure to thrive	High in protein, high in calories	Emotional and environmental support along with help to foster parents' capacity to nurture and protect their child
	Judgmental errors Low iron intake (see Chap. 7)	Iron-deficiency anemia	High iron with initial supplementation to replete iron stores	Mothers may need support in the following areas: 1 To encourage the use of iron-containing foods the child may be rejecting 2 To wean the child in order to decrease milk consumption (large amounts of milk decrease iron absorption)
	High sugar intake (see Chap. 17)	Dental caries	Low in concentrated carbohydrates (sugar, jams, jellies, honey, candy, cookies, cake)	Removal of sugar may cause conflict; mothers need positive reinforcement; frequency of sugar in the diet is as important as the total amount; if a sugar-containing food is allowed, it should be given once per day after a meal rather than throughout the day
Defective absorption	Gluten sensitivity (see Chap. 22)	Gluten-induced enteropathy	Low-gluten diet (avoidance of oats, wheat, rye, barley)	Offending grains are obvious in cereal forms but are also used in many commercial products as thickeners or fillers; need for careful reading of product labels should be discussed
	Surgery (see Chap. 28)	Surgical resection of small bowel (degree of malabsorption and general and specific nutrient deficiencies will depend on the amount and area of bowel resected)	Hyperalimentation, tube feedings, or high-energy, high-carbohydrate (mostly simple sugar) diet with small frequent feedings	Compensations for lack of oral satisfaction and necessity to provide normal food-related experiences; when solids are restarted, food rejection and emotional problems are common

Defective utilization	Inborn error of metabolism (see Chap. 27)	Galactosemia (absence of the enzyme galactose 1-phosphate uridyl transferase, one of three enzymes involved in the conversion of galactose to glucose)	Lactose-free diet (no milk or milk products)	A milk substitute must be used and careful attention must be paid to other food sources of lactose (drugs, breads, prepared mixes, etc.); careful reading of product labels should be discussed
Defective function of major organ system	Congenital anomalies (see Chap. 26)	Cleft lip and palate	Adequate for normal nutritional requirements, but needs special consideration regarding the presence of the cleft; also should provide for nutritional stores in anticipation of surgery; acid and spicy foods may irritate the mouth and nose and may need to be eliminated	Special attention to the feeding position and equipment (appropriate nipple) is necessary; allay parents' fears that child may choke; explain to parents that patience is necessary, as feeding is apt to be a long, drawn-out process
		Cyanotic heart disease	High in calories (150–200 kcal/kg) with small frequent feedings; need for sodium restriction depends on individual condition (normal diet for child contains 2–4 g Na^{2+}); adjustments in food texture may be necessary to prevent fatigue	Overdependence of child should be avoided; encourage normal age progression and independence in feeding
	Brain damage (see Chap. 26)	Cerebral palsy with or without mental retardation	Adapted to the degree of handicap and level of independence; child's feeding position, food texture, and special equipment are specific considerations; muscular contractions (if present) may increase caloric needs; immobile patients need supervision to prevent obesity	Same as for cyanotic heart disease

(Continued)

TABLE 13-8 CONTINUED

Cause	Example	Disease or condition	Therapeutic diet	Pediatric concerns
Increased loss of food substances	Diarrhea (see Chap. 22)	Ulcerative colitis	Nutritional management is primarily supportive, symptomatic, and nonspecific	Elimination diets are employed widely; despite occasional dramatic responses, there is no conclusive evidence that they are beneficial; when elimination diets are used, check to see that necessary nutrients have not also been eliminated
		Gastroenteritis (mild)	Reduction of food and formula (especially carbohydrate and fat) and restriction of liquids to water and clear fluids (broth, diluted apple juice, liquid gelatin)	A gradual return to a full diet should be stressed, and liquid gelatin in the bottle should be discontinued. Initially milk may be poorly tolerated and should be added slowly
Increased metabolism	Malignancy (see Chap. 29)	Leukemia	High in calories, high in protein (special frappes, eggnogs); nutrition status important to body's tolerance of drugs and immune response	Child's appetite may be poor due to general condition and drug treatment; the diet should begin at the level of his appetite and work upward; avoid cajoling him and forced feedings
Excessive food intake	Overeating (see Chap. 25)	Obesity	Appropriate for age, height, weight, and activity, with slight reduction in calories	Interdisciplinary approach: diet integrated with the psychologic factors and physical activity

Source: E. Gretchel and R. B. Howard, "Nutrition in Development," in G. Scipien et al., *Comprehensive Pediatric Nursing,* McGraw-Hill Book Company, New York, 1979.

TABLE 13-9 PRACTICAL APPROACHES TO INFANT FEEDING PROBLEMS

Problem	Signs and symptoms	Management
Intake of formula too large	Regurgitation Vomiting Diarrhea or frequent large stools Normal or excessive weight gain History of excessive intake for age	Reduce formula intake at feedings Explain the problem in detail to the parents and give reassurance
Intake of formula too small	Irritable Underweight Hungry Constipated History of inadequate intake for age	Increase the amount and frequency of formula and possibly the calorie content of the feedings
Improper technique of feeding	Any of the above signs and symptoms Following errors frequently encountered: 1 Hole in rubber nipple too small (providing too long feeding period) or too large (causing excessive swallowing of air, discomfort, and regurgitation)	A puncture with a needle will not increase the size of aperture; discard and use a new one
	2 Formula too hot	Moderately cold or room temperature formulas are well tolerated
	3 Improper placement of nipple in mouth	Place nipple far enough back in mouth
	4 Failure to bubble the infant	After feeding, hold the infant erect against shoulder to expel swallowed air
	5 Improper position of infant during feeding, such as horizontal or with propped pillow	The position should be inclined to at least a 45-degree angle
	6 Nursing from an empty bottle	Formula should fill the nipple throughout feeding, and ½ to 1 oz should be left in the bottle at termination of feeding
	7 Improper sterilization technique	Check sterilization technique Terminal sterilization technique consists of 1 Scrub bottles, nipples, equipment 2 Measure and mix formula 3 Pour mixture into bottles 4 Place bottle on rack in sterilizer and boil gently for 25 minutes 5 Store capped bottles in refrigerator
Improper composition of formula and/or infant's intolerance to a specific nutrient		
Carbohydrate	Excessive amounts may produce diarrhea and/or the infant with a disaccharidase deficiency will not tolerate normal amounts	Added carbohydrate in the form of corn syrup to evaporated milk formula need rarely exceed 1 oz or 2 tbsp per 24-hour volume; honey should not be used in infant formulas or feeding*
Protein	Allergy to protein in cow's milk; allergic infants may have vomiting, irritability, diarrhea, with or without blood in the stool; onset 2–4 weeks after initiating of formula; history in other family members is significant	A few days' trial with a cow's milk substitute such as soy formula, Nutramigen, or Cho-Free, with subsequent alleviation of symptoms, indicates milk allergy

(Continued)

*S. S. Arnon et al., "Honey and Other Environmental Risk Factors for Infant Botulism," *Journal of Pediatrics*, **94**(2):331–336, February 1979.

TABLE 13-9   CONTINUED

Problem	Signs and symptoms	Management
Improper composition of formula and/or infant's intolerance to a specific nutrient (continued)		
Fat	Improper fat digestion causes large bulky stools; digestion of cow's milk butterfat may be less complete than that of fat of breast milk	Substitute a formula free of butterfat, such as Similac, Enfamil, etc.
Emotional problems in the family	Irritability Colic Spitting up Vomiting Failure to gain weight	Explanation, education, patience, and understanding are needed along with constant reassurance and considerable tact

Source: E. Getchel and R. B. Howard, "Nutrition in Development," in G. Scipien et al., *Comprehensive Pediatric Nursing,* McGraw-Hill Book Company, New York, 1979, p. 164, adapted from W. T. Hughes and F. Falkner, "Infant Feeding Problems: A Practical Approach," *Clinical Pediatrics,* 3:65, 1964.

TODDLER (1 TO 3 YEARS)

As the rapid growth of the pre- and postnatal period subsides, the ego identity of the toddler becomes the thrust of this next developmental period. Decreasing energy requirements [90–100 kcal per kilogram (377–418 kJ) of body weight] and appetite reflect this period of slow progressive growth as mealtime negativism with food "jags" become the prevailing theme in the toddler's bid for autonomy. Protein needs are also less than in the first year, and recommended amounts are for 1.76 g per kilogram of body weight.

With the increasing refinement of hand and finger movements and the appearance of most of the primary teeth, the toddler can be allowed more independence at mealtimes and can be presented with most table foods. However, meat and stringy vegetables may still pose a problem, as good tongue lateralization and rotary chew-ing, skills necessary to facilitate good chewing, do not develop until somewhere between 18 and 21 months of age. Also, the ritualistic toddler may prefer plainer food to mixed dishes and may designate specific places for the various food items on his or her plate.

During this period, parents need to understand that the characteristic small, finicky appetite is part of this stage of development. Overreacting to the situation by forcing, bribing, or punishing to make the child eat only reinforces the child's negative behavior. Parents need help in maintaining reasonable limits on the child's behavior while allowing the child some personal control. The toddler's negativism can be met by phrasing questions so as to elicit a positive response; for example, "Do you want milk or juice first?" This approach maintains parental control yet fosters toddler independence. Servings of a reasonable size are also

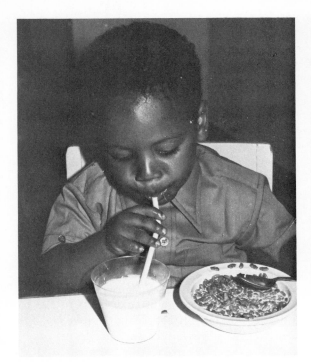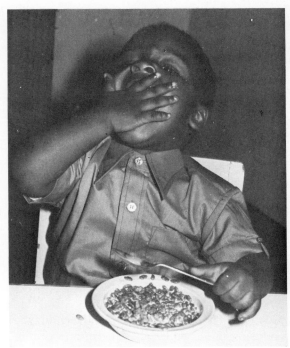

Figure 13-10 *The toddler: able to use a straw and a spoon but still apt to resort to the hands.*

Figure 13-11 *The difference between being (below, left) 22 months and (right) 36 months of age.*

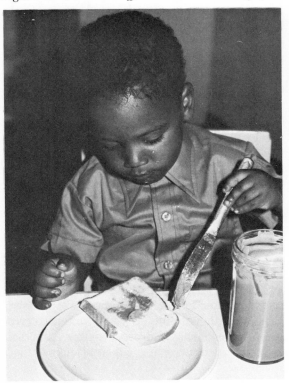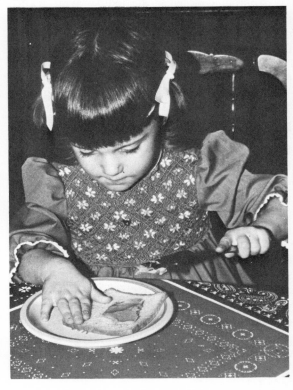

needed to encourage the toddler whose appetite is easily overwhelmed, especially by frequent drinks or between-meal snacks. Still-uncoordinated fine motor control makes spills a common occurrence, and unrealistic social expectations should not be made of the toddler at the family dinner table.

Frequent spills, finicky appetite, and underdeveloped chewing skills leave the toddler open to nutrient deficiencies. Vitamin A, calcium, phosphorus, riboflavin, and iron deficiencies are the concerns with a child who may be refusing to drink milk or who has difficulties in chewing meat. Meat and vegetables are the foods most frequently refused during this period, which further compromises the toddler's zinc and folate nutriture.

Powdered or evaporated milk, added to soups, can help as supplements for the child who is refusing milk, while wheat germ and peanut butter are folate-containing foods that are readily acceptable to the toddler. Meat that is easy to chew (chicken, turkey) and minced, moist meat can help to solve the meat dilemma.

Another concern is the toddler who drinks milk to the exclusion of solid foods, leaving the diet particularly deficient in iron, zinc, vitamin C, and folate. Iron-deficiency anemia (see Chap. 7) and encopresis (see Chap. 22) are common findings in this age group.

Pica

Increasing mobility leads to greater environmental exploration, and a great deal of exploration revolves around oral examination of both edible and nonedible objects. Pica, an aberration of appetite leading to the consumption of inedible objects such as dirt, soap, or paint chips, commonly occurs in young children between the ages of 18 and 24 months. The cause is unknown and seems related to environmental deprivation rather than to a deficiency of any specific nutrient, although diets of these children are often deficient in iron.[58,59] Pica can be the cause of lead poisoning from the ingestion of plaster or other objects that are saturated or coated with lead-based paint. Treatment includes the use of chelating agents. Many children are iron-deficient and may be receiving iron therapy when the diagnosis of lead poisoning is made. Iron binds the chelating agents, and must be discontinued during chelation therapy.

THE PRESCHOOL CHILD

The preschool child, now mostly independent at the table, continues to make slow, steady gains in weight and height of approximately 2 kg (4.5 lb) and 6 to 8 cm (2½ to 3½ in) per year. Although growth is at a slower rate, it imposes demands on the young body that are further enhanced by the constancy of activity. Psychosocially, the child struggles to develop a sense of initiative, taking an eager and inquisitive approach to the surroundings. Size, form, color, shape, time, and space now take on a new meaning.

As conversation skills improve, questions become more relevant and demand more than a simple response. The child mimics adult conversations and behaviors, television personalities, and advertisements. A nutrition education program that recognizes these influences and the psychosocial characteristics of the preschool child can help to form the basis of a lifetime of good eating practices. This type of program does not need the structure of a preschool, day-care, or head-start center but can be conducted by the parent in the kitchen during meal preparation, or at the table, or even in the aisles of the supermarket, a trip of special significance to the preschooler. In a survey of factors associated with children's food habits, parental attitudes and social factors were found to be the most important predictors of children's food preferences and dietary complexity.[60]

A survey of the nutritional status of the preschool child was conducted between 1968 and 1970. Evidence of nutritional risk, lower biochemical indices, smaller physical size for age, and lower dietary intake was found clustered among preschool children of lower socioeconomic status because of the insufficiency of food (see Chap. 18). Iron-deficiency anemia and dental caries crossed all socioeconomic barriers, however, although they showed a high preponderance in the lower socioeconomic group. Many preschool children continued to take a vitamin-mineral supplement despite an adequate diet—a waste, as large quantities of the water-soluble vitamins are excreted in the urine daily. Convenience foods such as frozen pot pies, canned beef stew, chili con carne, spaghetti, macaroni and cheese, pizza, and foods from fast-food establishments were identified by this survey as staples in the preschool diet to the extent that a broader selection of well-balanced foods may have been precluded.[61] In these circumstances vitamin-mineral supplements should be continued.

Figure 13-12
The preschool child: interested, inquisitive, and especially receptive to nutrition education when offered as part of meal-time preparation.

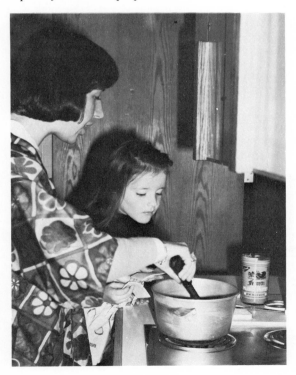

SCHOOL YEARS (6 TO 12 YEARS)

These years, described as middle childhood, are the product of early growth and development and the preparatory period for adolescence. Adaptation to the school experience and peer identification are significant developmental tasks as the child begins a life that is increasingly independent from the family.

Permanent teeth begin to appear and growth proceeds at a moderate rate of about 3 to 3.5 kg (7 lb) and 6 cm (2½ in) per year, as bodily resources are laid down in preparation for adolescence. Growth during these years is characterized by spurts and plateaus, with a pronounced spurt toward the end of this period. Energy needs decrease per kilogram of body weight, but total energy requirements continue to increase.

Although the child aspires to the adult world, some of the prerogatives of childhood are maintained and food behavior vacillates accordingly. School activities and pressing schedules impose stress, and hurried or skipped breakfasts and lunches are common complaints of this age group. These meals often go unnoticed, and replacement of needed nutrients is forgotten. School breakfast and lunch programs may mean new foods and ways of food preparation, and acceptance is now increasingly governed by peers, as food habits take on new social influences and the lure of the vending machines and the corner store is felt for the first time.

The hungriest time of the day for the school-age child is after school. Nutritious snacks (see Table 13-10, p. 279) should be made available to assuage hunger while maximizing nutrient intake. Forethought in snack preparation is particularly important for the working parent, since many children left to their own devices or in the care of a baby-sitter will forage for cookies and candy in attempts to satiate their appetite. Parents must consider themselves as "gatekeepers" who will only allow nutritious foods through the doors of their homes. They will need much support to withstand television, peer, and family pressures to buy certain foods.

It is during this period that childhood obe-

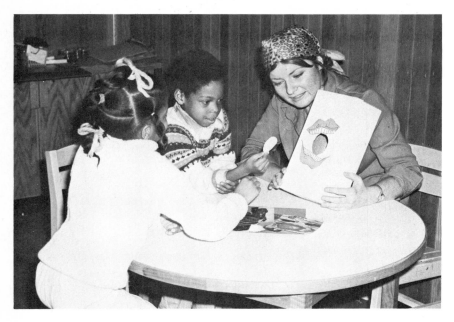

Figure 13-13
The school-aged child learns through this nutrition game that the "big mouth"
accepts only nutritious foods, with no room for junk foods.

Figure 13-14
In the aisles of the supermarkets. Parents need support to maintain their stance
as "gatekeepers" of their families' nutrition—parents who have no room in their
shopping carts for junk foods. How would you cope with this situation?

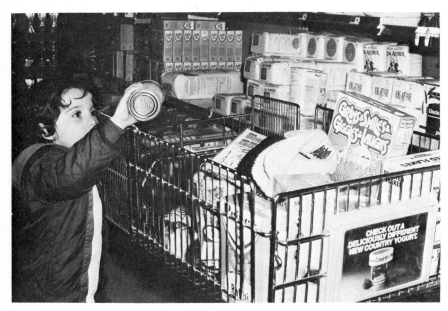

TABLE 13-10 NOURISHING SNACKS FOR CHILDREN

Thirst quenchers	Juices, milk, protein shake (½ cup milk, ½ cup orange juice, ¼ cup powdered milk)
Finger fruits	Orange, tangerine, banana disks, apple, pear, peach slices, pineapple wedges, dried apricots, dates, raisins, grapes, plums, cherries, berries
Finger vegetables	Cherry tomatoes, carrot and celery sticks, cucumber and zucchini wedges, green pepper strips
Spread-ons	Peanut butter, cream cheese, yogurt dips, butter
Other	Yogurt, cottage cheese, tofu, cold meat cubes, whole-grain crackers and cookies, whole-grain bread, fortified cereals

sity becomes apparent. Riding to school and sitting in front of the television after school for an average of 5 h per day afford little opportunity for physical expenditure. Children living in the inner city have even less opportunity for activity because of limited recreational programs and a high-crime environment that imposes risks on personal safety. Games and toys that require movement, family outings directed to exercise, and sports interests which rely more on individual than on team participation and which can be maintained throughout life (skating, swimming, tennis, jogging) should all be encouraged. Children must learn to program activity into their daily life-style, for herein lies the key to the prevention of adult obesity (see Chap. 25).

ADOLESCENCE: THE PREADULT YEARS

The developmental experience of adolescence and the increased velocity of growth are two characteristics shared by boys and girls, and both have nutritional consequences.

During this period the adolescent body undergoes a transition from immature to adult size and shape, changing the configuration of breasts in females and external genitalia in males. With this change in body image comes the new search for identity and the assertion of independence. Moods vacillate from passiveness to rebellion, which can be considered the hallmark of adolescence. *Confused, impatient, impulsive* are all adjectives that can describe the questioning adolescent.

Although emerging differences in growth and body composition alter the nutrient needs of the two sexes, boys and girls share an overriding concern for body image and peer group identification. New eating patterns may evolve, some of which are extreme, faddish, eccentric, or grossly restricted, and cola, chips, pizza, and doughnuts may become the mainstays of the diet. The adolescent vegetarian, fruitarian, macrobiotic, or "health-food freak" is a somewhat disruptive influence at the family meal table, causing both parental and, in some instances, professional concern. Nevertheless, the diet is the adolescent's own personal choice and should be treated accordingly. The preadult will be more receptive to information on how to incorporate the appropriate nutrients (e.g., vitamin B_{12} into the vegetarian's diet) into his or her chosen diet than to suggestions of a change in life-style in order to incorporate needed nutrients.

Drugs—marijuana, psychedelics, barbiturates, amphetamines, cocaine, volatile aerosol sprays, heroin, alcohol, tobacco—are mediums of rebellion, connoting feelings of status, pleasure, and comfort,[62] and also imparting nutritional risks, either directly through effects on nutrient metabolism or indirectly through effects on appetite. Nutritional therapy becomes a vital part of the rehabilitation of the drug- or alcohol-dependent adolescent.

At the time of puberty, there is an increased demand for thyroxine to support growth. Enlargement of the thyroid gland is indicative of iodine deficiency, a finding among the adolescent

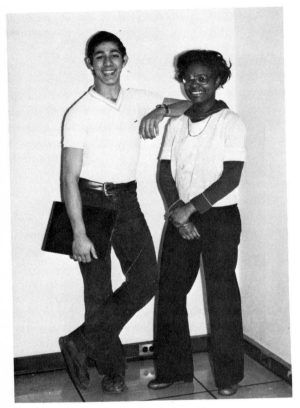

Figure 13-15
The adolescent: searching for identity, looking for answers. "Why should I eat a well-balanced diet? Prove it!" As a future health professional, are you able to?

hygiene may help to ameliorate symptoms but are without guarantee.

Adolescent Girls

For girls, the adolescent growth spurt occurs somewhere between 10 and 14 years. There is great variability in the patterns of growth and hormonal changes, and standards that are related only to age are misleading (see "Onset of Menarche" in Chap. 9).

During the active growth period between ages 10 and 14 years, energy requirements reach 48 kcal (200 kJ) per kilogram of body weight and thereafter drop to 39 kcal (163 kJ) per kilogram. Iron to replace menstrual losses and to provide for growth, along with protein in the vicinity of 1 g per kilogram, folate, and B vitamins, should be stressed.

The normal physiological fat deposition around the abdomen and pelvic girdle raises adolescent concerns about weight. Inactivity can accelerate normal deposition and can lead to an overweight condition which leaves the body-conscious girl an easy prey to fad diets. The aesthetic pursuit of thinness can then result in a malnourished state during the very period when her need for nutrients is the greatest and in some extreme cases leads to anorexia nervosa or bulimarexia, neurotic feeding disturbances (see Chap. 26).

In a study of energy intake of adolescent girls, a marked variation of intake was noted. Fluctuations were not related to mood, suggesting that this has less influence on dietary patterns than is usually supposed. While taking examinations, energy intake was reduced by an average of 12 percent. Energy intake was not changed during a field trip or menstruation. The study suggests that dietary patterns considered abnormal are regularly exhibited by and firmly entrenched in normal school girls.[64] Weight control programs appear to be more successful among girls either in the preadolescent period or after age 15. The years between 10 and 15 are fraught with change, and motivation becomes extremely complex.

population. In the Hanes survey of 1971–1972, both grade I and grade II goiters, indicators of moderate and high-risk deficiency states, were found in 11 percent of Negro youths between the ages of 12 and 17 years.[63] (See "Endemic Goiter" in Chap. 24.)

Acne, a consequence of changing hormones, adds but another stress to the adolescent experience. Treatment with drugs (e.g., tetracycline) and vitamins A or B₆ has a palliative effect and, in the case of vitamin A, can lead to toxicity. A prudent diet (see Chap. 2), with avoidance of caffeine (coffee, tea, cola, chocolate), and good

TABLE 13-11   THE BASIC FOUR FOOD GROUPS THROUGHOUT THE GROWING YEARS

Food group	Servings per day	Average-size servings for age			
		Toddler	Preschool	School	Adolescent
Milk or equivalent; ½ cup milk equals	4	½–¾ cup	¾ cup	¾–1 cup	1 cup
2 tbsp powdered milk					
1 oz of cheese					
¼ cup evaporated milk					
½ cup cottage cheese					
1 serving custard (4 servings from 1 pt milk)					
½ cup milk pudding					
½ cup yogurt					
Meat, fish, poultry, or equivalent; 1 oz meat equals	2 or more	3 tbsp	4 tbsp	3–4 oz (6–8 tbsp)	4 oz or more
1 egg, 1 frankfurter					
1 oz cheese,* 1 cold cut					
2 tbsp peanut butter, cut meat					
¼ cup tuna fish or cottage cheese*					
½ cup dried peas or beans					
Vegetables and fruits, to include	4 or more				
citrus fruit or equivalent	1 or more	4 oz	4 oz	4–6 oz	4–6 oz
1 citrus fruit serving equals					
½ cup orange or grapefruit juice					
½ grapefruit or cantaloupe					
¾ cup strawberries					
1 medium orange					
½ citrus fruit serving equals					
½ cup tomato juice or tomatoes, broccoli, chard, collards, greens, spinach, raw cabbage, brussels sprouts					
1 medium tomato, 1 wedge honeydew					
Yellow or green vegetable or equivalent; 1 serving equals	1 or more	4 tbsp	4 tbsp	⅓ cup	½ cup
½ cup broccoli, greens, spinach, carrots, squash, pumpkin					
5 apricot halves					
½ medium cantaloupe					
Other fruits and vegetables	2 or more				
Other vegetables including potatoes		2–3 tbsp	4 tbsp	⅓–½ cup	¾ cup
Other fruit including apples, banana, pears, peaches		½ med apple	½–1 med apple	1 med apple	1 med apple
Breads and cereals or whole grain or enriched equivalent;	4 or more				
1 slice bread equals		½ slice	1 slice	1–2 slices	2 slices
¾ cup dry cereal		½ cup	¾ cup	1 oz	1 oz
½ cup cooked cereal, rice, spaghetti, or macaroni; 1 roll, muffin, or biscuit		2 tbsp	¼–½ cup	½–1 cup	1 cup or more

*If cottage or cheddar cheese is used as a milk equivalent, it should not also be counted as a meat equivalent.

Source: Getchel and Howard, "Nutrition in Development," in G. Scipien et al., *Comprehensive Pediatric Nursing,* McGraw-Hill Book Company, New York, 1979, p. 166. Adapted from *Infant Feeding Guide,* for use by professional staffs, Washington State Department of Social and Health Services, Health Services Division, Local Health Services, Nutrition Unit, 1972.

The use of oral contraceptives and intra-uterine devices among the teenage population is an additional influence to be considered in determining nutritional needs. Despite the widespread use of contraceptives, teenage pregnancies are escalating, and the juvenile gravida is fast becoming the new obstetrical problem, as the developing fetus places additional demands on the body of the still-developing adolescent (see Chap. 15).

Adolescent Boys

Like their female counterparts, boys manifest adolescence with a great range of variability. Some begin early, usually by age 12, and have completed their sexual maturation when others are commencing, at 15. The adolescent male with greatly expanding muscle mass and energy needs has been identified as being at nutritional risk by the Ten-State Nutrition Survey of 1968–1970 (see Chap. 18). Prior to this time the adolescent male was largely overlooked in deference to the teenage girl.

Between the ages of 11 and 14 years, 60 kcal (251 kJ) per kilogram of body weight are needed to support growth, with a decrease to 42 kcal (175.7 kJ) per kilogram by age 15 to 18. As with girls, boys' energy needs must be interpreted according to physiological stage rather than chronological age. Sexual maturity ratings can help to identify the stage of development, a better indicator of energy needs than age. (The scale of sexual maturity ranges from 1 to 5; a rating of 1 represents the prepubertal stage and 5, adulthood.) Growth needs are further met by 1 g of high-biological-value protein per kilogram. Iron, folate, B vitamins, and iodine also merit attention.

The high school athlete is particularly interested in diet. Programs both to gain and to lose weight are undertaken in attempts to achieve a desired ratio of muscle strength to body weight. With weight loss a reduction only in body fat is desired and should be achieved at a rate of no more than 1 kg per week through a moderate decrease in food, accompanied by a moderate increase in exercise. Regimens to promote gains in weight should increase muscle but not fat. This is achieved through an increase in muscular exercise supported by an appropriate increment in food intake.[65]

There has been a particular mystique associated with the athlete's diet. In reality, a well-balanced, prudent diet (see Chap. 2) during the training period with sufficient energy to meet the athletic needs, which typically range to as much as 5000 to 6000 kcal (21 to 25.2 MJ) per day, is all that is necessary. The young athlete from an economically disadvantaged family will have difficulty in meeting these requirements and should be given special consideration, such as additional servings of the school breakfast or lunch (see Chap. 10).

CONCLUSION

Both the adolescent male and the adolescent female are particularly prone to nutritional insult. Nutritional education should be part of every student's curriculum. "Rap sessions" on food facts, fads, and foods in space science, and slide talks on food buying can help to stimulate a lifetime interest in nutrition that is needed to optimize adolescents' own health and their future families' health. However, a positive food interest is initially formulated as the infant is placed at the breast or given a bottle and is provided a nutrient feeding experience with self-expression and good models to follow. The infant, toddler, preschooler, school-aged child, and adolescent perpetuate the cycle in much the same way as their parents and their grandparents before them. Only through a family approach can nutritional education hope to be successful.

STUDY QUESTIONS

1   Describe the processes and mechanisms underlying growth.

2   What are the extrinsic factors influencing growth?

3 During which periods of development would you expect accelerated growth?

4 How would you go about the assessment of a child's growth pattern?

5 Through each stage—infant, toddler, preschooler, school-age child, adolescent—there are certain psychosocial traits which influence food and feeding. Identify and describe these traits and their influence on mealtime behavior.

6 The oral and neuromuscular development of an infant progresses rapidly in the first year of life. How would you associate this development with the progression of food and feeding during this time? What type of food would you offer to a 3-month-old, 6-month-old, and 1-year-old child?

7 What does the phrase "classic infant feeding problem" mean? How would you identify this problem area?

8 Which would you recommend, home-prepared or commercially prepared baby foods?

9 What adolescent characteristics could be utilized as motivational forces for a nutritional education program?

CLINICAL STUDY 13

Jennie, a 14-year-old girl, was brought to the adolescent unit of the Children's Hospital Medical Center by her parents, who were concerned about her attempts to control weight by periodic fasting at family meals and about her complaints of lethargy.

On physical examination, Jennie was found to be a pretty, healthy adolescent with a sexual maturity rating of stage 5, a height of 64 in and a weight of 114 lb. Of significance in the laboratory analysis was a hematocrit of 35.3.

The social worker noted that Jennie was a somewhat shy, confused adolescent with overprotective and anxious parents, who spent her time after school listening to records in her room. She had no friends. Because of conflicting reports between parents and daughter, no reliable diet history was obtained. On the basis of Jennie's withdrawal, the diagnosis of adjustment reaction to adolescence was made, and the family was referred to a local mental health facility for counseling. Before the family left the unit, the parents and Jennie were seen both alone and together by the nutritionist.

Clinical study questions

1 Judging from the information presented, does Jennie have a nutritional problem?

2 How would you associate Jennie's feeding behavior with the developmental experience of adolescence?

3 What would you recommend to Jennie, and to her parents, to normalize mealtimes?

REFERENCES

1 Donald B. Cheek, *Human Growth: Body Composition, Cell Growth, Energy and Intelligence,* Lea & Febiger, Philadelphia, 1968, p. 3.

2 Jean Sands, John Dobbing, and C. Gratrix, "Cell Number and Cell Size: a Reconsideration of Organ Growth and Development and the Control of Catch-up Growth," *Lancet,* **ii:**503–505, 1979.

3 John Dobbing and Jean Sands, "Vulnerability of Developing Brain Not Explained by Cell Number/Cell Size Hypothesis," *Early Human Development,* **5:**227–231, 1981.

4 G. J. Bowles, *New Types of Old Americans at Harvard,* Harvard University Press, Cambridge, Mass., 1932.

5 *NCHS Growth Charts, 1976, Monthly Vital Statistics Reports,* **25**, suppl. 3, U.S. Department of Health, Education, and Welfare Publication (HRA)76-1120, 1976.

6 C. Yarborough et al., "Length and Weight in Rural Guatemalan Ladino Children: Birth to Seven Years of Age," *American Journal of Physical Anthropology,* **42**:439–448, 1975.

7 A. Prader, J. M. Tanner, and G. A. Von Harnack, "Catch-up Growth Following Illness or Starvation: An Example of Developmental Canalization in Man," *Journal of Pediatrics,* **62**:646, 1963.

8 J. M. Tanner, *Fetus into Man: Physical Growth from Conception to Maturity,* Harvard University Press, Cambridge, Mass., 1978.

9 Ibid.

10 A. Prader et al., op. cit.

11 Donald B. Cheek and Donald Hill, "Changes in Somatic Growth after Placental Insufficiency and Maternal Protein Deprivation," in Donald B. Cheek (ed.), *Fetal and Postnatal Growth: Hormones and Nutrition,* John Wiley & Sons, Inc., New York, 1975, p. 299.

12 S. Babson and G. I. Benda, "Growth Graphs for the Clinical Assessment of Infants of Varying Gestational Age," *Journal of Pediatrics,* **89**:814–820, 1976.

13 L. O. Lubchenko et al., "Intrauterine Growth as Estimated from Live-born Birth Weight Data at 24 to 42 Weeks of Gestation," *Pediatrics,* **32**:793, 1963.

14 Myron Winick, "Malnutrition and Brain Development," *Journal of Pediatrics,* **74**:667–679, 1969.

15 John Dobbing, "Human Brain Development and Its Vulnerability," in *Mead Johnson Symposium on Perinatal and Developmental Medicine,* 6, Evansville, Indiana, 1974.

16 John Dobbing and Jean Sands, "Quantitative Growth and Development of Human Brain," *Archives of Disease in Childhood,* **48**:757, 1973.

17 Donald Cheek, A. B. Holt, and E. D. Mellits, "Malnutrition and the Nervous System," *Nutrition, the Nervous System and Behavior,* Pan American Health Organization Science Publication 251, Washington, 1972, pp. 3–14.

18 J. Hirsch, J. L. Knittle, and L. B. Salan, "Cell Lipid Content and Cell Number in Obese and Nonobese Human Adipose Tissue," *Journal of Clinical Investigation,* **45**:1023, 1966.

19 J. Knittle and J. Hirsch, "Infantile Nutrition as a Determinant of Adult Adipose Tissue Metabolism and Cellularity," *Clinical Research,* **15**:323, 1967.

20 Alex F. Roche, "The Adipocyte-Number Hypothesis," *Child Development,* **52**:31–43, 1981.

21 William Cameron Chumlea, Jerome Knittle, Alex Roche, Roger Siervogel, and Paul Webb, "Size and Number of Adipocytes and Measures of Body Fat in Boys and Girls 10 to 18 Years of Age," *American Journal of Clinical Nutrition* (in press).

22 William Cameron Chumlea, Jerome Knittle, Roger Siervogel, Alex Roche, and Paul Webb, "Adipocytes and Adiposity in Adults," *American Journal of Clinical Nutrition* (in press).

23 Christine Cronk, Alex Roche, William C. Chumlea, and R. Kent, "Longitudinal Trends of Weight/Stature^2 in Childhood in Relation to Status in Adulthood" (in preparation).

24 Alex Roche, Roger Siervogel, William Cameron Chumlea, and Paul Webb, "Grading of Body Fatness from Limited Anthropometric Data," *American Journal of Clinical Nutrition* (in press).

25 Virginia Knott, "Stature, Leg Girth and Body Weight of Puerto Rican Private School Children," *Growth,* **27**:157–174, 1963.

26 Noel Cameron, "The Methods of Auxological Anthropometry," in Frank Faulkner and James Tanner (eds.), *Human Growth II,* Plenum Press, New York, 1978, pp. 35–90.

27 A. R. Frisancho, "Triceps Skinfold and Upper Arm Muscle Size Norms for Assessment of Nutritional Status," *American Journal of Clinical Nutrition,* **27**:1052, 1974.

28 F. L. Trowbridge and N. Staehling, "Sensitivity and Specificity of Arm Cicumference Indicators in Identifying Malnourished Children," *American Journal of Clinical Nutrition,* **33**:687, 1980.

29 M. Zeitlin, "The Derivation of a Reference Standard for Maximum Thigh Circumference of Preschool Children Aged 0–5 Years," *Human Biology,* **51**:11, 1980.

30 Alex F. Roche and John H. Himes, "Incremental Growth Charts," *American Journal of Clinical Nutrition,* **33**:2041–2052, 1980.

31 *Skinfold Thickness of Children 6–11 Years, Vital and Health Statistics,* ser. 11, no. 120, U.S. Department of Health, Education, and Welfare Publication (HSM) 73-1602, 1974.

32 *Skinfold Thickness of Youths 12–17 Years, Vital and Health Statistics,* ser. 11, no. 132, U.S. Department of Health, Education, and Welfare Publication (HRA) 74-1614, 1974.

33 J. M. Tanner and R. H. Whitehouse, "Standards for Subcutaneous Fat in British Children," *British Medical Journal,* **1**:446, 1962.

34a John Himes, Alex Roche, and David Thissen, *Parent-Specific Adjustments for Assessment of Recumbent Length and Stature, Monographs in Paediatrics* (in press).

34b T. G. H. Drake, "Pap and Panada," *Annals of Medical History,* **3**:289–295, 1931.

35 W. Schmidt, "Health and Welfare of Colonial American Children," *American Journal of Diseases of Children,* **130**:694–701, 1976.

36 G. A. Martinez and J. P. Nalenziens, "Recent Trends in Breast Feeding," *Pediatrics* **64**:686, 1979.

37 Committee on Nutrition, "Commentary on Breast Feeding and Infant Formulas: Including Proposed Standards," *Pediatrics* **57**:278, 1976.

38 American Academy of Pediatrics, *Committee on Nutrition Handbook,* American Academy of Pediatrics, Evanston, Illinois, 1979.

39 Council on Scientific Affairs, American Medical Association, *Journal of the American Medical Association,* **242**:2335, 1979.

40 A.P.H.A. Position Paper, "Infant Feeding in the United States," *Nation's Health,* Sept. 7, 1979.

41 R. Kron, M. Stein, and K. Goddard, "Newborn Sucking Behavior Affected by Obstetric Sedation," *Pediatrics,* **37**:1012–1016, 1966.

42 Food and Nutrition Board, *Recommended Dietary Allowances,* 9th ed., National Academy of Sciences, National Research Council, Washington, 1980.

43 Committee on Nutrition, "Vitamin and Mineral Supplement Needs in Normal Children in the United States," *Pediatrics,* **66**:1015, 1980.

44 Committee on Nutrition, "Fluoride Supplementation," Revised Dosage Schedule, *Pediatrics* **63**:150, 1979.

45 S. J. Fomon, F. J. Filer, T. A. Anderson, and E. E. Ziegler, "Recommendations for Feeding Normal Infants," *Pediatrics* **63**:52, 1979.

46 American Academy of Pediatrics, *Committee on Nutrition Handbook,* op. cit.

47 V. Beal, "Termination of Night Feeding in Infancy," *Journal of Pediatrics,* **75**:690–692, 1969.

48 S. J. Fomon et al. (1979), op. cit.

49 S. Fomon, "What Are Infants Fed in the United States?" *Pediatrics,* **56**:350–354, 1975.

50 S. J. Fomon et al. (1979), op. cit.

51 C. M. Kerr, K. S. Reisinger, and F. W. Plankey, "Sodium Concentration of Homemade Baby Foods," *Pediatrics,* **62**:331, 1978.

52 S. J. Fomon, *Infant Nutrition,* W. B. Saunders Company, Philadelphia, 1974, p. 484.

53 R. Illingsworth and J. Lister, "The Critical or Sensitive Period with Special Reference to Certain Feeding Problems in Infants and Children," *Journal of Pediatrics,* **65**:839–848, 1964.

54 S. J. Fomon et al. (1979), op. cit.

55 C. Woodruff, "The Role of Fresh Cow's Milk in Iron Deficiency Anemia," *American Journal of Diseases of Children,* **124**:18–23, 1972.

56 S. J. Fomon et al. (1979), op. cit.

57 W. T. Hughes and F. Faulkner, "Infant Feeding Problems: A Practical Approach," *Clinical Pediatrics,* February 1964, pp. 65–67.

58 M. F. Gutelius et al., "Nutritional Studies of Children with Pica: 1. Controlled Study Evaluating Nutritional Status; 2. Treatment of Pica with Iron Given Intramuscularly," *Pediatrics,* June 1962, pp. 1012–1022.

59 S. Pueschel, S. Cullen, R. Howard, and M. Cullinane, "Pathogenic Considerations of Pica in Lead Poisoning," *International Journal of Psychiatry in Medicine* **8**:13, 1977–1978.

60 A. M. Yperman and J. A. Vermeersche, "Factors Associated with Children's Food Habits," *Journal of Nutrition Education,* **11**:72, 1979.

61 G. Owen et al., "A Study of Nutritional Status of Pre-School Children in the United States, 1968–1970," *Pediatrics,* **53**:597–646, 1974.

62 S. Blades, "Clinical Notes on Adolescent Drug Abuse," in G. Scipien and M. Barnard (eds.), *Issues of Comprehensive Pediatric Nursing,* McGraw-Hill Book Company, New York, 1976, pp. 60–64.

63 U.S. Department of Health, Education and Welfare: *Preliminary Findings of the First Health and Nutrition Examination Survey, United States, 1971–2. I. Anthropometric and Clinical Findings,* DHEW Publ. No. (HRA) 75-1229, 1973.

64 J. H. Lacey, C. Chadbund, A. H. Crisp, J. Whitehead, and J. Stordy, "Variations in Energy Intake of Adolescent School Girls," *Journal of Human Nutrition,* **32**:419, December 1979.

65 N. J. Smith, "Gaining and Losing Weight in Athletics," **236**:149–151, 1976.

CLINICAL DISCUSSION 13

Growth needs and the onset of menstruation have a negative effect upon iron stores and hemoglobin level, as evidenced by Jennie's low hematocrit, which is diagnostic of iron-deficiency anemia. However, anthropometric data (height/weight ratio) and the clinical state do not support the presence of other nutrient deficiencies.

Jennie has been surreptitious in her eating behavior and has been able to cache food without her parents' knowledge. She exhibits, through her manipulative food refusals, a desire to control—an exercise of the will, hitherto denied by her overly restrictive parents.

Normalization of mealtimes depended upon her parents' acceptance of the fact that Jennie's eating habits had evolved over a period of 14 years and at this point were no longer subject to their influence; and, furthermore, that her food choices were her own personal choices and that their reactions further reinforced Jennie's behavior.

Jennie was assured by the nutritionist that she was proportionate for her size and that she could improve an already good figure by exercise. She was further advised that her brittle nails and lethargy were related to the lack of iron, a result of her poor eating habits and increased menstrual losses. Her concern for her body image was used as the motivating force to encourage a better diet and exercise program. She was initially reluctant to join the program at the local youth club, but with counseling at the local mental health facility she overcame her fears of peer rejection. She was maintained on an iron supplement for the next six months.

CHAPTER 14

THE NUTRITIONAL CARE OF THE PREMATURE INFANT

James L. Sutphen

KEY WORDS
Metabolic Limitations
Intrauterine Growth
Intrauterine Nutrition
Nutrient Requirements
Feeding Rationale

INTRODUCTION

At one time in the evolution of neonatology, the initial feeding of preterm infants was delayed to allow the infant to "stabilize." In a retrospective analysis of children with birth weights of 1500 to 2500 g, Bacola et al. showed that the ultimate IQ scores were higher in those infants who received their first feedings at a younger age (28 vs. 37 hours).[1] Churchill demonstrated a correlation between the incidence of spastic diplegia among surviving prematures and the time required to regain birth weight.[2] Although the maximum increase in fetal brain cellularity occurs before the minimum age of extrauterine viability (approximately 25 weeks gestation), there is considerable increase in brain cellularity during the last trimester of pregnancy. Moreover, myelination and the establishment of synaptosomal connections proceed at maximal rates during this later period.[3] In Winick's studies of infants who died of malnutrition during the first year of life, the most marked decrease in brain cellularity was seen in an infant of low birth weight.[4] These data underscore the need for aggressive nutritional intervention.

Neonatal intensive care units now provide care for extremely small, fragile, metabolically immature infants with high metabolic requirements. Holliday et al. demonstrated that the basal metabolic rate per unit of body weight is higher in smaller children.[5] This reflects the higher percentage of body weight comprised by metabolically active organs in the younger child. Although the infant's metabolic requirement is high, the infant's body energy reserves (muscle, fat) are low. Heird et al. estimated that very-low-birth-weight infants have sufficient reserves to support their metabolic rate for only 4 days.[6] These infants with limited reserves, large metabolic requirements, and immature systems present a challenge to those providing nutritional support.

The morbidity rate of larger premature infants has declined over the last 50 years with the advent of improved respiratory care. However, now there is a greater percentage of very small,

287

high-risk infants successfully maintained. Infants with weights of less than 700 g frequently survive. The challenge of adequate metabolic support for this very-high-risk, fragile group often overwhelms present technology.[7] Rates of survival and morbidity hopefully will improve as effective methods of nutritional support evolve. At present, development of good nutritional techniques for these infants has lagged so far behind respiratory technology that starvation in various degrees is a major problem.

Principles of nutrition for the premature are presented in this chapter. The student is introduced to the preterm infant with an overview of intrauterine and postnatal growth—for intrauterine growth is the present standard for determination of nutrient requirements, and observed postnatal growth is an indicator of nutrient effectiveness.

DEFINITION

The World Health Organization defines as preterm those infants whose gestational age is less than 37 weeks (see Fig. 14-1). Prematurity is subdivided into low- and very-low-birth-weight classes. The term *low birth weight* was introduced to define a population with birth weight of less than 2500 g. This was clarified by the subsequent definition of a very-low-birth-weight subgroup with a weight of less than 1500 g.

GROWTH

Intrauterine Growth

Intrauterine growth and body composition data are used to project nutrient requirements for the premature infant. However, the intrauterine growth rate is not usually observed in extrauterine growth. Due to conditions of stress and/or infection, there may be increased metabolic demands on the infant that preclude growth at intrauterine rates. Accurate projection of nutritional requirements from fetal analyses of body composition is complicated by adjustments for nutrient retention and maintenance requirements. Also, the rate of growth per unit of body weight declines by 40 percent during the third trimester of pregnancy, thereby influencing the net accretion of nutrients per unit of body weight. Therefore, requirements may vary with the rate of growth, clinical status, and the quality of ingested nutrients.

Shaw has determined regression lines for rates of nutrient accumulation as a function of gestational age[8] (see Fig. 14-2). These accretion rates have also been determined by others.[9,10]

Fomon et al. estimated a 1200-g preterm infant's protein requirements to be 3.2g/kg per day, based on intrauterine accretion rates.[11] Similarly, other nutrient requirements can be derived from intrauterine accretion rates. In Fig. 14-2, note the marked acceleration of fetal fat deposition during the third trimester. The synthesis of fat constitutes a considerable energy requirement, which must be met by extrauterine nutritional support.

Postnatal Growth

The postnatal growth patterns of low-birth-weight infants have been the subject of a recent

Figure 14-1
A small, typical premature infant attached to life-support systems and lying under a radiant warmer.

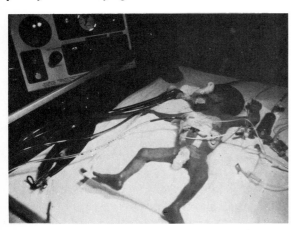

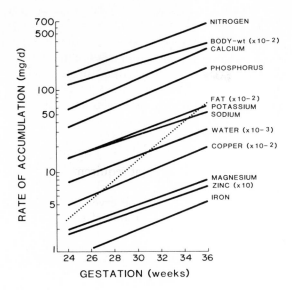

Figure 14-2
Rates of accretion of various constituents of the human
fetus in utero between 24 and 36 weeks' gestation.
[Reprinted from Shaw (1974) with permission.]

exhaustive review.[12] When plotting the infant's weight on standard growth charts, the weight must be adjusted downward by the number of months the infant is premature. By the time the premature infant reaches the age of 40 weeks (term), the weight of the age-adjusted premature infant is still less than the weight of the term infant. However, within 2 additional months of age, their weights are equal. By the time the infant reaches 2 years of age, the age adjustment for prematurity is no longer significant. Similarly, the length of the preterm infant (age-corrected for degree of prematurity) is less than that of the same age, term infant until the infant reaches 21 months of age. It is no longer necessary to correct for prematurity after the child reaches 3.5 years.[13] Finally, the head circumference of the premature infant (age-adjusted for degree of prematurity) is equal to that of the term infant by 40 weeks. Thus, the head circumference grows at the normal intrauterine rate, in contrast to the weight and length. When using standard head circumference growth charts, it is necessary to correct the age for the degree of prematurity until the age of 18 months. Thereafter, standard head circumference growth curves may be used without age correction.[14]

Brandt examined a special group of uniformly small-for-gestational-age (SGA) preterm infants and found a subgroup of these infants who underwent catch-up growth in head circumference. The following conclusions were made:[15]

1   Catch-up growth in head circumference occurs within the first 6 to 8 months of postnatal life. Thereafter, there seems to be little capacity for catch-up growth in head circumference.

2   Catch-up growth in weight and length may occur at a later age, independent of catch-up growth in head circumference.

3   The infants with the best catch-up growth were distinguished by better pre- and postnatal care. The initiation of early postnatal feeding was a major determinant in the attainment of catch-up growth.

This final conclusion again emphasizes the importance of aggressive nutritional support.

INTRAUTERINE NUTRITION

The fetus is provided a constant flow of metabolic substrate (carbohydrate, protein, fat, ketones) by the mother. With maternal fasting there is a rapid increase in maternal ketone levels and a coincident decline in glucose and insulin levels.[16] In contrast, feeding produces an exaggerated rise in insulin and glucose. Human placental lactogen (HPL) is postulated to be partially responsible for these observations. During pregnancy, HPL stimulates anabolism, maternal lipolysis, and insulin resistance.[17] Its synthesis is proportional to the total placental mass and is stimulated by maternal fasting.[18] This hormone may, in part, ensure the flow of metabolic substrate to the fetus. However, actual substrate transport takes place through several mechanisms.

Placental glucose transport proceeds by facilitated diffusion.[19] The amount of this transfer is estimated to be 20 mg per minute at term.[20] It appears that glucose transport satisfies most of the fetal energy demand. At term the fetal glucose levels parallel maternal levels,[21] and the infant's respiratory quotient at birth is 1 or greater,[22] implying fetal reliance on glucose as a major metabolic fuel.

With respect to fat transport, humans, like other mammals, do not transport intact triglycerides directly across the placenta.[23] Rather, component fatty acids are transported. The bidirectional transport of fatty acids across the placenta is demonstrated in vitro.[24] During the first trimester, fatty acid transfer is indicated by the similarity between fetal and maternal fatty acid profiles. Possibly there is less actual transfer at term.[25] It is during the last trimester of pregnancy that the major deposition of fetal fat occurs. Presumably this fat is synthesized primarily from glucose.

Placental amino acid transfer proceeds by an active transport mechanism. At birth, fetal plasma amino acid levels are 10 to 30 percent higher than the corresponding maternal level.[26] This suggests vigorous transport of substrate to the fetus. In sheep, the net transfer of amino acids to the fetus was documented in vivo by Davis et al., who demonstrated that glutamine accounted for 22 percent of the total nitrogen transfer to the fetus. Glutamate was the only amino acid with significant fetal-maternal transfer.[27] Also, in fetal sheep, urea production and excretion are documented.[28] Therefore, glutamate and urea may be vehicles for nitrogen transfer in the premature.

Data substantiating placental transport of ketones are inferential. Early in pregnancy, amniotic fluid ketone concentrations parallel maternal plasma levels.[29] During labor maternal ketone concentrations increase. There is a simultaneous rise in umbilical vein ketone levels with an umbilical artery-to-vein gradient consistent with fetal transfer.[30] These data suggest fetal ketone utilization. However, during an adequately nourished pregnancy, ketones probably constitute a minor energy source for the fetus.

Premature birth interrupts the transfer of metabolic substrate. The immature infant must suddenly ingest, digest, and assimilate nutrients to support metabolism and growth. Removal of the maternal thermoneutral, sterile environment abruptly creates new metabolic requirements for thermogenesis and immune function. These new nutrient demands stress the infant's capacity to the limit, and unfortunately often beyond that limit.

THE DEVELOPMENT OF GASTROINTESTINAL FUNCTION

Morphologic development of the fetal intestine proceeds throughout gestation with a coincident improvement in total absorptive area and intestinal function. The maturation of the fetal intestine is the subject of a review.[31] Intestinal maturation continues postnatally in full-term infants. The digestive limitations found in the premature are seen to a lesser extent in full-term infants. The nutritional implications of the morphologic development of the fetal intestine are significant.

The motor function of the gastrointestinal (GI) tract is limited in the premature infant. This often makes oral feeding difficult. Oral feeding involves the coordination of breathing, sucking, and swallowing. It is difficult for an infant under 34 weeks gestation to be able to obtain adequate nutrition by oral intake alone, although brief periods of oral feeding can be adequately coordinated in infants as young as 28 weeks.[32] If the infant is further compromised by respiratory disease or other stress, he or she may tire easily. These factors increase the danger of aspiration with nipple feeding. Thus, alternative feeding methods, such as intermittent gavage or continuous nasogastric or nasojejunal feedings, are used to supplement or replace nipple feedings in sick and immature infants. See Tables 14-1 (pp. 292–293) and 14-2 (p. 294).

The esophagus of the full-term and premature infant may demonstrate nonperistaltic waves and impaired lower esophageal sphincter function.[33] These compromised functions increase the likelihood of regurgitation and aspiration. Moreover, there may be decreased gastric emptying due to stress and increased pressure on the stomach as a result of rapid respirations. McLain radiographically demonstrated the swallowing of amniotic fluid in utero as early as 33 weeks gestation.[34] Intestinal motility was noted to improve throughout gestation, as evidenced by the subsequent rate of passage of radiocontrast material to the colon. The transit time from mouth to colon was noted to decrease by 50 percent between 32 weeks gestation and term. The clinical significance of poor intestinal transit may be in its contribution to the frequent intermittent periods of paralytic ileus, and in consequent abdominal distension observed in the very small premature infant. The exact mechanism of this distension is probably multifactorial, with hypoxia, bacterial overgrowth, stress, poor vascular perfusion, and an immature propulsive mechanism among the contributing causes. The net result is the interruption of enteral intake. Often, repeated regurgitation, intermittent ileus, and poor gastric emptying force the clinician to abandon the enteral route entirely. Parenteral nutrition may then be used as the total nutrient intake or as a supplement to inadequate enteral intake.

The absorptive function of the small intestinal mucosa improves during growth. This improvement is best documented in the case of carbohydrate absorption. The transport of D-glucose is saturated at low glucose loads in infants compared with adults. This observation has not been extended to the premature infant.[35] Presumably, the premature infant demonstrates at least an equivalent deficiency. Low intestinal disaccharidase activities were measured in human fetuses by Antonowicz and Lebenthal.[36] Between the ages of 26 and 34 weeks, sucrase and maltase reach activity levels that are 70 per-

cent of the enzyme activity of that found in the full-term infant. In contrast, lactase activity during the same interval increases by only 30 percent. From these data, it may be inferred that an infant might not tolerate lactose in the diet. However, feeding studies do not document superior growth with sucrose or maltose.[37,38] Also, the presence of lactose in the gastrointestinal lumen fosters the growth of a fermentative bacterial flora that may offer some protection against infection.[39] Lactose may improve intestinal calcium transport.[40] Finally, human milk contains large amounts of lactose. Therefore, a teleologic argument at least exists for its use in infant feeding. In spite of the paucity of data demonstrating its superiority, lactose is often employed as the carbohydrate source of choice in commercial formulas for premature infants.

Compared with the data available on mucosal carbohydrate transport in the premature, there are few data on the development of amino acid transport in the intestine. In vitro experiments demonstrate that amino acid transport in everted gut sacs does not vary with gestational age,[41] but this has not been shown in vivo.

Intact proteins are absorbed across the mucosal wall in humans. The relative capacity for this process may be greater in the premature infant.[42] Although the amount of this transfer is not nutritionally significant, it may constitute an antigenic stimulus in the infant. It is postulated that such stimuli are important in the development of allergic and autoimmune states. Human breast milk and colostrum may prevent this absorption because of their antibody content.[43] This theory is the subject of current research.

Fatty acid transport across intestinal mucosa may be linked to binding by a specific protein.[44] The capacity of this transport process has not been evaluated in the premature. Fat malabsorption is known to occur in the premature, but it is presently linked to deficiencies in the intraluminal phase of digestion. The large amount of unhydrolyzed intact triglyceride in the stool of premature infants suggests that the limiting step in fat digestion is the intraluminal phase.[45]

TABLE 14-1 COMPENDIUM OF FEEDING METHODS

Feeding method	Nutrient delivery	Technique	Complications*	Considerations	Advantage
Total intravenous alimentation by central line	Crystalline amino acids, 2.5 g/kg per day, 20% glucose solution. Electrolyte, vitamin, and mineral additives. Intralipid by Y connector.	Slow and continuous infusion of approximately 130 mL/kg per day into the superior vena cava via external or internal jugular vein. Gradual increase from 8 to 20% carbohydrate concentration required to establish tolerance.	+ + + + + Hyperglycemia, glycosuria, increased BUN and hyperammonemia with high protein intakes. Abnormal plasma aminograms. Cholestasis. Hyperchloremic metabolic acidosis with crystalline amino acids. With lipid: lipemia and increased risk of kernicterus and sepsis.	Frequent chemical monitoring. Meticulous aseptic technique in preparation of solutions, placement of catheter, and subsequent care. Intralipid contraindicated with jaundice.	Increased energy retention through elimination of digestion and absorption. Decreased risk of necrotizing enterocolitis.
Peripheral intravenous alimentation	Crystalline amino acids, 2.5 g/(kg·day). 10% glucose solution with or without Intralipid. Electrolyte, vitamin, and mineral additives.	Slow and continuous infusion into superficial scalp veins. Intralipid infused by Y connector.	+ + + + Sclerosis at infusion site. (See above.)	Unsuitable when poor venous access.	Avoids central line. Lower rate of sepsis.

Method		Complications		
Intravenous supplementation of tolerated oral feedings	Breast milk or formula given orally or enterally, plus 10% glucose with or without amino acids given by intravenous. Intralipid is useful as it is most calorically concentrated.	Peripheral infusion plus oral alimentation by gavage or nipple with increase in oral intake, concomitant decrease in IV.	+++ Includes complications of intravenous and enteral intake.	Maintain total protein at 8 to 15% of calories. Total fat at less than 60% of calories.	Reduced risk of aspiration due to small size of feeding. Early and gradual stimulation of natural digestive and absorptive processes. Immunological advantages with the use of breast milk.
Nasojejunal/nasogastric (continuous)	Initially glucose, breast milk, or formula.	Nasal insertion of small silastic catheter into the upper jejunum or stomach. Infuse at continuous rate. Amount increased slowly until the desired energy level is required.	++ Perforation reported with the use of polyvinyl tubing. Decreased effect of lingual lipase in nasojejunal feedings.	Formulas of high osmolality less well tolerated with nasojejunal feeding. Must aspirate stomach periodically with nasogastric feeding.	Nasojejunal bypasses problems of delayed gastric emptying. Nasogastric offers better absorption of dietary fat.
Oral-gastric gavage	Initially glucose, breast milk, or formula.	Oral insertion of polyvinyl chloride tube into stomach. Alternate with oral feeds.	+ Accidental tracheal intubation, choking.	Within reason, trial at conventional feeding precedes choice of other feeding methods.	

*+ Indicates degree of severity of complications.

TABLE 14-2   SUGGESTED EARLY FEEDING SCHEDULE (NIPPLE PLUS GAVAGE)

Body weight	Initial feeding, mL	Advancement, mL per feeding	Frequency
1000 g	3	1 to 10	q* 1–2 h
1.0–1.5 kg	5	2 to 15–20	q 2–3 h
1.5–2.0 kg	7	3 to 20–25	q 3 h
2.0–2.5 kg	9	3 to 25–30	q 3 h
2.5 kg	15	3–5 to 40–45	q 4 h

* q = every.

Note: Amounts may be supplemented by intravenous intake depending upon fluid balance. In the lowest-birth-weight classes there is increased, often exclusive, dependence on gavage. Nipple feedings are used increasingly in older infants. Gastric residual contents should be aspirated, measured, and reinfused prior to gavage feedings. The amount of the residual contents is subtracted from the total volume of the feeding.

Indeed, there is considerable fat malabsorption in the premature and, to a lesser extent, in the full-term infant. The lipids of human breast milk are better absorbed than other lipid sources for reasons which remain obscure.[46] Zoppi et al. assessed pancreatic function by duodenal intubation and measurement of amylase, trypsin, and lipase.[47] It was concluded that premature and full-term infants were deficient in pancreatic enzymes relative to older children. Although premature infants were more deficient than full-term infants at birth, by 1 week of age the premature infant actually exceeded the full-term infant in pancreatic output. Therefore, it is unlikely that impaired pancreatic function causes the premature's fat malabsorption.

A more likely etiology of poor intraluminal fat digestion involves bile salt deficiency. Watkins et al. measured the bile acid pool size and synthesis rate in premature infants and found them to be deficient.[48] The duodenal concentration of bile salts may be less than that required for micelle formation. This explanation for fat malabsorption underscores the possible importance of lingual lipase in intraluminal fat digestion. Lingual lipase is active in the absence of bile salts. It has kinetic properties more suited to the acid environment of the stomach. Hamosh et al. demonstrated active hydrolysis of triglyceride (by lingual lipase) in the stomachs of premature infants.[49] Products of this hydrolysis (free fatty acids and monoglycerides) are amphiphilic and may facilitate the solubilization of other more nonpolar lipids, thereby partially replacing deficient bile salt solubilization. Although lingual lipase output is possibly best stimulated by sucking and swallowing, it seems to be active during direct intragastric feedings.[50] It is interesting that Roy et al. demonstrated improved fat absorption with intragastric versus intrajejunal feedings.[51] This finding may be a clinical manifestation of a deficiency of lingual lipase activity during jejunal feeding. It suggests a theoretical advantage for intragastric over intrajejunal feeding.

Lingual lipase may hydrolyze medium chain length triglycerides (MCT) better than longer chain triglycerides.[52] The solubilizing properties of the amphiphilic products of MCT hydrolysis may improve the subsequent intestinal digestion of other fats. In fact, it was demonstrated that MCT improves the absorption of other long chain triglycerides (LCT) in the premature infant.[53] The activity of lingual lipase on MCT and the solubilizing properties of the products of this digestion offer a possible explanation for the activity of MCT in improving LCT absorption.

As a result of fat malabsorption, the absorption of fat-soluble vitamins may be impaired. This is documented in the case of vitamin E. Vitamin E is a highly polar molecule which must be solubilized for adequate absorption.[54] Vitamin E deficiency may lead to hemolysis in the premature. Vitamin E is postulated to aid the premature in the prevention of hemolysis and oxidative damage in the eye[55] and lung.[56] Deficiencies of vitamin D are also documented in the premature.[57] Vitamin K is routinely administered intramuscularly to full-term and premature infants at birth to prevent hemorrhagic disease. Ultimately, endogenous bacterial flora in the gut synthesize adequate amounts of vitamin K for the premature and full-term infant. However, if antibiotics are administered, parenteral vitamin K must be repeated, as its production by gut bacteria may be compromised. To date, there are no reports of vitamin A deficiency in the premature.

METABOLIC LIMITATIONS OF THE PREMATURE INFANT

The fetus has intrauterine metabolic adaptations which may become limitations in the extrauterine environment. The intrauterine environment accommodates these adaptations by integration with maternal-placental metabolism. The activities of fetal cystathionase and, to a lesser extent, cystathionine synthase and methionine-activating enzyme are depressed in the fetus relative to the adult.[58] These adaptations may elevate cysteine to the status of an essential or semiessential amino acid for the premature. Premature infants on low-cysteine diets were demonstrated by Snyderman to have poorer weight gain and nitrogen retention, but her data were not statistically analyzed.[59]

Taurine has been implicated as a putative neurotransmitter. It is present in high concentrations in human fetal brain and in breast milk.[60] Humans have a low capacity for taurine synthesis.[61] Taurine synthesis might be deficient in infants on regular cow's milk formulas containing little taurine. In fact, prematures maintained on regular 18 to 82 whey/casein ratio cow's milk have lower plasma taurine levels than those on breast milk.[62] To date, no formula manufacturer has added taurine. The question of the potential status of taurine as an essential or semiessential amino acid for the premature infant remains unresolved.

There are reported deficiencies of phenylalanine catabolism,[63] tyrosine aminotransferase,[64] and para-hydroxyphenylpyruvate oxidase.[65] Large doses of vitamin C and folic acid have been reported to aid tyrosine and phenylalanine catabolism,[66,67] although this has been recently disputed.[68,69] Plasma levels of phenylalanine and tyrosine are elevated in infants fed high-protein diets.[70,71] Low levels of plasma tyrosine are reported in infants receiving low tyrosine intakes during parenteral nutrition.[72]

The nutritional significance of abnormal plasma aromatic amino acid levels in the premature infant is undetermined. In utero, excess phenylalanine exposure is linked to mental retardation in offspring of phenylketonuric mothers.[73] High-phenylalanine diets induce changes in brain DNA, RNA, and protein in rat models.[74] Transient tyrosinemia of infancy has not been linked to mental retardation. However, Rassin and Gaull have noted that breast-fed infants maintain levels of plasma tyrosine much lower than the levels investigated in studies of possible neurological impairment from transient tyrosinemia.[75]

Abnormalities in ammonia handling are noted in the premature infant. Premature infants maintain higher plasma ammonia levels than full-term infants fed identical diets.[76] Premature infants fed cow's milk protein at 4.5 g per kilogram per day have elevated plasma ammonia levels relative to those fed 2.25 g per kilogram per day.[77] Elevated ammonia levels are implicated in the mental retardation observed in urea cycle disorders.[78] It is possible that chronic low-grade hyperammonia may be harmful to the infant. Visek has suggested that plasma ammonia concentration is only a fraction of the actual intracellular ammonia level and that its toxic effects may be more closely related to intracellular than to extracellular concentrations.[79] This hypothesis remains speculative. However, good utilization of administered protein may be expected to minimize ureagenesis and ammoniagenesis. To ensure good utilization of protein, it should be limited to 15 percent of the total calories.

NUTRIENT REQUIREMENTS OF THE PREMATURE INFANT

Fluid

In the first week of life, there is a contraction in the extracellular water compartment of the newborn. This contraction constitutes a fluid load for the infant to excrete over the first few days of life. Also, there are limitations in renal concentrating and diluting capacities. There may be additional insensible water losses due to phototherapy and radiant warmers which further complicate fluid balance. The occasional development of heart disease (patent ductus arteriosus) often necessitates a reduction in total fluid intake. Often older preterm infants suddenly develop fluid retention while thriving on presumably appropriate fluid and caloric intakes. The cause of this retention is obscure. One must constantly assess fluid balance by routine daily weights and measurement of intake and output.

Table 14-3 illustrates the range of neonatal fluid requirements. Generally, by the second week of life, the fluid requirement of the infant is known by monitoring his or her input and output. These requirements are relatively high, ranging from 150 to 200 mL per kilogram per day. Once the fluid requirement is determined, the nutritional content of the total volume is maximized. According to normal intrauterine growth patterns, rates of growth seldom exceed 20 to 30 g per day. Daily weight gain in excess of these figures may represent the gradual development of edema.

Energy

Energy requirements reflect both energy storage and expenditure. Expenditure is related to oxygen consumption. Minimal rates of oxygen consumption in preterm infants are obtained in the preprandial period; therefore, the available oxygen consumption data probably overestimate actual basal levels.[80] By 6 weeks of age, minimal rates of preprandial oxygen consumption per kilogram are similar in premature and full-term infants (approximately 7 mL per kilogram per day).[81] Cold stress in the premature increases the metabolic expenditure. The relatively mild stress of room temperature (20 to 22°C) induces a 35 percent rise in oxygen consumption in infants previously thermally supported at 33 to 36°C.[82] Although radiant warmers induce a considerable increase in evaporative water loss

TABLE 14-3   WATER REQUIREMENTS FOR LOW-BIRTH-WEIGHT INFANTS

	Water required, mL/(kg · 24 h)	
Water losses	1500 g body weight	1500–2500 g body weight
Urine	50–100	50–100
Stool	5–10	5–10
Insensible	30–60	15–35
Total	85–170	70–145
Increment for phototherapy	20	

Source: R. Neil Roy and J. C. Sinclair, "Hydration of the Low Birth-Weight Infant," *Clinics in Perinatology*, **2**(2):400, 1975.

over the standard incubator, this is not accompanied by a commensurate increase in oxygen consumption, suggesting that the evaporative energy is derived from the warmer, not the baby. Either form of thermal support is adequate. The isolette may decrease the rate of infection. There are no generally accepted estimates of the increases in energy expenditure induced by surgery and systemic infection in premature infants. It is assumed that the preterm infant responds to the stress with an increase in energy expenditure.

Brooke et al. have performed energy balance studies on premature infants.[83] The maintenance energy requirement determined by them was 65 kcal per kilogram (269 kJ per kilogram per day). The energy cost of growth was 5.7 kcal per gram weight gain. Therefore, to meet an intrauterine growth rate of 20 g per day, an infant must retain 179 kcal per kilogram per day (751 kJ per kilogram per day). It is possible that these requirements need to be further adjusted upward to allow for retention. These estimates of energy requirements are enormous. Although they may be in error, they represent the most carefully derived data available to date. Synderman and Holt compared growth on high-energy diets (155 to 180 kcal per kilogram per day) to normal-energy diets (120 to 130 kcal per kilogram per day).[84] The high-energy group gained 43.9 g per day vs. 26.7 g per day for the low-energy group. A higher mineral intake in the high-energy group may have contributed to their greater weight gain. These infants crossed weight growth lines and appeared unusually fat.

In summary, although forced calorie intakes over 150 kcal per kilogram per day may promote weight gain equivalent to the intrauterine rate, and are supported by recent energy balance data, these amounts cannot be unequivocally recommended, as body composition data do not exist to establish the normality of the observed weight gain. The present energy recommendation for the premature infant (120 to 150 kcal per kilogram per day, or 505 to 630 kJ per day) may not represent the optimum intake. However, it remains a reasonable estimate. Adequate

thermal support with radiant warmers or isolettes will lessen the energy expenditure of the infant, thereby allowing more energy for growth.

The infant under a radiant warmer often has a very large fluid requirement relative to the infant in an isolette. The fluid requirement can contribute significantly to the nutrient intake when given as a nutritional solution. When the infant is transferred from the warmer to an isolette, the fluid requirement decreases and the caloric intake must then also be decreased. The advantage of the isolette as a barrier against infection and casual, often unnecessary manipulation of the infant outweighs the advantage of higher calorie intakes under radiant warmers.

Protein

Studies in the literature have compared the effects of various protein intakes on growth. Davidson et al. compared several dietary levels of cow's milk protein (2, 3, 4, and 6 g per kilogram per day). Significant improvement in weight gain was observed in all groups compared with the low-protein intake (2 g per kilogram per day) group.[85] Other studies[86–88] compared protein intakes above and below Fomon's estimate of 3.2 g per kilogram per day, an amount estimated as the requirement to meet projected intrauterine growth needs. It has generally been supported as adequate by these feeding studies. Babson and Bramhall found a significant improvement in linear growth with diets containing 5.25 g cow's milk protein per kilogram per day vs. 2.25 g per kilogram per day,[89] but they did not compare intermediate levels of protein intake. Unfortunately, most studies are of insufficient length to allow adequate comparison of linear growth, which is a better assessment of nutrient adequacy than simple weight gain. Improved linear growth has not been documented when very high protein intakes are compared with Fomon's estimate.

Goldman et al. compared the clinical effects of high (6.0 to 7.2 g per kilogram per day) and low (3.0 to 3.6 g per kilogram per day) protein intakes.[90] Those infants receiving higher protein intakes had a greater incidence of fever, lethargy, and poor nipple feeding. They also had higher plasma proteins and a decreased incidence of edema. In a follow-up study at 5 and 6 years of age, the infants who received high protein intakes had a higher incidence of strabismus and significantly decreased mean IQ scores.[91] Poor growth has been documented in premature infants who receive greater than 8 g of cow's milk protein per kilogram per day.[92] It is prudent to advise milk formula protein intakes within the range of 3 to 5 g per kilogram per day, providing 8 to 15 percent of the total energy as protein. It is not customary to supplement breast milk with casein to increase the protein intake. This practice would, however, increase the protein content of human milk to the range of the presumed requirement. There may be some advantage to high protein intakes in the premature, but possible neurologic morbidity precludes this as a routine practice.

The relative benefit of "humanized" cow's milk protein was examined by Raiha et al.[93] "Humanized" cow's milk contains an adjusted 60 to 40 whey/casein ratio, whereas standard cow's milk has an 18 to 82 whey/casein ratio. Two dietary levels of both milk proteins (2.25 g per kilogram per day and 4.5 g per kilogram per day) were compared with one level of pooled human milk protein (1.63 g per kilogram per day). All formula-fed infants gained weight significantly faster than the breast-fed infants. Linear growth rates did not vary significantly among the dietary regimens. Human milk produced the lowest serum albumin of all groups. It should be noted that the human milk used in the study was milk pooled from mothers of term infants. The protein from milk of mothers of premature infants has a higher protein content than that of mothers of full-term infants.[94] Therefore, the poor growth and low serum albumin levels of breast-fed infants in the Raiha study do not preclude the use of breast milk in the premature infant. To date, there are no data comparing breast milk from the infant's own mother with "humanized" or standard cow's milk formulas. There are also no data on protein supplementation of the premature infant's mother's milk.

There are now special neonatal formulas with an adjusted "humanized" whey/casein ratio. These need careful assessment. Their higher protein content may be a cause of lactobezoars. Human milk contains many nonprotein nitrogen sources. These constituents have yet to be added to "humanized" formulas. "Humanized" milk contains none of the immunologic properties of actual human milk. Although soy formulas are sometimes used in infants who cannot tolerate other standard formulas, soy protein adequacy has not been demonstrated in preterm infants.[95]

Calcium, Phosphorus, Vitamin D

Hypocalcemia and rickets are vexing nutritional problems in the premature. Actual requirements for calcium and phosphorus are considerable if the requirements are based on intrauterine accretion data. After adjusting these accretion data for retention of ingested nutrients, the proposed requirements are enormous. It is difficult to meet these requirements using standard infant formulas. These requirements are above the level of solubility of these elements in intravenous solutions. Because of these problems, inadequate bone growth and demineralization are often consequences of prematurity, and may be even a greater problem when the infant is parenterally nourished. At present, the complex interplay of calcium, phosphorus, calcitonin, parahormone, and vitamin D (and hydroxylated forms) is poorly understood. A brief review of available data gives perspective to the present recommendations. However, extrapolation of precise requirements from these data awaits a better understanding of the premature's physiology.

Neonatal hypocalcemia is observed in full-term infants and, to a greater extent, in the premature infant. Hypocalcemia seen in the first 36 hours of life is associated with complications at delivery, with prematurity, and with maternal diabetes.[96] Another form of neonatal hypocalcemia occurs from 5 to 10 days of age. Both forms are associated with seizures; however, the neurologic prognosis in the latter form appears to be better.[97] The etiology of late hypocalcemia may be linked to any or all of the following:

1   A high dietary phosphate such as that provided in cow's milk[98]

2   A decreased parahormone secretion with consequent poor bone mobilization of calcium and low kidney excretion of phosphate[99]

3   A poor responsiveness of the kidney to parahormone as evidenced by decreased urinary excretion of cyclic AMP following parahormone injection[100]

The present poor understanding of the kidney hydroxylation step in infantile vitamin D metabolism makes it difficult to interpret available data.

Other possible nutrient interactions must be considered in the mineral balance of the premature infant.[101] Various dietary components may aggravate deficiencies of other nutrients.[102] In adult humans, high intake of dietary protein increases renal losses of calcium.[103] This effect is unexplored in the premature, although high protein intakes are sometimes used. Calcium absorption is also impaired by the addition of fat to the formula, presumably as a result of the malabsorption of fat-calcium complexes in the stool.[104] In the clinical setting, formulas are sometimes supplemented with dietary fat, protein, and carbohydrate. These supplements may have potential consequences on the requirement of related nutrients.

The American Academy of Pediatrics recommends calcium intakes of 50 mg per 100 kcal (420 kJ) and phosphorus intakes of 25 mg per 100 kcal (420 kJ). The ratio of calcium to phosphorus should be 1.1 : 1 to 2.0 : 1. These recommendations are less than those used in studies of calcium and phosphorus supplementation. The current low-birth-weight formulas contain levels substantially in excess of these recommendations. Rickets due to hypophosphatemia is reported with breast milk[105] and with PM 60/40.[106] These formulas may have inadequate phosphorus content to support normal growth in the premature infant. Since they are also low in calcium, phosphorus supplementation can precipitate hypocalcemia and must be undertaken with caution. Whenever calcium or phosphorus supplements are added to the diet, deficiency of the complementary element may result.

Vitamin E, Iron, and Polyunsaturated Fatty Acids (PUFA)

Premature infants have poor vitamin E absorption.[107] Provision of oral vitamin E in its water-soluble form may improve absorption.[108] The enteral absorption of iron, however, is relatively normal. Premature infants will develop depleted iron stores by about 2 months of age.[109] Therefore, it is recommended that iron be routinely given. However, in the presence of a high polyunsaturated fatty acid intake, iron, which is well absorbed, may paradoxically increase anemia, possibly as a result of peroxidation of red blood cell membrane PUFA.[110] Thus, the American Academy of Pediatrics recommends that premature infants receive 0.7 IU vitamin E per 100 kcalories (420 kJ) and 1 IU of vitamin E per gram of linoleic acid.[111] Although iron depletion may develop by 2 months of age, a therapeutic intake of iron (2 mg per kilogram per day) is usually not instituted until that time to prevent this potential hemolytic consequence. If supplemental iron is provided at birth, the diet should contain sufficient vitamin E and only moderate amounts of PUFA.

Folic Acid

Folate is well absorbed by the premature. However, the rapid growth of the low-birth-weight infant may precipitate low serum folic acid levels and hypersegmented neutrophils when folic acid intake is low.[112] Actual macrocytic anemia is uncommon. However, supplementation of folate, 50 mg per day, has been suggested to prevent laboratory signs of deficiency.[113]

Riboflavin

Riboflavin is photodegraded in infants exposed to phototherapy. Although this degradation is demonstrated in vivo, its clinical significance is unclear. At present, additional riboflavin is not recommended. When a standard multivitamin preparation is used, there is probably enough riboflavin to prevent deficiency, even in the face of potential increased requirements due to phototherapy.

Trace Elements

Present recommendations for zinc, copper, iodine, and manganese are derived from the content of human breast milk.[114] Deficiency is not documented in infants taking the recommended amount of these minerals.

FEEDING THE PREMATURE INFANT

Oral and Enteral Feedings

The formulation of an effective feeding strategy for the premature infant must include a consideration of the infant's gestational age and clinical status. In the oldest and most stable infants (usually over 34 weeks gestational age), complete nutritional support may be attained by nipple feedings alone. In less mature infants, a portion of the feeding may be gavaged until adequate intake is achieved. It is frequently necessary to use continuous nasogastric or nasojejunal feedings (see Table 14-1). In infants who cannot tolerate sufficient enteral intake, parenteral alimentation may be utilized to supplement or replace the enteral feeding.

In many centers intravenous dextrose is used exclusively for the initial day of life in sick infants unable to start oral feedings. If no oral intake is achieved, nasogastric or nasojejunal feedings are used by the second or third day of life. Frequently, in very sick infants, paralytic ileus, unstable respiratory status, and/or necrotizing enterocolitis prevent the use of the gastrointestinal tract altogether for a period of time. In these infants peripheral vein intravenous alimentation is frequently instituted. If it is known that poor or absent enteral intake will persist over several weeks to months, it is reasonable to consider central intravenous alimentation with an intravenous catheter placed in the right atrium. This alternative should be used only in large centers with hyperalimentation teams.

As discussed, infants under 34 weeks gestation may need supplemental gavage feedings. If a tired infant is forced to nipple feed for a long period of time, the danger of aspiration increases. It is acceptable to alternate nipple feedings with gavage feedings or gavage the remainder of a feeding initiated by nipple. It is often less traumatic and more nutritionally adequate to administer the feeding continuously by syringe pump.

Both nasogastric and nasojejunal continuous feedings have been used successfully in premature infants. Placement of a nasojejunal tube requires that a special weighted tube be passed through the pylorus. Both polyvinyl chloride and silicone rubber feeding tubes are used. Polyvinyl tubes are changed daily. They become stiff with prolonged use and may perforate the bowel.[115] Silicone rubber tubes are difficult to pass through the nasopharynx without a stylette or a polyvinyl sleave. However, once in place, the silicone rubber tube is nonirritative and does not need to be changed as frequently.[116] It is definitely superior for nasojejunal feedings. It is difficult to aspirate with a silicone rubber tube because the side walls collapse easily. When aspirating the gastric contents to assess the passage of nutrients, gentle suction should be used. Gastric contents are aspirated every 3 to 4 h or as indicated. Tube placement must be verified to prevent accidental intratracheal feedings.

Although both nasogastric and nasojejunal feedings are effective, the nasogastric route is technically easier. Moreover, it has the advantage of exposing dietary fat to lingual lipase action in the stomach. Improved fat absorption has been noted with the nasogastric technique compared with the nasojejunal route.[117] Nasojejunal feedings should be isosmolar to lessen the risk of dumping syndrome and necrotizing enterocolitis. Urine glucose should be monitored with any continuous feeding technique to prevent the development of hyperosmolar syndrome. Gradually, the continuous feedings are shifted to bolus feedings as the infant matures. This assures a smooth transition to bolus oral and/or gavage feedings.

A complete list of infant formulas for oral and nasoenteral use is presented in Chap. 13, Table 13-4.

The Use of Dietary Supplements in Enteral Feedings

Presently, there are three commonly used enteral dietary supplements: medium chain triglyceride (MCT), Polycose, and Casec. These supplements are added to the infant formula to increase the caloric or protein density of the feeds.

MCT has been used extensively in the nutritional care of the premature and is present in commercial premature infant formulas. When MCT is added to infant formulas to increase the energy content, the amount should be limited so that the amount of total fat in the diet contributes less than 60 percent of the total calories. This decreases the possibility of ketosis from excessive fat intake. Also, when using these dietary additives, it is possible to increase the nonprotein calories to the extent that protein constitutes too little of the total caloric intake. This, in turn, may precipitate hypoalbuminemia when such a formula is fed to the rapidly growing infant. Protein should provide 8 to 15 percent of the total calories.

Polycose is an enzymatic hydrolysate of cornstarch composed of 80 percent amylose and 20 percent amylopectin. Because it is a glucose polymer, it has approximately one-fifth the os-

molarity of an equal weight of glucose.[118] Polycose requires little or no amylase for digestion. This is supported by its effective absorption in children with cystic fibrosis who have little amylase.[119] Apparently, the premature infant utilizes Polycose effectively. Presently it is included as a partial carbohydrate source in one commercial premature infant formula (see Table 13-4, Chap. 13).

Casec, calcium caseinate, is used as a protein supplement. When used, care should be taken that the protein does not exceed 15 percent of the total calories, or 5 g per kilogram per day. Uremia, hyperammoniemia, and acidosis can result from overly aggressive protein supplementation. High concentrations of dietary protein have been correlated with lactobezoars.

Intravenous Alimentation

Intravenous alimentation has gained acceptance among neonatologists as a form of nutrition support for premature infants not able to tolerate an adequate enteral intake. The relatively high fluid requirement of the premature (150 to 200 mL per kilogram per day) can provide a volume capable of delivering significant amounts of intravenous nutrient. However, it is difficult to meet the total nutrition requirements of the premature for maintenance and normal growth when calorically dilute peripheral intravenous lines are used. Maintenance requirements and only a modest excess of calories for growth may be obtained by the peripheral route. This may be adequate for a period of several weeks, especially when supplemented by the gradual introduction of enteral nutrition. The sclerotic effects of high-osmolarity, peripheral intravenous feedings make them unsuitable for prolonged total support of infants. Infants who are unable to use their GI tract for more than a few weeks may be candidates for a central venous hyperalimentation line. Delivery of hypertonic nutrient solutions may be possible with this form of therapy. However, there are significant metabolic and infectious complications of central intravenous alimentation. Central hyperalimentation should be used only at centers where specialized intravenous alimentation programs exist.

Intravenous Nutritional Products

Glucose has been used as an intravenous nutrient for many years. Initially, it was used to prevent hypoglycemia and to decrease catabolism in starving infants. Now it is used with lipid and amino acids to provide calories in a "balanced" intravenous diet. These intravenous diets promote actual growth. In contrast, simple glucose infusions only decrease rates of catabolism. Glucose is the major osmolar component of intravenous alimentation solutions. A 10 percent glucose solution has an osmolarity of approximately 600 mosmol per liter. This can produce phlebitis in peripheral veins. Often it is difficult to achieve glucose tolerance in the premature infant. Hyperglycemia (plasma levels greater than 125 mg) increases the risk of intracerebral hemorrhage.[120]

The etiology of this abnormal glucose tolerance is probably multifactorial. It occurs in term and preterm infants. In the first few days of life, an infant responds to a bolus of glucose with a high peak level and slow decline. With advancing age glucose tolerance improves. Infants over 1 week of age show smaller peak glucose levels with more rapid decline.[121] Plasma insulin response to glucose increases during the first week of life.[122] Because of the infants' low renal glucose threshold, urines are often positive for glucose. Glycosuria can complicate fluid balance by producing an osmotic diuresis. When present, glycosuria is a signal to slow or stop the introduction of carbohydrate-containing solutions.

Most premature infants tolerate 5 percent dextrose solutions at maintenance fluid rates. The concentration in the infusate may be advanced to 10 percent over periods of time ranging from hours to several days. Peripheral veins do not tolerate glucose concentrations in excess

of 12 percent for prolonged periods. Ten percent glucose concentration is generally used in peripheral alimentation, as it is less injurious to the veins than 12 percent. Concentrations in excess of 12 percent must be administered through a central venous line.

There are two intravenous fat products licensed in the United States: Liposyn® and Intralipid®. Presently only Intralipid is approved for premature infants; however, approval is expected for Liposyn. Liposyn is derived from safflower oil; it contains no linolenic acid and contains a higher percentage of calories from linoleic acid than Intralipid. Intralipid may be given at rates up to 3 g per kilogram per day, or a maximum of 60 percent of the total calories. The emulsion produces a fall in the respiratory quotient consistent with the metabolic utilization of fat.[123] When lipid infusions are added to glucose infusions, a rise in the plasma glucose is observed.[124] This complicates glucose tolerance. Prior administration of calories as amino acid and glucose may lead to improved tolerance of lipid.[125] Therefore, amino acids and glucose are first instituted; subsequently, lipid is added.

Serum lipemia is monitored frequently when lipid products are used. Excessive lipemia may progress to fat overload (focal seizures, fever, leukocytosis, splenomegaly, and shock).[126] Lipid is instituted slowly and is advanced over several days. Lipid does not pass through an intravenous filter. Nothing may be added to the lipid emulsion, and the lipid-containing intravenous line should be separate from the amino acid–glucose line, or should join the line through a Y connector at the point closest to the patient.

Fatty acids from intravenous lipid may displace bilirubin from albumin binding sites, thereby exposing the newborn brain to bilirubin and the risk of kernicterus.[127] Recent data indicate that this effect may be overemphasized.[128] However, intravenous lipid is usually avoided during periods of hyperbilirubinemia. Heparin may transiently increase the clearance of triglyceride from the serum but simultaneously increases the total free fatty acid level.[129] If the premature infant is hyperbilirubinemic, heparin can possibly displace bilirubin from albumin by its effect on free fatty acids. Due to the unknown effects of chronic administration of heparin on fat metabolism, it is not recommended for routine use.

Intralipid is cleared more slowly in small-for-dates and premature infants. The continuous infusion of the lipid product may maximize its clearance.[130] Lipid products leach phthalate plasticizers from intravenous tubing. Therefore, it is recommended that they be used only with tubing that does not contain phthalate plasticizers.[131]

Intravenous protein supplements have been developed over the past two decades. The first products were protein hydrolysates. These were criticized for their relatively poor biologic value.[132] This may have been due to the clinical status of the subjects and not to the poor intrinsic value of the protein hydrolysates. In one infant study, the nitrogen retention of hydrolysates was comparable to the newer amino acid products.[133] The superiority of these newer amino acid products over hydrolysates is inadequately documented. Plasma amino acid analyses in patients receiving hydrolysates suggested that amino acid levels were related to the free amino acid content of the hydrolysate and not to peptide amino acids.[134] This was thought to imply that peptides were poorly utilized. However, subsequent animal studies suggested that intravenous peptide amino acids are utilized.[135] Hydrolysates may be associated with hyperammonemia. Therefore, amino acid products are generally preferred for the premature.

The amino acid composition of parenteral alimentation solutions is not optimal for the premature infant. Cystine and tyrosine are sparingly soluble and therefore are not provided in intravenous alimentation solutions. The consequences of an inadequate supply of these amino acids is unclear. However, as discussed, their synthesis is probably deficient in the premature infant. Taurine, aspartate, and glutamate are also not in the solutions. Although these amino acids are not essential in humans, the effect of their long-term dietary exclusion has not been assessed in the premature infant. Glycine and alanine comprise the bulk of the intravenous nonessential amino acids. The large glycine load produces enormous plasma levels in parenterally alimented infants.[136] Glycine is reputed to be a neurotransmitter.[137] The effect of chronic high intravenous doses on brain metabolism is unclear. Caution is advised in the prolonged use of large amounts of parenteral amino acids in the newborn. After 3 weeks of intravenous alimentation, the plasma aminogram should be monitored. Amino acid dose should be adjusted downward if excessive levels are observed.

Presently available intravenous amino acid products are clearly suboptimal for the nutrition support of the premature infant. They are used only when enteral protein intake is impossible. In order to minimize the amount of amino acids, maximization of their utilization is prudent. This is done by providing sufficient nonprotein calories to ensure good amino acid utilization. Intravenous amino acids should comprise between 8 and 15 percent of the total calories, or a maximum of 3 g per kilogram per day. The infant should be weaned to an oral intake as soon as possible.

In the newborn nursery at Children's Hospital Medical Center, Boston, Massachusetts, glucose–amino acid solutions are instituted on the second or third day of life if enteral intake has not been possible. Initial glucose concentrations vary between 5 and 10 percent, depending on the infant's fluid and glucose tolerance. If there is no hyperbilirubinemia, Intralipid is added to the regimen after 2 to 3 days. Both solutions are delivered by infusion pumps through a peripheral vein. Unless lipemia limits fat administration, lipid is advanced stepwise over several days to a maximum of 3 g per kilogram per day, or 60 percent of the total calories. Serum lipemia is monitored frequently during the increase in lipid dose and then daily. During periods of stress, lipemia is monitored more frequently. A 10 percent dextrose–1.5 percent amino acid solution, with added minerals, trace elements, and vitamins, is provided as a stock solution. Adjustments in glucose concentration are made by diluting this standard solution with an appropriate amount of the 5 percent dextrose or sterile water. This ensures a similar reduction in amino acid concentration to maintain amino acid between 8 and 15 percent of calories.

Infants are carefully monitored for metabolic abnormalities. All urines are checked for glucose. Serum levels of sodium, potassium, and chloride are monitored at least twice weekly. Serum, calcium, phosphorus, magnesium, liver function tests, and plasma ammonia are monitored at least weekly. More frequent monitoring is done when the clinical status merits closer attention. Due to underlying respiratory disease, blood gases are monitored frequently. Additional blood gas determinations to detect acid-base problems due to intravenous alimentation are therefore not necessary. When detected, metabolic acidosis is treated through the addition of acetate to the intravenous solutions. With prolonged alimentation, periodic mineral and nitrogen balances are recommended (see Table 14-4).

CONCLUSION

As mentioned, early fetal malnutrition may have lasting effects on subsequent brain development. Starvation occurs quickly owing to the infant's rapid metabolic rate and low nutrient stores. Providing adequate nutrition for neonates should be an important goal in all newborn nurseries. Nutrition for the premature infant is provided by various combinations of oral, direct enteral, and parenteral feedings. Special care must be given to the limited metabolic and gastrointestinal function of the premature. A delicate balance must be achieved between the appropriate amount of nutrients and that amount which constitutes an overload to the infant's immature system. The nutritional support of the premature infant is a challenge for the entire nursery staff. Proper instruction of parents in feeding techniques and special requirements is a vital part of anticipatory guidance at discharge. The nutritionist should continue to be involved following discharge to ensure continued good nutrition in the home.

TABLE 14-4 TENTATIVE SUGGESTED CONTENTS OF INTRAVENOUS NUTRIENT SOLUTION FOR THE PREMATURE INFANT

Amino acid	2.0 to 3.0 g/kg
Glucose	10 to 20 g/kg
Sodium*	3 to 4 meq/kg
Potassium*	2 to 3 meq/kg
Calcium*	0.5 to 1.5 meq/kg
Magnesium*	0.25 to 1.0 meq/kg
Phosphorus*	0.5 to 1.3 meq/kg
Multivitamins	5 mL/liter of solution
Folic acid	0.5 mg/liter of solution
Vitamin B-12	6.6 μg/liter of solution
Vitamin K	0.2 mg/liter of solution
Zinc*	300μg/kg
Copper*	20 μg/kg
Manganese	2–10 μg/kg
Chromium	0.14 to 0.2 μg/kg
Acetate†	variable

*The plasma levels of these elements must be periodically monitored.

†The amount added may be varied depending on acid-base status.

STUDY QUESTIONS

1 Why are intrauterine growth and body composition used to project the nutrient requirements of the premature?

2 What type of catch-up growth in length, weight, and head circumference would you expect in the premature infant?

3 Describe the gastrointestinal and metabolic limitations found in the premature infant.

4 How are nutrient requirements for energy, protein, vitamins, and minerals altered in the premature infant?

5 Nutrition for the premature infant is provided via oral, enteral, or parenteral routes or by a combination of these routes. Explain the rationale.

CLINICAL STUDY 14

A 964-g infant was delivered by cesarean section at 28 weeks due to abruptio placentae. Her birth weight placed her at the 25th percentile on Lubchenco's intrauterine weight chart. With an Apgar score of 1 at 1 minute, the infant was immediately intubated and placed on 100 percent oxygen, which was reduced to 35 percent within 8 hours. However, the infant was maintained on a respirator for 5 days, and during the early weeks of life continued to experience recurrent episodes of apnea and bradycardia. Her respiratory distress intermittently required nasal CPAP (contin-uous positive airway pressure), which compromised her ability to feed by mouth.

Clinical study questions

1   Would you recommend oral, enteral, or intravenous alimentation for this infant?

2   How would the nutritional effectiveness of the feeding program be determined?

3   How would the infant be monitored for metabolic abnormalities?

REFERENCES

1   E. Bacola, F. C. Behrle, L. de Schweinitz, H. C. Miller, and M. Mira, "Perinatal and Environmental Factors in Late Neurologic Sequelae," *American Journal of Diseases of Children*, **112**:369–374, 1966.

2   J. A. Churchill, "Weight Loss in Premature Infants Developing Spastic Diplegia," *Obstetrics and Gynecology*, **22**:601–605, 1963.

3   J. Dobbing and J. Sands, "Quantitative Growth and Development of Human Brain," *Archives of Disease in Childhood*, **48**:757–767, 1973.

4   M. Winick, "The Effect of Severe Early Malnutrition on Cellular Growth of the Human Brain," *Pediatric Research*, **3**:181–184, 1969.

5   M. A. Holliday, D. Potter, A. Jarrah, and S. Bearg, "The Relation of Metabolic Rate to Body Weight and Organ Size," *Pediatric Research*, **1**:185–195, 1967.

6   W. C. Heird, J. M. Driscoll, J. N. Schullinger, B. Grebin, and R. W. Winters, "Intravenous Alimentation in Pediatric Patients," *Journal of Pediatrics*, **80**:351–372, 1972.

7   M. Huck, A. A. Fanaroff, and I. R. Merkatz, "The Low-birth-weight Infant—Evolution of a Changing Outlook," *New England Journal of Medicine*, **301**:1162–1165, 1979.

8   J. C. L. Shaw, "Malnutrition in Very Low-birth-weight Pre-term Infants," *Proceedings of the Nutrition Society*, **33**:103–111, 1974.

9   G. B. Forbes, "Is Human Milk Best for Low-birth-weight Babies?" *Pediatric Research*, **12**:434, 1978.

10   E. E. Ziegler, R. L. Biga, and S. J. Fomon, "Nutrient Requirements of the Premature Infant," in R. M. Suskind (ed.), *Pediatric Nutrition*, Raven Press, New York, 1978.

11   S. J. Fomon, E. E. Ziegler, and H. D. Vasquez, "Human Milk and the Small Premature Infant," *American Journal of Diseases of Children*, **131**:463–467, 1977.

12   I. Brandt, "Growth Dynamics of Low-birth-weight Infants with Emphasis on the Perinatal Period," in F. Falkner and J. M. Tanner (eds.), *Human Growth*, vol. 2, *Postnatal Growth*, Plenum Press, New York, 1978, pp. 557–617.

13   Ibid., p. 576.

14   Ibid., p. 583.

15   Ibid., p. 610.

16   P. Felig and U. Lynch, "Starvation in Human Pregnancy: Hypoglycemia, Hypoinsulinemia and Hyperketonemia," *Science*, **170**:990–992, 1970.

17   M. M. Grumbach, S. J. Kaplan, J. J. Sciarra, and I. M. Burr, "Chorionic Growth Hormone, Prolactin Secretion, Disposition, Biological Activity in Man and Postulated Function as the 'Growth Hormone' of the Second Half of Pregnancy," *Annals of the New York Academy of Sciences*, **148**:501–531, 1968.

18   P. A. J. Adam and P. Felig, "Carbohydrate, Fat, and Amino Acid Metabolism in the Pregnant Woman and Fetus," in F. Falkner and J. Tanner (eds.), *Human Growth*, vol. 1, *Principles and Prenatal Growth*, Plenum Press, New York, 1978, pp. 461–546.

19   A. S. G. Hugget, "Carbohydrate Metabolism in

Placenta and Fetus," *British Medical Bulletin,* **17**:122, 1961.

20 E. W. Page, "Human Fetal Nutrition and Growth," *American Journal of Obstetrics and Gynecology,* **104**:378–387, 1969.

21 F. H. Morriss, E. L. Makowski, G. Meschia, and F. C. Battaglia, "The Glucose-Oxygen Quotient of the Term Fetus," *Biology of the Neonate,* **25**:44–52, 1975.

22 K. W. Cross, J. P. M. Tizard, and D. A. H. Trythall, "The Gaseous Metabolism of the Newborn Infant," *Acta Paediatrica Scandinavica,* **46**:265–285, 1957.

23 A. J. Szabo, R. D. Grimaldi, and W. F. Jung, "Palmitate Transport across Perfused Human Placenta," *Metabolism, Clinical and Experimental,* **18**:406–415, 1969.

24 Ibid., p. 414.

25 K. C. King, P. A. Adam, D. E. Laskowski, and R. Schwartz, "Sources of Fatty Acids in the Newborn," *Pediatrics,* **47**:192–198, 1971.

26 B. S. Lindblad and A. Baldesten, "The Normal Venous Plasma Free Amino Acid Levels of Nonpregnant Women and of Mother and Child during Delivery," *Acta Paediatrica Scandinavica,* **56**:37–48, 1967.

27 J. Davis, W. L. Money, D. Springer, and M. Levitz, "Transport of Amino Acids by Placenta," *American Journal of Obstetrics and Gynecology,* **101**:820–829, 1968.

28 E. L. Gresham, E. J. James, J. R. Raye, F. C. Battaglia, E. L. Makowski, and G. Meschia, "Production and Excretion of Urea by the Fetal Lamb," *Pediatrics,* **50**:372–379, 1972.

29 Y. K. K. Kim and P. Felig, "Maternal and Amniotic Fluid Substrate Levels during Calorie Deprivations in Human Pregnancy," *Metabolism, Clinical and Experimental,* **21**:507–512, 1972.

30 V. Sabata, H. Wolf, and S. Lausmann, "The Role of Free Fatty Acids, Glycerol, Ketone-bodies and Glucose in the Energy Metabolism of the Mother and Fetus during Delivery," *Biology of the Neonate,* **13**:7–17, 1968.

31 R. J. Grand, J. B. Watkins, and F. M. Torti, "Development of the Human Gastrointestinal Tract," *Gastroenterology,* **70**:790–810, 1976.

32 S. Saint-Anne Dargassies, "Neurological Maturation of the Premature Infant of 28–41 Weeks Gestational Age," in F. Falkner (ed.), *Human Development,* W. B. Saunders, Philadelphia, 1966, pp. 306–325.

33 J. D. Gryboski, "The Swallowing Mechanism of the Neonate: I. Esophageal and Gastric Motility," *Pediatrics,* **35**:445–452, 1965.

34 C. R. McLain, "Amniography Studies of Gastrointestinal Motility of the Human Fetus," *American Journal of Obstetrics and Gynecology,* **86**:1079–1087, 1963.

35 M. K. Younoszai, "Jejunal Absorption of Hexose in Infants and Adults," *Journal of Pediatrics,* **85**:446–448, 1974.

36 I. Antonowicz and E. Lebenthal, "Developmental Pattern of Small Intestinal Enterokinase and Disaccharidase Activities in the Human Fetus," *Gastroenterology,* **72**:1299–1303, 1977.

37 A. S. Fosbrooke and B. Wharton, " 'Added Lactose' and 'Added Sucrose' Cow's Milk Formulae in Nutrition of Low Birth Weight Babies," *Archives of Disease in Childhood,* **50**:409–418, 1975.

38 B. F. Andrews and L. N. Cook, "Low-birth-weight Infants Fed a New Carbohydrate-free Formula with Different Sugars," *American Journal of Clinical Nutrition,* **22**:845–850, 1969.

39 P. Gyorgy, R. Kuhn, C. S. Rose, and F. Zilliken, "Bifidus Factor in Milk from Different Species and in Other Natural Products," *Archives of Biochemistry and Biophysics,* **48**:202, 1954.

40 R. H. Wasserman and C. L. Comar, "Carbohydrates and Gastrointestinal Absorption of Radiostrontium and Radiocalcium in the Rat," *Proceedings of the Society for Experimental Biology and Medicine,* **101**, 314–317, 1959.

41 R. J. Levin, O. Koldovsky, J. Hoskova, et al., "Electrical Activity across Human Foetal Small Intestine Associated with Absorption Processes," *Gut,* **9**:206–213, 1968.

42 R. M. Rothberg, "Immunoglobulin and Specific Antibodies Synthesis during the First Weeks of Life of Premature Infants," *Journal of Pediatrics,* **75**:391–399, 1969.

43 J. N. Udall, K. Pang, N. S. Scrimshaw, and W. A. Walker, "The Effect of Early Nutrition on Intestinal Maturation," *Pediatric Research,* **13**:409, 1979.

44 R. K. Ockner and J. A. Manning, "Fatty Acid-binding Protein in Small Intestine," *Journal of Clinical Investigation,* **54**:326–338, 1974.

45 J. B. Watkins, C. M. Bliss, R. M. Donaldson, et al., "Characterization of Newborn Fecal Lipid," *Pediatrics,* **53**:511–515, 1974.

46 E. Signer, G. M. Murphy, S. Edkins, and C. M. Anderson, "Role of Bile Salts in Fat Malabsorption of Premature Infants," *Archives of Disease in Childhood,* **49**:174–180, 1974.

47 G. Zoppi, G. Andreotti, F. Pajnu-Ferrara, D. M. Njai, and D. Gaburro, "Exocrine Pancreas Function in Premature and Full-term Neonates," *Pediatric Research,* **6**:880–886, 1972.

48 J. B. Watkins, P. Szczepanik, J. B. Gould, P. Klein, and R. Lester, "Bile Salt Metabolism in the Human Premature Infant," *Gastroenterology,* **69**:706–713, 1975.

49 M. Hamosh, K. N. Sivasubramanian, C. Salzmon-Mann, and P. Hamosh, "Fat Digestion in the Stomach of Premature Infants," *Journal of Pediatrics*, **93**:674–679, 1978.

50 M. Hamosh, "The Role of Lingual Lipase in Neonatal Fat Digestion," in K. Elliott (ed.), *Development of Mammalian Absorptive Processes, Ciba Foundation Symposium 70* (new series), *Excerpta Medica*, New York, 1979, pp. 69–92.

51 R. N. Roy, R. P. Pollinitz, J. R. Hamilton, and G. W. Chance, "Impaired Assimilation of Nasojejunal Feeds in Healthy Low-birth-weight Newborn Infants," *Journal of Pediatrics*, **90**:431–434, 1977.

52 M. Hamosh et al., op. cit., p. 79.

53 P. Tantibhedhyangkul and S. A. Hashim, "Medium-chain Triglyceride Feeding in Premature Infants: Effects on Fat and Nitrogen Absorption," *Pediatrics*, **55**:359–370, 1975.

54 D. K. Melhorn and S. Gross, "Vitamin E Dependent Anemia in Premature Infants. II. Relationship between Gestational Age and Absorption of Vitamin E," *Journal of Pediatrics*, **79**:581–588, 1971.

55 L. Johnson, D. Schaffer, and R. Boggs, "The Premature Infant, Vitamin E Deficiency and Retrolental Fibroplasia," *American Journal of Clinical Nutrition*, **27**:1158–1173, 1974.

56 R. A. Ehrenkranz, B. W. Bonta, R. C. Ablow, and J. B. Warshaw, "Amelioration of Bronchopulmonary Dysplasia after Vitamin E Administration," *New England Journal of Medicine*, **299**:564–569, 1978.

57 L. S. Hillman and J. G. Haddad, "Human Perinatal Vitamin D Metabolism. I. 25-Hydroxyvitamin D in Maternal and Cord Blood," *Journal of Pediatrics*, **84**:742–749, 1974.

58 G. Gaul, J. A. Sturman, and N. C. R. Raita, "Absence of Cystathionase in Human Fetal Livers. Is Cystine Essential?" *Science*, **196**:74–76, 1970.

59 S. E. Snyderman, "The Protein and Amino Acid Requirements of the Premature Infant," in J. H. P. Jonxis, H. K. A. Visser, and J. A. Troelstra (eds.), *Nutrition Symposium, Metabolic Processes in the Fetus and Newborn Infant*, Stenfert Krosse, Leiden, 1971, pp. 129–143.

60 J. A. Sturman, D. K. Rassin, and G. E. Gaull, "Mini Review—Taurine in Development," *Life Sciences*, **21**:1–29, 1977.

61 G. E. Gaul, J. A. Sturman, and N. C. R. Raiha, "Development of Mammalian Sulfur Metabolism: Absence of Cystathionase in Human Fetal Tissues," *Pediatric Research*, **6**:538–547, 1972.

62 G. E. Gaul, D. K. Rassin, N. C. R. Raiha, and K. Heinonen, "Milk Protein Quantity and Quality in Low-birth-weight Infants. III. Effects on Sulfur Amino Acids in Plasma and Urine," *Journal of Pediatrics*, **90**:348–355, 1977.

63 A. McLean, M. J. Marwick, and B. E. Clayton, "Enzymes Involved in Phenylalanine Metabolism in the Human Fetus and Child," *Journal of Clinical Pathology*, **26**:678–683, 1973.

64 N. C. R. Raiha, A. L. Schwartz, and M. C. Lindroos, "Introduction of Tyrosine-alpha-ketoglutarate Transaminase in Fetal Rat and Fetal Human Liver in Organ Culture," *Pediatric Research*, **5**:70–76, 1971.

65 N. Kretchmer, S. L. Levine, H. McNamara, and H. L. Barnett, "Certain Aspects of Tyrosine Metabolism in the Young. I. The Development of the Tyrosine Oxidizing System in the Human Liver," *Journal of Clinical Investigation*, **35**:236–244, 1956.

66 M. E. Avery, C. L. Clow, J. H. Menko, A. Ramos, C. R. Scriver, L. Stern, and B. P. Wasserman, "Transient Tyrosinemia of the Newborn, Dietary and Clinical Aspects," *Pediatrics*, **39**:378–384, 1967.

67 J. Matthews and M. W. Partington, "The Plasma Tyrosine Levels of Premature Babies," *Archives of Disease in Childhood*, **39**:371–378, 1964.

68 M. W. Partington and J. Matthews, "The Prophylactic Use of Folic Acid in Neonatal Tyrosinemia," *Pediatrics*, **39**:776–778, 1967.

69 H. D. Bakker, S. K. Wadman, F. J. Van Sprang, C. Van Der Heiden, D. Ketting, and P. K. DeBree, "Tyrosinemia and Tyrosyluria in Healthy Prematures: Time Courses Not Vitamin C-Dependent," *Clinical Chimica Acta*, **61**:73–90, 1975.

70 S. Levine, E. Marples, and H. Gordon, "A Defect in the Metabolism of Tyrosine and Phenylalanine in Premature Infants: I. Identification and Assay of Intermediary Products," *Journal of Clinical Investigation*, **20**:199–207, 1941.

71 S. E. Snyderman, L. E. Holt, P. M. Norton, and S. V. Phansalkar, "Protein Requirement of the Premature Infant. II. Influence of Protein Intake on Free Amino Acid Content of Plasma and Red Blood Cells," *American Journal of Clinical Nutrition*, **23**:890–898, 1970.

72 R. W. Winters, W. C. Heird, R. Dell, and J. F. Nicholson, "Plasma Amino Acids in Infants Receiving Parenteral Nutrition," in H. L. Greene, M. A. Holliday, and H. N. Munro (eds.), *Clinical Nutrition Update—Amino Acids*, American Medical Association, Chicago, 1977, pp. 147–159.

73 R. A. MacCready and H. L. Levy, "The Problem of Maternal Phenylketonuria," *American Journal of Obstetrics and Gynecology*, **113**:121–128, 1972.

74 S. Costello, R. Zischka, and N. Addo, "Alteration in Composition of Deoxyribonucleic Acid, Ribonucleic Acid, Proteins and Amino Acids in Brain of Rats Fed High and Low Phenylalanine Diets," *Pediatric Research*, **5**:329–331, 1971.

75 D. K. Rassin and G. E. Gaull, "Protein Requirements and the Development of Amino Acid Metabolism in the Preterm Infant," in H. L. Greene, M. A. Holliday, and H. N. Munro (eds.), *Clinical Nutrition Update—Amino Acids,* American Medical Association, Chicago, 1977, pp. 147–159.

76 M. L. Batshaw and S. W. Brusilow, "Asymptomatic Hyperammonemia in Low-birth-weight Infants," *Pediatric Research,* **12**:221–224, 1978.

77 N. C. R. Raiha, K. Heinonen, D. K. Rassin, G. E. Gaull, "Milk Protein Quantity and Quality in Low-birth-weight Infants: I. Metabolic Responses and Effects on Growth," *Pediatrics,* **57**:659–674, 1977.

78 V. E. Shih and M. L. Efron, "Urea Cycle Disorders," in J. B. Stanbury, J. B. Wyngaarden, and D. S. Frederickson (eds.), *The Metabolic Basis of Inherited Disease,* McGraw-Hill Book Company, New York, 1972, pp. 370–392.

79 W. J. Visek, "Ammonia Metabolism, Urea Cycle Capacity and Their Biochemical Assessment," *Nutrition Review,* **37**:273–282, 1979.

80 V. A. Lee and A. I. Liff, "The Energy Metabolism of Infants and Young Children during Postprandial Sleep," *Pediatrics,* **18**:739–749, 1956.

81 J. W. Scopes and I. Ahmed, "Minimal Rates of Oxygen Consumption in Sick and Premature Newborn Infants," *Archives of Disease in Childhood,* **41**:407–416, 1966.

82 J. Mestyan, I. Darai, M. Kekete, and G. Soltesz, "Specific Dynamic Action in Premature Infants Kept at and below the Neutral Temperature," *Pediatric Research,* **3**:41–50, 1969.

83 O. G. Brooke, J. Alvear, and M. Arnold, "Energy Retention, Energy Expenditure and Growth in Healthy Immature Infants," *Pediatric Research,* **13**:215–220, 1979.

84 S. E. Snyderman and L. E. Holt, Jr., "The Effect of High-Caloric Feeding on the Growth of Premature Infants," *Journal of Pediatrics,* **58**:237–240, 1961.

85 M. Davidson, S. Z. Levine, and C. H. Bauer, "Feeding Studies in Low-birth-weight Infants. I. Relationships of Dietary Protein, Fat and Electrolyte to Rates of Weight Gain, Clinical Courses, and Serum Chemical Concentrations," *Journal of Pediatrics,* **70**:695–713, 1967.

86 B. M. Kagan, V. Stanincova, N. Felix, V. Hodgman, and D. Kalman, "Body Composition of Premature Infants: Relation to Nutrition," *American Journal of Clinical Nutrition,* **25**:1153–1164, 1972.

87 W. B. Omans, L. A. Barness, C. Rose, and P. Gyorgy, "Prolonged Feeding Studies in Premature Infants," *Journal of Pediatrics,* **59**:951–957, 1961.

88 H. H. Gordon, S. Z. Levine, and H. McNamara, "Feeding of Premature Infants: A Comparison of Human and Cow's Milk," *American Journal of Diseases of Children,* **73**:442–452, 1947.

89 S. G. Babson and J. L. Bramhall, "Diet and Growth in the Premature Infant," *Journal of Pediatrics,* **74**:890–900, 1969.

90 H. I. Goldman, R. Freudenthal, B. Holland, and S. Karelitz, "Clinical Effects of Two Different Levels of Protein Intake on Low-birth-weight Infants," *Journal of Pediatrics,* **74**:881–889, 1969.

91 H. I. Goldman, J. S. Goldman, I. Kaufman, and O. B. Liebman, "Late Effects of Early Dietary Protein Intake on Low-birth-weight Infants," *Journal of Pediatrics,* **85**:764–769, 1964.

92 W. B. Omans et al., op. cit., p. 956.

93 N. C. R. Raiha, K. Heinonem, D. K. Rassin, and G. E. Gaull, "Milk Protein Quantity and Quality in Low-birth-weight Infants: I. Metabolic Responses and Effects on Growth," *Pediatrics,* **57**:659–674, 1977.

94 S. J. Gross, R. J. Davia, L. Bauman, and R. M. Tomarelli, "Nutritional Composition of Milk Produced by Mothers Delivering Preterm," *Journal of Pediatrics,* **96**:641–644, 1980.

95 W. B. Omens, W. Leterer, and P. Gyorgy, "Feeding Value of Soy Milks for Premature Infants," *Journal of Pediatrics,* **62**:98–106, 1963.

96 A. Mizrahi, R. D. London, and D. Gribetz, "Neonatal Hypocalcemia—Its Causes and Treatment," *New England Journal of Medicine,* **278**:1163–1165, 1968.

97 J. K. Brown, F. Cockburn, and J. O. Forfar, "Clinical and Chemical Correlates in Convulsions of the Newborn," *Lancet,* **1**:135–139, 1972.

98 A. Mizrahi et al., op. cit., p. 1163.

99 L. David and C. S. Anast, "Calcium Metabolism in Newborn Infants. The Interrelationship of Parathyroid Function and Calcium, Magnesium, and Phosphorous Metabolism in Normal, 'Sick,' Hypocalcemic Newborns," *Journal of Clinical Investigation,* **54**:287–296, 1974.

100 L. G. Linarelli, J. Bobik, and C. Bobik, "Newborn Urinary Cyclic AMP and Developmental Renal Responsiveness to Parathyroid Hormone," *Pediatrics,* **50**:14–23, 1972.

101 G. M. Day, G. W. Chance, I. C. Radde, B. J. Reilly, E. Park, and J. Sheepers, "Growth and Mineral Metabolism in Very Low-birth-weight Infants. II. Effects of Calcium Supplementation on Growth and Divalent Cations," *Pediatric Research,* **9**:568–575, 1975.

102 P. K. Lewin, M. Reid, B. J. Reily, P. R. Swyer, and D. Fraser, "Iatrogenic Rickets in Low-birth-weight Infants," *Journal of Pediatrics,* **78**:207–210, 1971.

103 H. M. Linkswiler, C. L. Joyce, and C. R. Anand, "Calcium Retention of Young Adult Males as Af-

fected by Level of Protein and Calcium Intake," *Transactions of the New York Academy of Sciences,* **36**:333–340, 1974.

104 E. M. Widdowson, "Absorption and Excretion of Fat, Nitrogen, and Minerals from 'Filled' Milks by Babies One Week Old," *Lancet,* **2**:1099–1105, 1965.

105 J. C. Rowe, D. H. Wood, D. W. Rowe, and L. G. Raisz, "Nutritional Hypophosphatemia Rickets in a Premature Infant Fed Breast Milk," *New England Journal of Medicine,* **300**:293–296, 1979.

106 L. S. Hillman and J. G. Haddad, "Vitamin D Metabolism and Bone Mineralization in Premature and Small-for-gestional-age Infants," in H. F. DeLuca and C. S. Anast (eds.), *Pediatric Diseases Related to Calcium,* Elsevier North Holland Inc., New York, 1980, pp. 335–368.

107 D. K. Melhorn and S. Gross, op. cit., p. 581.

108 S. Gross and D. K. Melhorn, "Vitamin E Dependent Anemia in the Premature Infant," *Journal of Pediatrics,* **85**:753, 1974.

109 P. R. Dallman, "Iron, Vitamin E and Folate Nutrition," *Journal of Pediatrics,* **85**:742–752, 1974.

110 M. L. Williams, R. J. Shott, P. L. O'Neal, and F. Oski, "Role of Dietary Iron and Fat on Vitamin E Deficiency Anemia of Infancy," *New England Journal of Medicine,* **292**:887–890, 1975.

111 *Pediatric Nutrition Handbook.* American Society of Pediatrics, Evanston, Illinois, 1979, p. 108.

112 W. L. Burland, K. Simpson, and J. Lord, "Response of Low Birth Weight Infants to Treatment with Folic Acid," *Archives of Disease in Childhood,* **46**:189, 1971.

113 Ibid., p. 189.

114 S. J. Fomon et al., op. cit., p. 103.

115 S. C. Sun, S. Samuels, J. Lee, and J. R. Marguis, "Duodenal Perforation: A Rare Complication of Neonatal Nasojejunal Tube Feeding," *Pediatrics,* **55**:371–375, 1975.

116 J. W. Rhea, O. Ghazzawi, and W. Weidman, "Nasojejunal Feeding: An Improved Device and Intubation Technique," *Journal of Pediatrics,* **82**:951–954, 1973.

117 R. N. Roy et al., op cit., p. 431.

118 M. I. Cohen, "Polycose®: Chemical Properties of a New Caloric Preparation," in *Current Approaches to Nutrition of the Hospitalized Patient* (proceedings of a conference), Ross Laboratories, 1977, pp. 89–99.

119 H. Berry, F. W. Kellogg, M. M. Hunt, R. L. Ingberg, L. Richter, and C. Gutjahr, "Dietary Supplement and Nutrition in Children with Cystic Fibrosis," *American Journal of Diseases of Children,* **129**:165–171, 1975.

120 L. Finberg, "Dangers to Infants Caused by

Changes in Osmolal Concentrations," *Pediatrics,* **40**:1031, 1967.

121 M. Cornblath, S. H. Wybregt, and G. S. Baens, "Studies of Carbohydrate Tolerance in Premature Infants," *Pediatrics,* **32**:1007–1024, 1969.

122 S. Grasso, A. Messina, N. Saporito, and G. Reitano, "Serum Insulin Response to Glucose and Amino Acids in the Premature Infant," *Lancet,* **2**:755–758, 1968.

123 I. Rubecz and J. Mestyan, "Energy Metabolism and Intravenous Nutrition of Premature Infants. II. The Response of Oxygen Consumption, Respiratory Quotient, and Substrate Utilization to Infusion of Fat Emulsion," *Biology of the Neonate,* **30**:66–73, 1976.

124 J. Mestyan, I. Rubecz, and G. Soltesz, "Changes in Blood Glucose, Free Fatty Acids and Amino Acids in Low-birth-weight Infants Receiving Intravenous Fat Emulsion," *Biology of the Neonate,* **30**:74–79, 1976.

125 P. P. Forget, J. Fernandes, and P. Haverkamp Begeman, "Utilization of Fat Emulsion during Total Parenteral Nutrition in Children," *Acta Paediatrica Scandinavica,* **64**:377–384, 1975.

126 Cutter Laboratories, Inc., Berkeley, California, 94710, 1978.

127 G. Andrew, G. Chan, and D. Schiff, "Lipid Metabolism in the Neonate. II. The Effect of Intralipid on Bilirubin Binding in Vitro and in Vivo," *Journal of Pediatrics,* **88**:279, 1976.

128 M. M. Thaler and A. Pelger, "Influence of Intravenous Nutrients on Bilirubin Transport. III. Emulsified Fat Infusion," *Pediatric Research,* **11**:171–174, 1977.

129 R. Olegard, A. Gustafson, K. Ingemar, and L. Victorin, "Nutrition in Low Birth Weight Infants. III. Lipolysis and Free Fatty Acid Elimination after Intravenous Administration of Fat Emulsion," *Acta Paediatrica Scandinavica,* **64**:745–751, 1975.

130 H. Bryan, A. Shennan, E. Griffin, and A. Angel, "Intralipid—Its Rational Use in Parenteral Nutrition of the Newborn," *Pediatrics,* **58**:787–790, 1976.

131 Cutter Laboratories, op. cit.

132 G. H. Anderson, D. G. Patel, and K. N. Jeejeebhoy, "Design and Evaluation by Nitrogen Balance and Blood Aminograms of an Amino Acid Mixture for Total Parenteral Nutrition in Adults with Gastrointestinal Disease," *Journal of Clinical Investigation,* **53**:904–912, 1974.

133 G. H. Anderson, H. Bryan, K. N. Jeejeebhoy, and P. Corey, "Dose-response Relationships between Amino Acid Intake and Blood Levels in Newborn Infants," *American Journal of Clinical Nutrition,* **30**:1110–1121, 1977.

134 Ibid., p. 1110.

135   T. T. Daabees and L. D. Stegink, "Soluble Tyrosine Peptides during Total Parenteral Nutrition: Studies of Alanyl-tyrosine," *Federation Proceedings*, **36**:1164, 1977.

136   B. S. Lindblad, G. Settergren, H. Feychting, and B. Person, "Total Parenteral Nutrition in Infants," *Acta Paediatrica Scandinavica*, **66**:409–419, 1977.

137   S. H. Snyder, A. B. Young, J. P. Bennett, and A. H. Mulder, "Synaptic Biochemistry of Amino Acids," *Federation Proceedings*, **32**:2039–2047, 1973.

CLINICAL DISCUSSION 14

Initially 3 mL D_5W per gavage every 2 h was tolerated, with an IV ($D_{10}W$) running at 4 mL per hour. Elevated bilirubin, which peaked on day 5, was treated with phototherapy. Early episodes of apnea limited intake to less than maintenance energy; therefore, intravenous alimentation using 1.5 percent Aminosyn® and minerals in $D_{10}W$ was begun on the 3d day. Mother's milk, by gavage, augmented intake, and energy increased to 70 kcal (294 kJ) per kilogram. By day 6, weight had fallen to 850 g—a 12 percent loss of birth weight—and intake had reached a marginal 80 kcal (336 kJ) per kilogram.

Over the next few days, small increases in the intake of breast milk, along with the addition of MCT, raised energy over 100 kcal (420 kJ) per kilogram. A 2 percent amino acid IV infusate, along with the protein present in the milk, provided 2.5 g of protein per kilogram. However, respiratory problems requiring nasal CPAP continued, and missed feedings decreased total intake. Between the 10th and 15th days, consistent weight gain was not achieved, and the decision was made to institute Intralipid and discontinue gavage feedings. Intravenous alimentation with 5 mL per hour of a 2 percent Aminosyn solution in $D_{10}W$ was continued. Intralipid was started at 0.5 mL per hour and increased over several days to a maximum of 1.5 mL per hour. In this manner, 2.5 g of protein and approximately 95 kcal (399 kJ) per kilogram were ultimately achieved.

During the ensuing 5 days, feedings were withheld and gradual increases in total daily volumes of Intralipid were made. Gradual reinstitution of oral feedings was attempted using half-strength breast milk. Apnea, bradycardia, and abdominal distension required intermittent discontinuance of feedings.

At 5 weeks, with apnea apparently resolved, combined nipple and gavage feedings were sufficient to allow decreases in daily volumes of intravenous feeding.

Intralipid was discontinued on the 43d day. During intravenous fluid administration, weight increased by 560 g (960 to 1520), with an average daily gain of 16 g.

With the resolution of respiratory problems, increasing volumes of formula intake became possible. Within several days of Intralipid discontinuance, IV was replaced totally by premature formula 150 mL per kilogram per day, divided into q 2 h nipple or gavage feedings (120 kcal or 504 kJ per kilogram). Erratic weight gain was observed that averaged 15 to 30 g per day.

By the 50th day, the infant succeeded in taking 30 mL of formula by nipple and over the next 2 weeks managed to achieve total oral intake. At 72 days of life, the equivalent of 38 weeks' gestation, the infant weighed 2100 g and was progressing on her growth curve.

The infant was discharged on the above formula plus a daily supplement of Poly-Vi-Sol. One month following discharge the baby was switched to regular infant formula (20 kcal per ounce). Prior to discharge, and once the infant was tolerating oral feedings, the parents were encouraged to feed their infant on visits to the newborn nursery. Their involvement familiarized them with the feeding process and helped them to recognize the components of their infant's feeding behavior. They were able to approach what could have been a tense situation in a more relaxed state, a feeling they transmitted to the infant. After discharge, there was close follow-up with periodic formula adjustments and much support given to the parents.

CHAPTER 15

NUTRITION IN PREGNANCY, LACTATION, AND THE MIDDLE AND LATER YEARS

Nancie Harvey Herbold

KEY WORDS
Primigravida
Amniotic Fluid
Hydramnios
Toxemia
Preeclampsia
Fetal Alcohol Syndrome
Oxytocin
Colostrum
Aging

PREGNANCY

Introduction

Adequate nutrition during pregnancy has proven to be one of the most important factors influencing its outcome.

A restricted diet during pregnancy may lead to inadequate weight gain, intrauterine malnutrition, or a shorter gestational period, factors which may result in low-birth-weight infants (either small for gestational age or premature) and infants who have lower survival rates. The studies of Burke at the Boston Lying-In Hospital in the 1940s revealed that poor maternal nutrition was associated with a higher incidence of prematurity, stillbirths, neonatal deaths, and congenital malformations.[1] These findings were supported by prospective data from Leningrad and Holland, where fertility rates, birth rates, and perinatal survival were decreased after the starvation that was experienced in these areas during World War II.[2,3] Genetic, biological, social, and psychological factors affect the course and outcome of pregnancy as well as nutritional status, which is the focus of the first part of this chapter. The second part looks at nutritional status during the middle and later years.

Biochemical and Physiological Changes

During the course of pregnancy many biochemical and physiological changes take place.

1 Plasma volume begins to increase at the end of the third month of pregnancy.
2 Red cell volume begins to increase toward the end of the first trimester and continues to expand through the second trimester. However, the red cell volume does not increase proportionately to the plasma volume, so that an apparent hemodilution occurs, causing a decrease in the hemoglobin concentration. This is a normal physiological anemia of pregnancy, occurring in all women regardless of their previous iron nutriture. However, the effect of hemodilution will be more severe if the pregnant woman has low iron stores. Normal hemoglobin values for a nonpregnant woman are 12 to 15

g per 100 mL; during pregnancy the average values are 11 g per 100 mL or greater. Serum ferritin is a more sensitive indicator of iron. Serum ferritin indicates the depletion of iron stores, while hemoglobin will only indicate serum iron levels.[4] Normal values are from 36 μg/L.

3   Protein concentrations fall during pregnancy. One biochemical measure of protein is the serum albumin level. Normal serum albumin values for the nonpregnant female are 4 g per 100 mL, and for the pregnant female, 2.5 g per 100 mL. The reason for this decline in albumin is not known.

4   Serum cholesterol rises during pregnancy from a norm of 200 mg per 100 mL to 250 to 300 mg per 100 mL.

5   Cardiac output increases because of an accelerated heart rate and a larger stroke volume.

6   There is a rise in venous pressure. The high venous pressure in the legs may explain the lower leg edema that is commonly seen during pregnancy. While venous pressure is rising arterial blood pressure decreases, returning to normal during the last 2 to 3 months of pregnancy.

During pregnancy the heart enlarges; it is uncertain whether this enlargement is a true myocardial hypertrophy or is due to a greater diastolic filling. There is an increased blood flow to the uterus, skin, and kidneys. The glomerular filtration rate (GFR) increases, depressing the urea and creatinine levels in the plasma. Improved renal clearance causes waste products to be excreted more efficiently. Sugar is excreted more rapidly and is often seen in the urine of pregnant women, as a result of the increased GFR. Amino acids and iodine are excreted in the urine as well. This excretion of iodine lowers the circulating iodine, which in turn leads to an increase in the size of the thyroid gland. Folic acid deficiency during pregnancy may be the result of an increased loss of renal folate caused by the more efficient clearance of nutrients during pregnancy.

During the early stages of pregnancy there is an increased urine flow; however, by late pregnancy urine excretion is below normal. This decrease of flow is probably due to the pooling of water in the lower limbs. The water is mobilized when the woman is in the supine position, perhaps explaining the nocturia that many women experience. There is an increase in total body fluid of 8.5 L. All the water gained up to 30 weeks of pregnancy can be accounted for by products of conception and increase in blood volume. Increased appetite and thirst, particularly during the first trimester (and not necessarily inconsistent with nausea), are often reported once nausea has subsided.

Nutrient digestion and absorption are generally more efficient during pregnancy. There is no evidence that the old wives' tale of "a tooth for every child" is true. Scientific data do not support an increase in caries or a demineralization of the teeth. However, gum involvement may occur. Gingival edema with consequent gingivitis is not uncommon.

Many women complain of heartburn. This is due to a relaxation of the cardiac sphincter, which permits the stomach contents to reach the esophagus, thus causing heartburn. During pregnancy gastric acid and pepsin production is depressed, slowing the emptying time of the stomach; this accounts in part for the nausea associated with pregnancy. The relaxation of the smooth muscles in the large intestine may produce constipation (discussed under "Complications of Pregnancy," p. 318).

Weight Gain

In one study the following weight gains produced the lowest perinatal mortality:[5]

13.6 kg (30 lb)—very thin woman

9.1 kg (20 lbs)—normal-weight woman

7.3 kg (16 lbs)—overweight woman.

However, the study did not control for health, age, parity, or nutrition. Therefore, until further evidence is accumulated, the recommended weight gain for a pregnant woman continues to

TABLE 15-1   WEIGHT GAIN DURING PREGNANCY   **313**

Tissue	Weight	
	lb	kg
Fetus	7.5	3.4
Uterus	2.0	0.90
Placenta	1.5	0.68
Amniotic fluid	2.0	0.90
Blood volume	3.0	1.36
Extracellular fluid	2.0	0.90
Breast tissue	1.0	0.45
Fat	9.0	4.0
Total	28.0	12.59

be 10 to 13 kg (22 to 28 lb). This weight gain encompasses the fetus, uterus, placenta, amniotic fluid, expanded blood volume, extracellular fluid, breast tissue, and fat (see Table 15-1, opposite).

The lowest incidence of preeclampsia, prematurity, and perinatal mortality is seen with an average weight gain of 12.5 kg. The pattern of weight gain is most important. A gain of 1 to 2 kg during the first trimester followed by a gain of approximately 0.4 kg per week throughout the last two trimesters of pregnancy is the recommended pattern (see Figs. 15-1 and 15-2, below).

Equally important is the type of weight gained; i.e., tissue accretion vs. fluid retention. Restricting the diet in order to limit the weight

Figure 15-1
Normal weight gain pattern during pregnancy. [U.S. Department of Health, Education, and Welfare, Social and Rehabilitation Service, Children's Bureau. Reprinted from Clifford B. Lull and R. A. Kimbrough (eds.), *Clinical Obstetrics*, J. B. Lippincott Company, Philadelphia, 1953.]

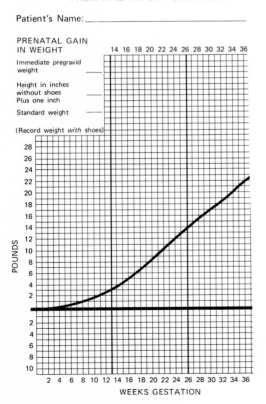

Figure 15-2
A weight gain of 1 to 2 kg during the first trimester and of 0.4 kg per week throughout the last two trimesters of pregnancy is recommended.

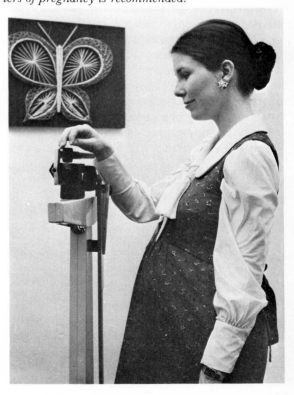

gain to less than 10 to 13 kg is not advisable. Limiting the weight gain increases the risk of a low-birth-weight infant's being born, especially if the regimen is instituted during the third trimester of pregnancy when the fetus is growing most rapidly in size.

Young pregnant women tend to gain more than 12.5 kg, whereas older women tend to gain less. Adolescent girls should gain the recommended 10 to 13 kg *plus* the amount of weight gained by nonpregnant girls of the same age.[6] Primigravidas (that is, women having their first pregnancy) gain slightly more than multigravidas, and thin women gain more than obese women.

Nutritional Requirements

The recommended daily dietary allowances (RDAs) for pregnancy are calculated for a semi-sedentary population. It should be remembered that the RDAs are not intended for evaluation of individual diets. They are meant to serve as guides for evaluating the diets of large populations.

Energy
Energy requirements vary, depending upon age, activity, height, prepregnancy weight, stage of pregnancy, and ambient temperature. Energy needs are greatest during the second and third trimesters of pregnancy because of the accelerated growth of the fetus. These needs are in part offset by the decrease in physical activity during late pregnancy. New tissue that is being laid down plus the storage of fat accounts for approximately 80,000 kcal (336 MJ). However, a decrease in energy expenditure by the mother, because of her heavier body weight, amounts to 40,000 kcal (168 MJ), leaving 40,000 kcal (168 MJ) as the total cost of pregnancy. The recommended *minimum* energy intake is 36 kcal per kilogram (151 kJ per kilogram) of ideal body weight, with a recommended *average* intake of 40 kcal per kilogram (168 kJ per kilogram) of ideal body weight. The pregnant woman does

not need to eat for two. She must increase her nutrient intake above the nonpregnant state, but she need only increase her energy consumption by 300 kcal (1260 kJ) per day.

Protein
The recommended protein intake[7] is an additional 30 g/per day above the nonpregnant recommendation or:

> 1.3 g per kilogram of ideal body weight for the mature woman
>
> 1.4 g per kilogram of ideal body weight for 15- to 18-year-olds
>
> 1.7 g per kilogram of ideal body weight for those younger than 15

Approximately two-thirds of the protein requirement should be of high biological value (meat, fish, eggs, cheese). An increased protein intake is needed for fetal growth and maintenance of maternal tissues. Low protein intakes may lead to nutritional edema. An adequate caloric intake is also essential, in order to avoid the utilization of protein for energy.

In a study of high-risk pregnant women, protein supplementation was investigated. A cohort of pregnant women received a beverage containing 40 g of protein and 470 kcal. These women were not protein-deficient and recieved this supplement in addition to their normal diet. The results, surprisingly, did not show an increase in infant birth weight, and furthermore, there was a greater incidence of premature birth and associated neonatal deaths in this population. It was also reported that growth retardation was significant up to 37 weeks gestation.[8,9] It is provident for the nutritionist to assess an individual's protein nutrition carefully before recommending additional protein.

Vitamins and Minerals
Studies have been carried out to investigate the effect of vitamin supplements on the outcome of pregnancy. There has been no evidence to suggest that pregnant women in developed countries benefit from vitamin supplementation.[10] In fact, in some cases supplements may be a detri-

ment, in that they provide a false sense of nutritional security. The pregnant woman may not realize that vitamin supplements do not contain all the nutrients obtained in a well-balanced diet. On the other hand, too much of a vitamin, especially the fat-soluble ones, can be harmful (see Chap. 6). Although vitamin supplementation as a routine practice has not been proven to be beneficial, there are some women for whom supplementation is necessary, such as the patient who is at nutritional risk because of her diet or previous nutritional status.

Iron   The amount of elemental iron needed for the full-term fetus is approximately 300 to 370 mg per 100 mL. The increase in maternal erythropoiesis requires approximately 300 to 500 mg of iron. The cessation of menstruation provides a saving of approximately 120 to 240 mg of iron. Therefore, the total amount of iron needed during pregnancy is approximately 480 to 630 mg.[11,12]

The amount of iron consumed in the diet is approximately 6 mg per 1000 kcal (6 mg per 4200 kJ). If a pregnant woman is consuming 2400 kcal per day (10,080 kJ per day), she is ingesting approximately 12 to 15 mg of iron. However, only 10 to 20 percent of dietary iron is absorbed. The RDA for a woman of childbearing age is 18 mg of iron. Since increased iron needs during pregnancy cannot usually be met by the diet, it is necessary to supplement dietary iron with other sources. The recommended daily supplementation is 30 to 60 mg of ferrous iron during the last two trimesters of pregnancy. Iron may cause black stools, constipation (see under "Complications," below), and, less frequently, diarrhea. Increased vitamin C intake has been shown to improve iron absorption. The pregnant woman should therefore be encouraged to include in her diet foods that are high in vitamin C. Also, heme sources of iron should be encouraged. (See Chap. 7.)

Folic acid   Folic acid deficiency during pregnancy is not as common as iron deficiency but may develop because of a low prepregancy folacin status (oral contraceptives can cause decreased serum folic acid), severe vomiting, or excess excretion. Some physicians and nutritionists recommend folic acid supplementation as a prophylactic measure. If a folate supplement is to be administered, the recommended dose is 400 to 800 μg per day. The RDA for folacin is 800 μg per day or an additional 400 μg above the nonpregnant requirement.

Calcium, phosphorus, and vitamin D   Calcium absorption is more efficient during pregnancy. The RDA for calcium is 1200 mg per day. When the pregnant woman is not ingesting sufficient amounts of calcium, the fetal requirements will be met by demineralization of maternal bones. Approximately 20 to 30 g of calcium is present in the infant at birth. If protein and calcium requirements are met, phosphorus requirements (1200 mg per day) will most likely be satisfied. The vitamin D requirement for pregnancy is an additional 5 mg (200 IU) above the nonpregnant allowance. It can usually be met with the use of vitamin D–fortified milk. However, if the pregnant woman is not consuming milk fortified with vitamin D, a supplement will be necessary.

Sodium   Sodium intake during pregnancy is not usually restricted. The kidneys are more efficient during pregnancy and maintain the body's sodium balance. *Excessive* sodium intake is not recommended for any individual as a general health measure. (See "Toxemia," below, for further discussion.)

Iodine   There is an increased need for iodine during pregnancy because of increased metabolic demands of the thyroid gland. The RDA (175 μg) can generally be met if the pregnant woman is using iodized salt. Other sources of iodine are seafoods, breads, and milk.

The Patient at Nutritional Risk

Nutritional risk during pregnancy is associated with age, socioeconomic status, and a history of past medical and obstetrical problems.

Not all the women within these risk groups

will have inadequate diets. However, nutritional screening and assessment will identify those who will need more intensified nutritional counseling and follow-up. Nutritional assessment should be carried out for each new prenatal patient seen in the clinic or health center. Assessment should be done as soon as possible, preferably during the patient's initial visit. This will allow the health professional to identify those patients at high nutritional risk and begin appropriate nutritional counseling.

Adolescence   By age nineteen, 25 percent of American girls have had at least one pregnancy. Ten percent of this total represents girls under the age of 15.[13] The metabolic demands for growth during adolescence plus the additional requirements of pregnancy place teenage mothers at high nutritional risk.

Age alone does not generally reflect obstetrical complications except with the very young (under the age of 14). Race and socioeconomic status are stronger determinants.[14] Adolescent mothers have a higher incidence of premature births and toxemia of pregnancy than older mothers have. When nonwhite race and low socioeconomic status are combined with adolescence, the incidence of prematurity and toxemia is greatly increased.[15] Neonatal mortality rates are higher for both white and nonwhite mothers under the age of 15 than for older women.

Even without the metabolic and physiologic demands of pregnancy, adolescent females are known to be a group vulnerable to poor nutrition. Many teenage girls are concerned about their weight and restrict their dietary intakes inappropriately; others have generally poor eating habits. Studies have revealed that the nutrients which are most poorly supplied by the pregnant teenager's diet are calcium, iron, vitamin A, and energy.[15,16,17,18]

The adolescent girl is subject to many psychological stresses during her pregnancy. Even though the number of teenage pregnancies is increasing, societal mores are not necessarily accepting of the adolescent girl who is pregnant and may need to leave school. These overriding concerns may cause her nutritional needs to be overlooked. Fortunately, more schools are attempting to be supportive of the pregnant adolescent. For example, nutrition services are being provided to pregnant teenagers within some school systems.[19]

High parity and frequency of conception (three or more pregnancies within 2 years)   It is necessary for women to have sufficient time to rebuild or replenish nutrient stores after pregnancy. High parity and frequency of conception can result in iron deficiency, premature labor, and low-birth-weight infants.

Low prepregnant weight   Low prepregnancy weight (10 percent or more below ideal weight for height) and inadequate weight gain during pregnancy (see Table 15-1) are associated with low-birth-weight infants. A recent study of women who were underweight and anemic prior to pregnancy but who gained sufficient amounts of weight during pregnancy revealed that they still delivered a high percentage of low-birth-weight infants.[20] This seems to suggest that prepregnancy weight is a significant factor in predicting the delivery of low-birth-weight infants. The woman who begins pregnancy 20 percent above her ideal weight for height is also at risk. (See "Complications," below.)

Medical complications   Medical problems may place a woman at nutritional risk. Nutrition may be compromised by malabsorption and poor utilization of nutrients as a consequence of the disease state. Anemia and diabetes are discussed under "Complications," below.

Obstetrical record   Particular attention should be paid to the past obstetrical record of the patient. Preeclampsia, miscarriage, anemia, premature labor, and bearing low-birth-weight infants are all conditions which can be associated with nutritional inadequacies.

Drug addiction, smoking, caffeine ingestion   The use of drugs may cause a decrease in nutrient intake as well as congenital anomalies and an altered metabolism.

Women who smoke deliver infants of lower birth weights than do nonsmokers. This may in part be due to a reduction in food intake as well as to the effects of nicotine.

Thus pregnant women are discouraged from smoking and are also discouraged from taking any form of medication.

The FDA is currently investigating the effect of caffeine on the developing fetus. Although the evidence is still inconclusive, the FDA recommends that pregnant women avoid caffeine-containing beverages.

*Fetal alcohol syndrome** The fetal alcohol syndrome has been described since early times. There has been a popular belief that alcoholic parents bear children who are undersized, malformed, and mentally retarded. During the late nineteenth and early twentieth centuries, investigators in England, France, and Germany reported an increased incidence of stillbirths, spontaneous abortions, and neonatal deaths among alcoholic women.[21,22]

For reasons that are not yet clear, the first reports of unusual yet characteristic features in the offspring of alcoholic mothers were not made until recently.[23,24,25,26] The spectrum of these features includes limb, cardiovascular, and facial anomalies; low birth weight; failure to thrive; and small cranial circumference with deficient intellectual performance and motor dysfunction.[27]

However, not all alcoholic mothers give birth to children with fetal alcohol syndrome. Authors suggest that the cause of pre- and postnatal growth retardation in some of these children may be secondary to factors other than alcohol per se. Alcoholic mothers usually have a history of other risk factors including poor diet, heavy smoking, high parity, and poor prenatal care, all of which are documented to contribute to the incidence of reproductive wastage. The fetal abnormalities resulting from the pregnancies of alcoholics may be related indirectly to alcohol consumption. For example, alcohol may affect the fetus adversely by modifying the integrity of the maternal fetal unit. Poor nutrition in alcoholic mothers may be due to the effects of alcohol on nutrient metabolism. This includes alterations in the absorption, the metabolism, and the excretion of specific vitamins and minerals.

Clinical and experimental animal research, thus far, has not established a safe level of ethanol intake during pregnancy. Individuals should be warned about the possible adverse effects of drinking during pregnancy. Expectant mothers should limit their alcohol intake. The safest course to follow during pregnancy is to avoid all alcoholic beverages. The health provider should assess inappropriate use of alcohol. Individuals with a drinking problem may have social and psychological problems as well as other forms of substance abuse which are often not subject to rational persuasion.[28]

A multidisciplinary approach to rehabilitation is essential. The nutritionist must monitor the alcoholic woman closely to ensure that alcohol is not replacing necessary nutrients. Particular attention should be paid to the B vitamins; especially thiamin, as it is not uncommon for the alcoholic to be deficient in this particular nutrient.

Inadequate income Women with inadequate income may not be able to purchase those foods needed to meet their nutritional requirements. If they are from another country, they may not be able to find culturally acceptable foods or to afford them once found and therefore may eat less nutritious substitutes. These pregnant women should be encouraged to utilize the Food Stamp Program and the Special Supplemental Feeding Program for Women, Infants, and Children (the WIC program) to help improve the quality of their diets (see the discussion of these programs in Chap. 16).

Pica Pica refers to the ingestion of nonfood substances. During pregnancy women may eat clay or dirt (geophagia) or laundry starch (amy-

*This section contributed by Rena A. Mendelson, DSc., Assistant Professor of Nutrition, University of Toronto, Toronto, Canada.

lophagia). These substances usually replace other nutrients in the diet and can interfere with iron absorption. Anemia can result if the amounts consumed are significant. Reasons for this particular behavior are usually custom, culture, superstition, or a liking for the taste, or a combination of these.

Psychological conditions Various kinds of psychological problems may also interfere with nutrient intake and may therefore place the woman at high nutritional risk.

Vegetarians Women who follow a vegan diet (no milk or milk products, and no meat, poultry, or fish) should have their dietary intakes assessed to ensure that all nutrient needs are met. Protein requirements can be met only if a variety of plant foods are eaten. Certain combinations of food are necessary in order to provide complete protein, containing all the essential amino acids in their proper proportions (see Chap. 3).

Vegetarians who do not eat any animal protein or drink cow's milk may need a vitamin B_{12} supplement, as these foods are the primary source of this nutrient.

Lacto-ovo-vegetarians (those who drink milk and eat eggs and milk products but do not eat meat) will have little difficulty in meeting most of the nutrient requirements of pregnancy. If the cow's milk that is consumed is not fortified with vitamin D, the diet should be supplemented, since vitamin D is necessary for the utilization of calcium.

Also, if no milk or milk products of any kind are consumed, calcium intake is likely to be inadequate. Plant foods contain some calcium, but its availability for absorption is limited, making supplementation necessary.

All types of vegetarian diets are likely to be inadequate in iron. A ferrous salt should therefore be prescribed for vegetarians.

Although riboflavin can be found in such foods as whole grains, enriched breads and cereals, legumes, nuts, and various vegetables, the vegetarian diet must be assessed to ensure an adequate intake of this vitamin, as milk and meat are ordinarily the chief sources of riboflavin.

The use of iodized salt should be encouraged. Sea salt does not contain iodine (see Chap. 16).

Food fads Individuals following food fads may not be consuming adequate amounts of all nutrients (see Chap. 16).

Saccharin The controversy regarding bladder cancer and saccharin ingestion remains unresolved. However, "when all the evidence of toxicity is weighed against the lack of objective evidence of benefit, any use by nondiabetic children or pregnant women [or by] young women of childbearing age, and excessive use by anyone, is ill-advised and should be actively discouraged by the medical community."[29]

Food Selection during Pregnancy

Daily Food Guide
The food guide (see Table 15-2) has been planned to meet the RDA for pregnancy. The foods are grouped according to the nutrients they provide.

The patient should be encouraged to eat the recommended number of servings in each food group daily. It is difficult to consume an adequate intake of iron and folic acid. Therefore, it is recommended that the diet be supplemented with 30 to 60 mg of iron and 400 to 800 μg of folacin.

Complications of Pregnancy with Nutritional Implications

Anemia
Iron-deficiency anemia is common in pregnancy. It should not be confused with the seeming hemodilution that occurs naturally during

TABLE 15-2 DAILY FOOD GUIDE

Food group	Amounts	
	Pregnancy	Lactation
Protein foods		
Animal protein foods also supply iron, riboflavin, niacin, B_6, B_{12}, phosphorus, zinc, and iodine	two 3-oz servings	two 3-oz servings
Vegetable protein (dried peas, beans, nuts, seeds) foods also supply iron, thiamin, folacin, B_6, E, phosphorus, magnesium, and zinc; should include at least 1 serving of legumes	(serving size varies; plan with nutritionist)	
*Milk and milk products**		
Supply calcium, phosphorus, vitamin D, riboflavin, A, E, B_6, B_{12}, magnesium, zinc, and protein	4 servings (serving equals 8 oz of milk or its equivalent)	4–5 servings
Grain products		
Supply thiamin, niacin, riboflavin, iron, phosphorus, zinc, magnesium (whole grains provide more magnesium and zinc and should be encouraged), and fiber	4 servings (serving equals 1 slice of enriched bread or ½ cup of enriched macaroni, rice, or hot cereal)	4 servings
Vitamin C–rich fruits and vegetables		
Supply ascorbic acid; when fresh, supply fiber	1 serving (serving equals approximately ½ cup fruit or ¾ cup of vegetables)	1 serving
Leafy green vegetables		
Supply folacin, vitamins A, E, B_6, riboflavin, iron, magnesium, and fiber	2 servings (serving equals approximately 1 cup raw or ¾ cup cooked)	2 servings
Other fruits and vegetables		
Include yellow fruits and vegetables, which supply large amounts of vitamin A as well as B complex, E, magnesium, phosphorus, zinc, and fiber	1 serving (serving equals approximately ½ cup)	1 serving

*Vitamin D is necessary for the utilization of calcium. Milk is fortified with vitamin D; most other sources of calcium are not. A supplement to ensure an adequate vitamin D intake may be necessary if milk is not consumed.

Source: Adapted from Maternal and Child Health Unit, California Department of Health, *Nutrition during Pregnancy and Lactation,* 1975, pp. 34–40.

pregnancy. Those patients who are found to have iron-deficiency anemia (hemoglobin less than 11 g per 100 mL or hematocrit less than 33 percent) are treated with 200 mg of iron per day as three 0.2-g tablets of either ferrous sulfate or ferrous fumarate. Women who are at higher risk of developing iron-deficiency anemia are those of high parity and a short interval between pregnancies. If the mother's iron intake is inadequate, the infant may have a low hemoglobin at birth and insufficient iron stores for use during the first several months of life. Such women should be counseled to increase not only the amount of iron-rich foods and heme-rich foods (see Chap. 17) in their diet, but also the protein sources, which provide amino acids for globin formation. An increase in vitamin C aids iron absorption.

Folic acid deficiency is sometimes seen during pregnancy. It is not as prevalent as iron-deficiency anemia. Folic acid supplementation may be needed by women with hemolytic anemia or multiple fetuses. Usually 400 to 800 μg is prescribed to decrease the likelihood of megaloblastic anemia of pregnancy.

Nausea and Vomiting

Women frequently complain of nausea during the first trimester of pregnancy. The nausea usually starts to subside after the twelfth week. A few women experience excessive vomiting (pernicious vomiting) which is severe enough to cause a weight loss. They must be followed closely to prevent dehydration and ketonuria (see Table 15-3)

Obesity

Weight reduction is *not* recommended during pregnancy. Research has shown that when maternal weight gain is limited, there is a greater chance of delivering a low-birth-weight infant, especially if the weight gain is restricted during the third trimester. Severe restriction of calories—to 1500 kcal (6300 kJ) or less per day—even with adequate protein, can result in the body's use of protein for energy requirements rather than for a growth and development of the

TABLE 15-3 DIETARY SUGGESTIONS FOR THE ALLEVIATION OF NAUSEA AND VOMITING

Frequent small meals*

Crackers or dry cereal at bedside to eat before rising

Drink liquids ½ to 1 h before or after meals*

Avoid heavy fried foods*

Avoid strongly flavored vegetables (onions, cabbage, turnips, etc.)*

Avoid highly spiced foods*

Use skim milk in place of whole milk if fat is not tolerated

Eat those nutrient-dense foods that stay down until intake can gradually be increased to a complete meal

*May also be suggested for patients suffering from heartburn

fetus. If fat stores are catabolized for energy, ketosis and acetonuria may result, leading to neuropsychological damage of the fetus.[30] The increased nutrient needs of pregnancy are difficult to meet when food is restricted.

Excessive weight gain, more than 7 lb per month, must be evaluated and edema ruled out. Excessive weight (fat) gain during pregnancy can lead to subsequent obesity. Weight reduction should only be initiated after delivery. The obese pregnant patient must be encouraged to consume the recommended amounts of food as specified in the food guide; to avoid or decrease such foods as candy, cake, soft drinks, potato chips, and other high-energy snack foods; and to eat snacks of fruit and fruit juice, vegetables, and yogurt instead.

Underweight

The woman who begins pregnancy with a low weight for her height and who gains less than 2 lb per month after the first trimester has an increased risk of delivering a low-birth-weight infant. Frequently, the underweight woman goes unnoticed by health professionals in their concern for the woman who is gaining excessively. Frequent meals and high-protein, high-energy snacks should be encouraged.

Constipation

Constipation is a common complaint of the pregnant woman. During the latter part of pregnancy constipation may be due to the pressure on the digestive tract exerted by the fetus. Also, many women experience constipation after iron therapy has been initiated. The diet should be evaluated for fiber content. Foods high in fiber and foods with a natural laxative effect should be increased as necessary. Fluid intake should be evaluated as well. A fluid intake of at least 6 or 8 glasses daily is recommended. However, if the woman is consuming 8 glasses of fluid per day, the efficacy of increasing intake beyond this amount for the treatment of constipation is questionable.

Diabetes and Pregnancy

There is a relatively high perinatal mortality among diabetics. It is important that prenatal care start as early as possible. The physician, nurse, and nutritionist must work together to maintain a "normoglycemic" patient. Early in pregnancy hypoglycemia may occur. This is due to the transfer of glucose to the fetus. The mother may develop hypoglycemic symptoms, and a reduction in insulin may be necessary.[31] This hypoglycemia is often intensified by the nausea and vomiting of early pregnancy and by a consequent decrease in food intake. Nausea and vomiting with a decrease in intake may produce "starvation ketosis." This is differentiated from diabetic ketoacidosis since hyperglycemia exists with diabetic ketoacidosis but is not present with starvation ketosis. Decreased mental development can occur in the offspring of mothers who developed starvation ketosis during pregnancy.[32]

Insulin requirements increase during the second half of pregnancy. There is an increase in placental hormones which are antagonistic to insulin and increase insulin needs. Ketoacidosis is more common during the second trimester of pregnancy and can be fatal to the fetus. During third trimester of pregnancy, ketoacidosis is less life-threatening to the fetus.

Hydramnios (excessive amniotic fluid accumulation) is often seen in the pregnant diabetic. This fluid accumulation represents an excessive urine output by the fetus, resulting from an overstimulation of the fetal kidneys caused by the mother's elevated blood sugar. Hydramnios can endanger the fetus by causing premature rupture of the membranes and, consequently, early delivery. Hydramnios has also been associated with preeclampsia and eclampsia.

The infant's birth weight tends to be higher than normal when the mother is diabetic. A relationship exists between maternal hyperglycemia and the infant's birth weight. Maternal hyperglycemia results in fetal hyperglycemia, which causes an excess of fetal insulin secretion. This increased insulin secretion in turn causes an increase in fat and glycogen storage, thus increasing fetal weight. A large baby can cause difficulties during labor or may necessitate a cesarean section.

The recommended nutrient requirements for the pregnant diabetic are the same as for the nondiabetic pregnant woman.

On the day of delivery nutrition is provided by intravenous glucose; 6 to 8 g of glucose per kilogram of body weight is administered.[33] After delivery the diabetic mother is gradually returned to her normal diet. Postpartum there is a brief remission of diabetes for 3 to 5 days.

Toxemia

Toxemia literally means "poison in the blood" and can be applied to any buildup of a toxic substance, although the term is generally associated with pregnancy. The cause of toxemia of pregnancy is not known, although many theories have been postulated, such as large weight gain, low weight gain, low protein intake, and lack of vitamin B_6.

Toxemia can be divided into two phases: preeclampsia and eclampsia.

Preeclampsia is defined by the American College of Obstetricians and Gynecologists as "hypertension with proteinuria or edema or both, appearing after the twentieth week of pregnancy."[34] *Eclampsia* is defined by the same group as "the occurrence of one or more convulsions in a patient with the criteria for the diagnosis of preeclampsia."[35]

Preeclampsia is associated with a rapid, sharp increase in weight after the twentieth week, caused by fluid retention. However, there is no evidence to suggest that a large, sharp weight gain, whether in the form of fat or water, will cause toxemia. Preeclampsia is more frequently seen in:

Primigravidas

Young adolescents

Women over the age of 30

Low-income populations

Women with multiple pregnancies

The important factor in the weight gain is the pattern of weight gain (see Fig. 15-1). Blood pressure rises to over 140/90 mmHg, albumin is present in the urine, and patients may complain of headaches and jitteriness.

The role of nutrition continues to be a controversial subject. The major controversy focuses on the issue of sodium restriction. Sodium has long been one of the elements restricted from the diets of women with preeclampsia. A reappraisal of the use of sodium-restricted diets has recently been conducted. One investigation has shown that during pregnancy there is an increased need for sodium, and even though sodium restriction may help to alleviate edema, a reduced sodium intake may actually exacerbate toxemia.[36] An adequate sodium intake is essential during the summer months, when greater amounts of sodium are being lost in the perspiration. Also, by restricting sodium in the pregnant woman's diet, one may inadvertently be restricting other nutrients as well.

An increased amount of sodium is needed during pregnancy to accommodate the expanded blood volume. If sodium is limited in the diet, the kidneys will try to conserve sodium via the renin-angiotensin system and sodium will be reabsorbed by the renal tubules.[37] (See Chap. 8.)

Studies altering the levels of sodium intake in women with toxemia of pregnancy have not demonstrated an improvement in their condition, and in light of the physiological need for increased amounts of sodium during pregnancy, sodium should be allowed ad libitum.[38] Nutritional treatment should continue to be a well-balanced diet, adequate in calories (joules) and all nutrients.

Fortunately, most cases of preeclampsia do not reach the eclampic stage. Eclampsia requires hospitalization and complete bed rest. Cesarean section is advisable in most cases. Nutritional treatment follows the guidelines outlined in Chap. 28 for surgery if a cesarean section is performed.

Diet during Labor

During the initial phases of labor carbohydrates may be allowed, as they remain in the stomach for the shortest amount of time. However, when active labor has begun, no food is usually allowed. This is to prevent the possibility of vomiting and aspiration. After delivery if a mother chooses to breast-feed, the infant can be placed to her breast and a unique feeding relationship develops as lactation commences.

LACTATION

Introduction

Whether or not to breast-feed should be decided by the parents during the prenatal period. Information, encouragement, and reassurance provided by the nurse, nutritionist, and obstetrician are extremely important factors in determining whether breast feeding will be the feeding method chosen. Breast feeding should be encouraged for any infant who has a strong familial history of allergy. The intestinal wall is more permeable to cow's milk than breast milk, thereby increasing the risk of allergy.

Only 1 percent of the women who decide to breast-feed are unsuccessful (see Table 15-4). In certain segments of the population—college-educated women and women in the upper middle class—breast feeding is gaining support. Findings from Cycle II of the National Survey of

TABLE 15-4 SUMMARY OF INFORMATION ABOUT BREAST FEEDING

Description	Advantages and contraindications	Additional information

ADVANTAGES

Water solids, and fat content similar to cow's milk. Protein and ash content only about one-third that of cow's milk. Lactose content approximately 1½ times that of cow's milk. Colostrum, a yellowish secretion which appears 2–4 days after delivery, is not mature milk.

Human milk is a natural food for infants; however, the psychological advantages are difficult to demonstrate.

Human milk is better tolerated; a small flocculent curd is formed instead of a large casein curd.

Protein utilization is somewhat higher because of the lactose content and amino acid pattern.

Lower renal solute load is due to lower levels of protein and minerals in human milk.

May prevent tendency to overfeed.

No sanitation or preparation problems.

Usually fewer and less serious feeding problems.

Constipation occurs less frequently.

Provides antibody immunization.

CONTRAINDICATIONS

A substance present in some women's milk appears to be responsible for persistent elevation of indirect-reacting bilirubin. In such cases breast feeding should be interrupted for 24–48 h, which generally permits the bilirubin concentration to fall below 10 mg per 100 mL with no increase in bilirubinemia on resumption of breast feeding.

Discontinue if mother supplies less than half the infant's needs.

Discontinue if mother has chronic illness (cardiac disease, tuberculosis, severe anemia, nephritis, chronic fevers).

May be necessary to discontinue if mother returns to work. However, with more places of employment providing child-care facilities, this may no longer prove problematic. Breast feeding prior to work and on returning from work with bottle supplements in between is another option.

Discontinue if infant is weak or unable to nurse because of oral anomalies.

Discontinue temporarily during acute maternal infections. milk should be pumbed so that supply will not dwindle.

Milk is more mature at the end of the first month than earlier.

Great variability in amount secreted by different women from one day to another, and from one breast to another; however, volume averages out over a period of time.

When a woman is poorly nourished, the volume of milk secreted will decrease, but the percent of carbohydrate, protein, and fat will be little affected. However, vitamin content does reflect intake.

Most drugs taken by a nursing mother, including anesthesia used in dental treatment, may inhibit milk production.

Cigarette smoking also reduces the amount of milk produced.

Due to the high bioavailability of breast iron, routine administration of supplementary iron to term infants may not be necessary, especially if iron-fortified foods are included in the diet after 3 to 5 months of age.[*]

Chocolate and cola drinks contain substantial amounts of theobromine, which has the same pharmacologic effect as caffeine.[†]

The La Leche League is an international organization supporting breast feeding. The league offers educational classes and support groups for nursing mothers.

[*]U. Saarinen, M. Slimes, and P. Dallman, "Iron Absorption in Infants: High Bioavailability of Breast Milk Iron as Indicated by the Extrinsic Tag Method of Iron Absorption and the Concentration of Serum Ferritin," *Journal of Pediatrics,* **91**(1):36–39, 1977.

[†]B. H. Resman, P. D. Blumenthal, and W. J. Jusko, "Breast Milk Distribution of Theobromine from Chocolate," *Journal of Pediatrics,* **91**(3):477–480, 1977.

Source: Adapted from G. M. Scipien et al., *Comprehensive Pediatric Nursing,* McGraw-Hill Book Company, New York, 1979, p. 156; chap. 10, Nutrition and Development, E. Getchel and R. Howard.

Family Growth show that breast feeding is twice as likely to occur with infants born to white mothers as with infants born to black mothers. Also, women who had 12 years or more of education were twice as likely to breast-feed their infants.[39]

Even though more infants are being breast-fed, the duration of breast feeding, in a majority of infants, is 3 months or less, which is shorter than the recommended 5 to 6 months.[40]

Many developing countries have had a falling off in the practice of breast feeding. Many people feel that this decline is due to the massive advertising of infant formula in third-world countries. The World Health Organization adopted an infant formula marketing code. (The United States cast the only vote against the code.) The code is designed to protect infants from unethical marketing and advertising practices.[41] In terms of national development and nutritional planning, this decline in breast feeding is a loss of a valuable natural resource that is a major force in the prevention of malnutrition (see Fig. 15-3).

The Physiology of Lactation

The female breast is composed of fat, glandular tissue, and connective tissue. The mammary glandular tissue contains many lobules which

Figure 15-3
Breast feeding, a natural resource, is a diminishing phenomenon in developing countries.
(Photo courtesy of Jane McCotter O'Toole.)

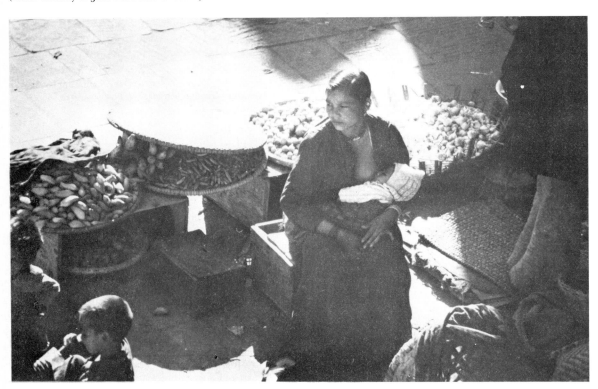

are composed of alveoli or acinar cells where the breast milk is actually formed.

The *letdown* of milk, or the *ejection reflex,* is a neurohumoral reflex brought about by the sucking of the infant. Proprioceptors in the nipple and areola are stimulated by the sucking. Nerve impulses are transmitted to the hypothalamus, which stimulates the anterior pituitary to secrete prolactin, the hormone needed for milk production. The posterior pituitary is stimulated to secrete oxytocin, which travels via the blood to the alveoli or acinar cells, causing them to rupture and contract, forcing the milk into the lactiferous ducts. The lactiferous ducts then transport the milk, first to storage spaces (ampullae) located under the areola, and finally out the nipple. The infant's continuous sucking empties these ducts of milk.

Women sometimes experience uterine cramps while first nursing. These cramps are caused by the contraction of the uterus brought about by the hormonal changes of lactation. These contractions are helpful to:

1   Expel the placenta if it has not already occurred
2   Reduce the chances of postpartum hemorrhage
3   Bring about involution of the uterus

Milk may be expelled from the breast at the mother's sight of the infant. Once nursing has begun, milk may drip from the breast that is not being suckled. A tingling sensation or nipple pain is experienced by some women but soon dissipates after nursing has begun.

Types of Milk

Breast milk can adequately nourish the infant for the first 4 to 6 months of life. (A fluoride supplement should be used in areas where the water supply is not fluoridated. See Chap. 17, Table 17-3.) For a comparison of nutrients in human milk and commercial formulas, see Chap. 13, Table 13-4.

Colostrum   Colostrum develops after the sixteenth week of pregnancy. It is produced for the first 2 to 4 days postpartum. Colostrum is thicker and more yellow than mature breast milk (milk produced after colostrum has ceased). Colostrum has less energy value (67 kcal per 100 mL or 281 kJ per 100 mL) than mature milk (75 kcal per 100 mL or 315 kJ per 100 mL) but has a higher protein, sodium, potassium, and chloride content. Colostrum contains secretory immunoglobins, i.e., antibodies to poliomyelitis and coliform microorganisms.

Mature milk   Mature milk is composed of foremilk and hindmilk. Foremilk is a low-fat milk that is secreted immediately at the initiation of feeding.[42] Hindmilk makes up approximately two-thirds of the total volume of milk produced and is secreted shortly after the infant commences sucking.[43]

Nutrient Needs during Lactation

Except in cases of extreme malnutrition, an inadequate maternal diet will affect the volume of milk produced but apparently will have little effect on the nutritional composition of the breast milk. Maternal nutrient stores are used to maintain the nutritional value of the milk

Table 15-2 lists the food groups and number of servings necessary to provide a nutritionally adequate diet for a lactating woman.

Energy   An additional 500 kcal (2100 kJ) per day is recommended for the lactating woman to produce 850 mL of milk (the average amount produced per day). This is based on the premise that 80 percent of maternal energy is converted to milk energy and that the production of 100 mL of milk requires 90 kcal (378 kJ). In addition, the 4 kg of body fat laid down during pregnancy will provide an additional 200 to 300 kcal (840 to 1260 kJ).[44] If a mother continues to breast-feed beyond 3 months (so that fat stores will be used up), or if she is underweight, or if she is breast-feeding more than one child at once, her energy needs will be further increased.

Protein   The recommended daily intake is 20 additional grams of high-biologic-value protein. Protein is necessary for maternal needs as well as to supply the amino acids in the breast milk.

Calcium   The requirement during lactation is an additional 400 mg per day or a total of 1200 mg per day; 1 L of breast milk contains approximately 300 mg of calcium. Since calcium absorption is not 100 percent efficient, an intake of 1200 mg is necessary to ensure sufficient absorption.

Iron   The recommended dietary iron intake for the lactating woman is not appreciably different than for the nonpregnant woman—approximately 18 mg per day. Iron stores may be depleted during pregnancy and after delivery. Therefore, iron supplementation initiated during pregnancy, should be continued for several months postpartum.

Fluids   The lactating woman should drink 2 to 3 qt of liquid per day. This increase in fluid intake is necessary to provide the liquid volume of breast milk.

Other Nutritional Concerns

Most foods, including spicy foods, do not need to be restricted from the mother's diet, as they are not gastrointestinal irritants to the infant.[45]

Both alcohol and coffee are excreted in the breast milk; therefore, moderation is recommended. (See Table 15-5 for a list of drugs excreted in human milk.)

How to Breast-Feed

Some authorities recommend breast massage and manual expression of milk during the last 2 months of pregnancy. This is thought to increase the protractibility of the nipple, which aids good nursing grasp by the infant. Infants can be breast-fed with the mother in either a sitting or a reclining position. If the mother is sitting while nursing, a chair with low arms is helpful. If the mother is reclining, she should lie on her right side to feed from the right breast. The baby should lie on its side, facing the mother and cradled in her arms.

When nursing is to begin the mother strokes the cheek of the infant with her nipple to produce the "rooting" reflex, which causes the infant to turn its head in that direction and open its mouth. Contact can then be made with the nipple. By grasping the nipple with her second and third fingers, the mother can increase the nipple's protractibility. This allows the infant to place its lips on the areola and not the nipple; room must be made between the breast and the infant's nose so that breathing is not hindered (see Fig. 15-4, p. 328).

In order to prevent sore nipples, the amount of time the infant is at the breast should be gradually increased. Maximum ejection of milk takes place approximately 2 to 3 min after sucking has begun; therefore a minimum of 5 min at the breast is essential, and feeding should continue for even longer, approximately 15 min. At the end of a feeding session the mother should place her little finger into the side of her infant's mouth. This releases the suction on the nipple and allows for easy removal. The infant should be nursed at both breasts to prevent engorgement. The subsequent nursing session should start with the breast that was sucked last to ensure emptying.

Sometimes it may be necessary for the mother to be away from her infant at feeding time. A supplementary bottle of formula or manually expressed breast milk can be introduced to the infant. Feedings should not be rushed, and a calm, pleasant environment is essential.

Nipple care   The sweat glands of the nipple provide sweat which mixes with the oils of the skin to produce an antibacterial agent; therefore nipples need only be washed with water. A nursing brassiere may provide support and comfort. However, plastic liners should not be used

TABLE 15-5 DRUGS EXCRETED IN HUMAN MILK*

Alcohol	Antibiotics and chemotherapeutics (cont.)	Estrogens	Metals, salts, minerals (cont.)
Allergens	Furadantin	Ethinamate (Valmid)	Potassium
Ambenonium chloride (Mytelase)	Isoniazid (more than twenty trade names)	Ethyl biscoumacetate (Tromexan)	Sodium
Aminophylline (theophylline with ethylenediamine)	Mandelic acid	Cyclophosphamide (Cytoxan)	Sulfur
Amphetamines	Neomycin (Mycifradin, Neobiotic)	DDT (chlorophenothane)	Nicotine
Amphetamine salts (Benzedrine and numerous other trade names)	Nitrofurantoins	Dicumarol (bishydroxycoumarin, Melitoxin)	Papaverine
Dextroamphetamine salts (Dexedrine and numerous other trade names)	Novobiocin (Albamycin, Cathomycin)	Ephedrine	Phenylbutazone (Butazolidin)
Analgesics (nonnarcotic)	Para-aminosalicylic acid and salts (numerous trade names)	Hexachlorobenzene	Phenytoin (diphenylhydantoin, Dilantin)
Acetaminophen (numerous trade names, including, Amdil, Anelix, Apamide, Elixodyne, Febrolin, Fendon, Lestemp, Lyteca Syrup, Metalid, Nacetyl, Nebs, Tempra, Tylenol)	Penicillin G	Imipramine hydrochloride (Tofranil)	Propylthiouracil
	Streptomycin	Iodides including ^{131}I	Pseudoephedrine (Sudafed)
	Sulfonamides (breast concentration may exceed maternal plasma level; this represents a small oral dose for infant)	Iopanoic acid (Telepaque)	Pyrimethamine (Daraprim)
Aspirin	Sulfamethoxazole (Ganthanol)	Laxatives and cathartics	Quinidine
Dextropropoxyphene (Darvon)	Sulfadimethoxine (Madribon)	Aloin	Quinine
Pehnacetin	Tetracycline	Calomel (mild mercurous chloride)	Reserpine (many trade names)
Sodium salicylate	Antihistamines (most pass into milk)	Cascara	Salicylates
Analgesics (narcotic)	Brompheniramine (Dimetane)	Danthron (Dionone, Dorbane, Istizin)	Scopolamine (hyoscine)
Mefenamic acid (Ponstel)	Diphenhydramine (Benadryl)	Rhubarb (said either not to pass or, conversely, to purge infant)	Sodium chloride
Methadone (Adanon, Althose syrup, Dolophine)	Methdilazine (Tacaryl)	Levopropoxyphene (Novrad)	Thiazides
Morphine (trace)	Atropine	Mephenoxalone (Trepidone)	Thiouracil
Heroin	Barbiturates	Methimazole (Tapazole)	Thyroid
Anesthetics	Amobarbital (Amytal)	Methocarbamol (Robaxin)	Tolbutamide
Chloroform	Methohexital (Brevital)	Metals, salts, minerals	Tranquilizers
Cyclopropane	Phenobarbital (Luminal)	Arsenic	Chlorpromazine (Thorazine)
Ether	Secobarbital (Seconal)	Calcium	Hydroxyzine (Atarax, Vistaril)
Antibiotics and chemotherapeutics	Thiopental (Pentohal)	Chloride	Phenaglycodol (Ultran)
Chloramphenicol (Chloromycetin)	Bromides	Copper	Trifluoperazine (Stelazine)
Cycloserine (Seromycin)	Caffeine	Iodides	Vitamins
Erythromycin	Chloral hydrate	Lead	A, B$_1$, B$_{12}$, D, C, E, K
Flabayl	Cortisone	Magnesium	Folic acid
	Ergot	Mercurous chloride (see Calomel)	Niacin
		Mercury	Pantothenic acid
		Phosphate	Riboflavin
			Thiamine

*Synonyms and combinations may be found in Charles O. Wilson and Tony E. Jones (eds.), *American Drug Index*, J. B. Lippincott Company, Philadelphia, 1975. Concentrations may be found in J. A. Knowles, "Excretion of Drugs in Milk—A Review," *Journal of Pediatrics*, **66**:1068, 1965.
Source: J. M. Arena, "Contamination of the Ideal Food," *Nutrition Today* magazine, 101 Ridgely Avenue, Annapolis, Maryland 21404, Winter 1970, p. 8.

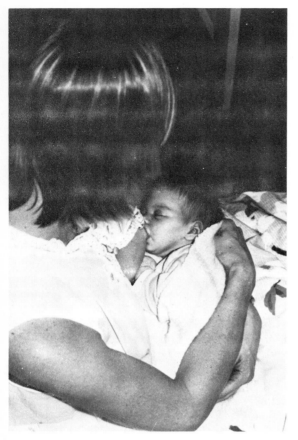

Figure 15-4
Proper technique ensures a positive feeding experience, which includes proper placement of the infant's lips on the areola and not on the nipple. (Photo courtesy of Jane McCotter O'Toole.)

since they hinder air circulation and hold in moisture, which can contribute to sore nipples.

Nipple engorgement Engorgement may be caused by a poor letdown reflex. If the milk is not ejected, the breasts are not adequately emptied and engorgement can result. This is generally the result of emotional influences or infrequent nursing. It may also be caused by an infant with poor sucking strength. Women who receive large amounts of anesthesia during childbirth may deliver infants who are not fully alert and who therefore initially have a weak suckle-swallow reflex. The discomfort of nipple engorgement can be relieved by applying ice packs to the breast.

Hyperbilirubinemia

Hyperbilirubinemia is a buildup of bilirubin in the blood, causing jaundice. Conjugation of bilirubin is essential for its excretion. In unconjugated hyperbilirubinemia there is a deficiency or an inadequacy of glucuronyl transferase, which is needed for bilirubin conjugation and hence its excretion. Maternal milk may contain an inhibitor of bilirubin conjugation. Therefore, if the breast-fed infant develops hyperbilirubinemia it will be necessary to discontinue breast feeding for several days until the infant's plasma bilirubin levels have returned to normal. Breast feeding can then be restarted without the return of elevated serum bilirubin. During the interim, the woman should manually express her milk to prevent breast engorgement.

Weaning

Most American women tend to discontinue breast feeding after the first 2 to 3 months. Weaning should be done gradually in order to prevent nipple engorgement and to allow the baby to become accustomed to the bottle. If breast feeding has continued until the baby is 6 months of age, weaning can proceed directly from the breast to a cup. Older babies may actually wean themselves (see Chap. 13). The period after pregnancy and lactation leads to emotional and nutritional adjustments as the individual moves into the middle and later years of the life cycle. The next section considers these changing needs.

NUTRITION THROUGH THE CONTINUING YEARS OF THE LIFE CYCLE

The Middle Years

The nutritional status of the adult in the middle years is a continuum of the early years of the life cycle. As with the infant, toddler, preschool child, school-age child, and adolescent, the adult is subject to physiological and psychological influences. Little research has been directed toward nutrition during this period nor to the psychological stresses inherent in working and rearing children. Unlike the well-documented turmoil of adolescence, the crisis of the middle years is only now being discovered. The middle-aged adult must integrate generativity and prevent stagnation in order to prepare for the later years of the life cycle.[46]

These are productive years when the adult makes a significant contribution to society. A person's type of employment may influence nutrient intake as hectic schedules leave little time to eat, and cocktails with clients over lunch greatly expand energy intake. Women who may no longer be part of the work force but may be at home caring for children now have ready access to the refrigerator and extra calories. The financial burden imposed by raising a family, especially with college-age children, in an inflation-ridden society, may necessitate an additional source of income from a second job. Busy schedules can lead to stress and mealtime disorganization. Increasingly, the family dinner is being replaced by snacks.

Both men and women need to decrease their energy intake at this stage of life; growth is complete, basal metabolic rate is decreasing, and activity is generally reduced. Because of this diminished energy requirement less food should be consumed and/or activity should be increased. Activity and exercise should be emphasized as an integral part of nutritional well-being. The amount and type of activity should be determined by past physical fitness and present tolerance. Many men and women begin to gain excessive amounts of weight during these years. Participation in sports diminishes, life-styles become more sedentary without a concomitant reduction in food energy intake, and hence weight gain occurs. Obesity has been associated with atherosclerosis and diabetes, which are already more prevalent during the adult years. Families with a history of these diseases should be carefully monitored. An increase in alcohol consumption can add unnecessary energy to the diet and can also lead to more serious problems such as liver disease. The nutritionist should counsel patients to select foods according to the dietary guidelines outlined in Chap. 2. Modifying diet and life-style during the early stages of the life cycle, before problems develop, may prevent or diminish the severity of degenerative diseases.

A special concern for women during these years is the effect of oral contraceptives on nutritional status. The woman using oral contraceptives may be at nutritional risk for the following vitamins: folic acid, vitamin B_6, and vitamin B_{12}.[47] She should be monitored accordingly. (See Table 15-6, p. 330, for observed modifications in nutritional status.) The use of an intrauterine device (IUD) can cause an increase in blood loss during menstruation, leading to iron-deficiency anemia. Women who are using the IUD for birth control should be monitored for iron status and iron nutriture.

Fibrocystic breast disease (benign breast cysts) has been associated with the consumption of methylxanthines (caffeine, theophylline, and theobromine). Methylxanthines are found in coffee, tea, chocolate, cola, and over-the-counter cold remedies. A study was conducted of individuals who had fibrocystic breast disease. A majority of these individuals showed distinct improvments when they stopped consuming any products containing methylxanthines.[48,49]

Careful selection of foods with the use of the daily food guide to ensure the prudent diet (see Chap. 2, Fig. 2-2) can help meet nutrient requirements and maintain a positive nutritional status for the continuing life cycle.

The Older Adult

Many older adults in the United States today are not adequately nourished. Reports from the Health and Nutrition Examination Survey report low energy intakes in the adult population, particularly among women over the age of 60. It is hypothesized that diet-deficiency diseases may arise if this decreased energy consumption continues.[50]

Approximately 14 percent of people over

TABLE 15-6 ORAL CONTRACEPTION AND NUTRITIONAL STATUS

Nutrient	Observed modification in nutritional status
Lipids	Increased plasma triglycerides.
	No consistent change in plasma cholesterol concentration; women with familial type II hyperlipoproteinemia show marked increases in plasma cholesterol.
Protein	Decreased plasma albumin.
	Increased plasma alpha and beta globulins and fibrinogen.
	Increased conversion of tryptophan to nicotinic acid.
	Increased early retention of dietary nitrogen (protein).
Carbohydrate	Small elevations of blood glucose and insulin levels; glucose tolerance curve shifted upward, but shape of curve unchanged.
Minerals	Decreased circulating levels of calcium, phosphorus, magnesium, and zinc; erythrocyte zinc levels simultaneously increase.
	Increased circulating levels of iron and copper; preceded by increase in serum levels of iron and copper transport proteins, suggesting that they induce alternations.
Vitamins	Increased circulating levels of vitamin A.
	Decreased circulating levels of carotene, vitamin E, folacin, vitamin B_{12}, vitamin B_6; early reports of decreased circulating levels of vitamin C have not been confirmed by more recent work.
	Increased in vitro stimulation of erythrocyte transketolase and glutathione reductase with thiamin and riboflavin, respectively; suggests availability of these vitamins is insufficient to maximize enzyme activity in vivo.
	Biochemical signs of B_6 deficiency in some women (low urinary pyridoxic acid, plasma phosphate, and erythrocyte aminotransferase); occasionally accompanied by depression which *may* be responsive to daily doses of 20 to 40 mg pyridoxine hydrochloride.

Source: Adapted from Bonnie S. Worthington, "Pregnancy, Lactation and Oral Conctraception," *Nursing Clinics of North America,* **14**(2):281, June 1979.

the age of 65 are part of the poverty population of the United States[51] Thirty-six percent of the elderly blacks have incomes below the poverty level.[52] Income is probably the strongest determinant affecting the nutritional status of the older adult.[53] If an older person does not have an adequate income or does not utilize food programs and resources appropriately, the diet can be inadequate. For many senior citizens, grocery shopping is difficult or inaccessible, and buying for one person is expensive. Other factors known to influence nutrition are nutritional knowledge, health, environment, and emotional status. Fre-

quently, older individuals do not like to cook a meal if they must eat alone.

Physiological and Psychological Aspects of Aging

Aging is not a process that begins late in life; it is initiated at conception and continues throughout life. Although the aging process is not thoroughly understood, we do know that reduced cell metabolism and cellular loss seem to play a role. Physiological changes that may be influenced by these phenomena are a decreased rate of nerve impulse transmission, decreased blood flow to the kidneys, and a decreased resting cardiac output. Also, protein tissue begins to be replaced by adipose tissue even in a person who is not overweight.[54]

Often the older adult will complain that food has no taste. An altered sense of taste and smell due to a decrease in the number of taste buds and/or to interference from a dental plate is a common problem. A recent theory has been postulated that this decrease in taste acuity may be the result of deficient zinc nutriture.[55] However, to date there is no evidence to support this hypothesis. Poor teeth or poorly fitting dentures, necessitating the use of soft, bland foods that are easy to chew, further exacerbate this problem. Some elderly may experience a decrease in saliva production, making the mastication and swallowing of food difficult.

Dental disease is common in the older population. It may be a result of natural loss of teeth due to the aging process, or may result from poor oral hygiene (see Chap. 17). In the population over the age of sixty-five, 50 percent have lost all their teeth and only 75 percent have adequate dentures.[56] This may be one factor in the development of malnutrition.

Gastric esophageal reflux (heartburn) and hiatus hernia are common in the older population as a result of dilatation of the esophagus. (see Chap. 22). The stomach may have a reduced acid secretion, making digestion more difficult. With age there is a decrease in enzyme production in the small intestine, leading to problems of malabsorption, obstruction, and diverticulitis. Diverticulitis is further aggravated by the lack of fiber in the diet since fibrous foods such as raw fruits and vegetables and whole grains are difficult to chew. The incidence of cholelithiasis (gallstones) increases with age, and a reduced secretion of bile results in a lower tolerance for fatty foods. The older adult also suffers from chronic disorders such as obesity, diabetes, atherosclerosis, hypertension, arthritis, and orthopedic problems.

Perhaps even more important than the physiological influences are the psychological factors which affect the nutritional well-being of the older adult. Many older adults experience feelings of inadequacy or loss of self-worth. Spouses and friends have died, and family members may no longer live near to provide needed emotional support during this stressful time.[57] Physical disabilities may prevent the individual from accomplishing activities once taken for granted. Isolation, loneliness, and fear of death are common among the elderly and frequently affect food intake. Many older adults will not prepare a meal for themselves or, having prepared one, will not eat if they must eat alone. In a study conducted by Davidson et al. the diets of isolated elderly persons were found to be much poorer than the diets of socially gregarious older adults.[58]

The fear of death and dying is often repressed because of the social stigma attached to it.[59] The older individual may need to discuss death, and frequently it is the health professional who is turned to, as the family finds the subject too painful and is unable to lend support.

The nutrition educator must respect the wishes of the older client and not adopt a condescending attitude. Dietary habits have developed over many years and are a source of security; therefore, it is important to initiate change gradually.

Nutrient Requirements

Energy As individuals grow older their basal metabolic rate decreases as well as their level of activity. Therefore, it is necessary to decrease dietary energy requirements. The RDA for males between the ages of 51 and 75 is approximately 2400 kcal (10.1 MJ); for those 76 and over it is 2050 kcal (8.6 MJ). The RDA for females between the ages of 51 and 75 is 1800 kcal (7.6 MJ); to those 76 and over it is 1600 kcal (6.7 MJ). However, this recommended allowance may be too high for the adult over the age of 60. A recent study revealed that 30 percent of the elderly persons surveyed were overweight, even though reported energy intakes were below the recommended dietary allowance.[60] The el-

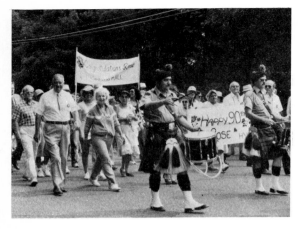

Figure 15-5
With a difference in stride illustrating the difference in aging, senior citizens march in Rose Kennedy's 90th birthday parade. While many older adults remain very active, energy requirements diminish owing to a decreased basal metabolic rate. Diet must be adjusted accordingly.

derly should be encouraged to remain physically active. (See Figure 15-5.)

Carbohydrate Carbohydrates such as breads, cakes, and cereals usually make up a large portion of the older individual's diet. Mildly flavored carbohydrate foods are generally easy to chew, easy to prepare, and packaged in small quantities, and the taste acuity for sweets is still strong among most older individuals, making these foods popular choices. Therefore, the substitution of whole grain breads and cereals for these foods should be encouraged to increase fiber intake.

Protein Protein foods may be scarce in the diets of the elderly. The cost of protein foods may make them prohibitive. Meat may be difficult to chew, and appropriate substitutions such as cheese, peanut butter, and eggs or tofu are often not made. Protein requirements for the older individual are the same as for the younger adult (44 g for females age 51 and over, 56 g for

males) since protein is needed to offset the catabolic processes of aging.[61]

Fat As an individual ages, there is an increased accumulation of fat in the blood and tissue. This is due to the diminishing ability of an elderly individual to synthesize, degrade, and excrete lipid.[62] Since many older individuals have coronary artery disease, the type of dietary fat may need to be modified and the amount decreased (see Chap. 21). Adults who are overweight should decrease the amount of fat in their diets.

Iron Elderly individuals are at nutritional risk for iron-deficiency anemia. Because their diet tends to be low in protein, it is also low in iron. Since there is a reduction in hydrochloric acid secretion and the intrinsic factor may be low, the likelihood of anemia due to poor iron and vitamin B_{12} absorption is increased.[63] The nutrition educator should recommend, as sources of iron and B_{12}, foods that are inexpensive and easy to chew, such as iron-fortified cereals, eggs, legumes, dark-green, leafy vegetables, chicken, and liver and red meat if affordable.

Calcium Diets low in calcium have been associated with osteoporosis, a disease of aging. Osteoporosis afflicts 25 percent of postmenopausal women.[64] Liberal amounts of high-calcium foods such as milk and milk products, which are easy to chew, are relatively inexpensive, and provide protein, should be encouraged. However, lactose intolerance may be a problem for some individuals, and other sources of calcium may have to be recommended, e.g., dark-green vegetables, beans, and nuts.

Antacids are a source of calcium carbonate and provide a potential source of calcium in the diet of elderly clients.

Vitamins Older adults make up a large percentage of the health food market. The use of vitamins and other "cure-alls" is a common practice among members of this age group. In one study, 30 percent of the elderly participants believed that in order to remain healthy, it was necessary to take vitamin and mineral supplements,[65] while 88 percent believed that natural vitamins were better than synthetic ones.[66] Vitamins C and E are frequently used by the older adult striving to remain young.

Vitamin E became known as an antiaging vitamin because of its property as a natural antioxidant. Antioxidants are protective forces against the effects of free radicals and oxygen, which cause normal cell aging. Vitamin C may act as a synergist to the antiperoxidative activity of vitamin E.[67] However, no evidence to date has shown that *increased* intakes of vitamin C or E will delay the aging process.

Many older individuals use mineral oil as a laxative, which is not recommended since vitamins A, D, E, and K will not be absorbed. Foods high in roughage and with natural laxative properties should be encouraged to aid in elimination. As previously discussed, senior citizens are an at-risk population due to physiological as well as psychological factors. Table 15-7 lists a variety of items which may influence older individuals' nutritional status when they are living in group homes or institutions. These factors should be important factors in menu and food service planning (see also Table 18-5 for the nutrition assessment of older adults).

Community Services for the Older Adult

Home-delivered meals ("Meals on Wheels") is one type of support service being offered to meet some of the special needs of the older adult and disabled individual. The program is designed for those persons who, for physical or mental reasons, are unable to prepare their own food. Meals prepared at a central location are delivered to the homes of the clients, thus enabling these individuals to remain in their own homes. Group meals for senior citizens are another service being offered by many communities under Title IIIc of the Older Americans Act (see Table 16-4). These programs are currently being run by councils on aging, antipoverty organizations, hospitals, and various volunteer groups.

The meals provided are planned to meet

TABLE 15-7   POSSIBLE DIETARY FACTORS AFFECTING THE NUTRITIONAL STATUS OF THE INSTITUTIONALIZED ADULT

1. Weekly cyclic menu or monotony of menu
2. Supper meal served too early
3. Lack of rapport between dietary staff and other health professionals
4. Residents' suggestions unheeded
5. Residents' needs for modified diets ignored
6. Inadequate or no contact between the dietary department and residents
7. Residents not allowed choice of portion size and/or second helpings
8. Little home-style cooking
9. No special occasions for food treats apart from Thanksgiving and Christmas dinner
10. Poor or no facilities for independence in providing food and drink
11. Hot foods served lukewarm or poor flavoring
12. Poor presentation of food including table setting and appearance of dining room
13. Unfriendly meal service, meal too rushed
14. No observation of weight changes
15. No help in feeding residents
16. Lengthy period between preparation, cooking, and serving
17. Lack of foods containing ascorbic acid and/or risk of unnecessary destruction of ascorbic acid
18. Inadequate vitamin D in the diet and lack of exposure to sunlight
19. Low-fiber diet

Source: Adapted from: Louise Davies and M. Diane Holdsworth, "An At-Risk Concept Used in Homes for the Elderly in the United Kingdom," *Journal of the American Dietetic Association,* **74:**265, March 1980.

part of the nutritional requirements of adults over the age of 60. Since the meal that is furnished only supplies one-third of the RDA, there is a need for nutritional education. The senior citizen should be taught how to augment the home-delivered meal or the congregate-site meal with other foods available in the home. Special educational emphasis should be given to those nutrients that are found to be low in the diets of the older adult. Meal planning, budgeting, and cooking for one are potential areas for nutritional education. The nutritional educator must help the senior citizen to plan and maintain a diet of adequate quality.

STUDY QUESTIONS

1 What is an appropriate weight gain for a pregnant woman? Why?

2 Why is an iron supplement recommended during pregnancy?

3 Why is the adolescent at nutritional risk during pregnancy?

4 What are the various types of milk produced by the lactating woman? How do they differ?

5 Why should the middle-aged and older adult decrease energy intake?

CLINICAL STUDY 15

C.P. is a 21-year-old primigravida at 30 weeks gestation. C.P. has had a weight gain of 10 lb in 1 month, bringing her total weight gain to 27 lb. Until this visit to the health center, C.P. had an appropriate weight gain for gestational date. Clinical examination and laboratory data revealed:

Blood pressure 140/98 mmHg

Proteinuria 2+

Edema 2+

Weight 145 lb

Height 5 ft 2 in

C.P. is experiencing symptoms of preeclampsia and is referred to the nutritionist.

Clinical study questions

1 *Should a weight-reducing program be instituted? What is an appropriate energy level?*

2 *Should sodium be restricted?*

3 *What other general nutritional recommendations would you make?*

REFERENCES

1 B. C. Burke et al., "Nutritional Studies During Pregnancy," *American Journal of Obstetrics and Gynecology,* **46**:38–52, 1943.

2 A. M. Antonov, "Children Born During the Siege of Leningrad in 1942," *Journal of Pediatrics,* **30**:250–259, 1947.

3 D. Baird, "Variations in Fertility Associated with a Change in Health Status," *Journal of Chronic Diseases,* **18**:1109–1124, 1965.

4 D. T. Jenkin, M. M. Wishart, and C. Schenberg, "Serum Ferritin in Pregnancy," *Australian and New Zealand Journal of Obstetrics and Gynaecology,* **18**(4):223–225, 1978.

5 R. I. Naeye, "Weight Gain and the Outcome of Pregnancy," *American Journal of Obstetrics and Gynecology,* **135**:3–9, 1979.

6 Food and Nutrition Board, *Recommended Dietary Allowances,* 9th ed., National Academy of Sciences, National Research Council, Washington, 1980, p. 26.

7 Ibid., p. 48.

8 Z. Stein, S. Mervyn, and D. Rush, "Prenatal Nutrition and Birth Weight: Experiments and Quasi-experiments in the Past Decade," *Journal of Reproductive Medicine,* **24**:287–297, 1978.

9 D. Rush, Z. Stein, and M. Susser, "A Randomized Control of Prenatal Nutrition Supplementation in New York City," *Pediatrics,* **65**(4):683–697, April 1980.

10 Food and Nutrition Board, Committee on Maternal Nutrition, *Nutrition and the Course of Pregnancy,* Summary Report, National Academy of Sciences, National Research Council, Washington, D.C., 1970, p. 133.

11 Ibid., p. 68.

12 American College of Obstetricians and Gynecologists, *Nutrition in Maternal Health Care,* 1974.

13 *Healthy People: The Surgeon General's Report on Health Promotion and Disease Prevention,* U.S. De-

335

partment of Health, Education, and Welfare Publication (PHS) 79-55071, 1979, p. 48.

14 John Grant and Felix Heald, "Complications of Adolescent Pregnancy. Survey of the Literature on Fetal Outcome in Adolescence," *Clinical Pediatrics,* **11**:567, October 1972.

15 Ibid., p. 567.

16 Harold Kamenetzky et al., "The Effects of Nutrition in Teenage Gravidas on Pregnancy and the Status of the Neonate," *American Journal of Obstetrics and Gynecology,* **115**:639–646, 1973.

17 Janet King, S. Cohenour, S. Calloway, and H. Jacobson, "Assessment of Nutritional Status of Teenage Pregnant Girls. I. Nutritional Intake and Pregnancy," *American Journal of Clinical Nutrition,* **25**:916, 1972.

18 W. J. McGanity et al., "Pregnancy in Adolescence. I. Preliminary Summary of Health Status," *American Journal of Obstetrics and Gynecology,* **103**:77, 1969.

19 Irene Alton, "Nutrition Services for Pregnant Adolescents Within a Public High School," *Journal of the American Dietetic Association,* **74**:667–669, June 1979.

20 Laura Edwards et al., "Pregnancy in the Underweight Woman: Course, Outcome and Growth of the Infant," *American Journal of Obstetrics and Gynecology,* **135**:297–301, 1979.

21 W. C. Sullivan, "The Children of the Female Drunkard," *Medical Temperance Reviews,* **3**:72, 1900.

22 H. W. Haggard and E. M. Jellinek, *Alcohol Explored,* Doubleday, Doran and Co., Ltd., Garden City, N.Y., 1942.

23 P. H. Lemoine, H. Harousseau, J. P. Bortegru, and J. C. Menuet, "Les Enfants De Parents Alcooliques," *Archives Francaises de Pediatrie,* **25**:830, 1967.

24 R. A Beargie, V. L. James, and J. W. Greene, "Growth and Development of Small-for-Date Newborns," *Pediatric Clinic of North America,* **17**:159, 1970.

25 C. N. Ulleland, "The Offspring of Alcoholic Mothers," *Annals of the New York Academy Of Sciences* **197**:167–169, 1972.

26 K. L. Jones, D. W. Smith, C. N. Ulleland, and A. P. Streissgath, "Patterns of Malformation in Offspring of Chronic Alcoholic Mothers," *Lancet,* **1**:1267, 1973.

27 K. L. Jones and D. W. Smith, "The Fetal Alcohol Syndrome," *Teratology,* **12**:1, 1975.

28 J. H. Mendelson, *The Fetal Alcohol Syndrome,* Advances in Alcoholism, Raleigh Hills Foundation, North Carolina, 1979.

29 Robert Hoover, "Saccharin—Bitter Aftertaste?" *New England Journal of Medicine,* **302**:574, 1980.

30 Food and Nutrition Boards, Committee on Maternal Nutrition, op. cit., p. 123.

31 J. Tyson and P. Felig, "Medical Aspects of Diabetes in Pregnancy and the Diabetogenic Effect of Oral Contraceptives," *Medical Clinics of North America,* **55**(4):952, 1971.

32 Ibid., p. 954.

33 R. Francois, "The Newborn of Diabetic Mothers," *Biology of the Neonate,* **24**:28, 1974.

34 American College of Obstetricians and Gynecologists, op. cit.

35 American College of Obstetricians and Gynecologists, op. cit.

36 Ruth Pike and H. Smiciklas, "A Reappraisal of Sodium Restriction during Pregnancy," *International Journal of Obstetrics and Gynecology,* **10**(1):1–8, 1972.

37 Ibid., p. 4.

38 Roy Pitkin et al., "Maternal Nutrition," *Journal of Obstetrics and Gynecology,* **40**:773–785, 1972.

39 Advance data from *Vital and Health Statistics,* no. 59, U.S. Department of Health, Education, and Welfare, Public Health Service, Health Resources Administration, Office of Health Research Statistics and Technology, March 28, 1980.

40 S. J. Fomon et al., "Recommendations for Feeding Normal Infants," *Pediatrics,* **63**(1):52–59, January 1979.

41 "Community Nutrition Institute Resolutions Favor Infant Formulas Code," *Community Nutrition Reports,* **XI**(17), April 23, 1981, p.6.

42 R. M. Applebaum, "The Modern Managment of Successful Breast Feeding," *Pediatric Clinics of North America,* **17**(1):222, 1970.

43 Ibid.

44 Food and Nutrition Board, *Recommended Dietary Allowances,* 8th ed., National Academy of Sciences, National Research Council, Washington, D.C., 1974, p. 32.

45 Applebaum, op. cit., p. 218.

46 E. H. Erikson, *Identity: Youth & Crisis,* W. W. Norton and Company, Inc., New York, 1968.

47 American College of Obstetricians and Gynecologists, op. cit.

48 J. P. Minton et al., "Caffeine, Cyclic Nucleotides and Breast Disease," *Surgery,* **86**:105–109, 1979.

49 J. P. Minton et al., "Response of Fibrocystic Disease to Caffeine Withdrawal and Correlation of Cyclic Nucleotides with Breast Disease," *American Journal of Obstetrics and Gynecology,* **135**:157–158, 1970.

50 U.S. Dept. of HEW, *Healthy People,* p. 129.

51 Ibid., p. 77.

52 Ibid., p. 77.

53 N. W. Shock, "Physiologic Aspects of Aging," *Journal of the American Dietetic Association,* **70**:491–496, 1970.

54   Joncier Green, "Nutritional Considerations of Older Americans," *Journal of the National Medical Association,* **71**(8)791–793, 1979.

55   J. L. Greger and B. S. Sciscae, "Zinc Nutriture of the Elderly," *Journal of the American Dietetic Association,* **70**(1):37–41, 1977.

56   R. A. Notzoid, "Geriatric Nutrition," *Osteopath Annals,* March 1974, pp. 32–47.

57   U.S. Dept. of HEW, *Healthy People,* p. 77.

58   S. Davidson et al., "The Nutrition of a Group of Apparently Healthy Aging Persons," *Journal of Clinical Nutrition,* **10**:191–199, 1962.

59   P. Cameron et al., "Consciousness of Death across the Life Span," *Journal of Gerontology,* **28**(1):92–95, 1973.

60   Joseph Carlin, "Nutritional Study of Elderly Women in the Inner City," paper presented at the American Dietetic Association annual meeting, Boston, Mass., October 1976.

61   A. Albanese, "Nutrition and the Health of the Elderly," *Nutrition News,* **39**(2):5,8; 1976.

62   David Kritchevsky, "Diet, Lipid Metabolism and Aging," *Federation Proceedings,* **38**(6):2001–2005, May 1979.

63   Myron Winnick, "Nutrition and Aging," *Contemporary Nutrition,* **2**:(6), July 1977.

64   A. Albanese, op. cit., p. 8.

65   J. Roundtree and M. Tinklin, "Food Beliefs and Practices of Selected Senior Citizens," *Gerontologists,* **16**:548, December 1975.

66   Ibid., p. 540.

67   A. Albanese, op. cit., p. 5

CLINICAL DISCUSSION 15

A weight-reducing regimen is not appropriate during pregnancy, especially during the third trimester when the fetus is growing most rapidly and energy demands are greatest.

An appropriate energy level would be approximately 40 kcal per kilogram (168 kJ per kilogram) of ideal body weight. C. P.'s ideal weight is 53 kg. Therefore, energy requirements would be

$$53 \text{ kg} \times 40 \text{ kcal} = 2120 \text{ kcal} = 8904 \text{ kJ}$$

There has been much controversy over sodium and its role in preeclampsia. However, it has been shown that there is an increased need for sodium during pregnancy. If sodium is not supplied via the diet, the renin-angiotensin system will conserve sodium and less will be excreted, thereby defeating the purpose. Sodium restriction may even exacerbate toxemia; therefore, no restriction should be initiated.

A thorough nutritional history should be taken to evaluate C. P.'s dietary intake, C. P. should be encouraged to consume the following if she is not already doing so:

4 servings of milk and milk products

2 servings of protein foods

4 servings of grain products

1 serving of vitamin C–rich fruits and vegetables

2 servings of leafy, green vegetables

1 serving of other fruits and vegetables

CHAPTER 16
COMMUNITY NUTRITION

Nancie Harvey Herbold

KEY WORDS
Food Patterns
Yin and Yang
Kashruth
Kosher
Food Stamps
WIC
Organically Grown Food
Zen Macrobiotics

INTRODUCTION

It is important for the nutrition educator to become familiar with the myriad of factors which affect the nutritional behavior of a community—factors such as cultural patterns and ethnic background, food fads, income and spending patterns, and community food programs (e.g., the Food Stamp and School Lunch programs). Before nutritional intervention programs are planned, a great deal of groundwork must be done. The nutrition educator should identify the diversified ethnic groups located in the community. It is important to understand the eating practices in the country of origin and the effect of immigration and Americanization on food habits. For example, foods available in the country of origin may have provided all necessary nutrients, but in the United States such foods, if imported, may be expensive or simply unavailable. Other foods are then substituted, often resulting in decreased nutritional quality.

The nutrition educator also needs to identify the major health problems in the community and to determine the areas where poor nutrition is adversely affecting health. Priorities for nutrition education can then be set, and nutrition intervention programs can be planned accordingly. For outreach programs to be effective, it is necessary to assess community needs. Identifying community leaders and obtaining input from community groups can be of great help in planning and implementing such programs.

CULTURAL FOOD PATTERNS

Every culture has an accepted standard of food practices. What is eaten, when, with whom, and how much are all factors which establish food patterns or food ways within a society. These food ways, which have developed over centuries (see Chap. 1) and have many meanings (religious, symbolic, emotional), are not easily changed. Food ways are influenced by a variety of conditions, such as food availability, economics, politics, food symbolism, and physiological and psychological needs (see Fig. 16-1). It is more difficult for older people to change long-established food habits than it is for younger people. When food practices are changing, it is important to consider the effect this may have on the nutritional quality of the diet.

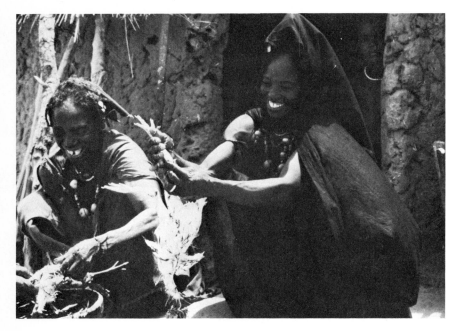

Figure 16-1
The plucking of a chicken is a social affair. (Bamako, Mali, West Africa. Photo courtesy of Jane McCotter O'Toole.)

Within a given culture there are subcultures with unique eating practices which differ from the typical diet. For example, within the United States, individuals who live in the north eat differently from individuals who live in the south. Differences may be due to climate, natural resources, and food availability. Food patterns may even differ within a family unit. An individual's food habits are the

characteristic and repetitive acts that he performs under the impetus of the need to provide himself with nourishment and simultaneously to meet an assortment of social and emotional needs.[1]

Individual food habits are learned and begin early. The child is influenced by the providers of food who already have preconceived ideas, values, beliefs, and attitudes regarding food and convey these to the child.

It is possible to say that the particular way children of any society are fed and weaned has significance for the food behavior of that society.[2]

The nutrition educator must be aware of those culturally accepted norms which affect food ways. Only by working within this established framework can the nutritionist make the appropriate recommendations that will bring about behavioral change. Change is a gradual process, and too many recommendations or too drastic a suggestion may overwhelm the individual. The nutrition educator must concentrate on the positive aspects of an individual's diet and strengthen these positive habits. The following section describes some of the common food patterns of several different cultures found within the United States. The student should be reminded, however, that the longer people have lived in the United States and have become acculturated to the country, the more their food ways will resemble those of the American diet.

Chinese

As with most peoples, the eating habits of the Chinese vary, depending upon the region of the country from which they originate. The northern area (Mandarin-style cooking) has many sweet and sour dishes, noodles, and steamed breads. Shanghai is coastal, and traditional meals include many fish and seafood dishes. Inland China (Szechwan-style cooking) is known for its "hot" foods seasoned with pepper. Southern China (Cantonese) uses pork, chicken, and dumplings with a variety of fillings, "dim sum."

The basic philosophy of Taoism is to obtain peace and harmony with one's environment. One concept of this Chinese philosophy is the duality of all things, as illustrated by the principles of yin and yang (see Table 16-1). Yin and

TABLE 16-1 CATEGORIZATION OF YIN AND YANG

	Yin	*Yang*
Attributes of personality	Female	Male
	Introversion of personality	Extroversion of personality
	Weakness of character	Strength of character
	Debilitating states	Strengthening states
	Cold	Hot
Symptoms related to yin and yang	Pallor, dry cough, dizziness, muscle cramps, diarrhea, menstrual periods	Dry throat, excess sweating, rash or hives, acne, dry lips, fissures at the corner of the mouth, constipation, spitting up blood, fevers
Yin and yang foods	Bananas	Chicken soup
	Winter melon	Wine
	Cold foods like salads	Liver
	Cold drinks	Lamb—soup meat
	Bamboo shoots	Pork
	Spinach	Beef—broth
	Cucumber	Ginger
	Grapefruit	Vinegar
	Lime	Honey
	Fruit juice	Bird's nest soup
	Mustard greens	Fish soup
	Asparagus	Garlic
	Bitter melon	Scallions
	Bean sprouts	Eggplant
	Bean curd	Lichee
	Pineapple	Black jujube
	Mung beans	Egg
	Celery	Nuts
	Papaya	Seeds
	Watermelon	Alcohol
	Lemon	

Source: Mabel Wang, M.Ed., R.D., South Cove Health Center, Boston, Massachusetts.

yang is probably the major influence on Chinese eating habits. Some foods are thought to be more yin (cold-feminine), and others more yang (hot-masculine). The hotness or coldness has no relationship to the actual temperature of the food. Foods are classified as yin and yang according to the degree of acid, salt, sweet, bitter, or pungent flavors they possess. In addition, the season of the year and the time of harvesting contribute to this classification. The theory is also used for medicinal purposes. When an individual is sick, more yin or more yang foods may be recommended, according to the ailment. Other medical practices within the Chinese community include acupuncture, Chinese chiropractic, heat treatments, and herbal medicine.

Milk and milk products   Milk is not used as a beverage but may be used on cereal. Cheese is not a common item in the Chinese diet, but ice cream is popular.

Protein   Bean curd (tofu) is used frequently and is a good source of protein and calcium. All types of meat are used but in smaller amounts than are found in the typical American diet. Meats are usually mixed with vegetables. Chicken, duck, and pigeon eggs are preserved or fermented, as well as used fresh in cooking.

Vegetables and fruits   A large variety of vegetables (see Fig. 16-2) are used: Chinese cabbage

Figure 16-2
Chinese vegetables—bok choy, upper right; winter melon, lower left. Recognition of the various cultural foods is important in nutritional planning for various ethnic groups. For example, vegetables such as bok choy and bitter melon are significant foods in the Chinese diet. (Photo courtesy of Richard F. Herbold.)

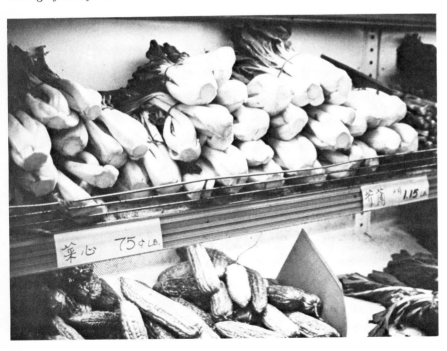

(bok choy), broccoli, spinach, bamboo shoots, bean sprouts, snow peas, bitter melon, mushrooms, and onions.

Fruits are usually eaten fresh, but some fruits are salted or dried. Plums, dates, pineapples, oranges, and litchi (lichee) nuts are among the fruits eaten.

Breads and cereals   Rice is the staple of the Chinese diet. Enriched rice should be encouraged. Noodles, millet, and steamed buns are also consumed.

Miscellaneous   Soy sauce, ginger, garlic, scallions, peppers, and vinegar are used for seasoning. Chinese restaurants frequently use monosodium glutamate in cooking. However, it is not generally used in the Chinese home.

Peanut oil, soybean oil, and lard are used in cooking. Green tea is the usual beverage of the Chinese.

Nutritional concerns   The Chinese use the stir-fry method of cooking and are therefore able to retain the maximum amount of nutrients in their food. The Chinese diet may be inadequate in calcium and vitamin D because of the low intake of milk and milk products. (This low intake may be due to the high prevalance of lactose intolerance among the east Asian population.) Bean curd, soybeans, mustard greens, and kale should be encouraged to improve calcium intake. A vitamin D supplement may be needed. Protein intake should be checked for adequacy, since the serving size of meats is ordinarily small.

Some individuals experience sensations of flushing, tingling, dizziness, and tachycardia after eating Chinese food. This is known as *Chinese restaurant syndrome* and is due to a sensitivity to monosodium glutamate, which dilates blood vessels, thereby causing the cited effects.

Vietnamese

Recently thousands of Vietnamese have resettled in the United States. The health professional needs to become familiar with their eating patterns and not confuse them with those of other Asian groups.

In Vietnam people usually shop daily, since refrigeration is almost nonexistent. The meal pattern of the Vietnamese includes breakfast, lunch, and dinner, with the latter two meals being the largest of the day. Breakfast may consist of soup (pho), which is made from rice noodles, thin slices of meat or poultry, bean sprouts, greens, and rice.[3]

Milk and milk products   Milk is not generally consumed as a beverage. This may be because of the high prevalence of lactose intolerance among the Vietnamese.[4] Sweetened condensed milk is sometimes used in beverages such as café au lait (which was introduced to the Vietnamese by the French).

Protein   Small amounts of meat and seafood are used in combination with rice and vegetables. Eggs are used by the Vietnamese and may be fried and eaten for breakfast. Dried beans are another source of protein that may typically be found in the diet.

Vegetables and fruits   Vegetables such as sweet potatoes, tomatoes, maize, manioc, squash, and spinach are consumed.

Many tropical fruits are included in the diet; they include bananas, pineapple, mango, custard apples, lichee nuts, jackfruit, and grapefruit.

Breads and cereal   Rice is the staple of the Vietnamese diet. Enriched rice should be encouraged. Noodles and french bread are also consumed.

Miscellaneous   Beverages such as tea, café au lait, soft drinks, and beer are frequently consumed. Hot peppers are a popular spice, and nuoc mam, a fermented fish sauce used as a condiment, contributes protein and iodine to the diet. It is also high in sodium.[5] Cooking methods include steaming, stir-frying, braising, and charcoal grilling.

Nutritional concerns   Generally, Vietnamese in the United States do not suffer from malnutrition, as may their relatives who remain in Vietnam. Their diet, however, may be low in calcium and vitamin D. Vegetables and beans that may improve calcium intake should be encouraged, such as mustard greens, kale, and soybeans. Depending upon the individual's exposure to sunlight, a vitamin D supplement may be necessary. The diet should also be assessed for protein adequacy since the serving size of meat is small.

Japanese

Many Japanese foods are similar to Chinese foods. Rice is a staple, and tea is the common beverage. Foods are marinated, broiled, and stir-fried.

Milk and milk products   Little milk or cheese is eaten; however, bean curd (tofu) is eaten.

Protein   The Japanese diet contains much seafood—fresh, smoked, and raw (sashimi). Meat is used in combination with vegetables and is spiced with soy sauce. Eggs may be used in soups as well as boiled or scrambled. Miso (soybean paste) is used in cooking.

Vegetables and fruits   Spinach, broccoli, mustard greens, snow peas, taro (Japanese sweet potato), cucumbers, tomatoes, and eggplant are eaten. vegetables may be steamed with soy sauce, pickled, or dipped in batter and fried in deep fat (tempura). Oranges, tangerines, and melons are eaten.

Breads and cereals   White rice (short-grained) is preferred. Wheat products, such as wheat noodles cooked in broth, are also used.

Miscellaneous   Dried seaweed is eaten as a snack food. Soy sauce, sweet and sour sauce, mustard sauce, and plum sauce are used in cooking.

Nutritional concerns   The Japanese diet, like the Chinese, may be low in milk and milk products, and the same nutritional concerns and suggestions apply.

Puerto Rican

The Puerto Rican people, like the Chinese, have a hot-cold theory related to food and health. Foods are grouped as either hot or cold (this varies with individual interpretation) and are eaten in different proportions depending upon the individual's state of health. The staples of the Puerto Rican diet are salted cod, lard, coffee, sugar, rice, and beans. For most Puerto Rican people the midday meal is a hot meal and the largest of the day.

Milk and milk products   Coffee with a large amount of hot milk added (café con leche) is the major source of milk in the Puerto Rican diet. Some cheese (queso blanco) is eaten; it is similar to farmer's cheese.

Protein   Chicken is frequently used, along with beef, pork, and salted cod (bacalao). Meat is used for seasoning in stews composed of vegetables rather than as a food by itself. Chickpeas, small black beans, and red kidney beans are mixed with rice and a sauce (sofrito, made from tomatoes, onion, garlic, green peppers, salt pork, and lard) and eaten almost daily.

Vegetables and fruits   Vianda is the name given to starchy vegetables common to the Puerto Rican diet. Examples of viandas are plantain (green starchy bananas), yucca (cassava), malanga, and ñame blanco (white sweet potato). Salads consisting of lettuce and tomatoes with olive oil and vinegar as dressing are served frequently. Fresh pineapples, bananas, oranges, and acerola cherries (an excellent source of vitamin C) are eaten, as well as canned fruits.

Breads and cereals Rice is a staple of the Puerto Rican diet. Although the use of breads and cereals is increasing, they are not yet generally accepted. Bread is sometimes eaten for breakfast.

Miscellaneous Lard and salt pork are common flavorings. Sugar is used in large amounts to sweeten beverages. Guava and mango paste may be eaten for snacks. Black malt beer (malta) is a nonalcoholic beverage believed to be very nourishing. It is given to pregnant women and underweight children.

Nutritional concerns Many pregnant Puerto Rican women develop megaloblastic anemia.[6] Generally, their diets meet the recommended dietary allowance (RDA) for folacin.[7] Therefore, they may require an intake which is higher than the RDA for folic acid. Foods high in folacin (see Chap. 6) should be encouraged.

Obesity is another problem among the Puerto Rican population. Decreasing the amount of fat used in cooking, as well as decreasing sugar consumption; also, increasing activity should be stressed.

Mexican-American

The Spanish-American eating habits are a blend of several different cultures—those of the Spanish settlers, the Indians, and the Anglos. The resulting food pattern is common among the Mexican-Americans living in the southwestern United States.

Milk and milk products Limited amounts of milk are used, usually in the form of custards or rice puddings. Cheese is a common item in the diet.

Protein Meat is eaten only a few times a week, usually as hamburger or chicken mixed with vegetables. Beans (pinto and garbanzo) are eaten at every meal. They may be prepared by boiling and then frying (refried beans—frijoles refritos) or may be boiled and added to hamburger seasoned with chili, peppers, and garlic (chili con carne).

Vegetables and fruits Chili peppers, tomatoes, and corn are the most popular vegetables. Oranges, apples, bananas, and some canned fruits may be used.

Breads and cereals Corn is the basic grain of the Mexican diet. Tortillas, a dietary staple, are flat cakes made from ground corn that is soaked in lime water and then baked on a griddle. Enchiladas and tacos are made by filling the tortillas with a variety of meat mixtures. Cornmeal gruel and oatmeal are sometimes eaten with milk.

Miscellaneous Lard is used freely. Seasonings include chili pepper, onion, garlic, oregano, and coriander.

Coffee is the common beverage and may be given to children.

Nutritional concerns The *Ten State Nutrition Survey* found a low vitamin A intake among the Mexican-American population;[8] however, this finding is now suspect of being a laboratory error. Until there is better documentation, foods that are high in vitamin A should be encouraged. The folacin content of the diet may be low, and dark green vegetables can be increased. There is a high incidence of obesity in the Mexican-American population. Decreasing the amount of fat used in cooking, as well as omitting any high-caloric foods which are low in nutrients and increasing exercise, should be suggested.

Black

Soul food, a name now associated with black eating habits, had its origins in the south, where both poor blacks and poor whites followed the same eating patterns.

Milk and milk products   Limited amounts of milk are used; this may be due to a high prevalence of lactose intolerance. Buttermilk (sour milk) is used in cooking and as a beverage. Cheese is eaten in dishes such as macaroni and cheese.

Protein   All types of meat, fish, and chicken are eaten and are frequently fried. Pig's feet, neck bones, ham hocks, chitterlings (intestines), hog maws (stomach), and spareribs are popular. Bacon and sausage are commonly eaten at breakfast.

Vegetables and fruits   Vegetables are cooked for long periods of time, with salt pork, ham hocks, or bacon fat used as seasoning. Water-soluble vitamins are lost in the cooking water. Therefore, individuals should be encouraged to decrease the amount of water and the cooking time in order to conserve nutrients. The liquid from these vegetables is known as *pot liquor* and is eaten with corn bread. Popular vegetables include turnips, mustard greens, collard greens, black-eyed peas, okra, green beans, corn, lima beans, white potatoes, and sweet potatoes. Sweet potatoes may be fried, baked, candied, or used to make pies. Oranges, apples, bananas, peaches, and watermelon are popular fruits.

Breads and cereals   Grits, corn bread, biscuits, and muffins are eaten. Rice is more frequently used than potatoes.

Miscellaneous   Gravies are used on rice, potatoes, and meat. Cakes and pies are popular desserts. Molasses is used as a sweetener. Large amounts of soft drinks and fruit drinks are consumed.

Nutritional concerns   Obesity is a problem among black women of lower socioeconomic status. Encouragement should be given to reduce snack foods, sweets, soft drinks, and fats. Increased activity should be recommended. The Health and Nutrition Examination Survey (HANES) found a high incidence of low hemoglobin values in black adults over the age of 60 and in children 6 to 17 years of age.[9] Foods high in iron should be encouraged. Hypertension is another health problem for this group. Foods high in sodium, such as salt pork, ham hocks, bacon, and sausage, should be limited as a preventive measure against hypertension.

Jewish

The Jewish dietary laws, kashruth, are observed by many members of the Jewish faith. The extent to which these laws are followed or interpreted will depend upon the religious group to which the individual may belong.

> *Orthodox Jews* observe the laws strictly.
> *Reform Jews* do not place great emphasis on the dietary rules.
> *Conservative Jews* are somewhere in the middle.[10]

Kosher, which means "clean" or "fit," includes foods such as grains, fruits, vegetables, tea, and coffee, which are considered naturally kosher foods. Those foods which are not naturally kosher (meats, poultry) must undergo a koshering process before they can be eaten by those individuals observing kashruth. In this process the animals must be slaughtered in accordance with a particular ritual; the meat is then soaked in salted water to remove all blood. Only certain types of animals can be koshered. Animals that are cloven-hoofed quadrupeds and chew a cud can be used (beef, lamb). Pork and pork products and fish without scales and fins (i.e., shellfish) are prohibited.

Milk and meat may not be eaten together. Milk should be consumed immediately before or

6 h after eating meat. Separate plates must be used for dairy and meat meals.

Many foods will have the emblem Ⓤ on the package, which signifies endorsement by the Union of Orthodox Jewish Congregations of America, indicating that the food was packed under rabbinical supervision. The letter K appearing on foods also indicates rabbinical supervision.

The Jewish sabbath starts at sundown Friday and continues until Saturday evening. No cooking is allowed on the sabbath; therefore food is prepared ahead to be used on Saturday.

Passover is a religious week when no leavened bread products are used. A special set of dishes is used during this week, again with different plates for meat and for dairy foods. Therefore, the Jew observing kashruth has four sets of dishes—everyday dishes for meat and for dairy, and a separate set for use during Passover.

Yom Kippur (Day of Atonement) is a religious holy day when fasting is observed for 24 h.

Milk and milk products   All types of milk and milk products are used.

Protein   Orthodox Jews will eat only the forequarters from allowed animals. All types of beef, lamb, chicken, and fish are used. A few specialties include chopped liver, lox (smoked salmon), gefilte fish (fish filet chopped and seasoned and stuffed), and herring.

Vegetables and fruits   All types of fruits and vegetables are eaten. Borscht (beet, cabbage, or spinach soup) is served hot or cold with sour cream. Potato pancakes (latkes), carrot pudding (tzimmes), and cooked dried fruits (prunes, raisins, and apricots) are other favorites.

Breads and cereals   Bagels, egg bread (challah), dark breads (which contain no milk and can be eaten with meat), and matzo (an unleav-

ened bread product eaten during Passover) are bread products commonly consumed.

Nutritional concerns   The Jewish diet contains many foods high in saturated fat and cholesterol. Individuals should be counseled to modify their intake of these foods.

NONTRADITIONAL FOOD PRACTICES

It is important for the student to remember that food fulfills a number of needs beyond physiological nourishment—psychological, emotional, religious, and symbolic (see Chap. 11). In this section nontraditional food practices are reviewed to sensitize the student of nutrition to the varied motivational factors that influence these eating practices. An understanding of these factors will enable the nutritional educator to counsel these clients better.

Food Fads

The public is exposed to many types of food misinformation via the media. Food fads usually meet one or more of the following criteria.[11]

1   Rapid rise and fall in popularity
2   Stretching facts or using them out of context
3   Special appeal to certain segments of the population
4   Simplistic
5   Promotion of special virtues of a food
6   Restriction of certain foods in the belief that they are harmful

In addition to characterizing the types of food fads, the individuals drawn to them can be described as well. Beal has grouped these individuals into eight categories that specify the type of need which their food practice fulfills.[12] They are as follows:

1   Miracle seeker—food fad fulfills the need for self-worth and stability regarding health.

2 Antiestablishmentarian—food provides a vehicle to express values.

3 Super-health seeker—food is used as an ego defense to delay the aging process.

4 Distruster of the medical profession—food is used to control one's own body and eliminate dependence upon others.

5 Fashion follower—food is used as a means for acceptance.

6 Authority seeker—food is used as an area of expertise.

7 Truth seeker—must experience first hand claims regarding food.

8 One concerned about the uncertainties of living—needs stability regarding the world.

It is important for the nutrition counselor to be aware of the various needs that food fads fulfill. In this way, food substitutions of a more nutritious nature can be suggested while the social and psychological needs of the individual are supported.[13] Table 16-2 outlines some of the more common food fads.

TABLE 16-2   COMMON FOOD FADS

Name	Description	Comment
Mayo Clinic diet (not related to the Mayo Clinic in Rochester, Minn.)	Promotes quick weight loss. High-protein diet consisting of grapefruit, meats, and vagetables.	Promotes grapefruit as having fat-burning properties. No scientific evidence to back up this claim.
Stillman diet	Promotes quick weight loss. High-protein, high-fat diet consisting of unlimited amounts of meat, fish, eggs, low-fat cheese, 8 glasses of water, plus a vitamin supplement.	Unbalanced. May be harmful for anyone with gout, diabetes, or kidney problems. High in cholesterol and saturated fat. No metabolic advantage over a well-balanced low-calorie diet.
Atkins diet	Promotes quick weight loss. No carbohydrate for first week, to produce ketosis; carbohydrate gradually added to reach a maximum of 50 g. Amount of protein and fat unlimited.	Unbalanced. High in saturated fat and cholesterol. May be harmful for anyone with gout, diabetes, or kidney problems. No metabolic advantage over a well-balanced low-calorie diet.
Scarsdale diet	Specific menus for 14 days are planned. Only foods on menu are allowed. No substitutions are to be made.	Mean caloric content of the diet is approximately 945 kcal. The diet is low in iron, calcium, and thiamin. (The diet cannot be calculated exactly as some portion sizes are left up to the dieter. This calculation is based on the following portion sizes: ½ grapefruit, 6–8 oz meats/fish, 1 cup fruit/vegetable).
Beverly Hills diet	Fruit is used as a staple of this diet. During the first week the diet is composed entirely of fruit. Other food items, such as potato, corn, chicken, steak, lobster, and some vegetables, are gradually introduced but make up a very limited portion of the diet plan. B-complex vitamins are recommended.	Diet is lacking in scientific foundation and is not balanced nutritionally.

TABLE 16-2 CONTINUED

Name	Description	Comment
Protein-sparing modified fast (liquid protein diet)	The use of liquid protein as the sole source of food or in combination with lean meat and fish.	FDA investigating several deaths thought to be associated with the liquid protein diet.
Simeon diet	Injections of the hormone human chorionic gonadatropin (HCG) plus a 500-kcal diet.	No scientific evidence to suggest HCG is useful for the treatment of obesity.
Mucusless diet	Allows only raw and cooked fruits, "starchless" vegetables, and cooked or raw leafy, green vegetables. All are considered "mucus" free. Diet, fasting, or both can cure all disease by preventing mucus formation.	Unbalanced. Claims are not substantiated scientifically.
Pritikin program for diet and exercise	Diet is low in protein, fat, and cholesterol, high in complex carbohydrate. Approximately 10% protein, 10% fat, and 80% complex carbohydrate. Dietary regimen also promotes exercise.	Suggests that by following the diet individuals will have more energy and that some symptoms of aging will disappear. Controlled scientific studies are needed to substantiate claims.
Adele Davis	Recommends massive doses of vitamins for all. Recommends a variety of foods to cure ills— brewer's yeast, dessicated liver, etc.	Scare tactics are used. Scientific information, often out of context, is mixed with author's own theories.
Hypoglycemia Foundation	Claims that millions of people have hypoglycemia and are undiagnosed. Advocates many expensive lab tests and use of injections of whole adrenocortical extracts to treat hypoglycemia.	According to the American Medical Association "these claims are not supported by medical evidence."*
Jerome Rodale	Owner of Rodale Press (which prints *Prevention Magazine* and *Organic Gardening and Farming*); makes such fallacious statements as that pumpkin seeds will cure prostatic disease;† opposed to organized medicine and the food industry.	Many erroneous statements with no scientific backup.
Orthomolecular therapy	Advocates use of megavitamins (large quantities, usually of the water-soluble type) for the treatment of a variety of mental disorders.	To date there is no evidence that this is an effective mode of treatment.

*American Medical Association, "Statement on Hypoglycemia," *Journal of the American Medical Association*, **223**:682, 1973.
†J. I. Rodale, *Prostate,* Rodale Press, Emmaus, Pa., 1969.

Natural, Organically Grown, and Health Foods

Natural foods The Federal Trade Commission (FTC) has established guidelines for the use of the term *natural* in advertising food.

Natural foods are generally regarded as those foods which remain in their original state. Natural foods have a minimum of processing (Freezing and canning are acceptable) and contain no artificial ingredients.

Organically grown foods The term *organic food* is a misnomer—all foods are organic. *Organically grown food* is more accurate. It refers to food grown without the use of pesticides, fumigants, or synthetic fertilizers, and containing no preservatives or synthetic coloring agents. Individuals who favor organically grown food may eat meats only from animals that receive no antibiotics or hormones and that are fed only organically grown grains.

There is no evidence that organically grown food offers any extra nutritional benefit. However, organic gardening includes a reduction of pollution and a concern for our environment, as well as a reminder of how many additives we are using in our food.[14] Growing food organically does not produce a large crop yield, and consequently the consumer must pay anywhere from 30 to 100 percent more for organically grown food.[15] Presently, there are no federal regulations governing the labeling of organic food. Therefore, it is important for those using organic foods to become acquainted with the stores in their neighborhood in order to know which ones are reputable and to be sure that the food is indeed organically grown.

Health foods A health food may or may not be natural or organically grown. It is a food that is usually thought to impart good health and is generally purchased in health food stores. Health foods may be advertised as preventing or curing illness. Some commonly used health foods include tiger's milk (dry skim milk powder, soy powder, and brewer's yeast with additional vitamins and minerals), brewer's yeast, blackstrap molasses, desiccated liver, kelp, and sea salt. Foods such as these are sources of nutrients but are not a panacea. For example, brewer's yeast is a good source of vitamin B_{12} and folic acid.

Natural and Synthetic Vitamins

There is no scientific or legal definition for the term *natural vitamin*. Two common fallacies associated with natural vitamins are as follows:

1 Natural vitamins are better than synthetic vitamins.
2 Natural vitamins contain no synthetic ingredients.[16]

The chemical properties of synthetic and natural vitamins are the same.[17] The body does not distinguish between the two. One manufacturer of a "natural" vitamin C compound uses rose hips with added chemical ascorbic acid; "natural" B vitamins have been made with brewer's yeast and synthetic B vitamins. Consumers may pay more for natural or organic vitamins since they are more difficult to produce than synthetic ones. They offer no extra nutritional benefit.

Zen Macrobiotics

Zen macrobiotics was introduced to the United States by George Ohsawa. Followers of the macrobiotic philosophy believe that the individual should live off his or her "natural" environment and achieve harmony by a healthful existence from the balance of yin and yang. Foods are grouped as having more yin or more yang:

Yang = meats—eggs—fish—grains—
   vegetables—fruits—dairy products—
   sugar—alcohol—drugs—chemicals = Yin

Yin and yang are used to determine appropriate food combinations. Climate and gender as well as the emotional, physical, and spiritual state of an individual influence the dietary proportions of yin and yang.

There are ten dietary stages incorporated into the macrobiotic philosophy which become progressively more restrictive (see Table 16-3). The lower-level diets contain cereals, vegetables, fruits, seafoods, and desserts; the higher-level diets consist of 100 percent cereal, usually brown rice. Fluids are limited at all levels. The higher-level diets are not nutritionally adequate. Scurvy, anemia, hypoproteinemia, hypercalcemia, emaciation due to starvation, and death can result.[18] Fortunately, most macrobiotic enthusiasts follow the lower-level diets, which can be planned to meet nutrient needs. Brown and Bergan, studying the intakes of macrobiotic individuals, found their diets to be adequate in most nutrients.[19] Those nutrients that were found to be limited were energy, calcium, riboflavin, and iron (in women only). They also studied a small group of children eating macrobiotic diets and found their energy and calcium intakes to be low.[20] Dwyer et al., studying pre-

school children consuming a macrobiotic diet, reported the diets to be marginal in vitamin D, calcium, and phosphorus. They also found that children following a macrobiotic diet were more likely to have possible signs of rickets when their health histories were studied.[21]

Followers of the macrobiotic philosophy believe that illness can be cured through proper eating. This is a dangerous assumption which can prove fatal if traditional medical care is not sought for an illness.

Vegetarianism

Although vegetarianism has been practiced for many years by Seventh-Day Adventists and Trappist monks, it is only within the past 15 years that it has gained popularity among young Americans.[22]

Individuals choose to become vegetarians for a number of reasons, the most common being:

Religious preference
Health concerns

TABLE 16-3   MACROBIOTIC DIET

	Content, %						
Diet level	Cereals	Vegetables	Soup	Animal products	Fruits, salads	Desserts	Drinking liquid
7	100	—	—	—	—	—	Sparingly
6	90	10*	—	—	—	—	Sparingly
5	80	20	—	—	—	—	Sparingly
4	70	20	10	—	—	—	Sparingly
3	60	30	10	—	—	—	Sparingly
2	50	30	10	10	—	—	Sparingly
1	40	30	10	20	—	—	Sparingly
−1	30	30	10	20	10	—	Sparingly
−2	20	30	10	25	10	5	Sparingly
−3	10	30	10	30	15	5	Sparingly

*Refined vegetables. In other regimens vegetables are not refined.
Source: R. Frankle and F. K. Heussenstamm, "Food Zealotry and Youth, New Dilemmas for Professionals," *American Journal of Public Health,* January 1974, p. 15.

Environmental considerations
Humanitarian issues
Economics
Political reasons

The term *vegetarian* is applied to those individuals whose diet consists primarily of plant foods. However, within this group there are several different types:

1 Vegans: strict vegetarians who eat or drink no animal or dairy products
2 Lacto-ovo-vegetarians: those who drink milk and eat eggs but consume no other animal product
3 Lacto-vegetarians: those whose only animal product is milk
4 Ovo-vegetarians: those who eat eggs but no other animal product
5 Pesco-vegetarians: those who eat fish but no other animal product
6 Partial or semivegetarians: those who eat fish and chicken but no red meat
7 Fruitarians: those whose diet is composed chiefly of fruits and nuts

Within the foregoing categories vegetarians can be considered traditional vegetarians or new vegetarians. Traditional vegetarians are those who adhere to a vegetarian pattern that has existed for generations. These are individuals who were raised within a culture or religious group that is vegetarian, for example, Seventh-Day Adventists. New vegetarians are individuals who were raised as omnivores but have now become vegetarians. Many of these vegetarians belong to a philosophical, quasi-religious, or religious groups which surfaced in the United States during the 1960s.[23] These new vegetarians are more likely to include natural, health, and organically grown foods in their diets. Table 16-4 lists a number of groups that are considered new vegetarians.[24]

Vegetarian diets are nutritionally sound if they include a wide variety of nuts, legumes, grains, fruits, vegetables, milk, and milk products (see Table 16-5). The diets of vegans and fruitarians are the only diets which offer no source of complete protein. It is important for the nutrition educator to teach these people the use of complementary proteins—beans and rice, tacos and beans, etc. (see Table 16-6, p. 352).

While vegans generally eat a variety of foods, fruitarians are more restrictive in their choices. Fruitarian diets require a great deal of expertise in planning nutritionally balanced regimens. Kwashiorkor has been reported in a 23-

TABLE 16-4   NEW VEGETARIANS

Group	Dietary characteristics
Yogic vegetarians (American Yogic sects such as Divine Light Mission, followers of Guru Maharaji and Baba Ram Dass, Ananda Marga Yogic sect, One Horse Commune, Health Happy Holy Yogic sect, and Transcendental Meditation groups)	Usually lacto-ovo-vegetarians but may be semivegetarians; use health, natural, and organic foods
Hare Krishnas (American Hindu sect)	Lacto-vegetarians; use natural foods
Sufis (American Moslem sect)	Lacto- or lacto-ovo-vegetarians
Sikhs (American sect based on teachings of East Indian religious group)	Lacto-vegetarians

Source: Adapted from "Position Paper on the Vegetarian Approach to Eating," *Journal of the American Dietetic Association,* **77**:61, July 1980.

TABLE 16-5 VEGETARIAN FOOD GUIDE

Food groups (servings per day)	Size of serving	Food sources or exchanges
I. Milk group (2 or more servings)	1 cup whole milk	½ cup evaporated milk 1 cup yogurt 1 cup skim milk 1 oz cheese ¼ cup cottage cheese 1 cup soymilk 4 tbsp powdered soymilk
II. Vegetable protein foods (2 or more servings)	1 cup legumes (beans, garbanzos, lentils, peas) 2–3 oz meat analogs	4 tbsp peanut butter 20–30 g dry textured vegetable proteins 4 oz soy "cheese" or curd 1½ tbsp nuts or oil seeds
III. Fruits and vegetables (4 or more servings)	½ cup cooked vegetables and/or fruits 1 cup raw vegetables ½ cup juice	1 serving vitamin C–rich foods; citrus, cabbage and tomatoes, melon, green pepper, strawberries 1–2 servings of green leafy vegetables and yellow vegetables and fruits (carotene-rich)

IV. Bread and cereals (4 or more servings)	1 slice of whole wheat or enriched bread
	½–¾ cup cooked cereal whole grain
	¾–1 cup dry cereal
		½–¾ cup enriched or whole rice
		½–¾ cup enriched noodles macaroni, or spaghetti
		½ cup granola
		½ hamburger bun
		Crackers
		  graham (2)
		  saltines (5)
		  wheat thins (8)

V. Other foods Eggs (3–4 per week) Fats (1 tbsp per day)	1 egg 1 tsp oil 1 tsp soft margarine	

Source: I. B. Vhymeister, U. D., Register and L. M. Sonnenberg, "Safe Vegetarian Diets for Children," *Pediatric Clinics of North America,* **24**(1):207, February 1977.

month-old infant fed a diet consisting almost solely of fruits.[25]

Most young vegetarians do not use textured vegetable protein, as it resembles meat in some products and the cost is prohibitive. Seventh-Day Adventists, however, may use these products.

Since red meats are not consumed and phytates found in whole grains inhibit iron absorption, iron deficiency can be a problem within the vegetarian population. Therefore, foods such as raisins, dried apricots, beans, peas, seeds, and blackstrap molasses should be incorporated into the diet to increase iron content.

TABLE 16-6   COMPLEMENTARY PROTEINS

Food group	Complementary proteins
Legumes	Legumes and rice
	Soybeans, rice, and wheat
	Beans and wheat
	Soybeans, corn, and milk
	Beans and corn
	Soybeans, wheat, and sesame seeds
	Soybeans, peanuts, and sesame seeds
	Soybeans, sesame seeds, and wheat
Grains	Rice and legumes
	Corn and legumes
	Wheat and legumes
	Rice and milk
	Wheat and cheese
	Wheat and milk
	Wheat, peanuts, and milk
	Wheat, sesame seeds, and soybeans
	Brewer's yeast and rice
Vegetables	Lima beans ⎫
	Peas ⎪ and sesame seeds
	Brussels sprouts ⎬ brazil nuts
	Cauliflower ⎪ mushrooms
	Broccoli ⎭
Nuts and seeds	Peanuts, sesame seeds, and soybeans
	Sesame seeds and beans
	Sesame seeds, soybeans, and wheat
	Peanuts and milk
	Peanuts and sunflower seeds
	Peanuts, wheat, and milk
	Sesame seeds, wheat, and soybeans

Source: Adapted from F. M. Lappe, *Diet for a Small Planet,* Friends of the Earth/Ballantine Books, Inc., New York, 1971.

A B_{12} deficiency was recently reported in a breast-fed infant of a strict vegetarian mother.[26,27] Although few cases of vitamin B_{12} deficiency are reported, presumably due to the body's vast reserves of this vitamin, vegetarians should be encouraged to use fermented soybean products and fortified soybean milks, which are high in vitamin B_{12}, since meat and meat prod-

ucts are the chief source of this nutrient. Calcium intake should be evaluated for adequacy. Dark green vegetables, especially kale, collards, mustard, turnip, and dandelion greens, and soybeans should be encouraged.

Milk is fortified with vitamin D and is the major dietary source of this nutrient. Vitamin D is also supplied by the action of the sun on the skin. If milk is not used and the individual is outdoors only occasionally, a vitamin D supplement may be needed.

Following a vegetarian diet offers several advantages. It is lower in cholesterol and saturated fat than the ordinary diet, and high in fiber. Most vegetarians are not overweight, perhaps because of the high fiber and water content of vegetables as well as the avoidance of high-fat snack foods.

It is important for the nutrition educator, when working with vegetarian children, to make sure that all nutrient needs are met for adequate growth. Studies have shown preschool vegetarian children to be lighter and shorter than omnivore children.[28]

COMMUNITY RESOURCES

Knowledge of food resources is essential, particularly in low-income communities. Helping clients to enroll in the Food Stamp program, the Special Supplemental Feeding Program for Women, Infants, and Children (WIC), or Elderly Feeding programs will help them to stretch limited incomes. Government programs and community agencies attempt to provide people with a minimum quality of life, and it is up to the health professional to help people, especially those with limited incomes, to utilize available resources to the utmost.

Addressed in this section are two examples of community resources, their purpose, their target population, and a general description of their function. These two examples are the Food Stamp program and the Special Supplementary Feeding Program for Women, Infants, and Children. Other programs are summarized in Tables 16-7 and 16-8. (See also the Appendix.)

TABLE 16-7 FEDERAL FOOD PROGRAMS

Program	Legislation	Funding	Eligibility	Services provided	Other
School Lunch program	National School Lunch Act of 1946 and Section II amendment to the National School Lunch Act and the Child Nutrition Act of 1966.	USDA reimbursement for partial cost of food.	All public and private nonprofit schools.	School lunch:* 8 oz milk 2 oz protein 1 starch serving ⅜ cup vegetable ¾ cup fruit Operates on a nonprofit basis. Provides free or reduced-price lunch for those eligible.	USDA authorized to buy food through the Surplus Removal and Price Support program to distribute to schools. Schools must agree to participate in school lunch program.
Child Care Food Program	Child Care Food Program, Section 17 of the National School Lunch Act 1975.	USDA reimburses participating agencies up to a prescribed amount for the cost of serving breakfast, lunch, and/or supper.	All public or private nonprofit institutions providing day-care services.	Provides meals which meet national requirements established by USDA. Provides free or reduced-price meals.	Can receive donated food or a cash reimbursement for each lunch and/or supper served to eligible children.
School Breakfast program	The Child Nutrition Act of 1966 funded the program for 2 years. An amendment in 1971 extended the program further.	USDA reimbursement for food cost.	All public and private non-profit schools.	Breakfast: 8 oz milk 1 slice of bread or equivalent grain product ½ cup fresh fruit or full-strength fruit or vegetable juice Schools are asked to provide a protein food as often as possible.	USDA authorized to buy food via the Surplus Removal and Price Support program.
Food Stamp programs	Food Stamp Act of 1964 (there had been pilot programs prior to this law).	USDA and state. At the state level, usually run by the welfare department.	All individuals who meet financial criteria.	Food Stamps or coupons that can be used like money to buy food. Increases purchasing power.	

*Owing to federal cutbacks, the school lunch may be revised.

(Continued)

TABLE 16-7 CONTINUED

Program	Legislation	Funding	Eligibility	Services provided	Other
The Special Supplemental Food Program for Women, Infants, and Children (WIC)	1972 amendment to the Child Nutrition Act of 1966.	Federal funds provide cash grants to states.	Health centers in areas of high risk because of inadequate nutrition and income. Individuals eligible—Pregnant women; mothers up to 6 months postpartum; nursing mothers up to 1 year; children to age 5; if a nutritional risk and income as determined by a professional.	WIC has 6 food package categories. Food Package I:Infants 0 through 3 months Food Package II:Infants 4 through 12 months Food Package III:Children/women with special dietary needs Food Package IV:Children 1 to 5 years Food Package V:Pregnant and breast-feeding women Food Package VI:Non-breast-feeding postpartum women	The amount and type of food varies with each package. Those foods included are: iron fortified formula; milk (whole, skim, buttermilk, evaporated whole or skim, dry whole or nonfat/lowfat); cheese (American, Monteray Jack, Colby, Natural Cheddar, Swiss, Brick, Muenster, Provolone, or Mozzerella); cereal (iron-enriched, no more than 21.2 g of sugar per 100 g of dry cereal); eggs (fresh or dried egg mix); legumes (peanut butter, mature dry beans, or peas); juice (at least 30 mg Vit C/100 mL of juice)†

Elderly Feeding program	Title III of the Older Americans Act.	USDA and state funds reimburse for partial cost of food.	All nonprofit organizations; all individuals over the age of 60.	Hot meal: Food to provide ⅓ of the RDA.	Health center must collect the following data: weight height head circumference hematocrit hemoglobin. May provide 10% of the meals served to home-bound elderly.

†*WIC Currents*, 7(1):1–4, January-February 1981 (Ross Laboratories, Columbus, Ohio).

TABLE 16-8 COMMUNITY RESOURCES*

Resource	Comment
Headstart program	Educational enrichment and nutritional services for children aged 3–5 years from low-income areas
Visiting Nurse Association	Provides nutritional information to clients—many have a nutritionist as a consultant
American Heart Association American Diabetes Association American Cancer Society	Local chapters run screening clinics, provide educational material for the public and professional
American Dietetic Association	Many state chapters sponser Dial-a-Dietitian whereby public may call and ask questions regarding nutrition
National Dairy Council	State branches provide educational material, run workshops in schools, employ nutritionists and home economists
Departments of Public Health (state and local)	Conduct clinics, health screening programs; provide educational materials; nutritionists work to set up needed nutritional programs in the community
Agricultural Extension Service	Provides nutrition education to the community; runs workshops and trains individuals from the community to work as nutrition aides
Consumer councils (state, voluntary)	Provide nutrition information and help individuals take legal action against misrepresentation
Schools, churches, agencies	May provide meals to special age groups

*See also Appendix.

Food Stamp Program

The Food Stamp program (see Table 16-7) began in 1964 and has grown to become a food program servicing a large segment of the population—approximately 21.3 million.[29] The number is sure to change with federal cutbacks and stricter eligibility criteria.

Food stamps are coupons that can be used in place of money to buy food. The individual is free to select any type of food (alcohol, tobacco, and pet food are excluded). Food stamps cannot be used to purchase cleaning items, soap, detergent, or paper goods. Food stamps can be used in any store, supermarket, or cooperative that has registered to accept food stamps. Almost all large grocery stores and many small stores are registered. Food stamps can also be used by the elderly to pay for authorized home-delivered meals or meals eaten at an elderly congregate meal site.

Individuals or families who are eligible for food stamps include anyone who receives public assistance and households where incomes and financial resources are limited. All households of the same size receive the same amount of food stamps. However, the cost of the food stamps will vary, depending upon income (i.e., the smaller the income, the less paid for the food stamps). For example, a family of four can receive approximately $155 worth of food stamps, but depending upon income one family might pay $100 while another family may only pay $50 for the same $155 worth of food stamps.

Individuals can apply for food stamps at a variety of locations which vary from state to state. As previously mentioned, those individuals or households receiving public assistance are automatically eligible, and fill out a simple application form. Members of non–public assistance households are required to complete a much more lengthy application and must be interviewed. This is necessary to verify income and financial resources, in order to determine how much must be paid for the food stamps. To facilitate the food stamp application procedure, the individual should bring proof of income (pay stubs) and proof of expenses (rent receipts, medical bills, utility bills, etc.) when applying. Once eligibility has been established, an identification card, which is needed for purchase and use of the food stamps, will be issued. Then an authorization-to-purchase card (ATP) will be received in the mail one or two times per month, notifying the individual of the amount of food stamps that can be purchased and how much they will cost.

Food stamps are issued in a variety of locations that differ from state to state. Some of the more common sites include banks, post offices, food stamp offices, and community action agencies. These organizations are paid by the government for each food stamp transaction. The individual goes to one of these locations, presents the identification card and the ATP card, pays the appropriate amount of money, and then receives the stamps. One of the problems encountered at the inception of the Food Stamp program was that recipients found it difficult to gather the full amount of money needed to purchase a month's food stamps. To help alleviate this problem, food stamp recipients can now buy all, three-fourths, one-half, or one-fourth of the monthly supply of stamps. Once the Food Stamps are purchased, they can then be used to buy food.

The Special Supplemental Feeding Program for Women, Infants, and Children

The Special Supplemental Feeding Program for Women, Infants, and Children (WIC) was established in 1972 as an amendment to the Child Nutrition Act of 1966. The purpose of the program is to prevent as well as correct nutritional deficiencies, thereby abating the physical and mental damage to infants that can be caused by malnutrition. To achieve this goal, approved health centers provide food to pregnant and lactating women (up to 1 year) postpartum women (up to 6 months), and infants and children (until age 5). Eligibility for the program is determined by the following criteria:

1   Individuals must reside in a low-income area serviced by an approved health care center which administers the WIC program. (This requirement may be waived by individual states.)

2   Individuals must be eligible for free or reduced-rate health care at this facility.

3   Individuals must be considered by a health professional to be at nutritional risk because of inadequate nutrition and income.

Nutritional risk has never been clearly defined; however, those criteria for pregnant women, postpartum women (up to 6 months), and lactating women (up to 1 year) usually include:

Nutritional anemia

Inadequate dietary intake

Inappropriate growth patterns (overweight, underweight, stunting)

High-risk pregnancy (premature or low-birth-weight infants, miscarriage, high parity, short interconceptual time)

The criteria for nutritional risk in an infant or child usually include:

Nutritional anemia

Inadequate dietary intake

Poor growth pattern (obesity, failure to thrive)

When a program has reached its enrollment capacity, a priority system is instituted. Priority is given to pregnant women, breast-feeding mothers, and infants. Persons with documented medical risk factors are ranked ahead of individuals with inadequate food intake.[30]

The foods that are provided by the program (see Table 16-7) were selected for their specific nutrient content: high-biological-value protein, iron, calcium, and vitamins A and C. These are nutrients known to be lacking in the diets of populations at nutritional risk.[31] Specific food packages are provided for infants with special needs, for example, infants with phenylkotonuria (PKU) or lactose intolerance.

Each WIC program center decides on the method it will use to provide these foods to the participants. The most commonly used method is the voucher system, whereby participants are given coupons that are redeemable for food at particular stores. Other methods include home delivery and warehousing by the health center (which then distributes the food items).

The participants in the program usually return monthly to receive their vouchers for food and return periodically for medical checkups. The minimal medical data that must be collected by the health center include height, weight, head circumference, hematocrit, and hemoglobin. It is hoped that having the participants return regularly will encourage and familiarize them with the use of the health care system.

If the community has a WIC program, it is important for the nutrition educator to initiate outreach. Federal funds are not provided for this activity; therefore the nutrition educator will need to publicize the program via word of mouth, media, community leaders, church groups, the Visiting Nurse Association, day-care centers, Head Start programs, and community action agencies. It should also be emphasized that the WIC program does not take the place of the Food Stamp program. Women who are participating in the WIC program may also be eligible for food stamps. The WIC program is designed to supplement the diet with food.

Evaluation is an important component of any program if effectiveness is to be achieved. There has been an evaluation of the WIC program; however, few conclusions can be reached. This is due to:[32]

1 A lack of uniformity in health and nutritional data collected by each WIC program
2 No universally accepted nutritional and health standards
3 Lack of exact determination of nutrient re-

quirements which will improve or maintain nutritional status
4 Inadequate indicators to determine an infant's mental development
5 Difficulty in finding and using a control group

The preliminary findings did reveal (though their accuracy is questionable because of the aforementioned problems) the following: an increase in height, weight, and head circumference among infants enrolled in the program; a decrease in anemia among both infants and mothers; an increase in the consumption of protein, calcium, phosphorus, iron, vitamin A, thiamin, riboflavin, niacin, ascorbic acid, and folacin; increased weight gain by pregnant women; and increased birth weight among minority-group infants.[33,34] Another study compared pregnant WIC participants with non-WIC participants. The results revealed a higher infant birth weight for infants born to women who were WIC participants. It also reported a lower incidence of low-birth-weight infants in the WIC group.[35]

STUDY QUESTIONS

1 Why is it important for the nutritional educator to understand cultural food patterns?
2 The Mexican-American, Chinese, Japanese, Vietnamese, Puerto Rican, and black diets may be inadequate in what nutrients?
3 If you were planning a diet for an Orthodox Jew, what dietary laws would you consider?
4 Differentiate between the WIC Program and the Food Stamp Program.
5 What are the various types of vegetarian diets? What nutrients may be inadequate in these diets?

CLINICAL STUDY 16

S. C. is a 3-month-postpartum. She immigrated to the United States from China 1 year ago. She is currently unemployed, as is her husband. This is her first visit to the health center, and she is referred to the nutritionist for dietary evaluation.

Her typical meal plan includes:

Breakfast
Roll
Tea

Lunch
Rice, with broth, celery, bitter melon, and broccoli

Orange
Tea

Supper
Chicken with bok choy, bamboo shoots, broccoli, and rice
Pineapple
Tea

Clinical study questions

1 *What nutrients appear to be inadequate in S. C.'s diet?*

2 *What recommendation would you make?*

3 *What food programs would you suggest?*

REFERENCES

1 H. Gifft et al., *Nutrition Behavior and Change,* Prentice-Hall, Inc., Englewood Cliffs, N.J., 1972, pp. 29–30.

2 M. Mead, "Food and the Family," in *Food and People,* UNESCO, New York, 1953, p. 7.

3 M. Kaufman, "Vietnam 1978: Crisis in Food, Nutrition, and Health," *Journal of the American Dietetic Association,* **74**:310–316, March 1979.

4 N. T. Ahn et al., "Lactose Malabsorption in Adult Vietnamese," *American Journal of Clinical Nutrition,* **30**:468, 1977.

5 M. Kaufman, op. cit., pp. 310–316.

6 V. Herbert, "Symposium: Folic Acid Deficiency," *American Journal of Clinical Nutrition,* **23**:841, 1970.

7 S. Parker and J. Bowery, "Folacin in Diets of Puerto Rican and Black Women in Relation to Food Practices," *Journal of Nutrition Education,* **8**(2):73–76, 1976.

8 *Ten State Nutrition Survey, 1968–1970,* U.S. Department of Health, Education, and Welfare Publication (HSM) 72-8133, 1970.

9 *Dietary Intake and Biochemical Findings, Preliminary Findings of the First Health and Nutrition Examination Survey, U.S., 1971–1972,* U.S. Department of Health, Education, and Welfare, Public Health Service, Health Resources Administration, National Center for Health Statistics, Rockville, Md., January 1974.

10 A. Natow et al., "Integrating the Jewish Dietary Laws into a Dietetic Program," *Journal of the American Dietetic Association,* **67**:14, 1975.

11 R. Schaffer and R. Yetley, "Social Psychology of Food Faddism," *Journal of the American Dietetic Association,* **69**:129, 1975.

12 V. Beal, "Food Faddism and Organic and Natural Foods," paper presented at the National Dairy Council Food Writers Conference, Newport, R.I., May 1972.

13 R. Schaffer and R. Yetley, op. cit., p. 133.

14 F. Clydesdale and F. J. Francis, *Food, Nutrition, and You,* Prentice-Hall, Inc., Englewood Cliffs, N.J., 1977, p. 89.

15 Review, *Nutrition Reviews,* **32**(Suppl.):53, July 1974.

16 Consumer's Union, *The Medicine Show,* Consumer's Union, Mt. Vernon, N.Y., 1974.

17 A. Kamil, "How Natural Are Those Natural Vitamins," *Nutrition Reviews,* **32**(Suppl.):34, July 1974.

18 Presentation of the Passaic, N.J., Grand Jury, "Zen Macrobiotic Diet Hazardous," *Public Health News,* New Jersey Department of Health, June 1966, pp. 132–135.

19 P. T. Brown and J. G. Bergan, "The Dietary Status of 'New' Vegetarians," *Journal of the American Dietetic Association,* **67**:455–459, 1975.

20 Ibid.

21 J. Dwyer et al., "Risk of Nutritional Rickets Among Vegetarian Children, *American Journal of Diseases of Children,* **133**:134–140, February 1979.

22 J. T. Dwyer et al., "New Vegetarians," *Journal of the American Dietetic Association*, **64**:376, 1974.

23 "Position Paper on the Vegetarian Approach to Eating," *Journal of the American Dietetic Association*, **77**:61, July 1980.

24 Ibid.

25 E. Klimek and C. Wharton, "Kwashiorkor as a Result of Food Faddism," *Journal of the American Osteopathic Association*, **78**:136/121–140/125, October, 1978.

26 M. Higginbottom et al., "A Syndrome of Methylmalonic Aciduria, Homocystinuria, Megaloblastic Anemia and Neurologic Abnormalities in a B_{12}-Deficient Breast Fed Infant of a Strict Vegetarian," **299**:317, 1978.

27 "Vitamin B_{12} Deficiency in the Breast-fed Infant of a Strict Vegetarian," *Nutrition Reviews, New England Journal of Medicine*, **37**:142–144, May 1979.

28 M. Shull et al., "Velocity of Growth in Vegetarian Preschool Children," **60**:410–417, 1977.

29 "Carter Budget Asks Cutbacks in Food Programs," *Community Nutrition Institute*, **X**(4):2, Jan. 24, 1980.

30 J. Berkenfield and J. Swartz, "Nutrition Intervention in the Community—The WIC Program," *New England Journal of Medicine*, **302**(11):580, 1980.

31 Comptroller General of the United States, *Report to Congress: Observation on Evaluation of the Special Supplemental Food Program*, Food and Nutrition Service, USDA RED-75-310, December 1974, pp. 2–3.

32 Ibid., pp. 23–24.

33 J. C. Edozien et al., *Medical Evaluation of the Special Supplemental Food Program for Women, Infants and Children*, vol. II, *Results*, University of North Carolina, Chapel Hill, N.C., School of Public Health, Department of Nutrition, July 15, 1976.

34 J. C. Endozien, B. R. Switzer, and R. B. Bryan, "Medical Evaluation of the Special Supplemental Food Program for Women, Infants and Children," *Journal of Clinical Nutrition*, **32**:677–692, 1979.

35 E. Kennedy, "Effects of WIC Supplemental Food on Birth Weight," Harvard School of Public Health, Boston, December 1978 (Doctoral Thesis).

CLINICAL DISCUSSION 16

Since S. C.'s diet contains no milk or milk products, it appears to be inadequate in calcium and vitamin D. Milk is not generally consumed as a beverage by many Chinese; however, it is acceptable when used on cereal. S. C. was also encouraged to use bean curd and soybeans, good sources of calcium and protein. Greens such as mustard greens and kale were also recommended for their calcium content.

By increasing the amount of milk in S. C.'s diet and by encouraging exposure to sunlight, the amount of vitamin D will most likely become adequate.

S. C.'s protein intake may be low, depending upon the amount of meat, fish, or chicken used in mixed dishes.

The nutritionist informed S. C. that she probably was eligible for food stamps and told her where she could apply. The nutritionist also enrolled S. C. and her baby in the WIC program at the health center, as she met the criteria for limited income and she also had an inadequate dietary intake.

CHAPTER 17

NUTRITION AND DENTAL HEALTH

T. Howard Howell

KEY WORDS
Odontogenesis
Plaque
Caries
Periodontal Disease
Fluoride
Calculus
Bottle Caries Syndrome

INTRODUCTION

The oral cavity is the initial segment of the gastrointestinal tract; there food is masticated, buffered, degluted (swallowed), and mechanically prepared for digestion. Thus, the covering tissues of the oral cavity are subjected to a wide spectrum of thermal, chemical, and mechanical stimuli. In order to perform their functions optimally and to maintain the structural integrity needed to withstand various insults, the tissues of the oral cavity must be given special care and adequate nourishment. Indeed, general health is dependent upon, as well as reflected in, the status of the oral mucosa and associated hard tissues. For this reason, it is necessary for the practicing health professional to understand the nutritional requirements for good general health and to be able to recognize pathological states derived from nutritional deficits.

STRUCTURE OF TEETH

Teeth develop as the result of several genetically determined, mutually inductive interactions of the embryonic ectoderm and mesoderm of the jaws. Fully differentiated teeth are composed of three calcified tissues: *enamel, dentin,* and *cementum.* Contained within and protected by these hard dental tissues is the delicate, highly vascular innervated connective tissue, the *dental pulp* (see Fig. 17-1, p. 362).

The *crown* is that portion of the tooth covered by enamel. As the hardest calcified tissue, *enamel* serves as a resistant overcasting for the relatively resilient underlying dentin. Enamel contains a very small percentage of organic matter; it is derived from ectodermal cells, the ameloblasts, which persist until the teeth erupt into the oral cavity. Ameloblasts must be present in order for dentin to be laid down by the mesodermally derived odontoblasts. *Dentin* determines the morphology of the tooth and is its main calcified component. It is the natural boundary of the pulp, and is maintained by the

Note: The author wishes to acknowledge the editorial assistance of Ellen Eisenberg, D.D.S., Assistant Professor in Oral Pathology.

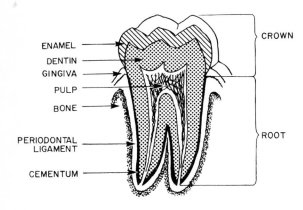

ENAMEL
DENTIN
GINGIVA
PULP
BONE
PERIODONTAL
LIGAMENT
CEMENTUM
CROWN
ROOT

Figure 17-1
The structure of the tooth.

persistent odontoblasts, located at the periphery of the pulp. Also of mesodermal origin is the *cementum*, a modified form of bone which is fabricated by the cementoblasts and deposited in layers which invest the dentin of the root. Cementum serves as the site of attachment for specialized fibers (the periodontal ligament) that anchor the teeth to the surrounding bone.

Giving vitality to these hard tissues is the *dental pulp*. Of mesodermal origin, it is a well-vascularized connective tissue which contains nerve endings with the capacity to transmit only the sensation of pain. Dental pulp houses the odontoblasts, the cells which secrete dentin matrix (the organic portion within which calcification takes place) and which have the propensity to do so continually as a protective response to minor tooth-directed insults of bacterial, mechanical, thermal, or chemical nature provided the tooth remains vital. As this secondary or separative dentin is laid down, the size of the pulp chamber and canal is progressively narrowed.

Communicating with the pulp and holding the teeth firmly in the alveolar processes of the maxilla and mandible is the specialized fibrous connective tissue, the *periodontal ligament*. Containing cells with multiple developmental potential, this ligament functions as a source of

new cementum and alveolar bone, supports the tooth in its bony socket, and has proprioceptive nerve endings and an ample blood supply.

It is apparent that the structural and supporting dental tissues are in an interdependent, dynamic relationship to one another and as such are sensitive to alterations in their environment. They are, as are all tissues, dependent upon an intact and adequate blood supply, which in turn is dependent upon well-balanced nutrition for maintenance of vitality.

GROWTH AND DEVELOPMENT OF TEETH (ODONTOGENESIS)

The growth and development of teeth are summarized in Figures 17-2 and 17-3 and Table 17-1.

Development of the primary teeth begins at 6 weeks in utero, and by 8 weeks in utero 20 tooth buds are evident. At birth, the established primary dentition continues to calcify, and development of the permanent first molars begins. By 6 months of age, odontogenesis and early calcification of all the permanent anterior teeth, except the upper lateral incisors has taken place. The eruption of the incisors occurs between 6 months and 1 year of age (see Fig. 17-2). The age of eruption will vary with race, sex, nutritional status, and systemic conditions of the child.

Slight deviation from the eruption dates is not cause for concern, since a broad time range is considered normal (see Table 17-1, p. 364). However, a significant delay in tooth eruption may be indicative of a nutritional or endocrine disturbance. Hereditary disorders of tooth and bone development and Down syndrome are among the other possible causes for delay in tooth eruption.

The primary dentition is composed of 20 teeth and is fully erupted by approximately 2 years of age. At 6 years, the permanent teeth begin to erupt, and the full complement of permanent teeth is usually established by 18 to 21 years of age (Fig. 17-3). Sixteen teeth are located in the maxilla and sixteen in the mandible.

Eruption and shedding of primary teeth

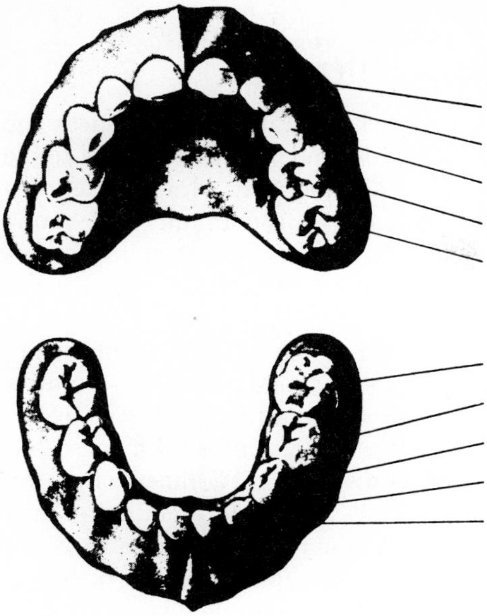

UPPER (MAXILLARY)	APPROXIMATE AGE OF ERUPTION	APPROXIMATE AGE OF SHEDDING
Central incisor	7½ mo.	7½ yr.
Lateral incisor	9 mo.	8 yr.
Cuspid	18 mo.	11½ yr.
First molar	14 mo.	10½ yr.
Second molar	24 mo.	10½ yr.
LOWER (MANDIBULAR)		
Second molar	20 mo.	11 yr.
First molar	12 mo.	10 yr.
Cuspid	16 mo.	9½ yr.
Lateral incisor	7 mo.	7 yr.
Central incisor	6 mo.	6 yr.

Figure 17-2
Eruption and shedding of primary teeth. (Photo courtesy of The New England Disabilities Communication Center.)

Figure 17-3
Eruption of permanent teeth. (Photo courtesy of The New England Disabilities Communication Center.)

Eruption of permanent teeth

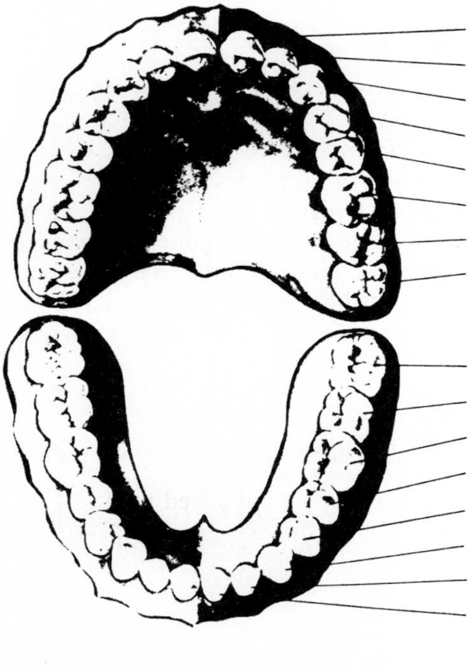

UPPER (MAXILLARY)	
Central incisor	7-8 yr.
Lateral incisor	8-9 yr.
Cuspid	11-12 yr.
First bicuspid	10-11 yr.
Second bicuspid	10-12 yr.
First molar	6-7 yr.
Second molar	12-13 yr.
Third molar	17-21 yr.
LOWER (MANDIBULAR)	
Third molar	17-21 yr.
Second molar	11-13 yr.
First molar	6-7 yr.
Second bicuspid	11-12 yr.
First bicuspid	10-12 yr.
Cuspid	9-10 yr.
Lateral incisor........................	7-8 yr.
Central incisor	6-7 yr.

TABLE 17-1   AGE AND STAGE OF TOOTH DEVELOPMENT

Age	Milestones
6 weeks in utero	Beginning of tooth development
8 weeks in utero	Twenty primary tooth buds present
20 weeks in utero	Beginning of permanent tooth development
16–24 weeks	Beginning of calcification of primary teeth
Birth–6 months	Development and calcification of the permanent first molars and anterior teeth (except the lateral incisors)
1–2 years	Eruption of the primary molars and cuspids
2–6 years	Gradual resorption of roots of primary teeth; continued development and calcification of permanent first molars and anterior teeth; beginning of development and calcification of crowns of permanent bicuspids and second molars
6–8 years	First permanent molars erupt; permanent incisors erupt
6–12 years	First permanent molars erupt; permanent incisors are shed
9–10 years	First biscuspids erupt; second bicuspids erupt
12–13 years	Permanent second molars erupt
18 years on	Permanent third molars erupt

Sources: M. Michael Cohen, *Pediatric Dentistry,* The C. V. Mosby Company, St. Louis, 1961; Tryphena Humphrey, *Pediatrics Digest,* December 1969; Isaac Schour and M. Massler, "The Developemnt of the Human Dentition," *Journal of the American Dental Association,* **28**:1153–1160, 1941.

NUTRITIONAL INFLUENCES ON ORAL HEALTH

The degree to which nutrition influences the oral structures is dependent on the type of tissue and its stage of development. Nutrition is particularly significant to the infant and young child, when most teeth are undergoing formation and calcification. Thereafter, nutritional factors assume a different role, in maintenance and growth of the gingiva, the alveolar bone, and and other periodontal structures. Nutritional deficiencies can affect the oral tissue, manifesting as frank deformities, an increased predisposition to disease, or an alteration of the response to disease. Adequate amounts of calcium, phosphorus, fluoride, and vitamins B, C, A, and D contribute to the formation of sound tooth structure and the maintenance of the oral tissues.

Calcium, Phosphorus, and Vitamin D

Vitamin D influences intestinal absorption of calcium and phosphorus, both components of the crystalline matrix of the teeth. Adequate amounts of these nutrients are therefore essential to tooth formation and calcification (see Chap. 7). However, once formed, teeth are not affected by the presence or absence of calcium or phosphorus in the diet.[1] Should the percentage of available calcium be lowered during development, the result will be enamel hypoplasia and irregular formation of the dentin, despite the fact that dentin receives calcium preferentially over bone.[2] Irregular markings that can be observed in the dentin may document periods of stress and malnutrition. Altered eruption patterns and decreased calcification of alveolar bone are other manifestations of vitamin D deficiency.

Vitamin A

The function of vitamin A is to maintain the integrity of structures of ectodermal origin such as the skin and the cornea (see Chap. 6). In tooth development, vitamin A is necessary for the normal differentiation and function of the ameloblasts, the cells of ectodermal origin that are responsible for enamel formation. Enamel hypoplasia has been reported in severe and prolonged vitamin A deficiency in both experimental animals[3] and in malnourished children.[4] The eruption rate is retarded and, in states of prolonged deficiency, ceases. In addition, the alveolar bone formation is defective, and the gingiva becomes hyperplastic and more susceptible to bacterial invasion.

Vitamin C

The promotion of collagen fibers and maintenance of odontoblastic function are among the basic roles of vitamin C (see Chap. 6). Since the deficiency of vitamin C affects the ability of connective tissue cells to elaborate their collagenous intracellular substances, formation of dentin by the odontoblasts is severely affected. In addition, weakness of the collagen fibers of supporting structures affects the ability of the teeth to withstand stress, resulting in increased mobility and loss. Vitamin C-deficient patients frequently exhibit severe gingivitis with tissue hyperplasia and bleeding. This condition may be affected by an altered response to local irritants. There appears to be an increase in capillary fragility and susceptibility to infection.

Protein

Since protein substances comprise the major organic components of enamel and dentin, states of protein malnutrition can affect the development of teeth. Kwashiorkor, a disease of protein deficiency, is associated with delayed eruption and hypoplasia of deciduous teeth.

B Complex Vitamins

Deficiencies in thiamin, pyridoxine, pantothenic acid, folic acid, and vitamin B_{12} may result in glossitis and stomatitis. Severe deficiencies may present as erosive and ulcerative lesions.

Tongues affected by these deficiencies generally show enlargement due to edema and papillary atrophy. A deficiency of riboflavin may result in angular cheilitis, an irritation of the corners of the mouth that frequently leads to erosion, ulceration, and fissure formation. Vitamin B_{12} and folic acid deficiencies produce anemic states, reflected by the oral soft tissues as generalized pallor and atrophy. These tissues become more susceptible to injury.

Fluoride

The most widely accepted theory concerning the effectiveness of fluoride in decreasing dental caries is that fluoride is incorporated into calcium crystals of the enamel hydroxyapatite, forming fluorapatite. This exchange renders the enamel more resistant to solubility in acid.[5]

$$CA_{10}(PO_4)_6(OH)_2 + 2F^- \longrightarrow$$
Hydroxyapatite fluoride ions

$$Ca_{10}F_2(PO_4)_6 + 2OH^-$$
Fluorapatite hydroxyl ions

Fluoride may also act to suppress the metabolic activity of the oral bacteria that are responsible for dental caries and periodontal disease. In addition, systemic fluoride at optimum levels (1 ppm) has been shown to alter the morphology of the teeth by reducing the depths of the pits and grooves on the occlusal surfaces of molar teeth, thereby reducing the area of mechanical retention of plaque. The use of fluoride is discussed further under "Fluoridation," below.

DENTAL CARIES

Dental caries is a disease characterized by destruction of the enamel, cementum, and dentin. The mechanism appears to be the demineralization of these calcified tissues by organic acid produced by bacteria in dental plaque (see Fig. 17-4).

Dental plaque is generally colorless and

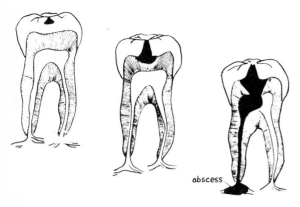

Figure 17-4
The progression of dental caries: (a) into the enamel;
(b) into the dentin; (c) into the pulp (nerve) of a
tooth, resulting in an abscess. (Photo courtesy of The New
England Disabilities Communication Center.)

transparent unless it has absorbed pigment from
foodstuff or is stained with disclosing solution.
The plaque complex adheres to the tooth surface
and can be detached only by mechanical cleaning. It is composed of mixed species of bacteria
which are embedded in an intracellular matrix
formed by bacterial and salivary polymers, epithelial cells, and leukocytes. Bacteria comprise
60 to 70 percent of the total plaque volume, and
this bacterial population is in constant state of
flux as the plaque ages. The change in the bacterial population is due to alteration in the environment of the plaque and to the availability
of factors necessary for the optimal growth of
some bacterial species (Fig. 17-5). Not only does
the composition of plaque change as it grows but
plaque composition also differs depending on its
location in the oral cavity. Thus, plaque found
in the pits and fissures of the occlusal surfaces
may differ greatly from plaque found at the gingival margins.

Certain acidogenic bacteria in dental plaque
such as streptococci and lactobacilli act upon
monosaccharides and disaccharides, producing
lactic acid which decalcifies the enamel. A
plaque pH of 5.5 or lower is necessary for the
initiation of a carious lesion. Pits and fissures on

the tooth surface are the most frequent sites of
caries attack, while smooth surfaces are less susceptible. Should the caries progress through the
enamel and into the dentin, pain may be felt.
Further progression of the carious lesion may
cause degeneration of the pulpal tissue. The
bone surrounding the apex of the root may subsequently be affected.

Studies have shown that carbohydrates are
an essential substrate for bacterial initiation of
dental caries. The decreasing order of cariogenicity of carbohydrates has been demonstrated to
be as follows: sucrose, glucose, maltose, lactose,
fructose, and sorbitol.[6]

Dentists often measure the extent of dental
caries by means of totaling the decayed (D),
missing (M), and filled (F) teeth. This DMF
score is useful as an epidemiologic tool to compare the incidence of dental caries in societies,
groups, or individuals.

Figure 17-5
The interaction between host and environment in the
production of dental caries. (Adapted from P. H. Keyes,
"Present and Future Measures for Dental Caries Control,"
Journal of the American Dental Association, **79:**1395–1404,
1969.)

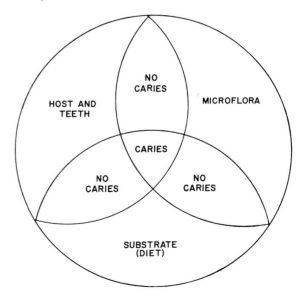

Prevalence

Dental caries appears to be a fairly recent disease. Studies of ancient human skulls reveal that dental caries was a relatively rare finding.[7] Indeed, in some parts of the world today dental caries is an uncommon disease.[8] Conversely, in the United States, dental caries is one of the most prevalent diseases of children. By 10 years of age, 80 percent of children in this country have dental caries, with the greatest carious activity in the primary teeth occurring between the ages of 4 and 8 years, and in the permanent teeth between 12 and 18 years. It has been estimated that the cost of treatment for dental caries in the United States exceeds the cost of treatment for any other single disease.[9]

During the past 10 years, three major surveys of our population have identified dental caries as a nutrition-influenced disease.[10-12]

Consumption of refined carbohydrates is the one significant factor directly correlated with the incidence of dental caries. In adolescent children of all races, the caries index rose progressively as refined carbohydrate in the diet increased. Present estimates now approximate sugar consumption at 100 lb per person per year.

Prevention

The key to treatment lies in the prevention of dental caries by a combined program of diet, fluoridation, and oral hygiene.

Diet

A nutritionally adequate diet of low cariogenicity is necessary for the prevention of dental caries. Sucrose is the most cariogenic sugar and should be restricted.[13] This may present problems of compliance because of the culturally ingrained use of sugar.

The more complex polysaccharides, such as starch, are less cariogenic and can be substituted in the diet for sugar. Starch is a very large molecule, relatively insoluble and practically non-diffusible through dental plaque; these physical and chemical properties of starch make it less caries-conducive.[14] In Guatemalan children fed a high-starch diet, a low caries rate was found. In contrast, neighboring children fed a diet containing sugar were found to have a higher caries rate.[15] However, cooked starch, when present in association with sugar (i.e., bread or cookies), lowers dental plaque pH to the same extent as does sucrose.[16] In vitro studies show that this decreased pH is maintained for a longer period of time; therefore, these starch/sugar products which are popular snack items can be as potentially cariogenic as sucrose.[17]

The frequency of food intake is considered a significant factor in caries formation since the teeth are exposed to acid for a greater length of time with frequent intake. Another factor is the retentiveness (sticky quality) of foods (e.g., peanut butter and jelly sandwiches) which causes them to adhere to the tooth surface. Since snacking is a prevalent American habit, people need information of low-cariogenic snack foods versus high-cariogenic foods. Snacks such as fresh fruit and vegetables, cheese, unsalted nuts, crackers, and popcorn are recommended (see Table 17-2). When consumed, the sugar-containing food should be part of the main meal, and time should be allowed for tooth brushing and the use of dental floss (flossing) afterward. Also, careful consideration should be given to between-meal drinks, since sugary liquids such as soft drinks and juices are frequently consumed between meals. One well-controlled study of children who were provided either 12 oz of a soft drink or water each day for 3 years showed that decay rates were higher in the soft-drink group than in the water group, and that in certain teeth 50 to 150 percent more decay was present.[18] Because of the fact that sweetened fruit juice contains both sugar and acid, feeding fruit juice to infants is not recommended until they can drink by cup, eliminating any possibility of its use in a bottle as a pacifier.[19] Also, sweet drinks and sweetened fruit juices are not recommended between meals for members of any age group.

Noncariogenic sweeteners offer promise for

TABLE 17-2   DIET GUIDELINES TO HELP PREVENT DENTAL CARIES

Avoid foods with high concentrations of sugar, especially the chewy, sticky varieties:

    Candy—especially caramels, gum drops, hard candy, lollipops, Life Savers, breath mints

    Sugar, honey, syrups

    Jams, jellies, preserves

    Marshmallows, marshmallow fluff

    Peanut butter and jelly or marshmallow fluff sandwich

    Cookies, cake, pies

    Sweet rolls, Danish pastry, sugar-coated doughnuts.

    Sugar-coated cereals

    Dried fruits (raisins, prunes, and apricots)

    Tonic, Kool-Aid, Zarex

    Popsicles, ice cream on sticks

    Caramel and taffy-coated apples, caramel-coated popcorn

    Space Food Sticks, Breakfast Bars

    Canned fruit

Eat a well-balanced diet (milk, bread and cereals, fruit and vegetables, protein), especially emphasizing foods with detergent action (such as raw fruits and vegetables):

    Snack foods—cold meats, hard-cooked eggs, cheese, cottage cheese, cheese spreads, raw vegetables (carrots, celery sticks), fresh or water-packed fruits, juices, pretzels, popcorn, unsalted crackers, unsalted nuts

    Dessert—fresh or water-packed fruit, yogurt plain or with added fresh fruit, cheese, and unsalted crackers

Decrease the amount of sugar in the diet and the frequency of eating sugar-containing foods.

Brush—floss—rinse mouth after eating.

Source: Children's Hospital Medical Center, Boston, Mass.

prevention of dental disease, but their long-term effect on the body is, as yet, unknown. Sugarless chewing gums commonly contain sorbitol, a nonnutritive sweetening agent, which appears to be less cariogenic than sucrose.

At present, xylitol is being investigated as a possible sweetening substitute for sucrose and fructose. In Scandinavia, marked caries reduction was observed in volunteers who substituted xylitol for sucrose over a period of 2 years as compared with subjects consuming foods containing sucrose and fructose.[20] The investigators concluded that xylitol was clearly noncariogenic. Further investigation concerning the relative cost and acceptability of xylitol as a sucrose substitute is needed.

Fluoridation

The prophylactic effect of fluorides in the prevention of dental caries has been well established. This effect is greatest during the period of calcification and is best accomplished through the fluoridation of local water supplies. (The benefit of prenatal exposure to fluoride is, however, equivocal.) Consumption of fluoridated water results in a 50 to 65 percent decrease in caries when the fluoride is provided at the optimal level of 1 ppm (1 mg per liter). Approximately 150 million people in more than 30 countries are drinking optimally fluoridated water; of these, 92 million live in the United States.[21]

Acute toxicity from fluorides in the drinking water is technically impossible because of the monitoring devices used in community water departments. One would have to consume 500 gallons of water containing 1 ppm fluoride to arrive at a toxic dose.

Dental fluorosis is caused by the ingestion of excessive amounts of fluorides (greater than 1 ppm of water) during the calcification of the developing teeth. It results in a mottled, opaque enamel which, in some instances, is chalky and crumbles easily. The fluorides usually come from artesian wells located in areas with a naturally high fluoride content.

Fluoride tablets or drops taken in amounts ranging from 0.25 to 1 mg daily provide both a preeruptive (endogenous) and posteruptive (topical) effect. Generally, a 30 percent reduction in tooth decay is produced.[22] Giving fluoride supplements to infants and children has raised concern over excessive intake. The newly recommended dosage schedule (see Table 17-3) allows for differences in age and in fluoride concentration of the community water supply.

Topical fluoride gels applied semiannually

TABLE 17-3 SUPPLEMENTARY FLUORIDE DOSAGE SCHEDULE (mg/day)

	Fluoride in drinking water (ppm)		
Age	<0.03	0.03–0.7	>0.7
2 weeks–2 years	0.25 mg	0	0
2–3 years	0.50 mg	0.25 mg	0
3–16 years	1.00 mg	0.50 mg	0

Source: American Academy of Pediatrics, Committee on Nutrition, "Fluoride Supplementation Revised Dosage Schedule," *Pediatrics,* **63**(1):150, January 1979.

to children's teeth by dentists have repeatedly been demonstrated to produce a 30 to 40 percent reduction in caries. Fluoride mouth rinses are also gaining use as a preventative.

Oral Hygiene

The presence of dental *plaque,* a mass of bacterial colonies surrounded by an intermicrobial matrix, is the most important etiologic factor in the development of dental caries and periodontal disease. Regular plaque removal is very effective

in reducing the prevalence and severity of these oral pathologies. At present, the most effective means for plaque removal are mechanical, such as toothbrushing and dental flossing. Since pellicle and plaque begin to form immediately on a clean tooth surface, thorough and efficient plaque removal is necessary on a daily basis. In addition to personal hygiene measures, professional cleaning is necessary to remove dental calculus and other local irritants.

PERIODONTAL DISEASE

Periodontal disease, a disease which affects the gingiva, bone, and other supporting structures of the teeth,[23] is primarily an inflammatory response to local irritants such as dental plaque, calculus, and food debris (Fig. 17-6). Poor oral hygiene which permits plaque and calculus to accumulate is the major factor responsible for this destructive disease. Food impaction, faulty restorations, missing teeth, mouth-breathing, and the use of tobacco influence the severity of pathologic periodontal conditions. In addition, systemic illnesses such as diabetes, hyper- or hypoparathyroidism, and leukemia alter the re-

Figure 17-6

Progression of periodontal disease: (a) slight calculus deposit; (b) moderate calculus deposit and gingival inflammation; (c) heavy calculus deposit, gingival inflammation, and loss of bony support; (d) advanced disease state with loss of tooth. (Photo courtesy of The New England Disabilities Communication Center.)

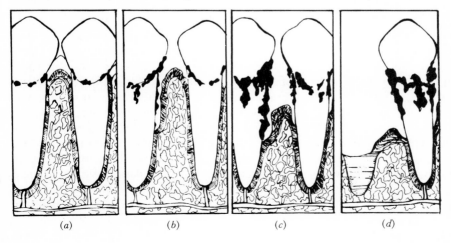

(a) (b) (c) (d)

sponse of the periodontal tissues to local irritants. The role of diet and nutrition in the causation of periodontal disease is ill-defined at present, although it has been demonstrated that the amount and composition of dental plaque and calculus are influenced by the diet.[24,25]

Calculus is a significant pathogenic factor which tends to perpetuate the inflammation of periodontal disease. There are many theories regarding calculus deposition, but none are totally acceptable. According to the physiochemical theory, *calculus* is dental plaque which has undergone calcification and mineralization. Saliva and fluid from the gingival crevice serve as the mineral sources for calcification. Epidemiologic studies of periodontal disease around the world strongly suggest that there is a direct relationship between the amount of plaque and calculus on the tooth surface and the severity of periodontal disease.[26]

In the United States approximately 66 million adults are affected with periodontal disease, and 20 million have lost all their natural teeth as a consequence of this disease.[27] Indeed, periodontal disease is the major cause of tooth loss in persons 35 years of age or older.[28] Although the adult population is the group most affected by periodontal disease, the onset may occur in childhood or puberty.

Prevention

Prevention of periodontal disease is accomplished by efficient removal of dental plaque. At present, the best method of controlling dental plaque formation is mechanical cleansing (flossing, brushing) by the patient. Alteration of the diet may be a necessary adjunct to plaque control.

Diet

The strong relationship of sucrose to plaque formation and consequent periodontal disease would necessitate reducing sucrose in the diet as part of any conscientious prevention program.

Studies have shown that firm or fibrous foods provide the following advantages in promoting good periodontal health:

1 They provide stimulation to the oral soft tissues.
2 They decrease calculus formation.
3 They promote keratinization (hardening of the epithelial tissue surrounding the tooth).

Firm foods (raw fruits, vegetables, and meats) require vigorous chewing, which prevents atrophy and degeneration of the oral hard and soft tissues. Detergent foods (raw fruits and vegetables) act as mechanical cleansers, helping to decrease plaque and calculus formation.[29] These foods promote keratinization by mechanically irritating the epithelium. Dietary treatment for periodontal disease involves:

1 Formulating a well-balanced diet with a reduction of sucrose-containing foods
2 Use of foods with firm consistency
3 Use of detergent foods at the end of a meal or as snacks

Successful prevention of periodontal disease is contingent upon the patient's following these fundamentals of food intake and oral hygiene.

SPECIAL CONCERNS

Bottle Caries Syndrome

Young children who habitually fall asleep while sucking a nursing bottle of juice or milk are candidates for *bottle caries*. During sleep, the rates of sucking, swallowing, and salivary secretion decrease so that carbohydrates present in the juice or milk tend to pool in the oral cavity, remaining in contact with the teeth for a prolonged period of time and promoting the formation of lactic acid. Thus, the caries process is enhanced, and rampant decay of the primary teeth is the result.

To prevent this serious oral health problem, it is recommended that children not be put to bed with a bottle. Should a diagnosis of bottle caries be made, it is imperative that the child's parents be educated about the cause of the disease and given guidance in methods of nontraumatically weaning the child from the bottle (see "Weaning" in Chap. 13).

Oral Hygiene in the Sick and Handicapped

Systemic disease or debilitating conditions may alter the quality and quantity of saliva. Since saliva is normally bacteriostatic, decreased secretion or changes in its chemical composition may permit greater oral bacterial activity, promoting the caries process. The individual who is caring for a debilitated patient must take the responsibility for the patient's oral hygiene by digitally removing debris from the mouth, gently cleansing the oral mucosa and teeth with a moistened gauze sponge, and flushing the oral cavity with noncaustic mouth rinses.

Oral health requirements of the handicapped or mentally retarded child are often superseded by more urgent medical concerns or are neglected because the parents, guardians, or health professionals are reluctant to tackle management-complicating problems such as hypersensitive gag or bite reflexes during the course of dental care. Specialized pedodontic methods are necessary for children with congenital anomalies of the oral cavity and associated structures or for children who have compromised function and coordination as a result of mental retardation syndromes.

Children who are physically incapable of carrying out personal oral hygiene techniques must be given daily custodial oral care. Parents or guardians must monitor the child's diet and must take charge of removing debris from the child's oral cavity by brushing and flossing the child's teeth. For those handicapped children who experience difficulty with a toothbrush, chewing on a cellulose sponge strip with tooth-

paste on both sides can facilitate cleansing. As the child chews, the sponge is forced around tooth surfaces. To ensure cleanliness, the sponge may be boiled after use.[30] Electric tooth brushing is also useful for those patients with inadequate dexterity.

Edentulous Patients

Although many elderly persons are fully or partially edentulous, it is apparent that tooth loss is *not* an age-related phenomenon. Proper nutrition and good oral hygiene, practiced throughout the lifetime of the individual, work in unison to maintain the health and integrity of the oral tissues.

Persons who are edentulous or who wear dentures may have problems with mastication and consequently with deglutition. Compensating for this difficulty, the individual may choose soft foods, such as breads and cereals which lack essential nutrients and fiber. To avoid the risk of inadequate nutrition, vitamin and mineral supplements, bran, and wheat germ may be incorporated into the diet to replace missing nutrients and fiber until the individual seeks dental care.

STUDY QUESTIONS

1 At what age would you expect complete eruption of the primary dentition? Of the permanent dentition?

2 What nutrients affect tooth development and calcification?

3 What factors are necessary for the development of dental caries?

4 Describe the combined program of diet, oral hygiene, and fluoridation that is necessary to prevent dental caries and periodontal disease.

5 What are the special dental concerns for the sick, the handicapped, and the elderly patient?

CLINICAL STUDY 17

Mary, a 2½-year-old child, was brought to the clinic by her mother with the complaint of food refusals and irritability.

The recent medical history revealed that aside from several colds, her overall health was good and she was up to date with her immunizations.

A diet history revealed that Mary was bottle-fed from birth. Baby and junior food additions were well tolerated. At the end of the first year, soft table foods were accepted, but Mary made little progress in moving toward more textured table foods. Increasingly, she became more selective with foods, refusing all that required chewing. Foods taken from the refrigerator and ice cream caused immediate rejection. Milk had to be served at room temperature. Mary's total intake of milk was 40 oz per day. She refused all meats, vegetables, and fruits except applesauce, preferring sugared cereal, spaghetti, and crackers.

The medical examination was normal except for a slight overweight condition, with height at the 50th percentile and weight at the 80th percentile on the NCHS growth grids, and iron deficiency that was revealed by the laboratory report (hemoglobin, 9.69 g

per 100 ml; hematocrit, 31 percent). The upper and lower primary molars were decayed, and a draining fistula above the central incisors was noted. Pain was elicited by touching the decayed teeth. Otherwise, the remaining teeth were noncarious, and the oral mucosa of the lips, cheek, tongue, floor of the mouth, and palate was within normal limits.

The diagnoses of bottle-caries syndrome, iron-deficiency anemia, and a slight overweight condition were made. The patient was referred to the dentist for extractions and restorative work and to the nutritionist for counseling and advice on weaning and on a diet suitable for Mary's age that would control weight and include proper foods.

Clinical study questions

1   What are the factors that have led to the development of bottle caries syndrome?

2   On the basis of the diet history, identify the missing nutrients. What are your recommendations for diet?

3   How could this have been prevented?

REFERENCES

1   A. Nizel, *Nutrition in Preventive Dentistry: Science and Practice,* W. B. Saunders Company, Philadelphia, 1960, p. 103.

2   Ibid., p. 104.

3   M. Goodhart and R. Shils, *Modern Nutrition in Health and Disease,* Lea and Febiger, Philadelphia, 1973, p. 740.

4   E. A. Sweeney et al., "Linear Hypoplasia of Deciduous Incisor Teeth in Malnourished Children," *American Journal of Clinical Nutrition,* 24:29, 1971.

5   F. Brudevold et al., "The Chemistry of Caries Inhibition: Problems and Challenges in Topical Treatments," *Journal of Dental Research,* 46:37–45, 1967.

6   E. Newbrun, "Sucrose, the Arch Criminal of Dental Caries," *Journal of Dentistry for Children,* 35:239, 1969.

7   L. I. Falin, "Histological and Histochemical Studies

of Human Teeth of the Bronze and Stone Age," *Archives of Oral Biology,* 5:5–13, September 1961.

8   A. L. Russell, "International Nutrition Surveys: A Summary of Preliminary Dental Findings," *Journal of Dental Research,* 42:233–244, 1963.

9   W. O. Young and D. F. Striffler, *The Dentist, His Practice and the Community,* W. B. Saunders Company, Philadelphia, 1969, p. 73.

10   *Ten State Nutrition Survey 1968–1970. V. Dietary,* U.S. Department of Health, Education, and Welfare, Publication (HSM) 72-8133, 1970.

11   G. Owen et al., "A Study of the Nutritional Status of Pre-School Children in the United States 1968–1970," *Pediatrics,* 54:597–646, 1974.

12   "Plan and Operation of the HANES (Health and Nutrition Examination Survey)," in *Vital and Health Statistics,* ser. 1, no. 10a, 10b, U.S. Depart-

ment of Health, Education, and Welfare, Public Health Service, Health Resources Administration, National Center for Health Statistics, February 1973.

13 Newbrun, op. cit., p. 239.

14 A. Nizel, op. cit., p. 36.

15 W. J. Loesche and C. A. Henry, "Intracellular Microbial Polysaccharide Production and Dental Caries in a Guatemalan Indian Village," *Archives of Oral Biology,* **12**:189–194, 1967.

16 I. Kleinberg and G. N. Jenkins, "Further Studies in the Effect of Carbohydrate Substrates on Plaque in Vivo," *Journal of Dental Research,* **38**:704, 1959.

17 T. G. Ludwig and B. G. Bibby, "Acid Production from Different Carbohydrate Foods in Plaque and Saliva," *Journal of Dental Research,* **36**:56–60, 1957.

18 A. D. Steinberg et al., "The Lincoln Dental Caries Study II. The Effect of Acidulated Carbonated Beverages on the Incidence of Dental Caries," *Journal of the American Dental Association,* **85**:81–89, 1972.

19 S. J. Fomon et al., "Recommendations for Feeding Normal Infants," *Pediatrics,* **63**:52–59, 1979.

20 A. Scheinin et al., "Turku Sugar Studies I. An Intermediate Report on the Effect of Sucrose, Fructose and Xylitol on the Caries Incidence in Man," *Acta Odontologica Scandinavica,* **32**:383–412, 1974.

21 J. M. Dunning, "Current Status of Fluoridation," *New England Journal of Medicine,* **27**:30–34, 84–88, 1965.

22 F. Brudevold, et al., op. cit., pp. 37–45.

23 *Research Explores Pyorrhea and Other Gum Diseases: Periodontal Disease,* U.S. Public Health Service Publication no. 1482, 1970.

24 J. Carlsson and J. Egelberg, "Effect of Diet on Early Plaque Formation in Man," *Odontologisk Revy,* **16**:112, 1965.

25 Bernier and Muhler, *Improving Dental Practice Through Preventive Measures,* The C. V. Mosby Company, St. Louis, 1971.

26 H. Loe, E. Theelache, and S. B. Jensen, "Experimental Gingivitis in Man," *Journal of Pedodontia,* **36**:177, 1965.

27 *Research Explores Pyorrhea,* op. cit.

28 H. M. Goldman, "Prevalence of Periodontal Disease in the United States," *International Dental Journal,* **5**:458, 1955.

29 A. Nizel, op. cit., pp. 372–374.

30 The New England Developmental Disabilities Communication Center, *Home Dental Care for the Handicapped Child,* Children's Hospital Center, Boston, Mass., 1976, p. 10.

CLINICAL DISCUSSION 17

The stagnation of milk, fruit juice, or sweetened beverages (Kool-Aid, cola) around Mary's teeth for a 10-h sleep interval led to lactic acid production and the subsequent destruction of the tooth structure, known as bottle-caries syndrome. Although brushing the teeth is not started before the third year of life because of the thin oral mucosa, Mary's parents could have cleansed her teeth with gauze pads to remove the plaque and prevent the problem.

Mary was 2½ and drinking well from a cup but, because of overdependency, continued to take a bottle to bed at nap and bedtime. Water was advised as a replacement for the milk in the bottle, along with a gradual reduction in the frequency of bottles. Milk was curtailed to 24 oz, given only by cup. Since Mary would only take milk from her bottle, an alternative source of calcium and phosphorus (yogurt, cheese) and the addition of small amounts of evaporated milk and dried milk solids to soups and puddings had to be utilized during this immediate period of adjustment. Because Mary refused vegetables, meats, and fruits, her diet was low in iron, folic acid, vitamin C, and zinc.

Iron medication was prescribed, and Mary's parents were given suggestions about including easy-to-chew foods containing the missing nutrients and about excluding sugar-containing ones. They were also counseled regarding food behavior problems, weight control, and the hazards of leaving the iron medication within easy reach of the child. They were advised to give the iron medication through a straw in order to prevent tooth stains.

Mary was scheduled for periodic dental visits at 6-month intervals, and topical fluoride treatments were given; a fluoride-containing toothpaste was recommended. She continued to take iron medication for the next 6 months, and during her well-child visits her parents periodically met with the nutritionist.

CHAPTER 18

THE EVALUATION OF NUTRITIONAL STATUS

Nancy S. Wellman

KEY WORDS
Nutritional Status
24-Hour Recall
Nutrition History
Problem-Oriented Medical Record (POMR)

The general term *nutritional status* describes one's overall state of nutrition. It is defined by Christakis (1973) as the "health condition of an individual as influenced by his intake and utilization of nutrients, determined from the correlation of information obtained from physical, biochemical, clinical, and dietary studies."

Assessment procedure levels are related to the nutritional needs of the individual and are somewhat influenced by the setting in which the evaluation takes place. Patients' dietary needs in long-term care facilities (nursing homes, psychiatric hospitals, etc.) may differ considerably from those in acute care facilities (hospital burn units, intensive care units, etc.) or from those seen in ambulatory care facilities [health departments, private offices, group sessions (weight control groups, community schools, health spas, etc)]. Thus an accurate screening, intervention, and monitoring process must be based upon appropriateness for the individual in relation to accepted standards of quality care. Tables 18-1 through 18-5 (pp. 375–381) provide levels of approach based upon age. Combinations of these levels of approach may be employed to best assess nutritional status of an individual or group at nutritional risk.

There is no single rapid reliable test which measures nutritional status. It is currently accepted that a true assessment of nutritional status requires collection of four types of data, *anthropometric, biochemical, clinical, and dietary* (see Fig. 18-1, p. 382). An unacceptable or deficient finding in any single area, such as short stature or a low serum ascorbic acid level, is not indicative of malnutrition per se. Detection of subclinical malnutrition remains difficult because of complexities in the definition of "optimal nutrition." Also, the progressive nature of deficiency diseases (from desaturation of blood stores, to a lesion at the molecular level, to the overt clinical lesion), the side range of individual nutrient requirements, the general inability of biochemical tests to assess body stores, and the lack of comparative standards further compound the problem. Therefore determination of nutritional status is dependent upon assessments of the total individual.

TABLE 18-1 LEVELS OF NUTRITIONAL ASSESSMENT FOR INFANTS AND CHILDREN

Level of approach*	History		Clinical evaluation	Laboratory evaluation
	Dietary	*Medical and socioeconomic*		
		For birth to 24 months		
Minimal level	1. Source of iron 2. Vitamin supplement 3. Milk intake (type and amount)	1. Birth weight 2. Length of gestation 3. Serious or chronic illness 4. Use of medicines	1. Body weight and length 2. Gross defects	1. Hematocrit 2. Hemoglobin
Mid-level	1. Semiquantitative (a) Iron-cereal, meat egg yolks, supplement (b) Energy nutrients (c) Micronutrients—calcium, niacin, riboflavin, vitamin C (d) Protein 2. Food intolerances 3. Baby foods—processed commercially; home-cooked	1. Family history: Diabetes Tuberculosis 2. Maternal: Height-weight Prenatal care 3. Infant: Immunizations Tuberculin test	1. Head circumference 2. Skin color, pallor, turgor 3. Subcutaneous tissue paucity, excess	1. RBC morphology 2. Serum iron 3. Total iron binding capacity 4. Sickle cell testing
In-depth level	1. Quantitative 24-h recall 2. Dietary history	1. Prenatal details 2. Complications of delivery 3. Regular health supervision	1. Cranial bossing 2. Epiphyseal enlargement 3. Costochondral beading 4. Ecchymoses	Same as above, plus vitamin and appropriate enzyme assays; protein and amino acids; hydroxyproline, etc., should be available
		For ages 2 to 5 years		
	Determine amount of intake	Probe about pica; medications	Add height at all levels Add arm circumference at all levels Add triceps skinfolds at in-depth level	Add serum lead at mid-level Add serum micronutrients (vitamins A, C, folate, etc.) at in-depth level
		For ages 6 to 12 years		
	Probe about snack foods Determine whether salt intake is excess	Ask about medications taken; drug abuse	Add blood pressure at mid-level Add description of changes in tongue, skin, eyes for in-depth level	All of above plus BUN

*It is understood that what is included at a minimal level would also be included or represented at successively more sophisticated levels of approach. However, it may be entirely appropriate to use a minimal level of approach to clinical evaluations and a maximal approach to laboratory evaluations.

Source: G. Christakis, "Nutritional Assessment in Health Programs," *American Journal of Public Health,* **63**, part 2, November 1973.

TABLE 18-2   LEVELS OF NUTRITIONAL ASSESSMENT FOR ADOLESCENTS

Level of approach	History		Clinical evaluation	Laboratory evaluation
	Dietary	*Medical and socioeconomic*		
Minimal level	1. Frequency of use of food groups 2. Habits-patterns 3. Snacks 4. Socioeconomic status	1. Previous diseases and allergies 2. Abbreviated system review 3. Family history	1. Height 2. Weight	1. Urine, protein and sugar 2. Hemoglobin
Mid-level	1. Above 2. Qualitative estimate 3. 24-hour recall	1. Above in more detail	1. Above 2. Arm circumference 3. Skinfold thickness 4. External appearance	1. Above 2. Blood taken by vein for albumin (serum), serum iron and TIBC; vitamins A and beta carotene; RBC indices; blood urea nitrogen (BUN); cholesterol; zinc
In-depth level	1. Above 2. Quantitative estimate by recall (3–7 days)	1. Above	1. Above 2. Per ICNND Manual 3. X-ray of wrist and bone density	1. Above 2. Blood tests: folate and vitamin C; alkaline phosphatase; RBC transketolase; RBC glutathione; lipids 3. Urine: creatinine; nitrogen; zinc; thiamin; robflavin; loading tests (xanthurenic acid/FIGLU) 4. Hair root: DNA; protein; zinc; other metals

Source: G. Christakis, "Nutritional Assessment in Health Programs," *American Journal of Public Health,* **63**, part 2, November 1973.

TABLE 18-3 LEVELS OF NUTRITIONAL ASSESSMENT FOR ADULTS

Level of approach	History — Dietary	History — Medical and socioeconomic	Clinical evaluation	Laboratory Evaluation

Minimal level	Present food habits
	Meal patterns
	"Empty calories"
	Dietary supplements
		Name, age, sex
		Address
		Socioeconomic level
		Number in family
		Brief medical
		  history (including
		  family)
			Height and weight
			Blood pressure
				Hemoglobin
				A simplified Dipstix
				  evaluation which
				  would identify
				  presence of protein
				  and glucose in
				  blood, urinary pH

Mid-level	Semiquantitative
	  determination of
	  food intake
		Sequential history
		  Present health,
		  past history,
		  review of
		  systems,
		  family history,
		  social history
		  (e.g., Cornell
		  Medical Index)
		  Smoking history
			Anthropometric
			  measurements
			  (skinfold thickness,
			  etc.)
			Brief examination by
			  M.D. or physician's
			  assistant
			Chest x-ray as
			  indicated
				Evaluations for
				  serum cholesterol,
				  vitamin A, vitamin
				  C, and folic acid
				Urine excretion for
				  thiamin

In-depth level	Household survey
	  data
	Quantitative 24-
	  h recall
	Dietary history
	Diet patterns as they
	  might influence
	  lipogenic
	  characteristics
		All of the above
		Personal interview
		  by physician
		Family history of
		  cardiovascular
		  disease
			Comprehensive health
			  status evaluation by an
			  appropriate health
			  team, by or under
			  supervision of a
			  physician
				Serum triglyceride
				  level, plus those
				  nutrients in mid-
				  level
				Urine or serum
				  evaluation of
				  pyridoxine status
				  (vitamin B_6,
				  nutriture)
				Evaluation of
				  protein nutriture by
				  height, weight, and
				  chronological age
				  indices
				Serum essentials and
				  nonessential amino
				  acid ratios
				Evaluation of
				  vitamin B_{12}
				  nutriture by serum
				  analysis
				Serum iron and
				  serum iron binding
				  capacity
				Adipose tissue
				  aspiration and fatty
				  acid analysis by
				  gas-liquid
				  chromatography

Source: G. Christakis, "Nutritional Assessment in Health Programs," *American Journal of Public Health,* **63**, part 2, November 1973.

TABLE 18-4   LEVELS OF MATERNAL NUTRITIONAL ASSESSMENT

Level of approach	History		Clinical evaluation	Laboratory evaluation
	Dietary	Medical and socioeconomic		
Minimal	Present basic diet; meal patterns; fad or abnormal diets; supplements	Obstetrical: Age: parity; interval between pregnancies; previous obstetrical history. Medical: Intercurrent diseases and illnesses; drug use; smoking history. Family and social: Size of family; "wanted" pregnancy; socioeconomic status	Pre-pregnancy weight; weight gain pattern during pregnancy; signs and symptoms of gross nutritional deficiencies	Hemoglobin; hematocrit
Mid-level	The above, plus semiquantitative determination of food intake	The above, plus occupational patterns; utilization of maternity care and family planning services	The above, plus screening for intercurrent disease	The above, plus blood smear; RBC indices; serum iron; sickle preparation
In-depth level	The above, plus household survey data; dietary history; quantitative 24-h recall		The above, plus special anthropometric measurements of skinfold, arm circumference, etc.	The above, plus folate and other vitamin levels

Source: G. Christakis, "Nutritional Assessment in Health Programs," *American Journal of Public Health,* **63**, part 2, November 1973.

TABLE 18-5 LEVELS OF NUTRITIONAL ASSESSMENT FOR THE ELDERLY

Level of approach	History		Clinical evaluation	Laboratory evaluation
	Dietary	*Medical and socioeconomic*		
Minimal level	1. Meals eaten per day, week; regularity	1. Chronic illness and/or disability; occupational hazard exposure; use of tobacco, alcohol, drugs	1. Height and weight; cachexia; obesity	1. Hemoglobin
	2. Frequency of ingestion of protective foods (four food groups)	2. Symptoms such as bleeding, fainting, loss of memory, dyspnea, headache, pain, changed bowel and/or bladder habits, altered sight and/or hearing, condition of teeth, and/or dentures	2. Blood pressure, pulse rate and rhythm	2. Blood and/or urine sugar
	3. Supplemental vitamins, protein concentrates, mineral mixes	3. Therapy (prescribed or self-administered) such as drugs, alcohol, vitamins, food fads, prescription items, eyeglasses, hearing aids	3. Pallor, skin color and texture	3. Urinalysis (color, odor, bile and sediment by gross inspection; pH, glucose, albumin blood, and ketones by stick test
	4. General knowledge of nutrition, sources of information	4. Names, addresses, and phone numbers of persons providing medical or health care; close family or friends	4. Condition of teeth and/or dentures and oral hygiene	4. Feces (color, texture, gross blood; occult blood by guaiac test)
		5. Lives alone, with spouse, or companion	5. Affect during interview and examination	
		6. Sources of income	6. Vision and hearing appraised subjectively and objectively by examiner	
			7. Any gross evidence of neglect	

(Continued)

TABLE 18-5 CONTINUED

Level of approach	History		Clinical evaluation	Laboratory evaluation
	Dietary	Medical and socioeconomic		
Mid-level*	In addition to the above: 1. Food preferences and rejections 2. Overt food fads 3. Meal preparation facilities and knowledge 4. Food budget 5. Usual daily diet: Protective foods (meats, dairy products, fruits and vegetables, cereals); nutrients (protein, fat, carbohydrates, iron, water- and fat-soluble vitamins, minerals, trace elements, and water); empty-calorie food (alcohol, candy, sucrose)	In addition to the above: 1. Family history of spouse, parents and siblings, other relatives, persons living in same household 2. Pain: Location, frequency, character, duration 3. Mental hygiene: Attitudes, fears prejudices, symptoms of psychoses, possible psychosomatic symptoms and signs. 4. Income: Amount and adequacy for nutrition, housing health, utilities, clothing, transportation, etc.	In addition include: 1. Head and neck examinations (otoscopic, ophthalmoscopic, dental and oral cavity, nose and throat) 2. Chest (inspection, palpation, auscultation and percussion, bimanual examination of breast tissue) 3. Abdomen (inspection, auscultation, percussion, and palpation) 4. Rectal and pelvic 5. Inspection and palpation of extremities (evaluation for temperature, edema, pulse, discoloration, ulcers) 6. Gross neurological evaluation; motor and sensory	In addition include: 1. Serum lipids (including β-lipoproteins) 2. Serum iron and iron binding capacity 3. Urinalysis 4. Electrocardiogram 5. Peripheral blood smear for differential white blood cell count and red cell morphology 6. Chest film 7. Post-voiding residual urine by catheterization (if indicated)
In-depth level*	In addition include: 1. 24-hour dietary recall, preferably for each of several widely separated days; analysis of nutrient intake; evaluation of adequacy, e.g., relate to activity, body weight, laboratory data, affect, etc. 2. History of past and present food preparation and practices 3. History of dining practices and facilities, including companionship	In addition include: 1. System review 2. Social history 3. Economic history including specifics on sources and amounts of income 4. Mental evaluation (attitudes toward aging)	If indicated, include: 1. Complete sensory and motor neurologic examination 2. Sigmoidoscopy 3. Ophthalmologic examination (ophthalmoscopic examination with pupils dilated, refraction, dark adaptation, color perception, visual field examination) 4. Audiometry	If indicated, include: 1. Serum total protein and albumin; serum creatinine and/or blood urea nitrogen (BUN) 2. Roentgenographic evaluation of bones and joints suspected of being fractured, harboring infection, and affected by rheumatic and/or metabolic bone disease and/or metastatic or primary neoplastic disease 3. Glucose tolerance tests

4. Blood and/or urine vitamin assays for water-soluble and fat-soluble vitamins

5. Trace element assays of blood, urine, and/or tissue

6. Kidney-ureter-bladder (KUB) film for stones in urinary tract or gallbladder

7. Bacteriologic cultures of any chronic infections

8. Barium enema, upper gastrointestinal series, gallbladder series and intravenous pyelography

9. Fluoroscopy of chest

10. Angiography for coronary arteries, aorta, peripheral vessels

11. Bone marrow for unexplained anemia

12. Renal clearance studies

13. Histologic evaluation of biopsies of tissue suspected of being neoplastic

*The aged, quite unlike children and youth, are the end result of lifetimes of physiologic aging, diseases, and disabilities and cannot be evaluated as if they belonged to younger cohorts. In the above table, it is assumed that mid-level evaluation procedures may be carried out in ambulatory care settings and that in-depth level procedures may be conducted as hospital or research procedures. The placement of these in actual practice will depend on availability of facilities and personnel.

Source: G. Christakis, "Nutritional Assessment in Health Programs," American Journal of Public Health, 63, part 2, November 1973.

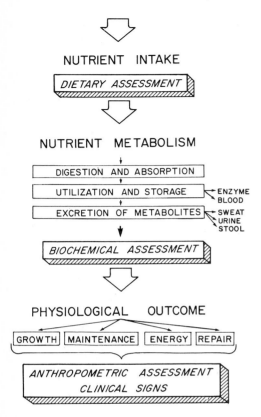

Figure 18-1
The evaluation of nutritional status includes dietary, biochemical, anthropometric, and clinical assessment.

ANTHROPOMETRIC METHODS

Taking body measurements constitutes a relatively simple assessment procedure that is useful in nutritional screening. Since physical measurements are partially dependent upon nutrient intake, they are of help in assessing nutritional status. In children, a fall-off or an acceleration in the rate of gain in both height and weight is a sensitive indicator of malnutrition (which may be due to either inadequate or excessive food intake) and of underlying disease conditions. In adults, weight is a useful indicator of change.

In addition to food intake, genetic and environmental factors influence growth and devel-

opment. However, nutrition is one of the critical factors, as evidenced by a significant dissimilarity in the growth of children in developed versus developing countries where there are differences in the availability of food.

Longitudinal measurements provide a system for monitoring nutrient effectiveness in infants, children, and adolescents, particularly when plotted on percentile curves. With care, measurements of body size, height, weight, and skinfold thickness can be taken efficiently and accurately. Standardized equipment and procedures should be used (see Chap. 13).

BIOCHEMICAL METHODS

Laboratory techniques have been developed to determine levels of various nutrients in the blood and urine and to examine some metabolic functions that depend on an adequate intake of certain nutrients. Such tests provide an objective means of monitoring aspects of nutritional status. The purpose of laboratory assessments is to detect subclinical deficiencies prior to the onset of overt clinical signs in order to allow early intervention for those at risk.

Blood constituents include nutritional, excretory, and intrinsic (functional) substances. *Nutritional substances* are either nutrients absorbed from the intestinal tract or intermediate products being transported for cellular utilization elsewhere. Examples include amino acids, glucose, minerals, vitamins, lipids, lactic acid, pyruvic acid, creatinine, and circulating hormones. Homeostasis controls their concentrations, which are therefore fairly stable under basal conditions. *Excretory substances* are en route for elimination by the kidneys, lungs, or liver. Examples include carbon dioxide, creatinine, urea, bilirubin, and some enzymes such as amylase and phosphatase. Normal concentrations may be influenced by food intake (urea), breakdown rate (bilirubin), or bodily content (creatinine). *Intrinsic* or *functional substances* are inherent fundamental blood components such as hemoglobin, glutathione, adenosine triphosphate (ATP), plasma proteins, fibrinogen, some minerals, hydrogen ions, and cations. They exhibit a narrow range of normal concentration, as in the case of electrolytes.

Three stages of gradual depletion take place in the body when nutrient intake is deficient over a prolonged period:

First, the nutrient or its metabolites are homeostatically conserved by a slight decrease in the urinary excretion level or the plasma concentration.

Second, tissue concentration and storage forms are reduced.

Third, as the internal nutrient supply is exhausted, clinical symptoms appear.

When considering the *normalcy* of circulating nutrient levels, it should be recognized that, in general, urinary excretion levels fluctuate more than plasma levels and reflect immediate rather than usual intake. Most circulating nutrient levels are not indicators of storage quantities. For example, a urinary ascorbic acid level is directly related to recent dietary intake and is, therefore, an unreliable indicator of nutritional status. On the other hand, some tests, such as serum protein, may reflect long-term dietary influences.

Tests which measure a step in the metabolism or use of a nutrient are commonly referred to as *functional tests*. They usually provide more sensitive indications of nutritional status. Measuring the erythrocyte activity of transketolase to determine thiamin status and measuring the level of glutathione reductase in red blood cells as a test of riboflavin are two examples of these newer, indirect, more specfic functional laboratory tests. For other nutrients (e.g., iron), the actual storage form level (ferritin) can now be determined. As standards are developed, early identification of decreasing levels of storage forms will aid in identifying inadequate dietary intakes, absorption, or utilization of specific nutrients. Depletion of some nutrients, such as water-soluble vitamins, is accurately reflected in

diminished plasma levels because the total body content is normally low in relation to utilization.

Attempts to find a single specific biochemical test to measure nutritional status have been unsuccessful. Some laboratory tests, such as the hydroxyproline index (urinary hydroxyproline to creatinine ratio), have no clear advantage over height and weight as an indicator of nutritional status. The biochemical tests that are chosen depend upon the situation. For a hospitalized patient, several routine laboratory procedures are readily available which can provide valuable information when integrated with data concerning the patient's condition and medicinal intake. Such tests include serum protein and albumin, creatinine and creatinine-height index, serum iron, transferrin saturation, plasma ascorbate, serum electrolytes, etc. The recoveries and/or lengths of stay of hospitalized patients are frequently compromised as a result of preexisting malnutrition caused by problems unrelated to food availability, such as anorexia, sepsis, gastrointestinal dysfunction, and various disease states. Laboratory analyses of serum albumin and total iron-binding capacity (TIBC) assess visceral protein; total white cell count, white blood cell differential, and specific skin antigen testing are useful in evaluating immune response (see Chap. 16). Iatrogenic malnutrition during hospitalization or institutionalization is a very real risk. Table 18-6 (p. 384) lists predisposing conditions which warrant close nutritional surveillance including periodic laboratory analyses.

In large-scale screening surveys, the laboratory analyses that are chosen should measure those nutrients which are suspected or known to be marginally available to the population group under investigation. For example, the high prevalence of iron-deficiency anemia among preschool children mandates measurement of iron, preferably in its storage form, for that population group.

Interpretation of biochemical data is not without problems. Assuming adequate laboratory quality control, neither dietary nor clinical findings may correlate with the laboratory find-

TABLE 18-6 CONDITIONS RESULTING IN NUTRITIONAL FAILURE

1. *Inadequate intake—quantity*
   Mechanical feeding problems or undeveloped feeding skills
   Anorexia (due to emotional problems, disease process, drugs)

2. *Inadequate intake—quality*
   Education of parents or caretaker
   Institutionalized setting
   Poor food habits
   Allergies

3. *Increased metabolism*
   Fever
   Infections
   Malignancy
   Hyperthyroidism
   Athetosis
   Surgery, stress, burns

4. *Increased loss*
   Vomiting
   Diarrhea
   Decreased food transit time through the gut

5. *Defective utilization*
   Metabolic diseases (aminoacidopathies, galactosemia, lipidoses)
   Disturbed metabolic states (hepatic insufficiency, renal tubular acidosis, nephrogenic diabetes insipidus, adrenal cortical hyperplasia with salt loss)
   Drug interference with nutrients

6. *Defective absorption*
   Intrinsic disease states (regional enteritis, Hirschsprung's disease)
   Exogenous states (intestinal parasitosis, celiac disease, surgical removal of the small bowel)
   Drugs

7. *Defects in the function of major organ systems*
   Severe congenital heart disease
   Severe chest disease
   Severe liver disease
   Kidney disease
   Brain damage

8. *Excessive food or vitamin intake*
   Obesity
   Vitamin intoxication—fat-soluble vitamins

ings. As previously indicated, reproducibility and reliability of results may be difficult to achieve even with one individual because of the relationship of findings to current dietary intake rather than to actual nutritional status. Coexisting illnesses, malabsorption, medications, and diurnal variation may also obscure results. Moreover, the classification of *normal* biochemical levels is not universally agreed upon. Standards for the lower limits of hemoglobin in children which indicate anemia vary between 10 and 12 g per 100 mL. Because hemoglobin levels may decrease because of protein insufficiency, the test is nonspecific for iron intake. Thus, immunoassays of serum ferritin are more valuable in detecting dietary deficiencies of iron. For some nutrients, normal limits are arbitrary decisions awaiting more sophisticated, specific laboratory procedures. Current guidelines for the interpretation of laboratory data for various nutrients are provided in Table 18-7.

Individuals can also be at nutritional risk for certain nutrients which can accumulate to toxic levels in the body. Blood levels of vitamin A greater than 100 mg per 100 mL are indicative of hypervitaminosis A. Vitamin D toxicity is evidenced by hypercalcemia (more than 12 mg per 100 mL).

CLINICAL METHODS

It is interesting to note that classical signs of malnutrition are practically nonexistent. Classic physical signs of deficiency disorders occur late in the continuum of events associated with malnutrition. Such signs of malnutrition may be nonspecific because they are often caused by multiple nutrient deficiencies or by nonnutritional factors such as poor hygiene or excessive sun exposure. Generally a malnourished person has multiple nutrient deficiencies. A clinical diagnosis alone is inadequate, and other nutritional status assessments (biochemical, anthropometric, dietary) must be given consideration. However, direct correlations may not be evident. For the diagnosis of mild deficiency, the clinical examination is ineffective. The low general

TABLE 18-7 CURRENT GUIDELINES FOR CRITERIA OF NUTRITIONAL STATUS FOR LABORATORY EVALUATION

Nutrient and units	Age of subject, years	Criteria of status		
		Deficient	Marginal	Acceptable
Hemoglobin* (g/100 mL)	6–23 months	Up to 90	9.0–9.9	10.0+
	2–5	Up to 100	10.0–10.9	11.0+
	6–12	Up to 100	10.0–11.4	11.5+
	13–16M	Up to 120	12.0–12.9	13.0+
	13–16F	Up to 100	10.0–11.4	11.5+
	16 + M	Up to 120	12.0–13.9	14.0+
	16 + F	Up to 100	10.0–11.9	12.0+
	Pregnant (after 6+ months)	Up to 95	9.5–10.9	11.0+
Hematocrit* (packed cell volume in percent)	Up to 2	Up to 28	28–30	31+
	2–5	Up to 30	30–33	34+
	6–12	Up to 30	30–35	36+
	13–16M	Up to 37	37–39	40+
	13–16F	Up to 31	31–35	36+
	16+ M	Up to 37	37–43	44+
	16+ F	Up to 31	31–37	33+
	Pregnant	Up to 30	30–32	33+
Serum albumin* (g/100 mL)	Up to 1	. . . .	Up to 2.5	2.5+
	1–5	. . . .	Up to 3.0	3.0+
	6–16	. . . .	Up to 3.5	3.5+
	16+	Up to 2.8	2.8–3.4	3.5+
	Pregnant	Up to 3.0	3.0–3.4	3.5+
Serum protein* (g/100 mL)	Up to 1	. . . .	Up to 5.0	5.0+
	1–5	. . . .	Up to 5.5	5.5+
	6–16	. . . .	Up to 6.0	6.0+
	16+	Up to 6.0	6.0–6.4	6.5+
	Pregnant	Up to 5.5	5.5–5.9	6.0+
Serum ascorbic acid* (mg/100 mL)	All ages	Up to 0.1	0.1–0.19	0.2+
Plasma vitamin A* (µg/100 mL)	All ages	Up to 10	10–19	20+
Plasma carotene* (µg/100 mL)	All ages	Up to 20	20–39	40+
	Pregnant	. . . .	40–79	80+
Serum iron* (µg/100 mL)	Up to 2	Up to 30	. . . .	30+
	2–5	Up to 40	. . . .	40+
	6–12	Up to 50	. . . .	50+
	12+M	Up to 60	. . . .	60+
	12+F	Up to 40	. . . .	40+
Transferrin saturation* (percent)	Up to 2	Up to 15.0	. . . .	15.0+
	2–12	Up to 20.0	. . . .	20.0+
	12+M	Up to 20.0	. . . .	20.0+
	12+F	Up to 15.0	. . . .	15.0+
Serum ferritin† (ng/mL)	16+M			77+
	16+F			36+

*†See notes on following page.

(Continued)

TABLE 18-7 CONTINUED

Nutrient and units	Age of subject, years	Criteria of status		
		Deficient	Marginal	Acceptable
Serum folacin† (ng/mL)	All ages	Up to 2.0	2.1–5.9	6.0+
Serum vitamin B_{12}† (ng/mL)	All ages	Up to 100	. . . .	100+
Thiamin in urine* (µg/g creatinine)	1–3	Up to 120	120–175	175+
	4–5	Up to 85	85–120	120+
	6–9	Up to 70	70–180	180+
	10–15	Up to 55	55–150	150+
	16+	Up to 27	27–65	65+
	Pregnant	Up to 21	21–49	50+
Riboflavin in urine* (µg/g creatinine)	1–3	Up to 150	150–499	500+
	4–5	Up to 100	100–299	300+
	6–9	Up to 85	85–269	270+
	10–16	Up to 70	70–199	200+
	16+	Up to 27	27–79	80+
	Pregnant	Up to 30	30–89	90+
RBC transketolase-TPP-effect† (ratio)	All ages	25+	15–25	Up to 15
RBC glutathione reductase-FAD-effect† (ratio)	All ages	1.2+	. . . .	Up to 1.2
Tryptophan load† (mg xanthurenic acid excreted)	Adults (Dose: 100 mg/kg body weight)	25+ (6 h) 75+ (24 h)	. . . .	Up to 25 Up to 75
Urinary pyridoxine† (µg/g creatinine)	1–3	Up to 90	. . . .	90+
	4–6	Up to 80	. . . .	80+
	7–9	Up to 60	. . . .	60+
	10–12	Up to 40	. . . .	40+
	13–15	Up to 30	. . . .	30+
	16+	Up to 20	. . . .	20+
Urinary N-methyl nicotinamide* (mg/g creatinine)	All ages	Up to 0.2	0.2–5.59	6.0+
	Pregnant	Up to 0.8	0.8–2.49	2.5+
Urinary pantothenic acid† (µg)	All ages	Up to 200	. . . .	200+
Plasma vitamin E† (mg/100 mL)	All ages	Up to 0.2	0.2–0.6	0.6+
Transaminase index† (ratio)				
SGOT‡	Adult	2.0+	. . . .	Up to 2.0
SGPT§	Adult	1.25+	. . . .	Up to 1.25

*Adapted from the *Ten State Nutrition Survey.*
†Criteria may vary with different methodology.
‡Serum glutamic oxalacetic transaminase.
§Serum glutamic pyruvic transaminase.
Source: G. Christakis, "Nutritional Assessment in Health Programs," *American Journal of Public Health,* **63**, part 2, November 1973.

prevalence of clinical signs of malnutrition in developed countries often means that such signs, when they do exist, are often overlooked or misinterpreted.

Certain characteristic physical signs which are associated with malnutrition, and which are valuable in nutritional assessment, are given in Table 18-8. Health care professionals should be able to recognize these dramatic signs, although there is some variation among population groups and according to age. Any suggestive physical finding should be pursued further through laboratory tests, dietary assessments, or other tests, such as x-rays for confirmatory evidence of rickets. The clinical examination should note other acute illnesses, chronic diseases, and disorders which could interfere with nutrient ingestion, absorption, or utilization. The oral cavity and teeth should be evaluated for signs of malnutrition and to note factors which may restrict the variety or amount of food intake, such as decayed or missing teeth, gum hypertrophy, ill-fitting dentures, or glossitis.

DIETARY METHODS

Information describing what an individual or a population group is in the habit of eating can help to determine dietary patterns that affect nutritional status and can enhance the understanding of socioeconomic and cultural influences involved in food selection. A variety of methods used in the collection of dietary information vary in reliability, validity, and depth. The method of choice depends upon whether information is being gathered for an individual diet assessment or a population survey, the extent of dietary information required, the time and money available, and the cooperation of the subjects.

Interviewing Techniques

Skillful interviewing is the foundation necessary for acquiring accurate information. Care must be taken to avoid distorting what is heard because of one's own perceptions, prejudices, and

TABLE 18-8   PHYSICAL SIGNS AND CAUSES OF MALNUTRITION

Body area	Signs associated with malnutrition	Nutrition-related causes
Hair	Lack of natural shine; dull, dry, sparse, straight, color changes (flag sign); easily plucked	Protein-calorie deficiency; often multiple coexistent nutrient deficiencies
Face	Dark skin over cheeks and under eyes (malar and supraorbital pigmentation), scaling of skin around nostrils (nasolabial seborrhea)	Inadequate coloric intake; lack of B complex vitamins, particularly niacin, riboflabin, pyridoxine
	Edematous (moon face)	Protein deficiency
	Color loss (pallor)	Iron deficiency, general undernutrition
Eyes	Pale conjunctivae	Iron deficiency
	Bitot's spots, conjunctival and corneal xerosis, soft cornea (keratomalacia)	Vitamin A deficiency
	Redness and fissuring of eyelid corners (angular palpebritis)	Niacin, riboflavin, pyridoxine deficiency

(Continued)

TABLE 18-8   CONTINUED

Body area	Signs associated with malnutrition	Nutrition-related causes
Lips	Redness and swelling of mouth or lips (cheilosis), angular fissure and scars	Niacin or riboflavin deficiency
Tongue	Red, raw and fissured, swollen (glossitis)	Folic acid, niacin, B_{12}, pyridoxine deficiency
	Magenta color	Riboflavin deficiency
	Pale, atrophic	Iron deficiency
	Filiform papillary atrophy	Niacin, folic acid, B_{12}, iron deficiency
	Fungiform papillary hypertrophy	General undernutrition
Teeth	Carious or missing	Excess sugar (and poor dental hygiene)
	Mottled enamel (fluorosis)	Excess fluoride
Gums	Spongy, bleeding, may be receding	Ascorbic acid deficiency
Glands	Thydroid enlargement (goiter)	Iodine deficiency
	Parotid enlargement	General undernutrition, particularly insufficient protein
Skin	Follicular hyperkeratosis, dryness (xerosis) with flaking	Vitamin A deficiency; insufficient unsaturated and essential fatty acids
	Hyperpigmentation	B_{12}, folic acid, niacin deficiency
	Petechiae	Ascorbic acid deficiency
	Pellagrous dermatitis	Niacin or tryptophan deficiency
	Scrotal and vulval dermatosis	Riboflavin deficiency
Nails	Spoon nails (koilonychia), brittle or ridged	Iron deficiency
Muscular and skeletal systems	Muscle wasting	Protein-calorie deficiency
	Frontal and parietal bossing; epiphyseal swelling; soft, thin infant skull bones (craniotabes), persistently open anterior fontanel; knock-knees or bow-legs	Vitamin D deficiency
	Beading of ribs (rachitic rosary)	Vitamin D and calcium deficiency
Internal systems		
Gastrointestinal	Hepatomegaly	Chronic malnutrition
Nervous	Mental confusion and irritability	Thiamin, niacin deficiency
	Sensory loss, motor weakness, loss of position sense, loss of vibration, loss of ankle and knee jerks, calf tenderness	Thiamin deficiency
Cardiac	Cardiac enlargement, tachycardia	Thiamin deficiency

assumptions. Questions which elicit meaningful responses should be asked. The questions and the tone of voice should not give clues to the expected answers. "Does your son drink a quart of milk every day?" and "How many eggs do you eat a week?" both imply positive answers. Even asking "What did you have for breakfast this morning?" includes an assumption. A better question is "What is the first thing you ate or drank today?" After a food item, such as bread, has been mentioned, follow-up questions should delineate the type, amount, and preparation method (such as "buttered"—which itself must be further defined). Assumptions should not be made about serving size. "A hamburger" and "a glass of milk" may each vary threefold in size. All glasses do not contain 8 oz or 1 cup. Food models of known sizes should be available to aid the interviewee in estimating portion sizes. The amount eaten may differ from the amount served.

The interviewer should be aware that distortion of amounts consumed may occur because those eating small amounts may think they should eat more and those eating large amounts may be well aware that they should eat less. Details may be missed when interviewers neglect to ask about food practices that are different from their own. Not everyone butters a hot dog roll, uses mayonnaise in sandwiches, or "cream" in coffee. Probing for details, such as snack habits and fluid intake, will often significantly change the day's reported total intake. Constant awareness of variables and biases which interviewers can introduce into data collection will help to control the problem.

THE NUTRITIONAL HISTORY

Eating patterns and nutrient requirements are influenced by factors such as age, dentition, economic situation, living conditions, physical activity level, nutrition knowledge, medication, allergies, chronic or acute illness, stress, and culture. These psychosocial, physical, and environmental factors must be considered when assessing the

nutritional status of an individual from the dietary perspective.

Depending upon the type of dietary problem under investigation, the nutritional history includes a food frequency section and may include a 24-h recall or daily food records, as described next and illustrated in the Appendix.

The Food Frequency

Information about overall food consumption patterns is obtained in the food frequency section of a dietary history. The number of times particular foods or food groups are eaten per day or per week is recorded, as are the foods seldom or never eaten. A food frequency enumeration is especially helpful when used to inquire about foods suspected of being deficient or excessive in a person's diet. Nutrients calculated from diet recalls or records which appear to be problematic can be correlated with the general frequency of intake of significant food sources to increase the validity of the dietary assessment.

The 24-Hour Recall

The most frequently used dietary survey procedure to measure current food intake is the 24-h recall. Collecting data via a 24-h recall requires a trained person to obtain accurate estimates of the quantity of all foods eaten during the previous 24 h or for the entire day preceding the interview. This simple, rapid method can be completed in 15 to 20 min. However, quantities consumed may be over- or underestimated, and food intake on a single day may not be representative of the usual intake. For these reasons, the information obtained from an individual will not necessarily correlate with physical or laboratory findings. When the 24-h recall is used as a screening tool in dietary surveys of population groups, the trends detected provide information about specific nutrient intake that is useful when measuring and comparing differences between large groups.

The interviewer should use glasses, spoons,

bowls, and food models of various sizes to help the respondent estimate the quantities consumed as accurately as possible. Some foods, such as beverages, margarine, gravy, sauces, and salad dressing, are often accidentally omitted, and the day's nutrient and caloric (kilojoule) totals may be underestimated.

The 3- or 7-Day Food Record

Another commonly used dietary tool is a written record of all food eaten, which is kept by an individual for a specified period of time. Instructions are given regarding weighing and measuring food and the need to indicate cooking methods and brand names. A standard set of measuring cups and spoons along with simple record forms should be provided to the recorder. Home visits by a trained person during the recording period will help to clarify serving portion size, recipes used, etc. As a minimum, the food record should be reviewed with the respondent to define the information provided. The accuracy of the record is dependent upon the cooperation and ability of the respondent, along with the adequacy and clarity of the instructions about how to complete the record.

The Household Survey

Household surveys measure all the food consumed by a family over a period of time, usually a week. The procedure includes initial weighing of all food in the home, recording all food purchases made during the period, and deducting any food remaining in the home at the end of the survey. Food wastage is also deducted. The age, sex, and occupation of household members are recorded, as is the number of meals eaten away from home. Nutrient intake can be calculated for the household as a group. Data are not available for any one individual because food distribution among family members is not distinguishable. The household survey is useful for differentiating food consumption patterns for varying economic and cultural groups. Marked seasonal variations may occur in some populations, particularly in developing countries.

EVALUATION OF DIETARY DATA

The records of foods that have been eaten are usually converted into nutrient quantities as a first step in the evaluation of dietary records. Food composition tables have become more comprehensive over the years because of improved laboratory analyses of nutrients in foods. Increased specificity of nutrient data and food products is reflected in the extensive revision of *Composition of Foods . . . Raw, Processed, Prepared* (U.S. Department of Agriculture Handbook No. 8, 1976), which is currently being issued by major food group sections to expedite release of newer data. *Nutritive Value of American Foods* (U.S. Department of Agriculture Handbook No. 456, 1975) and *Food Values of Portions Commonly Used* (J. B. Lipincott Company, Philadelphia, 1980) are frequently used to translate the amount of food eaten into nutrient intake. Boston research dietitians have compiled a manual to help locate nutrient data not commonly included in general food composition tables.

Problems are frequently encountered in the calculation of dietary data and may result in questionable validity. For this reason, there is often a poor correlation between dietary histories and other parameters studied in nutritional surveys. Common sources of error leading to miscalculation of dietary data include:

1   Mistakes in converting a household portion to a weighed amount (e.g., 1 cup to 100 g)

2   Arithmetic mistakes converting food intake into nutrient values

3   Use of food table values which are estimated rather than actual laboratory analysis amounts for nutrient content

4   Use of food table average values which may not reflect nutrient variations due to seasonal differences and methods of processing, cooking, and storage

5   Frequent ingredient changes in processed food products

6   Wide variability in combination-dish recipes (e.g., baked goods, casseroles).

In metabolic balance studies, laboratory analyses of an aliquot of all foods consumed can accurately measure the actual nutrient intake. This provides a basic knowledge of nutrient metabolism in order to establish minimum requirements or study metabolic disorders.

Calculating the nutrient content of dietary records by hand may be a lengthy, tedious process. Therefore, manual calculations usually include only a small number of nutrients. Deciding which nutrients to calculate is based upon other indices of nutritional problems of a population group or individual. For example, it would be appropriate to calculate the energy and protein intake for a failure-to-thrive infant, while estimating the usual energy intake would be adequate when counseling an obese adolescent.

Computer analysis of dietary records provides a rapid means of calculating a large number of nutrients. However, considerable time must be spent in preparing the dietary record information for computer processing. Programs have been devised for use with a data bank of the known nutrient content in foods. Updating the nutrient data bank is necessary at frequent intervals. The USDA Nutrient Data Bank, begun in 1972, is compiling data on approximately one hundred nutrients and over two hundred other constituents in foods according to universal food codes for use in the computer analysis of dietary intake. The limitations and sources of error with computer analysis are similar to those for manual calculations.

To assess the adequacy of dietary intake, it is necessary to compare dietary data with established standards. Comparing the record of foods consumed with the recommended number of daily servings from each of the food groups (see Chap. 2) helps to provide a general impression regarding the nutritional adequacy of the diet. Consistent omission of one or more food groups focuses attention on a group of nutrients whose intake may be suboptimal.

The international standards that are used to judge dietary adequacy vary widely in their levels of recommended intake. The standard most frequently used in the United States is the Recommended Dietary Allowances (RDA) of the National Academy of Sciences–National Research Council. The inherent limitations of the RDA must be recognized when comparing it to an individual's intake (see Chap. 2). A person's nutrient intake may be expressed as the percentage of that nutrient's RDA, qualified for the age and sex of the individual. Certain nutrient intakes are evaluated on the basis of body size, such as calories and protein per kilogram of body weight in infants, or on the basis of quantity per 1000 kcal (4200 kJ) for niacin and thiamin. Such measurement standards indicate metabolic relationships which may vary considerably.

Since the RDA includes a margin of safety, a person not consuming 100 percent of all the RDA nutrients may not necessarily be deficient in a nutrient and should not be considered malnourished without the support of biochemical, clinical, and anthropometric data.

NUTRITIONAL STATUS OF THE UNITED STATES POPULATION

Since 1967, nutrition surveys have attempted to define the nutritional problems that beset our population. The first of these, the *Ten State Nutrition Survey* (1968–1970) was mandated by the U.S. Congress in response to testimony on the existence of hunger in America. The demographic, dietary, clinical, anthropometric, and biochemical data collected in this survey revealed that undernutrition was causing growth failure in children and that it tended to be more prevalent in low-income populations. Iron-deficiency anemia, obesity, dental caries, and hyperlipidemia were additional findings. Groups at risk of developing malnutrition were noted to include elderly and adolescent males, in addition to infants, children, and pregnant women. The relatively high prevalence of vitamin A deficiency found among low-income Spanish-Americans is now suspected of having been a laboratory error. As a result of this survey, federal food programs were initiated and/or expanded.

Other surveys include the Pre-School Nutrition Survey (1968–1970), the Health and Nutrition Examination Survey (HANES) (1971–72), the U.S. Nationwide Food Consumption Survey, and the National Center for Disease Control Surveillance. This surveillance by the National Center for Disease Control utilizes already existing data (e.g., height, weight, hemoglobin, hematocrit) from agencies such as the Early Periodic Screening, Diagnosis, and Treatment (EPSDT) programs, Headstart, Special Supplemental Feeding Program for Women, Infants, and Children (WIC), well-baby clinics, and family planning clinics. The participating states and counties submit the data for computer analysis and comparison with standards. These enable the states and counties to identify and follow-up individuals and target populations and then to allocate services to areas with a high prevalence of nutritional risk.

Preliminary nutritional surveillance has shown that iron-deficiency anemia, as measured by hemoglobin and hematocrit, continues to be a major problem, as are obesity and poor growth in a number of children. In the United States, the surveillance program has yet to identify third-degree malnutrition.

PROBLEM-ORIENTED MEDICAL RECORD

The *problem-oriented medical record system* (POMR) developed by Weed is a modern professional tool. It provides a logically organized method for recognition of all of a patient's problems. The POMR coordinates members of the entire health team with the potential to improve patient care. The *data base* includes the patient's chief complaints, present illness, past medical history, patient profile, physical examination findings, and basic laboratory studies. Following completion of the data base, a numbered *master problem list* is drawn up, composed of items demanding attention of a diagnostic, therapeutic, or educational nature. A problem may be a symptom, a physiologic abnormality, an abnormal laboratory test, a diagnosis, or a social, nutritional, psychiatric, or demographic factor. A plan is developed as part of each problem's analysis. The acronym SOAP, derived from the first letters of the words *subjective, objective, assessment,* and *plans,* provides the format for the problem formulation, as follows:

> Date, Problem Number, Title
> *Subjective* Brief summary of pertinent history for this problem
> *Objective* Pertinent hard facts such as physical findings, laboratory data
> *Assessment* Precise interpretation of the problem and related factors
> *Plans* Diagnostic, therapeutic, and patient education plans

Progress notes, which follow the same SOAP format, document further developments.

An example follows, showing the original problem formulations by the physician and the dietitian of a child seen in a pediatric clinic.

7-9-77 #2 Nutritional Anemia

S   17-month-old girl appears pale to mother recently—drinks 1½ qt milk daily—no history of pica—child still eats mainly pureed foods; doesn't like to chew.

O   Questionably pale, no hepatomegaly or splenomegaly. Hemoglobin 9.1 g per 100 mL, white blood cells and platelets normal, reticulocytes 1.4 percent. Height, 80 cm; weight, 10.5 kg.

A   History and findings compatible with iron-deficiency anemia.

P   Rx Fer-In-Sol 1.2 mL bid for 1 month (approximately 5 mg elemental iron per kilogram body weight per day).
Patient education:
1 Mother instructed to decrease daily milk intake and to increase iron-containing foods.
2 Appointment made for counseling by dietitian regarding poor iron intake.
Follow-up:
Repeat hemoglobin at return visit in 1 month.
_____M.D.

7-9-77 #2 Nutritional Anemia

S Large intake of milk daily, questionable iron intake from food sources, diagnosis of iron-deficiency anemia confirmed; mother considers the child underweight.

Daily food intake consists of 48 oz milk, one 4½-oz jar strained cereal with fruit, and one 7-oz jar junior vegetables and meat. More than 90 percent of total calories comes from milk.

O Child observed eating: drinks liquids from a bottle, is spoon-fed, does not chew well. No other developmental delays. Dentition is normal for age. Height, weight, and weight-for-stature are at the 25th percentile.

A 1 Iron deficiency appears to be caused by low iron intake, which is less than one-third the RDA.

2 Delayed feeding skills related to parental overprotectiveness.

3 Intake of other nutrients such as ascorbic acid is suboptimal because of limited dietary variety. Appetite for other foods is diminished by the excessive intake of milk.

P Parent education:

Nutritional counseling included

1 Explanation of average milk requirements for young children

2 Discussion of normal feeding skills for age

3 Demonstration of techniques to encourage development of self-feeding skills

4 Discussion of iron-rich sources of culturally acceptable foods and suggestions to increase food variety

5 Reassurance regarding the child's adequate physical development, utilizing anthropometric graph for visual enhancement

6 Reinforcement of the need to give the prescribed medicinal iron as directed

Follow-up:

Appointment with dietitian at time of return clinic visit in 1 month.

_____R.D.

The POMR has interesting implications for health care professionals. The team approach is encouraged by the use of the medical record as a communication vehicle which focuses on the patient's problems. All health professionals involved in the patient's diagnosis, therapy, or education document their input in the patient's record. The "total patient" is more likely to receive care in a facility utilizing the POMR since the anthropometric, biochemical, clinical, and dietary data are clearly observable and readily available to determine nutritional status. Close nutritional surveillance is expedited by the use of the POMR for the hospitalized or institutionalized patient.

STUDY QUESTIONS

1 Define the term *nutritional status.*

2 Identify the type of information obtained in each of the four assessment areas which is helpful when evaluating the nutritional status of a person or a population group.

3 Despite the difficulty in diagnosing subclinical malnutrition, explain why it is important to identify persons at nutritional risk prior to the onset of clinical signs.

4 Discuss the factors involved in the calculation and interpretation of dietary data which affect the reliability and validity of the data.

5 List the most common nutritional problems of the American population.

6 In the problem-oriented medical record system, explain the type of information contained in each area of the SOAP format.

7 Choose a clinical study from a previous chapter, and identify the nutrition-related problem(s) for inclusion on the patient's master problem list. Rewrite each problem in SOAP format to comply with charting procedures in a hospital or clinic setting using the Problem-Oriented Medical Record system. Write a progress note in SOAP format for one problem to document an improvement you could anticipate following your therapeutic intervention.

CLINICAL STUDY 18

The nutritional problems of a hospitalized cancer patient are written in a SOAP format below. The Subjective and Objective sections provide anthropometric, biochemical, clinical, and dietary data related to the patient's nutritional status. Complete the Assessment and Planning portions for the patient's nutrition-related problems as you would enter them in the chart.

#1 Poor nutritional status due to resectable cancer of the pancreas.

Subjective: Elderly famale patient, very fearful about eating because of constant diarrhea following surgery. Patient reports decreased appetite and has noticed that "even ice cream makes her run."

Objective: Hospital diet prescription is 1800 kcal (7560 kJ) with 100 g fat. Patient's height is 160 cm; weight on hospital admission was 82 kg; weight prior to surgery was 68.5 kg; weight at present is 59 kg. Serum potassium is 3.0 meq per liter; sodium, 120 meq per liter. Fasting blood glucose was 175 mg per 100 mL; patient currently receiving NPH insulin. Appears lethargic and exhibits overall weakness.

Assessment:

Plan:

Clinical study question

1 On the basis of subjective and objective data presented, develop both the assessment and plans section of the problem-oriented record.

BIBLIOGRAPHY

American Dietetic Association: Patient Care Audit—A Quality Assurance Procedure Manual for Dietitians, The American Dietetic Association, Chicago, 1980.

American Dietetic Association: Patient Nutritional Care in Long-Term Care Facilities, The American Dietetic Association, Chicago, 1977.

Boston Area Research Dietitians: Nutrient Composition of Foods: Selected References and Tables, Massachusetts Dietetic Association, Boston, 1978.

Butterworth, C. E., and G. L. Blackburn: "Hospital Malnutrition," Nutrition Today, 10:8–18, March–April 1975.

Christakis, G.: "Nutritional Assessment in Health Programs," American Journal of Public Health, 63: 80–82, November 1973.

Hertzler, A. A., and L. W. Hoover: "Development of Food Tables and Use with Computers," Journal of the American Dietetic Association, 70:20–31, 1977.

Hoffman, W. S.: The Biochemistry of Clinical Medicine, 4th ed., Year Book Medical Publishers, Inc., Chicago, 1970, chaps. 1 and 7.

Madden, J. P., S. J. Goodman, and H. A. Guthrie: "Validity of the 24-hour Recall," Journal of the American Dietetic Association, 68:143–147, 1976.

Nichaman, M. Z.: "Developing a Nutritional Surveillance System," Journal of the American Dietetic Association, 65:15–17, 1974.

Owen, G. M., K. M. Kram, P. J. Garry, J. E. Lowe, and A. H. Lubin: "A Study of Nutritional Status of Preschool Children in the United States, 1968–1970," Pediatrics, 53: 597–646, April 1974.

U.S. Department of Health, Education, and Welfare: Highlights, Ten State Nutrition Survey, 1968–1970, DHEW Publ. no. (HSM) 72-8134.

U.S. Department of Health, Education, and Welfare: Preliminary Findings of the First Health and Nutrition Examination Survey, United States, 1971–72, I. Anthropometric and Clinical Findings, DHEW Publication no. (HRA) 75-1229; II. Dietary Intake and Biochemical Findings, DHEW Publication no. (HRA) 76-1219-1.

U.S. Department of Health, Education, and Welfare: Screening Children for Nutritional Status: Suggestions for Child Health Programs, DHEW Publication no. (PHS) 2158, 1971.

Voytovich, A. E., F. M. Walters, and M. DeMarco: "The Dietitian/Nutritionist and the Problem-oriented Medical Record," Journal of the American Dietetic Association, 63: 639–643, 1973.

Weed, L. L.: Medical Records, Medical Education and Patient Care, The Press of Case Western Reserve University, Cleveland, 1970.

Willcutts, H. D., and G. L. Blackburn: Nutritional Assessment: The Challenge of Malnutrition in Comminity Medicine and Techniques of Nutritional Assessment, Cutter Medical Teaching Monograph, Cutter Laboratories, Inc., Berkeley, California, 1980.

CLINICAL DISCUSSION 18

#1 Poor nutritional status due to resectable cancer of the pancreas

Assessment

1 Significant weight loss due to inadequate food intake and malabsorption.
2 Diarrhea caused by lactose intake which exacerbates the electrolyte imbalance; also related to malabsorption of fat.
3 Elevated blood glucose resulting from postoperative diabetes.

Plan

1 Recommend 2200-kcal (9240 kJ), lactose-free, 100-g-fat diet, six small feedings. Gradual reintroduction of milk products to determine tolerance.
2 Increase potassium-rich foods. Push fluids.
3 Carefully chart food and fluid intake for review by doctor.
4 Continual dietary counseling during hospitalization in preparation for discharge.
Follow-up:
Counseling during outpatient visits, especially upon initiation of radiation therapy.

_____R.D.

PART THREE

THE CONSEQUENCES
OF DISEASE ON
NUTRITIONAL CARE

Advances in technology have tempered the effect of disease in many cases, but unfortunately the routine and policies of hospitals and clinics have allowed little change in the total care of the patient. Upon hospitalization, patients lose their individual control as they face the ever-present threat of death and dying. Subsequent mood swings, from withdrawal to denial, to anger, to bargaining, to depression, and, in children, acceptance with regression, are all characteristic of this process.

It is in the midst of conflict and in the maze of hospital or clinic routines—laboratory tests, x-rays, physical examinations, medications—that you will interact with your client. This person, who is in a debilitated state conditioned by age, emotions, culture, and past general health, must marshal physiological and psychological resources to offset the disease and adapt to being sick, being treated, and possibly being hospitalized (see "The Psychology of Diet," in Chap. 11).

The individual's response to food, both physiological and psychological, is altered by the disease state. The disease itself or the drugs used in treatment may interfere with nutrient effectiveness or alter taste sensations (see the table on pages 400–401), and the food presented or the special therapeutic diet may now be rejected as the patient maintains his or her last vestige of control. Nutrition is essential in the treatment and rehabilitation of the patient and the cause of indifferent appetite and food complaints (legitimate in some instances) must be discerned. A number of factors should be explored to ensure the success of a nutritional care plan;* these factors are listed on the opposite page.

*E. Getchel and R. Howard, "Nutrition in Development," in G. Scipien et al., *Comprehensive Pediatric Nursing,* McGraw-Hill Book Company, New York, 1975, p. 239.

Physical factors

General physical condition (too weak or too ill to eat)

Position in which the patient is fed

Comfort (need to void, comfortable dress, cleanliness of hands and teeth, treatments given before or after meals, environment with unpleasant objects in sight, odors or inappropriate room temperature)

Presentation of food (unattractive tray, inappropriately sized utensils, rushed meals with too little time to chew and swallow)

Medications (some cause drowsiness, nausea, alterations of taste and appetite—e.g., amphetamines decreases appetite, steroids increase it)

Forced feedings

Emotional factors

Anxiety

Depression

Stress

Loneliness

Because of the multiplicity of factors a team approach becomes essential. Increasingly medical centers are forming primary care teams, composed of doctor, nurse, dietitian or nutritionist, social worker, and physical therapist (see "Nutrition Support Team" in Chap. 28).

This last part of the book is directed to the effect of disease on the human condition. Diseases, like nutrients, do not operate in a vacuum, and the total patient, along with his or her family, must be considered in planning the special diet, for there are no special diets, only special people.

COMMONLY USED DRUGS WITH NUTRITIONAL IMPLICATIONS

Drug	Potential nutrient interference	Side effects with nutritional implications
Adrenal corticosteriods	Decreased absorption of calcium, phosphorus.	Gastric inflammation; may produce ulcers.
	Increased excretion of urinary ascorbic acid, potassium, zinc, nitrogen.	Stimulate protein catabolism and depress protein synthesis, delay wound healing.
	Increased blood glucose, serum triglycerides, serum cholesterol.	
Antibiotics		
Choramphenical	Increased serum iron.	Aplastic and hypoplastic anemia, nausea, vomiting, diarrhea may occur; glossitis and stomatitis.
	May increase need for riboflavin, pyridoxine, vitamin B_{12}.	
	Can interfere with response to folate, iron, and B_{12} therapy.	
Erythromyocin		Inhibits protein synthesis; gastrointestinal discomfort, cramping. Nausea, vomiting, and diarrhea occur occasionally. May form salts with acids—avoid orange, lemon, cranberry juices, and other acid drinks.
Neomycin	Decreased absorption of fat, nitrogen, carotene, MCT, glucose, amino acids, lactose, sodium, potassium, calcium, iron, vitamins B_{12}, A, D, K.	Glossitis, stomatitis, nausea, vomiting, diarrhea. May produce malabsorption with increased fecal fat.
Penicillin	Increased excretion of urinary potassium.	Nausea, vomiting, occasionally hemolytic anemia.
Tetracycline	Decreased absorption of calcium, iron, magnesium, zinc, amino acids, and fat.	If used during tooth development may cause permanent staining. May cause increased blood urea nitrogen, anorexia, nausea, vomiting, diarrhea, glossitis, dysphagia, hemolytic anemia. Should not be taken with milk, since calcium impairs absorption.
	Decreased synthesis of vitamin K by intestinal bacteria.	
	Increased excretion of urinary ascorbic acid, riboflavin, nitrogen, amino acids, folic acid, and niacin.	
Anticoagulants		
Coumarin derivatives	Antagonist of vitamin K.	Gastrointestinal bleeding, nausea, vomiting, diarrhea, mouth ulcers.
Anticonvulsants	See Chap. 26.	
Phenobarbitol		
Dilantin		
Antidepressants (monoamine oxidase inhibitors) Thenelzine Tranylcypromine	See Chap. 26.	Foods high in tyramine should be avoided as they may precipitate a hypertensive crisis. Foods to avoid: aged cheddar cheese, alcohol, yogurt, sour cream, yeast, bananas, broad beans, canned figs, raisins, chicken liver, chocolate, cola, coffee, tea, pickled herring, licorice.

Drug	Potential nutrient interference	Side effects with nutritional implications
Antihypertensives		
Diuretics Chlorothiazides	Increased urinary excretion of potassium, magnesium, zinc, and riboflavin. Decreased carbohydrate intolerance.	Fluid and electrolyte imbalance.
Furosemide		Oral and gastric burning, nausea, vomiting and diarrhea, fluid and electrolyte imbalance.
Hydralazine		Anorexia, nausea, vomiting, diarrhea, constipation, reduction in hemoglobin.
Antilipemic agents		
Cholestyramine	Decreased serum calcium and B_{12}.	Binds bile acids, may interfere with normal fat absorption.
	Decreased absorption of vitamins A, D, K, B_{12}, folate, fat, glucose, iron, carotene.	Constipation, flatulence, nausea, diarrhea.
Clofibrate	Decreased absorption of carotene, glucose, iron, MCT, B_{12}, and electrolytes.	Nausea, diarrhea, vomiting, anemia, decreased taste activity.
Cardiac glycosides		
Digitalis	Increased excretion of urinary magnesium and calcium.	Nausea, vomiting, diarrhea, anorexia.
Levodopa	Decreased absorption of tryptophan and other amino acids.	Nausea, vomiting, diarrhea, anorexia.
	Increased excretion of urinary sodium and potassium antagonize pyridoxine.	Drug effectiveness decreased by increased intakes of protein. Anorexia, nausea, vomiting, burning sensation of the tongue, bitter taste.
Uricosuric agents		
Allopurinol Probenecid	Increased urinary excretion of riboflavin, calcium, magnesium, sodium, potassium, phosphate and chloride. Decreased urinary excretion of pantothenic acid. Decreased intestinal absorption of riboflavin and amino acids.	Increased fluid intake is desirable. Nausea, vomiting, diarrhea. Anorexia, nausea, vomiting, anemia, sore gums.

Source: D. C. March, *Handbook: Interactions of Selected Drugs with Nutritional Status in Man,* 2d ed. American Dietetic Association, 1978; *Physicians' Desk Reference,* 35th ed., Medical Economics Company, Oradell, N.J., 1981.

CHAPTER 19

MALNUTRITION AND THE IMMUNE RESPONSE

Robert M. Suskind

KEY WORDS
Marasmus
Kwashiorkor
Antigen
Cell-Mediated Immune Response
Humoral Immunity
Polymorphonuclear Leukocytes
Complement System

INTRODUCTION

A study of childhood mortality in Latin American countries cited malnutrition as either the direct or the indirect cause of death of over one-third of the children under 5 years of age.[1] Up to 80 percent of over 190,000 children surveyed in 46 Asian, African, and South American communities between 1963 and 1972 suffered moderate or severe forms of protein-calorie malnutrition (PCM).[2] Judging from these figures, roughly 100 million children under 5 years of age are now severely or moderately malnourished.

Malnutrition is found in both adults and children of developed nations as well as in the developing world. It is in urban as well as rural areas and is also, surprisingly, found in hospitals. Primary protein-calorie malnutrition is not commonly seen in American hospitals. However, physicians are becoming aware that malnutrition may develop from other disease states such as renal, liver, or cardiopulmonary illness. A nutrition survey at a pediatric referral center reported that one-third of the patients had signs of acute malnutrition.[3] When epidemiological studies of malnutrition are conducted, those hospitalized individuals suffering from disease states leading to malnutrition must be included.

Although this chapter focuses on the malnourished child, malnutrition in the adult is also a concern. The effect on the adult is less devastating because of the body's nutrient reserves and the fact there are not the additional demands of growth. However, the same effect on the body's immune response will be found in the adult (see "The Malnourished Adult," in Chap. 28).

ETIOLOGY OF MALNUTRITION

The development of malnutrition depends on a complex of interactions among nutrient, host, and environment.[4]

In deficiency states, nutrients act as if they were present in insufficient quantities at a cellular level to satisfy metabolic needs.[5] When considering protein intake, it is important to determine whether the composition of essential amino acids is adequate for body requirements. If the dietary protein lacks one essential amino acid, the body reacts as if all essential amino acids were deficient in the food. The biological value of a protein food depends not only on its amino acid composition, but on the degree to which the amino acids are liberated during digestion, since complete protein utilization will not occur until all the essential amino acids are available at approximately the same time.[6] In addition, the energy value of the diet affects the biological value of the protein. If the diet lacks energy, protein will be used, with the eventual result being similar to the effects of a protein-deficient diet. Conversely, excess calories will spare the utilization of protein for energy. In many parts of the world, the foods children consume for energy, such as cassava or sweet potato, are grossly deficient in essential nutrients and contribute to protein deficiency.[7,8]

Host factors affecting nutritional status include age, sex, activity, growth, pregnancy, lactation, and various pathological states. The nutrient requirements of a growing child are much different from those of an adult. Pregnancy and lactation increase the nutrient requirements. Activity and genetic variability must also be considered. Environmental factors which affect the availability of nutrients include food production, cost, processing, distribution, and population density.[9] Temperature, humidity, and sunlight affect nutrient requirements.

Cultural influences are among the most important environmental determinants of what an individual eats.[10] For example, northern Thai children from birth are started on supplemental rice and bananas, which are often given prior to breast feeding. This practice leads to a decreased consumption of breast milk. As a result, these children often develop permanent protein deficits from early infancy. Prejudices such as withholding cow's milk from young infants for fear that it causes diarrhea lead to decreased utilization of important protein sources in certain parts of the world. Religious taboos, such as the Hindu prohibition of beef in India, have greatly

affected efforts to improve nutritional status. When a child has acute diarrhea or an infection and parents withdraw food, kwashiorkor (protein malnutrition) often develops from the metabolic loss of nitrogen. The nutritional status of the child further deteriorates when he/she receives strong purgatives to eliminate parasites which the mother believes are causing the diarrhea.

CLASSIFICATION OF PROTEIN-CALORIE MALNUTRITION

In 1955, Gomez et al.[11] defined childhood malnutrition in terms of deficits in the weight that would be appropriate for the child's age (weight for age). Using local standards, they categorized first-, second-, and third-degree malnutrition in terms of 75 to 90 percent of weight for age, 60 to 75 percent of weight for age, and less than 60 percent of weight for age, respectively. Today Gomez's classification has been modified to use internationally accepted standards derived from the mean weights and heights of healthy children from North America or Europe.[12] Since genetic differences apparently do not affect growth potential during the early years of life,[13] norms from developed countries also apply to communities with widespread malnutrition.

Height for age and weight for height are often more useful tools for defining an individual's nutritional status than weight for age, which fails to consider the height deficit caused by chronic malnutrition. The child with a decreased weight for height is wasted or acutely malnourished, while the child with a decreased height for age is stunted or chronically malnourished. Often the malnourished child is both wasted and stunted.

Waterlow's table classifies children according to their degree of malnutrition and retardation (Table 19-1).[14] Studies from several developing countries commonly show both wasting and stunting in children between the ages of 1 and 2 years. By age 3 or 4, underweight-for-age children are chiefly stunted rather than wasted.[15] In other words, they have stopped growing lin-

TABLE 19-1 CLASSIFICATION ACCORDING TO DEGREE OF MALNUTRITION AND RETARDATION

Malnutrition grade	Expected height* for age, percent	Expected weight† for height, percent
0	> 95	> 90
1	< 95	< 90
2	< 90	< 80
3	< 85	< 70

*Expected values = Boston 50th percentile; 95% expected height for age = approximately Boston 3d percentile.
†Expected values = Boston 50th percentile; 90% expected weight for height = approximately Boston 3d percentile.
Source: Adapted from J. C. Waterlow, "Some Aspects of Childhood Malnutrition as a Public Health Problem," *British Medical Journal*, 4:88, 1974.

TABLE 19-2 THE EFFECT OF MALNUTRITION ON HEIGHT AND WEIGHT

Type of malnutrition	Weight for age	Height for age	Weight for height
Chronic (past, long-term)	Decreased	Decreased	Normal
Current acute	Decreased	Normal	Decreased
Chronic and acute	Decreased	Decreased	Decreased

early but have a normal weight for height. Table 19-2 summarizes the effects of malnutrition on height and weight. The above classification of wasting and stunting provides a guide for use in the development of public health or community intervention programs. Wasted children require nutritional rehabilitation, either as inpatients or as outpatients, while stunted children need a total community program with public health intervention and child-feeding programs.

SEVERE MALNUTRITION: MARASMUS AND KWASHIORKOR

Children develop *marasmus* following severe deprivation of both protein and calories, resulting in growth retardation, weight loss, muscular atrophy, and severe loss of subcutaneous tissue (Fig. 19-1). Children with *kwashiorkor,* caused by acute protein loss or deprivation, are char-

acterized by edema, skin lesions, hair changes, apathy, anorexia, an enlarged fatty liver, and decreased total serum protein and serum albumin (Fig. 19-2). These children have abundant subcutaneous fat and recover rapidly on a high-protein diet.[16] (See illustrations, p. 406.)

Marasmus and kwashiorkor may be superimposed on one another at any stage. Patients with combined marasmus-kwashiorkor are undersized and underweight, with markedly diminished subcutaneous fat, mild to moderate fatty infiltration of the liver, and a greater degree of muscular wasting than is seen with kwashiorkor alone. They may have mild to moderate edema which disappears within a few days of nutritional therapy, leaving only signs of marasmus. Children with marasmic kwashiorkor have considerably lower total serum protein and serum albumin values than marasmic children, whose values are usually only slightly below normal.

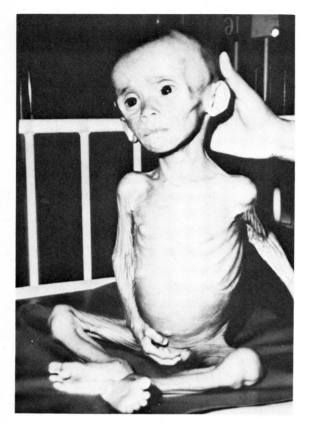

Figure 19-1
Marasmic child with evidence of growth retardation, weight loss, muscular atrophy, and severe decrease of subcutaneous tissue. [Courtesy of Medical Staff, Anemia and Malnutrition Research Center, Chiang Mai, Thailand. From R. M. Suskind, O. Thanangkul, D. Damrongsak, C. Leitzmann, L. Suskind, and R. E. Olson, "The Malnourished Child: Clinical, Biochemical, and Hematological Changes," in R. M. Suskind (ed.), *Malnutrition and the Immune Response,* Raven Press, New York, 1977.]

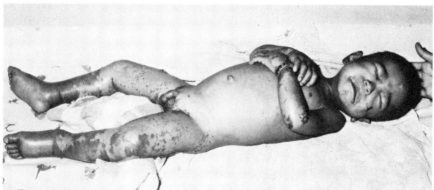

Figure 19-2
Child with kwashiorkor, with evidence of edema, skin lesions, hair changes, and apathy. Anorexia, an enlarged fatty liver, and decreased serum total protein and albumin are also present. [Courtesy of Medical Staff, Anemia and Malnutrition Research Center, Chiang Mai, Thailand. From R. M. Suskind, O. Thanangkul, D. Damrongsak, C. Leitzmann, L. Suskind, and R. E. Olson, "The Malnourished Child: Clinical, Biochemical, and Hematological Changes," in R. M. Suskind (ed.), *Malnutrition and the Immune Response,* Raven Press, New York, 1977.]

TABLE 19-3   CLINICAL AND BIOCHEMICAL DETERMINANTS OF MARASMUS AND KWASHIORKOR

	Marasmus	Kwashiorkor
Age of maximal incidence	6–18 months	12–48 months
Emaciation	3+	1–2+
Edema	None	1–3+
Fatty infiltration of liver	None to 1+	3+
Skin changes	Infrequent	Frequent
Serum albumin	Almost normal	Markedly decreased
Serum enzymes		
Lipase	Normal	Markedly decreased
Amylase	Normal	Decreased
Esterase	Slightly decreased	Decreased

Source: Adapted from C. Gopalan, "Kwashiorkor and Marasmus: Evolution and Distinguishing Features," in R. A. McCance and E. M. Widdowson (eds.), *Calorie Deficiencies and Protein Deficiencies*, Little, Brown and Company, Boston, 1968.

Because of variations in feeding practices and nutritional requirements, the various states of malnutrition have characteristic age distributions. Marasmus usually occurs in children under 1 year of age when the mother's breast milk provides insufficient protein and calories for the growing child and when the supplementary feeding is inadequate.[17] Kwashiorkor, on the other hand, most commonly occurs after age 1 when a borderline diet becomes deficient in protein relative to calories, as a result of superimposed infection.[18] Gopalan has outlined the differences between children with marasmus and kwashiorkor[19] (Table 19-3). His observations are similar to those of others who have described these syndromes from various parts of the world. Table 19-4 is an example of a nutritional assessment system developed by the Cleveland Clinic Foundation based on a point system to determine protein-calorie status.[20]

TABLE 19-4   NUTRITIONAL ASSESSMENT-OBJECTIVE MEASUREMENT STANDARDS, CLEVELAND CLINIC FOUNDATION

1. Percent weight loss:

$$\frac{\text{Usual weight} - \text{current weight}}{\text{usual weight}} \times 100 = \% \text{ weight loss}$$

Weight loss:

    0–5% = 0 points (normal)

    6–15% = 1 point (depleted)

    > 15% = 2 points (severely depleted)

2. Creatinine-height index (CHI):

$$\frac{\text{Actual urinary creatinine excretion (mg)}}{\text{Ideal urinary creatinine excretion (mg)}} = \text{CHI}$$

Creatinine-height index:

    ≥ 0.75 = 0 points

    0.50–0.75 = 1 point

    < 0.50 = 2 points

3. Serum albumin:

    ≥ 3.5 g/dL = 0 points

    3.0–3.4 g/dL = 1 point

    < 3.0 g/dL = 2 points

4. Serum transferrin:

    ≥ 190 mg/dL = 0 points

    100–190 mg/dL = 1 point

    < 100 mg/dL = 2 points

5. Delayed hypersensitivity skin tests:

    Two or more positive skin tests = 0 points

    One positive skin test = 1 point

    Zero positive skin tests = 2 points

6. Nutritional status (with respect to somatic and visceral protein status):

    Normal = 0–2 points

    Moderate depletion = 3–5 points

    Severe depletion = 6–10 points

Source: Ruth Hooley, "Clinical Nutrition Assessment: A Perspective," *Journal of the American Dietetic Association*, **77**(6):683, December 1980.

INFECTION AND MALNUTRITION

Scrimshaw et al.[21] noted that infection worsens the individual's nutritional status by reducing appetite, creating a tendency for solid foods to be withdrawn (especially those of animal origin), increasing metabolic losses of nitrogen, and (when infection involves the gastrointestinal tract) decreasing nitrogen absorption. Purgatives and various home remedies may also adversely affect absorption.[22]

The prevalence rates for infectious disease range from 50 to 60 percent during the 6- to 24-month age period.

The child who gains weight more or less normally during the first 4 to 6 months but thereafter develops recurrent infectious diseases will show a leveling off in both weight and height gain. During the period of no significant weight gain there is usually no increase in height, leaving the child's weight for height unchanged. However, if an intercurrent infection develops, a resultant decrease in weight for height occurs simultaneously as the child's nutritional status deteriorates.

Reyna-Barrios et al.[23] evaluated the frequency of infectious diseases in an Indian village in the Guatemalan highlands. Upper respiratory infections and acute diarrheal diseases were major problems for some children up to 7 years old, with both diseases peaking between 6 and 24 months of age. Other researchers report similar observations on the frequency of infectious diseases in developing countries. Scrimshaw et al.[24] outlined very clearly the consequences of infection on human nutritional status. Even the mildest infectious diseases increase urinary nitrogen excretion,[25] because of an increased mobilization of amino acids from peripheral muscle for gluconeogenesis in the liver, with deamination and the excretion of nitrogen in the form of urea. Unless an augmented dietary intake compensates for the lost nitrogen, the depletion will precipitate a syndrome like that characterizing kwashkiakior.

Besides nitrogen, metabolic losses also include potassium, magnesium, zinc, phosphorus, sulfur, and vitamins A, C, and B$_2$.[26] There is increased utilization, sequestration, or diversion from normal metabolic pathways of several nutrients. In spite of the mobilization of amino acids from the peripheral muscle, whole-blood amino acids decrease after exposure to an infectious agent.[27] Increased gluconeogenesis is accompanied by an increased diversion of amino acids for the synthesis of acute-phase proteins such as haptoglobin, C-reactive protein, alpha$_1$-antitrypsin, and alpha$_2$-macroglobulin in response to the infection.

MALNUTRITION AND THE IMMUNE RESPONSE

The term *immune* is derived from the Latin word *immunis*, meaning "safety." Several immune defenses have been shown to be affected in the malnourished host: these include the cell-mediated immune response, antibody production, phagocytic and killing function of the leukocytes, and the complement system. They are discussed below.

Cell-Mediated Immunity

The malnourished child is susceptible to recurrent infections because the child's immune defense system is depressed. The child's already poor nutritional status further deteriorates after the infection, making the child more susceptible to a secondary infection.

The cell-mediated immune response is controlled through the *thymus-dependent lymphocytes* (T cells). It plays a major role in the body's defense against viruses, mycobacteria, and fungi.[29] Thymus-dependent lymphocytes are present in the peripheral blood, thymus, spleen, and peripheral lymph nodes.

Jackson was the first to call attention to lymphoid atrophy associated with severe protein-calorie malnutrition (PCM) when he noted at autopsy that the thymus glands of children with kwashiorkor were reduced to only a few strands of tissue.[30] In addition to atrophy of the thymus, lymph nodes, and tonsils, the spleen appeared smaller in malnourished children.[31-33] Malnourished children have fewer circulating T cells,[34,35] but this thymus-dependent lymphopenia improves with nutritional recovery.[36] Lymphocytes account for 30 percent of the normal differential white count (6.300 per mm³ average value for a 2-year-old child).[37] A lymphocyte count below this value in a child of 2 may indicate an impaired cellular immune defense mechanism.

The cell-mediated immune response is evaluated in individuals by intradermal skin testing and in vitro by enumeration of T lymphocytes and by the antigen and mitogen stimulation of isolated lymphocytes. When an individual is exposed to a new antigen such as mycobacteria or BCG, the uncommitted lymphocytes become sensitized to the new antigen. With reexposure to the antigen, the lymphocytes proliferate, releasing lymphokines which produce the inflammatory response and a positive skin test.

Several investigators have noted decreased numbers of positive tuberculin skin tests in children with PCM, although the defective skin test response improves after nutritional rehabilitation.[38] The depressed reactivity to skin test antigens in the malnourished child correlates well with depression of lymphocyte function in culture medium. This in vitro evaluation of lymphocytes reveals a decreased rate of DNA synthesis. After nutritional recovery, in vitro lymphocyte transformation also becomes normal.[39]

The depressed cell-mediated immune response may be secondary to deficiencies of protein, calories, vitamins, or minerals, or may be due to the suppressive effect of the superimposed infection. These nutritional factors interact with and depress the cell-mediated immune system, leading to increased susceptibility to those infections which the system normally handles.

Polymorphonuclear Leukocytes and Macrophages

The polymorphonuclear leukocytes (PMNs) and macrophages are phagocytic cells with functions related to three major areas.[40]

1 Chemotaxis (the ability of the cell to be attracted to a foreign object)
2 Phagocytosis (engulfment of particles)
3 Postphagocytotic events, including:
   a Phagocytic vacuole formation and degranulation
   b Microbial killing
   c Concomitant metabolic changes

Under normal conditions, PMNs constitute 65 percent of the differential leukocyte count, of which 59 percent are segmented polymorphs and 5 percent are nonsegmented. With certain infections a polymorpholeukocytosis occurs and the number of nonsegmented polymorphs increases. In vivo chemotaxis of PMNs in malnourished children is not depressed.

Phagocytosis and killing function of various organisms by the PMNs are not significantly affected by the child's nutritional state.[41,42] In addition the opsonic activity of the plasma in protein-calorie malnutrition does not appear depressed.[43] (Opsonic activity refers to the presence of opsonins in the serum, which attack bacteria, rendering them more susceptible to phagocytosis.)

Humoral Immunity: Immunoglobulin and Antibody Response

A second population of circulating lymphocytes, the B cells (bursa cells) or thymus-independent lymphocytes, is responsible for immunoglobulin production. In humans there are five major structural types or classes of immunoglobulins called IgG, IgM, IgA, IgD, and IgE.

Although the majority of malnourished children have elevated circulating immunoglobulins secondary to an intercurrent infection, many children are unable to respond to various antigenic stimuli when they enter the hospital.[44] In addition to the depressed antibody response to foreign antigens, the malnourished child has depressed secretory IgA in nasopharyngeal and salivary secretions.[45] Chandra et al. have demonstrated that malnourished children have a reduced secretory IgA antibody response to poliomyelitis vaccine. Other changes accompanying the decreased secretory immunoglobulins include reduced digestive enzymes, atrophy of the intestinal wall, and an impaired hepatic reticuloendothelial system, all of which affect the body's susceptibility to gram-negative organisms, especially those from the gastrointestinal tract.[46]

It has not been determined which of the specific nutrient deficiencies in malnourished children is responsible for the depressed antibody response.

Complement System

This system comprises several protein fractions, known as *complement* components, which interact and are involved in several host defenses.[47]

Viral neutralization
Chemotaxis of leukocytes, monocytes, eosinophils

Opsonization of fungi (a process related to opsonin activity)
Endotoxin inactivation
Lysis of virus-infected cells
Bacteriolysis

Sirisinha et al. found that most of the complement components and the serum hemolytic activity were depressed in children with PCM. In addition, malnourished children had evidence of anticomplementary activity in their serum.[48] It is well known that several substances, including endotoxin and immune complexes, activate complement or have anticomplementary activity. Circulating endotoxin has also been found in 50 percent of the hospitalized children with PCM on hospital admission.[49] (Table 19-5 summarizes the changes in the immune system in PCM.)

INTRAUTERINE MALNUTRITION

Severe nutritional deficits during pregnancy affect intrauterine growth. Intrauterine growth is indicative of maternal well-being as well as socioeconomic status.[50] The effects of malnutrition on fetal growth depend on the timing, severity, and duration of the nutritional insult. Subacute fetal distress occurs when the fetus is overdue

TABLE 19-5   CHANGES IN THE IMMUNE SYSTEM IN PROTEIN-CALORIE MALNUTRITION

A. Cell-mediated immunity (T-cell-mediated)	Depressed
B. Humoral immunity (B-cell-mediated)	
1 Serum immunoglobulins	Normal or elevated
2 Antibody response	Depressed
3 Secretory immunoglobulins	Depressed
C. Polymorphonuclear leukocyte response	
1 In vivo chemotaxis	Normal
2 Phagocytosis	Normal
3 Killing function	Normal
D. Complement system	
1 Complement proteins	Depressed
2 Hemolytic complement activity	Depressed

and is deprived of appropriate supplementation for days prior to birth; this leads to a wasted infant of normal length. In chronic fetal distress, deprivation extends over weeks and arrests growth at an earlier period. Inasmuch as the fetus has not acquired any excess body fat, deficits occur in weight proportional to length. The post-term sequelae of chronic fetal intrauterine malnutrition include height and weight retardation, in which the neonate tends to remain small for his age, in addition to defects in immunocompetency similar to those seen in postnatally malnourished children.

Several etiologic factors contribute to the development of intrauterine malnutrition. The influence of maternal nutrition on ultimate fetal weight has been pointed out by Lechtig et al.,[51] who found that when short women from the lower socioeconomic group were given caloric supplementation during pregnancy, neonatal birth weight was significantly increased. However, supplementation during pregnancy must be undertaken judiciously. (See Chap. 15.)

THE TREATMENT OF THE MALNOURISHED CHILD

Severely malnourished children usually have either diarrhea, pneumonia, otitis media, urinary tract infection, or septicemia. It is important to determine the site of infection and the etiologic agent. The malnourished child should have a complete blood count; serum electrolyte determination; and cultures of stool, urine (by suprapubic tap), blood, ear exudate, throat and nasopharnygeal specimens, and cerebrospinal fluid where clinically indicated. Therapy should be rigorous in the treatment of infection.

Initial intravenous rehydration is with Ringer's lactate with 50 percent dextrose added to make a 10 percent solution. A child with severe potassium depletion should receive up to 6 to 7 meq of supplemental potassium per kg of body weight per day. Intravenous fluids may contain up to 40 meq per L of potassium. The remainder of the potassium supplementation is

given orally. A severely dehydrated child may receive up to 20 mL of fluids per kg during the first hour of therapy in order to increase the intravascular volume and renal blood flow. Following initial rehydration, the patient's fluid balance can be maintained through the use of ¼ normal saline–10 percent dextrose solution.

After initial rehydration, the patient continues to receive supplemental potassium at a maintenance dose of 5 meq per kg per day. Magnesium is given at a dose of 0.4 meq per kg intramuscularly daily for 7 days, followed by daily oral magnesium doses of 1.4 meq per kg. Once a patient has reached a daily oral intake of 175 kcal (735 kJ) per kg and 4 g of protein per kg, magnesium and potassium are usually met by diet alone.

Patients with severe diarrhea are kept NPO (nothing per os—by mouth) for up to 24 to 48 h. Following the first 24 to 48 h, the patient is placed on gradually increasing protein and energy intakes. By the end of the first week, the patient usually tolerates 100 kcal (420 kJ) per kg and 4 g of protein per kg of body weight. Initially, the needed energy and protein may be supplied by a diluted milk-based formula supplemented with Dextri-Maltose and corn oil, which can be readily given by tube feeding. A formula which provides 175 kcal (735 kJ) per kg and 4 g of protein per kg would have 9.5 g of fat and 18.3 g of carbohydrate. When cow's milk is used as a formula base it is important to consider the addition of essential vitamins and minerals[52] (Table 19-6). Iron supplementation should be given when indicated.[53]

After the patient's course has stabilized, solid food may be gradually introduced into the diet. When children with protein-calorie malnutrition are offered solid food ad lib., they soon take up to 160 to 180 kcal (672 to 756 kJ) per kg by the second or third week of hospitalization. This intake is maintained for the first month and then gradually is decreased to 140 to 150 kcal (588 to 630 kJ) per kg. After the child has reached the optimal weight for height, intake usually decreases to 110 to 120 kcal (462 to 504 kJ) per kg of body weight per day.

TABLE 19-6 SUPPLEMENTATION OF COW'S MILK
FORMULA BASE WITH VITAMINS AND MINERALS

Formula (g per kilogram body weight)			
Calories	Protein	Fat	CHO
175	4	9.5	18.3

Vitamin supplementation			
Vitamin	Unit	Daily initial therapy IM or IV for 3 days beginning on day 2	Daily maintenance therapy from the fifth day until the end of week 10
Thiamin	mg	5.0	0.6
Riboflavin	mg	5.0	1.0
Pyridoxine	mg	2.5	1.0
Nicotinamide	mg	37.5	11.0
Pantothenate	mg	5	5.0
Ascorbic acid	mg	200	30.0
Folic acid	mg	1.5	0.1
Vitamin B_{12}	μg	7.5	5.0
Vitamin A	IU*	5000	2500
Vitamin D	IU*	400	400
Vitamin E	IU		50
Vitamin K	μg*	300	100

Mineral content of formula and supplement trace minerals	
Mineral	Dose (meq per kilogram per day)
Na	2.7
K	5.0
Ca	7.3
Mg	1.4
Zn	0.014
Mn	0.018
Cu	0.0028
I	0.00008
F	0.006
Al	0.070
Mo	0.001
Cr	0.366
Se	0.003

*Therapeutic doses of the fat-soluble vitamins are given as indicated to combat overt deficiency disease.

Source: Adapted from R. Suskind, "The In-Patient and Out-Patient Treatment of the Child with Severe Protein Calorie Malnutrition," in R. E. Olson (ed.), *Protein-Calorie Malnutrition,* Academic Press, New York, 1975.

THE PREVENTION OF MALNUTRITION

Before initiating preventive measures, one must define the objectives of such a program, such as:[54]

1 Detection of early signs of malnutrition in order to take remedial action
2 Reduction of the frequency and severity of infectious disease
3 Improvement of the nutritional status of women of childbearing age, particularly through adolescence, pregnancy, and lactation
4 Reduction in the number of low-birth-weight infants and in perinatal mortality and morbidity
5 Spacing pregnancies at reasonable intervals

Ignorance of nutritional requirements and of the nutritive value of foods often plays an important role in the etiology of malnutrition.[55] Nutritional information should be included in all educational activities. However, if educational measures ignore the population's existing food habits and prejudices, proposed nutritional changes are likely to be unrealistic and unacceptable.[56] Improvements through relatively small alterations in established food habits are easier to institute than radical changes. Nutrition education programs should recommend locally available foods.

To prevent malnutrition, the basic principles of nutrition must be taught to teachers, nurses, social workers, agricultural extension workers, home economists, and other professionals who use their knowledge in community activities.[57] In addition, political authorities and professionals at the university level in medicine, public health, biological sciences, agriculture, economics, and other subjects directly or indirectly related to health and nutrition should be included in educational programs.

Education and intervention programs should be aimed at improving the children's nutritional status. Early weaning risks in developing countries[58] arise largely from infection associated with poor hygiene, especially in formula preparation, and from the lack of knowledge and money to prepare a nutritious substitute for breast milk. Mothers should be encouraged to breast-feed for as long as possible.

Supplementary feeding programs have been widely used for improving nutrition. (See "WIC," Chap. 16.) Pregnant and lactating women are frequently the recipients of such food distribution. School lunch programs and nutritional rehabilitation centers help to carry out supplementary feeding programs.[59] These low-cost day-care center programs are particularly intended to rehabilitate malnourished children without the expense of full hospitalization. Day-care centers have also been set up in different parts of the world for children over 2 years of age; they receive supplementation at these centers as well as in home visits. In terms of maternal- and family-child interaction, the supplemented child often receives more stimulation, rewards, and deferences than the unsupplemented child, and becomes an active, independent, playful youngster who frequently verbalizes and demands. This behavior appears to stimulate the parent, resulting in more frequent and varied two-way interaction between child and parent, and between child and environment.

Adding a relatively small quantity of animal products to the diet of predominantly vegetarian populations can be beneficial. Animal protein supplementation corrects the lysine deficiency of wheat and the tryptophan and lysine deficiency in corn. INCAP studies demonstrated that adequate combinations of vegetable products result in protein values that are comparable to the protein content of animal foods.[60]

Control of infectious disease should be given the highest priority because infection adversely affects the nutritional status of the child. Two essential programs for preventing the consequences of infection are immunization programs and the rehydration of children with diarrhea to minimize the detrimental metabolic response.

Family planning is of paramount importance in most developing countries,[61] since a strong relationship exists between malnutrition and close spacing of pregnancies.[62] The cumulative effect of multiple pregnancies starting very early in life often leads to maternal nutritional depletion. Therefore, family planning should be given its proper role in the prevention of protein-calorie malnutrition.[63]

Successful implementation of the above programs should decrease the prevalence of protein-calorie malnutrition.

CONCLUSION

The synergism between poor nutritional status, the body's depressed immune response, and infection has been established. There remains now the need to establish a program which combines food, medicine, nutritional education, and sanitation in such a way as to interrupt this continuous synergetic interaction and to ensure total health and well-being. This particularly applies to the developing nations where hundreds of

millions of subsistence farmers and many millions of the absolute poor living in exploding cities are constantly menaced by hunger and malnutrition. Closer to home, it means identifying the at-risk population within hospitals and institutions, giving special attention to the indigent poor in rural and urban areas, and providing extra support and attention to the elderly.

STUDY QUESTIONS

1 Distinguish between the clinical states of kwashiorkor and marasmus.
2 How does infection affect the individual's nutritional status?
3 Explain the cell-mediated immune response. What effect does protein-calorie malnutrition have on this response?
4 Explain humoral immunity. How is it affected by protein-calorie malnutrition?
5 Describe the functions of the complement system and the way in which the child is affected by protein-calorie malnutrition.

CLINICAL STUDY 19

The following history is that of a severely malnourished infant whose clinical picture, course, and treatment may be used as a model to better understand the significance of malnutrition in pediatrics today.

The patient was a 26-day-old malnourished white male admitted to the Boston Children's Hospital Medical Center with severe isotonic dehydration, shock, and apnea. He was born to a gravida 2, para 1, 25-year-old woman after a normal pregnancy, labor, and delivery. The baby was breast-fed 10 or 12 times daily at home and was given no supplemental foods or vitamins. The mother denied any feeding problems, but noted that the baby was often fussy. Eventually the parents did realize that the baby was thin, but he still seemed to be feeding well. On the day before hospitalization, the infant began sleeping longer than usual, and by the time of admission

he was limp and unresponsive. He had no history of fever or vomiting, but several loose stools were noted during the week prior to admission. Admission data showed the following.

Anthropometric measurements:

Birth weight	*3270 g*
Admission weight	*2280 g (69% of birth weight)*
Length	*50 cm*
Head circumference	*34 cm (after rehydration)*

Laboratory values:
Hematology
  Hematocrit   *46%*

White blood cells   10,000
(included 13 PMNs, 15 band cells, 56 lymphocytes, 11 monocytes, 3 myelocytes, and 2 metamyelocytes)

Platelets	Increased on peripheral smear
Urinalysis	
Specific gravity	1.013
Protein	1+
Glucose	Negative
Red blood cells	0
White blood cells	5–10
Hyaline casts	1–2
Chemistries	
Sodium	142 meq per L
Potassium	6.0 meq per L
Chloride	115 meq per L
Bicarbonate	17 meq per L
Blood urea nitrogen	136 mg per 100 mL
Creatinine	1.7 mg per 100 mL
Calcium	6.8 mg per 100 mL
Phosphorus	12.0 mg per 100 mL
Total protein	4.8 g per 100 mL

After initial resuscitation in the emergency clinic, the pale, emaciated, moribund infant was transferred to the intensive care nursery, and an indwelling central venous cannula was inserted. Following initial emergency hydration, his blood pressure was measured at 98/66 mmHg and central venous pressure at 5 cmH₂O. He had loose, wrinkled skin and decreased subcutaneous tissue. His anterior fontanelle was depressed and his sutures were overriding. Additional physical findings on admission included decreased breath sounds over the left lung field, decreased cardiac sounds, lethargy, and limp reflexes.

Blood, urine, cerebrospinal fluid, and nasopharyngeal, throat, and stool cultures were all negative for pathogens. A chest x-ray revealed a partial left pneumothorax secondary to the attempted placement of the central venous pressure catheter. Long bone x-rays and an upper gastrointestinal x-ray series were normal.

Clinical study questions

1 What criteria would you use to classify this infant nutritionally?

2 How may infection have compromised his nutritional status?

3 Explain the way in which the patient's nutritional status may have affected his immune response and ability to combat infection.

REFERENCES

1 Pan American Health Organization, *Inter-American Investigation of Mortality in Childhood, First Year of Investigation, Provisional Report,* Pan American Health Organization, Washington, D.C., 1971.

2 J. M. Bengoa, "The Problem of Malnutrition," *WHO Chronicle,* 28:3, 1974.

3 R. J. Merritt and R. M. Suskind, "Nutritional Survey of Hospitalized Pediatric Patients," *American Journal of Clinical Nutrition,* 32:1320, 1979.

4 N. S. Scrimshaw, "Causes and Prevention of Malnutrition," in G. H. Beaton (ed.), *Nutrition, a Comprehensive Treatise,* Academic Press, New York, 1964.

5 Ibid.

6 Ibid.

7 D. B. Jelliffe, "Infant Nutrition in the Subtropics and Tropics," World Health Organization Monograph Series, no. 25, 1955.

8 M. Behar, "Principles of Treatment and Prevention of Severe Protein Malnutrition in Children (Kwashiorkor)," *Annals of the New York Academy of Science,* 69:954, 1958.

9 Scrimshaw, op. cit.

10 Scrimshaw, op. cit.

11 F. Gomez, "Malnutrition in Infancy and Childhood with Special Reference to Kwashiorkor," *Advances in Pediatrics,* 7:131, 1955.

12 J. C. Waterlow, "Some Aspects of Childhood Malnutrition as a Public Health Problem," *British Medical Journal,* 4:88, 1974.

13 J. P. Habicht, "Height and Weight Standards for Preschool Children—How Relevant are Ethnic Differences in Growth Potential?" *Lancet,* 1:611, 1974.

14 Waterlow, op. cit., p. 88.

15 Habicht, op. cit., p. 611.

16 Behar, op. cit., p. 954.

17 C. J. Waterlow, *Advances in Protein Chemistry,* 15:138, 1960.

18 Scrimshaw, op. cit.

19 C. Gopalan, "Kwashiorkor and Marasmus: Evolution and Distinguishing Features," in R. A. McCance and E. M. Widdowson (eds.), *Calorie Deficiencies and Protein Deficiencies,* Little, Brown and Company, Boston, 1968.

20 R. Hooley, "Clinical Nutrition Assessment: A Perspective," *Journal of the American Dietetic Association,* 77:683, December 1980.

21 N. S. Scrimshaw, C. E. Taylor, and J. E. Gordon, "Interactions of Malnutrition and Infection: Advances in Understanding," World Health Organization Monograph Series, no. 57, 1968.

22 Ibid.

23 J. M. Reyna-Barrios, "Methods to Increase Coverage and Improve the Quality of Ambulatory Patient Care in Rural Areas of Guatemala, Using Medical Auxiliaries," *Revista del Colegio Medico de Guatemala,* 22:134, 1971.

24 N. S. Scrimshaw, C. E. Taylor, and J. E. Gordon, op. cit.

25 W. R. Beisel, "Malnutrition as a Consequence of Stress" in R. M. Suskind (ed.), *Malnutrition and the Immune Response,* Raven Press, New York, 1977.

26 W. R. Beisel, "Non-Specific Host Defense Factors," in R. M. Suskind (ed.), op. cit.

27 R. D. Feigin, "Whole Blood Amino Acids in Experimentally Induced Typhoid Fever in Man," *New England Journal of Medicine,* 278:293, 1968.

28 W. R. Beisel, "Nutritional Effects on the Responsiveness of Plasma Acute Phase Reactant Glycoproteins," in R. M. Suskind (ed.), op. cit.

29 R. Edelman, "Cell Mediated Immune Function," in R. M. Suskind (ed.), op. cit.

30 C. M. Jackson, *The Effects of Inanition and Malnutrition upon Growth and Structure,* P. Blakiston's Son and Co., Philadelphia, 1925, p. 285.

31 J. W. Mugerwa, "Lymphoreticular System in Kwashiorkor," *Journal of Pathology,* 105:105, 1971.

32 T. H. Work, "Tropical Problems in Nutrition," *Annals of Internal Medicine,* 70:701, 1973.

33 P. M. Smythe, "Thymic Lymphatic Deficiency and Depression of Cell Mediated Immunity in Protein Calorie Malnutrition," *Lancet,* 2:939, 1971.

34 R. K. Chandra, "Rosette-Forming T Lymphocytes and Cell-Mediated Immunity in Malnutrition," *British Medical Journal* 3:608, 1974.

35 P. Kulapongs, "In Vitro Cellular Immune Response in Thai Children with Protein Calorie Malnutrition," in R. M. Suskind (ed.), op. cit.

36 Ibid.

37 J. Wallach, *Interpretaton of Diagnostic Tests,* Little, Brown and Company, Boston, 1974, p. 5.

38 R. Edelman, "Cell-Mediated Immune Function," in R. M. Suskind (ed.), op. cit.

39 Ibid.

40 S. D. Douglas, "Disorders of Phagocyte Formation; Analytical Review," *Blood,* 35:851–866, 1970.

41 E. U. Rosen, "Leukocyte Function in Children with Kwashiorkor," *Archives of Diseases of Children* 50:220, 1975.

42 A. Seth, "Opsonic Activity of Phagocytosis and Bactericidal Capacity of Polymorphs in Undernutrition," *Archives of Diseases of Children,* 47:282, 1972.

43 Ibid.

44 R. K. Chandra, "Immunoglobulins and Antibody Response in Malnutrition," in R. M. Suskind (ed.), op. cit.

45 S. Sirisinha, "Secretory and Serum IgA in Children with Protein Calorie Malnutrition," *Pediatrics,* 55:166, 1975.

46 R. K. Chandra et al., "Reduced Secretory Antibody Response to Live Attenuated Measles and Polio Virus Vaccines in Malnourished Children," *British Medical Journal,* 2:583, 1975.

47 R. B. Johnston, "The Biology of the Complement System," in R. M. Suskind (ed.), op. cit.

48 S. Sirisinha et al., "The Complement System in Protein Calorie Malnutrition," in R. M. Suskind (ed.), op. cit.

49 R. M. Suskind, "Endotoxemia, A Possible Cause of Decreased Complement Activity in Thai Children with Protein Calorie Malnutrition," in R. M. Suskind (ed.), op. cit.

50 P. Gruenwald, "Fetal Growth as an Indicator of Socioeconomic Change," *Public Health Reports,* 83:867, 1968.

51 A. Lechtig et al., "Influence of Maternal Nutrition on Birth Weight," *American Journal of Clinical Nutrition,* 28:1223, 1975.

52 R. Suskind, "The In-Patient and Out-Patient Treatment of the Child with Severe Protein-Calorie Malnutrition," in R. E. Olson (ed.), *Protein Calorie Malnutrition,* Academic Press, New York, 1975.

53 Ibid.

54 J. M. Bengoa, op. cit.

55 N. S. Scrimshaw, "Causes and Prevention of Malnutrition," op. cit.

56 Ibid.

57 J. C. Waterlow, *Advances in Protein Chemistry,* op. cit.

58 J. M. Bengoa, "Prevention of Protein Calorie Malnutrition," in R. E. Olson (ed.), op. cit.

59 Ibid.

60 N. W. Scrimshaw, "All Vegetable Protein Mixture for Human Feeding. V. Clinical Trials with INCAP Mixtures 8 & 9 and with Corn and Beans," *American Journal of Clinical Nutrition*, **9**:196, 1961.

61 J. M. Bengoa, "Prevention of Protein Calorie Malnutrition," op. cit.

62 R. Bisewara, "Nutrition and Family Size," *Journal of Nutrition and Diet*, 1969, p. 258.

63 J. M. Bengoa, "The Problem of Malnutrition," op. cit.

CLINICAL DISCUSSION 19

According to Waterlow's standards the infant was classified as having third-degree malnutrition since his weight for height was 79 percent of the expected value and his weight had dropped significantly from his birth weight because of an inadequate supply of breast milk, although the child was placed at the breast every 2 h throughout the day.

On admission, the child was rehydrated with Ringer's lactate and subsequently with 5 percent dextrose and 0.2% saline, and was given potassium supplementation and magnesium intramuscularly. He was also treated with ampicillin and gentamicin for 10 days because of clinical suspicion of sepsis. After 48 h, he was started on one-half-strength Similac with Iron and then gradually advanced to full-strength Similac with Iron. He was also given additional vitamins and minerals (B complex, K, multivitamins, folic acid, and iron). After 4 weeks of hospitalization, the infant was discharged weighing 3160 g. Parents were advised on the amount of formula to give per feeding (4½ to 5 oz). They were given suggestions about the type of nipple to use (since the infant was formerly breast-fed, he initially experienced difficulties getting accustomed to the bottle). Additional information was provided on the introduction of baby food. The child was followed up routinely in the well-child clinic and after 1 month the supplementary vitamins were discontinued.

Malnutrition occurring during this critical period of rapid brain and body growth placed this child at risk. In addition his condition was further compromised by the depression of the immune response system, leaving him susceptible to infection and allowing the sepsis to develop. This child shows the effect of the synergism between nutritional status, the body's immune response, and infection.

CHAPTER 20

THE ALLERGIC RESPONSE AND DIET

Mary Alice Marino

KEY WORDS
Antigen
Antibody
Allergen

INTRODUCTION

A problem specific to childhood but occurring at all ages is that of *food allergy*. Because of the possible effect of food allergy on nutrient utilization and the physiological stress imposed by the allergy, individuals are placed at nutritional risk, with the growth and development of children particularly threatened. Good management is imperative and includes strict avoidance of the offending foods, and awareness of the age-specific nutritional needs.

An *allergy* is the immunologically mediated reaction or hypersensitivity to a substance which produces symptoms in the allergic individual. Although the allergy can appear at any age, the incidence is highest in infants and young children. The sensitivity to a particular food often diminishes with increasing age, but the tendency may never be completely outgrown. It has been estimated that approximately half of adult allergies begin in childhood.[1]

IMMUNOLOGICAL BASIS OF ALLERGY

To understand food allergy, it is necessary to consider the allergic reaction as a response of the body's immune defense system, whereby the body guards against the intrusion of a foreign substance, the *antigen* (see Chap. 19). In the case of food allergy, the antigens are natural products, usually protein, that are ingested in food. Since the body regards these as intruding substances, it produces an *antibody* which binds the antigen. Antibodies, also known as *immunoglobulins,* are found in the blood or tissues of all healthy persons. However, the allergic individual often produces a greater quantity than normal of a particular immunoglobulin, IgE, which creates an overreaction of this protective mechanism. IgE is present in high concentration in the mucosa of the gastrointestinal tract, bronchial tubes, and nose. These are referred to as the allergy "shock organs" and are very frequently the sites for the antigen-antibody reactions of food allergy.

During the process of digestion, most food

antigens are destroyed by the gastrointestinal tract. Because the protein molecules are very large, they rarely enter the bloodstream. The higher incidence of food allergy in infants is thought to be related to the lower efficiency of their immature gastrointestinal systems. This allows more incompletely digested food and consequently more antigens or food allergens to penetrate the mucosa. When allergens do cross the mucosa and enter the bloodstream, antibody production is stimulated, thus sensitizing the individual. On reexposure to the same antigen, an antigen-antibody reaction occurs locally at the mucosa or at various end-organ sites. If the allergic reaction is intense enough, there will be a clinical manifestation with symptoms.

SYMPTOMS

Because the symptoms are often varied and nonspecific, the topic of food allergy is a subject of much confusion and debate. There are no immunological methods for accurately confirming or predicting the allergic symptoms that may follow ingestion of any food.[2] The reactions may occur in almost any body system—gastrointestinal, respiratory, cutaneous, urinary, or nervous system, mucous glands, and mucous membranes.

Table 20-1 shows the diversity of the symptoms which have been attributed to food allergy. Although the allergy may be as localized in manifestation as the appearance of eczema on the hands, it often occurs as a generalized and diffuse reaction with such symptoms as headache, vomiting, and urticaria (hives), involving many body systems. One particular food may be responsible for a variety of symptoms in the same individual.

The immunological responses to foods often duplicate the symptoms of other disorders. Conditions which produce similar symptoms include: intestinal enzyme deficiency, bacterial or viral infections, chemical and drug contamination, neurological problems, and psychological disturbances.[3]

The reaction to an ingested food may be immediate (within the first hour), intermediate (1 to 24 h), or delayed (after 24 h). Although the foods causing immediate symptoms are easy to identify, those which produce intermediate or delayed responses often make diagnosis difficult.[4] It is thought that intact proteins crossing the gastrointestinal mucosa are responsible for the rapidly occurring symptoms, whereas the later reactions are caused by products formed during the digestive process.

TABLE 20-1   COMMON ALLERGIC SYMPTOMS

System	Symptoms
Gastrointestinal	Canker sores, cheilitis, colic, colitis, diarrhea, malabsorption, enteropathy, vomiting
Respiratory	Rhinitis, cough, asthma, bronchitis
Cutaneous	Angioedema, eczema, pruritus, purpura, urticaria
Central nervous system	Headache, neuralgias, irritability, personality change
Miscellaneous	Pallor, enuresis, retarded growth, menstrual irregularity

FOOD ALLERGENS

Although almost any food could be the cause of an allergic reaction, certain foods are known to be particularly potent allergens. Some of the most common offenders are milk, eggs, wheat, chocolate, nuts, fish and shellfish, citrus fruit, tomatoes, legumes, and corn. It is the protein component of the foods which is considered to be the cause of the allergy.

Milk Allergy

Hypersensitivity to cow's milk is usually considered to be the most common allergy in infants and young children.[5,6] Part of the reason that cow's milk is such a frequent offender is its high level of consumption, particularly in infancy. The estimated frequency of occurrence in infants ranges from less than 1 to 7.5 percent, depending on the method used for diagnosis.[7-9] The sensitivity may be due to one of three proteins found in milk: lactalbumin, lactoglobulin, and casein. Lactalbumin plays the primary role in allergic reactions. Symptoms often related to milk allergy are eczema, colic, mucous and bloody diarrhea, and asthma.

The protein in cow's milk has also been implicated as a cause of an acquired carbohydrate intolerance in young infants.[10,11] Some infants with gastrointestinal symptoms resulting in hypersensitivity to cow's milk demonstrate small-bowel mucosal damage and decreased levels of lactase.

Iron-deficiency anemia and intestinal loss of blood and protein have been noted to result from high intakes of pasteurized milk. These conditions occur primarily in infants under 1 year of age whose milk intake is over 1 L per day. Heat treatment of commercially prepared formulas seems to alleviate this problem, thus making heat-labile protein the suspected cause of the difficulty. This problem does not, however, have a demonstrated immunologic basis. It is, therefore, more appropriately classified as a protein- and cell-losing enteropathy than as an allergy.[12]

Wheat Allergy

Wheat contains several proteins which are potential antigens and is the cereal grain responsible for most allergic responses. Gluten, a protein found in wheat, but also occurring in barley, rye, and oats, is responsible for celiac disease in children and nontropical sprue in adults. It is speculated that antibodies produced following the ingestion of gluten cause an immune response which injures the mucosa and results in the malabsorption of protein, fat, carbohydrate, vitamins, and minerals [see "Gluten-Sensitive Enteropathy (Celiac Sprue)," in Chap. 22]. Although both corn and rice are low in gluten, many individuals are also sensitive to corn. Rice is the grain that is least likely to produce an allergic manifestation.

Egg Allergy

Egg is an important allergen, frequently causing violent and almost instantaneous reactions. Egg allergy, often manifesting as eczema or urticaria, is most common in infancy and early childhood. The sensitivity is in response to *albumin,* the protein in the egg white, and may even be induced by inhaling the odor of cooking eggs. Although not as common a problem as the albumin of the egg white, the egg yolk can also cause symptoms. Because many vaccines are often grown on egg or chick embryo, the egg-sensitive child must be guarded against such inoculations, which may have dangerous effects.

Other Allergies

The vegetable most commonly producing an allergic response is tomato. Legumes (including peanuts) are also important allergens. Citrus fruits and melons are the fruits associated with the highest incidence of allergies. Urticaria is a symptom frequently observed in fruit allergies. Botanical group allergies are common. For example, an individual who is allergic to oranges will often be sensitive to other citrus fruits: grapefruit, lemon, and lime.

Fish and seafood are also potent allergens. Some individuals are sensitive to fish but can tolerate shellfish, whereas others have a generalized allergy to all types of seafood. Symptoms often reported from fish allergy include urticaria, gastrointestinal problems, and migraine headaches. Beef, pork, and poultry may cause cutaneous and respiratory problems. Of all the meats, lamb is the least common offender.

Nuts, chocolate and cocoa, mustard, black pepper, cloves, and food additives are other reported sources of food allergy. Food additives have been implicated as a causative factor in hyperactivity, although there is no definitive evidence for this (see "Food Additives and Hyperactivity" in Chap. 26).

DIAGNOSIS

By using the fundamentals of immunology and observing the requirements of scientific method, an orderly approach to diagnosing food allergy is possible.[13] The steps involved in the diagnostic process include: clinical study, dietary study, food challenge, and identification of an immunologic basis for the problem.

Clinical Study

Family history, medical history, and differential diagnosis are important areas of the clinical study. There are hereditary factors present in food allergies in terms of both the offending foods and the symptoms that occur. It has been noted that a child has nearly a 75 percent chance of having a food allergy if both parents have allergies, and a 50 percent chance if one parent is affected.[14] A medical history can help identify the symptoms as to time of appearance, severity, and any accompanying physiological or psychological stress. Infection and emotional stress can precipitate an allergic response to food in a previously nonallergic individual. Because adverse reactions to foods may be associated with various medical problems, it is necessary to rule out these other conditions before a definitive diag-

nosis of food allergy can be made. The history and physical findings are utilized as the basis for determining the appropriate diagnostic procedures. For example, if ulcerative colitis is suspected, a sigmoidoscopy may be indicated; or if lactase deficiency is a possibility, a lactose tolerance test, a breath hydrogen test, or a small intestinal biopsy may be performed. (See Chap. 22.) These diagnostic procedures must be used discerningly if an accurate clinical appraisal is to be made. During the evaluation phase, objectivity on the part of the patient and physician must be maintained.

Dietary Study

A dietary history and a food diary are useful diagnostic tools. The dietary history can be utilized to correlate the individual's food intake with the clinical manifestation of the symptoms. It will provide information regarding the kinds and amounts of foods usually eaten. In addition, the individual may be asked to keep a food diary for a 3- to 14-day period. (See Chap. 18.) The diary should include the kinds and amounts of all foods and beverages consumed as well as the symptoms that occur.

Food Challenge

If the clinical and dietary studies positively suggest food allergy, the next step in the diagnostic process is a food challenge. This is necessary to verify that the adverse reaction noted is caused by food.[15] For 2 weeks prior to the challenge, all suspected foods are avoided. If it is not clear which foods are responsible for the symptoms, an elimination diet may be used (see Table 20-2). The elimination diet excludes all foods which commonly cause allergic responses.

In the challenge period one particular suspected food is given in gradually increasing amounts. The effects are then observed for 1 week before another food is added. It is suggested that for optimal clinical accuracy, especially with subjective complaints, the dou-

TABLE 20-2   ELIMINATION DIET

Foods allowed at mealtime	Snacks	Avoid
Rice	1 box rice cereal	Any food and drink
Puffed rice	midmorning	suspected to cause
Rice flakes	and	reactions or not
Rice Krispies	midafternoon	on this list
Pineapple		Pepper and spices
Apricots		
Cranberries		Coffee
Peaches		Tea
Pears		
		Chewing gum
Lamb		
Chicken		
Asparagus		
Beets		
Carrots		
Lettuce		
Sweet potato		
White vinegar		
Olive oil		
Honey, 2 oz per day		
Cane sugar		
Salt		
Oleomargarine without milk (Mazola margarine)		
Crisco, Spry		
Tapioca		
Bubble Up (a carbonated, dye-free beverage)		

Source: C. D. May and S. A. Bock, "Adverse Reactions to Food Due to Hypersensitivity," in E. Middleton, Jr., C. E. Reed, and F. E. Elliot (eds.), *Allergy Principles and Practice,* vol. 2, The C. V. Mosby Company, St. Louis, 1978, p. 1164.

ble-blind technique be utilized in the food challenge.[16] Neither the patient nor the observer should know what food is being challenged. The food should be disguised in some way or fed in opaque colorless capsules.

Identification of Immunologic Basis

The use of objective measurements to identify the immunologic basis for an adverse reaction to food is another important diagnostic step. Because of the primary role of IgE (gamma-E globulin) antibodies in initiating the allergic re-

sponse, diagnostic procedures are often directed at identifying either antigen-specific IgE or total IgE. The skin test and the radioallergosorbent test (RAST) are two techniques which may be useful to verify foods causing an IgE-mediated response.

Skin Test

In skin testing the patient's skin is exposed to extracts of the suspected food by the scratch, prick, or intradermal techniques. The appearance of localized edema or of a wheal within 20 min of the challenge is considered a positive test. This swelling, which is sometimes accompanied by erythema, indicates that a specific antigen-antibody reaction has occurred. The skin test is not always reliable, however, in diagnosing food allergies. Hill et al. demonstrated that 10 out of 17 infants with clinically documented cow's-milk allergy had a negative skin test to cow's milk.[17] On the other hand, hypersensitivity noted on skin testing of food often is false positive and has no clinical significance.[18]

RAST

The RAST is a relatively simple and convenient test for measuring circulating levels of allergen-specific IgE antibodies in a patient's serum. The RAST method has some of the same reliability problems as the skin test, since levels of IgE to a particular food may or may not correlate with clinical problems.[19,20] However, a recent study by Wraith et al. demonstrated the RAST technique to be particularly useful in diagnosing food allergy in patients with immediate as well as with nonimmediate symptoms.[21]

TREATMENT

Once the source of the allergy is determined, treatment is that of strict avoidance. A second, and as important, aspect of management involves a careful assessment of the nutritional adequacy of the modified diet. Comparable foods must be substituted for the foods eliminated, particularly when they represent important sources of energy, protein, vitamins, and minerals. The three allergens which require the most aggressive management in relation to both ensuring optimal nutrition and maintaining consistent avoidance are milk, wheat, and egg.

Milk-Free Diet

Since milk is the primary source of nutrients in infancy and continues to function as a valuable contributor of protein, energy, calcium, riboflavin, and vitamin D during childhood and into adult life, the individual with milk allergy requires special consideration. The milk-sensitive infant may be given one of the soybean or hypoallergenic milk substitutes (see Table 20-3). Also available on the market is Gerber's Meat Base Formula, a combination of strained beef hearts, sucrose, sesame oil, tapioca, calcium ascorbate, and vitamins A and D. This is perhaps useful for infants who are allergic to both cow's milk and soybean milk. Some children who are sensitive to the lactalbumin in milk may be able to tolerate goat's milk as a substitute because the

TABLE 20-3   SOY AND HYPOALLERGENIC FORMULAS* SUBSTITUTED FOR MILK

Formula	Company	Protein Source
Isomil	Ross Laboratories	Soy protein isolate
Meat Base Formula	Gerber Products Co.	Beef hearts
Mull-Soy	Borden Inc.	Soy protein isolate
Nutramigen	Mead Johnson & Co.	Hydrolyzed casein
ProSobee	Mead Johnson & Co.	Soy protein isolate
Sobee	Mead Johnson & Co.	Soy protein isolate
Soyalac	Loma Linda Food Co.	Soy protein isolate

*For more composition information, refer to Table 13-4.

whey portion, which is the lactalbumin portion, is different in goat's and cow's milk. It is important to note, however, that a macrocytic anemia due to a deficiency of vitamin B_{12} in goat's milk sometimes occurs in the children receiving this substitute.

In older children and adults, adherence to a milk-free diet is more difficult, since milk is such a common ingredient in foods. Some individuals are able to tolerate milk after it is heated, and therefore are allowed custards, puddings, cakes, breads, and soups made with milk. For others, however, heat treatment has no effect on the allergic response to milk. Table 20-4 presents a milk-free diet, which would be necessary for the management of this allergy.

TABLE 20-4   MILK-FREE DIET

Type of food	Foods allowed	Foods avoided
Beverages	Carbonated drinks, Kool-Aid, fruit juices, cocoa made with water, lemonade, tea Special formulas: See Table 20-3	Fresh, dried, or evaporated milk, malted milk, cocoa made with milk solids
Bread and crackers	French bread, rye bread, RyKrisp, homemade bread made without milk, pretzels, Ritz crackers, Triscuit, graham crackers, saltines, soda, Premium, Uneeda	Bread unless made without milk; hot breads (pancakes, waffles, griddle cakes, muffins, biscuits)
Cereals	Any cereal served with fruit juice or milk substitute	Cereals if served with milk or cream
Meat, fish, and poultry	All, if prepared without sauces made with milk or cream	Wieners and bologna if milk solids added in processing (check labels)
Eggs	In any form, if milk is not added	None, if milk is not added
Cheese	None	In all forms
Desserts	Fruit, Popsicles, fruited Jello, homemade puddings made without milk (tapioca, junket, cornstarch pudding), fruit ice, water ice, homemade pies, cakes, cookies made without milk	Ice cream, sherbet, all puddings, custards, cakes, pies, and cookies made with milk, yogurt
Fats	Vegetable oils, lard, margarines without added milk solids (kosher margarine)	Butter, cream, sour cream, margarine with added milk solids, salad dressings with milk added
Potato and substitutes	Potato, rice, pastas (spaghetti, macaroni, noodles) if milk or cheese is not added	None, if milk, cream, butter, or cheese is not added
Soups	Broth, clear consommé, bouillon, broth-based	Creamed soups
Vegetables	All	None, if milk, cream, butter, or cheese is not added
Fruits	All	None
Miscellaneous	Moderate amounts of sugar, jams, jellies, lollipops, hard candies, peanut butter, nuts, corn chips, potato chips, popcorn (without butter added), pickles, olives, meat juice gravy	Candy made with milk (caramels, milk chocolate, fondant, nougat), hollandaise sauce

Wheat-Free Diet

Since most baked and commercial products use wheat flour as an important ingredient, strict adherence to a wheat-free diet is a particular challenge. Obtaining an adequate energy intake is often difficult on this regimen (see Table 20-5). The avoidance of enriched wheat flour removes a source of iron, thiamin, niacin, and riboflavin, and care must be taken to ensure that these nutrients are provided from other sources. Rice flour may be substituted in most recipes, in the proportion of ¾ cup of rice flour for 1 cup of regular wheat flour.

Egg-Free Diet

Egg has many uses in cooking, and therefore its presence in foods is extremely common. Other

TABLE 20-5   WHEAT-FREE DIET

Type of food	Foods allowed	Foods avoided
Beverages	Milk, carbonated drinks, Kool-Aid, fruit juices, lemonade, hot chocolate	Postum, Ovaltine
Breads and crackers	Rye bread if 100% rye, RyKrisp, corn bread or muffins, rice flour bread or muffins if made at home without wheat flour added	All other breads, rolls, crackers
Cereals	Any corn, oat, or rice cereal	Wheat cereals—farina, bran, puffed wheat, shredded wheat
Meat, fish, and poultry	Plain meats, fish, and poultry prepared without breading and without gravy made with flour	Breaded meats, processed meats (wieners, hot dogs) if bread fillers added, meat loaf, croquettes, meatballs if bread added
Eggs	Fried, poached, boiled, scrambled, baked	None
Cheese	Cheddar, American, Swiss, cottage, farmer	None, unless flour is added to processed cheese foods
Desserts	Fruits, Jello, fruit ice, sherbet, ice cream, custard, Junket, puddings made from rice or cornstarch	Cakes, pies, cookies, doughnuts (except if made with rice flour)
Fats	Vegetable oils, butter, margarine, lard	Salad dressings, gravy, if thickened with flour
Potato and substitutes	Potato, rice	Spaghetti, noodles, macaroni, stuffing unless made with rice, dumplings
Soups	Homemade soups, consomme, made without flour	All canned soups
Vegetables	All	Only if sauce made with flour is added
Fruits	All	None
Miscellaneous	Moderate amounts of sugar, jams, jellies, peanut butter, nuts, potato chips, pickles, olives, meat juice gravy	Beer, pretzels

foods with protein and iron, such as meat, fish, and poultry, can be substituted for egg. The primary nutritional concern in the growing child who is egg-sensitive relates to ensuring adequate calories, since a great majority of baked goods contain egg and need to be avoided. Egg binds and adds volume to cakes, thickens creamed dishes and sauces, helps pies and cookies brown, and glazes breads. To replace egg as the binding substance in cakes, an equal amount of mashed banana may be substituted. An extra ½ teaspoon of baking powder can also be added to the egg-free cake recipe to make up for the loss of volume. In creamed dishes and sauces, extra flour or cornstarch can be added to replace the thick-

ening action of the egg. Table 20-6 lists the allowable foods and those which must be avoided by the egg-sensitive individual.

DIET COUNSELING

Successful treatment of food allergy depends on good diet counseling based on the following considerations:

1 A thorough diet history accompanied by a 24-h recall must serve as the basis for counseling. These techniques are useful in identifying adherence to the diet as well as nutritional problems. When an important

TABLE 20-6 EGG-FREE DIET

Type of food	Foods allowed	Foods avoided
Beverages	All except those which have egg added	Eggnog
Breads and crackers	Saltine crackers, soda crackers, graham crackers, white, wheat, rye, French, pumpernickel breads	Hot breads or any breads and crackers made with egg, French toast
Cereals	Any	None
Meat, fish, and poultry	All except those with egg added	Any prepared or coated with egg; sausage, croquettes, meat loaf
Eggs	None	All
Cheese	All	None
Desserts	Fruits, Jello, fruit ice, sherbet, ice cream, puddings if made without egg, pies if made without egg	Cakes, cookies, frostings, French ice cream made with eggs, meringue, custards, Bavarian creams
Fats	Vegetable oils, butter, margarine, lard	Salad dressing if egg added
Potato and substitutes	Potato, rice, noodles except those with added egg, macaroni, spaghetti	Egg noodles
Soups	All except those with egg or egg noodles added	Soups with egg or egg noodles
Vegetables	All	None
Fruits	All	None
Miscellaneous	Moderate amounts of sugar, jams, jellies, lollipops, hard candy, candies made without egg, peanut butter, nuts, potato chips, corn chips, pretzels, pickles, olives	Hollandaise sauce, candies made with egg

nutrient source or an entire food group must be eliminated because of the allergy, alternative food sources must be included. In certain instances it may be necessary to supplement the diet with vitamins and/or minerals, if other food sources cannot be successfully added.

2 An important habit to foster in proper management of food allergy is reading the labels of all prepared and processed foods. The offending allergen may be present in unexpected sources and may be listed in unfamiliar terms. The following ingredients indicate that milk or a milk derivative has been added: lactose, caseinate, sodium caseinate, casein, lactalbumin, curds, and whey. Eggs may be added to foods in the following forms: albumin, vitellin, livetin, yolk, powdered or dried egg, globulin, ovomucoid, and ovomucin.

3 Advice regarding recipes appropriate for milk-free, wheat-free, and egg-free diets is helpful (see Table 20-7).

4 Guidelines for restaurant choices and other meals eaten away from home are also important considerations in diet counseling.

Strict avoidance of the food allergen and relief of the troublesome symptoms are vital concerns in the management of food allergy, but also necessary is a sensitivity to the nutritional and emotional needs of the patient. Nutritional adequacy and variety are important goals in the food allergy diet.

PREVENTION OF FOOD ALLERGY

There has been much interest in recent years concerning the usefulness of dietary measures to prevent food allergy.[22,23] These prophylactic techniques have particular importance to infants of parents with a history of allergies. Because there is an increased vulnerability in early infancy to the passage of intact food protein across the gastrointestinal mucosa, methods to prevent this sensitization in infants with a family history of allergy have been studied.[24,25] These studies

TABLE 20-7 SOURCES OF RECIPES FOR ALLERGY DIETS*

Allergy Recipes
> The American Dietetic Association
> 430 North Michigan Avenue
> Chicago, IL 60611

Baking for People with Food Allergy
> Superintendent of Documents
> U.S. Government Printing Office
> Washington, DC 20402

Carnival Recipes (party food ideas for egg-free, wheat-free, and milk-free diets)
> General Foods
> Box 130
> Coubourg, Ont., Canada

Low Gluten Diet with Tested Recipes and a List of Gluten-Free Commercial Products
> A. B. Frence
> Clinical Research Unit
> University Hospital
> Ann Arbor, MI 48104

Milk-Free, Egg-Free, Wheat-Free, Milk-Egg-Wheat-Free Diets
> Ralston Purina Co.
> Consumer Services
> St. Louis, MO 63188

125 Recipes for Allergy Diet
> Good Housekeeping
> 959 Eighth Avenue
> New York, NY 10019

Wheat, Milk, and Eggfree Recipes from Mary Alden
> Quaker Oats Co.
> Merchandise Mart Plaza
> Chicago, IL 60654

*Although many recipes are free, some do require a fee. It is best to contact the individual company for a current cost policy.

have focused on delaying the introduction of foods known to be potent allergens. Johnstone and Dutton demonstrated a decreased incidence of allergic responses in infants who for the first nine months of life did not receive cow's milk, chicken, egg, or wheat.[26] In a study by Matthew et al. exclusively breast feeding infants for at least the first 3 months of life resulted in fewer cases of infantile eczema.[27] Although the routine use of these prophylactic dietary measures is still subject to debate,[28] they may have value in preventing the occurrence of allergic reactions in susceptible infants.

STUDY QUESTIONS

1 What is an allergic reaction?
2 What are some of the common allergic symptoms related to food allergy?
3 What are the four steps in diagnosing a food allergy?
4 What are the nutritional concerns for an individual with milk allergy? Wheat allergy? Egg allergy?
5 List four considerations that are important when one is counseling the allergy patient.

CLINICAL STUDY 20

Julie, a 7-month-old infant girl, was seen by her pediatrician with a 2½-week history of diarrhea and vomiting. Her weight had dropped from 7.3 kg (50th percentile) at age 6 months to a present weight of 7.0 kg (10th to 25th percentile). Julie's length at 6 months was 67 cm (75th percentile), and at this visit it was measured at 68 cm (50th to 75th percentile).

Julie's early history was unremarkable, having had no significant problems before the current onset of symptoms. She had been breast-fed from birth and had always been a good feeder. At 3½ months her mother had introduced cereals (rice, oats, and barley); at 4 months, strained fruits (applesauce, bananas, peaches, and pears); and at 5 months, strained vegetables (green beans, carrots, beets, and spinach). Julie's mother had been careful to introduce each new food gradually and to wait several days before trying another new food. The solids had all been well accepted without any problems. Approximately 3 weeks prior to this visit, Julie's mother had begun weaning her from the breast. She had introduced one 6-oz bottle of cow's milk each day for the first three days and then had increased the amount to two 6-oz bottles each day.

Julie's family history was positive for food allergy, since her mother was allergic to shellfish and strawberries. Because the presenting symptoms and the family, medical, and dietary histories suggested a possible hypersensitivity to food, further diagnostic procedures were conducted. For two weeks Julie was placed on an elimination diet, including only the following foods: breast milk, rice cereal, peaches, pears, carrots, and beets. After three days on this diet, her symptoms disappeared. At the end of the 2-week period, Julie was brought into the hospital for food challenge and further testing. A cow's milk challenge was conducted, and two days later, the vomiting and diarrhea recurred. Skin test and RAST were negative for cow's milk. A biopsy of the small intestine showed normal levels of disaccharidase enzymes and no structural defects in the mucosa.

Clinical study questions

1 *What condition would you diagnose in this infant? Relate the dietary history, clinical findings, and diagnostic procedures to the suspected problem.*
2 *Why was the biopsy performed?*
3 *How do you explain the negative skin test and RAST?*
4 *What would be the appropriate dietary intervention, considering the diagnosis?*
5 *What specific nutritional concerns would you have for this infant?*

REFERENCES

1 C. A. Frazier, *Coping with Food Allergy,* Quadrangle Books, The New York Times Company, New York, 1974, p. 6.

2 S. J. Fomon, *Infant Nutrition,* 2d ed., W. B. Saunders Company, Philadelphia, 1974, p. 414.

3 C. D. May and S. A. Bock, "Adverse Reactions to Food Due to Hypersensitivity," In E. Middleton, Jr., C. E. Reed, and F. E. Elliot (eds.), *Allergy, Principles and Practice,* vol. 2, The C. V. Mosby Company, St. Louis, 1978, p. 1160.

4 Ibid., p. 1161.

5 C. A. Frazier, op. cit., p. 9.

6 G. B. Goldstein and D. C. Heiner, "Clinical and Immunological Perspectives in Food Sensitivity," *Journal of Allergy,* **46**(5):270, 1970.

7 C. D. May and S. A. Bock, op. cit., p. 1160.

8 E. J. Eastham and W. A. Walker, "Effect of Cow's Milk on the Gastrointestinal Tract: A Persistent Dilemma for the Pediatrician," *Pediatrics,* **60**(4):477, 1977.

9 J. W. Gerrard et al., "Cow's Milk Allergy: Prevalence and Manifestations in an Unselected Series of Newborns," *Acta Paediatrica Scandinavica Supplement,* 234, 1973.

10 N. Iyngkaran et al., "Acquired Carbohydrate Intolerance and Cow Milk Protein-Sensitive Enteropathy in Young Infants," *The Journal of Pediatrics,* **95**(3):373, 1979.

11 D. J. Hill et al., "The Spectrum of Cow's Milk Allergy in Childhood," *Acta Paediatrica Scandinavica,* **68**:847, 1979.

12 C. D. May and S. A. Bock, op. cit., p. 1167.

13 Ibid., p. 1159.

14 C. A. Frazier, op. cit., p. 4.

15 C. D. May and S. A. Bock, op. cit., p. 1163.

16 Ibid., pp. 1163–1165.

17 D. J. Hill et al., op. cit.

18 L. H. Criep, *Allergy and Clinical Immunology,* Grune and Stratton, New York, 1976, p. 171.

19 D. J. Hill et al., op. cit.

20 C. D. May and S. A. Bock, op. cit., p. 1166.

21 D. G. Wraith et al., "Recognition of Food-Allergic Patients and Their Allergens by the RAST Technique and Clinical Investigation," *Clinical Allergy,* **9**:25, 1979.

22 "Breast Feeding and Avoidance of Food Antigens in the Prevention and Management of Allergic Disease," *Nutrition Reviews,* **36**(6):181, 1978.

23 D. J. Atherton et al., "Double-Blind Controlled Crossover Trial of an Antigen-Avoidance Diet in Atopic Eczema," *Lancet,* **1**:401, 1978.

24 D. E. Johnstone and A. M. Dutton, "Dietary Prophylaxis of Allergic Disease in Children," *New England Journal of Medicine,* **274**(13):715, 1966.

25 D. J. Matthew et al., "Prevention of Eczema," *Lancet,* **1**:321, 1977.

26 D. E. Johnstone and A. M. Dutton, op. cit.

27 D. J. Matthew et al., op. cit.

28 S. J. Fomon, op. cit., p. 456.

CLINICAL DISCUSSION 20

On the bases of the symptoms, the family, medical, and dietary histories, and food challenge, the diagnosis of cow's-milk allergy was made. Because Julie had had no reaction at the time the various cereals, fruits, and vegetables were introduced, challenges to these foods were not considered necessary. The biopsy ruled out celiac disease and intestinal enzyme deficiencies. This test had further usefulness in determining that no mucosal damage or lactase deficiency had occurred secondary to the cow's-milk allergy. Skin test and RAST often show poor correlation to food allergies. The false negative results are common in cow's-milk allergy which manifests as gastrointestinal symptoms.

All cow's milk was excluded from the infant's diet. Julie's mother decided to proceed with weaning Julie from the breast, but soy protein formula (processed with supplements of vitamins and iron) was used in place of cow's milk. The soy formula provided an essential source of protein, calories, calcium, vitamin D, and riboflavin.

One month later, Julie was seen for follow-up in the allergy clinic. She had made excellent gains in both weight and length, and her parents reported that she was again a contented baby with none of the former symptoms. She was taking approximately 28 oz of soy formula each day and tolerated it without problems. Her mother had begun introducing meats, which were well-accepted. Julie was also enjoying a variety of cereals, fruits, and vegetables. Her caloric intake averaged 825 cal (3465 kJ) per day, or 105 kcal (441 kJ) per kilogram of body weight. It was decided that the milk-free diet should be continued and that Julie should receive regular medical follow-up with a periodic review of the diet.

CHAPTER 21

THE CARDIOVASCULAR SYSTEM

Margaret L. Mikkola

KEY WORDS
Ischemic Heart Disease
Atherosclerosis
Cholesterol
Hyperlipoproteinemia
Hypertension
Congestive Heart Failure
Diuretic

INTRODUCTION

The heart and blood vessels make up the cardiovascular system, and together establish and maintain the circulation. The heart is a muscular organ which functions as a pump. The blood vessels are a successively dividing series of progressively smaller tubes beginning with the aorta, progressing to arteries, then to arterioles, and finally reaching the capillaries. At this point they gather successively into venules, veins, and the vena cava to return to the heart. The aorta is primarily an elastic structure; the arteries and arterioles, muscular; and the capillaries, thin-walled (one-celled) structures. The venules, veins, and vena cava lack, in large part, the elastic and muscular tissue of the arteries. The heart and blood vessels are so arranged as to link the systemic circulation (peripheral blood vessels) and the pulmonary circulation (blood vessels of the lungs) in series, thus providing a continuous system for blood flow (Fig. 21-1).

The primary functions of the cardiovascular system are to deliver oxygen, required for aerobic metabolism, from the lungs to the other organs (brain, kidneys, liver, skeletal muscle), and, on return, to transport carbon dioxide, as metabolic waste, back to the lungs. These functions are autoregulated by a complex feedback mechanism between the heart and blood vessels on the one hand and the metabolic demands of the organism for oxygen on the other hand.

Diseases of the cardiovascular system affect the heart and its components (heart valves, conduction system, and myocardium) and the blood vessels, primarily the arteries.

In 1977, disease of the cardiovascular system accounted for over 700,000 deaths in the United States.[1] This figure represents deaths; there are many people alive who are affected by one or more of these diseases. Many of these people are asymptomatic and undiagnosed, while others are handicapped. Because of the high incidence of cardiovascular diseases, many investigations have been initiated to develop effective and feasible means of prevention and treatment.

Blood flow	*Area*
Blood returns from the general systemic circulation through the inferior and superior venae cava to the right atrium	Inferior and superior venae cava Right atrium
It then flows to the right ventricle through the tricuspid valve and then is ejected by the right ventricle through the pulmonary valve into the pulmonary artery and to the lungs.	Right ventricle Pulmonary arteries ↓ Lungs
Oxygenated blood returns to the left atrium via the pulmonary veins. It then passes through the bicuspid valve to the left ventricle and is pumped through the aortic valve into systemic circulation through the systemic capillary beds where the oxygen and nutrients are distributed.	Pulmonary veins Left atrium Left ventricle Aorta ↓ Systemic capillary beds

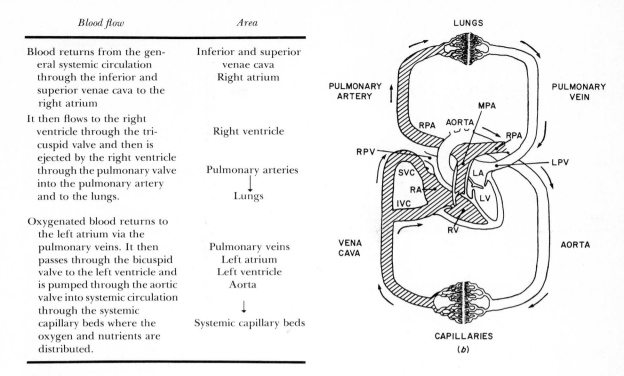

Figure 21-1
Diagram of the cardiovascular system. The heart and blood vessels are so arranged as to link the systemic circulation and the pulmonary circulation in a series, thus providing a continuous system for blood flow.

Cardiovascular disorders that affect human morbidity and mortality in the United States are ischemic heart disease, hypertensive heart disease, congestive heart failure, rheumatic heart disease, and congenital heart disease. In this chapter, ischemic heart disease will be emphasized both because of its high incidence and because of the direct implications for dietary management in prevention and treatment. *Ischemic heart disease* and *coronary artery disease* are inclusive terms that imply deprivation of the blood supply to the heart and include atherosclerosis, angina pectoris, and myocardial infarction.

ISCHEMIC HEART DISEASE

Atherosclerosis is a degenerative disease of the large and medium arteries. It results from a loss of elasticity *(sclerosis)* that occurs when the inner layer of the arterial wall becomes thickened by atheromatous plaques, consisting first of lipid (mainly cholesterol) followed by fibrous tissue. As these plaques increase in size they may inhibit blood flow through the affected arteries, leading to the clinical manifestations of the disease, primarily ischemic (deprived of blood supply) heart disease. The mechanisms by which these plaques progress is not completely understood. The suspected mechanisms are:[2]

1 Thrombus formation (clot formation on the surface of the plaque followed by fibrous organization of the thrombus)
2 Continued lipid accumulation
3 Hemorrhage into the plaque

A question frequently posed in regard to plaque formation and atherosclerosis is whether atherosclerosis is a pediatric problem. Fatty streaks in the major arteries have been identified in the first years of life.[3-5] (A fatty streak is a superficial yellowish-gray lesion, similar in composition to the lipids in blood and the earliest accumulation of lipid found in the intima of medium-sized and large arteries.) However, because these streaks have been shown to have about the same severity and prevalence in the first decades of life among many races and countries no matter what the incidence of ischemic heart disease in these countries, their causative role in the later formation of adult lesions is not clear. Adult lesions evolve from fatty streaks, but the streaks found in the early decades of life do not necessarily predict liability to the disease. Presently, this question must await further research before it can be answered. Figure 21-2 is a diagrammatic illustration of the natural history of atherosclerosis.

Anticoagulants are often used in the treatment of atherosclerosis in addition to diet therapy. The purpose of anticoagulants is to prevent clot formation. The most commonly used anticoagulants are Heparin, Warfarin, and Dicumarol. When an individual is receiving anticoagulant therapy, specifically Dicumarol, the dietary intake of vitamin K and supplements providing this vitamin should be monitored. This monitoring is necessary since vitamin K promotes clotting of the blood by increasing hepatic synthesis of prothrombin. (Vitamin K sources include spinach, alfalfa, cabbage, and egg yolk.)

The most serious form of atherosclerosis is ischemic heart disease. Its major clinical manifestations are angina pectoris, acute myocardial infarction, sudden death, disturbance in heart rhythm, and congestive heart failure.

Angina pectoris may be defined as a symptom complex consisting of acute substernal chest pain, usually with a characteristic radiation to the left arm, resulting from transient ischemic deprivation of blood flow to the subendocardial layers of the ventricular myocardium. This may

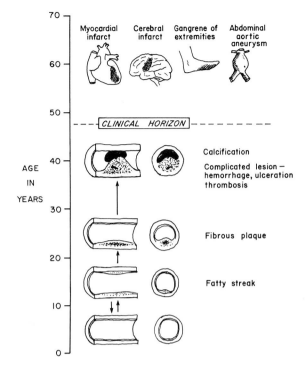

Figure 21-2
Diagram of the natural history of atherosclerosis.
[Adapted from H. C. McGill, J. C. Geer, and J. P. Strong, "Natural History of Human Atherosclerotic Lesions," in M. Sandler and G. H. Bourne (eds.), *Atherosclerosis and Its Origins,* Academic Press, New York, 1963, p. 42.]

occur when the blood supply to the heart is diminished by stenotic obstructive atheromatous lesions in the walls of the coronary arteries. The symptoms of angina frequently may be precipitated by exertion or exercise, when the coronary blood flow, because of the atheromatous plaques, is unable to meet the oxygen requirements of the exercising heart. Angina pectoris is a common warning signal of coronary artery disease. It can exist for many years in a stable form or may be altered and thus signal the onset of a myocardial infarction.

Myocardial infarction (heart attack) is the extension of diminished coronary blood flow from a transient phenomenon to a state of total permanent deprivation of blood supply to various areas of the heart by complete obstruction of the coronary artery. The severity of the heart attack is related to the site and extent of the interruption of coronary flow, the state of unaffected coronary arteries (the collateral circulation), and the condition of the heart muscle (e.g., from previous heart attacks).

Treatment for angina pectoris includes avoidance of activities which produce its occurrence (often excessive exertion), the use of nitroglycerin and other drugs, maintenance of ideal body weight, and appropriate prescribed exercise. Intractable angina pectoris (unresponsive to nitroglycerin or propranolol), with operative stenotic lesions demonstrated by coronary angiography, has been surgically treated by inserting an autogenous saphenous vein graft from the aorta to the involved coronary artery, bypassing the obstructive lesions. Symptomatic results are encouraging although a certain percentage of the grafts have become obstructed after surgery.

Treatment for myocardial infarction requires hospitalization for proper management. This will include diet therapy when the patient's condition is stable. The emphasis of dietary therapy immediately after hospitalization is of course to aid in attaining a stable condition by utilizing a nutritionally adequate diet which is usually soft, bland, and easily tolerated. If this can be done with the type of diet (i.e., fat-controlled, low-cholesterol) that the patient will be following after discharge, dietary teaching will be more effective.

Complications that may develop after a myocardial infarction are cardiovascular shock, arrhythmias, and congestive heart failure. These complications are treated with medical therapy, which includes digitalis, anticoagulants, diuretics, and dietary salt restriction as well as mechanical methods to aid the pumping function of the heart.

Sudden death may occur during an acute myocardial infarction but also may occur in a patient with no symptoms or with stable angina, or when there has been a previous myocardial infarction. The immediate mechanism is probably ventricular fibrillation (total disorganization of heart contractions). Recently mortality from myocardial infarction has been decreasing in areas where there are mobile and hospital coronary care units.

It is important that patients be educated about the warning signs of myocardial infarction (for example, chest pain) and about the risk factors, which are discussed below.

Cerebrovascular disease is another major form of atherosclerosis. It includes the complex clinical symptoms of *transient cerebral ischemic attacks* and *strokes*. The symptoms that occur depend on the artery involved, the area of the brain supplied, the nature of the collateral circulation, and the pathologic process in the artery. Strokes may be associated with atherosclerosis, resulting in cerebral infarction (the brain is deprived of blood), or may be associated with hypertensive disease, resulting in brain hemorrhage.

Other types of atherosclerosis include aortic, renovascular, peripheral vascular, and pulmonic. Each type has symptoms manifested in the organ or area supplied by the affected arteries. Treatment depends on the extent and location of the plaque and may consist of medical therapy, including medication, diet (e.g., weight reduction, sodium restriction), and exercise, or surgical intervention.

Risk Factors

Several risk factors, identified through extensive epidemiologic studies, have been associated with an increased rate of atherosclerosis and ischemic heart disease. Of the factors identified none is believed to be solely responsible; they are thought to be multiple causal, each playing an interrelated role. The risk factors cited by the American Heart Association can be separated into (1) overt problems and personal attributes, and (2) environmental factors (see Table 21-1). From the factors identified in the table one can separate into groups those which cannot be modified, those which are difficult to adjust, and those which can be altered or are subject to intervention (see Table 21-2). In the future, epidemiologic studies of populations in whom these

TABLE 21-1   RISK FACTORS AND CORONARY DISEASE

Overt problems and personal attributes	Environmental factors
Familial occurrence of coronary disease at an early age	Cigarette smoking
Hypertension	Lack of physical activity
Electrocardiographic abnormalities	Emotionally stressful situations
Diabetes mellitus	
Lipid abnormalities involving serum cholesterol and triglycerides and their lipoprotein vehicles	
Obesity	
Gout (hyperuricemia)	
Certain personality and behavior patterns	

Source: Risk Factors and Coronary Heart Disease: A Statement for Physicians, American Heart Association Publication EM451, 1968. Reprinted with permission.

risk factors have been changed may define the extent to which the progression of atherosclerosis and ischemic heart disease can be altered.

Dietary intervention is especially important in the adjustment of three risk factors, namely, *obesity, hypertension,* and *hyperlipidemia.* Since hyperlipidemia has been identified as one of the major risk factors and is particularly responsive to diet therapy, its role in ischemic heart disease will now be considered.

Hyperlipidemia

Hyperlipidemia is an elevation of serum cholesterol, triglycerides, or both. Cholesterol, triglycerides, and phospholipids are carried in the plasma bound to specific proteins, the alpha-globulin and beta-globulin fractions of plasma protein. These lipoproteins vary as to the amount of protein and fat they contain and can be identified according to their density and electrophoretic mobility. The four major classes of lipoproteins are:

> Chylomicrons
> Pre-beta (very-low-density) lipoprotein (VLDL)
> Beta (low-density) lipoprotein (LDL)
> Alpha (high-density) lipoprotein (HDL)

Figure 21-3 shows the composition of the various lipoproteins. Low-density lipoproteins (LDL) and very-low-density lipoproteins (VLDL) are those lipoproteins which contain the most lipid and the least protein; high-density lipoproteins (HDL) are those containing the most protein and the least lipid. Table 21-3 gives the normal limits of the plasma lipids and lipoproteins. Generally, the HDL level is higher in women than in men,[6] and the level has been thought to remain relatively constant in all individuals. Studies, however, have indicated a link between increased physical activity and high levels of HDL, but this is still unconfirmed in general population studies. Other factors believed to affect an individual's HDL and pres-

TABLE 21-2   ALTERABILITY OF RISK FACTORS IN ATHEROSCLEROSIS AND ISCHEMIC HEART DISEASE

Possible	Difficult	Impossible
Hyperlipidemia*	Underlying disease	Heredity
Hypertension*	Stress	Advancing age
Obesity*	Personality	Sex
Smoking		
Exercise		

*Dietary implications.

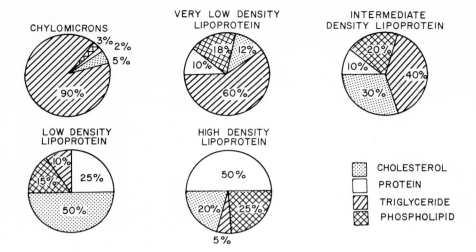

Figure 21-3
Composition of lipoproteins. (Adapted from R. I. Levy, "Drug Therapy Treatment of Hyperlipidemia," *New England Journal of Medicine,* **290**:1296, 1974.)

TABLE 21-3 PLASMA LIPID AND LIPOPROTEIN CONCENTRATIONS
Suggested normal limits*

Age	Total cholesterol, mg/100 mL	Triglyceride, mg/100 mL	Pre-beta cholesterol, mg/100 mL	Beta cholesterol, mg/100 mL	Alpha cholesterol, mg/100 mL Males	Alpha cholesterol, mg/100 mL Females
0–19	120–230	10–140	5–25	50–170	30–65	30–70
20–29	120–240	10–140	5–25	60–170	35–70	35–75
30–39	140–270	10–150	5–35	70–190	30–65	35–80
40–49	150–310	10–160	5–35	80–190	30–65	40–85
50–59	160–330	10–190	10–40	80–210	30–65	35–85

*Based on 95 percent fiducial limits calculated for small samples—all values rounded to nearest 5 mg. (It will be noted that, for practical purposes, differences between the sexes have been ignored except for alpha-lipoprotein concentrations.)
Source: D. S. Fredrickson, "Fat Transport in Lipoproteins—An Integrated Approach to Mechanisms and Disorders," *New England Journal of Medicine,* **276**:151, 1967.

ently being investigated include diet, alcohol consumption, and medications. At present there is considerable emphasis being placed on an individual's HDL level as a result of several population studies which have demonstrated an inverse association between HDL cholesterol and coronary heart disease.[7,8]

The occurrence of another lipoprotein has been proposed, that of a transient intermediate-low-density lipoprotein (ILDL) appearing during conversion of VLDL to LDL.[9] This lipoprotein has not been shown to have any dietary significance at this time.

Electrophoresis enables the lipoprotein to be separated by charge, on paper or agarose gel, to a nonmigrating lipoprotein band (Fig. 21-4).

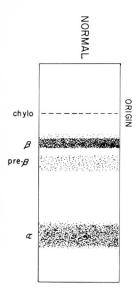

Figure 21-4
Normal lipoprotein band on electrophoresis.

The lipoproteins can also be identified by ultracentrifugation, which separates them according to their density. These two methods have been used to determine the lipoprotein values in plasma and to identify five major types of hyperlipoproteinemias, which are discussed in detail below.

Since diet is essential in the treatment of the hyperlipoproteinemias, those dietary factors influencing the lipoproteins will now be discussed.

Dietary treatment involves alteration in the following dietary components: cholesterol, fat, saturated fat, polyunsaturated fat, carbohydrate, and alcohol.

Cholesterol

Changes in the diet can cause predictable changes in the plasma cholesterol level. The cholesterol level in the red blood cells remains very constant, approximately 138 mg per 100 mL of cells, and the effects of diet exert their influence on the serum.[10] Most of the cholesterol in the plasma is carried in the LDL. Keys has reported that the usual American diet averages approxi-

mately 250 mg cholesterol per 1000 kcal (or 250 mg cholesterol per 4200 kJ) and that at this level of intake substantial changes in the serum cholesterol level are difficult to detect.[11] Table 21-4 gives the average amount of cholesterol in some common foods.

Fat

The normal metabolic pathways of fat are described in Chap. 5. The ingested long-chain free fatty acids (chain length of C_{12} or greater) are reesterified with glycerol to form triglycerides in the intestinal mucosa. These triglycerides combine with cholesterol esters, phospholipids, and protein to form the chylomicrons of plasma. These macroparticles serve as a vehicle for transport of fatty acids within the plasma. In the human body chylomicron levels rise after meals; the amount of chylomicron formation is determined by the amount of fat ingested. Chylomicrons eventually move from the plasma into the body's fat depot, a process facilitated by the enzyme lipoprotein lipase. There are certain individuals who do not adequately clear the chylomicrons and even after a 12 to 16 hour fast their plasma levels remain elevated. This is known as *exogenous hyperlipidemia* and indicates a deficient clearing mechanism, possibly resulting from decreased lipoprotein lipase activity.

Dietary fat has a less understood effect on the VLDL. Both the liver and intestine synthesize VLDL from glucose and free fatty acids. An elevation of VLDL from this source is known as *endogenous hyperlipidemia*. The availability of free fatty acid is determined by several factors, one of which—and of primary importance—is obesity.

Saturated Fats

Saturated fatty acids, primarily those with 12 through 17 carbon atoms and especially lauric acid, elevate the plasma cholesterol. Saturated fats are primarily of animal origin, although several nonanimal sources are highly saturated, for example, coconut oil. Table 21-4 lists some of the common sources of saturated fats.

TABLE 21-4   CHOLESTEROL AND FAT CONTENT OF SELECTED FOODS

Food	Measure	Weight, g	Fat, g	SFA, g	Linoleic acid, g	Oleic acid, g	Cholesterol, mg
Egg yolk	1 large	50*	5.6	1.7	0.6	2.0	274
Liver (beef, calf, lamb, pork)		100					438
Kidney		100					804
Brains, raw		100					>2000
Veal (lean only)		100	2.4	0.7	0.1	0.6	99
Beef, round (lean only)		100	6.4	2.7	0.25	2.3	91
Lamb, leg (lean only)		100	9.6	4.0	0.4	3.4	100
Pork							
Loin (lean only)		100	13.9	4.7	1.15	5.8	88
Cured ham		100	8.8	3.0	0.7	3.7	
Poultry (chicken, turkey)							
Light (flesh only)		100	3.9	1.1	0.7	1.0	77
Dark		100	10.1	2.9	2.1	2.8	90
Fish							
Flounder (raw)		100					50
Haddock		100	1.0	0.6	tr	0.3	60
Halibut		100					60
Tuna, canned water pack		100	0.8	0.2	0.01	0.1	63
Salmon, canned pink		100	5.2	0.85	0.1	0.8	35
Shellfish							45–150 (varies widely)
Milk							
3.7% fat	1 cup	244	8.9	5.6	0.3	2.3	35
1% fat	1 cup	244	2.6	1.6	0.1	0.7	10
Skim	1 cup	245	0.4	0.3	tr	0.1	4
Butter	1 tbsp	14	11.4	7.1	0.3	2.8	31
Cream							
Light	1 tbsp	15	2.9	1.8	0.1	0.7	10
Half & half		15	1.7	1.1	0.04	0.4	6
Heavy		15	5.5	3.5	0.2	1.4	21
Sour		12	2.5	1.6	0.1	0.6	5
Cottage cheese							
4% fat	½ cup	113	5.1	3.2	0.1	1.5	17
1% fat	½ cup	113	1.2	0.7	0.02	0.3	5
Cheddar cheese	1 oz	28	9.4	6.0	0.2	2.2	30
American cheese	1 oz	28	8.9	5.6	0.3	2.1	27
Cream cheese	1 oz	28	9.9	6.2	0.2	2.4	31

SFA = saturated fatty acids; tr = trace; > = more than; < = less than.

*Whole egg.

(Continued)

TABLE 21-4 CONTINUED

Food	Measure	Weight, g	Fat, g	SFA, g	Linoleic acid, g	Oleic acid, g	Cholesterol, mg
Yogurt							
Whole milk	½ cup	113	3.7	2.4	0.1	0.8	14
Partially skim	½ cup	113	1.8	1.1	0.05	0.4	7
Ice cream 16% fat	1 cup	148	23.7	14.7	0.9	6.0	88
Sherbet, orange	1 cup	193	3.8	2.4	0.1	1.0	14
Oils							
Safflower		100	100	9.1	74.5	11.7	
Sunflower		100	100	10.3	65.7	19.5	
Corn		100	100	12.7	58.7	24.2	
Soybean		100	100	14.4	51.0	22.8	
Cottonseed		100	100	25.9	51.9	17.0	
Olive		100	100	13.5	7.9	72.5	
Peanut		100	100	16.9	32.0	44.8	
Coconut		100	100	86.5	1.8	5.8	
Nuts							
Walnuts	1 cup	100	63.4	6.9	34.9	9.7	
Peanuts	⅔ cup	100	49.7	9.4	14.4	22.9	
Cashews	⅔ cup	100	45.6	9.2	7.3	26.2	
Margarines							
Corn oil (average)							
Tub	1 tbsp	14	11.8	2.1	4.2	4.5	
Stick	1 tbsp	14	11.8	2.1	3.3	5.4	
Shortening, Vegetable	1 tbsp	12.8	12.8	3.2	3.1	5.7	
Mayonnaise	1 tbsp	13.8	11.2	1.6	5.1	3.1	8
Avocado	⅔ cup	100	16.4	3.3	2.1	7.4	
Chocolate	1 oz	28	15.0	8.4	0.3	5.6	
Lard		100	100	39.2	10.2	41.2	95

SFA = saturated fatty acids; tr = trace; > = more than; < = less than.

Sources:
1 R. M. Feeley, "Cholesterol Content of Foods," *Journal of the American Dietetic Association,* **61**:134–149, 1972.
2 L. P. Posati, *Comprehensive Evaluation of Fatty Acids in Foods—Dairy and Egg Products,* U.S. Department of Agriculture Handbook 8-1, November 1976.
3 B. A. Anderson, "Comprehensive Evaluation of Fatty Acids in Foods. II. Beef Products," *Journal of the American Dietetic Association,* **67**:35–41, 1975.
4 J. B. Reeves III, *Composition of Foods: Fats and Oils,* U.S. Department of Agriculture Handbook 8-4, June 1979.
5 G. A. Fristrom, "Comprehensive Evaluation of Fatty Acids in Foods. IV. Nuts, Peanuts and Soups," *Journal of the American Dietetic Association,* **67**:351–355, 1975.
6 L. P. Posati, *Composition of Foods: Poultry Products,* U.S. Department of Agriculture Handbook 8-5, August 1979.
7 B. A. Anderson, "Comprehensive Evaluation of Fatty Acids in Foods. VII. Pork Products," *Journal of the American Dietetic Association,* **69**:44–49, 1976.
8 J. Exler, "Comprehensive Evaluation of Fatty Acids in Foods. VIII. Finfish," *Journal of the American Dietetic Association,* **69**:243–248, 1976.
9 C. F. Adams, *Nutritive Value of American Foods,* U.S. Department of Agriculture Handbook 456, November 1975.
10 B. K. Watt, *Composition of Foods,* U.S. Department of Agriculture Handbook 8, December 1963.
11 R. M. Leverton, *Fats in Food and Diet,* U.S. Department of Agriculture Information Bulletin 361, January 1974.
12 B. A. Anderson, "Comprehensive Evaluation of Fatty Acids in Foods. X. Lamb and Veal," *Journal of the American Dietetic Association,* **70**:53–58, January 1977.

Polyunsaturated Fats

Polyunsaturated fatty acids, primarily linoleic acid, in contrast to saturated fatty acids, have a lowering effect on the plasma cholesterol, but approximately 2 g of polyunsaturates are needed to counteract the effect of 1 g of saturates; thus, a dietary ratio of 2 to 1 (polyunsaturates to saturates) is sometimes recommended. (This is a point of controversy; see p. 446.) Polyunsaturates are primarily of vegetable origin, the greatest source being vegetable oil. Table 21-4 lists the linoleic fatty acid content of some selected foods.

Food processing may induce partial hydrogenation of polyunsaturated fat, decreasing the total amount available. Another change that may occur following food processing is isomerization of some of the naturally occurring cis fatty acids into trans fatty acids.

The effect of larger amounts of trans fatty acids in the diet is controversial; there are conflicting reports of their effect on plasma lipids, on essential fatty acid requirements, and on cell membranes.[12] Other questions have been raised regarding possible adverse effects of diets with high levels of polyunsaturated fats on the incidence of cancer,[13] but the evidence about this is inconclusive.

Vitamin E requirements are thought to be increased with higher intakes of polyunsaturated fats.[14] The vitamin E requirement for men is 10 mg α-tocopherol equivalents and for women 8 mg α-tocopherol equivalents.[15] Some sources high in polyunsaturated fats also have higher levels of the vitamin, but many do not.

Studies in adults living at home and eating diets high in polyunsaturated fat have not demonstrated a decrease in serum vitamin E levels or conclusive evidence of any harmful effect. The effects on populations who have consumed large amounts of polyunsaturated fats for extended time periods are unknown.

One needs to exert clinical judgment in the amount of polyunsaturated fat to be recommended.

Monounsaturated Fats

Monounsaturated fatty acids, primarily oleic and erucic acids, have no known effect on plasma cholesterol levels. Table 21-4 lists some of the most common oleic acid food sources.

Carbohydrate

The liver and intestine make VLDL from glucose and free fatty acids. It is believed that the primary effect of excess carbohydrate on plasma lipids is the elevation of VLDL. Normal individuals, when on a high-carbohydrate diet, will exhibit a degree of elevated plasma VLDL but this will usually disappear gradually. However, some persons have persistently elevated VLDL levels. Low-carbohydrate diets cause a significant reduction in the mean levels of triglyceride and VLDL in men who previously exhibited elevated levels. There remains controversy as to the effect of simple carbohydrates (sugars) versus more complex carbohydrates (starches) on the plasma lipids. It is generally accepted that simple sugars seem more lipemic (increasing the VLDL) in patients who have hyperlipoproteinemia. This is most likely because of the increased quantity that is frequently ingested.

Alcohol

In many types of hyperlipoproteinemia alcohol produces or exacerbates hyperglyceridemia,[16,17] but the exact mechanisms are unclear.

Hyperlipoproteinemias

Having presented the dietary factors which affect the lipoproteins, the five major types of hyperlipoproteinemia (Table 21-5, p. 440) will now be discussed, with emphasis on the dietary treatment as recommended in Table 21-6 (p. 441).

Type I Hyperlipoproteinemia

Type I hyperlipoproteinemia is manifested by the inability to clear chylomicrons from the plasma. It is believed to be due to a deficiency of the enzyme lipoprotein lipase. It is usually diagnosed in childhood.

TABLE 21-5   THE TYPES OF PRIMARY HYPERLIPOPROTEINEMIA

Type	Lipoprotein abnormalities	Usual age of expression	Familial forms	Some clinical features
I	Severe chylomicronemia	Infancy and childhood	Rare and usually familial (recessive)	Bouts of abdominal pain, pancreatitis, eruptive xanthomas, hepatosplenomegaly
IIa	LDL increased	At birth, if genetic	Most obvious genetic form is expressed in heterozygote, but is more severe in homozygote; many mild examples are not obviously familial	Premature vascular disease; in familial forms, tendon and tuberous xanthomas
IIb	LDL and VLDL increased	At birth, if genetic	Pattern alternates with IIa in families affected with "monogenic" type II; milder defects are sporadic or due to other genetic defects	Severe forms are like IIa; milder IIb patterns tend to be accompanied by glucose intolerance, obesity
III	VLDL and LDL of abnormal composition	Third decade; often after menopause in women	Frequently familial, genetic mode uncertain	Glucose intolerance, tuberoeruptive or planar xanthomas, premature vascular disease (especially peripheral vascular disease); worsened by alcohol excess
IV	VLDL increased	Usually third decade or later, can occur in children	Often half of adult close relatives will also have type IV; number of mutants or frequency of familial involvement unknown	Glucose intolerance in about 50%, excess caloric intake common; occasionally eruptive xanthomas, hyperuricemia; worsened by alcohol excess
V	VLDL increased, chylomicrons present	Adulthood, very rare in children	When familial, more than half of close relatives have either type IV or type V	Bouts of abdominal pain and pancreatitis, eruptive xanthomas, hepatosplenomegaly, excess caloric intake common, hyperuricemia; most patients have glucose intolerance; worsened by alcohol excess

LDL = low-density lipoproteins; VLDL = very-low-density lipoproteins.
Source: R. I. Levy, "Dietary and Drug Treatment of Primary Hyperlipoproteinemia," *Annals of Internal Medicine,* **77**:273, 1972.

TABLE 21-6   SUMMARY OF DIETS FOR TYPES I–V HYPERLIPOPROTEINEMIA

	Type I	Type IIa	Type IIb & Type III	Type IV	Type V
Diet prescription	Low-fat (25–35 g)	Low-cholesterol; polyunsaturated fat increased	Low-cholesterol calories approx. 20% from protein 40% from fat 40% from carbohydrate	Controlled carbohydrate—approx. 45% of calories; moderately restricted cholesterol	Restricted fat—30% of calories; controlled carbohydrate —50% of calories; moderately restricted cholesterol
Calories	Not restricted	Not restricted	Achieve and maintain "ideal" weight; i.e., reduction diet if necessary	Achieve and maintain "ideal" weight; i.e., reduction diet if necessary	Achieve and maintain "ideal" weight; i.e., reduction diet if necessary
Protein	Total protein intake is not limited	Total protein intake is not limited	High protein intake*	Not limited other than control of patient's weight	High protein intake*
Fat	Restricted to 25–35 g; type of fat not important	Saturated fat intake limited; polyunsaturated fat intake increased	Controlled to 40% of calories (polyunsaturated fats recommended in preference to saturated fats)	Not limited other than control of patient's weight (polyunsaturated fats recommended in preference to saturated fats)	Restricted to 30% of calories (polyunsaturated fats recommended in preference to saturated fats)
Cholesterol	Not restricted	As low as possible; only source of cholesterol is the meat in the diet	Less than 300 mg; only source of cholesterol is the meat in the diet	Moderately restricted to 300–500 mg	Moderately restricted to 300–500 mg
Carbohydrate	Not limited	Not limited	Controlled; concentrated sweets restricted	Controlled; concentrated sweets restricted	Controlled; concentrated sweets restricted
Alcohol	Not recommended	May be used with discretion	Not more than 2 servings (substituted for carbohydrate)	Not more than 2 servings (substituted for carbohydrates)	Not recommended

*High protein: 18–21% of calories in type IIb and III, 21–24% type V. This is well above the recommended allowances for protein and is aimed at keeping the total fat and carbohydrate in the diet restricted.

Source: D. S. Fredrickson, *Dietary Management of Hyperlipoproteinemia, A Handbook for Physicians and Dietitians,* Dept. Health, Education, and Welfare Publication (NIH) 76-110.

Clinical and laboratory signs   Chylomicrons are present in the serum (expressed in a triglyceride value often in the thousands) and give a creamy appearance to the blood. Eruptive xanthomas may be seen. Patients may complain of abdominal pain and suffer from pancreatitis.

Dietary treatment   Type I is treated with a diet very low in fat (25 to 35 g in adults, 10 to 15 g in infants),[18,19] to aid in keeping the plasma chy-lomicron level low. Medium-chain triglycerides (MCT), i.e., fatty acids of 8 to 10 carbon atoms in length, are available commercially and are often used to make the diet more palatable. MCT are absorbed directly via the portal circulation and do not increase chylomicron formation. Calories, carbohydrate, protein, and cholesterol are not restricted, but alcohol should be avoided as it may produce hypertriglyceridemia (the exact mechanism by which this is produced is unclear).

Type II Hyperlipoproteinemia

Type II hyperlipoproteinemia, also known as familial hyperbetalipoproteinemia or familial hypercholesterolemia, is characterized by an elevated cholesterol of LDL origin. Type II is one of the severest types in regard to its arterial involvement and is believed to account for a large degree of premature morbidity and mortality from ischemic (coronary) heart disease. Familial hypercholesterolemia can be diagnosed in childhood and there is considerable controversy regarding diagnosis. There are proponents for testing all children in the general population; since the cost factor is prohibitive, most are recommending screening of those infants and children who have positive family history for myocardial infarction or coronary heart disease at an early age. Also debated are the diagnostic tests to determine the at-risk population in terms of total cholesterol and triglyceride or total lipoprotein quantification. Glueck and other investigators recommend analysis of total cholesterol, triglyceride, and HDL cholesterol levels. Because elevated HDL cholesterol has been found in a significant number of children screened (up to 16 percent in some studies), the elevated HDL cholesterol may have an inverse association with coronary heart disease.[20]

Type II is further differentiated into types IIa and IIb. In type IIa triglycerides are normal while in type IIb they are elevated, as shown by increased VLDL. The fundamental defect, which appears to be inherited, is unknown.

Clinical and laboratory signs In type IIa serum cholesterol is elevated, frequently to 300 to 600 mg per 100 mL, and on electrophoresis the beta-lipoprotein band is enlarged. The homozygous child may exhibit clinical signs at birth or within the first few years of life, but the heterozygous child often is not diagnosed until environmental factors such as diet have exacerbated the clinical symptoms in later years or adulthood. The clinical signs include corneal arcus (cholesterol deposits surrounding the cornea), xanthelasma (cholesterol deposits around the eye such as on the eyelid), tendinous and tuberous xanthomas (cholesterol deposits on tendons, heel, and elbow), and premature vascular disease involving the coronary, lower limb, and cerebral arteries.

In type IIb triglycerides of VLDL origin as well as cholesterol of LDL origin are found to be elevated. Severe forms of type IIb may exhibit the same clinical features as type IIa; however, IIb is often of a milder form. Patients with mild IIb tend to be obese and glucose-intolerant.

Dietary treatment Cholesterol intake is restricted to less than 300 mg per day, ideally to 100 to 150 mg per day in children and 200 mg per day in adults when possible.[21,22] Saturated fats should be restricted to 6 to 10 percent of total calories, and the polyunsaturated fats should be adjusted to attain a polyunsaturates/saturates ratio of 1 to 1 or higher. Maintenance of ideal body weight, which may require weight reduction, is recommended. Protein, carbohydrate, and total fat from the allowed sources are not limited in type IIa if ideal body weight is maintained, and alcohol may be used with discretion. In type IIb, concentrated sweets should be restricted as well as alcohol since both have an effect on the triglyceride level.

Type III Hyperlipoproteinemia

Type III hyperlipoproteinemia is characterized by an abnormal lipoprotein with the electrophoretic mobility of a beta-lipoprotein but with a very low density. The defect is thought to be in the conversion of VLDL to LDL.

Clinical and laboratory signs Both the cholesterol and triglycerides are elevated and both are close to the same value. The plasma often appears lipemic. A "broad beta" band is found on electrophoresis. Clinical signs include planar xanthomas, tuberoeruptive lesions, xanthelasma, premature corneal arcus, and tendon xanthomas. Abnormal glucose tolerance and hyperuricemia may be found. Ischemic coronary artery disease and peripheral vascular disease are common.

Dietary treatment   Maintenance of ideal body weight is very important, so that weight reduction is frequently necessary. Dietary cholesterol should be restricted to approximately 300 mg per day or less with a concurrent substitution of polyunsaturated for saturated fats.[23] Concentrated sweets and alcohol intake should be restricted and total carbohydrate intake should make up approximately 40 percent of calories.

Type IV Hyperlipoproteinemia

Type IV or hypertriglyceridemia is characterized by an elevation of endogenous pre-beta-lipoprotein (VLDL).

Clinical and laboratory signs   Triglycerides are elevated and a slight elevation of cholesterol may be found. Plasma may appear clear, cloudy, or milky depending on the degree of triglyceride elevation. A pre-beta-lipoprotein band appears on electrophoresis. Individuals with type IV hyperlipoproteinemia often have eruptive xanthomas. Obesity, hyperuricemia, and glucose intolerance are frequently present.

Dietary treatment   Type IV responds well to attainment of ideal body weight, controlled carbohydrate intake (specifically restriction of concentrated sweets), alcohol limitation, moderate cholesterol restriction (usually 300 to 500 mg per day), and substitution of polyunsaturated for saturated fats.[24]

Type V Hyperlipoproteinemia

Type V hyperlipoproteinemia is characterized by an increased concentration of pre-beta-lipoprotein (VLDL) and an increase in chylomicrons in the fasting patient, which results in a lipemic plasma.

Clinical and laboratory signs   Triglycerides are elevated, frequently into the thousands, and concurrent elevated cholesterol is often found. Patients with type V may have eruptive xanthomas, lipemia retinalis, recurrent abdominal pain, acute and chronic pancreatitis, and hepatosplenomegaly. Type V is frequently associated with obesity and hyperuricemia, and glucose intolerance is common.

Dietary treatment   Restriction of total fat is recommended because of the appearance of some chylomicrons and the high VLDL levels. Type V requires a moderate restriction of carbohydrate since both fat and the glycerol from carbohydrate metabolism influence VLDL formation. Cholesterol is usually moderately restricted, and maintenance of ideal weight is stressed.[25] Alcohol is not recommended. The use of MCT is not recommended for type V because it also increases the VLDL levels.

Dietary Principles for Reducing Blood Lipids

Since there are some conflicting views regarding the age at which diet therapy should be started, questions arise regarding the role of cholesterol in the developing infant and whether a low-cholesterol diet could be harmful. Since maternal milk is much higher in cholesterol than many infant formulas, the advisability of a low-cholesterol diet is even more complicated because mother's milk is the prototype in infant feeding.

Fears concerning harmful effects of a low-cholesterol diet during infancy have generally been dispelled due to the significant number of newborns presently receiving commercially prepared formulas (i.e., Similac, Enfamil, SMA), which are low in cholesterol and high in polyunsaturated fat. However, there is still a concern that a high polyunsaturated fat diet could lead to the formation of gallstones.

Glueck has been able to demonstrate that infants with familial type II hyperlipoproteinemia can have their cholesterol normalized in the first year of life with dietary intervention;[27] however, it is not yet known what effect this early normalization of cholesterol means in terms of general health or of preventing the development of atherosclerosis.

Typing of the hyperlipoproteinemias has helped to determine the best treatment. There are rare occasions when typing may not be feasible. In these situations, general recommendations common to all types of hyperlipoprotein-emia may be justified.

The nutrient composition and energy patterns of the American Heart Association's preventive and therapeutic diets are shown in Table 21-7.

The American Heart Association's recommendations to physicians and health professionals are:[28]

1 Adjustment of the caloric content of the diet to achieve and maintain optimal weight

2 Reduction of the total fat content of the diet to no more than 35 percent of total calories, with restriction of saturated fat to less than 10 percent of total calories and inclusion of polyunsaturated fat to comprise up to 10 percent of total calories

3 Restriction of dietary cholesterol to less than 300 mg per day

4 Increase in carbohydrate to be derived from vegetables, fruits, and cereals

5 "Prudent" use of salt until its role in hypertension is defined

These recommendations are in accordance with the 1979 U.S. dietary goals (see Chap. 2).

The American Heart Association has also addressed the increased incidence of hyperlipidemia in childhood and adolescence and made recommendations for its diagnosis and treatment.[29]

Table 21-8 lists recommendations for one week's intake that is low in cholesterol and saturated fat. Egg yolks are the highest common source of cholesterol; persons on cholesterol-re-

TABLE 21-7   COMPOSITION OF FAT-CONTROLLED DIETS RECOMMENDED BY THE AMERICAN HEART ASSOCIATION

	Preventive diet (3) *	Therapeutic diets			
		1200 kcal (5.04 MJ)	1800 kcal (7.56 MJ)	2000–2200 kcal (8.4–9.24 MJ)	2400–2600 kcal (10.08–10.92 MJ)
Nutrients					
Carbohydrate, g	273	120	200	270	335
Protein, g	114	75	85	95	110
Fat, g	83	42	68	70	84
Saturated fatty acids, g	18	7	10	11	12
Linoleic, g	26	14	26	26	33
Cholesterol, mg	356	258	258	279	286
Iron, mg	21.6	14	14	17	19
Dietary patterns					
% energy from carbohydrate	47	41	45	51	52
% energy from protein	20	26	20	18	17
% energy from fat	33	32	35	30	30
% energy from saturated fatty acids	7	5	5	4	4
% energy from linoleic acid	10	10	13	11	11
P/S ratio†	1.4:1	2:1	2.6:1	2.4:1	2.8:1

*2300 kcal (9.66 MJ).

†Ratio of linoleic acid to saturated fatty acids.

Source: J. F. Mueller, "A Dietary Approach to Coronary Artery Disease," *Journal of the American Dietetic Association,* **62**:614, 1973.

TABLE 21-8   RECOMMENDATIONS FOR ONE WEEK'S LOW-CHOLESTEROL,
LOW-SATURATED-FAT DIETARY INTAKE

2 eggs per week (egg whites freely)

42 oz meat, fish and poultry to include: 16 oz meat
                                          14 oz poultry
                                          12 oz fish

3 oz cheddar cheese or equivalent

2 cups low-fat (1%) cottage cheese

14 cups skim milk

Approximate cholesterol content: 1650 mg per week

Approximate fatty acid content:

Saturated fatty acids	Linoleic acid
50.8 g	8.9 g

Polyunsaturated fats (safflower, sunflower, corn oil, etc., and margarines made from
these oils)—add to give the desired polyunsaturated/saturated (P/S) ratio; the amount
will also depend on the energy level desired, that is:

	Saturated fatty acids	Linoleic acid
14 tsp corn oil	8.9 g	41.1 g
14 tsp corn oil tub margarine	10.5	21.0
Total	19.4 g	62.1 g
plus fat from above items	50.8	8.9
Total	70.2 g	71.0 g
Approximate P/S ratio = 1/1		

Note: The P/S ratio can be increased by the use of safflower or sunflower oil rather than corn oil if
desired. *A minimum of 4 servings from the fruit/vegetable group and 4 servings from the bread/
cereal group should be included with the above foods to give a nutritionally balanced diet yielding
approximately 1200 calories.* For higher energy allowances more foods from the vegetable/fruit,
bread/cereal and polyunsaturated fat groups should be added accordingly.

stricted diets should either limit or avoid them
and use various egg substitutes if necessary. If
egg yolks are avoided the diet can offer much
more variety by including other cholesterol-con-
taining foods.

Meat (lamb, pork, beef) and dairy products
(whole milk, butter, cream, cheese, etc.) are the
primary sources of saturated fats and need to be
controlled. In addition, there are some highly
saturated vegetable fats, such as coconut oil and
shortenings, that are found in many prepared
products which need to be avoided. Animal
meats, because of their saturated fat content,
should be limited, and greater emphasis should
be placed on the inclusion of fish, poultry, low-
fat diary products, and vegetables as protein
sources. Table 21-9 lists those foods which
should be avoided on a low-cholesterol, low-saturated-fat diet.

The method of preparing allowed meats, by

TABLE 21-9   FOODS TO AVOID ON LOW-CHOLESTEROL, LOW-SATURATED FAT DIETS

Egg yolks—except as allowed on diet

Organ meats

Fatty meats, luncheon meats, frankfurter, bacon, sausage, poultry skin, duck, caviar

Whole milk, evaporated and condensed whole milk, filled milks with coconut oil, cream, ice cream, sour cream, whole milk cheeses and yogurt

Butter, lard, gravies made with animal fat, hydrogenated vegetable shortenings

Coconut, chocolate, palm oil

Mixed nuts, cashews, potato chips

Commercially prepared baked goods which may contain the above foods

---

trimming of fat and by baking or broiling, is essential to fat control. Several cheeses made partially or totally from skim milk as well as skim, nonfat, and fat-free milks in powdered, liquid, and evaporated forms are encouraged in the diet. An individual should be made aware of the difference between the many fat-free and low-fat products available. When making these changes in the diet, such as avoiding egg yolks and limiting red meats, the diet should be checked for nutrient adequacy since in this case the excluded foods may cause the diet to be low in vitamin A and iron content.

The most common sources of polyunsaturated fats are safflower, sunflower, corn, soybean, and cottonseed oils, and the margarines made from these oils (see Table 21-4). There are many textured vegetable-protein products being marketed today which are good sources of polyunsaturated fat. The use of oils in cooking and the use of margarines only when spreads are desired ensures a higher polyunsaturates/saturates ratio without the consumption of large amounts of fats and calories. For those people who dine out frequently, close adherence to a low-cholesterol, low-saturated-fat diet is difficult. More restaurants are willing to cater to the requests of those requiring special diets. An entrée which is broiled or baked without the addition of saturated fat and/or sauces can be requested. There is usually an adequate selection of vegetables and fruits for appetizers, salads, and desserts. As a beverage, skim milk, fruit, or vegetable juices may be possibilities. It is important to ask what menu items would be suitable for the required diet.

Many investigators are in disagreement regarding the 2 to 1 polyunsaturates/saturates ratio previously recommended. Often it is not considered necessary when the total saturated fat intake can be kept very low; moreover, with weight-reduction diets that necessitate the control of total fat intake, the use of large amounts of polyunsaturates is impossible. In the future, changing the fat composition of beef by means of variations in the feed of cattle, leading to a product that is higher in polyunsaturated fat and lower in saturated fat, may be the solution to the problem of providing variety on a fat-controlled diet.

The client should be made aware of the product label as a source of information (see "Labeling" in Chap. 2). Local and regional heart associations can be contacted for dietary booklets dealing with commercial products for fat-controlled diets.

There are several other dietary factors receiving attention in the search for causes of ischemic heart disease and hyperlipidemia. These include coffee and hard water. However, there has been no conclusive evidence of any harmful effects of these factors. Lack of dietary fiber has been proposed as a factor in atherosclerosis. It has been postulated that dietary fiber may exert a cholesterol-lowering effect. Various investigations have demonstrated a hypocholesterolemic effect with a high-fiber diet but it is not known whether this effect is due to an increase in the fiber or to the complex carbohydrate content of the diet. Trowell has presented data to support the hypothesis that dietary fiber decreases reabsorption of bile salts, increases fecal excretion, and reduces hyperlipidemia.[30]

Medical Treatment of Hyperlipidemia

Diet is the cornerstone of therapy for any of the primary or familial disorders. Diet therapy should al-

ways be tried before any drug is used. If the addition of drugs proves necessary, diet should be continued, for in essentially all cases, the effects of diet and drugs are additive and more effective than either alone.[31]

Unfortunately there are those patients in whom diet alone cannot normalize the lipid abnormalities and those who fail to comply with the dietary recommendations advised. The effects of adequate diet and medication are additive, so the client who adheres to a diet is more successfully treated with medication. If the individual chooses not to follow a diet, medical management is usually more difficult because of the compliance problems.

Each type of hyperlipoproteinemia responds most effectively to specific medications. However, different patients with the same type of hyperlipidemia often respond differently to medications, so each patient needs to be considered individually to achieve optimal benefit. There are several medications available which have been shown to treat certain lipid abnormalities effectively. These are usually grouped into two types: those that decrease lipoprotein synthesis and whose primary site of action is systemic (nicotinic acid, clofibrate), and those that increase lipoprotein catabolism and whose primary site of action is intestinal (cholestyramine, sitosterol and D-thyroxine).[32,33]

HYPERTENSION AND HYPERTENSIVE HEART DISEASE

Hypertension is defined as a sustained increase in the arterial blood pressure, either diastolic, systolic, or both. The prevalence of hypertension in adults is estimated to be somewhere between 15 and 20 percent of the population. Disparities in this estimate occur because of observer bias, because of inappropriate equipment, and because many people remain undiagnosed. Furthermore, there is not a natural cutoff point between normal and elevated blood pressures. Table 21-10 gives the generally accepted upper limits of "normal" blood pressure for different age groups. A hypertensive individual is one who has had at least three consecutive blood

TABLE 21-10 UPPER LIMITS OF NORMAL BLOOD PRESSURE BY AGE GROUP

Age group, years	Blood pressure, mmHg
Infants	90/60
3–6	110/70
7–10	120/80
11–17	130/80
18–44	140/90
45–64	150/95
65 and older	160/95

Source: B. Batterman, "Hypertension, Part 1: Detection and Evaluation," *Cardiovascular Nursing,* **11:**38, July–August 1975.

pressure values which are elevated by two or more standard deviations above the normal for the appropriate age group. Blood pressure readings should be done while the person is at rest and the values should be taken several days apart. Even the normotensive person may have elevated blood pressure at times of excitement or when involved in physical activity. Labile hypertension is diagnosed if the blood pressure is intermittently elevated. (*Labile:* subject to free and rapid change.)

There are several factors which influence the prognosis of the hypertensive patient. The factors of primary importance are age, sex, and race. The prevalence of hypertension among blacks in the United States is almost twice as high as it is in whites. Blacks also have more severe hypertension and under the age of 50 have a death rate approximately 6 to 7 times higher than whites. This rate decreases to about 2½ times higher after the age of 50.[34] At any age level the hypertensive individual has a worse prognosis than the normotensive person of the same age. More adult men have hypertension than adult women until age 50. After menopause the incidence of elevated blood pressure in women rises and remains higher. Women have a better prognosis than men at any level of blood pressure.[35] Any elevation of blood pressure, systolic or diastolic, is associated with an increased risk of morbidity and mortality from cardiovascular disease.[36,37]

Hypertension may either be *essential* (of unknown cause) or *secondary* (of known cause). Essential hypertension, i.e., without any known cause, accounts for about 90 percent of hypertensive patients. Causes of secondary hypertension include renal parenchymal disorders, peripheral vascular disease, endocrine abnormalities, and coarctation of the aorta. The family history of hypertensives suggests genetic factors; however, the bulk of evidence indicates that in the origin of hypertension genetic tendencies are modified by environmental factors. Obesity, cigarette smoking, stress, and sedentary life-styles have all been associated with the occurrence of hypertension,[38] although none of these factors alone has been shown to cause hypertension. Morbidity from cardiovascular diseases also increases when hypertension occurs in conjunction with these conditions.

Diet, specifically sodium intake, is receiving more attention in the search for the cause of essential hypertension.[39,40,41] Many studies, both in human populations and in animal experiments, have implicated a high sodium intake as a causative factor.[42] The Committee on Nutrition of the American Academy of Pediatrics has estimated that approximately 20 percent of the children in the United States are at risk of developing hypertension when they reach adulthood.[43] Because of this high number, much attention has focused on the dietary sodium intake of infants and children. When solid foods are introduced early into the infant's diet, sodium intake increases substantially and exceeds by severalfold the minimum requirements of the amount provided by human milk. In the last few years manufacturers have reduced the salt content of baby foods, and solid foods have been delayed until 5 to 6 months of age (see Chap. 13). The diets of older children and adolescents continue to exceed the minimum daily requirement for sodium,[44] since we consume much commercially prepared food high in sodium content. Also, certain food patterns, such as kosher and Chinese, provide large amounts of sodium.

Hypertension may occur in mild forms and often remains undiagnosed for years. When undiagnosed or left untreated, hypertension, if severe, may result in damage to the heart, eyes, kidneys, or brain. If the hypertension is diagnosed before complications occur, treatment may delay end-organ manifestations. As in the hyperlipidemia syndrome, the problem of early treatment in the child with a predisposition for essential hypertension remains a quandary. Treatment of children with elevated blood pressure is based on the hypothesis that therapy will reduce morbidity and mortality rates later in life. Studies have recently been established that will follow up early hypertensive children into adulthood to determine if this is correct. Factors such as obesity, diet, and life-style of the adolescent probably play a role.

Treatment

Treatment of the hypertensive individual includes both medications and diet. Diet may include sodium restriction and weight reduction, depending on the condition of the patient.

Sodium Restriction

Sodium restriction lowers arterial blood pressure by producing a negative salt and water balance, which prevents the development of sodium and water retention. Currently there is much discussion in the literature with respect to the appropriate level of sodium restriction. While various levels of sodium restriction are often advised, most advocates of sodium deprivation agree that to be effective in long-term treatment of essential hypertension, dietary sodium intake must be limited to 200 to 250 mg (approximately 9 to 10 meq) per day.[45,46,47] There are individuals with hypertension who respond well to milder sodium restriction, so that its value should not be discounted. An intake of 250 mg is very restricted and often impractical when renal function is adequate enough to allow diuretic drugs to be effective. Strict sodium restriction is advised at the beginning of diuretic treatment in patients with cardiac failure or decreased kidney function, in order to hasten the establishment of negative sodium and water balance. Any treatment of hypertension should include the avoidance of obviously salted foods and other forms of excessive sodium intake. This is advised to avoid overriding the ability of the diuretic to prevent sodium retention.

For help in planning a sodium-restricted diet, Table 21-11 lists the sodium content of selected foods and suggested amounts for use in sodium-restricted diet plans. Cultural food habits with predilections for salt may prevail, along with acquired taste from years of usage, so that diet planning may not be easy. Salt substitutes may help to make diets more appetizing and various herbs and spices (see Table 23-6) can be used in food preparation; however, this is a difficult transition for any patient. Salt is one of the primary tastes—taste buds specific for salt are located on each side of the tongue. Individuals accustomed to receiving a lot of taste stimulation from these centers need to be highly motivated and given much support to help them refrain from this basic instinct.

Generally, animal foods and dairy products have a sodium content which varies with the protein content: the higher the protein content, the higher the sodium. Thus, skim milk products and leaner meats have a higher sodium content than whole milk products and fatty meats. Most cheeses and dairy products contain high levels of sodium.

Kosher meats are generally quite high in sodium (approximately 600 to 1000 mg sodium per 3 oz). This can be altered to an extent by the type of koshering. Low-sodium meats may be koshered by broiling rather than salting. This permits the blood to drip away from the meat. The sodium content of other fresh meats and fish can be reduced by boiling them in water and discarding the liquid.

The amount of sodium in the drinking water varies considerably. Water treated in most water-softening equipment is often much higher in sodium because the conditioners add sodium to replace calcium and magnesium in harder water.

There are many medications which contain considerable amounts of sodium and should be avoided on sodium-restricted diets. These include many antacids, laxatives, and bromides, such as Alka-Seltzer and Brioschi (see Table 23-7).

Many high-sodium compounds are used in food manufacturing and in food preservation. These commonly include baking powder, sodium bicarbonate, sodium propionate, sodium alginate (found in chocolate milk drinks and ice cream), sodium nitrate, and monosodium glutamate.

Table 21-12 (p. 451) lists the most common foods that should be avoided on sodium-restricted diets.

Weight Reduction

Weight rduction is advised in the treatment of the hypertensive patient. The intent is to decrease the extra cardiac load imposed by obesity. It is not clear whether there is a direct relationship between body weight or obesity and blood pressure. However, obese individuals have an increased tendency to develop diabetes or hyperlipidemia, which may influence the morbidity and mortality of the hypertensive patient.

Medications

The medications used in the treatment of hypertension are numerous. The first ones usually employed are the oral diuretics, including the thiazides, ethacrynic acid, and furosemide. Both sodium restriction and these medications produce saluresis (salt loss) and diuresis (water loss), resulting in a reduction in extracellular fluid volume, plasma volume, and total exchangeable sodium, with the desired fall in blood pressure. An associated decrease in cardiac output then occurs. After several weeks of this therapy these factors rise to their previous normal levels but blood pressure usually remains lower. The exact mechanisms which maintain the lowered blood pressure are not known.

Side effects of these diuretics include hypokalemia (low serum potassium), hyperuricemia (high serum uric acid), and hyperglycemia (high

TABLE 21-11 SODIUM CONTENT OF SELECTED FOODS AND SODIUM-RESTRICTED DIET PLANS*

Food	Amount	Sodium, mg (approximate values)	Levels of sodium restriction (amounts per day)			
			500 mg	1000 mg	2000 mg	4000 mg
Milk						
Regular	8 oz (240 g)	125	2 cups	2 cups	2 cups	2 cups
Low-sodium		less than 5				
Egg	1 average	60	†	†	†	†
Butter, margarine	1 tsp (5 g)					
Salted		50	...	2	4	4
Unsalted		0-1	4	4	freely	freely
Cheese‡	1 oz (28 g)	200-300	...	...	...	1
Meat, fish, poultry	1 oz					
Salted		300	...	...	...	5
Unsalted		20	5	5	5	
Vegetables	½ cup					
Salted		250	...	...	...	1
Unsalted		10	3	3	3	3
Fruit	½ cup	0-5	4	4	4	4
Bread						
Salted	1 slice	125-150	...	2	6	6
Unsalted	(approx. 25 g)	5-10	6	4		
Cereals:						
Salted	1 cup	200-300	...	...	1	1
Unsalted		5	1	1		
Beverages (beer, wine, distilled spirits, carbonated beverages, coffee, tea)	8 oz	0-20				
Desserts						
Gelatin (made from dessert powder)	½ cup	60	...	...	...	1
Ice cream	½ cup	55	...	...	...	
Baked goods	Varies widely. Any containing baking powder or baking soda should be omitted on sodium-restricted diets.					

*The above amounts are those needed to provide recommended dietary allowances for various nutrients. For unrestricted caloric diets, unsalted foods from any of the food groups may be used to make up the required caloric intake.

†1 egg may be substituted for 1 oz of meat, poultry, or fish (limit to 1 egg per day).

‡¼ cup unsalted cottage cheese of 1 oz low-sodium cheese may be substituted for 1 oz of meat, poultry, or fish.

Source: C. F. Adams, *Nutritive Value of American Foods*, U.S. Department of Agriculture Handbook 456, November 1975.

TABLE 21-12 FOODS TO AVOID ON SODIUM-RESTRICTED DIETS*

Salt

Obviously salty foods such as salted crackers, potato chips, pretzels, salted nuts, pickles, olives, sauerkraut

Smoked, cured, or pickled meats and fish such as ham, bacon, frankfurters, bologna, salami, other cold cuts, salted fish and pork, corned beef

Seasonings such as catsup, prepared mustard, Worcestershire sauce, celery salt, onion salt, garlic salt, soy sauce, barbecue sauce, monosodium glutamate

Bouillon cubes, concentrated, canned, or frozen soups, dried soup mixes

Baking soda, seltzers, or antacids

Most commercial salad dressings

*See Table 23-5 for a more complete list of high-sodium foods.

TABLE 21-13 POTASSIUM-CONTAINING FOOD*

Food	Amount	Potassium, mg
Banana	1 small	350
Broccoli	1 cup	415
Canteloupe	¼ of 5-in melon	340
Grapefruit juice	1 cup	400
Orange	1 medium	270
Orange juice	1 cup	495
Potato	1 medium	555

*See Table 23-8 for potassium content of common foods.
Source: C. F. Adams, *Nutritive Value of American Foods*, U.S. Dept. of Agriculture Handbook No. 456, November 1975.

blood sugar). Hypokalemia is especially common and can be treated with diet or potassium supplements. When possible, dietary sources of potassium are preferred because of the unpleasant taste of most potassium supplements.

Table 21-13 lists some food sources that are relatively high in their potassium content. (Table 23-8 gives the potassium content of other foods commonly found in the American diet.) If potassium depletion becomes a problem, there are several potassium-sparing diuretics available. Both potassium tablets and some of the potassium-sparing diuretics may irritate the gastric

mucosa, so that caution must be exerted with their usage. There are also various salt substitutes on the market which substitute potassium for sodium. These may be contraindicated if there are any kidney problems, so patients are encouraged to check with their physicians before using these regularly in their diet.

Chloride depletion may also be a problem for patients taking diuretics. Both the salt substitutes and potassium elixir (one of the common supplements) provide a source of chloride in addition to potassium.

Other antihypertensive medications used include hydralazine, methyldopa, and guanethidine. These drugs and the diuretics are often used in combination to achieve a maximum reduction of blood pressure with a minimum of side effects. These agents, in contrast to the diuretics, produce a decrease in blood pressure by reducing peripheral vascular resistance through blocking of the sympathetic receptor sites in the arterioles and the sympathetic nervous system. Medications should be chosen on an individual basis with respect to dosage, frequency, and side effects, just as diet should be tailored to the individual need by the health professional, with respect to the patient's cultural, physical, and emotional background.

RHEUMATIC HEART DISEASE

Rheumatic fever is an inflammatory disease affecting the heart, connective tissues, and brain that occurs in 3 percent of patients after untreated pharyngitis caused by the group A beta-hemolytic streptococcus. It may be prevented by adequate treatment of "strep throat" (streptococcal pharyngitis) with penicillin. Malnutrition may result in increased rates of infection and therefore may correlate with a higher incidence of rheumatic fever among those that are malnourished. Major complications result from inflammation of the heart valves and heart muscle, leading to chronic rheumatic heart disease. The main nutritional concern in treatment is the provision of a diet with adequate nutrients to eliminate a prior state of malnutrition and to compensate for losses due to the stress of illness and increased temperature.

CONGENITAL HEART DISEASE*

Congenital heart defects may take many forms—ventricular septal defect, coarctation of the aorta, transposition of the great arteries, tetralogy of Fallot, and aortic stenosis, to name a few (see Table 21-14)—and often may not be diagnosed or detectable at birth. The only known causative factor is maternal rubella, which results in a specific syndrome in approximately 20 percent of affected infants. The many other malformations are probably multifactorial in origin, involving both unidentified genetic and unidentified prenatal environmental factors. Cyanosis (decreased oxygen in the blood), congestive heart failure, pulmonary hypertension, bacterial endocarditis, repeated respiratory infections, and poor physical growth frequently complicate the lives of children with these malformations.

Surgery is frequently performed, with relief of many of the symptoms. Recent trends in cardiac surgery have been aimed at correction of the defects during infancy, particularly in those with cyanotic ("blue baby") lesions. Survival and relief of symptoms are the immediate goals of treatment. Long-term goals are the provision of optimal physical, intellectual, and emotional growth.[48]

Growth retardation is common in children with congenital heart disease (Fig. 21-5). The mechanism of growth failure is most likely multifactorial in origin, with genetic, intrauterine, hemodynamic, nutritional, and other postnatal factors playing a role.[49] A number of hypotheses have been proposed to explain this altered pattern. These include congestive heart failure, chronic hypoxia with acidosis, pulmonary hypertension, repeated infections, or some combination of these. Traditionally, these factors have been grouped into three general categories: (1) abnormal metabolism of ingested food sub-

*Contributed by Rosanne B. Howard.

TABLE 21-14   COMMON CONGENITAL HEART DEFECTS

Type	Description
Ventricular septal defect (VSD)	A malformation resulting in a hole in the septum between the right and left ventricles.
Coarctation of the aorta	Constriction of the lumen of the aorta at any point—usually at the junction of the aortic arch and descending aorta.
Transposition of the great arteries	A defect in the anatomic relationship of the pulmonary artery and the aorta such that the aorta arises above the right ventricle and the pulmonary artery above the left ventricle.
Tetralogy of Fallot	A combination of four defects: (1) Interventricular septal defect (2) Stenosis of the pulmonary artery (3) Hypertrophy of the right ventricle (4) Dextroposition of the aorta so that it overrides the VSD
Aortic stenosis	A congenital narrowing of the aortic valve, usually with a unicuspid or bicuspid configuration rather than the normal tricuspid morphology.

stances, (2) an excessive loss of nutrients via the urine and feces, or by removal of body fluids, and (3) quantitatively poor intake.[50]

Hypermetabolism has been proposed as a cause for failure to thrive in these infants on the theory that the following conditions may possibly prevent a basal state: increased metabolic demands of specific tissues, an elevated body temperature, and a level of thyroid activity in-

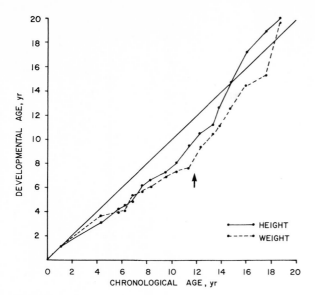

Figure 21-5

Growth curve in congenital heart disease. Growth curve shows catch-up growth after surgery with subsequent normal growth. (A. Rosenthal and A. Castaneda, "Growth and Development after Cardiovascular Surgery in Infants and Children," *Progress in Cardiovascular Diseases,* **18**:27–37, 1975.)

compatible with a reduction in cardiac reserve and energy intake.[51]

However, there is research to show that hypermetabolism may be the effect rather than the cause of growth failure.[52] Some investigators have found that infants with congenital heart disease were not hypermetabolic when oxygen consumption was related to lean body mass rather than determined per kilogram of body weight. Huse suggests that the growth failure seen in these infants appears more directly related to chronically inadequate intake rather than to any other factor studied.[53]

Although the question of a hypermetabolic state is unresolved, it is a well-established fact that many affected infants do not accept a normal volume of food. Voluntary reduction of food is so common that some researchers ascribe this to a compensatory role whereby infants reduce their food intake in order to prevent the additional strain on the failing myocardium that a large meal with its resulting increase in splanchnic (visceral) blood flow would impose.[54] Additional factors causing a decrease in intake are the rapid fatigue with feeding and labored respiration. Respiration takes precedence over alimentation, so when the infant cannot breathe, there is a concomitant decrease in oral intake. This limited intake, with a questionable state of hypermetabolism, malabsorption, or both, causes these children to be at risk nutritionally.[55] At even greater risk for failure to thrive are children with heart defects which result in cyanosis or congestive failure. Early intervention is dependent on considering the nature of the cardiac lesion, monitoring growth performance, and the effects of psychosocial influences.

It has been estimated that these children need somewhere in the vicinity of 29 to 59 extra calories (122 to 248 kJ) per kilogram of body weight over the recommended dietary allowances (RDA) for their age to achieve increments in weight.[56] For example, an infant requiring 117 kcal (491 kJ) per kilogram of body weight daily according to the RDA would then require 148 to 178 kcal (622 to 748 kJ) per kilogram of body weight or a midpoint of approximately 160 kcal (672 kJ) per kilogram.

The normal infant formula, after dilution, provides 20 kcal (84 kJ) per oz. To achieve a diet of high energy density without increasing the renal solute load, infant formulas with low electrolyte and protein values (10 to 11 percent protein) can be supplemented with Karo syrup, Polycose, or medium-chain triglycerides to provide 25 to 30 kcal (105 to 126 kJ) per oz (see Table 21-15). Dietary management for these children needs careful supervision to determine their ability to tolerate increasing levels of carbohydrate without developing diarrhea. Since often the total volume the infant consumes is low, the amount of protein may be deficient. In those instances when the intake is increased by adding less water to the formulas, the renal solute load must be monitored closely.

Nutritional management of infants with severe congenital heart disease involves providing essential nutrients in a form of food or formula

TABLE 21-15   ENERGY SUPPLEMENTS FOR DIETS OF CHILDREN WITH CONGENITAL HEART DISEASE

Product	Calories/tbsp (kJ/tbsp)	Description
Karo syrup (carbohydrate)	57 (239)	Corn sugar (mainly glucose) in syrup form Taste—sweet
Lipomul Oral Upjohn (fat)	90 (378)	Corn-oil emulsion White liquid Taste—perfumelike
Polycose, Ross (carbohydrate)	30 (126)	Glucose polymer in powdered and liquid forms with low osmolarity; rapidly absorbed as glucose Taste—less sweet than most sugars
MCT Oil, Mead Johnson (medium-chain triglycerides)	115 (483)	MCT Oil made from fractionated coconut oil containing triglycerides of medium-chain fatty acids; these are rapidly hydrolyzed and absorbed into the intestinal mucosa, not depending on bile salts, chylomicron formation, or lymphatic transport; they travel directly to the liver via the portal circulation Taste—bland

Amount to be added to formulas to make 25 kcal (105 kJ)/oz:

To 1 qt of SMA* or Similac PM 60/40* add

   3 tbsp Karo syrup or
   6 tbsp Polycose or
   1½ tbsp MCT Oil

*See Table 21-16.

that is easily digestible, without presenting an excessive renal load. The possibility of excessive fecal loss of fat should be considered, and the use of formulas providing fat in the form of easily absorbed vegetable oils is recommended. Formulas that provide a low renal solute load and a form of easily digestible fat are SMA (Wyeth) and Similac PM 60/40 (Ross) (see Table 21-16). It is recommended that the formulas used have an energy distribution of approximately 8 to 10 percent protein, 35 to 65 percent carbohydrate, and 35 to 50 percent fat in order to attain an adequate intake without incurring a high renal solute load.[57] When foods other than formulas are fed, they should be given with attention to their energy density (calories per teaspoon or tablespoon), sodium content, renal solute load, and digestibility.

The renal solute load is based on the dietary intake of nitrogen and three major minerals—

TABLE 21-16 FORMULAS PROVIDING A LOW RENAL SOLUTE LOAD AND EASILY DIGESTED FAT

Type	Fat sources	Protein, g/100 mL	Carbohydrate, g/100 mL	Fat, g/100 mL	Na, meq/L	K, meq/L	Cl, g/100 mL	Estimated renal solute load,* mosmol/L
SMA	Oleo (desterarinated beef fat), coconut oil	1.5	7.2	3.6	6.5	14.4	10.4	91
Similac PM 60/40	Safflower and soybean oil	1.6	7.6	3.5	7	15	7	92

Na = sodium; K = potassium; Cl = chloride.

*Using Fomon's simplified method (see reference 56) to calculate renal solute load, 1 g protein equals 4 mosmol; each meq, Na, K, Cl equals 1 mosmol.

sodium, potassium, and chloride. Fomon has developed a simplified method for calculating the renal solute load whereby each gram of dietary protein is considered to yield 4 mosmol of renal solute load, and each milliequivalent of sodium, potassium, and chloride is assumed to contribute 1 mosmol.[58]

Small amounts of energy supplements can be added to foods without appreciably changing the renal solute load since those which are recommended are pure fat or carbohydrate and have only trace electrolyte values. These energy supplements (Table 21-15) have a high satiety value and should only be given in small amounts. Large amounts of supplements can decrease the appetite for meals and produce diarrhea.

The sodium content of the diet should not exceed that of normal infants (7 to 8 meq per day).[59] Since commercially prepared strained foods contribute substantial amounts of sodium (see Table 21-17), supervision of both the type and amount used is necessary. With home-prepared baby food the amount of added salt can be controlled; however, foods low in sodium must be selected for preparation.

Water balance must be maintained to compensate for losses through the lungs due to tachypnea and for losses from the skin and lungs during illness or high environmental temperatures. (Normal estimated water requirements for infants range between 80 and 160 mL per kilogram of body weight depending upon age. The range of average water requirements for children between the ages of 2 and 10 years is 40 to 125 mL per kilogram of body weight).[60] Determinations of urine osmolarity can be used to monitor the renal solute load, and dietary adjustments can be made accordingly. Fomon suggests that urine osmolarity be maintained below 400 mosmol per liter.[61]

As mentioned earlier, children with congenital heart disease fatigue with feeding. It may be the result of cardiac decompensation or may be due to psychological factors in both the parent and the child. In the presence of chronic and life-threatening disease, the child may be forced

TABLE 21-17   SODIUM CONTENT OF COMMONLY USED BABY FOODS

Product	Measure	Sodium, mg
Baby ready-to-serve dry cereal	6 tbsp (14.2 g)	3.3–4.8
Baby dry cereal with fruit	6 tbsp (14.2 g)	14.2–16.8
Strained cereal with fruit (jar)	7 tbsp (100 g)	2–5
Strained fruit (pure fruit)	7 tbsp (100 g)	1–3
Strained fruit with tapioca	7 tbsp (100 g)	4–7
Strained dessert	7 tbsp (100 g)	7–61
Strained vegetables	7 tbsp (100 g)	1–79
Strained meat	7 tbsp (100 g)	41–63
Strained egg yolk	7 tbsp (100 g)	57
Strained dinners (vegetable and meat)	7 tbsp (100 g)	12–47
Strained high meat dinners	7 tbsp (100 g)	21–31
Baby fruit juice (strained orange)	1 oz	0.6–1.9
Orange juice (fresh)	1 oz	0.7
Whole milk	1 oz	15.5
Teething biscuit	1	39.8

Source: Gerber Products Company, 1979.

to eat by anxious parents who equate food intake with their child's survival, with the child in turn reacting negatively to food. Feeding a child with congenital heart disease brings into play many uncertainties, leading some parents to respond to their unpredictable child by being unpredictable themselves. Parents may find it difficult to set consistent limits with a child who "turns blue" with prolonged crying. Inconsistent parental management and the child's loss of pleasure in the function of eating may pave the way for neurotic feeding disturbances.

Anticipatory guidance centered around feeding and mealtime management should be provided to all parents of children with congenital heart disease. They need to have an understanding of feeding behavior (see Chap. 12 and Chap. 13) so that they can develop a consistent approach that fosters independence at the level appropriate to the child's physical and mental capabilities (e.g., increasing texture in the diet; encouraging self-feeding, weaning, drinking from a cup, etc.). Overprotection thwarts the child's psychosocial development and causes him or her to react negatively and manipulatively toward food. However, it must be remembered that the infant who has had early difficulties coordinating breathing with swallowing is not necessarily enamored of mealtimes. It takes time and patience to help reestablish trust in feeding and reduce the associated mealtime anxiety that may exist in both the parent and child.

An explanation of the child's tolerance levels by the physician and nurse along with a few simple directives for mealtime management can help to alleviate feeding problems. For example, the parents can learn to reinforce positive food behaviors, using the same words of praise while giving a lot of attention. Usually, it is the crying that receives the attention; this can best be met by withholding attention through calmly and quietly ignoring it without comment. The parents' approach needs to be consistent and in some instances behavior reinforcements other than praise must be found. Also, the parents need the support of all professionals in setting the appropriate limits and in distinguishing real food problems (vomiting, gagging, regurgitation) associated with their child's condition from those related to behavior. The following questions can help to determine difficulties in infant feeding:

Does the infant tire easily with feeding?

Does the infant need to rest while feeding?

Does the infant vomit frequently?

Does the infant consume approximately 3 to 4 oz of formula over a 20- to 30-minute period?

Does the infant's color become increasingly gray with feeding?

The child should be observed in the feeding situation so that these questions can be answered objectively.

Positioning for feeding is an important consideration. The child should be upright and well supported. Also, oral-pharyngeal stimulation of the lips, tongue, and gums can help to improve sucking ability, as can the selection of nipples that allow the infant to suck more easily (e.g., premie nipple).

CONGESTIVE HEART FAILURE

When the various cardiovascular disease states (ischemic, hypertensive, rheumatic, congenital) are sufficiently severe, the patient may manifest a constellation of symptoms and physical signs called *congestive heart failure*. This syndrome may be either acute, occurring over a short period when the insult is sudden and severe (as in massive myocardial infarction), or chronic, developing over a long period of time (this can occur in all forms of heart disease). The primary characteristic of congestive heart failure is the decreased efficiency of the heart as a pump, or decreased contractility of the myocardium. In order to maintain an adequate cardiac output, the heart compensates by increasing both its size (cardiomegaly) and its rate (tachycardia). Despite this effort at compensation, the cardiac output may fall, decreasing in turn the renal blood flow and glomerular filtration rate. Normal excretion of sodium and water is thus impaired, leading to retention of excess salt (sodium) and water; peripheral edema, pulmonary edema, and ascites are the physical signs of the retained solute and fluid. Acute pulmonary edema, related primarily to left ventricular failure, is a medical emergency requiring prompt treatment to prevent the patient from drowning in his or her own fluids. Other signs and symptoms of cardiac failure are fatigue, shortness of breath (dyspnea), paroxysmal nocturnal dyspnea, rales (abnormal respiratory sounds), hepatic enlargement (hepatomegaly), and weakness.

Treatment of congestive heart failure involves proper use of digitalis, diuretics, and oxygen; sodium restriction; and bed rest. Reduction in body weight decreases the metabolic demands of the patient and thus reduces the work imposed on the failing heart. The objectives of diet therapy in the patient with congestive heart failure are:

1 *Prevention or elimination of edema.* This involves diuretic therapy along with sodium and fluid restriction where indicated.

  a *Sodium restriction.* The range of sodium intake for the acute stage of congestive heart failure is 250 to 1000 mg. In the acute stage, a dietary restriction of 500 mg can be effective, although a lower level of 250 mg of sodium or a higher level of 1000 mg may be indicated. As edema is eliminated, the diet may be liberalized to permit a sodium intake ranging from 1000 to 1500 mg.

  b *Fluid restriction.* Usually necessary. If the kidneys have not been injured, fluid restriction does not have to be severe, since the mechanisms regulating sodium concentration in the extracellular fluid do not allow for retention of fluid without sodium. The aim is to avoid causing extra work for the kidneys by the administration of excessive fluids or by restricting sodium so severely that the kidneys cannot adequately excrete waste products (see Chap. 8). All food in liquid form and those foods that are liquid at room temperature (e.g., Jello, ice cream, gruel) should be considered as part of the fluid intake, in addition to some fruits with a high water content (e.g., orange, grapefruit, baby-food fruits). These may have to be limited, depending on the severity of the restriction on fluid intake.

2 *Provision of easily digestible foods to avoid excessive strain on the heart during digestion.* Foods should be soft in texture (to minimize chewing) and easily digested, although some foods containing fiber (fruits, vegetables, whole-grain breads, and cereals) and foods with laxative effect (prunes, prune juice, raisins, apricots) should be included to prevent constipation. Foods should also be bland and those containing significant amounts of caffeine should be avoided, especially in intensive cardiac care units. Foods that produce flatulence (cauliflower, onions, cabbage, etc.) should be restricted in order to prevent confusion resulting from symptoms of heartburn. Meals should be divided into small, frequent feedings to prevent exertion. The patient should be positioned to prevent aspiration.

3 *Maintenance of nutritional well-being.* During periods of stress such as that imposed by congestive heart failure, the provision of adequate calories, protein, vitamins, and minerals is essential but often difficult to achieve because of loss of appetite and restricted diets. Supplements of vitamins and minerals and the use of high-energy foods (e.g., concentrated carbohydrates such as jams, jellies, and syrups; and polyunsaturated fats) may be indicated. When foods to increase energy are included, those foods known to be lipogenic, such as fried foods, butter, and rich pastries, should be avoided.

EDUCATION OF PATIENTS

There are many cookbooks available for fat-controlled, low-cholesterol, or sodium-restricted diets. Suggestions for altering recipes and information about commercially available products for use in cooking should be given to the patient. Public libraries often carry a varied selection of cookbooks that can be recommended (*The American Heart Association Cookbook, The Fat and Sodium Controlled Cookbook, The Low-Fat–Low-Cholesterol Diet*). Another point that should be presented to individuals with heart disease is that their diet can be successfully used for the entire family and that they need not prepare separate meals for themselves. When possible, the husband, wife, and other family members should be taught the diet together so that both those who cook and those being served understand the reason for the dietary limitations. If the diet is very restrictive, "extras" can then be added for the rest of the family.

STUDY QUESTIONS

1 What are the three major risk factors of coronary heart disease that have dietary implications and what three major dietary components do they involve?

2 For patients who are at their ideal weight, what difference would the amount and type of fat make if they had type I hyperlipoproteinemia? Type II?

3 List the American Heart Association's recommendations to physicians and health professionals.

4 Why might it be difficult for an individual on a low-sodium diet to get an adequate calcium intake?

5 Why are many patients with hypertension told to have a large glass of orange juice or a banana every day?

6 What energy requirement might a 10-kg infant with congenital heart disease require? How would this differ from the energy requirement of a normal infant? What type of feeding problems might be encountered?

CLINICAL STUDY 21

Past history

Mr. Smith, a professor of electrical engineering, was 30 years old when he first developed chest pressure. This pressure was without pain and was brought on by physical exercise and anxiety, and occasionally occurred after eating. After these initial episodes of chest pressure he started a fairly active physical exercise program. Over the next few years the chest pressure gradually became less frequent. At age 47, while still remaining very active, he developed a recurrence of these chest symptoms. Approximately 1 year later Mr. Smith suffered an acute myocardial infarction with ventricular fibrillation and cardiac arrest requiring resuscitation. After discharge from the hospital, his course was stable for the next 5 years. He continued to be physically active by taking nitroglycerin prophylactically before extensive physical exertion and during periods of stress. Mr. Smith's family history was positive for coronary heart disease.

Mr. Smith smoked two packs of cigarettes per day for 16 or 17 years, stopping at approximately age 36. He drank five to six cups of coffee per day and occasional alcoholic beverages.

Diet

He had been limiting the amount of eggs and shellfish he was eating, and used oil and margarine as his primary fat sources. His diet was normal, without excessive fat, protein, or carbohydrate.

Initial physical examination

Three months after the myocardial infarction a physical examination was unremarkable except for a mild left facial weakness.

Laboratory findings

All values were within normal limits except for the serum cholesterol and triglycerides, which were 316 mg per 100 mL and 139 mg per 100 mL respectively.

Clinical study questions

1 What risk factors for coronary disease did Mr. Smith have?

2 Is it possible to classify the type of hyperlipoproteinemia Mr. Smith had? If so, what type was it? If not, what further information is needed?

3 What type of diet would be likely to be advised, considering that Mr. Smith was at his ideal body weight? Is it critical that the type of hyperlipoproteinemia be identified in order to advise him regarding his diet?

REFERENCES

1   U.S. Department of Health, Education, and Welfare, *Healthy People, The Surgeon General's Report on Health Promotion and Disease Prevention*, Publication (PHS) 79-55071, 1979, p. 56.

2   Natioal Heart and Lung Institute Task Force on Arteriosclerosis, *Arteriosclerosis,* vol. 1, U.S. Department Health, Education, and Welfare Publication (NIH) 72-137, June 1971, p. 3.

3   W. B. Kannel, "Atherosclerosis as a Pediatric Problem," *Journal of Pediatrics, 80*:544–554, 1972.

4   G. C. McMillan, "Development of Arteriosclerosis," *American Journal of Cardiology, 31*:543–546, 1973.

5   J. P. Strong, "The Pediatric Aspects of Atherosclerosis," *Journal of Atherosclerosis Research, 9*:251–265, 1969.

6   A. Keys, "Blood Lipids in Man—A Brief Review," *Journal of The American Dietetic Association, 51*:508–516, 1967.

7   W. P. Castelli, "HDL Cholesterol and Other Lipids in Coronary Heart Disease," *Circulation, 55*:767–772, 1977.

8   T. Gordon, "High Density Lipoprotein as a Protective Factor against Coronary Heart Disease—The Framingham Study," *The American Journal of Medicine, 62*:707–713, 1977.

9   R. I. Levy, "Drug Therapy—Treatment of Hyperlipidemia," *New England Journal of Medicine, 290*:1295–1301, 1974.

10 A. Keys, op. cit., pp. 508–516.

11 A. Keys, op. cit., pp. 508–516.

12 National Dairy Council, "The Biological Effects of Polyunsaturated Fatty Acids," *Dairy Council Digest, 46* (6):31–35, 1975.

13 F. Ederer, "Cancer Among Men on Cholesterol-Lowering Diets," *Lancet 2*:203, 1971.

14 M. M. Christiansen, "Dietary Polyunsaturates and Serum Alpha-Tocopherol in Adults," *Journal of the American Dietetic Association, 63*:138, 1973.

15 Food and Nutrition Board, *Recommended Dietary Allowances,* 1980.

16 R. I. Levy, "Dietary Management of Hyperlipoproteinemia," *Journal of The American Dietetic Association, 58*:406–416, 1971.

17 D. S. Fredrickson, "Fat Transport in Lipoproteins—An Integrated Approach to Mechanisms and Disorders," *New England Journal of Medicine 276*:32–33, 93–103, 148–156, 215–226, 273–281, 1967.

18 D. S. Fredrickson, *Dietary Management of Hyperlipoproteinemia—A Handbook for Physicians and Dietitians,* U.S. Department Health, Education, and Welfare Publication (NIH) 76–110.

19 R. I. Levy, "Diagnosis and Management of Hyperlipoproteinemia in Infants and Children," *American Journal of Cardiology, 31*:547–556, 1973.

20 C. J. Glueck, "Hyperlipoproteinemia in Children," *Primary Cardiology,* January 1980, pp. 106–115.

21 Ibid.

22 R. S. Lees, "Therapy of the Hyperlipidemias," *Postgraduate Medicine, 60*:99–107, 1976.

23 D. S. Fredrickson, *Dietary Management of Hyperlipoproteinemia—A Handbook for Physicians and Dietitians,* op.cit.

24 Ibid.

25 Ibid.

26 J. L. Breslow, "Pediatric Aspects of Hyperlipidemia," *Pediatrics, 62*:510–520, 1978.

27 C. J. Glueck, "Pediatric Familial Type II Hyperlipoproteinemia; Effects of Diet on Plasma Cholesterol in the First Year of Life," *American Journal of Clinical Nutrition, 25*:224–230, 1972.

28 American Heart Association Committee on Nutrition, Diet and Coronary Heart Disease, *A Statement for Physicians and Other Health Professionals,* 1978.

29 American Heart Association, *The Value and Safety of Diet Modification to Control Hyperlipidemia in Childhood and Adolescence, A Statement for Physicians and Other Health Professionals,* 1978.

30 H. Trowell, "Ischemic Heart Disease and Dietary Fiber," *American Journal of Clinical Nutrition, 25*:926–932, 1972.

31 R. I. Levy, "Dietary Management of Hyperlipoproteinemia," op. cit., pp. 406–416.

32 R. I. Levy, "Drug Therapy—Treatment of Hyperlipoproteinemia," op. cit., pp. 1295–1301.

33 R. S. Lees, op. cit., pp. 99–107.

34 E. D. Freis, "Age, Race, Sex and Other Indices of Risk in Hypertension," *American Journal of Medicine, 55*:275–280, 1973.

35 Ibid.

36 L. B. Page, "Medical Management of Primary Hypertension," *New England Journal of Medicine, 287*:960–965, 1018–1023, 1074–1081, 1972.

37 W. B. Kannel, "Systolic versus Diastolic Blood Pressure and Risk of Coronary Heart Disease," *American Journal of Cardiology, 27*:335–346, 1971.

38 B. Batterman, "Hypertension. Part I: Detection and Evaluation," *Cardiovascular Nursing, 11*:38, July-August 1975.

39 American Academy of Pediatrics Committee on Nutrition, "Salt Intake and Eating Patterns of Infants and Children in Relation to Blood Pressure," *Pediatrics, 53*:115, 1974.

40 H. A. Guthrie, "Infant Feeding Practice—A Predisposing Factor in Hypertension?" *American Journal of Clinical Nutrition, 21*:863–867, 1968.

41 E. D. Freis, "Salt, Volume and the Prevention of Hypertension," *Circulation, 53*:589–595, 1976.

42 L. K. Dahl, "Salt and Hypertension," *American Journal of Clinical Nutrition, 25*:231–244, 1972.

43 American Academy of Pediatrics Committee on Nutrition, op. cit., p. 115.

44 Ibid.

45 H. R. Dustan, "Diuretic and Diet Treatment of Hypertension," *Archive of Internal Medicine,* **133**:1007–1013, 1974.

46 A. N. Brest, "Therapeutic Aspects of Hypertension," *Angiology,* September 1975, pp. 584–591.

47 Food and Nutrition Board, *Sodium-Restricted Diets and the Use of Diuretics,* National Research Council, National Academy of Sciences, Washington, 1979.

48 A. Rosenthal, "The Patient with Congenital Heart Disease after Surgical Repair: An Overview," *Progress in Cardiovascular Disease,* **17**:401–402, 1975.

49 K. H. Ehlers, "Growth Failure in Association with Congenital Heart Disease," *Pediatric Annals,* **7**:11, November 1978, pp. 750–759.

50 J. G. Pittman, "The Pathogenesis of Cardiac Cachexia," *New England Journal of Medicine,* **271**:403, 1964.

51 L. Martin, "Relative Hypermetabolism in Infants with Congenital Heart Disease and Undernutrition," *Pediatrics,* **26**:183, 1965.

52 I. Krieger, "Growth Failure and Congenital Heart Disease," *American Journal of Diseases of Children,* **120**:497–502, 1970.

53 D. Huse, "Infants with Congenital Heart Disase," *American Journal of Diseases of Children,* **129**:65–69, 1975.

54 J. G. Pittman, op. cit., p. 403.

55 J. Hakkilia, "Absorption of 1 Triolein in Congestive Heart Failure," *American Journal of Cardiology,* **5**:295, 1960.

56 S. Fomon, "Nutritional Management of Infants with Congenital Heart Disease," *American Heart Journal,* **83**:581–588, 1972.

57 Ibid.

58 S. Fomon, op. cit., pp. 581–588.

59 Ibid.

60 W. E. Nelson, *Textbook of Pediatrics,* W. B. Saunders Company, Philadelphia, 1979, p. 175.

61 S. Fomon, op. cit., pp. 581–588.

CLINICAL DISCUSSION 21

Mr. Smith was diagnosed as having type II hyperlipoproteinemia after base-line cholesterol, triglyceride, and electrophoresis results were determined. Other risk factors present included smoking, lack of activity (until he had initial feelings of chest pressure), and a positive family history.

After Mr. Smith's physician diagnosed his hypercholesterolemia he referred Mr. Smith for a dietary consultation. A dietary history revealed that he had already made several alterations in his dietary intake but still needed to decrease his cholesterol and saturated fat intake further. He was instructed on a diet low in cholesterol (250 mg or less) and low in saturated fat (less than 10 percent of caloric intake and inclusion of polyunsaturated fat to comprise up to 10 percent of the total energy), with calories unrestricted as long as he maintained a lean body weight. Mr. Smith had a drop of approximately 20 percent in both serum cholesterol and triglycerides with strict adherence to this diet.

Drug therapy was instituted when Mr. Smith's plasma lipids were not lowered to the desired level with diet alone. The importance of continued dietary restriction was emphasized also. Several different doses and forms of medication were prescribed to achieve an optimal lowering of his plasma lipids to acceptable levels.

Mr. Smith was referred to an exercise physiologist for evaluation of his exercise capabilities. He has had several cardiac stress tests to help determine the appropriate level of exercise for him. He continues to be very physically active but must take medication for relief of angina.

Mr. Smith has continued to be seen regularly by his physician with yearly lipid determinations. He has adhered strictly to his diet and was able to discontinue lipid lowering medications; however, a weight gain of approximately 10 lb has elevated his lipid values slightly.

Mr. Smith will continue to be followed periodically with review of his diet. He knows and understands the dietary principles involved. He has good support from his family and does not feel that the diet imposes restrictions on them. He has found many of the new dietary products for fat-controlled diets very useful, such as egg substitutes and textured vegetable proteins. His continued adherence to his diet and exercise program will be monitored by the combined efforts of his health care team, consisting of the nutritionist, nurse, exercise physiologist, and physician.

CHAPTER 22

THE GASTROINTESTINAL SYSTEM

Christine Adamow Murray
Nancie Harvey Herbold
Rosanne Beatrice Howard

KEY WORDS
Bland Diet
Cystic Fibrosis
Diarrhea
Disaccharidase Deficiency
Diverticulosis
Gastritis
Hiatus Hernia
Lactase Deficiency
Pancreatitis
Regional Enteritis (Crohn's Disease)
Tropical Sprue
Ulcerative Colitis
Ulcer

INTRODUCTION

The gastrointestinal tract is subject to disorders and disease states, many of which are first manifested by symptoms of digestive complaints. Often, the individual's complaints first appear during periods of stress or emotional conflict, and arise from changes in gastrointestinal motility. Symptoms such as dysphagia (difficulty with swallowing), nausea, vomiting, abdominal pain, diarrhea, or constipation appear. These alterations in intestinal function which occur under stress are far from understood, although we are now able to associate the relationship of these symptoms with psychogenic changes in the gut. The question of why the gut is sensitive to symptom formation in some individuals during stress remains unanswered. In the past, much speculation has been offered, based upon psychiatric theories. For example, the psychoanalytic school of thought associates the etiology of peptic ulcers to reaction patterns persisting from the first stage of personality development or the "oral phase." Disorders of the colon are similarly related to the persistence of the "anal phase." Diarrhea is seen as an attempt to appease parents and constipation is attributed to the desire to withhold affection.[1] Although anecdotal evidence occasionally supports this theory in individual patients, the lack of solid evidence has tended to discourage attention to this field by the trained clinician.[2]

Traditionally, the failure to find a reason for these complaints on clinical examination has led to an artificial classification of disorders into those that are "functional" and those that are "organic" diseases. This classification does not account for the fact that often symptoms caused by an "organic lesion," such as a neoplasm of the bowel or disaccharidase deficiency, and those caused by emotional reaction to the disease, such as diarrhea or colitis, are additive and intertwined. In some disease states emotional factors

Note: The authors wish to acknowledge the assistance of Cynthia Taft Bayrl, M.S., R.D., in revising the section on cystic fibrosis.

appear to be significant elements in the etiology of the disease, and the choice of therapy includes treatment of the psychosomatic components of the illness.

The differential diagnosis between so-called functional and organic conditions, then is less often a matter of "either-or" than "how much of each."[3]

It is important to consider together the psychophysiological aspect of the illness with all pathogenetic mechanisms.

The confusion that exists over classification of diseases of the gastrointestinal tract carries over to the role of diet treatment of gastrointestinal disturbances. For the most part, excluding those conditions where there is a clear physiological basis for dietary modification, dietary regulation is based on tradition and on unsubstantiated information. It is the purpose of this chapter to examine the current use of diet and the clinical expression of the diseases of the gastrointestinal system.

Since there is evidence that many common gastrointestinal symptoms are often produced by biologically ingrained patterns of defense and adaptations to stress,[4] there are strong implications for psychotherapeutic management for many patients. When psychogenic factors predominate in the etiology of the disease, the therapeutic treatment plan should include psychiatric intervention as a priority. Therapeutic diets should be used as a tool within this framework of understanding, and the diet should be individually tailored to the patient's tolerance as well as the severity of the disease state. The diet should not act as a target for the patient's manipulation by placing unwarranted restrictions on the patient; rather, the dietary regimen should help toward the reestablishment of coping power, as the person learns to identify his or her own level of food tolerance.

The gastrointestinal system begins with the lips, which serve as a gateway of the system. The finely coordinated movement of the lips, mouth, and tongue prepare and propel food in the waves of muscular contraction that constitute swallowing. An understanding of swallowing is essential to the health professional who is studying the gastrointestinal system, since many patients with gastrointestinal diseases, especially those with esophageal disorders, present with complaints of dysphagia (difficult swallowing) in addition to heartburn, regurgitation, and vomiting. Certain neurological disorders with damage to those cranial nerves that control swallowing will also present with the same complaint (see Chap. 26).

THE PHYSIOLOGY OF SWALLOWING

Swallowing can be considered in three separate stages: the *oral stage,* which is initially under voluntary control, and the *pharyngeal* and the *esophageal* stages, which are reflexive and involuntary.[5]

Oral stage. A masticated bolus of food is gathered on the upper surface of the tongue, which rises at the tip. A contraction of the tongue flows backward, pushing the bolus toward the pharynx. At this point the swallowing becomes involuntary and nerve impulses emanating from the fifth, ninth, and tenth cranial nerves produce a series of reflexes that propel the food backward and downward.

Pharyngeal stage. In this phase the pharyngeal muscles contract, squeezing the contents downward into the esophagus. Simultaneous reflexes close the mouth, nasopharynx, and respiratory passages. The posterior part of the tongue is pressed upward against the roof of the mouth; the soft palate is elevated, and the posterior wall of the nasopharynx bulges forward. Respiration is halted and the air passages are isolated by elevation of the larynx. Swallowing and voluntary inhalation are virtually impossible when the mouth is open. Therefore, patients who cannot properly seal their lips or close the mouth cannot be expected to swallow.

Esophageal stage. During this phase the food is passed along the length of the esophagus and into the stomach. Esophageal contractions commence at the upper end of the esophagus with each conscious swallow and travel uninterruptedly to the lower esophageal sphincter at a rate of approximately 4 to 5 cm per second.[6,7] A second wave of peristaltic contractions then takes over if the primary effort fails to empty the esophagus. A third wave, considered to be segmental and nonpropulsive, plays little part in the normal swallowing reflex. For the most part, esophageal peristalsis is not required for swallowing fluids, as the initial phase of swallowing, along with the action of gravity, is sufficient to deliver food to the stomach.

The reverse of this process, vomiting, begins with the opening of the gastroesophageal sphincter. This is caused by contraction of the pyloric sphincter, which induces the stomach and the esophagus to relax. Respiration is then halted, with a fixation of the diaphragm in the inspiratory position. The air passages are isolated, with closure of the glossitis and elevation of the pharynx. Violent contractions of the abdominal muscles expel the contents of the stomach.[8]

Normally, once food is delivered to the stomach, it becomes the primary function of the lower esophageal sphincter to prevent the reflux of the acid gastric contents. Failure of this mechanism produces symptoms associated with two disorders of the esophagus, namely, achalasia and hiatus hernia.

Diagnosis of disorders of the esophagus can be made by plain x-ray, barium swallow x-ray studies, endoscopy, and pressure recordings of the sphincters and muscle walls of the esophagus.

DISEASES INVOLVING THE ESOPHAGUS

Achalasia

Achalasia is a motor disorder involving the smooth muscle of the esophagus. It causes a dou-

ble defect in esophageal function. Passage of food and fluids from the esophagus to the stomach is impeded by the lower esophageal sphincter, and there is a failure of the normal progressive peristalsis in the upper two-thirds of the esophagus. The individual experiences dysphagia without pain and a feeling of fullness in the chest after meals. The onset is insidious, developing over a period of time, and the age of onset is nonspecific. However, there is a tendency for the disorder to occur in young individuals.[9]

Regurgitation is another symptom; it is exacerbated by changes in position or by physical exercise. It is interesting to note that true heartburn is an uncommon manifestation of achalasia, yet this frequent regurgitation of material from the esophagus leads to a marked pulmonary change.

Presently, the etiology of the disease is unknown. The original hypothesis of a psychosomatic origin of the disease has been discarded and the disorder is considered to be primarily neural in origin and to represent a muscular adaptation to a primary nerve disorder. Microscopic examination shows fewer ganglion cells in the body of the esophagus and those present may be engulfed by chronic inflammatory cells. The disturbance dilates the esophagus above the stricture. As the disease progresses, the esophagus assumes a sigmoid configuration. This, coupled with the absence of peristalsis and the failure of the lower sphincter to open, is the combination of events that causes the individual to experience difficulties in swallowing.

Treatment The treatment of achalasia is aimed at weakening the lower esophageal sphincter so that gravity can facilitate emptying. This is usually accomplished by hydrostatic or pneumatic dilation. In some cases surgery is necessary, involving the incising of the circular muscle fibers down to the mucosa.

Prior to treatment, liquids may present as much of a problem in swallowing as solids because of the closed esophageal stricture. However, since fluids do not require esophageal peristalsis, small, frequent feedings of semisolid food at moderate temperature will be tolerated better.

In some, alcohol is reported to help food pass into the stomach.[10] Whether this effect is due to the demonstrated ability of alcohol to decrease esophageal pressure[11] or is due to the psychic effect is unknown. Since the competence of the sphincter is now felt to be controlled by gastrointestinal hormones and in particular by gastrin,[12,13] and since individuals with achalasia are known to be hypersensitive to gastrin, a diet that would reduce gastrin production might be helpful for patients awaiting medical treatment.

Foods containing protein and carbohydrate liberate gastrin and therefore may be responsible for increasing sphincter pressure. In view of this association, a moderate reduction in such foods may be helpful. Fat stimulates the production of cholecystokinin, a duodenal hormone responsible for lowering sphincter pressure either directly or through competition with gastrin. Therefore, foods with a high fat content (e.g., whole milk rather than skim milk) may be encouraged. Babka and Costell also report[14] that chocolate and coffee are known to decrease sphincter pressure and may therefore be included. Spicy foods and citrus and tomato juice should be avoided to prevent direct insult to the esophageal mucosa.

Weight loss may be noted, especially with advanced esophageal stasis associated with bronchopulmonary aspiration and bouts of bronchopneumonia. In these individuals diet considerations should allow for the repletion of nutrient stores.

Hiatus Hernia

A diaphragmatic or hiatus hernia is the condition resulting from a defect in the diaphragm muscle, around the opening in the diaphragm where the esophagus continues into the abdomen. This allows the stomach to protrude upward or herniate into the thoracic cavity (see Fig. 22-1). Symptoms are related to the esophagitis produced by the reflux of gastric juice into the lower esophagus,[15] and include heartburn, acid regurgitation, vomiting, dysphagia (diffi-

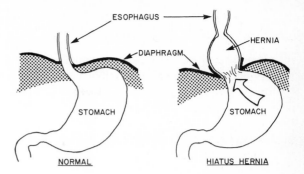

Figure 22-1

The normal esophagus and the mechanism of a hiatus hernia. The diaphragm muscle stretches across the midpoint of the abdomen and the chest cavity. The hernia occurs at the juncture of the stomach and the esophagus as a result of weakness or relaxation of the opening in the diaphragm. (Adapted from J. Pullock, *Gaseous Digestive Conditions,* Charles C Thomas, Publishers, Springfield, Ill., 1967.)

culty in swallowing), and odynophagia (painful swallowing).

The etiologic factors are confusing. Congenital weakness of the diaphragmatic muscle, trauma, and the aging process have been considered to contribute to the cause. In addition structural or postural change, as observed in kyphoscoliosis, and conditions that increase abdominal pressure such as obesity, pregnancy, ascites, and tight-fitting clothes have been associated with the etiology.[16] There is evidence suggesting that there is a direct relationship between long-term ingestion of a low-fiber diet and the incidence of hiatal hernia.[17]

There are several different types of hiatus hernia (sliding hernia, rolling or parietal hernia, short-esophagus hernia), all of which can be small or large; however, these distinctions are not significant from a clinical nutrition standpoint. Diagnosis depends on radiologic examination.

Treatment Medical treatment is successful in 80 percent of the patients with hiatal hernias. Treatment is aimed at reducing factors which promote reflux of acid juice into the esophagus and at neutralization of the acid.[18] To reduce factors promoting reflux the following measures are recommended:

>Removal of tight-fitting garments
>Weight reduction (if the individual is obese)
>Separation of meals from sleeping time (patient should not eat before retiring—2½ to 3 h should elapse to allow the meal to be digested)
>Elevating the head of the bed by placing the bed legs on blocks (the head of the bed should not be elevated in a jackknife position such as occurs in hospital beds)
>Giving small meals rather than large meals (6 small feedings are recommended instead of 3 meals)
>Small amounts of fluids should be sipped at meals rather than large amounts gulped
>Gum chewing should be discouraged to prevent swallowing large amounts of air

To neutralize acid, treatment akin to peptic ulcer management is recommended (see "Gastric and Duodenal Ulcers," below). The following nutritional management is recommended:

>Bland diet, which strictly avoids those foods that reduce lower esophageal sphincter pressure, such as coffee, peppermint and chocolate, and foods that irritate the esophageal mucosa, such as orange, grapefruit, and tomato juice. In addition, since fat lowers pressure of the sphincter, a diet which controls fat may be better tolerated.
>Small feedings, as described above.
>Antacids (Maalox, Amphogel).
>Anticholinergic drugs (drugs which slow gastric emptying time).

Surgical treatment is indicated when medical treatment fails and complications arise.

Special Feeding Considerations

There are other conditions which may impede the function of the esophagus or certain congenital problems such as esophageal atresia (congenital abnormality of the esophagus with or without tracheoesophageal fistula) which do not necessarily require a special diet per se, but do require special feeding techniques. Special tube feeding (see Chap. 28) is required to maintain or improve nutritional status in conditions that restrict feeding by the oral route. An infant with esophageal atresia requires surgery during the newborn period, and gastrostomy feedings are employed until the function of the esophagus is restored. Children born with congenital abnormalities that affect normal feeding may be maintained until they are as much as 2 years of age on gastrostomy feedings along with amounts of oral food, which are added as tolerated. These children may present further feeding problems after surgical repair because of their lack of food-related experiences. During the period of food introduction, parents need anticipatory guidance on the types, the amount, and the texture of the food to be presented to the infant. They need to understand that the infant's acceptance of food will take time and patience. Some of the techniques of behavior modification may be useful in establishing a positive, well-accepted feeding routine (see Chap. 11).

The same type of feeding problem may also be encountered in the child who has swallowed a corrosive substance such as lye. The recuperative period following ingestion of a caustic agent requires a child to go for long periods without food by mouth. After surgical repair to the damaged esophagus, the child often continues to experience discomfort on swallowing after food ingestion, further slowing the return to oral feeding and increasing reliance on special tube preparations.

DISEASES OF THE STOMACH

The function of the stomach is threefold: (1) The stomach is a major storage organ in the body, holding large quantities of food until the partially digested mass can be accommodated by the lower portion of the gastrointestinal tract. (2) The organ mixes gastric solutions of hydrochloric acid and food to form a semifluid substance called *chyme*. (3) The stomach regulates the flow of chyme into the intestine to allow for optimal digestion and absorption of ingested nutrients.

Pathologic disorders that affect stomach function will interfere with the breakdown of food entering the organ, with the formation of chyme, or with the passage of the chyme to the intestines for further action by intestinal secretions and bacteria.

Gastritis

Gastritis is an acute or chronic inflammation of the stomach mucosa. The individual may experience anorexia, nausea, vomiting, epigastric pain, and a feeling of fullness. Acute gastritis may be caused by the ingestion of certain drugs (salicylates, antibiotics), excessive intake of alcohol, allergic reaction to foods, food poisoning, and bacterial and viral infections. The etiology of chronic gastritis is unknown.

Treatment For the first day or two during the acute state of the disease no food is given by mouth (NPO) and parenteral nutrition should be used for nutritional support (see Chap. 28). Liquids are gradually added to the diet as tolerated by the individual patient. When symptom-free the patient can then progress to a bland diet (see page 468 for a discussion of bland diets).

Gastric and Duodenal Ulcers

An ulcer is a circumscribed erosion of mucosal tissue that can occur at various sites in the gastrointestinal tract which are exposed to gastric juice. An ulcer may occur at any of the following sites: esophagus, stomach (gastric ulcer), duodenum (duodenal ulcer), and the jejunum when a gastrojejunostomy has been performed. All ulcers will be considered together, as nutritional intervention and medical treatment are basically similar wherever the lesion is located.

The exact etiology of peptic ulcers is unclear but hypersecretion of gastric acid (hydrochloric

acid, pepsin, and water) by the parietal cells of the stomach has been implicated. Hypersecretion of gastric acid is seen in individuals with duodenal ulcers; however, patients with gastric ulcers tend to secrete less acid than normal individuals. The tissue insult in gastric ulcer disease may be due to weakened resistance of the mucosa rather than to the increased amount of gastric acid.

Gastrin, a hormone that is stimulated by the presence of food in the stomach, promotes acid secretion. Investigators have found that fasting levels of gastrin are similar in both normal and ulcer patients. However, ulcer patients had elevated levels of gastrin postprandially, perhaps indicating that hormonal response may be an influencing factor in the development of ulcer disease. Many drugs are known to be "ulcerogenic," for example, salicylates and steroids. These drugs increase gastric acid secretion as well as decreasing mucosal resistance.

Ulcers are more frequently seen in males than females, usually in nervous, tense, aggressive individuals, supporting the theory that the etiology of the disease may be related to emotional factors.

Pain is the major symptom of ulcer disease and is often accompanied by a feeling of hunger. A barium swallow x-ray study is a common procedure used in the diagnosis of ulcer disease. Barium is an opaque dye that will appear on x-rays and reveal a "crater" if an ulcer is present.

Treatment The major medical treatment for the ulcer patient is rest, both physical and mental, and the use of antacid therapy.

Healing of the ulcer is aided when hydrochloric acid is neutralized or suppressed. Ideally gastric secretions should be between a pH of 4.0 and 5.0.[19] Initially, antacids may be prescribed as frequently as every hour, with subsequent administration reduced to between meals and at bedtime. There are a variety of antacids that may be used. Calcium carbonate, magnesium hydroxide, and aluminum hydroxide are the preferred drugs as they are more palatable and their side effects (constipation and diarrhea) are easier to regulate[20] than those of the other antacids. In addition, the milk-alkali syndrome is a complication that may arise from the excessive intake of milk while on antacid therapy. Besides antacid, antispasmodics or anticholinergic drugs may be used to relieve pain and decrease secretion of acid.

The *bland diet* is the common terminology used in describing the dietary treatment of ulcer disease. For many years the dietary treatment for ulcer disease was based on the premise that all foods which are chemically, mechanically, and thermally irritating to the stomach were to be avoided. However, the foods that were restricted had never been scientifically tested to establish their effect on the stomach. Therefore, different hospitals, physicians, and nutritionists had their own ideas of what should or should not be allowed on a "bland" diet. In the acute phase of ulcer disease it was common practice to provide the patient with small frequent feedings of milk, cream, and antacids. This was known as the *Sippy diet,* named after the physician who introduced it in 1915.[21] The patient slowly progressed to other easily tolerated foods, such as creamed soups, gelatin, and poached eggs, and finally to a "bland" diet. (See Table 22-1.) This regimen is still used in some hospitals. The atherogenic nature of the diet is a concern which can be altered by substituting skim milk and polyunsaturated fats for whole milk and cream.

Milk is used in the treatment of the ulcer patient because milk protein, as well as other proteins, neutralizes gastric acid and acts as a buffer. The buffering action of protein is only temporarily effective and necessitates frequent feedings. However, other research indicates that proteins are also gastric stimulants and therefore should be limited. For example, histidine, an amino acid, is decarboxylated to histamine, a gastric stimulant. Fats, on the other hand, are gastric inhibitors and decrease gastric motility, allowing more neutralization of gastric acid; they are therefore encouraged. Large volumes of food can also cause an increase in gastric secre-

tion; hence the need for small meals. Foods and condiments that are presumed to increase secretion, and/or cause mucosal irritation—such as black and red pepper, chili powder, cocoa, cola beverages, alcohol, caffeine and decaffeinated beverages—are avoided. Smoking is discouraged since nicotine has this same effect. Traditionally, gas-forming foods (cabbage, onions, brussels sprouts, turnips) and fiber have been eliminated from the daily diet of the individual patient.

However, opinions[22-24] exist suggesting that the ulcer patient, as well as the patient diagnosed with irritable bowel syndrome, can tolerate a wide range of foods and that healing is not aided by the avoidance of foods traditionally listed as irritating, such as foods high in fiber or caffeine. The American Dietetic Association revised the list of foods to avoid for bland diets. Now added to the list are red pepper, decaffeinated coffee, and cola beverages.[25]

The use of decaffeinated coffee in place of regular coffee to decrease acid production may be unwarranted. Studies have demonstrated that decaffeinated coffee stimulates 75 percent as much hydrochloric acid production as regular coffee.[26,27] This evidence suggests that there are no increased benefits derived from the use of decaffeinated coffee.

It is difficult to generalize treatment for any patient and all diet therapy must be individualized. Those factors which will influence the nutritional management of the ulcer patient are:

Stage of ulcer disease
Other medical complications
Nutritional status
Food tolerances

The bland diet is used to prevent exacerbation of the ulcer condition resulting from foods that are not well tolerated. The individual is instructed to avoid any foods that are not well tolerated; a diet as tolerated is prescribed. Foods which may cause stress to patients recuperating from ulcer disease include the gas-forming vegetables, fried foods, and very spicy foods.

TABLE 22-1 PROGRESSIVE BLAND DIET FOR TREATMENT OF ULCER DISEASE

| Type of food | Foods allowed | | Foods to be avoided |
	Gastric I	Gastric II	
Beverage	Milk (skim) at room temperature, 1½ oz each waking hour or at intervals prescribed by the doctor	Gastric I with only these additions: buttermilk, eggnog, milk, milk drinks at room temperature; hot water; and hot milk (fat content may be altered by use of polyunsaturated cream substitute)	Carbonated beverages; coffee; coffee substitute; ice and iced beverages; cocoa; tea
Bread	None	White and toasted; rusk; crackers made with refined flours; saltines	Bread and crackers containing whole-grain flour or bran
Cereal	None	Cooked refined corn, rice, and wheat cereals; strained oatmeal	Dry cereals; whole-grain cereals
Desserts	None	Angel, plain, or sponge cake; plain cookies; custard, gelatin, and rennet desserts; rice, tapioca, and vanilla puddings; melting vanilla ice cream (all desserts must be made without fruits, nuts, or spices)	
Fat	None	Butter, sweet and sour cream, cream cheese, oil	All other
Fruits	None	Cooked and strained: apples, apricots, prunes, plums, pears, peaches, fruit cocktail, ripe bananas; apple, apricot, prune, and orange juices with or after lunch and dinner only	
Meats, fish, poultry, eggs, cheese	None	Eggs baked, boiled, poached, or scrambled in double boiler; cottage or cream cheese; tender chicken and turkey; fresh or frozen fish; canned tuna or salmon, water packed, with bones removed	Fried eggs; any meat or cheese not included on allowed list

(Continued)

TABLE 22-1 CONTINUED

| Type of food | Foods allowed | | Foods to be avoided |
	Gastric I	Gastric II	
Potato or potato substitute	None	Baked or boiled potatoes (without skin) macaroni, noodles, refined rice, spaghetti	Fried potato, potato chips, hominy, whole-grain rice
Soup	None	Cream soup made with pureed vegetables: asparagus, green or wax beans, beets, carrots, peas (not dried), potato, spinach, squash	All soups prepared from meat, fish, or poultry
Sweets	None	Sugar and jelly in moderation	All other
Vegetables	None	Canned, cooked, and strained: beets, green or wax beans, carrots, peas, pumpkin, squash, whole asparagus tips	All other
Miscellaneous	None	Moderate amount of salt; white sauce	Alcohol, condiments; gravy, herbs, ice, nuts, olives, pickles, popcorn, relishes, spices, vinegar, chocolate

Type of food	Foods allowed, strict bland	Foods to be avoided
Beverage	Buttermilk; milk; milk drinks (all at room temperature)	Carbonated beverages, coffee, strong tea, cocoa, decaffeinated beverages
Bread	White, well toasted; rusk; crackers made with refined flours	Whole-grain breads
Cereals	Cooked refined corn, rice, and wheat cereals; strained oatmeal	Whole-grain cereals
Dessert	Angel, plain, or sponge cake; plain cookies; custard, gelatin, and rennet desserts; ice cream and sherbets; rice, tapioca, and vanilla pudding (all without fruits, seeds, nuts, spices, or coconut)	All other pastries
Fat	Margarine, butter; sweet and sour cream; cream cheese	All other
Fruits	Cooked and strained: apples, prunes, plums, fruit cocktail; ripe bananas; whole cooked or canned peaches, pears, and peeled apricots; all fruit juices, including orange juice (strained and diluted) and other citrus juices, taken with lunch and supper meals only	All other

470

TABLE 22-1 CONTINUED

Type of food	Foods allowed, strict bland	Foods to be avoided
Meat, fish, poultry, eggs, cheese	Eggs creamed, baked, boiled, poached, or scrambled in a double boiler; cottage, cream, mild American cheese; ground or tender beef, lamb, liver, veal; tender or ground chicken and turkey; fresh or frozen fish; canned tuna or salmon, water packed (baked, boiled, or broiled)	Fried eggs, meat, fish, fowl; any not included on allowed list; clams
Potato or potato substitute	Potato; macaroni; noodle; refined rice; spaghetti	Fried potato; potato chips; hominy; whole-grain rice
Soup	Cream soup made with pureed vegetables: asparagus, green or wax beans, beets, carrots, peas (not dried), potato, spinach, squash	
Sweets	Jelly; sugar in moderation; syrup	Jam; marmalade; coconut, candy with nuts
Vegetables	Canned or cooked: asparagus tips; strained: beets, green or wax beans, beans, carrots, peas, pumpkin, squash; limit to 1 serving daily	Gas-forming vegetables: onions, turnips, brussels sprouts, cabbage, broccoli, garlic
Miscellaneous	Moderate amount of salt; white sauce	Alcohol, condiments, gravy, herbs, ice, nuts, olives, pickles, popcorn, relishes, spices, vinegar

Type of food	Foods allowed, liberal bland	Foods to be avoided*
Beverage	Buttermilk, milk, milk drinks, fruit drinks, carbonated beverages	Caffeine-containing beverages (coffee, tea), cocoa, alcohol, decaffeinated coffee, cola beverages
Bread	All types	
Cereals	All types	
Desserts	All types	
Fats	All types	
Fruits	All types	
Meat, fish, poultry, eggs, cheese	All types	
Potato or potato substitute	All types	
Soup	All types	
Sweets	All types	
Vegetables	All types	
Miscellaneous		Black pepper, red pepper, chili powder

*Any food that the individual finds irritating should be avoided.
Source: Adapted from Beth Israel Hospital, *Diet Manual,* Boston, Mass.

DISEASES OF THE LOWER GASTROINTESTINAL TRACT

The small bowel is the primary site of nutrient absorption. Partially digested food in the form of chyme is emptied from the stomach into the duodenum for further enzymatic action by brush border enzymes and ultimate absorption by the intestinal mucosa.

However, many conditions can alter mucosal function and result in nutrient malabsorption and consequent nutrient imbalance. A review of Chap. 9 is recommended to enhance understanding of normal nutrient digestion and absorption as related to the malabsorption that is characteristic of gastrointestinal diseases of the small bowel.

Diarrhea

Major developments within the last 10 years relate to defining the pathogenesis of the condition. Treatment has changed very little.[28] Diarrhea results in the passage of loose, frequent stools. Diarrhea stools consist of water, sodium, potassium, and frequently undigested food.

Diarrhea may occur as an acute or chronic condition. Frequently, the intestines may be exposed to mucosal irritants such as spices, foodstuffs, or drugs. Overeating, nervous irritability, fermentation of carbohydrates in the gut, and bacterial overgrowth in the gut may result in functional diarrhea. Bacterial food spoilage is also a common cause.

Acute diarrhea is the most common classification. Most cases do not require medical intervention and usually remit within 24 to 48 h. Chronic diarrhea is defined as diarrhea of 2 weeks' or longer duration. This condition can be symptomatic of a primary illness.

The etiology of chronic diarrhea is the result of pathogenic bacterial action on the gut. It is often associated with such diseases as celiac disease, typhoid fever, dysentery, chronic ulcerative colitis, viral diseases, or tuberculosis. Enzyme-deficient states or disease conditions that cause intestinal lesions can also result in chronic diarrhea.

Treatment Generally, minimal or no treatment is necessary for mild acute attacks of diarrhea. In most cases elimination of the food suspected to have irritated the gut will resolve the acute condition. Clear fluids and nonirritating, soft, bland foods such as refined breadstuffs or soups are often tolerated until the condition is completely resolved.

The etiology of chronic diarrhea must be determined before effective intervention can occur. Because of the rapid passage of the feces through the colon and the resulting water and electrolyte losses, replacement of lost nutrients is crucial to prevent dehydration and fluid and electrolyte imbalances. Fluid replacement is essential to compensate for the osmotic shift of water into the intestinal lumen and rapid excretion in the liquid stools.

In the first 24 to 48 h of severe diarrhea it is beneficial to rest the gastrointestinal tract. Giving intravenous therapy to replace fluids and electrolyte losses while allowing nothing by mouth will permit the bowel to rest.[29] When the diarrhea subsides, a clear liquid regimen should be started, with progression to a full liquid diet and then to a diet as tolerated. If the diarrhea persists after the initial 48-h period, continuing nothing by mouth and initiating parenteral administration of an amino acid infusion in conjunction with intravenous glucose therapy will achieve bowel rest while supplying the patient with nutrition parenterally.

When oral feeding is allowed, the inclusion of food items containing pectin, a hydrophilic polysaccharide, can prove beneficial. Applesauce made with skins and peeled raw apple contain pectin and are often given every 2 to 4 h to improve the uptake of free water and the consistency of the stools.

The most common dietary treatment is to eliminate the food known to have irritated the intestine. Institution of a low-residue diet decreases intestinal irritation. (See Table 22-8, page 485.) The use of hydrophilic vegetable protein compounds that absorb water in the gut may be beneficial in returning the stool to a soft consistency without the loss of free water.

Steatorrhea

Steatorrhea is a diarrhea characterized by excessive fat in the stools and the presence of loose, foul-smelling, infrequent stools that float. Steatorrhea is indicative of the presence of an organic disease and is commonly found as a secondary problem in (1) intestinal mucosal lesions (e.g., celiac disease); (2) structural lesions of the intestine such as short gut, Crohn's disease, or lymphoma; (3) infections such as enteritis; (4) maldigestion, such as occurs with bile acid deficiency, cystic fibrosis, or pancreatitis; or (5) after gastrointestinal surgery such as intestinal resection or gastric surgery.

Steatorrhea results in decreased absorption of most nutrients, and weight loss. Increased loss of fecal nitrogen is common and can contribute to hypoalbuminemia. Fecal fat losses result in concomitant losses of fat-soluble vitamins. Excess loss of vitamin D can interfere with calcium metabolism. This mechanism, coupled with the loss of the calcium that is bound as soaps in the greasy stool, makes calcium depletion a real problem in the patient with severe steatorrhea.

Treatment   Since steatorrhea is a symptom of many organic diseases, treatment of the primary disease will bring secondary relief from fatty stools. It is important to remember that severe losses of fluid, electrolytes, vitamins, minerals, and other nutrients can occur if the underlying disease is not properly treated to ensure a decrease in fecal fat losses.

The use of medium-chain triglycerides (MCT) as an energy supplement provides an available source of energy in the form of short-chain fatty acids. MCT can be directly absorbed and utilized and seems to be well tolerated in patients experiencing severe loss of fat through steatorrhea (see Chap. 5).

Malabsorption Syndromes

Malabsorption syndromes are classified according to the age of onset of the disease, and the characteristics of the patient's stools. There is some evidence that malabsorption can occur in the newborn, in relation to congenital abnormalities affecting gastrointestinal structure and function.[30] However, it is more commonly manifested in early infancy and is considered to result from damage to the absorptive areas of the small bowel by enteropathogenic bacteria, viruses, parasites, congenital abnormalities of the gut, or genetic enzymatic malfunctions. Diseases of the small intestine, liver, pancreas, and gall bladder result in primary or secondary malabsorptive states and require specific medical and nutritional therapy.

Malabsorption syndromes clinically present with weight loss, anorexia, abdominal distention, borborygmi (loud bowel sounds), muscle wasting, and passage of abnormal stools. The stools have been described as light yellow to grey, greasy, soft, bulky, bubbling, and glistening, with a tendency to float. Long-standing malabsorption can result in edema, ascites, skeletal disorders, paresthesia, tetany, bleeding, glossitis, cheilosis, and generalized protein-calorie malnutrition. The etiology of these symptoms will be examined here in relation to specific diseases resulting in malabsorptive states.

Gluten-Sensitive Enteropathy (Celiac Sprue)

Dicke[31] first recognized the relationship between dietary wheat products and the course of celiac disease in 1950. Further investigations have demonstrated the efficacy of the gluten-free diet on the anatomy and physiology of the diseased small bowel of patients with this disorder. Therefore, the term *gluten-sensitive enteropathy* best describes the etiological and functional abnormalities found in afflicted patients. Synonymous terms such as *celiac disease, nontropical sprue,* and *idiopathic steatorrhea* have been coined; however, they can be considered to be as accurately descriptive of the disease as the term gluten-sensitive enteropathy.

Gluten-sensitive enteropathy (GSE) is a disease of the intestinal mucosa affecting the proximal portion of the small bowel. Vitamin

B_{12} malabsorption may occur because of the severity of steatorrhea and also the severity of the ileal mucosal lesion.

The mechanism whereby gluten causes damage to the intestinal mucosa, resulting in lesions, is not known. However, there are two possible mechanisms which have been proposed.[32] One is that GSE is due to an inborn error of metabolism with a peptidase deficiency, resulting in an accumulation of undigested gluten peptides and consequent mucosal damage. The other suggestion is that an abnormal immune reaction to gluten might be responsible for the damage to the intestinal mucosa.[33] However, neither of these two theories is completely without criticism.

Celiac disease affects both children and adults and seems to have two peaks in the onset of symptoms. The first is in the very young child, primarily the 1- to 5-year-old, and the other is in the third to fourth decade of life.[34]

The major clinical finding associated with gluten-sensitive enteropathy is diarrhea, characterized by bulky, offensive, greasy, loose, watery stools and caused by the lack of mucosal surface area housing the intestinal enzymes. Green and Wollanger[35] report that 90 percent of patients experience diarrhea at some time during the course of the disease. Edema, nonspecific gastrointestinal symptoms, prolonged pain in the bones due to calcium losses in the stools, osteomalacia, malnutrition, tetany, and hemorrhage from vitamin K malabsorption have been reported. Classic symptoms in afflicted children are failure to gain weight, resulting in failure to thrive; diarrhea; muscle wasting; irritability; and increased appetite due to nutrient depletion. Following treatment there is generally good catch-up growth. Symptoms result from impaired absorption of fat, protein, carbohydrate, fat-soluble vitamins, minerals, electrolytes, and even water. Pregnancy, infection, gastric surgery, and emotional stress may exacerbate the condition.

Common diagnostic tests for gluten-sensitive enteropathy are stool fat determinations, oral tolerance tests, and jejunal biopsy.

Stool fat. A 72-h stool collection while the patient is taking a measured fat intake is useful in determining the amount of fat lost in the stool and consequently is assaying the extent of fat malabsorption. Fecal fat excretion is higher in individuals with various degrees of malabsorption than in normal subjects. (See Chap. 5.)

Oral tolerance tests. A glucose tolerance test is a useful indicator of mucosal functioning if no metabolic abnormalities such as diabetes exist. A xylose tolerance test is performed in some centers and is felt to be a valuable diagnostic tool when jejunal biopsy is not available. Glucose and xylose uptake in the cells can be correlated to mucosal integrity and the presence or absence of mucosal lesions.

Intestinal biopsy. Jejunal biopsy is the only definite method for making a diagnosis of mucosal abnormality and is the preferred diagnostic tool. Jejunal biopsy reveals an abnormal jejunal mucosa with a loss of the intestinal villi. The intestinal surface resembles tanned pigskin.

A diagnosis of celiac disease is made on the basis of (1) demonstration of impaired intestinal absorption, (2) finding of histological changes in the duodenal-jejunal mucosa, and (3) definite clinical response to withdrawal of dietary gluten.

Treatment The treatment of gluten-sensitive enteropathy is complete withdrawal of gluten from the diet. Gluten is the glutamine-bound fraction (glutenin and gliadin) of protein. In this diet, wheat, rye, barley, oats, and all products containing any of these grains are eliminated. These grains contain a large amount of gluten, which is responsible for the malabsorption associated with the disease. Corn and rice are the only grains permitted on the gluten-free regimen. Table 22-2 gives a diet plan omitting wheat, rye, and oats from the daily intake. It may take several weeks to restore normal jejunal integrity and for symptoms to disappear com-

TABLE 22-2   GLUTEN-FREE DIET FOR TREATMENT OF CELIAC DISEASE

Type of food	Foods allowed	Foods to avoid
Beverage	Milk (skim may be better tolerated at first) Fruit juice, cocoa (read label to see that no wheat flour has been added) Slowly add: carbonated beverages, coffee, tea, distilled alcoholic beverage	Postum, malted milk, Ovaltine, instant coffee, beer, ale, whiskey, chocolate dairy drink, root beer
Bread	Only those made from rice, corn, soybean, wheat-starch (gluten-free), potato, lima bean flours, rice wafers	All bread, rolls, crackers made from wheat, oats, rye, barley, wheat graham flours; RyKrisp, muffins, biscuits, waffles, pancakes, dumplings, rusk, zwieback, baked goods from forbidden grains
Cereals	Cornmeal, hominy, rice, puffed rice, pre-cooked rice	All wheat, rye, oats, barley, wheat cereal, Grapenuts, bran, kasha, corn flakes, Rice Krispies, malt
Desserts	Gelatins, fruit gelatin, ice, or sherbet; homemade ice cream, custard, Junket, rice or cornstarch pudding, tapioca, cakes or cookies made from allowed flours	Commercial pies, cookies, pastries, ice cream, ice cream cones, prepared mixes, puddings
Fat	Oil, corn oil margarine, olive oil (unsaturated fats may be better tolerated initially); later additions: butter, cream, vegetable shortening, bacon, lard	Commercial salad dressings except pure mayonnaise (read labels)
Fruits	All cooked and canned juices and fruit; include citrus fruit at least once/day; initially avoid: skins, seeds, frozen fruits, prunes, plums, and their juices	Canned fruit pie filling
Meats, fish, poultry	All lean cuts; better tolerated if baked, broiled, boiled, or roasted	Breaded creamed meat, fish, poultry (e.g., croquette); processed meats (unless pure)
Eggs	As desired; initially avoid frying	
Cheese	All types; add slowly to diet	
Potato or potato substitute	Potato, rice	Noodles, spaghetti, macaroni, some packaged rice mixes
Soups	All clear and vegetable soups, cream soups if thickened with cornstarch or allowed flours	Commercially prepared soups; soups thickened with wheat, rye, oat, barley flours

(Continued)

TABLE 22-2 CONTINUED

Type of food	Foods allowed	Foods to avoid
Vegetables	All cooked and canned; slowly add: raw vegetables	Creamed if thickened with wheat, oat, rye, barley products
Miscellaneous	Gravies and sauces thickened with cornstarch or allowed flours; vegetable gum	Gravies and sauces thickened with wheat, rye, oat, barley flours

pletely. However, subjective improvement usually occurs within the first few days after gluten withdrawal.

Because the diet is a restrictive one, it is important to provide the individual with a variety of recipes to prevent boredom and lack of compliance. Adequate energy intake may be a problem since the restricted grains are found most often in high-caloric, baked products. Skill is required in meal planning and the importance of label reading needs to be stressed to ensure that commercial products do not contain restricted grains. Close cooperation between the physician, nutritionist, and patient is necessary to increase the probability of strict compliance with the diet. Vitamin and mineral supplements may be prescribed to augment the diet and correct deficient states.

Tropical Sprue

Another of the malabsorption syndromes, most common to tropical and subtropical areas, is tropical sprue. Although the etiology of the disease is unknown, it has been postulated that bacteria[36] or a diet deficient in folic acid may be responsible for the damage to intestinal absorption of vitamin B_{12}, for megaloblastic anemia and for bacterial overgrowth in the proximal small intestine. Because of the extensive microbial overgrowth abdominal distention and loud borborygmia are present; anorexia and vomiting occur frequently. Characteristically, the stools are semiformed or watery and may contain blood and mucus.

Tropical sprue and celiac disease are somewhat related in that both diseases present with villous atrophy of the intestinal mucosa.

Treatment There is a rapid clinical improvement with folic acid and broad-spectrum antibiotic therapy. Vitamin B_{12} therapy is often started because of the megaloblastic anemia. There is prompt response to this treatment.

A gluten-restricted diet does not relieve the symptoms. Rather, a high-energy, high-protein diet in conjunction with vitamin and mineral supplements will counteract the malnutrition and depleted nutrient stores associated with the disease. With treatment patients become asymptomatic and the intestinal mucosa returns to normal.

Disaccharidase Deficiencies

In the western world a large portion of the daily energy consumed comes from carbohydrates.

Kirschmann[37] reports that in the second year of life infants consume an average of 165 g of carbohydrate per day, and by the age of 12 years, the average consumption reaches approximately 350 g of carbohydrate daily. Approximately 60 percent of the carbohydrate ingested is starch while sucrose accounts for 30 percent and lactose 10 percent of the total amount ingested.[38]

The oligosaccharides and disaccharides (sucrose, lactose, maltose) are hydrolyzed by specific enzymes called disaccharidases which are located in the brush border of the intestinal mucosa. Hydrolysis results in the release of the monosaccharides (glucose, galactose, and fructose) which are absorbed by the mucosa.

When disaccharidases are absent from the

brush border, ingested carbohydrates cannot be absorbed and utilized by the body. "Fermentative diarrhea" results—the stools become frequent and are liquid and acidic in character. Abdominal pain and flatulence occur concomitantly with the abnormal stool pattern. The severity of the malabsorption varies with the amount and type of sugar ingested. Symptoms are relieved when a diet free of the problem sugar (e.g., a lactose-free diet) is prescribed.

Disaccharidase deficiencies may be either primary or secondary. Primary deficiencies, which are usually congenital, result in the absence of enzymes although the small intestinal mucosa is normal. Primary lactose and sucrose deficiencies have been described.[39]

Secondary disaccharidase deficiency may occur in any disease involving damage to the small bowel mucosa, such as celiac disease, ulcerative colitis, and cystic fibrosis. Most commonly, secondary disaccharidase deficiency involves lactase.

Lactase Deficiency

Lactose intolerance may be the result of a congenital inborn error of metabolism, resulting in the absence of the enzyme lactase from the intestinal mucosa. Secondary lactase deficiency may result from damage to the small bowel mucosa, as in protein-calorie malnutrition, celiac disease, and infections, or from the administration of colchicine or the antibiotics neomycin and kanamycin.[40]

Lactase deficiency seems most common in black, oriental, and Jewish populations, suggesting that the enzyme-deficient state may be inherited as a recessive trait. Lactose malabsorption may appear as early as the first few days of life or as late as 20 years of age. Clinically, children fail to thrive and appear weak, frail, and irritable, with muscle wasting, chronic diarrhea, vomiting, and dehydration. Stools are characterized as loose, watery, and acid. Adults with the enzyme deficiency experience diarrhea, abdominal discomfort, borborygmi, flatulence, nausea, and general discomfort.

When dietary lactose is not absorbed it re-

mains in the lumen and increases the osmotic load of the contents in the small bowel. As a result, intestinal bacteria act on the sugar, which causes the accumulation of lactic acid in the bowel, giving the stool its characteristic acidity and aiding the production of gas in the gut. In response to the increased osmotic load, fluid is attracted into the bowel in order to decrease the concentration of sugar in the gut, resulting in increased intestinal motility and diarrhea (see Fig. 22-2).

The increased fluid load is responsible for the watery, acid stools characterized as having an offensive odor and a pH of less than 6. As a result of the increased peristalsis, malabsorption of protein, fats, carbohydrates, and drugs occurs.

A preliminary screening test can be accomplished by testing the stools for reducing sub-

Figure 22-2

The development of lactose intolerance. Unabsorbed lactose remains in the intestinal lumen and increases the osmotic load. Bacterial fermentation results in the production of lactic acid and gas in the gut. Increased peristalsis and malabsorption occur in consequence.

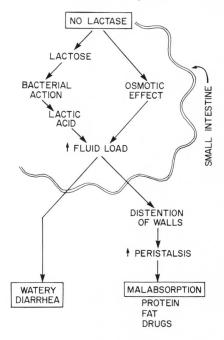

stances with a Clinitest tablet. The presence of 0.5 percent or more of reducing substance in the stool is considered abnormal.

Diagnosis of lactose intolerance can be made by giving a lactose load of 2 g per kilogram of body weight (up to a total of 50 g) and then drawing periodic blood samples. A finding of 20 mg or less of glucose indicates decreased enzyme activity. Often an exaggeration of symptoms resulting from the lactose load will also indicate a lactase-deficient state. Oral tolerance tests are less satisfactory than a biopsy assay. A small intestinal biopsy taken from the area of the ligament of Trietz can be analyzed for mucosal disaccharidases.[41] This technique is the most accurate and definitive test for disaccharidase deficiency states.

The diagnostic tests previously described may be invasive, unreliable, and not feasible for the diagnosis of lactose malabsorption, particularly in the pediatric population. Recently, measurement of breath hydrogen has been used successfully to identify lactase deficiency in children and adults.[42-45] Bacterial fermentation of nonabsorbed carbohydrate results in intraluminal hydrogen production. The collection of expired air followed by a measurement of breath hydrogen via gas chromatography provides a noninvasive and reliable index of lactose malabsorption. For example, an increase in breath hydrogen excretion following a lactose load indicates lactase deficiency. The test is based on the principle that hydrogen in expired air is proportional to intraluminal gas production, and calculation of hydrogen excretion permits an estimation of the amount of lactose not absorbed in the small intestine.

Treatment   Elimination of lactose from the diet brings relief from the symptoms of lactase deficiency. Lactose is primarily found in dairy products. In severe cases of lactose intolerance a totally lactose-free diet is warranted. The elimination of all dairy products increases the susceptibility to calcium deficiency, since dairy products are the best sources of calcium in the daily diet. Birge et al.[46] suggest that the restric-

tion of calcium-rich dairy foods as treatment for lactose intolerance may possibly explain the etiology of at least one type of osteoporosis. The increase in fecal calcium excretion as a result of the chronic diarrhea also suggests that an alternative source of calcium is necessary.

The value of total exclusion of dairy products for the lactose-intolerant individual is under debate. Through the process of fermentation, lactose is removed from aged cheese. The lactose content of cottage cheese is also low because the lactose in the whey is lost during processing (see Table 22-3). Gallagher et al.[47] report that when fermented dairy products are added to the diet a decrease in fecal calcium excretion follows. This suggests that these dairy products may be used as food sources of calcium in the lactose-free diet. However, calcium supplements are recommended in the absence of adequate dietary sources of the mineral.

Infants who are lactose intolerant are given lactose-free formula (e.g., Isomil, Cho-Free) until they are able to tolerate a formula containing the sugar. Certain medications also contain lactose and need to be avoided.

Cystic Fibrosis

Cystic fibrosis (CF) is a chronic disease inherited as an autosomal recessive disorder. The disease afflicts 1 out of every 2000 live births and is evident early in infancy.

The disease affects the mucosa and sweat glands of the body. The mucosal glands secrete thick mucus and the sweat glands secrete abnormally high concentrations of sodium chloride. Chronic pulmonary disease results from the extensive mucus secretions in airways of the lungs. Fat malabsorption occurs as a result of mucus plugs blocking the pancreatic duct, preventing secretion of pancreatic enzymes. Hypoproteinemia may be seen in childhood because of the expanded plasma volume, which decreases the concentration of protein circulating in the blood. If the pancreatic insufficiency is not treated, chronic malnutrition will ensue because of the malabsorption associated with the disease.

TABLE 22-3   LACTOSE AND PROTEIN CONTENT OF SELECTED DAIRY PRODUCTS

Product	Unit	Lactose content, g	Protein, g
Whole milk	1 cup	11	8
Low-fat milk (2%)	1 cup	9–13	8
Skim milk	1 cup	12–14	8
Chocolate milk	1 cup	10–12	8
Buttermilk	1 cup	9–11	8
Light cream	1 tbsp	0.6	0.3
Low-fat yogurts	1 cup	11–15	8
Cheddar cheese	1 oz	0.4–0.6	8
Cream cheese	1 oz	0.8	2.2
Processed cheese	1 oz	0.5	8
Cottage cheese	1 cup	5–6	15-0
Butter	1 tbsp	0.15	0.1
Oleomargarine	1 tbsp	0	0.1
Ice cream	1 cup	9	3.5
Sherbert	1 cup	4	2.8

Source: American Journal of Clinica Nutrition, **31**:595, 1978

The majority of patients diagnosed as having cystic fibrosis have some degree of pancreatic involvement. However, the extent of pancreatic insufficiency depends on the nature and severity of the disease. Shwachman[48] reports that over 10 percent of neonates with CF have meconium ileus, pancreatic insufficiency, steatorrhea, rectal prolapse, growth retardation, and glucose intolerance. Less common but indicative of the cystic condition is liver cirrhosis, esophageal varices, diabetes, fat-soluble vitamin deficiencies, and lactase deficiency.

A diagnosis of cystic fibrosis requires a positive sweat test plus one of the following: (1) documented family history of the disease, (2) chronic pulmonary disease, or (3) pancreatic insufficiency.

Children with cystic fibrosis have been described as having voracious appetites. Although this may be true of the patient with untreated malabsorption, some clinical observations would indicate that the child with cystic fibrosis consumes fewer calories than healthy peers.[49]

Pancreatic insufficiency is the major cause of nutritional deficiency in the typical individual with CF. Inadequate secretion of bicarbonate and digestive enzymes results in maldigestion and malabsorption. Digestion and absorption of fat appear to be affected, resulting in as much as 80 percent incidence of steatorrhea in patients who are not supplemented with pancreatic enzyme.[50]

Fat maldigestion and malabsorption is associated with increased fecal losses of other nutrients including protein. Protein digestion and malabsorption, although affected by pancreatic insufficiency, does not present as complex a clinical course as fat malabsorption.[51]

Glucose homeostasis is a problem in a significant proportion of CF patients. Approximately 25 percent of the population develops diabetes mellitus.[52]

Meconium ileus, an obstruction of the small intestine by sticky meconium, occurs in 15 percent of all babies with cystic fibrosis and can be considered diagnostic of the disease. However, the most reliable diagnostic test for cystic fibrosis is a quantitative analysis of the sweat for sodium and chloride. Elevation of sodium and chloride routinely occurs in cystic fibrosis because of abnormal function of the sweat glands. Finger- and toenail analysis for increased levels of sodium and potassium provides an accuracy of 90 percent and is also useful in diagnosing cystic fibrosis. Hair analysis may prove to be of even greater accuracy for sodium and chloride analysis.

Treatment Involvement of the respiratory and digestive systems and the sweat glands forms the basis for medical management of the disease. (See Table 22-4.) Immediately after diagnosis, the patient will frequently require an intense period of hospitalization to stabilize the pulmonary condition and to allow the development of a comprehensive medical care plan to treat the primary systems involved. Antibiotic therapy aids in the treatment of pulmonary lesions and has significantly increased the life expectancy of CF patients. The pulmonary care program includes the use of inhalation therapy and physical therapy for additional treatment and prevention of the pulmonary lesions.

Dietary regulation and pancreatic replace-

TABLE 22-4 SUMMARY OF MEDICAL PROBLEMS CONFRONTING THE CHILD WITH CYSTIC FIBROSIS AND THE ACCEPTED TREATMENT FOR EACH

Problem	Treatment
Bronchial obstruction	Inhalation therapy Physical therapy
Pulmonary infection	Long-term or intermittent antibiotic therapy
Exocrine gland dysfunction	Sodium replacement during periods of stress or high environmental temperature
Pancreatic deficiency	Enzyme replacement
Nutritional deficiency	High-caloric, high-protein, modified fat diet; vitamin and mineral supplements

ment therapy are aimed at minimizing the extent of the malabsorption that is likely to occur as a result of the lack of pancreatic enzymes (lipase, amylase, peptidase, cholesterolase). Fat malabsorption seems to present a greater problem than the difficulty in digestion and absorption of carbohydrates and protein caused by the pancreatic insufficiency. In infancy, a formula containing predigested proteins and medium-chain triglycerides (MCT) rather than long-chain fats (e.g., Pregestimil and Portagen; see Table 13-4) is more readily tolerated.

For the infant, strained or pureed meats are a better source of protein than vegetable and meat combinations. High-protein infant cereals should be given in small amounts because cereals tend to fill the infant and are a lower biological source of protein.

The diet should be adjusted to the age and tolerance level of the individual. Nutrient guides as recommended by the Cystic Fibrosis Foundation are listed in Table 22-5. Calories should be increased 50 to 100 percent above the normal requirements for age. Recent studies have described the increased caloric requirements of the child with cystic fibrosis.[53] The high energy needs have been attributed to (1) a 30 to 50 percent increase in basal metabolic rate (BMR), (2) chronic lung disease, (3) increased oxygen consumption, and (4) malabsorption. Protein requirements are 2 to 2½ times the normal recommended amounts, while fat intake varies with age, caloric intake, and degree of fat intolerance. Restriction of excess fatty foods is usually desirable in view of the extensive fat malabsorption associated with the disease. A modified fat diet (Table 22-6, pp. 482–483) is best tolerated, but should be individually tailored. For example, one child may not be able to tolerate the fat in chocolate or peanut butter, while another child may. Likewise, gastrointestinal tolerance of the gas-producing vegetables is highly individual. When planning a diet for the CF child, individual food tolerance must be a primary consideration. Owing to the decreased pancreatic enzyme secretion, simple carbohydrate sources and protein may be better tolerated.

TABLE 22-5 NUTRIENT GUIDELINES FOR CHILDREN WITH CYSTIC FIBROSIS

Age, years	Kilocalories (kilojoules)
Infants (to 1)	150–200 kcal/kg/day (630–840 kJ/kg/day)
Children (1–9)	130–180 kcal/kg/day (545–755 kJ/kg/day)
Males (9–18)	100–130 kcal/kg/day (420–545 kJ/kg/day)
Females (9–18)	80–110 kcal/kg/day (335–460 kJ/kg/day)

Age	Protein
Infants	4 g/kg/day
Older children	3 g/kg/day
Young adults	2½–3 g/kg/day

Age	Fat*
Infants	
Normal	6+ g/kg/day
Moderate	4.5–6 g/kg/day
Low-fat	4.5 g/kg/day
Older children	
Normal	3+ g/kg/day
Moderate	2–3 g/kg/day
Low-fat	1–2 g/kg/day

*Cystic Fibrosis Clinic, Children's Hospital, Boston, 1980.
Source: Adapted from *Guide to Diagnosis and Management of Cystic Fibrosis,* Cystic Fibrosis Foundation, 1974.

Vitamin supplementation is necessary. A multivitamin supplement in a water-miscible solution is suggested. The fat-soluble vitamins, especially vitamins A and D, are prescribed in twice the usually recommended doses. Water-soluble forms of Vitamin E are routinely prescribed although hypovitaminosis E secondary to cystic fibrosis has not been reported. Vitamin B complex is recommended, especially for patients with cheilosis and those taking broad-spectrum antibiotics. In areas where the local water supply is unfluoridated, fluoride supplementation is also recommended.

Dietary supplements have recently been introduced as a means of increasing the energy intake of the child with cystic fibrosis. Allan et al.[54] report on the use of a nutritional supplement consisting of beef serum protein hydrolysate, a glucose polymer, and medium-chain triglycerides in a group of 17 patients with cystic fibrosis. Increased rates of weight gain and linear growth were seen in 11 of the children as a result of the increased energy intake from these supplements.

MCT (medium-chain triglycerides, Drew Chemical Company) provides 8.3 kcal per mL (38 kJ per mL) and has been used to facilitate the direct absorption of fatty acids in the cystic fibrosis population at Children's Hospital Medical Center in Boston. More recently, Polycose (Ross Laboratories), a glucose polymer, has also been employed as a carbohydrate supplement in the diet of these children. It provides 0.67 kcal per mL (2.8 kJ per mL) and is tasteless, and colorless when dissolved in solution.

Parenteral hyperalimentation with an amino acid infusion has been used in acute periods of illness when appetite is poor or the function of the gastrointestinal tract is questionable. Elliot[55] used Intralipid hyperalimentation in 7 children with cystic fibrosis. A weight gain was experienced by all 7 children during the period of infusion and a feeling of well-being was reported concomitantly with the intravenous therapy. The levels of essential fatty acids (linoleic and arachidonic) rose during this time period, suggesting that fatty acid deficiency may be a concern in the cystic fibrosis population because of fat malabsorption.

Pancreatic enzyme replacement is needed with meals to improve the digestion and absorption of fat and protein. The dosage and the enzyme preparation selected are determined by the individual's fat tolerance and response to the enzyme therapy. Pancreatic enzymes should be taken with all meals and snacks. The quantity is determined by age and body size. In infants, the powdered enzyme is mixed in a small amount of baby fruit and is fed immediately; otherwise enzyme breakdown of the fruit occurs.

TABLE 22-6   MODIFIED FAT DIET PROVIDING APPROXIMATELY 45 TO 50 g OF FAT PER DAY*

Type of food	Food permitted	Foods to avoid
Beverages	Coffee, tea, decaffeinated coffee, cereal beverage, skim milk, skim buttermilk, carbonated beverages	Any others
Breads and cereals	Enriched or whole-grain bread, crackers, plain hard rolls, plain dinner rolls	Very rich breads made with large amounts of eggs or fat, such as quick breads, pancakes, waffles
Desserts	Angel food cake, fruit whips made with foods permitted, gelatin desserts, sherbet, fruit ices, puddings made with skim milk	Pastries and very rich desserts, ice cream, desserts made with egg yolk, chocolate, cream, fat, or whole milk
Eggs, meats, and cheeses	*Lean* beef, lamb, liver, veal, poultry, fish, canned tuna or salmon (wash off oil carefully); limit eggs to 1 per day (egg whites as desired); uncreamed cottage cheese, pot cheese	Pork; skin of poultry; fried meat, fish, or poultry; fish preserved in oil; bacon; fried eggs; other cheese
Fats	Limit to 1 tsp per meal: butter, fortified margarine, salad oil, cream	Peanut butter, lard, salad dressing, shortening
Fruit and juices	All fruits except those listed under *Foods to avoid,* all juices	Fruits possibly causing gastric distress include: avocado, watermelon, cantaloupe, honeydew melon, raw apple
Potatoes and substitutes	White or sweet potatoes, hominy, macaroni, noodles, rice, spaghetti, pretzels	Potato chips; fried rice, noodles or potatoes; highly seasoned sauces with fat
Soups	Fat-free broth or bouillon, vegetable soup made with allowed vegetables, tomato bouillon, cream soups made with skim milk and allowed vegetables and meat	Cream soups made with whole milk, cream, or butter
Sweets	Sugar, honey, jelly, jam, plain hard candy, syrups	Candy made with cream fat, nuts, or chocolate

*This diet should be adapted to individual needs and may not need to be this restrictive.

TABLE 22-6 CONTINUED

Type of food	Food permitted	Foods to avoid
Vegetables	All vegetables except those listed under *Foods to avoid*	Vegetables causing gastric distress† such as onion, radishes, sauerkraut, green or red peppers, kohlrabi, cabbage, corn, cucumbers, broccoli, brussels sprouts, turnips, lima beans, dried peas and beans, rutabagas
Miscellaneous	Salt, vinegar, lemon, juice, fat-free gravy	Chocolate, condiments, spices† nuts, olives, pepper†

†May be tolerated unless there is presence of severe abdominal cramping and steatorrhea.

The most common preparations in use in the United States are Viokase, Cotazym, and Pancrease. However, several other preparations are also in use (see Table 22-7). The enzymes are available in powder, tablet, and capsule forms and are made from beef or pork sources.

Clinical signs and symptoms of inadequate pancreatic replacement or excessive fat intake may include the following: abdominal cramps; abdominal distention; light-colored, frequent, mushy stools; foul-smelling flatus; rectal prolapse; and failure to thrive.

TABLE 22-7 PREPARATIONS AVAILABLE FOR PANCREATIC ENZYME REPLACEMENT IN CYSTIC FIBROSIS

Enzyme preparation (manufacturer)	Source	Dosage*
Cotazym (Organon)	Whole hog pancreas	1–5 capsules/meal ¼–2 pks. powder/meal
Viokase (Viobin)	Whole hog pancreas	2–10 tablets/meal ½–2 tsp/meal
Pancrease (Johnson & Johnson)	Whole hog pancreas	1–2 capsules/meal
Panteric granules & enteric tablets (Parke-Davis)	Whole hog pancreas	¼–1 tsp granules or 3–5 tablets/meal
Papase tablets (Warner-Chilcott)	Whole hog pancreas	½–3 tablets/meal
Piget-Aide† (Johnson & Johnson)	Whole hog pancreas	1–3 capsules/meal
Ilozyme (Warren-Teed)	Whole hog pancreas	1–5 tablets/meal

*Related to meal or snack size, and age.
†Not available in United States.

DISEASES OF THE LARGE BOWEL

The large intestine functions in the absorption of water and crystalloids from the gut and aids in the passage of the feces to the rectum for excretion.

The large bowel is located in the lower abdomen and starts with the caecum. The appendix projects from this segment. From the lower right quadrant of the abdomen, the large intestine extends upward (ascending colon), crosses underneath the liver and stomach to the spleen (tranverse colon), and turns downward (descending colon) on the left side. The sigmoid segment connects the large bowel to the rectum.

Ulcerative Colitis

Ulcerative colitis is an organic inflammatory disease of the mucosal and submucosal linings of the large bowel. Characteristic lesions or ulcerations are apparent in the left colon and rectum, and often in the entire organ.

Colonic motility is greatly increased, resulting in rapid movements of the small bowel and increased secretions by the colon. The patient has frequent diarrhea, and the stools often contain blood and mucus. Nausea, abdominal pain, anorexia, tachycardia, and anemia are common symptoms.

The etiology of the disease is not known. However, several theories have been proposed. The disease may be due to a nutritional deficiency state, particularly of vitamin B_{12} or protein; or it may be of infectious origin. Many researchers claim that psychogenic disturbances resulting in increased stress will result in the disease. Fried et al.[56] suggest that the disease may be inherited as an autosomal recessive trait.

Ulcerative colitis results in serious local and systemic complications. The disease is characterized by remissions and exacerbations and most frequently appears in youth and early middle age. The disease occurs more frequently among females than males and appears to be predominantly a disease of the Caucasian race with a high incidence in the Jewish population.

The diagnosis of ulcerative colitis is most often based on clinical symptoms. Sigmoidoscopy reveals an abnormal, inflamed colonic mucosa and seems to be the best tool available for diagnosis of the disease. The diagnosis can be supported by rectal biopsy and x-ray examination.

Treatment Medical treatment of the disease includes fluid and electrolyte replacement for the dehydration and water losses from the diarrhea. Blood transfusion, for replacement of losses through rectal bleeding, has decreased the morbidity and mortality associated with the disease. Because ulcerative colitis is an inflammatory bowel disease, administration of the anti-inflammatory drugs ACTH and cortisone has been used to effect a remission during an acute attack.

Dietary treatment should aim to (1) decrease stool frequency through elimination of irritants to the bowel; (2) provide adequate protein for tissue regeneration and enteric protein losses; (3) provide adequate energy in response to increased catabolic rates; and (4) exclude food substances which careful history reveals may worsen the diarrhea.

Cady et al.[57] have demonstrated a lactase-deficient state in 46 percent of their study population. Therefore a low-lactose diet may improve weight gain in the patient with secondary lactose intolerance.

In general, the diet for patients with ulcerative colitis should be appealing in order to overcome the anorexia associated with the disease. A diet low in residue (Table 22-8) will eliminate mechanical irritants to the inflamed bowel, while an increased protein and energy intake will improve clinical response to the chronic diarrhea and tissue breakdown associated with the disease. Elimination of particular food items, especially lactose-containing foods, will improve nutrient absorption and decrease malabsorption due to the inflammatory condition.

High-fiber diets as a maintenance treatment of ulcerative colitis in remission have been studied.[58] In a small sample of these patients, the use of a high-fiber diet with discontinuation of maintenance drug therapy was not well toler-

TABLE 22-8 LOW-RESIDUE DIET

Type of food	Foods permitted	Foods to avoid
Beverages, milk	Coffee, tea, decaffeinated coffee, cereal beverages, carbonated beverages; 2 cups milk per day (to drink or in cooking)	Milk in excess of 2 cups
Bread and cereals	Enriched white or light rye bread without seeds; cooked refined corn, rice or wheat cereals	Whole-grain or bran flour and cereals
Desserts	Cakes with plain icing, plain cookies, gelatin desserts (all without nuts, coconut, or fruits not listed under *Foods permitted*); smooth and milk-flavored sherbet and ice cream	Pastries, any other not listed
Fats	Butter, margarine, mayonnaise, salad oil, cream	None
Fruits and juices	Strained fruit juice; ripe banana; strained, cooked, and peeled fruits without seeds	Any others
Meats, fish, poultry, eggs, cheese	Crisp bacon; roasted, baked, broiled, or boiled tender beef, ham, lamb, liver, veal, fish, chicken, or turkey; cottage, cream, and mild American cheese; eggs any way except fried	Tough meats, fried meats, highly seasoned meats, skins of poultry, strong-flavored fish, shellfish, cheese other than those permitted
Potatoes or substitutes	White and sweet potatoes, pasta	Skins of potatoes, fried potatoes, potato chips
Soups	Bouillon, broth, strained cream soups made with foods permitted and within daily milk allowance	Any others
Sweets	Candy without nuts or chocolate, honey, clear jelly, sugar, molasses, syrup, smooth chocolate in moderation	Candy containing fruits or nuts; jam, marmalade
Vegetables	Tomato juice, canned or cooked pureed vegetables	Any others
Miscellaneous	Gravy, herbs (except garlic), spices in moderation, vinegar, white sauce, smooth peanut butter	Garlic, nuts, olives, pickles, popcorn, pepper, relishes, fried foods, highly seasoned sauces

ated. It seems that a small subgroup of colitis patients who develop colonic stasis with clinical relapse of the disease may benefit by a high-fiber diet. Terminating drug therapy in lieu of a maintenance high-fiber diet has not been proven to be a consistent therapeutic approach.

Regional Enteritis (Crohn's Disease)

Enteritis is an inflammation of the bowel of varying degrees. The condition may be the result of a mechanical or chemical irritation at some point in the bowel. Overeating, poisoning, or bacterial invasion can cause the inflammation. The exact etiology is not known.

When the colon is involved, the resulting disease state is called *regional enteritis* or *Crohn's disease*. However, Crohn's disease has been reported to occur in any portion of the gastrointestinal tract.[59]

Inflammation of the bowel results in a shift of water into the intestine to act as a cleansing and diluting solution. Cramping results from increased intestinal motility. Diarrhea, weight loss, fatigue, and irritability are characteristics of the disease. Frequently steatorrhea will occur, resulting in a loss of large quantities of ingested fat in the stools. Characteristic stools often contain mucus, blood, and pus.

Treatment   Dietary principles for the treatment of regional enteritis include a low-residue diet that is high in protein and rich in vitamins and minerals to promote tissue regeneration. Elimination of residue in the diet reduces mechanical irritation to the gut and provides rest. Low-residue liquid feedings may be incorporated into the diet (see Chap. 28, Table 28-6).

Restriction of fat in the diet will aid in controlling the fecal fat losses that occur in steatorrhea. Fat absorption may be improved through the use of medium-chain triglycerides as a source of increased calories.

Diverticulosis

Diverticula are acquired herniations or pocketings of the mucosa through the layers of the bowel wall. *Diverticulosis* is the presence of diverticula which are not inflamed. Infection often occurs as a result of the accumulation of fecal matter within the diverticula, which can become ulcerated or perforated. Inflammation of diverticula is called *diverticulitis*.

Diverticular disease is the most common colonic disease of the western nations. The increased incidence of diverticulosis has been attributed to a diet low in fiber. The deficiency of dietary fiber alters the consistency of the feces, causing the sigmoid colon to segment more rapidly. The increased segmentation propels the feces, which generates increased intraluminal pressure, causing herniation of the colonic mucosa. The development of diverticula follows.

Treatment   For many years a low-residue diet had been prescribed to help eliminate irritation of the bowel. In view of the recent findings that hypersegmentation of the colonic mucosa is a result of increased intraluminal pressure,[60] a diet high in fiber is the current trend of dietary treatment for the disease, since fiber lowers the intraluminal pressure and shortens the intestinal transit time by providing bulk to the stool. (See Chap. 4 for fiber content of foods.)

Kirwan et al.[61] found that unprocessed bran was successful in shortening gastrointestinal transit time. Bran resists digestion by absorbing water, resulting in a soft, bulky stool which is easily passed.

The increased intraluminal pressure associated with diverticular disease develops as a result of increased force exerted by the muscle, increased diameter of the intestinal lumen, and decreased viscosity of the intestinal contents. Burkitt et al.[62] suggest the use of bran in relieving the symptoms associated with diverticular disease that result from increased intraluminal pressure. Findlay et al.[63] report the positive effects of ingesting 20 g of unprocessed bran per day in their population suffering from diverticular disease. Their findings clearly point to the use of coarse bran as therapeutic for (1) shortening intestinal transit time in diverticular disease, (2) increasing stool weight in normal people and to a lesser extent in patients with diverticular disease, (3) modifying fecal flow patterns, and (4) providing a vehicle for interstitial water. They demonstrated a decrease in the intraluminal pressure in response to the bran's stimulus to the distal colon, thus relieving the symptoms associated with increased intraluminal pressure in patients with diverticular disease.

Increased fiber intake is considered the most appropriate dietary treatment for diverticular disease. However, as many treatments for gastrointestinal disease change, so it is with dietary management of diverticular disease and the dispute over the effectiveness of a low-fiber versus a high-fiber diet.

Bowel Resection

Surgical removal of a section of the ileum (ileectomy) or the colon (colectomy) may be indicated in chronic conditions such as carcinoma, intestinal obstruction, lesions, or ulcerative colitis. Following removal of the bowel segment a permanent opening is made in the abdominal wall to provide for elimination of digestive wastes.

An *ileostomy* results from attaching the proximal end of the ileum to the opening in the abdominal wall. Because the absorptive capacity of the ileum is reduced as a result of the decreased surface area, the ileostomy continuously drains fluid which is often irritating to the surrounding tissue. Proper hygiene and use of a well-fitted appliance is necessary to prevent tissue erosion around the stoma.

Initially, large sodium and water losses occur following an ileostomy procedure because the absorptive capacity of the ileum has been disturbed by the surgery. However within 7 to 10 days postoperatively the losses are adjusted to within normal limits. Extensive resection of the ileum results in fat malabsorption requiring a dietary restriction in fat. Vitamin B_{12} absorption is permanently decreased and is often totally lost. Therefore intravenous fluid and electrolyte replacement is necessary during the convalescent period, while vitamin B_{12} injections are necessary for life to compensate for the isolated defect in vitamin B_{12} absorption. The diet is aug-

mented progressively as tolerated. After complete recovery postoperatively, the ileostomy patient is able to resume a regular diet. However, ingestion of excessive dietary roughage may obstruct the stoma and result in discomfort to the patient.

A *colostomy* results from attaching the proximal end of the colon to the opening in the abdominal wall. The colon retains some capacity to absorb water; therefore, the stools are semiformed. The patient is able to learn to control bowel movements through the colostomy, thus enabling reestablishment of bowel regularity.

Diet is increased progressively as tolerated. The colostomy patient should observe the stools to determine individual tolerances to particular food items and should regulate the diet accordingly. The dietary management of colostomy patients aims to provide adequate energy and nutrition and to allow for good control of bowel movements.

Therapeutic dietary management of ostomy patients must be individualized. The greater the extent of intestinal resection, the greater the degree of secondary malabsorption. In all cases, diet is aimed at providing optimal nutrition through vitamin and mineral replacement and nutrient supplementation in response to the degree of malabsorption. (See Chap. 28.)

Constipation

Constipation is a disorder of the colon characterized by infrequent or difficult evacuation of feces. Stools are hard and have a dry consistency. Symptoms include dull headache, lazy feeling, lassitude, anorexia, low-back pain, and weakness. Diagnosis is most often made by physical examination of the colon through an anoscope or by a digital rectal examination and proctoscopy.

There are three classifications of constipation: imagined, rectal, and colonic.

Imagined constipation can occur in response to a skipped regular bowel movement. An individual assumes that without a daily bowel movement, constipation exists and treatment must follow. However, skipping a daily defecation may not be a result of constipation but might suggest a reaction to a change in diet or to stress.

Rectal constipation results from delayed elimination and is the most common form of constipation. Most often a routine elimination pattern is formed to coincide with the daily work and life schedule. However, routine elimination schedules may become disturbed, and the change may affect the conditioned bowel reflexes. Thus constipation develops.

Colonic constipation is the result of a delay in the passage of residue through the colon. The stool is hard, dry, and difficult to eliminate. Inadequate water intake or a diet rich in food items that are not well tolerated by the individual can result in constipation.

Mechanical obstruction of the colon by a tumor of anal stricture can also influence fecal elimination. Extracolonic pressures during pregnancy, a fibroid uterus, and the aging process can result in poor muscle tone and constipation.

Treatment   Drug therapy with a variety of laxatives can improve fecal consistency or increase transit time, thus relieving symptoms associated with constipation. Table 22-9 outlines common types of medications currently in use for the treatment of constipation and their mode of action. Enemas give immediate relief from constipation by softening feces and increasing peristalsis. Increased exercise and the development of regular bowel habits can aid in relieving symptoms of constipation.

Dietary treatment includes the use of a high-fiber diet with increased liquids to promote soft, passable stools. Benson[64] suggests an intake of approximately 1500 mL of water per day to help improve stool consistency. Inclusion of food items known to have a laxative effect such as prunes, figs, raisins, apricots, whole grains, and bran can increase stool bulk and bring relief from constipation.

Highly sugared foods will increase fermentation in the gut and aid in the formation of

TABLE 22-9   MEDICATIONS COMMONLY PRESCRIBED FOR TREATMENT OF CONSTIPATION AND THEIR MODE OF ACTION

Type of medication	Action
Stimulants	
Cascara, senna Phenolphthalein (Ex-Lax)	Affects intestinal muscle, increasing motility
Castor oil	Interferes with water absorption thus affecting intestinal motility
Saline cathartics	
Milk of magnesia Magnesium citrate	Acts as osmotic force in lumen; stimulates peristalsis
Emollient laxatives	
Mineral oil	Coats stool, prevents absorption of fecal water (Note: interferes with absorption of fat-soluble vitamins)
Dioctyl sodium sulfosuccinate (Colace, Disonate)	Lowers surface tension, allowing water to penetrate feces, thus softening the stool
Bulk-forming laxatives	
Methycellulose	Absorbs water; softens, thus increases peristalsis
Psyllium hydrophilic mucilloid (Metamucil)	
Osmotic loads	
Sugar syrup Brown sugar Malt soup (Maltsupex)	Increases fermentation; draws fluid into the gut, distending rectum and leading to defecation

Source: Adapted from L. Olney, *American Family Physician,* March 1976, p. 89.

small-chain acids. The resulting acids act as osmotic forces and draw fluid into the gut lumen, thus distending the rectum and leading to defecation.

Encopresis
Encopresis is the voluntary withholding of stools, resulting in chronic constipation and rec-

tal leakage of watery fecal matter. The condition occurs in the young child and often arises around issues of bowel training.

Treatment includes education of the parent and child, training of muscles, and the development of a routine toilet regimen. The use of a high-fiber diet in conjunction with mineral oil (known to inhibit absorption of fat-soluble vitamins) is begun and continued until bowel movements are regulated.

Hemorrhoids

Hemorrhoids are ruptured blood vessels located around the anal sphincter. They may be internal or external and may or may not cause pain. Most often hemorrhoids are a result of straining at defecation, of constipation, of prolonged use of cathartics or enemas, or of strain during childbearing.

Treatment Surgical removal is recommended if the condition does not improve.

Dietary modifications are aimed at providing relief from the symptoms rather than at treatment. A low-fiber diet with increased fluid intake and the inclusion of stewed fruits and vegetables most often will prevent constipation and reduce the irritation that may occur from a high-fiber diet. Foods such as spices known to cause individual discomfort should be avoided.

GASTROINTESTINAL CONDITIONS IN INFANCY

A host of conditions occur in infancy that require immediate surgical repair. These congenital conditions affecting the gastrointestinal tract can ultimately alter the nutritional status of the infant and cause failure to thrive as a result of gastric dumping syndromes or intestinal malabsorption.

Many clinical features are common among these conditions, especially the demand for increased nutrients and energy as a result of malabsorption and the metabolic trauma of surgery.

These conditions often cause gastric, intestinal, or colonic obstruction, which requires immediate surgical intervention. Suggested nutritional therapy includes the introduction of a central venous catheter for delivery of total parenteral nutrition (see Chap. 28). The goal of the nutritional plan is to have the infant progress to an oral formula as soon as the bowel has recuperated and the infant can tolerate the oral feeding. Oral motor stimulation in the child who is fed through the extended use of parenteral alimentation is critical. The use of a pacifier or manual oral stimulation will help the parenterally fed child to develop normal feeding patterns.

Table 22-10 is a summary of the special nutritional problems associated with gastrointestinal conditions in the newborn. A full discus-

TABLE 22-10 GASTROINTESTINAL CONDITIONS CAUSING NUTRITIONAL PROBLEMS IN INFANTS

Condition	Secondary nutritional problem
Gastric	
Gastroschisis	Dumping syndrome
Omphalocele	Diarrhea
Intestinal	
Small bowel obstruction	Malabsorption
Intestinal atresia	Diarrhea
Meconium ileus	Steatorrhea
Colonic	
Necrotizing enterocolitis	Water malabsorption
Hirschsprung's disease	Difficulty with fecal passage
Imperforate anus	Difficulty with fecal passage

sion of these gastrointestinal conditions and their treatment is, however, beyond the scope of this chapter.

DISEASES OF THE LIVER AND BILIARY TRACT

The liver is the largest organ in the body, with an approximate weight of 1300 g. The normal liver is not palpable; however, when it becomes diseased the liver increases in size and can be palpated. The liver plays an important role in determining an individual's nutritional status as many of its functions relate to nutrient metabolism. The functions of the liver can be summarized as follows:

Formation of bile. Bile is synthesized by the liver and stored in the gallbladder. The major function of bile is to aid in the digestion and absorption of fat and fatlike substances. The primary constituent of bile is water. Other components are bile salts (sodium and potassium), bile pigments (biliverdin, bilirubin), cholesterol, fatty acids, lecithin, fat, and alkaline phosphatase.

2 *Detoxification of metabolic by-products, poisons ingested in foods, and drugs.*

3 *Carbohydrate metabolism.* Synthesis of glucose, storage of glycogen, and blood glucose homeostasis.

4 *Protein metabolism.* Formation of plasma protein and urea.

5 *Fat metabolism.* Synthesis of lipoprotein and ketones.

6 *Vitamin and mineral storage.* Storage of fat-soluble vitamins, B complex, vitamin C, iron, and copper.

A brief description of the more common liver function tests and laboratory indices is summarized in Table 22-11. Familiarization with the diagnostic criteria for liver disease will aid the student in understanding the clinical manifestations of the disease condition.

TABLE 22-11 LABORATORY TESTS AND INDICES FOR DIAGNOSIS OF LIVER AND BILIARY DISEASE

Diagnostic test	Findings in liver and biliary disease
Bilirubin (serum, urinary)	Elevated
Alkaline phosphatase	Elevated
Cholesterol	Elevated (cholesterol cannot be properly metabolized to bile acids)
Prothrombin time	Decreased (prothrombin and fibrinogen production reduced)
Serum glutamic oxalacetic transamminase (SGOT)	Elevated (as a result of dying liver cells)
Sulfobromophthale in Bromsulphalein (BSP)	Elevated (diseased liver is unable to filter at normal rate)
Albumin (serum)	Decreased (protein synthesis is depressed)

Diseases of the Liver

Hepatitis

Hepatitis is an inflammation of the liver caused by toxins (chloroform, carbon tetrachloride) and infectious microbes (viruses and bacteria). The term viral hepatitis refers to two conditions: (1) Infectious hepatitis can be transmitted via the oral-fecal route. Other sources of contamination include drinking water, food (many times seafood), and sewage. (2) Serum hepatitis, on the other hand, is transmitted parenterally, from syringes, tubing, and blood. The clinical manifestations are similar for both types; therefore, they can be considered as a clinical entity.

Common clinical symptoms of hepatitis include anorexia, malaise, headache, nausea, vomiting, and the loss of the desire to smoke or drink alcohol. Several days later, jaundice (yellow-appearing skin and eyes) may develop and the urine becomes dark because of the increase in the circulating bilirubin. The liver becomes enlarged (hepatomegaly) and, in some cases, the spleen enlarges (splenomegaly) as well. Laboratory analysis reveals that bilirubin, alkaline phosphatase, and serum glutamic oxalacetic transaminase (SGOT) are elevated.

Treatment   Bed rest and diet therapy are the two major components of treatment. In the acute stages of hepatitis when vomiting is severe an intravenous solution of 5 to 10 percent dextrose and water must be administered. If this stage is prolonged hydrolysates must be added to the intravenous solution. Parenteral nutrition must be supplied until the patient is able to consume sufficient energy by mouth. (See Chap. 28 for a more detailed explanation of parenteral nutrition.) Since the patient is anorexic and becomes easily nauseated, frequent small meals must be encouraged.

The energy intake should be 3000 to 4000 kcal (12.6 to 16.8 MJ), of which carbohydrate comprises 300 to 400 g in order to promote glycogen synthesis and spare protein. Protein should be planned to provide 1.4 to 2.0 g per kilogram of body weight to maintain positive nitrogen balance. This is often difficult to accomplish since the patient has a lack of appetite and may complain of nausea. Fat restriction, once a common practice for hepatitis patients, is no longer indicated. Use of high-caloric drinks and the addition of dry powdered skim milk to regular milk, hot cereals, mashed potatoes and creamed soups not only help to increase energy but protein as well. The use of margarine wherever possible—on vegetables, potatoes, hot cereals, in soups—will also help to increase the energy content of the diet. Vitamin and mineral supplements may or may not be warranted, depending upon the nutrient intake of the patient. Alcohol is to be avoided by all hepatitis patients to prevent any further liver cell necrosis. Disposal precaution trays and dishes should be used during the infectious stages of the disease.

Cirrhosis

Cirrhosis is the end stage of liver injury and is characterized by fibrosis of the connective tissue and degeneration of liver cells with a resultant loss of liver function. The pathophysiologic etiology of cirrhosis is unknown but it is commonly seen in chronic alcoholism and malnutrition as well as in biliary obstruction and infection. The accumulation of fat in the liver (steatosis) may be the first stage of cirrhosis, though some authorities feel that this is not necessarily a sequel of the disease. Fatty liver, which is commonly seen in alcoholics, was originally thought to be due to the accompanying malnutrition rather than to alcoholic consumption. However, Lieber has demonstrated that subjects fed alcohol plus a nutritionally adequate diet still developed fatty liver.[65] Therefore, fatty liver in alcoholics seems to be due to the direct effect of alcohol on the liver and only by the withdrawal of alcohol can the condition be corrected.

The etiology of the injury to the liver in the alcoholic patient has been attributed to (1) alcohol toxicity, (2) genetic predisposition to the disease, (3) malnutrition, or (4) a combination of all these factors.[66] Malnutrition in chronic liver disease can result from malabsorption, decreased hepatic nutrient storage, inadequate dietary intake, and disturbed nutrient metabolism.

Nutritional assessment of the cirrhotic patient is difficult since changes in weight secondary to edema may nullify the use of anthropometric weight data. Also, plasma proteins are reduced and serum ribonuclease activity is increased. Therefore, plasma amino acid profiles are of limited use in determining protein-nitrogen status.[67]

The most common form of cirrhosis is Laennec's cirrhosis. It is generally associated with alcoholism, although not all alcoholics will develop Laennec's cirrhosis and it may be seen in nonalcoholics. A variety of metabolic activities are impaired in Laennec's cirrhosis. Scar tissue forms in the liver, and the conversion of fat to lipoproteins is impaired, hence the accumulation of fat in the liver. Portal hypertension may develop and blood flow becomes obstructed, with esophageal varices (varicose veins in the esophagus) the end result. Esophageal varices are a serious complication since the danger of rupture with ensuing hemorrhage is an imminent possibility.

The cirrhosis patient has an enlarged liver as a result of fat accumulation and necrosis of the liver cells. Ascites (accumulation of fluid in the abdomen) and edema of the extremities may be present since hepatic filtering is impaired and serum protein levels are low. SGOT is elevated and BSP (sulfobromophthalein) clearing time is reduced resulting in elevated levels. Vitamin deficiencies and depressed hematocrit and hemoglobin values are commonly seen and may be due to malnutrition, gastrointestinal bleeding, or both. Patients may appear jaundiced, may lack appetite, and may have delirium tremens (DTs).

Collection of clinical, biochemical, and dietary data will provide a data base for the development of a nutrition care plan.

Treatment Providing a diet which will improve the malnutrition associated with liver disease is the goal of nutritional therapy. A high-energy diet is recommended—approximately 45 to 50 kcal per kg (189 to 210 kJ per kg) of ideal body weight per day. Table 22-12 lists recommended guidelines for dietary therapy of liver disease.

Protein of high biological value must be provided to enable repair of damaged liver cells. An intake of 1 g of protein per kg of body weight is the ultimate goal. However, optimal protein intake must be attained gradually in response to the patient's tolerance as measured by neurological status. Increased protein intake is contrain-

dicated if hepatic coma is present or imminent (see below).

A diet high in carbohydrate must be provided in order to achieve the desired energy levels and to spare the body protein. A moderately high fat intake is necessary to provide palatable meals and aid in increasing energy. Fat may need to be reduced if there is biliary obstruction or a decrease in bile salt production, or if evidence of fatty liver is present. Medium-chain triglycerides are useful to incorporate into the diet if there is a problem with obstruction and bile salt production; however, in advanced cirrhosis the use is contraindicated. A therapeutic vitamin and mineral preparation is needed. Vitamin B deficiencies, particularly of thiamin, are commonly seen in alcoholic patients. Other nutrients that are inadequately supplied are iron and folic acid. Vitamin K supplementation may be necessary if the prothrombin time is prolonged. Supplementation of other fat-soluble vitamins may also be necessary if there is a problem with fat absorption.

If ascites is present, sodium should be restricted to 10 meq (230 mg) per day. Some physicians may be reluctant to initiate a low-sodium dietary regimen, especially if the patient's serum sodium is low. However, a low-sodium intake will promote water excretion, thereby increasing the serum sodium.[68] A diet restricted to this degree will need careful planning in order to incorporate all needed nutrients within the constraints of the sodium limitation. Low-sodium milk such as Lonalac can be a useful adjunct, as are commercially produced supplements which

TABLE 22-12   DIETARY GUIDELINES FOR LIVER DISEASE

	Hepatitis	*Cirrhosis*
Protein	1.4–2.0 g/kg	1.0 g/kg
Fat	Moderate 35–50 g	Moderate 35–50g
Carbohydrate	300–400+ g	300–400+ g
Energy	45–50 kcal/kg (3000–4000 kcal)	45–50 kcal/kg (3000–4000 kcal)

are low in sodium and high in protein and energy. (See Chap. 23, Table 23-4.) Sodium intake can be gradually liberalized as diuresis occurs. Fluids may need to be restricted (1200 to 1500 mL per day) if the patient's weight does not decrease or if a weight gain is seen.

The use of salt substitutes may be contraindicated depending upon the chemical composition of the preparation. Ammonia chloride preparation will contribute to the high ammonia levels secondary to liver disease and should not be substituted for sodium chloride. Other salt substitutes should be evaluated on the basis of the client's clinical and biochemical status and the chemical composition of the preparation (see Chap. 23).

If esophageal varices are present, it is important that small frequent feedings in conjunction with antacids be instituted in order to prevent or minimize bleeding.[69] Nicotine and foods which are known to be gastrointestinal irritants (caffeine, pepper, chili) should be avoided. Foods of a soft or semisolid nature are easier for the patient to swallow and should be incorporated into the diet. Many cirrhotic patients have altered carbohydrate metabolism, and a high incidence of diabetes is seen,[70,71] necessitating carbohydrate control.

Hepatic Coma

Hepatic coma can develop in patients with severe liver disease because the entrance of ammonia into the cerebral circulation causes intoxication. This may be caused by portacaval shunting or by severe damage to the liver cells. Ammonia is produced in the gastrointestinal tract, probably from bacterial action.[72] Davidson reports that other toxic substances such as indoles and amines derived from tyrosine and tryptophan may also play a role in the pathogenesis. He suggests that these substances bypass the liver where they normally are detoxified and affect the brain tissue, perhaps causing the euphoria that commonly characterizes this condition.[73]

Altered sleep patterns may be present; patients sleep during the day and remain awake at night. Alternating states of depression and mania may occur.[74] Serum ammonia levels are elevated. Administration of protein to these patients will precipitate coma.

Treatment The usual treatment is the administration of antibiotics to decrease intestinal bacteria and thereby reduce ammonia production.[75] If this proves ineffective, reducing the dietary protein of high biological value to 30 g or less will be necessary. This protein restriction should be maintained for as short a time as possible since protein is needed for tissue regeneration. Foods which yield high amounts of ammonia and should be avoided are cheeses, meats, and vegetables.[76] Patients who are comatose must be nourished parenterally, with minimal protein intake and in some cases with protein completely eliminated. (See Chap. 28 for further discussion of parenteral nutrition.)

DISEASES OF THE PANCREAS

The pancreas is located in the upper abdomen, behind the stomach. This organ is responsible for the production of the hormone insulin and several important digestive enzymes (see Chap. 9) that aid in protein, fat, and carbohydrate digestion. The pancreatic duct allows the flow of pancreatic juices to join with bile in the common bile duct, from which they drain into the duodenum. See Chap 24, "Diabetes Mellitus."

Pancreatitis

The presence of stones in the common bile duct or spasm of the sphincter may result in a backflow of pancreatic secretions and bile into the pancreas. Inflammation of pancreatic tissue, known as *pancreatitis,* may result. Pancreatitis brings bouts of moderate to severe pain in the upper abdomen that can last for hours or days. Jaundice is usually present. Weight loss, steatorrhea, malabsorption, diabetes mellitus, and pancreatic calcification may occur, depending on the degree of severity of the disease. Serum and urine amylase are increased and are used as diagnostic criteria for pancreatitis.

The acute form of pancreatitis may or may not progress to the chronic form. There are several theories accounting for the etiology of pancreatitis. Obstruction of the pancreatic duct, alcoholism leading to disease of the biliary tract, and reflux of duodenal contents into the pancreatic duct with regurgitation of bile from the common duct up the pancreatic duct have been proposed.

Duodenal intubation allows the collection of stimulated pancreatic juice for analysis of electrolytes and enzymes. The majority of patients with pancreatitis exhibit increased serum amylase.

Treatment Pancreatic secretions are stimulated by the products of protein digestion and fat in the duodenum, and therefore these nutrients are restricted in the diet. In acute episodes of pancreatitis, intravenous feedings of fluids, electrolytes, and glucose are given. When oral feedings are tolerated, clear liquids containing simple carbohydrates are started. The diet is augmented progressively as tolerated, with the addition of protein and limited fat sources. Fat remains restricted until there is no evidence of steatorrhea (which results from decreased pancreatic lipase). Chronic pancreatitis is treated with a high-protein, high-carbohydrate, low-fat diet. Protein is necessary for optimal pancreatic function and should be encouraged. Simple carbohydrates are needed to provide energy and to prevent hypoglycemia. A diet low in fat may be initiated to inhibit pancreatic secretion.

Parenteral hyperalimentation may be started if the patient's intake is poor because of decreased appetite and constant pain. In all cases, alcohol should be restricted because the inflamed pancreas is unable to utilize it.

DISEASES OF THE GALLBLADDER

The gallbladder is a pear-shaped organ attached to the underside of the liver. The main function of the organ is to store and concentrate bile secreted by the liver. The gallbladder is usually full and relaxed between meals. Upon stimula-tion by secretion of the hormone cholecystokinin from the intestinal mucosa, the gallbladder contracts, releasing concentrated bile into the duodenum via the common bile duct.

Cholecystitis

The gallbladder may become infected by bacteria traveling from various parts of the body. Inflammation of the gallbladder is known as *cholecystitis*. Abnormal function of the organ may also result from pregnancy, overweight, constipation, or digestion upsets. Cholecystitis is accompanied by epigastric pain in the area of the gallbladder, vomiting, flatulence, and soreness in the upper right quadrant. Jaundice may appear in some cases.

Gallstones often develop as a result of infection or changes in bile composition. Diet, heredity, and female hormones are implicated in the disease. The formation of stones is called *cholelithiasis*. When stones occur in the prescence of infection the condition is known as *cholecystolithiasis*. *Choledocholithiasis* develops when the stones slip into the common bile duct, resulting in obstruction. Ductal stones are found in 10 to 20 percent of all patients with stones in the gallbladder. Gallstones are composed of cholesterol, bile salt, and pigment, or a combination of these.

Diagnosis can be made by means of oral cholecystography. Failure to visualize the contrast agent is definitive for gallbladder disease. Intravenous cholangiography gives visualization of the bilary tract and can reveal stones in the common bile duct.

Treatment Administration of chenodeoxycholic acid is effective in dissolving small gallstones. However, surgical removal of the gallbladder may be necessary in the presence of stones that are large in either number or size.

Nutritional therapy for gallbladder disease must be individualized. Patients soon learn their particular food intolerances. Generally, most gallbladder patients complain of distention and epigastric pain on ingestion of rich pastries, fatty foods, vegetables from the "gas-forming" group, and chocolate.

Fat stimulates the gallbladder and bile duct to contract; therefore, a low-fat diet (25 to 40 g) is recommended. In acute attacks the use of a low-fat clear liquid regimen is advisable, with parenteral supplementation if a state of malnutrition exists. Starches and lean meats may be added as soon as they are tolerated. It is advisable for the patient to follow a low-fat diet until the gallbladder is removed surgically.

If the patient is overweight, a low-caloric diet is recommended to achieve ideal weight. Protein sources should be relatively low in fat. Gastrointestinal disease represents a major threat to the nutritional status of the patient. Disease affecting the esophagus interferes with the mechanics of feeding, requiring an alternative route for nutrition such as enteral (tube) or parenteral feedings.

Diseases of the stomach and bowel interfere with enzyme function and consequently result in malabsorption and the loss of nutrients through diarrhea or steatorrhea. Vitamin and mineral depletion often occurs. Elemental liquid diets or parenteral hyperalimentation may be used for nutritional support in conditions affecting the absorptive capacity of the gut.

Water losses and consequent fluid and electrolyte problems occur with diseases of the lower bowel. As with the small intestine, conditions affecting the colon and the rectum most often will improve with a diet modified in consistency and texture; in severe cases, intravenous hyperalimentation can help to meet the increased nutrient needs.

This increased energy need may be met with a special diet supplement of an elemental nature. See Table 28-4.

CONCLUSION

It is important for the student health professional to recognize and appreciate the significant impact on nutrient requirements that gastrointestinal diseases present, since an individual's nutritional status is an ultimate factor in the recovery from an acute or chronic gastrointestinal condition.

STUDY QUESTIONS

1 What is the rationale for a bland diet regimen in ulcer therapy? List those foods that should be eliminated from the diet of an ulcer patient.

2 Compare and contrast the malabsorption that is seen in celiac disease with that seen in cystic fibrosis.

3 What enzymes may be affected in ulcerative colitis? Why?

4 Explain the rationale for a high-fiber diet in the treatment of diverticulitis.

5 Why is protein restricted in the patient with hepatic coma?

CLINICAL STUDY 22-1

S. is a 12-year-old white male admitted to the Children's Hospital after a 1-month episode of diarrhea, crampy abdominal pain, and bloody stools. The intake interview revealed a history of a 6- to 8-kg weight loss over the last year, complicated by acute attacks of abdominal cramps relieved by bowel movements numbering 6 to 20 loose stools daily. Physical examination revealed a pale, thin, hyperkinetic *young boy. The abdomen was soft, with guarding on the right and mid quadrant. The spleen was palpable to 6 cm. Height and weight on admission were 152 cm and 35.7 kg respectively. An upper gastrointestinal x-ray study showed normal findings but a barium enema revealed a loss of haustration from the transverse colon to the rectum with diffuse small ulcerations, findings consistent with a diagnosis of co-*

litis. Sigmoidoscopy findings were consistent with a diagnosis of ulcerative colitis, and a rectal biopsy revealed an inflamed, edematous mucosa with dilated crypts filled with polymorphonuclea leukocytes. Significant laboratory data on admission were as follows:

Blood pressure 108/76 mmHg

Temperature 98.2° F

Blood urea nitrogen, sugar, electrolytes normal

Serum calcium 9.8 mg per 100 mL

Serum magnesium 2.0 meq per mL

Serum phosphorus 4.4 mg per 100 mL

Serum alkaline phosphatase 6.3 units

Serum vitamin B $_{12}$ 925 pg per mL

Serum folic acid 24 ng per mL

Serum iron 22 μg per 100 mL

Total iron-binding capacity 344 mg per 100 mL

Prothrombin time 12.4 s

Hemoglobin 10.4 g per 100 mL

Hematocrit 32.6%

Mean corpuscular volume (MCV) 24 μm^3

Platelets 630,000/mm^3

The diagnosis was ulcerative colitis, with iron-deficiency anemia secondary to chronic blood loss.

Orders were to start S. on prednisone 20 mg twice daily; multivitamins once daily; ferrous sulfate 300 mg TID; folate 1 mg daily; and Tums 3 tablets TID. A dietary prescription for a 6-meal bland, low-residue, high-protein, limited-dairy-product (480 mL of whole milk or equivalent daily) diet was ordered.

S. progressed during the following several weeks of hospitalization. The number of bowel movements decreased significantly to 3 or 4 daily and were described as blood-free and loosely formed. Significant laboratory data after 3 weeks of hospital treatment were as follows:

Height 152.25 cm

Weight 37 kg

Hemoglobin 13.9 g per 100 mL

Hematocrit 43.3%

MCV 82 μm^3

Serum calcium 10 mg per 100 mL

S. was discharged with orders to continue taking multivitamins, ferrous sulfate, folate, Tums, and prednisone, and to follow a 6-meal bland, low-residue, restricted-dairy-products (480 mL whole milk or equivalent) dietary plan

Clinical study questions

1   How does ulcerative colitis affect absorption of key nutrients? What are the implications of this malabsorption?

2   With ulceration of the small bowel, what enzyme secretions might be affected? Relate this problem to the absorption of the associated nutrients.

3   Explain the rationale for the elimination of roughage, spices, and dairy products and the inclusion of a 6-meal dietary regimen in the treatment of ulcerative colitis.

CLINICAL STUDY 22-2

Past history

S. J. is a 35-year-old woman with obesity, elevated blood pressure, and increased triglyceride levels. Past history reveals a sedentary life style with an early diagnosis of obesity in childhood. At age 15, S. J. weighted 170 lb (77 kg) and was 5 ft 5 in (165 cm) tall. Past attempts to control weight gain were without success.

Present history

A physical examination reveals an adult woman in no apparent distress. Her height is 5 ft 7 in (170 cm) *and her weight is 280 lb (127 kg). Blood pressure is recorded at 190/110. Other significant laboratory data include:*

Serum cholesterol	*260 mg per 100 mL*
Serum triglycerides	*200 mg per 100 mL*
SGOT (serum glutamic oxalacetic transaminase)	*30 units per mL*
Alkaline phosphatase	*10 king-Armstrong units*
Serum glucose (after 24-h fast)	*70 mg per 100 mL*

Present food intake is 3700 kcal/day (15,481 kJ) (250 g protein, 400 g carbohydrates, 125 g fat). Because of the increased stress to the cardiovascular system and the threat to S. J.'s general health, a jejunoileal bypass was performed. This is an extraordinary procedure reserved for extreme cases of intractable obesity. It has been replaced by the gastric by-pass (see Chap. 25).

The procedure creates a surgical bypass of the jejunal and ileal segments of the small intestine, resulting in direct passage of nutrients from the duodenum to the colon.

The postoperative course was complicated by diarrhea, steatorrhea, and electrolyte imbalance. Progressive weight loss followed.

Clinical study questions*

1 *Describe the function of the jejunum and ileum in nutrient absorption.*

2 *Relate this function to the problems of diarrhea and steatorrhea that S. J. encountered postoperatively.*

3 *Which nutrients are most likely to be affected by the jejunoileal bypass? Why?*

* The student should refer back to Chap. 9.

REFERENCES

1 F. Alexander, "Psychological Factors in Gastrointestinal Disturbances," in F. Alexander and T. M. French (eds.), *Studies in Psychosomatic Medicine,* The Ronald Press Company, New York, 1948.

2 M. Sleisenger and J. Fordtran, *Gastrointestinal Disease,* 2d ed., W. B. Saunders Company, Philadelphia, 1978, p. 3.

3 Ibid., p. 13.

4 Ibid., p. 14.

5 Ian Gillespie and T. J. Thompson, *Gastroenterology, An Integrated Course,* Churchill Livingston, London, 1972, pp. 12–32.

6 Ibid.

7 W. Gangon, *Review of Medical Physiology,* Lange Medical Publications, Los Altos, Calif., 1969, p. 292.

8 Gillespie and Thompson, op. cit., p. 14.

9 Sleisenger anf Fordtran, op. cit., p. 520.

10 Ibid.

11 W. J. Hogan, S. R. V. de Andrade, and D. H. Winship, "Ethanol-Induced Human Esophageal Motor Dysfunction," *Journal of Applied Physiology,* **32**:755–760, 1972.

12 D. Q. Castell, "Hormonal Control of the Gastroesophageal Sphincter Strength," *New England Journal of Medicine,* **282**:886–889, 1970.

13 C. Cohen and W. Lipslutz, "Hormonal Regulation of Human Lower Esophageal Sphincter Competence," *Journal of Clinical Investigation,* **50**:449–454, 1971.

14 J. Babka and D. O. Costell, "Effects of Specific Foods on the Lower Esophageal Sphincter," *Digestive Disease,* **18**:391, 1973.

15 M. Paulson, *Gastroenterologic Medicine,* Lea and Fabiger, Philadelphia, 1969, pp. 662–663.

16 M. Greenberger and D. Winship, *Gastrointestinal Disorders; A Pathophysiologic Yearbook,* Medical Publications, Inc., Chicago, 1976, p. 24.

17 D. P. Burkitt, "Mechanical Effects of Fibre with Reference to Appendicitis, Hiatus Hernia, Haemorrhoids and Varicose Veins," *Journal of Plant Foods,* **3**(1,2):35–40, 1978.

18 Paulson, op. cit., p. 663.

19 P. B. Beeson and W. McDermott, *Cecil-Loeb Textbook of Medicine,* 13th ed., W. B. Saunders Company, Philadelphia, 1971, p. 1274.

20 Ibid.

21 B. W. Sippy, "Gastric and Duodenal Ulcers; Medical Care by an Efficient Removal of Gastric Juice Erosion," *Journal of the American Medical Association,* 64:1625, 1915.

22 J. Soltroft, E. Gudmand-Hyer, B. Kray, E. Kristensen, and H. Wuiff, "A Double-Blind Trial of the Effect of Wheat Bran on Symptoms of Irritable Bowel Syndrome," *Lancet,* 1:270, 276.

23 W. E. Anderson, "The Therapy of Peptic Ulcer Disease," *West Virginia Medical Journal,* 74:57, 1978.

24 D. A. Drossman, D. W. Powell, and J. T. Sessions, "The Irritable Bowel Syndrome," *Gastroenterology,* 73:811, 1977.

25 "Position Paper on Bland Diet in the Treatment of Chronic Duodenal Ulcer Disease," *Journal of the American Dietetic Association,* 60:306, 1971.

26 J. A. Roth and A. Ivy, "Effect of Caffeine upon Gastric Secretion in the Dog, Cat and Man," *American Journal of Physiology,* 141:454, 1944.

27 S. Cohen and G. H. Booth, "Gastric Acid Secretion and Lower Esophageal Sphincter Pressure in Response to Coffee and Caffeine," *New England Journal of Medicine,* 293:897, 1975.

28 C. V. Netchbolodoff and M. D. Hargrove, "Recent Advances in the Treatment of Diarrhea," *Archives of Internal Medicine,* 139:813–816, 1979.

29 R. B. Sack, N. F. Pierce, and N. Hirschorn, "The Current Status of Oral Therapy in the Treatment of Acute Diarrheal Illness," *The American Journal of Clinical Nutrition,* 31:2251–2257, 1978.

30 M. E. Ament, "Malabsorption Syndromes in Infancy and Childhood," *Journal of Pediatrics,* 81:685–697, 867–884, 1972.

31 W. K. Dicke, "Coeliac Disease: Investigation of Harmful Effects of Certain Types of Cereal on Patients with Coeliac Disease," thesis, University of Utrecht, Netherlands, 1950.

32 A. Ferguson, "Coeliac Disease (Gluten Hypersensitivity)," *Journal of Human Nutrition,* 30:193, 1976.

33 K. G. Kenrick and J. A. Walker-Smith, "Immunoglobulins and Dietary Protein Antibodies in Childhood Coeliac Disease," *Gut,* 11:635, 1970.

34 P. A. Green and E. D. Wollanger, "Clinical Behavior of Sprue in the United States," *Gastroenterology,* 38:399, 1960.

35 Ibid.

36 M. E. Ament, op. cit., p. 875.

37 J. D. Kirschmann, "Nutrition Research," in *Nutrition Almanac,* South Minneapolis, 1974.

38 G. M. Gray, "Carbohydrate Digestion and Absorption," *New England Journal of Medicine,* 292:1225, 1975.

39 A. Holzel, "Sugar Malabsorption and Sugar Intolerance in Childhood," *Proceedings of the Royal Society of Medicine,* 61:1095, 1968.

40 A. D. Newcomer, "Disaccharidase Deficiencies," *Mayo Clinic Proceedings,* 48:638–652, 1973.

41 A. Dahlquist, "Method for Assay of Intestinal Disaccharidases," *Analytical Biochemistry,* 7:18, 1964.

42 A. D. Newcomer, D. B. McGill, P. J. Thomas, et al., "Prospective Comparison of Indirect Methods for Detecting Lactase Deficiency," *New England Journal of Medicine,* 293:1232, 1975.

43 J. Perman, R. Barr, and J. Watkins, "Sucrose Malabsorption in Children: Noninvasive Diagnosis by Interval Breath Hydrogen Determination," *The Journal of Pediatrics,* 93(1):17–22, 1978.

44 D. H. Calloway, E. L. Murphy, D. Bauer, "Determination of Lactose Intolerance by Breath Analysis," *American Journal of Digestive Diseases,* 14:811, 1969.

45 H. V. Maffei, G. Metz, V. Bampoe, M. Shiner, S. Herman, and C. G. Brook. "Lactose Intolerance, Detected by the Hydrogen Breath Test in Infants and Children with Chronic Diarrhea," *Archives of Disease in Childhood,* 52:766–771, 1977.

46 S. J. Birge, H. T. Kaufman, P. Cuatresas, and G. D. Whedon, "Osteoporosis, Intestinal Lactase Deficiency and Low Dietary Calcium Intake," *New England Journal of Medicine,* 276:445, 1969.

47 C. Gallagher, Molleson, and J. H. Caldwell, "Lactose Intolerance and Fermented Dairy Products," *Journal of the American Society of Agronomy,* 65:18–19, 1974.

48 H. Shwachman, "Gastrointestinal Manifestations of Cystic Fibrosis," *Pediatric Clinics of North America,* 22: 787–805, 1975.

49 C. Taft-Bayerl, personal communication, 1980.

50 R. Wood, T. Boat, and C. Doershuk, "Cystic Fibrosis, State of the Art," *American Review of Respiratory Disease,* 113:833–878, 1976.

51 A. Lapey, J. Kahwinkel, P. diSant'Agnese, and L. Laster, "Steatorrhea and Ozotorrhea and Their Relation to Growth and Nutrition in Adolescents and Young Adults with C. F.," *Journal of Pediatrics,* 84:328–334, 1974.

52 J. Palmer, C. Dulon, S. Capasso, B. Hearne, et al. "Why Do Children with Cystic Fibrosis (CF) Develop Diabetes Mellitus?" *Perspectives in Cystic Fibrosis, Proceedings of the Eighth International Congress on Cystic Fibrosis,* Toronto, May 1980.

53 S. Adeniyi-Jones, R. Suskind, B. Kean, J. Polombo, and K. T. Khaw, "Growth, Energy, Metabolism, and T_3 levels in Malnutrition in Cystic Fibrosis," *Cystic Fibrosis Club Abstract,* Atlanta, 1979, p. 22.

54 J. D. Allan, A. Mason, and A. Moss, "Nutritional Supplementation in Treatment of Cystic Fibrosis of the Pancreas," *American Journal of Diseases of Children,* **126**: 1973.

55 R. B. Elliot, "Therapeutic Trial of Fatty Acid Supplementation in Cystic Fibrosis," *Pediatrics,* **57**:474–479, 1976.

56 K. Fired and E. Vare, "Lethal Autosomal Recessive Enterocolitis of Early Infancy," *Clinical Genetics,* **6**:418–419.

57 A. B. Cady, J. B. Rhodes, A. Littman, and R. K. Kane, "Significance of Lactase Deficit in Ulcerative Colitis," *Journal of Laboratory and Clinical Medicine,* **70**:279, 1976.

58 P. S. Davies and J. Rhodes, "Maintenance of Remission in Ulcerative Colitis with Sulphasalazine or a High-Fibre Diet; A Clinical Trial," *Journal of Plant Foods,* **3**(1,2):125–127, 1978.

59 K. Zetzel, "Granulomatous (Ileo) Colitis," *New England Journal of Medicine,* **282**:600–605, 1970.

60 P. Plumey and B. Francis, "Dietary Management of Diverticular Disease," *Journal of the American Dietetic Association,* **63**:527–530, 1973.

61 W. O. Kirwan, A. N. Smith, A. A. McConnell, W. D. Mitchell, and M. A. Eastwood, "Action of Different Bran Preparations on Colonic Function," *British Medical Journal,* **4**:187–189, 1974.

62 D. P. Burkitt, A. R. P. Walker, and N. S. Painter, "Dietary Fiber and Diseases," *Journal of the American Medical Association,* **229**:1068, 1974.

63 J. M. Findlay et al., "Effects of Unprocessed Bran on Colon Function in Normal Subjects and in Diverticular Disease," *Lancet,* **1**:146–149, 1974.

64 J. A. Benson, "Simple Chronic Constipation," *Postgraduate Medicine,* **57**(1): 1975.

65 C. Lieber, "Liver Disease and Alcohol: Fatty Liver Alcoholic Hepatitis, Cirrhosis and Their Interrelationships," *Annals of the New York Academy of Sciences,* **252**, 1975.

66 M. A. Morgan, "Alcohol and the Liver," *Journal of Human Nutrition,* **33**:350–356, 1979.

67 A. Shenkin, "Assessment of Nutritional Status: The Biochemical Approach and its Problems in Liver Disease," *Journal of Human Nutrition,* **33**:341–349, 1979.

68 C. Davidson, "Dietary Treatment of Hepatic Disease," *Journal of the American Dietetic Association,* p. 517, May 1976.

69 Ibid., p. 68.

70 G. Sereny, L. Endrenyl, and P. Denenyl, "Glucose Intolerance in Alcoholics," *Journal of Studies in Alcohol,* **36**:359–364, 1975.

71 H. O. Conn, W. M. Schreiber, S. G. Elkington, and T. R. Johnson, "Cirrhosis and Diabetes: Increased Incidence of Diabetes in Patients with Laennec's Cirrhosis," *American Journal of Digestive Diseases,* 1969, p. 837–852.

72 G. J. Gabuzda, "Ammonium Metabolism and Hepatic Coma," *Gastroenterology,* **53**:806, 1967.

73 Davidson, op. cit., p. 518.

74 Ibid.

75 C. J. Fischer and W. W. Faloon, "Blood Ammonia Levels in Hepatic Cirrhosis. Their Control by the Oral Administration of Neomycin," *New England Journal of Medicine,* **256**:1030, 1957.

76 D. Rudman, R. Smith, A. Solom, D. Warren, J. Galambas, and J. Wenger, "Ammonia Content of Food," *American Journal of Clinical Nutrition,* **26**:487–490, 1973.

CLINICAL DISCUSSION 22-1

S. suffered from ulcerative colitis, an illness affecting the transit time of the small bowel and the absorptive capacities of the colon, with consequent malabsorption, of ingested vitamins, minerals, and some nutrients.

Characteristic of ulcerative colitis is the presence of an inflamed intestinal mucosa with the occurrence of lesions and haustrations in the colon. Evident from S.'s admission laboratory data is a significant loss of red blood cells because of these lesions, resulting in a secondary anemia. There is no interference with the initial process of digestion, nor are amylase and gastric secretions affected in ulcerative colitis. However, the malabsorption and diarrhea have caused the low serum calcium, magnesium, and folic acid levels, and the generalized malnourished state. S. experienced an 8-kg weight loss during the early stages of his disease due primarily to a loss of healthy, functioning intestinal mucosa and consequent malabsorption of ingested nutrients. Dehydration developed as a result of the massive stooling and dysfunctioning colon; however, not in significant enough degree to affect the fluid and electrolyte characteristics.

The presence of a diseased intestinal mucosa often interferes with the colitis patient's ability to properly digest and absorb lactose because of interference with the production and functioning of the intestinal disaccharidases. However, mucosal damage does not usually affect sucrose hydrolysis, probably because of the high levels of sucrase that usually are present. Lactase deficiency is commonly believed to be responsible for the colitis patient's intolerance to dairy products. S. is in a critical period for growth and development of skeletal tissue. He requires a high supply of dietary calcium, which is perhaps the greatest mineral contribution of the dairy and milk food group (his recommended dietary allowance is 1200 mg of calcium daily). Therefore, Tums, an antacid containing calcium bicarbonate, was prescribed to compensate for the decreased dietary calcium intake. One tablet provides 195 mg of utilizable calcium.

Dietary fiber and spices such as black pepper and chili powder have been found to affect the absorptive capacity of the normal intestinal mucosa, and therefore aggravate the diseased mucosa of the colitis patient. Elimination of these items from the diet and establishment of a bland low-residue regimen achieves the purpose of resting the small bowel and eliminating potential mucosal irritation. However, with the elimination of all raw and most processed fruits and vegetables because of their fiber content, the dietary supply of water-soluble vitamins and minerals is critically low. Since the nutritional status of the colitis patient is significant in recuperation from the illness, multivitamins were necessary to compensate for decreased cellular resistance to infection and to help in the regulatory process during the healing stage.

To aid in tissue regeneration of the inflamed mucosa and colonic lesions, as well as to improve hemoglobin levels, a high-protein diet was ordered simultaneously with the administration of ferrous sulfate, folate, and prednisone. High-protein snacks coupled with high-protein meals of low fat constitution will improve the body's ability to regenerate diseased cells and expedite the recuperative process. Consequently, with improved absorption because of decreased stress to the small bowel, S. was able to gain in height and weight.

Recuperation from the initial onset of colitis is a slow process requiring strict dietary monitoring and compliance with the drug regimen. As the patient's symptoms subside, food items are gradually reintroduced into the daily diet and the individual is able to liberalize the diet as tolerated. The ultimate dietary restrictions depend on the status of mucosal integrity and functioning.

CLINICAL DISCUSSION 22-2

The most active site of nutrient absorption in the gastrointestinal tract is the small intestine. Disaccharidases, peptidases, and intestinal lipase are secreted by the mucosa of the small intestine and are responsible for nutrient breakdown. Intestinal absorption of most nutrients occurs in the upper portion of the intestine where the mucosal enzymes are able to act on complex carbohydrate, protein, and fat molecules and break them into more easily absorbable forms.

However, the jejunal and ileal mucosa is active in the absorption of monosaccharides, amino acids, monoglycerides, and some diglycerides. In the presence of a diseased mucosa, or with a bypass of the jejunum and ileum as in the case of S. J., nutrient absorption becomes incomplete for two reasons:

1   Although some breakdown of nutrients occurs at the gastric level and in the duodenum, the lack of contact with enzymes from the lower section of the small bowel results in incomplete nutrient breakdown.

2   Malabsorption results in the quick loss of partially digested nutrients in the form of diarrhea. Because fats require a longer time in the small bowel for enzymatic breakdown and are considered to be the most complex nutrient molecules for digestion, the consequent lack of mucosal surface contact results in a massive loss of partially digested fats in the form of steatorrhea.

Because of the contribution of carbohydrate-, protein-, and fat-specific enzymes, all nutrients are affected in a bypass of the jejunum and ileum. The absorption of water, vitamins, and minerals is also affected. Rapid loss of partially digested fats results in the loss of significant fat-soluble vitamins and warrants close attention in malabsorption.

In lieu of surgical intervention for obesity, many authorities recommend a balanced calorie-deficient diet that will result in weight loss and prevent further weight gain.

CHAPTER 23

THE KIDNEYS AND URINARY TRACT

Roberta Ruhf Henry

KEY WORDS
Nephron
Blood Urea Nitrogen
Creatinine
Oliguric
Anuric
Acute Renal Failure
Chronic Renal Failure
Uremia
Azotemia
End-Stage Renal Disease
Dialysis

During the past several decades, much progress has been made in the field of nephrology. Great advances have been made in the understanding of both normal renal physiology and the treatment of renal diseases. However, even with the development of artificial kidney machines and improved methods of kidney transplantation, nutritional support and diet therapy continue to be an important aspect of the management of the individual with malfunctioning kidneys.

The primary focus of this chapter is the nutritional management of renal disease. Included also is a review of normal kidney anatomy and physiology, to enable the student to appreciate the effect of disease on kidney function.

NORMAL RENAL FUNCTION

Physiology

Normally, the two bean-shaped kidneys are located behind the peritoneum, one on each side of the spinal column. Each kidney, about the size of an adult fist, weighs approximately 150 g, or 5 oz, which is only 2 to 4 percent of the total body weight. The kidney is a very vascular organ, with its primary blood supply being the renal artery, a large branch of the aorta. Ordinarily, 180 L of blood—20 to 25 percent of the total cardiac output—perfuses the kidneys each day. This results in an average daily urine volume of 1 to 2 L for an 80-kg adult male.

Each kidney contains approximately 1 million microscopic functioning units called *nephrons,* and each nephron, although quite complex, can be looked at in its five basic segments. Figure 23-1 shows these segments and their respective functions. They are presented in the order found in the nephron unit, progressing from the first segment, which is intimately associated with its blood supply, to the end of the nephron where it ultimately elicits urine. This urine then passes into the renal pelvis, through the ureters, and into the bladder for excretion.

When the specific functions of the major segments of the nephron are examined (filtration, reabsorption, and secretion), the overall physiological activities of the kidneys should be apparent. These life-sustaining functions can be categorized according to role: those which are related to homeostasis and those which can be related to the endocrine system.

Description	*Primary Functions*
Glomerulus The glomerulus is a capillary tuft, freely permeable to metabolic end products, other potentially toxic substances in the blood, and almost all other constituents of plasma except for most plasma proteins.	*Filtration* Initial site of plasma filtration where the so-called "ultrafiltrate" of plasma is created. (This glomerular filtrate contains no cells or proteins.)
Proximal tubule A highly convoluted section, the proximal tubule is the first tubular section of the nephron and is found almost totally in the outer cortex of the kidney. It is one cell layer thick; however, these cells are highly specialized in their functions. (ADH is not required.)	*Reabsorption and secretion* The proximal tubule isotonically reabsorbs 60–80% of the glomular filtrate; 80–90% of the filtered Na^+, Cl^- and H_2O is reabsorbed. Glucose, amino acids, urate, potassium phosphate, bicarbonate and any remaining proteins are reabsorbed. NH_4, H^+, organic acids and bases are secreted.
Loop of Henle The loop of Henle is a U-shaped and therefore relatively straight segment, dipping into the inner portion of the kidney, the medulla.	*Reabsorption* Na^+ is reabsorbed by a complex mechanism that allows the kidney to control urine Na^+ (the countercurrent mechanism, see p. 160), and a hypotonic fluid is the result.
Distal tubule Anatomically similar to the proximal tubule, the distal tubule is predominantly in the renal cortex. (ADH from the pituitary makes this segment more permeable to water in the presence of dehydration.)	*Secretion and acidification* Acid-base balance is regulated; H^+ and NH_3 are secreted into the filtrate. Urine becomes isotonic. Remaining Na, Cl, and H_2O are reabsorbed according to the physiologic state of the body.
Collecting duct The distal-most portion of the distal tubule is the collecting duct. A specialized segment, where "fine tuning" takes place and formed urine passes into the pelvis of the kidney.	*Concentration of filtrate* The remaining Na^+, Cl^- and H_2O are reabsorbed. Further H^+ and NH_4 are secreted (as required by the physiologic state of the body).

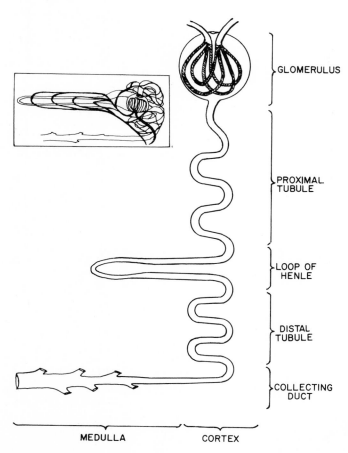

GLOMERULUS

PROXIMAL TUBULE

LOOP OF HENLE

DISTAL TUBULE

COLLECTING DUCT

MEDULLA   CORTEX

Figure 23-1

The functioning nephron. Above: a description of each nephron segment and its primary function; left: a schematic view.

Homeostatic Functions

1   *Waste excretion.*   The end products of metabolism, such as urea, creatinine, uric acid, and sulfates, as well as various drugs and potentially toxic substances, are excreted by the kidneys.

2   *Acid-base balance* (see Chap. 8). Hydrogen ions and bicarbonate are either excreted or retained to maintain the proper pH of the body's fluids.

3   *Water and electrolyte balance* (see Chap. 8).   Water, sodium, potassium, and chloride, as well as electrolyte and solute levels of the body, are regulated by renal excretion when they are in excess and by retention when deficient.

Endocrine Functions

Another very important function is not readily apparent from review of the nephron structure. That is its vital role as an endocrine gland.

1   When oxygen delivery to the kidneys is diminished, the kidneys secrete the hormone *erythropoietin* into the bloodstream. This hormone stimulates the bone marrow to produce red blood cells.

2   The kidneys play an important role in blood pressure regulation by secreting the proteolytic enzyme *renin* into the bloodstream when blood pressure is low. Renin, in turn, splits the plasma protein *angiotensinogen* into a smaller molecule, *angiotensin* I. A converting enzyme further splits angiotensin I to angiotensin II which acts to constrict the arterioles and increase blood pressure. This stimulates the secretion of *aldosterone* from the adrenal cortex which causes the kidneys to retain sodium and water, thus increasing blood pressure even further. Renin, therefore, has a very profound effect upon the cardiovascular system.

3   The kidneys are influential in calcium and phosphate metabolism, bone structure, and parathyroid function by converting the inactive form of vitamin D, which is produced by the body (from the skin) or found in food, to its effective form, 1,25-$(OH)_2D_3$ or 1,25-dihydroxycholecalciferol. This *active form of Vitamin D* is essential for normal calcium absorption from the gastrointestinal tract and is now considered to be a hormone.[1,2]

With their homeostatic and endocrine functions intact in almost all of the nephrons, the kidneys will efficiently regulate the body's physiological state. Therefore, at any age, under normal conditions, the variety and amounts of nutrients that can be safely consumed are limitless and the kidneys easily dispose of excess or waste produced by a full and varied diet.

RENAL FAILURE

Renal failure denotes the loss of nephron function severe enough to interfere with homeostatic and endocrine functions of the kidneys. This failure may occur rapidly or progressively but as the number of functioning nephrons decreases, regardless of the cause, the kidneys become less able to eliminate the multitude of wastes produced from an unrestricted diet.

When the number of functioning nephrons decreases significantly, laboratory tests will detect this change in renal function. The biochemical indices are either increased, decreased, or altered by the disease state (see Table 23-1).

When greater than 60 to 75 percent of the total nephron mass is destroyed by disease (see Table 23-2 for the etiology of kidney diseases),

TABLE 23-1   BIOCHEMICAL INDICES OF KIDNEY FUNCTION

Increased	Decreased	Altered (distribution)
Serum creatinine	Glomerular filtration rate	Sodium
Blood urea nitrogen	Creatinine clearance	Potassium
Serum uric acid	Urea clearance	Calcium/phosphorus ratio
	Urine concentrating ability (not necessarily volume)	Glucose metabolism Acid-base balance
Hematocrit	Fluid balance	

TABLE 23-2   ETIOLOGY AND CLINICAL MANIFESTATIONS OF SPECIFIC RENAL DISORDERS*

Condition	Etiology	Clinical manifestations
Acute glomerulonephritis	Usually follows an infection such as beta-hemolytic streptococcal infection.	Lethargy, malaise, anorexia, weakness, Hypertension, circulatory congestion, hematuria. Edema of face and eyelids is common.
Chronic glomerulonephritis	May occur after acute disease above. Frequently, etiology unknown.	Proteinuria, edema; may have hypertension and associated headache; anemia. As disease progresses, azotemia and uremia occur.
Nephrotic syndrome	May occur during chronic glomerulonephritis, metabolic diseases, systemic sensitivity diseases.	Edema; massive proteinuria with decreased serum albumin and increased cholesterol.
Polycystic kidney disease	Familial disease in which cysts develop in the parenchyma of both kidneys. Mean age of onset, 40 years.	Hypertension, intermittent hematuria, slight proteinuria, lumbar pain and/or tenderness, pyuria, and bacturia may be present. Palpable renal mass.
Acute chronic pyelonephritis	May follow urinary tract infection or be due to obstruction.	Chills, fever, abdominal pain, backache, nausea, vomiting, urinary frequency, dysuria.
Fanconi's syndrome	May be inherited or acquired. Proximal renal tubular transport function is impaired. Substances usually absorbed by the proximal tubule are lost.	Failure to reabsorb phosphate, with hypophosphatemia; renal rickets; glycosuria; aminoaciduria.
Cystinosis	Genetic metabolic anomaly affecting renal transport. Cystine is deposited in organs.	Similar to Fanconi's syndrome.
Renal tubular acidosis	Defective urinary acidification or reabsorption of bicarbonate. Cause is unknown.	Hypokalemia; osteomalacia may be present; hypophosphatemia, hypercalciuria.
Chronic potassium depletion	May result from renal tubular disorders, Cushing's syndrome, aldosteronism. Most common abnormality is the kidney's inability to concentrate urine.	Nocturia, polyuria, polydypsia, slight proteinuria.
Tuberculosis of the kidney	Bacterial infection of the kidney via the bloodstream. Can result in renal scarring and destruction.	Frequently there are no clinical manifestations. However, there may be dysuria and intermittent hematuria.

*Partial listing of known renal disorders.

and kidney function has decreased as evidenced by changes in the biochemical indices, dietary intervention and nutritional support become an essential part of the patient's care.

Nutritional Considerations

The primary nutritional goal is to maintain or achieve optimal nutritional status. Within the framework of renal disease, the minimization of protein catabolism, the maintenance of fluid balance, and the maintenance of electroyte balance are the goals of treatment. These are achieved by altering the intake of water, protein, calories, sodium, potassium, phosphorus, or calcium (see Table 23-3). From these goals, and from individualized assessment of the patient, an appropriate diet can be prescribed.

The control of protein, calories, sodium, water (fluids), potassium, and phosphorus is extremely important in the nutritional management of adults and children with renal disease. However, it is incorrect to assume that every patient with renal disease needs diet modification of all of these nutrients. Diet therapy for patients with renal failure should be individualized.

We will now consider the relevance of the dietary constituents—protein, carbohydrate, fat, sodium, potassium, phosphorus, and water—to the diet of the patient with renal disease.

Protein

The three major constituents of food—carbohydrates, proteins, and fats—contain carbon, hydrogen, and oxygen, and are metabolized to carbon dioxide and water, but *only* the proteins contain nitrogen. Protein is 16 percent nitrogen; i.e., 1 g of nitrogen is found in each 6.25 g of protein.

The metabolism of the amino acids in dietary protein produces nitrogenous waste products. Of these, approximately 70 percent are normally excreted in the urine and the remainder in the feces and through skin losses.[3] Furthermore, 80 to 90 percent of these amino acid catabolites, or breakdown products, are excreted in the urine as urea, with approximately 4 to 5 percent as creatinine, 3 percent as ammonia, and 1 to 2 percent as uric acid.

When the kidneys fail, urea and other nitrogenous wastes produced from the normal diet cannot be properly excreted. The inability of the kidneys to excrete urea is most evident by an elevation of the blood urea nitrogen (BUN). Normal range for BUN is 8 to 25 mg per 100 mL. However, because of the great influence of dietary protein intake on BUN, and the fact that abnormal physiological states such as gastrointestinal bleeding, dehydration, and others, alter this measurement, BUN is not usually considered a reliable tool for assessing kidney function.

A more accurate assessment of renal func-

TABLE 23-3 GOALS OF NUTRITIONAL MANAGEMENT OF THE RENAL PATIENT

Nutritional goal	Nutrients altered to achieve goal
To minimize protein catabolism (adults and children)	Protein
To promote anabolism, i.e., growth (children)	Energy Carbohydrates Fats
To maintain fluid balance (adults and children)	Sodium, water (fluids)
To maintain electrolyte balance (adults and children)	Sodium, potassium, phosphorus (and calcium) water (fluids)

tion is a measurement of urine creatinine clearance or of serum creatinine, since these are less influenced by dietary protein. Serum creatinine measures the kidney's ability to filter this product of muscle metabolism. Normal serum creatinine is relatively constant and is in the range of 0.5 to 1.4 mg per 100 mL, while normal creatinine clearance is 120 mL per min.

Since one of the goals of the nutritional management of renal disease is to prevent catabolism and promote anabolism while maintaining or achieving nitrogen balance, dietary protein restriction is not usually imposed until the patient begins to develop the signs and symptoms related to a high protein intake. These may include the following: a BUN of greater than 100 mg per 100 mL, a creatinine clearance below 30 mL per min, severe acidosis, nausea, vomiting, lethargy, or anorexia.

The optimum level of protein intake for people with renal failure has been the subject of intensive research for many years and still remains quite controversial. However, there is general agreement that dietary protein intake should be individualized in an attempt to achieve or maintain nitrogen balance and prevent catabolism which leads to the wasting syndrome so frequently seen in the renal failure population. Therefore, protein restriction should not be arbitrary; the quantity of protein permitted should be prescribed in accord with the current level of renal function. This can be accomplished by judicious and knowledgeable monitoring of laboratory data and clinical conditions.

A new approach to prescribing dietary protein intake from clinical data has much promise. The principles of mass balance (accumulation of a substance is equal to its input minus its output) can be used to quantitatively describe a person's protein catabolic rate. When calculated accurately, this data can be used to prescribe the dietary protein intake with far greater accuracy than has been possible in the past. Additionally, this method allows prediction of actual dietary protein intake in the stable patient population. The principles of mass balance can be employed for the predialysis population[4] as well as for people receiving hemodialysis therapy.[5,6,7]

The quality as well as quantity of protein in the diets of patients with renal disease is also important. When protein is restricted, a minimum of 50 to 60 percent of the total protein intake should be from foods of high biological value, such as milk, eggs, and meats, which contain the essential amino acids (see Chap. 3).

Of interest to note is the fact that a remarkable number of patients automatically reduce their own dietary protein intake prior to any formal diet instruction. In so doing, they may be affecting the quality of protein and the total energy intake. Therefore nutrition counseling is directed toward the protein quality and quantity and energy intake needed to prevent unwanted weight loss or breakdown of muscle mass, while at the same time controlling for undesirable gastrointestinal symptoms. (For more specific recommendations on protein intake, see the discussion of stages of chronic renal failure, p. 521.)

Energy

Energy intake is an important component of the meal plans for people with renal disease. In general, calories should not be restricted and every effort should be made to maintain or achieve ideal body weight. Although no current standard for energy requirements exists, 35 to 45 kcal (147 to 189 kJ) per kilogram of ideal weight is frequently recommended for adults with renal failure. Children and adolescents require as much as 100 to 150 kcal (420 to 630 kJ) per kilogram in order to support or enhance growth. The energy needs will vary according to age, sex, activity, height, and weight.

Nonprotein calories are especially important when individuals are following a protein-restricted diet.[8] Calories from concentrated carbohydrates (sugar, honey, sour balls or other hard candies, jelly, etc.) and fats (oils, margarine, butter) may be encouraged in order to spare endogenous protein breakdown and enable the body to utilize the dietary protein for anabolism. (See Table 23-4.)

TABLE 23-4   HIGH-ENERGY, LOW-ELECTROLYTE, LOW-PROTEIN SUPPLEMENTS

Product	Manufacturer	Composition and form	Approximate calories (joules)
Cal Power	General Mills	Deionized glucose; liquid (fruit-flavored)	2 kcal per mL (8.4 kJ per mL) (295 kcal per 240 mL; 1239 kJ per 240 mL)
Polycose	Ross laboratories	Glucose polymers (from hydrolysis of cornstarch); liquid or powder	Liquid: 2 kcal per mL (8.4 kJ per mL) Powder: 4 kcal per g (16.8 kJ per g)
Controlyte	Doyle Pharmaceutical Co.	Polysaccharides and vegetable oil; powder	5 kcal per g (21 kJ per g)
HyCal	Beecham-Massengill Pharmaceuticals	Demineralized glucose; liquid (fruit-flavored)	2 kcal per mL (8.4 kJ per mL)
Lipomul Oral	Upjohn Co.	Corn oil; liquid	3 kcal per mL (12.6 kJ per mL)

Carbohydrates and Fats

In addition to protein, the individual with renal disease may also have difficulty in tolerating carbohydrate and fat because of abnormal metabolism.

Carbohydrate and fat metabolism   In renal patients without any previous history of diabetes, glucose intolerance frequently occurs. This abnormality is not totally understood and is rarely of clinical significance. Fasting blood sugars are usually slightly elevated, as reflected by an abnormal glucose tolerance curve. In most instances this alteration in carbohydrate metabolism is not a contraindication to encouraging a high dietary intake of carbohydrate calories. This abnormal state may be corrected by dialysis.

Individuals with overt diabetes mellitus who were receiving hypoglycemic agents or insulin prior to the onset of renal disease frequently display a decreased need for insulin. However, this does allow more liberal amounts of carbohydrate calories in the diet. A liberal carbohydrate diet without concentrated sweets is usually tolerated.

Fat metabolism is also altered in renal failure. While cholesterol levels are usually normal, except in nephrotic syndrome (see discussion below) and posttransplantation, plasma triglyceride levels are elevated in both undialyzed and dialyzed people with renal failure.[9] This phenomenon is not generally improved with dialytic therapy and a significant percentage of these people present a type IV hyperlipoproteinemia pattern (see Chap. 21). This may be related to metabolic abnormalities of insulin and glucose and/or a defective triglyceride removal.[10] Some researchers feel that this is, at least in part, the result of the high carbohydrate and fat intake which results when one attempts to increase calories while maintaining a moderate or low dietary protein intake. Controversy still exists regarding the effectiveness of dietary manipulation for the treatment of the hyperlipidemia of renal failure but a low-carbohydrate, low-cholesterol, high-polyunsaturated-fat diet may be effective.[11] While this type of diet therapy is not routinely used for the treatment of hypertriglyceridemia, most agree that when the patient is stable medically, weight reduction should be encouraged.

Sodium

Normal renal function permits the urinary sodium output to approximate dietary sodium intake. While renal dysfunction does limit the ability of the kidneys to properly handle sodium, not every patient with renal failure requires a sodium-restricted diet. Ideally, the amount of sodium a patient requires is that amount which will prevent or control hypertension and heart failure and concurrently maintain a state of normal hydration.

An excellent method for determining a patient's hydration status is measurement of daily weight. When an individual is receiving sufficient sodium, this should be reflected by a stable body weight. An excessive intake of sodium will lead to excessive fluid retention and weight gain, while a low intake of sodium will lead to an abnormal weight loss. Daily weights should routinely be recorded for all hospitalized renal patients. Sodium and fluid intake should be modified accordingly.

Restricting the sodium in the diets of some patients with renal failure can lead to sodium depletion, as manifested by dehydration, with symptoms of orthostatic hypotension and leg cramps, as well as by worsening renal function. (The state of dehydration is accompanied by low blood pressure, caused by the reduced blood volume, and results in diminished renal function and a decrease in the glomerular filtration rate.) Unfortunately, sodium depletion, as a result of vigorous sodium restriction, is quite common in patients with renal failure. This is especially true in patients with polycystic kidney disease, medullary cystic kidney disease, and pyelonephritis (see Table 23-2). Since these disease states tend to cause polyuria and excessive urinary sodium loss, patients may be referred to as "salt wasters" or "salt losers."

Another common, preventable cause of sodium depletion and its resultant deterioration of renal function is the concurrent use of diuretic therapy and a diet which is severely restricted in sodium. The deleterious effect can be prevented if sodium losses are carefully monitored and dietary sodium intake is individualized.

However, sodium-restricted diets are useful in preventing fluid retention, and thereby controlling blood pressure and preventing heart failure. Since the sodium needs of patients with decreasing renal function are not static but variable, the need for sodium restriction changes.

Even patients with salt-losing nephropathy may develop edema and circulatory congestion and require some degree of sodium restriction.

Patients with advanced renal disease who are prone to sodium retention seem to have difficulty with extremes of sodium intake (too high or too low) and appear to do well with an intake in the range of 800 mg (35 meq) to 1600 mg (70 meq) per day;[12] however, sodium modification may vary from as little as 500 mg (22 meq) per day to as much as 4000 mg (173 meq) or more per day.

Sodium and food   Certain canned or processed foods must be avoided in most sodium-restricted diets (see Table 23-5, p. 510). Whether or not special dietetic low-sodium food products (e.g., low-sodium bread, margarine, etc.) are required depends on the level of sodium restriction. There are herbs, spices, and seasonings which can help to lend palatability to the patient's diet (see Table 23-6, p. 511).

Sodium and medications   Certain medications contribute a significant amount of sodium to a patient's total daily intake (see Table 23-7, pp. 511–512). When these medications are prescribed, the sodium content of the patient's diet should be altered accordingly. For example, if an individual requires a 2-g sodium diet (2000 mg or 87 meq sodium) and 2 g of sodium bicarbonate ($NaHCO_3$) is required to treat acidosis, the sodium content of the $NaHCO_3$, which is approximately 550 mg (24 meq sodium), must be subtracted from the dietary allowance. The diet should contain 1500 mg (65 meq) sodium per day. Instructions should be given to the patient and family members regarding the sodium content of both the diet and drugs.

Sodium (Na) conversion:
1 meq Na = 23 mg Na
1 g NaCl (table salt) = 400 mg Na
1 tsp table salt = 2300 mg Na
(100 meq Na)
1 g Na = 1000 mg Na
(43 meq Na)
Na = approximately 40% of NaCl

TABLE 23-5 HIGH-SODIUM SOURCES
(Usually avoided when a modified sodium intake is prescribed)

Seasonings

Baking soda	Monosodium glutamate	Steak sauce
Baking powder	Prepared mustard	Tabasco sauce
Catsup	Salt	Tartar sauce
Celery salt	Salt brine	Worcestershire sauce
Chili sauce	Sea salt	
Garlic salt	Seasoned salt	
Meat tenderizers	Soy sauce	

Meats and fish (smoked, cured, or dried)

Anchovies	Frankfurters
Bacon, Canadian and regular	Ham
Caviar	Luncheon meats
Corned beef	Pastrami
Corned beef hash	Salt pork
Dried beef	Sardines
	Tuna (packed in oil)
	TV dinners (frozen)

Cheese

American cheddar	Processed, all varieties: includes cheese spreads and cheese foods
Blue	
Feta	
Gouda	Romano (hard)
Parmesan (hard)	Roquefort

Snack foods (all with obvious salt on them)

Corn chips and corn curls	Pretzels
Crackers (salted)	Salted nuts
Party mixes	Salted popcorn
Potato chips	

Miscellaneous

Bouillon	Salad dressings
Ethnic foods: e.g., Chinese, Italian, and Kosher	Sauces and gravies (commercially prepared)
Olives, green and ripe	Sauerkraut
	Soups, canned, dried, frozen
	Relishes

TABLE 23-6   LOW-SODIUM HERBS, SPICES, AND SEASONINGS

Allspice
Almond extract
Basil*
Bouillon, low sodium†
Cardamon
Caraway seed*
Catsup, salt-free*
Chili powder*
Chives
Cinnamon
Cloves
Curry powder
Dill
Fennel
Garlic (fresh, juice, or powder)
Horseradish (without added salt)*
Honey
Juniper†
Lemon juice
Mace
Maple extract
Marjoram
Meat extract, low-sodium
Meat tenderizer, low-sodium
Mustard, dried or seed
Mint

Nutmeg
Oregano
Onion (fresh, juice, powder)
Parsely (fresh, flaked, dried)
Paprika*
Pepper, black, red, white
Pepper, fresh, red or green
Peppermint extract
Pimento peppers†
Poppy seeds
Purslane†
Rosemary
Saccharin
Saffron
Sage
Savory
Sesame seed
Sorrel†
Sugar, white or brown
Sugar syrups
Tarragon*
Thyme
Tumeric*
Vanilla extract
Vinegar

*Contain > 34 mg of potassium per level teaspoon and should be limited if a potassium-restricted meal plan is prescribed.

†Potassium content unknown.

Source: U.S. Department of Agriculture Handbook, "Spices and Herbs, Raw, Processed, Prepared," revised, 1977.

TABLE 23-7   SELECTED MEDICATIONS WITH THEIR SODIUM CONTENT

Medication	Dosage	Sodium content, mg
Fleet's enema	1 container	5000*
Citrocarbonates	1 oz	5100
Viokase powder	100 g	2400
Bisodol powder	10 g	1540
Sal Hepatica	1 rounded tsp	1000
Eno salts	1 tsp	738
Bromo-Seltzer	80 gr	717
Fizrin	1 packet	673
Kayexalate, powder	15 g	550
Nervine effervescent	1 tablet	544
Calcium carbonate and soda	1 tablet	543
Alka-Seltzer	1 tablet	521
Citrasulfas improved liquid	30 mL	400
Sodium chloride, tablet	15 g	393

*Average absorption.

(*Continued*)

TABLE 23-7   CONTINUED

Medication	Dosage	Sodium content, mg
Mucomyst 1%	10 mL	280
Keflin	4 g vial	249
Diaquel liquid	5 mL	75
Pektamalt	5 mL	75
Vick's Formula 44 Syrup	5 mL	68
Phenergan V.C. Expectorant	5 mL	51

Antacids†	Dosage	Sodium content, mg
Rolaids	1 tablet	53
Phosphajel	15 mL	39
Mylanta II liquid	15 mL	30
Robalate liquid	15 mL	27
Basajel	15 mL	27
A-M-T Suspension	15 mL	27
Amphojel suspension	15 mL	15
Gelusil	1 tablet	15

†Although the sodium content of these antacids does not seem appreciable, if they are taken frequently or in large quantities, the sodium from this source could be significant.
Source: Sodium in Medicinals, Tables of Sodium Values, San Francisco Heart Association, Inc., 1966, 1973 (revised).

Potassium

Most patients with renal failure and adequate urine volumes (1000 mL or more per day) are able to eliminate a "normal" intake of dietary potassium of 2 to 6 g (51 to 154 meq) per day without difficulty. Normal serum potassium levels are 3.5 to 5.0 meq per L and in the early stages of renal failure *hypokalemia,* a serum potassium level of less than 3.5 meq per L, may develop especially if "potassium-losing" diuretics are prescribed. In these instances a relatively high-potassium diet may be prescribed. Even so, a high load of potassium, whether given orally or intravenously, may be poorly tolerated by any patient with deteriorating renal function. For this reason, serum potassium levels and dietary intake of potassium should be cautiously monitored.

It is interesting to note that patients with *advanced* renal failure seem to tolerate *hyperkalemia,* a serum potassium level greater than 5.0 meq per L, better than normal, healthy people. In fact, these patients seem to encounter few problems with chronic potassium levels in the 5.0 to 6.5 meq per L range for prolonged periods of time. However, if the serum potassium level rises too rapidly or reaches an extremely high level, even in these patients, potassium intoxication and its associated side effects of cardiac arrhythmia, abnormal electrocardiogram, and ultimate cardiac arrest can occur. The exact level at which these side effects occur cannot be defined, since it is extremely variable from patient to patient. Therefore, the more limited potassium restrictions of 1.5 to 2.5 g (38 to 64 meq) per day may be prescribed.

Potassium and food Essentially all foods contain potassium (except pure sugar and pure fat), and a potassium-restricted diet can be calculated to include almost any food in certain amounts; however, generally, to promote the patient's understanding, only certain foods that are very high in potassium are eliminated when potassium-restricted diets are prescribed (see Table 23-8, below, which lists selected high-potassium foods).

TABLE 23-8 SELECTED HIGH-POTASSIUM FOODS
(Usually limited or avoided on potassium-restricted diets)

Fruits [containing 200 mg or more potassium per 100-g (3½-oz) portion]

Apricots, fresh or canned	Nectarines
Avocado	Papayas
Banana	Peaches, fresh
Cantaloupe	Prunes, dried (*all* dried fruit)
Casaba melon	Prune juice
Currants, black, red, white	Raisins
Dates	Rhubarb
Elderberries	Oranges
Honeydew	Orange juice

Vegetables [containing 300 mg or more potassium per 100-g (3½-oz) portion]

Artichokes	Dark green, leafy vegetables:
Acorn squash	Beet greens
Butternut squash	Chicory
Carrots, raw	Collards
Celery, raw	Dandelion greens
Cowpeas	Kale
Lima beans	Mustard greens
Parsnips	Parsley
Potato, baked or French fried	Spinach
Potato chips	Swiss chard
Winter squash	

Miscellaneous	*Amount, portion size*	*Potassium content, mg*
Pumpernickel bread	1 slice	113
Bran	¾ oz	214
Coffee	5-oz cup	80–169 (depending upon strength and brand)
Molasses	3½ oz	1000–2000 (depending upon type)
Peanuts and other nuts	3½ oz	600
Salt substitute	¼ tsp	400
Chocolate and cocoa		variable
Coconut, dried, sweetened dried, or unsweetened fresh	3½ oz	250–590
Low-sodium milk	8 oz	600
Milk, whole or skim	8 oz	350
Meat, fish, poultry	1 oz	100 (average)

Source: Based on figures from U.S. Department of Agriculture Handbook 8, revised, 1963, and Handbook No. 456, 1976.

High-protein foods, such as meat, fish, poultry, and milk, contribute a significant amount of potassium. For example, 1 oz of meat, fish, or poultry contains approximately 100 mg of potassium and if an individual consumes 1 lb of meat, fish, or poultry (approximately 1600 mg of potassium), a significant quantity of potassium would be obtained from meat alone. As a result, if a protein restriction is imposed, the potassium intake will simultaneously be reduced. When a patient's protein intake is not limited and a potassium-restricted diet is required, special food allowances (exchanges, portion sizes, etc.) should be stated.

Other sources of potassium Potassium from food is not the only source of potassium which will influence the patient's serum potassium level. Other contributory factors must be assessed when an elevated serum potassium level exists. There are both endogenous and exogenous factors requiring careful consideration. They are as follows:

Exogenous factors

1 Blood transfusions
2 Potassium salts, e.g., potassium chloride per se, or salt substitutes are intentionally prescribed in anticipation of potassium loss when diuretics are used
3 Medications
4 Severely restricted sodium intake (see endogenous factor #2)

Endogenous factors

1 Catabolism (potassium "leakage" from cell breakdown)
2 Severe vomiting and diarrhea (causing salt depletion, which in turn causes decreased glomerular filtration and retention of potassium)
3 Metabolic acidosis (presumably due to potassium leaving cells and hydrogen entering)

While dietary control of potassium is an extremely important consideration in maintaining or achieving a normal serum potassium level, these other factors must also be well controlled or hyperkalemia will persist. Furthermore, when diet control is ineffective or when potassium levels become extremely difficult to control, sodium polystyrene sulfonate resin (Kayexalate) may be used to reduce serum potassium levels. This resin is considered unpalatable by most people but can be prepared as a candy to improve palatability.[13] The primary action of this ion exchange resin is to exchange sodium for the potassium in the gastrointestinal tract.

Potassium (K) conversion:
1 meq K = 39 mg K
40 meq K = 1560 mg K (approx. 1.5 g)
51 meq K = 1989 mg K (approx. 2 g)
1 g KCl = 507 mg K (13 meq K)
K = approx. 50% of KCl

Phosphorus and Calcium

Altered calcium and phosphorus metabolism in renal failure causes secondary hyperparathyroidism and bone disease (renal osteodystrophy).[14] The condition is seen in children and adults. Recently the complex mechanisms involved have become more clearly understood, although they have not yet been fully elucidated. The condition evolves in the following steps:

1 *Phosphorus is retained.* Normally, 60 percent of the phosphorus ingested from food is excreted by the kidneys and 40 percent is excreted via the gastrointestinal tract. When the kidneys begin to fail, phosphorus retention occurs and a process which can lead to secondary hyperparathyroidism begins. A homeostasis naturally exists between serum calcium and phosphorus (see Chap. 7). Therefore, when phosphorus is retained and the serum phosphate rises, the serum calcium falls in an attempt to maintain their equilibrium. (The reverse is also true as seen in tetany.) This reduction in serum calcium,

coupled with the high serum phosphate, triggers the parathyroid glands to elaborate parathyroid hormone. This hormone raises the serum calcium by mobilizing calcium and phosphate from bone. Because phosphate is also liberated from bone by the action of parathyroid hormone, the serum phosphate level rises again and a vicious cycle develops.

Initially, blood tests detect this process, rather than the presence of overt symptoms. If this process is allowed to continue for a prolonged period of time, demineralization of bone (evident on radiological examination) can occur to the extent that the patient does become symptomatic, suffering from severe bone pain, and may experience spontaneous fractures and irreversible bone disease.

2   *Calcium absorption is decreased and vitamin D metabolism is impaired.* Patients with renal insufficiency require a much higher than normal amount of vitamin D to enhance calcium absorption. (Vitamin D is found in natural and fortified foods and is made in the skin on exposure to sunlight. See Chap. 6.) Without the active form of vitamin D, which is normally formed in the kidney, the calcium from food or medication will be poorly absorbed and instead will be excreted via the gastrointestinal tract. This results in a low serum calcium and again parathyroid hormone is elaborated by the parathyroid glands. Eventually because of phosphorus retention and impaired vitamin D metabolism, the parathyroid glands hypertrophy, producing excessive amounts of parathyroid hormone even if serum calcium and phosphate level become normal.

When serum phosphate and calcium are not well controlled, a situation can arise in which calcium and phosphate precipitate to form calcium phosphate, which is deposited at sites other than bone, such as soft tissue and blood vessels. This condition is known as metastatic calcification (see Fig. 23-2).

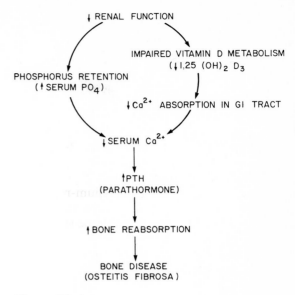

Figure 23-2
The development of bone disease secondary to decreased renal function.

Control of serum phosphate   Both medications and diet are employed to control serum phosphate levels:

1   Phosphate binders, in the form of aluminum-containing antacids (e.g., Amphogel, Basajel, Alucaps, Alternagel, Dialume), are prescribed. These are taken immediately after meals, since the aluminum in these preparations binds the phosphorus from the ingested food in the gastrointestinal tract.[15] Too frequently the hospitalized patient experiences a rise in serum phosphate simply because the phosphate binders were not given in conjunction with meals.

Magnesium-containing antacids, such as Maalox or Mylanta, which are more palatable, are not generally prescribed for patients with renal failure, since magnesium cannot be excreted by the abnormal kidneys and an elevated serum magnesium can be toxic to the central nervous system. The medical team should be aware of the contents of any antacids the patient receives. The quantity of antacids prescribed will vary according to the patient's serum phosphate level. Normal serum phosphate is 2.5 to 4.5 mg per 100 mL.

2   Calcium supplements and vitamin D preparations might be prescribed, if serum phosphate is appropriately controlled.

The serum phosphate level is influenced by diet as well as by the efficacy of the phosphate binders. The patient may be advised to avoid or limit high-phosphorous foods such as milk (and all milk products), organ meats, nuts (and nut products), cocoa, chocolate, whole grains, dried beans, and dried fruits. Meats, fish, poultry, and eggs, in large quantities, can also contribute a significant amount of phosphorus to the patient's diet.

Problems encountered with phosphate control
It must be noted that constipation is a frequent side effect of the phosphate-binding agents prescribed to control serum phosphate. Stool softeners or laxatives are used to correct this problem, since the often necessary multirestricted diets (fluid and potassium in particular) interfere with the usual dietary treatment of constipation. The patient should be cautioned against home remedies for constipation. Milk of magnesia, for example, contains a significant amount of magnesium, which can be harmful to the patient with renal failure.

Children frequently (and adults on occasion) have difficulty taking their prescribed phosphate binders. It therefore is often necessary to crush the medications and add them to foods or dissolve them in small amounts of their favorite (permitted) beverage. Special cookies containing these antacids can also be prepared and used in lieu of the large pills or capsules.

Patients need to be reminded to carry their phosphate binders with them at all times, for they are to be taken after *all* meals or large snacks, even if the patient is dining out.

Fluid

Normally a person's fluid intake and output are in equilibrium.

Sources of fluid intake include

1   Overt fluids
2   Water content of solid foods (see Table 23-9)
3   Water of oxidation of solid foods [approximately 100 mL for every 1000 kcal (4200 kJ)]

Modes of fluid output include

1   Respiration
2   Perspiration
3   Gastrointestinal (emesis, stool, drainage, etc.)
4   Urine
5   Breast milk (not usually present in patients with renal failure)

A person with kidney disease has precisely the same methods of fluid gain or loss (except as noted above) as a healthy person does; however, some patients with renal disease lose their abil-

TABLE 23-9   APPROXIMATE WATER CONTENT OF FOODS

Food	Amount of water per 100 g portion, mL
Fruits Vegetables	50–96
Cooked cereal Cooked rice, noodles Other pastas	80–90
Meat, fish, poultry, eggs	50–75
Breads, cheeses	30–40
Butter, margarine	15–20
Dry cereal Crackers Sugars Oils	0–14

ity to produce urine volumes sufficient to maintain fluid balance when a normal fluid intake is continued. When urine volume decreases, attempts should be made to adjust the fluid intake to ensure that fluid intake equals fluid output, thereby preventing overhydration and dehydration.

An *oliguric* (diminished urine volumes) or *anuric* (without urine) adult patient is usually advised to decrease fluid intake to 500 to 800 mL per day, to replace insensible loss. Children will be more severely restricted (200 to 500 mL per day), because of their smaller total body volume.

Patients should be carefully taught how to measure their fluid intake and output. Encouraging patients to record their own fluid intake and output while in the hospital, with the close supervision of a staff person, is a very helpful teaching tool. All of the following factors need to be considered as part of fluid control.

Considerations for fluid control

1 Fluids have weight. *Weigh hospitalized patients daily.*
  (1 L = 1000 mL = 2.2 lb = 1 kg)
  (1 lb = 16 oz = 2 cups = 480 mL = 1 pt)

2 Fluid weight gains or losses occur at a much more rapid rate than solid weight changes do.

3 If fluid intake equals fluid output, there will be little or no change in weight from day to day, providing the patient is receiving sufficient calories to maintain solid weight.

4 For patient teaching purposes, and for accurate intake and output records, fluids are generally considered to be anything which is liquid at room temperature:

  Ice
  Water (including that taken with medications)
  Sherbets
  Popsicles
  Ice cream
  Tonics (sodas)
  Soups and broths
  All liquid medications including intravenous ones
  Gelatin
  Other beverages (tea, coffee, juice)
  Milk
  Syrups or water from canned fruits and vegetables

5 The water content of solid foods must be borne in mind (refer back to Table 23-9).

6 Extensive fluid losses occur when the abnormal states of diarrhea, vomiting, or excessive perspiration exist. Whenever these occur, fluid losses should be replaced.

7 A high dietary sodium intake will cause increased thirst which makes it difficult to control fluids.

Teaching patients to carefully and accurately measure their fluid intake and urine output is extremely important.

Renal Failure and Other Disease States

Occasionally a patient with renal failure has other disease entities requiring diet therapy, such as cardiovascular disease, ulcer disease, or diabetes mellitus. In these cases, the priorities have to be set according to the immediate needs of the patient. For example, if a patient with diabetes mellitus develops markedly elevated blood levels of urea nitrogen and creatinine, and has associated nausea, vomiting, and gastrointestinal distress, a decreased protein intake and a high-energy diet would be prescribed. The dietetic priority would be the renal failure and its associated symptoms, rather than the diabetes mellitus. In this example, the protein intake would be decreased and energy intake encouraged, using carbohydrates and fats. The patient's blood sugar would then be controlled by insulin therapy.

Acute Renal Failure

Acute renal failure is generally considered to be the sudden loss of renal function with a consequent decrease in urine volumes to oliguric levels of (200 to 600 mL per day), usually without a previous history of renal impairment. (Acute renal failure on occasion does occur without oliguria, and in fact with urine volumes of 1500 mL or more. However, oliguric acute renal failure is most common. Also, acute renal failure can develop in patients with chronic renal impairment.) A continuation of the oliguric state for more than 24 to 48 h without treatment will result in the rapid accumulation of metabolic waste products (urea, uric acid, sulfates, creatinine, organic acids), and the rapid development of the symptoms of uremia. (See the section on uremia, p. 521.) Therefore, if oliguria persists and serum creatinine continues to rise above normal levels, peritoneal dialysis or hemodialysis is usually instituted (see pp. 525–527.)

Causes of Acute Renal Failure

The causes of actue renal failure are numerous, but include damage due to hypotension, nephrotoxins, or obstructions:

1   Hypotension may be secondary to hemorrhage, severe dehydration, postoperative shock, septic abortion, crushing injury, or any other trauma causing shock (see Fig. 23-3).
2   Nephrotoxins are substances with a direct toxic effect on the kidneys. Examples are gold, mercuric chloride, carbon tetrachloride, a variety of medications, and ethylene glycol (antifreeze).
3   Obstruction to the outflow of urine from the kidney is usually secondary to renal stones or prostate enlargement.
4   Obstruction of blood supply to the kidneys is usually secondary to renal artery thrombosis.

Obstructive renal failure is frequently totally correctable with surgical intervention.

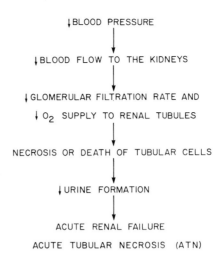

Figure 23-3
The physiological sequelae of acute renal failure as caused by hypertension.

Acute renal failure is seen more frequently in adults than in infants or children and is usually a self-limiting, potentially reversible disease entity, since the renal tubular cells are capable of regeneration. The length of time needed for total resolution of the renal failure is, however, variable and unpredictable, and the primary cause of the renal failure does often conceal and interfere with its clinical course.

Nutritional Considerations in Patients with Acute Renal Failure

Energy intake   Inasmuch as acute renal failure is usually seen in conjunction with another major medical problem, most patients suffering from this type of renal failure are critically ill, severely catabolic, and unable to take oral nourishment. At the same time, the energy needs of these patients are increased. This is related to the rate and degree of catabolism which accompanies the major predisposing insult. Therefore, the energy intake is increased either intravenously or orally, as soon as possible. Estimates of the energy requirements of these patients range from 2000 to 5000 kcal (8.4 to 21 MJ) per day.

In the initial anuric or oliguric phase of acute renal failure, when fluid intake must be severely limited, intravenous glucose is administered to supply sufficient energy to

1   Support basal metabolic needs
2   Lessen endogenous protein breakdown
3   Prevent ketosis from fat catabolism

Hypertonic glucose solutions, 25 to 70 percent glucose, may be administered through large cannulated major vessels to supply needed energy (see Chap. 28).

When the patient is able to tolerate oral feedings, energy intake can be increased markedly by the addition of concentrated carbohydrates, fats, or both. In addition to butterballs (a butter and sugar mixture which can be flavored for somewhat improved palatability) and hard sugar candies, an increasing number of protein-free, high-energy, low-electrolyte food supplements and additives are currently available. (See Table 23-4 for examples of these supplements.)

Protein   The protein intake of patients in acute renal failure is severely limited if they are unable to take oral feedings. Indeed in an anuric or oliguric patient with a rapidly rising blood urea nitrogen this might be considered advantageous, since protein or protein-containing foods will contribute to the urea nitrogen pool, thus enhancing the onset of uremia. However, malnutrition will develop after prolonged deficit of protein and attention must be given to maintaining or achieving nitrogen balance. When oral intakes are tolerated and resumed, a diet of 20 to 40 g of high-biological-value protein (0.3 to 0.6 g protein per kilogram body weight) is usually recommended, if the patient is not receiving supportive peritoneal or hemodialysis therapy. If dialytic therapy is being given, the protein intake should be liberalized accordingly.

Fluids and sodium   An important priority is the restoration of proper fluid and sodium balance, since dehydration may be a causative fac-

tor in oliguric acute renal failure. Once normal fluid balance has been restored, additional intravenous fluids may be administered in quantities sufficient to maintain balance. Maintenance is best accomplished by allowing the patient quantities of fluid equal to basal requirements (300 to 500 mL per day) *plus* amounts sufficient to replace urine volumes, gastrointestinal losses, increased respiratory losses, or losses from excessive perspiration. The patient must be monitored for dehydration and overhydration (see Chap. 8).

Assessment of proper fluid balance should be made by charted daily weights. It is important to realize that when energy intake is severely limited, a weight loss of 0.2 to 0.3 kg per day should be expected.[16] In these instances, if this loss is not obvious to the daily weight chart, or if in fact the patient gains weight, one may assume that the patient's fluid intake has been excessive.

Potassium hyperkalemia   Potassium hyperkalemia is a serum potassium of greater than 5 meq per L. It is a problem in acute renal failure and exists because (1) potassium excretion is severely limited by the decreased urine volumes, and (2) potassium is being released from cells at a fairly rapid rate by tissue breakdown. The presence of undrained blood or infection can also contribute to an elevated serum potassium level. The hyperkalemia of acute renal failure is frequently more life-threatening than that seen in chronic renal failure because of its rapid onset. Under these conditions potassium intake must be kept as low as possible, and a patient who is receiving intravenous feedings should not have potassium added. When the patient is able to tolerate oral feedings, the diet should be limited to practical levels of 1 to 1.5 g (maximum) per day until urine volumes begin to increase and the serum potassium levels are maintained within normal limits. At that time the potassium content of the diet can be liberalized.

Peritoneal dialysis or hemodialysis controls serum potassium levels and allows for a more liberal intake of dietary potassium; however, the patient's serum potassium levels need to be monitored frequently, with the food adjusted accordingly.

Phosphorus   In acute renal failure, phosphorus levels should also be carefully monitored and steps should be taken to keep the serum phosphate level as close to normal as possible.

The Diuretic Phase of Acute Renal Failure
As kidney function begins to improve, the patient enters what is commonly called the *diuretic* or *high-output phase* of the renal failure. During the recovery phase, fluids should be increased to equal the daily urine volumes plus gastrointestinal, respiratory, and other losses. Serum sodium and potassium levels are closely monitored and help to determine the dietary needs of these minerals. Generally if the patient is alert and able to tolerate food and fluids, salt and water are permitted as desired. Thirst is frequently used as a guide to fluid intake. Potassium can be liberalized at this time, and frequently high-potassium intakes are required to replace the quantities lost and prevent depletion.

As blood urea nitrogen and creatinine begin their downward trend (which does not necessarily occur at the same time as or immediately following diuresis), dietary protein intake can gradually be increased, eventually returning to unlimited quantities.

Total Parenteral Nutrition in Acute Renal Failure
Despite the increased availability of hemodialysis, as well as the use of improved antibiotics, diuretics, anesthesia, and modern intensive care units, the mortality in acute renal failure remains quite high. Recent research suggests that the mortality rate can be decreased if adequate nutritional support is provided. To this end, the use of intravenous solutions containing the eight essential amino acids plus histidine and other essential nutrients in hypertonic glucose solution, administered by catheterization of the superior vena cava, has been tried successfully.[17-20] The mortality rate decreases and patients' general nutritional status, electrolyte balance,

uremic symptoms, and wound healing improve. This type of total parenteral nutrition uses the rationale of the Giordano-Giovannetti diet (see p. 524) and provides proteins of high biological value with sufficient energy to permit the body to utilize urea for synthesis of the nonessential amino acids (see the discussion of uremia on p. 521).

This method has not been widely used because of inherent problems of hyperalimentation (i.e., sepsis, solutions mixtures); however, it does have merit for patients who are unable to eat for prolonged periods of time. (See Chap. 28 for more specific details about parenteral nutrition.)

Chronic Renal Failure

Chronic renal failure is the term used to describe the gradual, progressive deterioration of the functioning nephron mass. There are a wide variety of diverse etiologies associated with chronic renal failure (see Table 23-2). The many disease processes which can cause renal disease and ultimate failure differ in their clinical course, but all eventually cause regulatory and excretory dysfunction of the kidneys which can result in the uremic syndrome if permitted to progress without appropriate treatment. Specifically, treatment with some form of dialysis is usually indicated just prior to the onset of frank uremia.

In addition to the numerous causes of chronic renal failure, unlike the case in acute renal failure, there are various levels or stages of chronic renal failure which may or may not develop, depending upon the nature of the primary cause. As the disease state changes, compensatory changes in diet are made.

Stages of Chronic Renal Disease with Guidelines for Diet Modifications*
For the purposes of this chapter, chronic renal failure will be categorized into four stages of decreasing renal function:

1   Decreased renal reserve or renal impairment
2   Renal insufficiency (mild azotemia)

*Adapted from Peter Bent Brigham Hospital, *Diet Manual,* Boston, Mass.

3 Renal failure (moderate to severe azotemia)
4 End-stage renal disease

In the first stage, *decreased renal reserve,* there can be a loss of up to 50 to 60 percent of nephron function without significant loss of homeostatic function or easily detected abnormalities. There is usually no diet restriction; sodium may be restricted in the hypertensive patient and energy adjusted to attain ideal weight.

In the second stage of renal insufficiency, *mild azotemia,* a decrease in homeostatic function is noted, with an accumulation of nitrogenous waste products as indicated by slight elevations of BUN, creatinine, and uric acid, as well as an ensuing mild anemia. Only under conditions of marked metabolic stress of dietary excess is there a derangement of body fluids with associated symptoms. Dietary modifications of sodium are made, depending on the degree of hydration and the presence of hypertension. Potassium is restricted in accordance with serum levels, and phosphorus modification is dependent upon serum phosphate levels and the efficacy of phosphate binders. Fluid control is regulated according to urine output and the degree of hydration. There is usually no protein restriction and calories are adjusted to weight.

In the next progressive stage of renal failure, *moderate severe azotemia,* there is a significant decrease in the homeostatic functions of the kidneys, with a decrease in concentrating ability, markedly elevated BUN and creatinine, and a striking anemia. However, symptoms of uremia are not present. There is usually no immediate need for dialysis treatment.

The following diet modifications are made:

Protein: 0.6 to 1.0 g per kilogram ideal weight (40 to 60 g average), with at least 50 to 60 percent of the total allowance from high-biological-value proteins.
Sodium: Amount prescribed depends upon the degree of hydration and blood pressure.
Potassium: Amount prescribed depends upon serum potassium levels.
Phosphorus: Amount prescribed depends upon serum phosphate levels (these are frequently elevated and 1.5 to 1 g or less of dietary phosphorus is usually recommended).
Fluid: When weight is stable (the patient is neither dehydrated nor overloaded) fluid intake should be either (1) 300 to 500 mL; or (2) a quantity sufficient to replace insensible loss *plus* fluid equivalent to the urine volume from the previous day; or (3) the quantity sufficient to maintain the desired stable daily weight.
Energy: Sufficient to prevent catabolism [Average for adults: 30 to 40 kcal per kilogram of body weight (126 to 168 kJ per kg); average for children: 100 to 150 kcal per kg (420 to 630 kJ per kg)].
Multivitamins: Usually prescribed.

In the last or *terminal stage* of renal failure, discussed below, which is permanent and irreversible, there is a severe decrease in homeostasis, with the clinical picture of uremia developing if dialysis (hemo- or peritoneal dialysis) is not initiated. (See Table 23-10.)

Uremia (End-Stage Renal Disease without Dialysis Intervention)

Regardless of the stage of renal failure, an extremely important aspect of diet is individualization. This can be accomplished only after judicious assessment of laboratory data and the overall medical-nutritional status of the patient. It is incorrect to assume that every person with renal disease will require restriction of all of the generally associated nutrients. Overzealous diet therapy can, in fact, be harmful in this patient population.

Uremia or the *uremic syndrome,* per se, is not a renal disease, but rather the complex of symptoms associated with untreated end-stage renal disease. It is characterized by numerous symptoms which can include any or all of the following, in addition to the biochemical abnormalities previously mentioned: anemia (secondary to decreased production of erythropoietin—B_{12} and folate levels are usually within normal limits); hypertension; gastrointestinal symptoms of anorexia, nausea, vomiting, hiccups, and

TABLE 23-10 GUIDELINES FOR DIET MODIFICATIONS DURING THE STAGES OF CHRONIC RENAL FAILURE

Renal stage	Energy	Protein	Sodium (Na)	Potassium (K)	Phosphorus (P)	Fluids	Vitamins
			Diet treatment				
Decreasing renal reserve	Sufficient to maintain ideal body weight	Usually no restrictions	Usually no restrictions	Usually no restrictions	Usually no restrictions	Usually no restrictions	With well-balanced diet, supplementation may not be necessary
Renal insufficiency (mild azotemia)	Sufficient to maintain ideal body weight	Usually no restrictions	Dependent upon degree of hydration and presence of hypertension	Dependent upon serum levels	Dependent upon serum levels and efficacy of phosphate binders	Dependent upon urine volumes and degree of hydration	
Renal failure (moderate—severe azotemia)	Sufficient to prevent catabolism; average: adults 30–40 kcal (126–168 kJ)/kg; children 100–150 kcal (420–630 kJ)/kg	0.6–1.0 g/kg ideal weight. Average 40–60 g at least 50–60% from HBV* protein	As for renal insufficiency	As for renal insufficiency	Dependent upon serum levels (frequently elevated); average 1–1.5 g is recommended	With stable weight, no dehydration or overload: 300–500 mL or amount sufficient to replace insensible loss and fluid equivalent to urine volume from previous day	Multivitamins prescribed
End-stage renal disease (uremia without dialysis)	Sufficient to prevent catabolism; average: 35–45 (147–189 kJ)/kg	18–25 g; almost entire allowance is from HBV* protein	Dependent upon state of hydration and blood pressure; average: 1000 mg (43 meq)	Dependent upon serum levels; average: 1500–1800 mg/kg (38–46 meq)	Dependent upon serum levels and efficacy of phosphate binders	Dependent upon state of hydration; manipulated according to daily weight	†
Peritoneal dialysis	35–45 kcal (147–189 kJ)/kg	Liberal or unrestricted	Liberal	Dependent upon serum levels	Dependent upon serum levels	Dependent upon state of hydration	

Hemodialysis: Children	100–150 kcal (420–630 kJ)/kg (cal are encouraged to enhance growth, which is usually stunted with renal disease)	2 g/kg to encourage growth permitted amount is limited by the need for **K** and **P** modification since both of these are elevated in protein foods)	Dependent upon state of hydration and blood pressure; average: 2000 mg (87 meq)	Dependent upon serum levels; average: 2000 mg (51 meq)	As low as possible, with dairy products and milk limited to 120 mL/day; dependent upon serum levels and efficacy of phosphate binders	20 mL/kg of body weight and fluid equivalent to previous day's urine volume
Adults	30–45 kcal (126–189 kJ)/kg of ideal weight	1–1½ g/kg of ideal body weight; 50% from **HBV*** protein	Average 1500–2000 mg (65–87 meq) unless patient is producing large volume of urine containing Na; then regulated accordingly	Dependent upon serum levels; average: 2000–2500 mg (52–64 meq)	1500 mg or less/day; dependent upon serum levels and efficacy of phosphate binders	Quantity to allow for 1½–2 kg fluid weight gain between treatments; 800–1000 mL and fluid equivalent to urine volume from previous day

*HBV = high biological value.

†Water-soluble or multivitamin preparations with folic acid are usually prescribed.

bleeding; neuromuscular disorders such as twitching and seizures; coma; and eventual death. In fact, uremia has appropriately been called "the total body disease."[21]

Diet Modification

Diets low in protein, but high in essential amino acids, e.g., the selected protein diet[22] or the Giordano-Giovannetti diet (G-G Diet),[23,24] are used.

The rationale for this low protein is that the small quantities of high-biological-value (HBV) proteins, with sufficient energy, will allow the excess urea in the blood to be used for synthesis of the nonessential amino acids, thus reducing the BUN and utilizing the essential amino acids from the permitted HBV protein foods. Today, this type of diet is less frequently required, with the increased availability of dialysis treatment. Patients rarely reach the stage at which this diet would be needed, since dialysis is usually initiated prior to the onset of the florid uremic syndrome.

It is very important to realize that this diet does not improve the function of the kidneys. It merely serves to reduce the BUN and decrease the gastrointestinal symptoms of uremia. A patient can maintain a positive nitrogen balance while following this diet, provided the permitted HBV protein foods and sufficient energy are ingested. The diet is a very stringent one, and it is expensive because of the need for the special low-protein products. Patients' compliance is also frequently a problem. Table 23-11 gives a sample meal plan for this type of diet.

In recent years, the use of keto analogues of essential amino acids (keto acids) have been studied as possible supplements to low-protein diets in an effort to alter the course of chronic renal failure.[25,26,27] Again, current research is inconclusive, but several investigators have reported varied improvement in nitrogen balance using this mode of nutritional support.

In end-stage renal disease without dialysis intervention, the following nutrients are restricted accordingly:

Protein: 0.26 g per kilogram of body weight (average, 18 to 25 g total protein per day).

TABLE 23-11 SAMPLE MENU FOR LOW-PROTEIN DIET

Breakfast
  100 mL cranberry juice
  1 ounce cream of rice cereal
  2 teaspoons margarine (salt-free, if necessary)
  2 teaspoons brown sugar
  1 slice low-protein bread
  1 teaspoon jelly
  120 mL milk
  1 teaspoon regular sugar
  100 mL tea

Lunch
  Fruit plate:
    1 medium apple
    2 canned peach halves
    2 canned pear halves
  1 slice low-protein bread
  1 teaspoon margarine (salt-free, if necessary)
  1 teaspoon jelly
  Water ice, sherbet, or special low-protein dessert
  210 mL ginger ale with Karo syrup
  100 mL tea
  30 mL milk

Dinner
  Vegetable plate:
    1 medium egg, any style
    ½ cup cooked green peas
    ½ cup cooked wax beans
    1 medium boiled potato
  1 slice low-protein bread
  2 teaspoons margarine (salt-free, if necessary)
  1 teaspoon jelly
  210 mL ginger ale with Karo syrup
  100 mL decaffeinated coffee
  30 mL milk
  1 teaspoon sugar
  Total calories: approximately 2100 to 2200 (8820 to 9240 kJ)
  Total protein: approximately 23 g

Notes: 1 Energy can be increased by adding additional sugar, other concentrated sweets, and salt-free margarine or oil or by incorporating the supplements listed in Table 23-4.
2 Desired potassium levels can be attained in this meal plan by altering the type of fruits and vegetables permitted.
3 Desired sodium levels can be attained by the addition of salt, per se, and/or sodium-containing foods.
4 The calcium and phosphorus content of this meal plan is low.
5 Multivitamins are recommended.

Almost the entire protein allowance is from HBV protein, as 6½ oz of milk and 1 egg. This contains approximately 14 g of HBV protein. The remaining 4 to 6 g is obtained from the low-biological-value proteins in fruits, vegetables, and starches. Special low-protein products are necessary.

Sodium: Amount prescribed is individualized and depends upon the state of hydration and the blood pressure (average, 1 g sodium per day).

Potassium: Amount depends upon serum potassium levels (average, 1500 to 1800 mg potassium).

Phosphorus: Amount depends upon serum phosphate levels and efficacy of phosphate binders.

Fluid: Amount depends upon the state of hydration and is manipulated according to daily needs.

Energy: In excess of 2000 kcal (8400 kJ) per day [35 to 45 kcal (147 to 189 kJ) per kilogram of body weight].

Multivitamins: Routinely prescribed.

End-Stage Renal Disease (Treatment with Dialysis)

Dialysis can be defined as the removal of the toxic substances contained in body fluids by diffusion and osmosis across a semipermeable membrane. This is accomplished by using a dialysis solution (dialysate) that is similar in composition to normal blood plasma. Two types of dialysis therapy currently exist: peritoneal dialysis (intracorporeal dialysis, using the peritoneal membrane as the semipermeable membrane) and hemodialysis (extracorporeal dialysis, using an artificial kidney employing synthetic semipermeable membranes).

Peritoneal Dialysis

Peritoneal dialysis is not a new procedure. It actually preceded hemodialysis by many decades, being reported in the literature as early as the 1920s and 1930s. However, in the 1960s hemo-dialysis became the widespread treatment of choice due to the technological advances and increased understanding of the procedure, and peritoneal dialysis became a secondary treatment used primarily for emergencies or cases where hemodialysis was not suitable.

Today, however, there is a resurgence of the use of peritoneal dialysis.[28] An increasing number of people with chronic renal failure are being treated with chronic peritoneal dialysis in centers and at home. A new form of peritoneal dialysis, continuous ambulatory peritoneal dialysis (CAPD), has been developed and is being used more extensively.[29,30]

Diet modifications A patient receiving peritoneal dialysis may experience the following dietary limitations:

Protein: Protein is usually liberalized or unrestricted since large amounts of protein and amino acids are lost into the dialysis solution and must be replaced.

Sodium: The amount allowed depends upon the degree of hydration during the peritoneal dialysis, the rate of sodium and fluid removal during the treatment, and the blood pressure response to the treatment; again, allowance is frequently quite liberal during the procedure.

Potassium: Amount depends upon serum potassium levels but is usually liberal.

Phosphorus: Amount depends upon serum phosphate levels.

Fluid: Amount depends upon the patient's state of hydration, as per sodium above.

Energy: In excess of 2000 kcal (8400 kJ) per day [35 to 45 kcal (147 to 189 kJ) per kilogram of body weight].

Vitamin supplements: Multivitamins are routinely prescribed.

Hemodialysis

Hemodialysis is now a common treatment for patients with end-stage renal disease and is usually performed three times per week. The length of each treatment varies from 4 to 6 h, depending upon the institution, its philosophy, the type of equipment used, the patient's body size, existing biochemical abnormalities, and the patient's general state of well-being. Similarly, standards of diet modification for the hemodialysis patient are controversial and vary from institution to institution. Most would agree, however, that diet modifications should be individualized according to each patient's specific needs at any given time.

Diet modifications for adults receiving hemodialysis[31]

Protein: 1 to 1½ g per kilogram g of ideal body weight; at least 50 percent of total protein should be obtained from high-biological-value protein foods.

Sodium: Usually limited to 1500 to 2000 mg (65 to 87 meq) per day, unless the patient is still producing large volumes of urine containing significant amounts of sodium, in which case sodium should be regulated accordingly.

Potassium: Usually limited to 2000 to 2500 mg (52 to 64 meq) per day, but quantity depends upon serum potassium levels.*

Phosphorus: Quantity depends upon serum phosphate levels and effectiveness of phosphate binders. Usually limited to 1 g or less per day.

Fluid: Quantity sufficient to allow for a 1- to 1½-kg weight gain between dialysis treatments. Most frequently the range for adults is 500 to 1000 mL *plus* an amount equivalent to the urine volume.

---

*Predialysis potassium levels are the reference levels that should be used, since postdialysis potassium levels are an unreliable reference. Dialysis very effectively removes potassium from serum, which is reflected in an abnormally low potassium level immediately postdialysis. After dialytic treatment there is a shift of potassium from the intracellular compartments where it normally is predominantly found to the extracellular compartments where it can be measured, thus effectively raising the serum potassium level in a relatively short period of time.

Energy: 30 to 45 kcal (126 to 189 kJ) per kilogram of ideal body weight or the quantity sufficient to attain ideal "dry" body weight. (*Dry weight* is generally considered to be the weight at which there is little or no excess fluid available for removal by dialysis. This is usually evident by a severe drop in blood pressure or severe cramping during the dialysis treatment.)

Vitamin supplements: Routinely prescribed, with emphasis on the water-soluble vitamins, which are partially removed during dialysis therapy.[32] Folic acid is also usually prescribed.

Diet modifications for children receiving hemodialysis[33,34]

Protein: 2 g per kilogram of body weight, to encourage growth. (The amount of protein permitted the pediatric patient receiving hemodialysis may be somewhat limited by the need for restriction of potassium and phosphorus, since both of these are plentiful in high-protein foods.)

Sodium: Average 2000 mg (87 meq) per day. Quantity depends upon the patient's state of hydration and blood pressure.

Potassium: Average 2000 mg (51 meq) per day. Quantity depends upon predialysis serum potassium levels, as for adults.

Phosphorus: As low as possible, with dairy products and milk limited to 120 mL per day. Quantity depends upon serum phosphate levels and effectiveness of phosphate binders.

Fluid: 20 mL per kg of body weight plus fluid equivalent to the previous day's urine volume.

Energy: 100 to 150 kcal (420 to 630 kJ) per kg. (Calories are encouraged in effort to enhance growth, which is usually stunted in children with renal disease.)

Vitamin supplements: Routinely prescribed, with the addition of folic acid.

The Dialysis Patient—A Total Person

The guidelines and recommendations for diet modification as outlined above are certainly necessary for most patients receiving dialysis treatments; however, there is one other extremely important consideration, namely, that the patient is undergoing a significant psychological adjustment further complicated by the prescribed multirestricted diet.

The psychological impact of a chronic, irreversible, and potentially terminal disease, especially one which makes the individual "machine dependent," is understandably overwhelming and can lead to chronic noncompliance with the prescribed medical and nutritional regimens.[35,36] Indeed, the patient requiring dialysis treatments has been called a "marginal man."[37]

In the case of children, this is particularly disruptive to development since both child and parents must now adjust to the trauma of a chronic life-threatening disease. Also, children may be greatly restricted in their customary motor and exploratory activities which normally help them to gain mastery over their bodies and establish psychosocial independence (see Table 23-12).

Prior to any diet instruction, a thorough diet history should be obtained and meals should be calculated to allow for as many of the patient's preferred foods as possible. Both the patient and the family should receive thorough diet instruction. While the responsibility of teaching the renal diet should fall to the dietitian, it is essential that the entire patient-care team be aware of the information being given. To be most useful, diet instructions should include food lists, meal planning guides, and other written or visual materials which will serve to clarify this multifaceted, potentially confusing topic. In addition, a concise explanation of the rationale for each nutrient involved, as related to the renal disease, its treatment (dialysis or transplantation), and the patient as a person, should be given. While the diet prescription should be individualized according to laboratory values and clinical conditions, diet therapy and instruction

TABLE 23-12 ISSUES OF MANAGEMENT OF PEDIATRIC RENAL PATIENTS*

I. Pediatric dialysis patients
  A. Fear of death
  B. Limited activity
    1. Access—fistual vs. shunt
    2. Chronically anemic
    3. Time—dialysis takes 3 to 5 h, 3 times/week
  C. Dependency vs. denial
  D. Limited peer contact
    1. Time of dialysis plus travel time—lost school days
    2. Hospitalizations
    3. Illness may cause below-average school achievement, resulting in need to repeat grades or semesters (classmates not the same age)
  E. Appearance
    1. Short stature (bone disease)
    2. Fistula/shunt
    3. Pale, less energy
    4. Delayed puberty, immature emotionally
  F. Home management
    1. Control of fluid intake—weight charts, prizes for best weights
    2. Dietary acceptance and compliance
    3. Care of access
  G. Medical crises leading to hospitalizations

II. Pediatric transplant patients†
  A. Reintegration—of a presumably healthy child who had been chronically ill
    1. Into family
    2. Return to school and peers—identity and body image problems
  B. Dependency leading to behavior problems
    1. Relationship of donor and patient
    2. Acute rejection leading to anxiety reactions
  C. Complications leading to fear of return to dialysis

*Contributed by Nancy Spinozzi, R.D., Renal Dietitian, Children's Hospital Medical Center, Boston, Mass.
†*Source:* D. M. Bernstein, "After Transplantation—The Child's Emotional Reactions," *American Journal of Psychiatry,* **127**:9, 1971.

must also be individualized according to each patient's interest, motivation, and learning abilities. Teaching pediatric patients will, for example, involve a variety of teaching skills which may not be appropriate for the adult.[38]

Unfortunately, diet instructions are frequently given during a very stressful time when the patient and family members are being given a great deal of new information by many unfamiliar people, in what is perceived as a very threatening setting. Furthermore, this quite often is the time when the patient and family members are attempting to adjust to and deal with the chronicity of the disease process. All of this, undoubtedly, will have a profound effect upon the patient's ability to listen and comprehend details of any instruction. For these reasons, reinforcement by repetition will, in most cases, be imperative and worthwhile.

Transplantation

Transplantation is a possible treatment for chronic renal failure but, unlike dialysis, a successful kidney transplant can restore normal renal function. However, not every dialysis patient is a candidate for kidney transplantation. There are several reasons, which include the following:

1   A suitable donor may not be available.
2   Medical reasons deem the patient unsuitable for transplantation (e.g., age, other concurrent illness, presensitization to donor antibodies).
3   The patient, having been given all pertinent information about transplantation and its associated problems, decides that dialysis is an acceptable way of life, and does not wish to have a transplant.

On the other hand, because of the bone and growth problems associated with renal failure, attempts are made to perform a transplant in pediatric patients as soon as possible. Growth does seem to improve if transplantation is performed prior to the onset of puberty, when the epiphyses have not yet closed. This is not to imply the transplantation in children is without its complications, for the complications are quite similar to those seen in adults.[39,40]

Nutritional Considerations

The nutritional management of people posttransplantation primarily depends upon how well the transplanted kidney functions; i.e., if the kidney functions perfectly, an ad lib diet is usually permitted, but if the kidney does not function well, the diet is adjusted as it would be for renal failure or dialysis.

In addition to adjusting the diet according to the status of the new kidney, there are other extremely important factors which influence the patient's nutritional needs. All patients receiving a kidney transplant (except for identical twins) are routinely required to take immunosuppressive medications such as azathioprine (Imuran) and corticosteroids such as prednisone, to reduce the risk of the body's rejection of the transplanted kidney. These medications, unfortunately, have potential adverse side effects which can affect the patient's nutritional status. Some of these and their consequent nutritional considerations are listed in Table 23-13. A high-protein, low-carbohydrate, 2-g sodium, 800–1200 mg calcium diet has been recommended for adult patients after transplantation. This regimen reportedly lessens the metabolic side effects associated with the corticosteroid treatment.[41]

Obesity and a "cushingoid" appearance are frequently observed side effects of the steroid therapy, especially when very high doses are used to treat a rejection episode. Since obesity is a common problem, patients should be given anticipatory guidance. They should be advised to use much common sense and discretion in food selection and portion size. (This concept is frustrating to the patient who has always been thin; however, eventually, in most cases even thin patients taking steroids will gain a substantial amount of weight when not watching their diet.) "Preventive dietetics" is strongly recommended since the psychological stress of an altered body image can become problematic to both children and adults.

Another important nutritional consideration is that, since dialysis does impose some inconvenience to the patient (usually including a modified diet), many patients view transplanta-

TABLE 23-13 IMMUNOSUPPRESSION: SOME ASSOCIATED SIDE EFFECTS AND POSSIBLE NUTRITIONAL IMPLICATIONS*

Side effects†	Common dietetic considerations
Azathioprine (Imuran)	
Severe bone marrow depression	All foods served by reverse precaution or precaution technique
Infection (fungal, protozoal, viral, and uncommon bacteria)	Small frequent feedings—high energy, high-protein foods
Toxic hepatitis or biliary stasis	Modified fat diet
Nausea, anorexia	Small frequent feedings
Diarrhea, vomiting	Fluid and electrolyte replacement
Steatorrhea	Low-fat diet
Negative nitrogen balance	High-protein, high-energy foods
Prednisone	
Sodium retention	Moderate to low sodium intake
Potassium loss	High-potassium foods
Peptic ulcer	Liberal bland diet, unless actively bleeding
Pancreatitis	Moderate to low fat intake
Abdominal distention	Small frequent feedings
Ulcerative esophagitis	Modified food consistency
Altered carbohydrate metabolism, manifestation of latent diabetes mellitus, higher insulin needs in patients with previous diabetes	Decreased concentrated sweets or American Diabetes Association diets
Negative nitrogen balance (secondary to protein catabolism)	High-energy, high-protein foods
Altered fat metabolism	Low-cholesterol or appropriate diet for specific type of hyperlipidemia

*The nutritional considerations stated here are quite general. As always, diets should be modified on an individual basis. Kidney function will, of course, also influence the diet prescribed.

†*Source: Physicians' Desk Reference,* 34th ed, Medical Economics Company, Oradell, N.J. 1980, pp. 752, 1388–1389.

tion as the only means of achieving a "normal" life and a normal diet. After transplantation, if complications arise and a modified diet is prescribed, depression, anger, and anxiety may result. Patients need the continuing support of the health care team to achieve a realistic expectation of kidney function following transplantation. Diet modifications might be necessary even after the transplant is performed and patients should be prepared for this.

NEPHROTIC SYNDROME

The nephrotic syndrome is not a disease, but rather a group of symptoms—biochemical and clinical—which can result from a variety of disease states. Glomerulonephritis is the most common cause of nephrotic syndrome, but it is also seen in metabolic diseases, systemic sensitivity diseases, circulatory disease, allergic states, and infective processes. The major symptoms include edema, massive proteinuria, hypoalbuminemia, and hyperlipidemia (as hypercholesterolemia). These symptoms occur primarily because of glomerular injury, which causes the loss of plasma protein in the urine while, at least initially, other blood chemistries such as BUN and creatinine are within normal limits.

Depending upon the cause and the patient's response to medical treatment (usually steroids) some patients with nephrotic syndrome can develop end-stage renal disease and require dialysis treatments or transplantation.

Diet Modifications

Protein: Normal or high intake, unless the patient is azotemic. (The exact amount of protein needed is still controversial. Certain physicians prescribe 150 g or more of protein per day and others suggest, on the premise that the more protein ingested, the greater the protein loss in the urine, and an ad-lib protein intake is sufficient. Since the edema seen in nephrotic syndrome is primarily due to the change in oncotic pressure occurring because of the large quantities of protein lost in the urine, the patient is usually encouraged to consume a well-balanced "high" protein diet.)

Sodium: An intake of 1000 to 2000 mg per day is frequently prescribed. (Once again, the philosophy of the primary physician is an important factor, as is the patient's clinical response to medical therapy.)

Potassium: Usually not restricted, but individualized according to each patient's serum levels.

Phosphate: Usually not restricted, but quantity depends upon serum levels.

Energy: Ad lib, or the quantity sufficient to achieve ideal weight. (Because of the edematous state, the patient's actual weight is difficult to determine.)

Cholesterol: Low-cholesterol diet, if serum level is elevated.

Vitamin supplements: Might be prescribed.

Childhood Nephrosis (Childhood Nephrotic Syndrome)

Childhood nephrosis is a primary renal disease which usually occurs in children between the ages of 1½ and 5 but is on occasion seen in older children and adults. It is not common and affects females more frequently than males. The cause is unknown. It does develop without other concurrent renal disease. The symptoms are very similar to those of nephrotic syndrome, although perhaps more pronounced. Basically the same dietary management outlined for nephrotic syndrome is utilized for childhood nephrosis.

URINARY TRACT INFECTIONS

The most common kidney-related disorders are urinary tract infections. These infections are common in women, because of their anatomy, but on occasion are seen in men and in children.

Urinary tract infections can be potentially damaging to the kidneys, and if allowed to go untreated can possibly lead to chronic pyelonephritis, which is potentially irreversible and can lead to end-stage renal failure. Causes of urinary tract infection include congenital obstructions or other obstructive processes such as kidney stones, injury to the urinary tract, or chronic inflammation from bacteria.

Nutritional Considerations

Nutritional management usually involves:

1 Push fluids: 2 L or more per day
2 Acid-ash diet: High-protein foods, such as meats, fish, eggs, and gelatin products, are encouraged. Only specific fruits—cranberries, plums, and prunes—are permitted. (This diet increases the acidity of the urine.*)

or

3 Alkali-ash diet: High intake of milk and milk products, most vegetables, citrus fruits

*Normal urine pH is 6 (range, 4.8 to 8.5).

(and their juices), and all other juices or fruits which are not permitted on the acid-ash diet. (This diet decreases the acidity of the urine and thereby produces a more alkaline urine.*)

NEPHROLITHIASIS (RENAL STONES OR CALCULI)

Nephrolithiasis is quite common in the United States, primarily affecting people 20 to 55 years of age, although children and older adults can develop renal stone disease. Calculi can occur as either single or multiple stones and can develop anywhere along the urinary tract. They are usually caused by the precipitation of urine salts, although the details of the mechanisms of stone formation are quite complex and not fully understood.[42] Factors which may promote the formation of renal calculi are numerous but generally are those conditions which increase the concentration of the urine, the quantity of urine excreted, or both. Examples of these conditions include dehydration, which increases urine concentration; excessive intake of vitamin D; milk-alkali syndrome; primary hyperparathyroidism and prolonged immobilization, which cause calcium loss from bone and thus increase calcium excretion; and the other metabolic diseases which characteristically increase the excretion of uric acid, oxalate, glycine, or cystine. In addition, anatomic factors such as infection, obstruction, and other abnormalities of the urinary tract may play a role in renal stone formation.

Of the major constituents of renal calculi—calcium, uric acid, oxalate, cystine, and glycine—calcium stones are by far the most common, with the largest percentage of these stones consisting of calcium oxalate. A slightly smaller percentage are a combination of calcium oxalate and calcium phosphate. (These can occur with or without excessive calcium excretion.) Uric acid stones are less common than calcium-containing stones, and cystine or glycine stones are rare.

*Normal urine pH is 6 (range, 4.8 to 8.5).

Nephrolithiasis, per se, can damage the kidneys by causing either a pressure necrosis, an obstruction, or a predisposition to infection. For this reason, removal or passage of renal stones is extremely important. The three most common methods of treating nephrolithiasis and preventing it from causing permanent damage to the kidneys are:

1 Encouraging spontaneous passage
2 Surgical or urological removal
3 Medications; examples for specific types of stones are:
   a Calcium stones—phosphate preparations or cellulose phosphate[43]
   b Uric acid stones—allopurinol, which prevents uric acid synthesis and lowers serum and urine uric acid levels
   c Cystine stones—D-penicillamine, which combines with cystine to form a soluble product

Nutritional Considerations

Diet modification was not listed above as a means of preventing or treating renal calculi, even though various diets have been used through the years, since much controversy exists about this mode of therapy. The efficacy of these diets has been less than optimal. However, there is agreement that there are instances when changes in a person's eating patterns will be helpful, regardless of the etiology of the renal calculi. For example, all individuals should be encouraged to maintain or achieve a nutritionally well-balanced diet. With a history of renal stone disease fluids should be forced to 3 to 4 L per day. (Since calculi are caused by precipitation of urine salts, increasing the fluid intake will increase urine volume and therefore dilute the precipitating salts.)

In specific instances, diet modifications based on the etiology of the stone formation may be somewhat helpful. Examples of such diet modifications include the following:

1 Calcium stones with idiopathic (of unknown cause) hypercalciuria: low-calcium diets or

avoidance of dairy products; acid-ash diet* (see p. 530), since calcium stones tend to be insoluble in alkaline urine.

2 Oxalate stones with hyperoxaluria (as in ileal disease): low-oxalate diet. (Foods commonly avoided include rhubarb, spinach, dandelion greens, asparagus, cranberries, almonds, cashew nuts, chocolate, cocoa, and tea.)

3 Uric acid stones with hyperuricosuria: Low-purine diets are rarely used today since medications are quite effective (foods which would be avoided include all organ meats, anchovies, meat extracts, gravies, and alcoholic beverages); alkali-ash diet (see p. 530), since uric acid stones tend to be insoluble in acid urine.

4 Cystine stones with cystinuria: low-methionine diet (foods frequently avoided include milk and milk products, eggs, cheese, fish,

*Acid- and alkali-ash diets are used less frequently today, apparently because medications which are relatively harmless serve the same or better purpose; however, on occasion, these diets might be prescribed.

and certain fruits and vegetables); alkali-ash diet, since cystine stones tend to be insoluble in acid urine.

Although there is no general agreement about the efficacy of diet modifications for renal stones, all seem to concur that *forcing fluids* and a well-balanced diet are essential and beneficial.

STUDY QUESTIONS

1 Describe the nutritional goals which should be achieved by diet therapy for individuals with renal failure.

2 What nutrients are frequently controlled in the food intake of the patient with kidney failure?

3 What biochemical and clinical information would you use to monitor kidney function?

4 Why is the protein intake decreased in end-stage renal disease when the patient is not being treated by chronic hemodialysis?

5 Differentiate between the diets of a posttransplant patient and a patient being maintained on chronic hemodialysis.

CLINICAL STUDY 23

Sara is a 20-year-old student with end-stage renal disease secondary to chronic glomerulonephritis. She has been receiving hemodialysis treatments 3 times per week, 5 h per treatment, for approximately 6 months, and is essentially anuric. She has resumed her status as a full-time student and is maintaining above-average grades. She is 5 ft 2 in tall, and normally weighs 52 kg, which approximates her ideal weight. Her average fluid weight gains between dialysis treatments have been 2 to 2½ kg. However, on occasion she has had weight gains of up to 3 kg between dialysis treatments. She was recently hospitalized with shortness of breath and a preliminary diagnosis of fluid overload. Her weight on admission was 60 kg and her blood pressure was 220/120

mmHg. Her admission followed an extended weekend trip to her hometown for a class reunion. Laboratory values were as follows:

BUN—100 mg per 100 mL
Serum creatinine 7.8 mg per 100 mL
Serum potassium—6.0 meq per L
Serum phosphorus—5.5 mg per 100 mL

Clinical study questions
1 How much fluid should Sara be allowed?
2 What energy level would be appropriate? How much protein should be planned in Sara's diet?
3 Should dietary sodium be restricted? If so, to what level?

REFERENCES

1 A. J. Vander, *Renal Physiology*, McGraw-Hill Book Company, New York, 1975, pp. 128–129.

2 H. F. DeLuca, "The Kidney as an Endocrine Organ Involved in The Function of Vitamin D," *American Journal of Medicine,* 58:39–47, 1975.

3 C. F. Anderson, R. A. Nelson, J. D. Margie, W. J. Johnson, and J. D. Hunt, "Nutritional Therapy for Adults with Renal Disease," *Journal of the American Medical Association,* 222:69, 1973.

4 J. A. Sargent and F. A. Gotch, "Mass Balance: A Quantitative Guide to Clinical Nutritional Therapy: I. The Predialysis Patient with Renal Disease," *Journal of the American Dietetic Association,* 75: 547–551, 1979.

5 J. A. Sargent, F. A. Gotch, R. R. Henry, and N. Bennett, "Mass Balance: A Quantitative Guide to Clinical Nutritional Therapy: II. The Dialyzed Patient," *Journal of the American Deitetic Association,* 75: 551–555, 1979.

6 J. Sargent, F. Gotch, M. Borah, L. Piercy, N. Spinozzi, P. Schoenfeld, and M. Humphreys, "Urea Kinetics: A Guide to Nutritional Management of Renal Failure," *American Journal of Clinical Nutrition,* 31: 1696, 1978.

7 F. A. Gotch, "Urea Guided Dialysis Therapy Current Clinical Results," *Dialysis and Transplantation*, October–November 1976.

8 J. S. Cost, "Diet in Chronic Renal Disease: A Focus on Calories," *Journal of the American Dietetic Association,* 64:2, 186–187, 1974.

9 J. Bagdade, A. Casaretto, J. Albers, "Effects of Chronic Uremia, Hemo-Dialysis and Renal Transplantation on Plasma Lipids and Lipoproteins in Man," *Journal of Laboratory Clinical Medicine,* 87: 37–48, 1976.

10 D. C. Cattran, S. S. A. Fenton, D. R. Wilson, and G. Steiner, "Defective Triglyceride Removal in Lipemia Associated with Peritoneal Dialysis and Haemodialysis," *Annals of Internal Medicine,* 85:20–33, 1976.

11 M. L. Sanfelippo, R. S. Swenson and G. M. Reaven, "Reduction of Plasma Triglycerides by Diet in Subjects with Chronic Renal Failure," *Kidney International,* 11:54–61, 1977.

12 D. W. Seldin, N. W. Carter, and F. C. Rector, Jr., "Consequences of Renal Failure and Their Management," in M. B. Strauss and L. G. Welt (eds.), *Diseases of the Kidney,* 2d ed., Little, Brown and Co., Boston, 1971, p. 654.

13 K. Johnson, "Review of Amphojel Cookies and Kayexalate Candy," *Dialysis and Transplantation,* 8: 145–178, 1979.

14 A. C. Schoolwerth, and J. E. Engle, "Calcium and Phosphorus in Diet Therapy of Uremia," *Journal of*
The American Dietetic Association, 66:460–464, 1975.

15 P. Fulkerson, "Phosphate Binders—Is Time of Ingestion Important?" *Dialysis and Transplantation,* 8(1):89–90, 1979.

16 J. P. Merrill, "Acute Renal Failure," M. B. Strauss and L. G. Welt, op. cit., p. 654.

17 R. M. Abel, C. H. Beck, W. M. Abbott, J. A. Ryan, Jr., C. O. Barnett, and J. E. Fischer, "Improved Survival from Acute Renal Failure After Treatment with Intravenous Essential L-Amino Acids and Glucose; Results of a Prospective, Double Blind Study," *New England Journal of Medicine,* 288:695–699, 1973.

18 S. J. Dudrick, E. Steiger, and J. M. Long, "Renal Failure in Surgical Patients, Treatment with Essential Amino Acids and Hypertonic Glucose," *Surgery,* 68:180–186, 1970.

19 R. M. Abel, W. M. Abbott, C. H. Beck, Jr., J. A. Ryan, and J. E. Fischer, "Essential L-Amino Acids for Hyperalimentation in Patients with Disordered Nitrogen Metabolism," *American Journal of Surgery,* 128:314–323, 1974.

20 M. J. Blumenkrantz, J. D. Kopple, A. Koffler, K. Kamdar, M. D. Healy, E. I Feinstein, and S. G. Massry, "Total Parenteral Nutrition in the Management of Acute Renal Failure," *American Journal of Clinical Nutrition,* 31:1831–1840, 1978.

21 G. L. Bailey, *Hemodialysis Principles and Practice,* Academic Press, Inc., New York, 1972, Chap. 1.

22 G. L. Bailey, and N. R. Sullivan, "Selected Protein Diet in Terminal Uremia," *Journal of The American Dietetic Association,* 52:125–259, 1968.

23 C. Giordano, "Use of Exogenous and Endogenous Urea for Protein Synthesis in Normal and Uremic Subjects," *Journal of Laboratory and Clinical Medicine,* 62:231.

24 S. Giovannetti, and Q. Maggiore, "A Low Nitrogen Diet with Protein of High Biological Value for Severe Chronic Uremia," *Lancet,* 1:1000, 1964.

25 M. Walser, W. E. Mitch, and V. U. Collier, "The Effect of Nutritional Therapy on the Course of Chronic Renal Failure," *Clinical Nephrology,* 11:66–70, 1979.

26 J. Bergstrom, M. Ahlberg, A. Alvestrand, and P. Furst, "Metabolic Studies with Keto Acids in Uremia," *American Journal of Clinical Nutrition,* 31: 1761–1766, 1978.

27 M. Walser, "Principles of Keto Acid Therapy in Uremia," *American Journal of Clinical Nutrition,* 31: 1756–1760, 1978.

28 D. G. Oreopoulos, "Peritoneal Dialysis Is Here to Stay," *Nephron,* 24: 7–9, 1979.

29 J. W. Moncrief and R. P. Popovich, "Continuous Ambulatory Peritoneal Dialysis," *The Kidney,* The National Kidney Foundation, **12**(3):9–12, 1979.

30 D. G. Oreopoulos, "The Coming of Age of Continuous Ambulatory Peritoneal Dialysis (CAPD)," *Dialysis and Transplantation,* **8**(6):480–482, 1979.

31 B. T. Burton, "Current Concepts of Nutrition and Diet in Diseases of the Kidney, Part II, Dietary Regimen in Specific Kidney Disorders, *Journal of the American Dietetic Association,* **65**:631, 1974.

32 J. Burge, "Vitamin Requirements of Hemodialysis Patients," *Dialysis and Transplanations,* October/November 1974.

33 N. S. Spinozzi, personal communication, 1976. (Renal Dietitian, Children's Hospital Medical Center, Boston, Mass.)

34 C. Chantler and M. A. Holliday, "Growth in Children with Renal Disease with Particular Reference to the Effects of Calorie Malnnutrition: A Review," *Clinical Nephrology,* **1**:230–242, 1975.

35 N. B. Levy (ed.), *Living or Dying, Adaptation to Hemodialysis,* Charles C Thomas, Publisher, Springfield, Ill., 1974.

36 C. J. Brown, "Chronic Non-Compliance in End-Stage Renal Disease: Assessment and Intervention," *Dialysis and Transplantation,* **8**(12): 1210–1214, 1979.

37 M. K. Landsman, "The Patient with Chronic Renal Failure: A Marginal Man," *Annals of Internal Medicine,* **82**:268–270, 1975.

38 N. S. Spinozzi, "Teaching Nutritional Management to Children on Chronic Hemodialysis," *Journal of The American Dietetic Association,* **75**(2):157–159, 1979.

39 F. N. Fine and B. M. Korsch, "Renal Transplantation in Children," *Hospital Practice,* March 1974, pp. 61–69.

40 M. A. Topor, "Kidney Transplantation, Especially in Pediatric Patients," *Nursing Clinics of North America,* **10**:503–516, 1975.

41 V. R. Liddle and P. J. Walker, "Diet in Transplantation," *Dialysis and Transplantation,* 9–11, May 1977.

42 H. E. Williams, "Nephrolithiasis; Physiology in Medicine," *New England Journal of Medicine,* **290**:33, 1974.

43 C. Y. C. Pak, C. S. Delea, and F. C. Bartter, "Successful Treatment of Recurrent Nephrolithiasis (Calcium Stones) with Cellulose Phosphate," *New England Journal of Medicine,* **290**:175–180, 1974.

CLINICAL DISCUSSION 23

Sara's problem of fluid overload is evident by three criteria: shortness of breath, hypertension, and an admission weight 8 kg above her normal weight. Dialysis was initiated immediately in an attempt to reduce Sara's fluid weight, and there were important routine procedures, relating to her admission diagnosis, which the nursing staff also initiated.

Daily weights were obtained every morning with accurately recorded intake and output records. (A fluid restriction of 500 to 800 mL total per 24 h was ordered since Sara is essentially anuric and fluid-overloaded.) With fluids identified precisely as to the percentage of the total fluid allowance to be sent on the patient's tray, the nursing staff was then responsible for administering the remaining fluids with medications and as nourishments (although Sara was not receiving intravenous therapy; this would have been another avenue of fluid entry). The dietitian determined from the diet history that Sara had overindulged in both sodium and fluid while at a weekend party and attempted to understand the reason for this indiscretion and to motivate Sara accordingly.

Diet prescription included 2100 kcal (882 kJ), 52 to 68 g of protein, 2 g of Na, 2 g of K, 1 g phosphorus, and 800 mL fluid. This was determined by using the energy requirements for an adult receiving hemodialysis: 35 to 45 kcal (126–189 kJ) per kg of ideal body weight. Sara's dry weight was 52 kg [52 kg × 40 kcal per kg = 2080 kcal (8736 kJ) or, rounded off, 2100 kcal (8820 kJ)]. Her protein requirements were 1 to 1½ g per kg of body weight or 52 g (52 × 1 g). Sodium was restricted to 1.5 to 2 g since she manifested symptoms of fluid overload and fluid was restricted to 800 mL. Since Sara was anuric, her diet was also limited in potassium and phosphorus.

CHAPTER 24

THE ENDOCRINE SYSTEM AND SKELETAL DISORDERS

Susan K. Golovin

KEY WORDS
Hyperthyroidism
Goiter
Myxedema
Addisonian Crisis
Growth Hormone
Polyuria
Cortisol
Corticosteroids
Polyuria
Polyphagia
Polydipsia
Ketosis
Hypoglycemia
Gouty Attack

INTRODUCTION

The endocrine system consists of a series of ductless glands scattered throughout the body: thyroid, parathyroids, pituitary, adrenals, and pancreas, the reproductive organs, and (with some dispute) the thymus. (See Figure 24-1, p. 536.) The pineal body is also recognized as an endocrine gland, acting as a neuroendocrine modulator of hypothalamic function. The endocrine system is one of the two major control systems of the body. The nervous system is functionally interrelated. The level of hormone secretion is under the control of the nervous system and the level of hormones affects the nervous system. The endocrine system primarily controls metabolic processes, growth, maturation, and reproduction and integrates the body's response to stress.

The hormones secreted by the endocrine glands either follow a rhythmic pattern or are secreted in response to blood levels of a specific substance, such as sodium, water, sugar, calcium, or another hormone. Disease of the endocrine glands may cause shift in hormone secretion. The resultant symptoms of dysfunction are those of increased or decreased regulation of the bodily processes that are normally controlled by the gland and its specific hormone.

This chapter will consider the physiology and the malfunction of those glands of the endocrine system where diet therapy is involved, with particular focus on diabetes mellitus. In addition, the role of diet therapy in diseases of the bones and joints will be considered.

THYROID

Physiology

The thyroid gland is located below the larynx on both sides, and anterior to the trachea. The function of the thyroid gland is twofold: (1) It maintains an optimal metabolic level in the tissues by stimulating the oxygen consumption of most body cells and by helping to regulate lipid and carbohydrate metabolism, and (2) it estab-

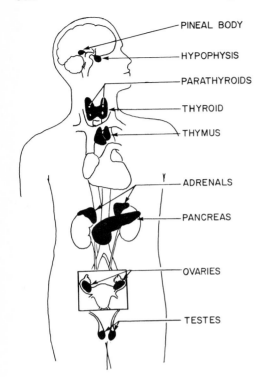

PINEAL BODY

HYPOPHYSIS

PARATHYROIDS

THYROID

THYMUS

ADRENALS

PANCREAS

OVARIES

TESTES

Figure 24-1
The glands of the endocrine system.

lishes or permits the long-term functions of growth and promotes skeletal maturation.

In order to accomplish these functions, the thyroid secretes three hormones, thyroxine (T_4), triiodothyronine (T_3), and thyrocalcitonin. The raw material essential for thyroid hormone synthesis is iodine. Iodine, once ingested, is converted to iodide and is absorbed, remaining chiefly in the extracellular fluids except for that portion taken up by the thyroid gland. Small amounts of excess iodide not taken up by the thyroid gland are excreted in the urine. A minimum daily intake of 100 to 150 μg of iodine is needed to maintain normal thyroid function.

The thyroid gland collects and concentrates iodide from the blood, converts iodide to thyroid hormone, and stores some of these hormones and secretes the remainder into the blood for distribution to all cells of the body. The function of the thyroid gland is controlled by a secretion of

the anterior lobe of the pituitary known as thyroid-stimulating hormone or TSH. TSH secretion is regulated in part by the pituitary, which is sensitive to high levels of circulating thyroid hormone, and in part by neural mechanisms mediated through the hypothalamus.

Thyroid hormone has an effect on many of the biochemical processes within the body:

1 *Metabolic rate.* Increases oxygen consumption by tissues that are metabolically active.
2 *Metabolism of protein, lipids, and carbohydrates.*
   a Protein. Favors protein anabolism; however, in large doses thyroid hormone stimulates protein catabolism, leading to negative nitrogen balance.
   b Lipids. Increases the oxidative processes of fat metabolism and increases the rate of both the biosynthesis and catabolism of cholesterol in the liver and extrahepatic tissue.
   c Carbohydrates. Increases the rate of glucose absorption from the gastrointestinal tract and increases utilization of glucose by the cells.

3 *Cardiovascular function.* Increases the blood flow, cardiac output, and heart rate, stimulates myocardial metabolism, and maintains hematopoiesis.
4 *Central nervous system.* Increases mental acuity.
5 *Growth and tissue differentiation.* Essential for normal growth.
6 *Vitamin metabolism.* Increases the quantity of enzymes and thereby causes an increased need for vitamins, since vitamins are an essential part of enzymes or coenzymes.

The consequence of thyroid dysfunction is reflected in the secretion of too much or too little thyroid hormone, which in turn affects all or some of the above functions. Table 24-1 summarizes the tests most commonly used to evaluate thyroid function.

TABLE 24-1 THYROID FUNCTION TESTS

Test	Description	Average values*
Radioactive iodine uptake (RAI)	Tracer doses of ^{131}I are given orally and thyroid uptake is measured by a gamma-ray counter. Used in diagnosing hyperthyroidism.	9–19% in 1 h 7–25% in 6 h 10–50% in 24 h
Thyroxine (T_4) (concentration)	Measures free thyroxine which determines metabolic status. Used in diagnosing both hyper- and hypothyroidism.	4.8–13.2 μg/100 mL serum (mean = 8.6, radio immunoassay)
Triiodothyronine (T_3) (concentration)	Measures triiodothyronine. Used in diagnosing hyper- and hypothyroidism.	50–210 ng/100 mL serum (radio immunoassay)
Thyroid-stimulating hormone (TSH)	TSH blood levels are valuable in providing a differential diagnosis. Elevated TSH levels are seen in hypothyroidism due to primary thyroid failure. Decreased TSH levels are seen in secondary hypothyroidism due to hypothalamic or pituitary disease.	$\leqq 0.2$ μU/mL

*Source: J. Wallach, *Interpretation of Diagnostic Tests,* 3d ed., Little, Brown and Company, Boston, 1978.

Hypothyroidism

Hypothyroidism is an endocrine disorder manifested by a decrease in thyroxine activity. Thyroxine (T_4) may be suppressed by a number of factors:

1 Inadequate consumption of iodine
2 High intake of goitrogens
3 An inborn error of metabolism

The first few months of life constitute a critical period at which time T_4 and T_3 must be present for normal cerebral development, and the lack of hormone results in defective myelinization and severely retarded mental development.

Cretinism is a condition resulting from early hypothyroidism. Children with cretinism are dwarfed, with large protruding tongues and bellies. They are the product of a prolonged pregnancy and at birth have an above-normal birth weight and length, are puffy and cyanotic, and show retarded prenatal osseous development and prolonged neonatal jaundice. Treatment begun after the first few months of life for the most part is ineffective and does not prevent mental retardation.

Those who develop hypothyroidism as children grow slowly and show delayed epiphyseal closure. Hypothyroid children may exhibit the following: lack of energy, respiratory infection, constipation due to decreased peristalsis, decreased linear growth, thick scaly skin with a yellow tinge and some mottling, cardiac enlargement, bradycardia, and depressed thyroid function tests [T_3, T_4, and radioactive iodine (RAI) uptake].

Also, because of an abnormality in nitrogen metabolism there is deposition of mucoprotein in subcutaneous and extracellular spaces. This material is osmotically active and results in fluid retention. This watery, mucuslike substance is responsible for dry swelling with abnormal mucin deposits in the skin, giving a puffy look to the face.

Since thyroid hormones must be present for heat production, hypothyroid individuals usually experience cold intolerance. Also, T_4 and T_3 promote catabolism of carbohydrate and fat; therefore, hypothyroidism results in a decreased rate of cholesterol breakdown, causing an increase in serum cholesterol to over 300 mg per 100 mL in a large proportion of patients.

Obesity is not a problem related to the condition, for even though catabolism is low, appetite also becomes depressed. There may be moderate anemia as a result of decreased bone marrow metabolism and poor vitamin B_{12} absorption from the intestine.

Hormone therapy is used for treatment. In children a delicate balance must be maintained in order to provide sufficient hormones to maintain positive nitrogen balance without precipitating protein catabolism and growth deficits.

Endemic Goiter

When exogenous iodine intake falls below 10 μg per day, thyroxine levels are insufficient. This results in increased TSH secretion and ultimately in thyroid hypertrophy. This condition, known as *iodine-deficiency goiter,* was common in the United States, in the Great Lakes area, before the advent of iodized salt. The classic cases of these endemic goiters occur in regions where iodine is lacking (and therefore iodine intake is low) because of low environmental soil and water resources. Another cause of endemic goiter is attributed to goitrogens. *Goitrogens* are vegetables of the Brassicaceae family, notably cabbage, rutabagas, and turnips, which contain progoitrin, as well as a substance which converts progoitrin into goitrin, an active antithyroid agent. Progoitrin activator is heat-labile, yet some activators remain even if the vegetables are cooked. Usually, these goitrins present no problems. However, large consumption by those with low iodine intake could possibly result in the so-called "cabbage goiter."

Goiter, for some unknown reason, will sometimes develop in people with normal thyroid function (euthyroids) who take cough medicines that are high in iodine. There is some possibility that goiter can be induced by a high iodine intake since large surveys in the United States found high urinary iodine and high iodine intake in people with goiters living in goiter-prevalent areas. This is of interest, since the average American diet can consist of high-iodine foods such as seafood, iodized salt, milk, bread made with iodate dough conditioners, and foods with iodine-containing dyes, not to mention iodine residues from compounds used to sterilize commercial processing equipment. These incidental sources of iodine such as dyes, alginates, and dough conditioners should be replaced by compounds with limited or no iodine to prevent overabundance of iodine in the diet. A varied United States diet, containing 2 to 6 g of iodized salt, provides approximately 500 μg of iodine per day.

Hypothyroidism sometimes accompanies endemic goiter, while hyperthyroidism is rarely identified with the condition. If the goiter is progressive and multinodular, iodine will be of little help. However, in the early hyperplastic state, endemic goiter will regress with iodine intake.

A daily intake of 100 μg of iodine is recommended for adults, with somewhat higher levels for adolescents and pregnant and lactating women.

Graves' Disease

Graves' disease is a combination of goiter, hyperthyroidism, and exophthalmos (protruding eyeballs). The occurrence of the disease is rare before age 10 and unlikely in the elderly. The condition is more prevalent among females than males (seven to one).

General symptoms include nervousness, exophthalmos, hyperexcitability, irritability, restlessness, emotional instability, weight loss, increased bowel motility, tremor, sweating, and heat intolerance. T_4, T_3, and RAI uptake are increased. When the metabolic rate increases, the need for all vitamins increases. Despite this, documentation of actual vitamin deficiencies is infrequent. However, endogenous protein and fat stores are catabolized, and weight loss persists even though the patient has an excessive appetite.

The excess of T_4 and T_3 results in bone demineralization, and therefore high urinary and fecal loss of calcium and phosphorus. Also, hyperthyroidism puts a heavy load on the cardiovascular system. Cardiac output increases, as does pulse rate, while circulation time decreases, thus producing tachycardia and tremor, and a rise in body temperature. In addition, the excess of T_4 and T_3 increases carbohydrate absorption from the intestine, causing a rise in blood sugar after a carbohydrate meal and possibly glycosuria if the renal threshold is exceeded.

Treatment

Diet therapy   Until the hyperthyroidism is controlled, ample energy intake is necessary to protect body tissues and to prevent weight loss. Mild hyperthyroidism calls for a 15 to 25 percent increase above the normal recommended dietary energy allowance, and severe hyperthyroidism, a 50 to 75 percent increase, which may mean a diet containing 4500 to 5000 kcal (18.9 to 21 MJ). In addition, protein allowance should be liberal: approximately 1 to 2 g per kilogram of ideal body weight. Carbohydrate intake should be increased to compensate for disturbed carbohydrate metabolism, to provide energy, and to spare protein; the increased carbohydrate intake necessitates an increased thiamin intake, which is essential for energy metabolism. Water should be adequate to compensate for losses incurred by the increased metabolic rate, sweating, and heavy breathing. The mineral and vitamin requirements—especially calcium, phosphorus, and the B vitamins—may have to be supplemented. One quart of milk per day can help to enhance calcium balance and will provide protein.

Stimulants, such as coffee, tea, other caffeine-containing beverages, and tobacco, should be eliminated, as they further aggravate symptoms of nervousness. Alcohol should receive a doctor's clearance before being incorporated into the diet, as individual tolerances differ.

It is necessary to counsel the patient to be conscious of the fact that once hyperthyroidism is treated, obesity could be a problem if the excessive intake established during the hyperthyroid period continues.

Drug therapy   Drug therapy consists of agents which block the oxidation of iodide to iodine and therefore prevent thyroid hormone synthesis. PTU (propylthiouracil) a synthetic goitrogen, is one such drug.

Exogenous thyroid hormone has not been documented to have any general usefulness for weight reduction. In fact, it can make one nervous and heat-intolerant; i.e., it can cause symptoms similar to hyperthyroidism. Short-term weight loss may occur if the individual's activity level increases in response to these symptoms. Exogenous thyroid hormone is contraindicated for those with cardiovascular disorders. Further, the hypermetabolism caused by excess thyroid hormone increases the body's demand for adrenal hormones. Thus, thyroid hormone administration may result in an acute adrenal insufficiency, especially if the patient already has adrenal insufficiency or hypopituitarism. Also, thyroid hormone may increase appetite.

THYMUS

The thymus gland, located in the chest cavity just above the heart, is large in infancy, and undergoes progressive atrophy after puberty. It is primarily a lymphoid organ, producing the antibodies necessary for the body's immune response (see Chap. 19).

PARATHYROID

Physiology

Although location and number may vary, in general, humans have four parathyroids, two located in the superior poles and two in the inferior poles of the thyroid. The main function of the glands is maintenance of a constant ionized calcium level in the extracellular fluid, which is necessary for blood coagulation, normal cardiac and skeletal muscle contraction, and nerve function. The circulating level of ionized calcium acts directly on the parathyroid glands in feedback fashion to regulate parathyroid hormone excretion. When plasma calcium is high, hormone secretion falls, and calcium is absorbed by the bones. When plasma calcium falls, parathyroid hormone increases, and calcium is mobilized from the bone. Further, the parathyroid stimulates the intestinal mucosa to increase calcium absorption and excrete phosphate. This mechanism is yet to be clearly defined. Also, the serum phosphorus is maintained via a homeostatic mechanism controlled by the parathyroid gland. As the serum phosphorus increases, the parathyroid hormone acts to inhibit the kidney from reabsorbing phosphorus. Phosphorus excretion (in the urine) increases, and the normal serum calcium/phosphorus ratio returns.

Tetany

Tetany is a condition caused by a disturbance of calcium and phosphorus metabolism, or by inadvertent parathyroidectomy during thyroid surgery. Tetany can be classified as:

1 Alkalotic tetany, usually due to hyperventilation or vomiting.
2 Hypocalcemic tetany, associated with rickets, osteomalacia, steatorrhea, and renal insufficiency; in newborns, temporary hypofunction of the parathyroid, causing tetany, may be precipitated by feeding an overload of phosphate, in the form of cow's milk.

Symptoms of tetany include convulsions, cramps, and muscle twitching. Total plasma calcium may fall as low as 4 mg per 100 mL (normal 8.5 to 10.5 mg per 100 mL).

The major goal of treatment is to restore plasma calcium without precipitating marked hypercalcemia or hypercalciuria. Dietary recommendation is for a high-calcium (1800 to 2400 mg), low-phosphorus diet. This is difficult to achieve, however, since most foods high in calcium, for example, milk, also contain high levels of phosphorus. Aluminum salts are used to decrease the absorption of dietary phosphorus.

A vitamin D supplement of 100,000 international units or 250 mg cholecalciferol is recommended (to enhance calcium absorption); however, the patient must be carefully monitored to avoid hypervitaminosis D (see Chap. 6). A more practical approach is to limit the intake of milk and milk products, and to use calcium supplements as an adjunct to diet (see Table 24-2). This allows a normal complement of calcium, yet avoids increasing the phosphorus levels.

ADRENALS

The adrenals are small, paired structures lying on either side of the midline of the abdominal cavity, above the kidneys. Each gland consists of an outer cortex and inner medulla. The cortex secretes the following steroids (analogues, known as *corticosteroids*): cortisol and corticosterone, which are referred to as *glucocorticoids,* secreted in response to physical and emotional stress; and aldosterone, a *mineralocorticoid,* which maintains sodium balance and extracel-

TABLE 24-2 CALCIUM SUPPLEMENTS

Compound	Calcium content, %	Possible route	Oral dose
Calcium gluconate	9	Oral, IV, IM	15 g daily in divided doses
Calcium lactate	13	Oral	5 g 3 times a day
Calcium chloride	27	Oral, IV	6–8 g in divided doses; best with milk
Calcium levulinate	13	Oral, IV	4–5 g 3 times a day with meals
Calcium carbonate	40	Oral	1 g 4 times a day

IV = intravenous; IM = intramuscular.

lular fluid volume. The adrenal medulla secretes the catecholamines epinephrine and norepinephrine, which, although not life-sustaining, help to integrate the body's reaction to stress.

Cushing's Syndrome

Cushing's syndrome (or disease) is glucocorticoid excess caused by lesions in the hypothalamus; adrenocorticotropic hormone (ACTH)–secreting tumors of the pituitary, lung, or elsewhere; tumors of the adrenal cortex; idiopathic adrenal hyperplasia; or excess corticosteroid therapy.

Since glucocorticoids increase protein catabolism, the patient with uncontrolled Cushing's syndrome is protein-depleted. The amino acids from catabolism are converted into glucose by the liver, causing blood sugar to rise. This, coupled with the anti-insulin effect of glucocorticoids on the peripheral tissues, causes a decrease in the body's use of glucose, and diabetes mellitus may develop. Of those with Cushing's disease 80 percent have an abnormal glucose tolerance test and 20 percent have overt diabetes mellitus. Other symptoms include thin skin and subcutaneous tissues, poorly developed muscles, and thin, scraggly hair. Minor injuries result in bruises and ecchymoses, and wounds heal poorly. Growth is inhibited in children.

Significant mineralocorticoid excess is responsible for the characteristic "moon face," as it causes considerable sodium and water retention. Potassium depletion and weakness are also part of the pathology. Eighty-five percent of these individuals have high blood pressure, which can be attributed to the glucocorticoid effect on blood vessels.

There is not necessarily a weight gain, but there is a redistribution of fat to the back of the neck ("buffalo hump") and supraclavicular regions. Relatively thin extremities accentuate an enlarged abdomen. Purple striae are common, and are located over the abdomen, thighs, and upper arms.

A high-protein diet (1 g per kilogram of body weight) is recommended to prevent or correct negative nitrogen balance. Sodium restriction may be useful in decreasing fluid retention.

The steroid used to treat Cushing's syndrome can result in osteoporosis (a softening and demineralization of the bone). The osteoporosis is caused by protein catabolism which inhibits new bone formation and breaks down existing bone matrix. Further, glucocorticoids not only have an anti-vitamin D action, but also increase the glomerular filtration rate, thus increasing calcium secretion.

Total adrenalectomy is the treatment of choice for progressive Cushing's disease. Partial adrenalectomy does not eliminate the possible recurrence of the syndrome. Of course, a total adrenalectomy results in adrenocortical insufficiency, or Addison's disease, which is easier to treat.

Addison's Disease

Addison's disease, or adrenocortical insufficiency, can be due to destruction of the adrenal glands by tuberculosis (now a rare cause), adrenal atrophy due to unknown (probably immunological) damage, corticosteroid withdrawal after long-term treatment, or surgical removal of the adrenals to treat Cushing's syndrome. Currently, metastatic malignancy is increasingly the cause.

In normal individuals, aldosterone maintains extracellular fluid volume. With adrenal insufficiency, there is decreased sodium absorption and increased sodium ion excretion by the kidneys as a result of insufficient secretion of aldosterone by the adrenals. Chloride ions and water are secreted into the urine in large quantities, causing decreased extracellular volume and low blood pressure. The body responds by retaining potassium, causing high serum potassium levels. If the disease is untreated, blood volume falls, precipitating what is called the *Addisonian crisis*.

Classic symptoms of Addisonian crisis include shock, low serum sodium, high serum potassium, and low serum glucose. Other symptoms, precrisis, include poor heat tolerance from high levels of sodium in the perspiration, and abdominal discomfort and diarrhea, because of the inability to reabsorb fluid from the intestinal lumen at normal rates. Also, there may be a low serum glucose, anorexia, vomiting, weight loss, and dermal pigmentation due to high levels of certain hormones, namely melanocyte-stimulating hormone (MSH) and adrenocorticotropic hormone (ACTH).

Treatment consists of replacement of adrenocortical hormones. This is accomplished with cortisol, which should be taken with meals to minimize gastric irritation. Weight gain is a complication of this therapy.

Individuals taking cortisol should be monitored for a high salt intake. The sodium intake should approximate 10 g per day. High-salt foods (such as condiments, potato chips, and cold cuts) plus 3 or 4 salt tablets with meals are recommended to achieve this level. Nevertheless, about 70 percent of patients require a sodium-retaining hormone, such as the mineralocorticoid deoxycorticosterone, to prevent orthostatic hypotension. In a few cases only salt therapy is required.

The low blood sugar necessitates small, frequent, high-protein, low-carbohydrate meals, as well as a bedtime snack. Fasting can lead to hypoglycemic episodes. A high fluid intake will help to alleviate the threat of dehydration. Foods extremely high in potassium, such as bananas and orange juice, should be avoided, but there is no reason for severe restriction. (See Chap. 23, Table 23-8, for a list of potassium-containing foods.) If mineralocorticoid therapy is prolonged, symptoms such as cardiac arrhythmias and headaches can occur because of potassium depletion. In this case, supplemental potassium is required, and salt intake should be decreased until sodium balance is achieved.

Corticosteroid Therapy

Since glucocorticoids have an antiinflammatory and antiallergenic effect, they are used to treat a host of diseases or conditions that have an allergic or autoimmune component (e.g., hives, rheumatoid arthritis.) With such therapy, it is important to consider interrelationships between diet and drugs.

An adjunct of corticosteroid therapy is weight gain due to appetite stimulation and fluid retention. If there is no need to increase sodium intake (as there is with Addison's disease), sodium should be restricted (some recommend less than 500 mg per day).

Therapeutic cortisone may result in negative nitrogen balance. Therefore the diet for patients taking this medication should be high in protein and high in carbohydrate to spare protein. Cortisone therapy can also precipitate hypokalemia, in which case supplemental potassium must be taken with meals.

Adrenocortical steroid therapy, including

ACTH and glucocorticoids, increases gastric acid and pepsin secretion, and may alter the resistance of the mucosa to these secretions and cause irritation. This may induce peptic ulcers which could ultimately hemorrhage. Therefore, patients on this therapy must be advised to take frequent (small) meals.

The diet for someone on prolonged ACTH therapy is high in protein (100 g), high in carbohydrate (200 to 300 g), and low in sodium (1000 mg), is divided into frequent small feedings, and includes a vitamin C supplement, since ACTH depletes the adrenal tissue of vitamin C.

PITUITARY

The pituitary gland (also called the hypophysis) is about the size of a large pea, and lies just beneath the hypothalamus of the brain, to which it is connected by the pituitary or hypophyseal stalk. Although small, it is a complex structure composed of two lobes, the anterior lobe and the posterior lobe, each separately responsible for the secretion of hormones (see Table 24-3, below).

These hormones are released from the anterior pituitary in response to *neurohormones* (formerly called *releasing factors*) which are produced in the hypothalamus in response to nervous, hormonal, and other influences. In certain disease states or conditions, this feedback mechanism between the hypothalamus and the pituitary becomes altered. This fact has caused some authorities to relate this mechanism to the etiology of nonorganic failure to thrive, a condition in which the child, despite adequate food intake, fails to grow. They regard these children as having clinical findings suggestive of idiopathic hypopituitarism, and raise the question of whether these children respond to an adverse family environment and emotional deprivation

TABLE 24-3   PITUITARY HORMONES AND THEIR FUNCTION

Hormone	Function
Anterior pituitary hormones	
Growth hormone (somatotropin)	Promotes growth by influencing metabolic functions, especially protein formation
	Decreases the rate of carbohydrate utilization throughout the body
	Increases the mobilization of fats and the use of fats for energy
Corticotropin (adrenocorticotropic hormone, ACTH)	Affects the secretion of the adrenocortical hormones which affect metabolism of protein, carbohydrate, and fat
Thyrotropin	Controls the amount of thyroxine secreted by the thyroid gland
Gonadotropins	Influences reproductive activities
Posterior pituitary hormones	
Antidiuretic hormone (vasopressin)	Affects the rate of water excretion
Oxytocin	Helps to mobilize milk from the glands to the nipple during lactation upon suckling

by an altered release of growth hormone from the pituitary. These children present with a perverted or voracious appetite and are either excessively passive or aggressive in behavior. Improvement is noted with changes in parental management or placement in a stimulating environment (see Chap. 26).

Growth hormone (somatotropic hormone or somatotropin) plays a significant role in the normal growth and development of the human body by promoting protein synthesis in all body organs through the transport of amino acids into the cell; it thus aids in determining the rate of organ enlargement. Also, growth hormone controls growth in bone length by controlling cartilage production in the ends of long bones, a process known as *chondrogenesis*.

The secretion of growth hormone is related to a person's nutritional status. Growth hormone increases during the hypoglycemia that is seen in states of starvation and fasting as protein stores are depleted. During these periods, an inverse relationship is noted, with growth hormone secretion increasing as protein stores decrease. This has clinical application in the treatment of kwashiorkor: when adequate protein is provided, a reversal in growth hormone secretion occurs, thereby normalizing carbohydrate and fat metabolism. Adequate calories alone are not sufficient to correct the excess production of growth hormone.

The conditions resulting from altered pituitary function are summarized in Table 24-4; for the most part these do not necessitate dietary intervention.

PANCREAS

The pancreas is a carrot-shaped gland located along the greater curvature of the stomach. It is a double gland with an *exocrine portion* producing the digestive enzymes (amylase, lipase, trypsin) and an *endocrine portion* producing the

TABLE 24-4   CONDITIONS RESULTING FROM ALTERED PITUITARY FUNCTION

Condition	Mechanism	Diet commentary
Acromegaly	↑ Growth hormone	Diabetes is a complication and diet is part of the treatment
Pituitary dwarfism	↓ Overall pituitary hormones ↓ Thyroid function ↓ Adrenal function	
Diabetes insipidus	↓ Antidiuretic hormone	Weight loss can be a problem because of patient's fear of drinking fluids and a lack of sleep due to increased urination
Precocious puberty	The hypothalamic mechanism which initiates puberty is activated earlier than usual, and stimulates pituitary to release gonadotropic hormones	

↑ = increased; ↓ = decreased.

hormones glucagon and insulin, on which we will focus. (The role of the pancreas in digestion is discussed in Chap. 9.)

Small islets of endocrine tissue known as the islets of Langerhans (islets are small masses of one type of tissue within another) are found in the pancreas. Their numbers have been estimated to be between 500,000 and 2 million. Each islet is well supplied with blood vessels and contains two types of cells, *alpha cells* and *beta cells,* each responsible for hormone production:

> *Alpha cells.* Secrete *glucagon,* a hormone that speeds the conversion of glycogen to glucose and thereby raises blood glucose level; thus, glucagon has a *hyperglycemic effect.*
>
> *Beta cells.* Secrete *insulin,* a hormone that is necessary for cellular uptake of glucose and also speeds the synthesis of glycogen in the liver—both actions draw sugar from the blood; therefore, insulin has a *hypoglycemic effect.*

The secretion of both glucagon and insulin is controlled by the blood glucose level. When blood sugar falls, glucagon is secreted; when blood sugar rises, insulin is secreted, causing blood sugar to be maintained within the narrow limits of 80 to 100 mg per 100 mL.

Presently, there is no named disease associated with glucagon secretion, although there are reports of patients with chronic low blood sugar associated with a lack or deficiency of alpha cells, an apparently hereditary disorder. The disease impairing insulin secretion, diabetes mellitus, will be considered in detail, since this disease now affects 5 percent of the population in the United States (also a decline in glucose tolerance is now a recognized phenomenon of aging) and diet is the cornerstone of treatment.

Diabetes Mellitus

Diabetes was first noted by the Egyptians in the year 1500 B.C. During the first century a Greek physician described a condition in which the body excreted large quantities of urine. He called this phenomenon *diabetes* from the Greek word meaning "to flow through." Centuries later the Latin word *mellitus,* "honeyed," was added to describe the glucose-laden urine.

In 1922 F. G. Banting and C. H. Best discovered insulin. Although its exact action is not clear it is believed to serve in the following functions:

1 Transportation of glucose through cell membranes

2 Conversion of glucose to glycogen and storage in the liver (glycogenesis)

3 Conversion of glucose to fat (lipogenesis)

4 Oxidation of glucose via the glycolytic pathway by phosphorylation catalyzed by glucokinase

The symptoms of diabetes mellitus show how these metabolic processes are affected by insulin deficiency. The sequence of symptoms is as follows:

> *Hyperglycemia.* An abnormally high blood sugar. The blood sugar may reach between 300 and 1200 mg per 100 mL from failure of the liver to synthesize glycogen and failure of the cells throughout the body to utilize glucose. This causes the blood sugar to rise and the kidneys to exceed their capacity to reabsorb glucose (i.e., glucose levels reach the renal threshold), which means that glucose spills into the urine. When blood sugar exceeds 180 mg per 100 mL, sugar spills into the urine, causing *glycosuria.*
> ↓
> *Glycosuria.* Sugar in the urine. The excretion of large amounts of glucose, which is osmotically attracted to water, means that large amounts of water are excreted (osmotic diuresis), along with the loss of urinary sodium and potassium. Glycosuria causes *polyuria.*
> ↓
> *Polyuria.* The secretion of large amounts of urine. The excessive water loss, along with excretion of electrolytes from the extracel-

lular fluid, affect the intracellular fluid, with the net effect of intracellular and extracellular dehydration, stimulating *polydipsia.*

↓

Polydipsia. Increased or excessive thirst due to water loss.

Because of the body's inability to utilize glucose for energy and the loss of glucose in the urine (every gram of glucose lost represents 4.1 kcal or 17.2 kJ), the body is left in a state of starvation manifested by an excessive appetite and excessive food intake, known as *polyphagia.*

Polyphagia. Excessive food intake. Despite excessive food intake, the body's inability to utilize glucose causes protein and fat stores to be mobilized for energy, resulting in muscle wasting and *weight loss.* The body's reliance on fat stores for an energy source causes an accumulation of ketones and the state of *ketosis* develops.

↓

Ketosis. During the body's accelerated lipolysis of fats, an increase of fatty acids is sent to the liver, resulting in an accelerated formation of ketone bodies (β-hydroxybutyric acid, acetoacetic acid, acetone). These ketone bodies are released into the bloodstream and are metabolized to some extent but are then excreted in the urine as a result of overproduction. (The presence of ketone bodies in the urine is detected by a positive Acetest reaction.) Since these ketoacids have a low threshold for excretion and about one-half need sodium for excretion, sodium is drawn from the extracellular fluid. As a result, the sodium concentration in the extracellular fluid usually decreases, and the loss of this basic ion adds to the acidosis already caused by the excessive ketoacids in the extracellular fluid. Subsequently, all the reactions that take place in metabolic acidosis take place in diabetic acidosis (see Chap. 8). These include *Kussmaul respiration* (rapid and deep breathing), causing excessive expiration of carbon dioxide; a marked de-

crease in the bicarbonate content of the extracellular fluids; and excretion of chloride ions by the kidneys. The resultant shift in the fluid compartment causes hypovolemia (low blood pressure) leading to *diabetic coma* and death. These extreme effects occur only in the most severe degrees of untreated diabetes.

(Note: The breath of poorly controlled diabetics smells fruity because of the expired ketone bodies. This helps to differentiate between diabetic coma and insulin reaction.)

Polyuria (excessive elimination of urine), *polydipsia* (excessive thirst), *polyphagia* (excessive eating), *weight loss,* and *asthenia* (lack of energy) are the earliest symptoms of diabetes. The diagnosis of diabetes is established by the following procedures.

Diagnosis of Diabetes Mellitus

If a physician suspects that an individual is manifesting symptoms characteristic of diabetes, an oral glucose tolerance test (OGTT) may be ordered to confirm the diagnosis (see Table 24-5, opposite). When a diabetic is given a glucose load, the blood sugar will rise higher and return to normal more slowly than occurs in a nondiabetic. If a patient has experienced symptoms of diabetes and has had an elevated 2-h postprandial blood sugar determination (postprandial = after meals), it is not necessary to tax the body further with a glucose load. It is not recommended that a glucose tolerance test be administered during hospitalization, as the imposed sedentary life results in a blood sugar level that is higher than normal because of the lack of activity.

The nurse or nutritionist can assist by explaining the diet preceding the test, the administration of the glucose, and the collection of blood samples. With children, commercially prepared glucose solutions might be more acceptable if given in their own cup or through a straw, and special games or some entertainment should be planned to amuse the child during the period of blood sample collection. Blood sugar values are taken during fasting and at ½, 1, 2,

TABLE 24-5 ADMINISTRATION OF THE ORAL GLUCOSE TOLERANCE TEST

Glucose dose		Diet	Special consideration
Child	Adult		
1.75 g/kg of ideal body weight: up to a maximum of 75 g; under the age of 18 months, 3 g/kg	1.75 g/kg of body weight or approximately 75-g of glucose	150-g carbohydrate diet for 3 days prior to the test. Patient fasts for at least 10 h, but not more than 16. No caffeine or nicotine for 12 h prior to the test.	The following medications may influence results: Dilantin Thiazide diuretics Glucocorticoids Oral contraceptives Ascorbic acid

and 3 h after glucose administration, and urine samples are collected for sugar determinations.

Another possible future diagnostic tool is the determination of hemoglobin A_{1C}, a glycoprotein which is the most abundant minor hemoglobin component in human erythrocytes. Research interest was sparked by the finding that hemoglobin A_{1C} levels are twice as high in diabetics as in nondiabetics. Hemoglobin A_{1C} determinations are potentially an excellent screening method for diabetes. They are not only highly reproducible, but also require no restriction on sampling time. Since these determinations are highly sensitive to minor fluctuations in glucose tolerance abnormalities, they may very well prove a better diagnostic tool than random glucose samples.

The diagnosis of diabetes in nonpregnant adults is limited to:

1 Those who exhibit the classic symptoms of diabetes and unquestionable hyperglycemia.

2 Those with fasting plasma glucose concentrations which equal or exceed 140 mg per dL on more than one testing.

3 Those who, even if fasting plasma glucose is less than 140 mg per dL, maintain elevated venous plasma glucose values during the oral glucose tolerance test (greater than or equivalent to 200 mg per dL, not only at 2 h after glucose ingestion, but also at some other interval between 0 and 2 h).

The diagnosis of a diabetic child can be made for those who display the classic diabetic symptoms (polyuria, polyphagia, polydipsia, and glycosuria), and who have a random plasma glucose greater than 200 mg per dL. An oral glucose tolerance test (OGTT) is unnecessary under these circumstances. If an OGTT is indicated, diagnosis is predicated upon a fasting plasma glucose which exceeds 140 mg per dL, the 2-h value which exceeds or equals 200 mg per dL, *and* a value between 0 and 2 h which exceeds or equals 200 mg per dL.

Due to the many factors which could influence a fasting plasma glucose value, or an oral glucose tolerance test (stress, drugs, inactivity, etc.), it is imperative that diagnosis be based on at least two different test determinations.

Classification of Diabetes Mellitus
An international team, sponsored by the National Diabetes Data Group of the National Institutes of Health, convened in 1978 and reorganized and extended the previous classifications for diabetes mellitus. Their recommendations, outlined here, have been endorsed by the American Diabetes Association and accepted by the Expert Committee on Diabetes of the World Health Organization. The classification includes:

Type I insulin-dependent diabetes mellitus (IDDM)

Type II noninsulin-dependent diabetes mellitus (NIDDM) which is further categorized into: gestational diabetes mellitus (GDM), impaired glucose tolerance (IGT), and previous abnormality of glucose tolerance (PrevAGT).

Type I Insulin-dependent, ketosis-prone diabetes mellitus, or IDDM, was formerly termed *juvenile diabetes;* however, since it can occur at any age, the new nomenclature seems more appropriate. Onset is sudden with a presentation of the full spectrum of symptoms. The body's total dependence on an exogenous supply of insulin causes this diabetic to be ketosis prone. Islet-cell antibodies are often present at diagnosis.

Type II Non-insulin-dependent diabetes mellitus, or NIDDM, for the most part occurs after age 40. However, it is diagnosed in young people, and hence the recommendation to abandon the *adult-onset* nomenclature.

The person with NIDDM is not dependent on insulin, and is not ketosis-prone. However, ketosis may occur under severe stress, such as infection or trauma. In the United States, 60 to 90 percent of all those with NIDDM are obese, and characteristically present with one or two mild symptoms, such as nocturnal polyuria and fatigue.

NIDDM has a genetic basis stronger than that found in IDDM; the familial pattern is more frequent. As mentioned above, NIDDM also includes:

Gestational diabetes (GDM)

Impaired glucose tolerance (IGT)

Previous abnormality of glucose tolerance (Prev AGT)

Gestational diabetes (GDM), as the name suggests, is glucose intolerance recognized during pregnancy. (Diabetics who become pregnant do not fall into this category.) Although insulin resistance may play an etiological role, GDM is not completely understood, However, it is known that these women are at higher risk of perinatal morbidity and mortality, and have a higher frequency of viable-fetus loss. With early detection, therapy can moderate such risks.

About 30 percent of women with gestational diabetes develop diabetes within 5 to 10 years; some, revert post partum to normoglycemia and remain so. However, during the period which they display normal plasma glucose, they are classified as PrevAGT: previous abnormality of glucose tolerance.

Impaired glucose tolerance (IGT), formerly referred to as *asymptomatic diabetes, chemical diabetes, borderline diabetes,* or *latent diabetes,* refers to those with plasma glucose intermediate between normal and diabetic. The mild glucose intolerance found in a person with IGT may be due to the normal variation of glucose tolerance found within a population, or it may be a step along the way in the development of NIDDM or IDDM. The majority of these individuals can be so classified for many years, or revert to normal glucose tolerance. Therefore, the term *diabetic* should not be used for those within this category.

Previous abnormality of glucose tolerance (PrevAGT), formerly known as *latent diabetes* or *prediabetes,* refers to those who previously demonstrated elevated plasma glucose, but who currently have normal values. The most common case is the person with gestational diabetes who reverts to normal glucose levels after delivery. Other examples include obese diabetics whose glucose tolerance normalizes when they achieve ideal body weight, or those whose plasma glucose is elevated during the acute phase of a myocardial infarction.

Potential abnormality of glucose tolerance (PotAGT), formerly termed *prediabetes* or *potential diabetes,* includes those who have never exhibited glucose intolerance, but who are at high risk for developing diabetes. Those who fall into such a category for developing NIDDM include (in descending order of risk): a monozygotic twin of an NIDDM diabetic; a first-degree relative of a NIDDM diabetic, such as a brother, sister, parent or offspring; a mother of a greater than 9-lb newborn; obese people; and those who belong to a highly susceptible racial or ethnic group. Those at increased risk for developing IDDM diabetes include (in descending order of risk): persons with islet-cell antibodies; a monozygotic twin of an IDDM diabetic; a brother or sister of an IDDM diabetic; an offspring of an IDDM diabetic.

It should be noted that it is often difficult to classify an individual. Classification should be avoided until the complete diagnostic information is available. Table 24-6 (pp. 550–551) summarizes the diagnostic criteria for diabetes mellitus; Table 24-7 (p. 552) shows normal glucose concentrations for children and nonpregnant adults.

Insulin-Dependent Diabetes Mellitus (IDDM)*

It is important to remember that IDDM can occur in adulthood and that treatment (insulin, diet, exercise) recommended is often similar to that for children. The focus of this section is on children because they represent the majority of those who develop IDDM. Also, they require special consideration due to age of onset. The onset is sudden. The individual is likely to be underweight and is unresponsive to oral hypoglycemic drugs, and insulin is required.

A child is frequently brought to medical attention because of growth failure in spite of a voracious appetite. Bed-wetting in a previously trained child may be noted. The diagnosis is confirmed by laboratory data (see Table 24-7).

The high incidence of vascular changes is considered to be the most important problem in IDDM. Eighty-five percent of patients are reported to show such changes occurring within 12 to 13 years from the date of diagnosis. One area of important potential research is the examination of impaired glucose tolerance in children, and its relationship to overt diabetes and its complications.

The overall growth of diabetic children appears to be related to the control of diabetes; however, to what extent the degree of control should approximate normoglycemia is not known. Slight delays of growth in stature have

*Contributed by Rosanne Beatrice Howard.

been noted but the tendency is to approximate adult height after a prolonged growth period. The onset of diabetes just prior to a growth spurt has been noted to interfere with adult height.

Since the onset of vascular changes and life expectancy have been considered to be independent of clinical control, many different opinions have evolved as to whether strict clinical control and strict adherence to the prescribed diet should even be a consideration for a growing child, whose psychosocial development may be thwarted by such treatment. However, the facts that poor control seems to intensify vascular disorders and interferes with growth, and that good control necessitates a balance of food and insulin, lead us to consider that diet is an essential component of treatment.

Treatment

The goals of treatment are as follows:

Insulin to approximate glycemic equilibrium

Diet for normal growth and activity (based on a child's likes and dislikes, with allowances made for self-expression and independence)

Restoration of the diabetic child to average physical and emotional well-being, which necessitates an acceptance on the part of the child and family that he or she is a "normal child" who happens to have diabetes, not a "diabetic child" constricted by the disease

Since diabetes in children is often first manifested as the state of ketoacidosis, initial treatment is a medical emergency requiring constant attention. A sample of blood is immediately drawn for determination of a blood glucose, pH, carbon dioxide, blood urea nitrogen, and total and differential white blood cell count, and urine is taken (by catheterization if necessary) for sugar and acetone tests. On the basis of the results a plan for fluid and electrolyte and insulin therapy is initiated.

After this period, the long-term establishment of glycemic equilibrium begins through

TABLE 24-6 DIAGNOSTIC CRITERIA FOR DIABETES MELLITUS

Classification	Symptoms	Fasting glucose concentration	Oral glucose tolerance test (OGTT)
Type I (IDDM), diabetes mellitus in nonpregnant adults	Presence of the classic symptoms of diabetes, such as polyuria, polydipsia, ketonuria, and rapid weight loss, together with gross and unequivocal elevation of plasma glucose.	Elevated fasting glucose concentration on more than one occasion: Venous plasma ≥ 140 mg/dL Venous whole blood ≥ 120 mg/dL Capillary whole blood ≥ 120 mg/dL If the fasting glucose concentration meets these criteria, the OGTT is *not required*. Indeed, virtually all persons with FBG 140 mg/dL will exhibit an OGTT that meets or exceeds the criteria in the next column.	Fasting glucose concentration less than that which is diagnostic of diabetes, but sustained elevated glucose concentration during the OGTT on more than one occasion. Both the 2-h sample *and* some other sample taken between administration of the 75-g glucose dose and 2 h later must meet the following criteria: Venous plasma ≥ 200 mg/dL Venous whole blood ≥ 180 mg/dL Capillary whole blood ≥ 200 mg/dL
Diabetes mellitus in children	Presence of the classic symptoms of diabetes, such as polyuria, polydipsia, ketonuria, and rapid weight loss, together with a random plasma glucose 200 mg/dL.	Fasting value: Venous plasma ≥ 140 mg/dL Venous whole blood ≥ 120 mg/dL Capillary whole blood ≥ 120 mg/dL	In asymptomatic individuals, both an elevated fasting glucose concentration and a sustained elevated glucose concentration during the OGTT on more than one occasion. Both the 2-h sample and some other sample taken between administration of the glucose dose (1.75 g/kg ideal body weight, up to a maximum of 75 g) and 2 h later must meet the criteria below. 2-h OGTT value and an intervening value: Venous plasma ≥ 200 mg/dL Venous whole blood ≥ 180 mg/dL Capillary whole blood ≥ 200 mg/dL

Type II (NIDDM), gestational diabetes

Nonsymptomatic except for elevated glucose levels.

Fasting value:
- Venous plasma ≥ 105 mg/dL
- Venous whole blood ≥ 90 mg/dL
- Capillary whole blood ≥ 90 mg/dL

Two or more of the following values after a 100-g oral glucose challenge must be met or exceeded:

	Venous plasma	Venous whole blood	Capillary whole blood
1 h	190 mg/dL	170 mg/dL	170 mg/dL
2 h	185 mg/dL ±	145 mg/dL	145 mg/dL
3 h	145 mg/dL	125 mg/dL	125 mg/dL

Impaired glucose tolerance (IGT) in nonpregnant adults

Three criteria must be met: the fasting glucose concentration must be below the value that is diagnostic for diabetes; the glucose concentration 2 h after a 75-g oral glucose challenge must be elevated between ½ h, 1 h, or 1½ h; the OGTT value later must be unequivocally elevated.

Nonsymptomatic except for elevated glucose levels.

Fasting value:
- Venous plasma < 140 mg/dL
- Venous whole blood < 120 mg/dL
- Capillary whole blood < 120 mg/dL

½-h, 1-h, or 1½-h OGTT value:
- Venous plasma ≥ 200 mg/dL
- Venous whole blood ≥ 180 mg/dL
- Capillary whole blood ≥ 200 mg/dL

2-h OGTT value:
- Venous plasma of between 140 and 200 mg/dL
- Venous whole blood of between 120 and 180 mg/dL
- Capillary whole blood of between 140 and 200 mg/dL

Impaired glucose tolerance (IGT) in children

Two criteria must be met: the fasting glucose concentration must be below the value that is diagnostic of diabetes; and the glucose concentration 2 h after an oral glucose concentration must be elevated.

Nonsymptomatic except for elevated glucose levels.

Fasting value:
- Venous plasma < 140 mg/dL
- Venous whole blood < 120 mg/dL
- Capillary whole blood < 120 mg/dL

2-h OGTT value:
- Venous plasma > 140 mg/dL
- Venous whole blood > 120 mg/dL
- Capillary whole blood > 120 mg/dL

Source: National Diabetes Data Group, "Classification and Diagnosis of Diabetes Mellitus and Other Categories of Glucose Intolerance," *Diabetes,* **28:**1039, December 1979.

TABLE 24-7 NORMAL GLUCOSE LEVELS

Age	Fasting glucose concentration	Oral glucose tolerance test (OGTT)
Children	Venous plasma < 130 mg/dL	2-h OGTT value
	Venous whole blood < 115 mg/dL	Venous plasma < 140 mg/dL
	Capillary whole blood < 115 mg/dL	Venous whole blood < 120 mg/dL
		Capillary whole blood < 140 mg/dL
Adults (nonpregnant)	Venous plasma < 115 mg/dL	2-h OGTT value
	Venous whole blood < 100 mg/dL	Venous plasma < 140 mg/dL
	Capillary whole blood < 100 mg/dL	Venous whole blood < 120 mg/dL
		Capillary whole blood < 140 mg/dL

diet and insulin control. This control is often brittle because of the variation in physical activity, emotional stresses at home and school, and the effects of maturation and growth.

As the child grows, he or she will need more insulin. This concept is somewhat confusing to parent and child alike, who sometimes think that the increase in insulin means that the disease state is worsening. Insulin requirements are based on body size and approximate 0.5 to 1 unit per kilogram of body weight. However, initially, the insulin requirement may be low because the pancreas is still capable of producing insulin. This period is known as the "honeymoon period" and could last 6 to 18 months. During this period the insulin is continued in homeopathic doses because of the problem encountered in reintroducing insulin. Usually, a combination of two types of insulin is used: an intermediate-acting insulin such as NPH and a short-term or regular crystalline insulin. *Two-thirds* of the required dose is administered in the form of intermediate insulin, given before breakfast, and *one-third* of the dose in the form of regular insulin, given before dinner. A rotation of insulin injection sites between the upper arm, the thigh, buttocks, back, and abdomen is necessary to prevent signs of induration or lipoatrophy at the sites of injection.

The use of a combination of insulins with different periods of onset and peak action (see Table 24-8) helps to approximate glycemic equilibrium throughout the day. However, food must be given in amounts to match these same periods of insulin activity. The *balance of food to insulin and exercise* is the goal of diet therapy. This is accomplished by a weighed diet or by the "middle of the road approach," in which the child is given an exchange diet based on age and energy needs. A helpful analogy in understanding this approach is that of a baseball game: this diet places the child in the right ball park but allows the child the freedom to move from base to base. The child, by learning the food groups comprising the exchange system—milk, meat, bread, fruit, vegetables, fat—learns to choose the foods in the amounts that can be effectively utilized by the body. For the most part, all foods that contain sugar are eliminated. Although some physicians do allow the limited use of ice cream or cookies on a once-per-week basis, this practice is generally not agreed upon. Others contend that if the child had an allergy to sugar, sugar would be avoided, and that this same principle should follow for the diabetic child. Furthermore, it is argued that allowing sugar foods on a once-per-week basis places special significance on the sugar-containing food, reinforcing the child's feeling of being deprived at other times. It is felt that the emphasis should be on a natural food diet without sugar.

A preschool-age child is capable of understanding the foods appropriate for his or her body. On the average, children are taught to give their own insulin injections around the age of 7 or 8 years. As they approach school age they are capable of daily urine testing which, along with an occasional blood sugar determination, forms

TABLE 24-8 COMMERCIALLY AVAILABLE INSULINS*

Type	Duration of blood-sugar-lowering effect, h	Peak of action, h
Regular	5–7	2–3
Neutral soluble	1½–8	1¼–4
Actrapid MC	1½–8	1¼–4
Insulin Leo Neutral RI	1½–8	1¼–4
Semilente	1½–8	1¼–4
Semitard MC	1½–8	1¼–4
NPH	24–28	8–12
Leo Mixtard RI	24	4–12
Globin zinc insulin BP	24	4–12
Rapitard MC	24	4–12
Lente	24	6–14
Lentard MC	24	6–14
Monotard MC	24	6–14
Isophane	24	4–12
Leo Retard	24	4–12
PZI	30	10–20
Ultralente	30	10–20
Ultratard	30	10–20

*Insulins are available in different units of strength per milliliter, e.g., U-80, U-100. The syringe used must be calibrated to the strength of insulin. There is a trend toward using only U-100 insulin.

TABLE 24-9 URINE TESTS FOR GLUCOSE

Test	Results
Benedict's solution	Blue (negative) → dark orange (2% glucose)
Clinitest tablets	Blue (negative) → orange (4+ or 2% glucose)
Testape	Yellow (negative) → blue (4+)
Clinistix	Red (negative) → purple (positive)

(Similar tests are available for testing the urine for acetone and albumin.)

the basis for determining diabetic control (see Table 24-9).

It should be noted that certain drugs can cause false-negative and false-positive reactions in various tests for glycosuria. Large quantities of ascorbic acid can also cause a false-positive test.

Urine tests are taken before meals. Before breakfast a second voided urine is taken because the accumulation of sugar in the bladder from the night causes the urine sample to be misleading. Periodically, fractional (or block) urine specimens are collected over a 24-h period, which represents the amount of glucose excreted in the urine at different periods during the day. The amount of carbohydrate lost in the urine—the total grams of glucose—should not exceed 20 percent of the total carbohydrate intake and some diabetologists consider control good only at 10 percent. (For example, a 5-year-old child consuming 150 g of carbohydrate per day would be allowed to spill 10 to 15 g of glucose in the urine, depending on the physician's definition of good control.) A new monitoring development is Chemstrip bG, a chemically treated strip that will allow diabetics to monitor their own blood sugar. By pricking a finger to draw blood and smearing it on the strip an individual can obtain a blood sugar reading and adjust diet and/or insulin accordingly.

Spilling some sugar, or 1+ on a urine test, is considered essential in order to prevent hypoglycemic periods resulting from too much insulin or too much exercise, which cause a lack of available glucose, especially to the brain, which is dependent on a continuous source of glucose. These periods are upsetting to the child and frequent occurrences can cause damage to the central nervous system. When the blood sugar falls to 50 mg per 100 mL, headaches, nervousness, sweating, trembling, confusion, and incoordination result, known as an *insulin reaction*. Immediate treatment by giving a readily available source of glucose—sugar in water, or fruit juices—is essential. If the child is unconscious, glucagon is administered. (A glucagon emergency kit is available, and some physicians suggest keeping one in the home.) Candy or sugar should be carried by the child so that it can be taken when the first symptoms appear. Children who participate in sports activities or vigorous play should learn to increase their food intake in anticipation of a busy day. However, a meal taken just prior to an event can cause discomfort in the best of athletes, and the diabetic child who has not prepared in advance would be better advised to eat a source of concentrated carbohydrate than to eat or drink a lot in preparation for the event.

In interpreting a period of hypoglycemia, the *Somogyi effect* must be considered. This effect consists of subclinical hypoglycemia (subclinical = too mild to cause symptoms), followed by a reactive hyperglycemia and ketonuria despite high levels of circulating insulin. The explanation is probably that the subclinical low blood sugar stimulates the secretion of insulin antagonists, such as catecholamines and glucagon, whereby insulin is made ineffective. The condition is recognized when, despite an increasing dose of insulin, there is a concomitant rise in blood sugar and a continued spillage of sugar in the urine. Treatment consists of splitting the insulin dose or reducing the total dose, or both.

Another problem encountered in interpreting hypoglycemic periods is presented by the adolescent patient who has a low blood sugar and yet has a urine that is positive for acetone. This biochemical profile is one of a teenager who is attempting to lose weight by severe food reduction. As a child approaches adolescence, the problem of weight control is one of many issues. This concern with body image, and the peer pressure to smoke and drink, is often reflected in poor diabetic control. The natural tendency to rebel appears heightened in adolescent diabetics, whose anger and denial are interpreted as a subconscious mourning process for the intact bodies they do not have. The problem-age period is between the ages of 12 and 15 years and is exhibited in the following vignette:

Betty is a 14½-year-old ninth-grader from the inner city whose diabetes was diagnosed at age 11 years, 2 months. At that time she was admitted to the hospital in mild acidosis following a 3-week history of lethargy, polydipsia, and polyuria. Discharged 1 week later taking 30 units of NPH and 10 units of regular insulin, her requirement fell to 4 units of NPH 4 months later. During the second year of her diabetes, she became increasingly resentful, particularly over the lipoatrophy in her thighs. She has been reluctant to discuss her condition with anyone but her closest friends. On several occasions she has admitted to not taking her insulin at all but has, so far, escaped severe ketoacidosis. While she tests her urine erratically and makes little attempt to adhere to a prescribed diet, she *has become more conscientious about her clinic visits and has been able to discuss her problems with the social worker and the nurse in the Diabetes Clinic.**

The management of the adolescent just described has begun to be facilitated by the nurse and social worker who have obviously been able to develop a helping relationship (see Chap. 11). During adolescence, youths must consolidate their own identity by integrating their own sexuality and separating from parents; the diabetic adolescent must also integrate the disease into his or her identity formation. Low self-esteem may become the catalyst for poor adjustment, difficulties, and rebellion seen in many teenage diabetics. The adolescent is concerned with the here and now and cannot be prodded into diet adherence by the threat of long-term complications.

The parents of both the young child and the adolescent need support incorporated into the diet counseling session, to deal with the anxiety experienced in having a child with a potentially life-threatening disease. The differences in child-rearing practices must be considered, as there is a continuum ranging from restrictive to permissive. Some ordinarily permissive parents will find it difficult to set limits, feeling sorry for the child. This easily leads to the child's using food as a tool with which to manipulate parents. Restrictive parents may find it difficult to foster independence in diabetic management. It is important to widen the angle of dietary vision to include the needs of both the child and parents as described by Stitt.†

In dealing with chronic illness, we must think of special dietary requirements for the particular chronically ill child at his particular age, and then consider to what extent those requirements can be derived from family care that would be suitable for the whole fam-

ily. Additions, deletions, and modifications may then have to be made for the child—or perhaps for the rest of the family—but the part of food which they can all share needs to be clearly established, for that becomes the foundation on which salutary influences can be built.

To widen the angle of dietary vision, a team approach is recommended with total family involvement.

Non-Insulin-Dependent Diabetes Mellitus (NIDDM)

The maturity-onset type of diabetic has beta cells with a normal morphology and a normal insulin content but the beta cells are "sluggish" and therefore cannot produce an adequate amount of insulin for the body, especially when the person is overweight, a common condition among this population.

The most important goal in the treatment of NIDDM is to achieve ideal body weight while maintaining optimum nutrition.

Achievement of this goal [weight reduction] may be associated with the reduction or disappearance of the requirements for exogenous insulin, improvement or correction of fasting hyperglycemia and glucose intolerance, and reduction of known risk factors for atherosclerotic vascular disease such as obesity, hypertension, hyperlipidemia and hyperglycemia.*

It is desirable for patients to be slightly leaner than their ideal body weight since insulin requirements are based on body size. A second goal of treatment is to prevent excessive glycosuria and hyperglycemia, while the final goal is to prevent the secondary complications of retinopathy, neuropathy, and nephropathy.

Peripheral vascular disease and coronary artery disease occur much more frequently in the diabetic. Nearly 75 percent of diabetic deaths in the United States are attributable to vascular disease. The onset and progression of vascular disease may be independent of diabetic

---

*Norman Spacks, Case Presentation, Grand Rounds, Children's Hospital Medical Center, Boston, Mass., Spring, 1975.
†Pauline Stitt, "The Family Approach to Feeding Chronically Ill Children," *Children,* **5**:215, November-December 1958.

*Committee on Food and Nutrition American Diabetics Association: *Diabetes,* **20**:633, 1971.

control. However, it is generally agreed that lack of control may intensify vascular disorders. Atherosclerosis may be accelerated by high circulating fat levels and the deposition of fat in the walls of blood vessels. This clogging of the blood vessels can cause a decrease of blood flow to tissues. If this happens tissue may die and gangrene can develop.

Treatment

The first treatment of choice for those with NIDDM is control by diet. However, if this proves ineffective, an oral antidiabetic agent may be prescribed.

The oral antidiabetic agents are not insulin (insulin is a protein, and if ingested would be digested) but, rather, consist of two classes of drugs:

1 *Sulfonylureas.* These sensitize the beta cells to glucose. For any given blood sugar level, the rate of insulin release is greater; thus, blood sugar is lowered. These drugs are effective only if the pancreas functions and are therefore prescribed only for maturity-type diabetics. Examples: Orinase (tolbutamide), Diabinese (chlorpropamide).

2 *Biguanides.* These do not depend on endogenous insulin, but cannot replace insulin. Their mode of action is not clear. They were most often prescribed for non-insulin-dependent patients, but because of the lactic acidosis side effect they have been removed from the market.

There has been much debate regarding the use of oral agents, since one study (University Group Diabetes Program) found a higher cardiovascular mortality rate in the groups treated with tolbutamide (a sulfonylurea) or with phenformin (a biguanide) than in the placebo- and insulin-treated groups.

An FDA audit did uphold the basic UGDP findings linking tolbutamide with a high risk of heart disease and stroke. The FDA further stated that although the UGDP study included errors and discrepancies, the fundamental conclusions of the study are valid. However, the FDA study itself has been criticized as based on faulty reports.

As for the alleged cardiotoxicity of tolbutamide and phenformin which the UGDP study claims, the results have not been confirmed in six other random trials of the oral hypoglycemic agents.

Type of Diet: IDDM and NIDDM

There are several different philosophies regarding the type of diabetic diet prescribed: the weighed diet, the measured diet, and the unmeasured or "free" diet. Whatever the philosophy, the nutritional care plan should always be individualized to meet the needs of each patient.

The *weighed diet* consists of weighing all food to comply with gram specifications. It is a rigid diet and allows little flexibility in lifestyle.

The *unmeasured diet* for individuals with IDDM entails flexibility of daily caloric intake to match energy demands. Meals and snacks are geared to activity and growth, with close attention paid to timing so as to avoid drastic swings in blood sugar.

The *measured diet* is probably advisable for the majority of NIDDM obese diabetics, who require a fixed energy intake. It is also appropriate for many adults with IDDM. Once the patient's energy and other nutrient requirements have been calculated, the food allowance is divided into "exchanges," depending on its carbohydrate, protein, and fat content. All exchanges within a food group contain approximately the same caloric content, and a certain number of exchanges per day are allowed within each group. The individual is taught to exchange within, and not between, groups; for example, a bread exchange and a meat exchange are not of similar nutrient composition and therefore cannot be exchanged or substituted for one another. The American Diabetic and Dietetic Associations have compiled a list of food exchanges (see Table 24-10 on the following pages, pp. 557–560).

TABLE 24-10 DIABETIC EXCHANGE LISTS

List 1: Milk exchanges
(includes nonfat, low-fat, and whole milk)

This list shows the kinds and amounts of milk or milk products to use for one milk exchange. Those appearing in **bold type** are **nonfat**. Low-fat and whole milk contain saturated fat. One exchange of milk contains 12 g of carbohydrate, 8 g of protein, a trace of fat, and 80 kcal (336 kJ).

Nonfat fortified milk

Skim or nonfat milk	1 cup (8 oz)
Powdered (nonfat dry, before adding liquid)	⅓ cup
Canned evaporated skim milk	½ cup
Buttermilk made from skim milk	1 cup
Yogurt made from skim milk (plain, unflavored)	1 cup

Low-fat fortified milk

1%-fat milk (omit ½ fat exchange)	1 cup
2%-fat milk (omit 1 fat exchange)	1 cup
Yogurt made from 2% fat milk (plain, unflavored) (omit 1 fat exchange)	1 cup

Whole milk (omit 2 fat exchanges)

Whole milk	1 cup
Canned evaporated whole milk	½ cup
Buttermilk made from whole milk	1 cup
Yogurt made from whole milk (plain, unflavored)	1 cup

List 2: Vegetable exchanges

This list shows the kinds of vegetables to use for one vegetable exchange. One exchange is ½ cup and contains about 5 g of carbohydrate, 2 g of protein, and 25 kcal (105 kJ).

Asparagus	Green pepper	Okra
Bean sprouts	Greens	Onions
Beets	Beet	Rhubarb
Broccoli	Chard	Rutabaga
Brussels sprouts	Collard	Sauerkraut
Cabbage	Dandelion	String beans, green or yellow
Carrots	Kale	
Cauliflower	Mustard	Summer squash
Celery	Turnip	Tomatoes
Cucumbers	Mushrooms	Tomato juice
Eggplant		Turnips
		Vegetable juice cocktail
		Zucchini

List 2: Vegetable exchanges
(continued)

The following raw vegetables may be used as desired

Chicory	Escarole	Radishes
Chinese cabbage	Lettuce	Watercress
Endive	Parsley	

(starchy vegetables are found in the bread exchange list.)

List 3: Fruit exchanges

This list shows the kinds and amounts of fruits to use for one fruit exchange. One exchange of fruit contains 10 g of carbohydrate and 40 kcal (168 kJ).

Apple	1 small
Apple juice	⅓ cup
Applesauce (unsweetened)	½ cup
Apricots (fresh)	2 medium
Apricots (dried)	4 halves
Banana	½ small
Berries	
Blackberries	½ cup
Blueberries	½ cup
Raspberries	½ cup
Strawberries	¾ cup
Cherries	10 large
Cider	⅓ cup
Dates	2
Figs (fresh)	1
Figs (dried)	1
Grapefruit	½
Grapefruit juice	½ cup
Grapes	12
Grape juice	¼ cup
Mango	½ small
Melon	
Cantaloupe	¼ small
Honeydew	⅛ medium
Watermelon	1 cup
Nectarine	1 small
Orange	1 small
Orange juice	½ cup
Papaya	¾ cup
Peach	1 medium
Pear	1 small
Persimmon, native	1 medium
Pineapple	½ cup

(Continued)

TABLE 24-10   CONTINUED

List 3: Fruit exchanges (continued)		*List 4: Bread exchanges (continued)*	
Pineapple juice	⅓ cup	*Crackers:*	
Plums	2 medium	**Arrowroot**	3
Prunes	2 medium	**Graham, 2½ × 2 in sq**	2
Prune juice	¼ cup	**Matzo, 4 × 6 in**	½
Raisins	2 tbsp	**Oyster**	20
Tangerine	1 medium	**Pretzels, 3⅛ in long by ⅛ in diameter**	25
(Cranberries may be used as desired if no sugar is added.)		**Rye wafers, 2 × 3½ in**	3
		Saltines	6
		Soda, 2½ × 2 in sq	4

List 4: Bread exchanges
(includes bread, cereal and starchy vegetables)

This list shows the kinds and amounts of breads, cereals, starchy vegetables and prepared foods to use for one bread exchange. Those appearing in **bold type** are **low-fat.** One exchange of bread contains 15 g of carbohydrate, 2 g of protein, and 70 kcal (294 kJ).

Bread

White (including French and Italian)	1 slice
Whole wheat	1 slice
Rye or pumpernickel	1 slice
Raisin	1 slice
Bagel, small	½
English muffin, small	½
Plain roll, bread	1
Frankfurter roll	½
Hamburger bun	½
Dried bread crumbs	3 tbsp
Tortilla, 6 in	1

Cereal

Bran flakes	½ cup
Other ready-to-eat unsweetened cereal	¾ cup
Puffed cereal (unfrosted)	1 cup
Cereal (cooked)	½ cup
Grits (cooked)	½ cup
Rice or barley (cooked)	½ cup
Pasta (cooked)	½ cup
Spaghetti, noodles, macaroni	
Popcorn (popped, no fat added)	3 cups
Cornmeal (dry)	2 tbsp
Flour	2½ tbsp
Wheat germ	¼ cup

Dried beans, peas, and lentils

Beans, peas, lentils (dried and cooked)	½ cup
Baked beans, no pork (canned)	¼ cup

Starchy vegetables

Corn	⅓ cup
Corn on the cob	1 small
Lima beans	½ cup
Parsnips	⅔ cup
Peas, green (canned or frozen)	½ cup
Potato, white	1 small
Potato (mashed)	½ cup
Pumpkin	¾ cup
Winter squash, acorn or butternut	½ cup
Yam or sweet potato	¼ cup

Prepared foods

Biscuit, 2 in diameter (omit 1 fat exchange)	1
Corn bread, 2 × 2 × 1 in (omit 1 fat exchange)	1
Corn muffin, 2 in diameter (omit 1 fat exchange)	1
Crackers, round, butter type (omit 1 fat exchange)	5
Muffin, plain small (omit 1 fat exchange)	1
Potatoes, french fried, length 2 to 3½ in (omit 1 fat exchange)	8
Potato or corn chips (omit 2 fat exchanges)	15
Pancake, 5 × ½ in (omit 1 fat exchange)	1
Waffle, 5 × ½ in (omit 1 fat exchange)	1

TABLE 24-10 CONTINUED

List 5(a): Meat exchages (lean meat)

This list shows the kinds and amounts of lean meat and other protein-rich foods to use for one low-fat meat exchange. One exchange of lean meat (1 oz) contains 7 g of protein, 3 g of fat, and 55 kcal (231 kJ).

Beef
Baby beef (very lean), chipped beef, chuck, flank steak, tenderloin, plate ribs, plate skirt steak, round (bottom, top), all cuts rump, spare ribs, tripe — 1 oz

Lamb
Leg, rib, sirloin, loin (roast and chops), shank, shoulder — 1 oz

Pork
Leg (whole rump, center shank), ham, smoked (center slices) — 1 oz

Veal
Leg, loin, rib, shank, shoulder, cutlets — 1 oz

Poultry
Meat without skin of chicken, turkey, cornish hen, guinea hen, pheasant — 1 oz

Fish
Any fresh or frozen — 1 oz
Canned salmon, tuna, mackerel, crab, lobster — ¼ cup
Clams, oysters, scallops, shrimp — 5 or 1 oz
sardines, drained — 3

Cheeses
Cheeses containing less than 5% butterfat — 1 oz
Cottage cheese, dry, 2% butterfat — ¼ cup

Legumes
Dried beans and peas (omit 1 bread exchange) — ½ cup

List 5(b): Meat exchanges (medium-fat meat)

This list shows the kinds and amounts of medium-fat meat and other protein-rich foods to use for one medium-fat meat exchange. For each exchange of medium-fat meat omit ½ fat exchange.

Beef
Ground (15% fat), corned beef (canned), rib eye, round (ground commercial) — 1 oz

List 5(b): Meat exchanges (medium-fat meat) (continued)

Pork
Loin (all cuts tenderloin), shoulder arm (picnic), shoulder blade, Boston butt, Canadian bacon, boiled ham — 1 oz

Liver
Heart, kidney, sweetbreads (these are high in cholesterol) — 1 oz

Cheeses
Cottage cheese, creamed — ¼ cup
Mozzarella, ricotta, farmer's, neufchatel, parmesan — 3 tbsp

Eggs and peanuts
Egg (high in cholesterol) — 1
Peanut butter (omit 2 additional fat exchanges) — 2 tbsp

List 5(c): Meat exchanges (high-fat meat)

This list shows the kinds and amounts of high-fat meat and other protein-rich foods to use for one high-fat meat exchange. For each exchange of high-fat meat omit 1 fat exchange.

Beef
Brisket, corned beef (brisket), ground beef (more than 20% fat), hamburger (commercial), chuck (ground commercial), roasts (rib), steaks (club and rib) — 1 oz

Lamb
Breast — 1 oz

Pork
Spare ribs, loin (back ribs), pork (ground), country style ham, deviled ham — 1 oz

Veal
Breast — 1 oz

Poultry
Capon, duck (domestic), goose — 1 oz

Cheese
Cheddar types — 1 oz

Processed meats
Cold cuts — 4½ × ⅛ in slice
Frankfurter — 1 small

(Continued)

TABLE 24-10 CONTINUED

List 6: Fat exchanges

This list shows the kinds and amounts of fat-containing foods to use for fat exchange. To plan a diet low in saturated fat select only those exchanges which appear in **bold type.** They are **polyunsaturated.** One exchange of fat contains 5 g of fat and 45 kcal (189 kJ).		Mayonnaise†	1 tsp
		Olives*	5 small
		Oil	
		Corn, cottonseed, safflower, soy, or sunflower	1 tsp
Avocado (4 in diameter)*	⅛	Olive*	1 tsp
Butter	1 tsp	Peanut*	1 tsp
Bacon, fat	1 tsp	Nuts	
Bacon, crisp	1 strip	Almonds*	10 whole
Cream, light	2 tbsp	Pecans*	2 large whole
Cream, sour	2 tbsp	Peanuts*	
Cream, heavy	1 tbsp	Spanish	20 whole
Cream cheese	1 tbsp	Virginia	10 whole
French dressing†	1 tbsp	Walnuts	6 small
Italian dressing†	1 tbsp	Nuts, other*	6 small
Lard	1 tsp	Salad dressing, mayonnaise type†	2 tsp
Margarine, tub or stick‡	1 tsp	Salt pork	¾ in cube

*Fat content is primarily monounsaturated.

†If made with corn, cottonseed, safflower, soy, or sunflower oil can be used on fat-modified diet.

‡Made with corn, cottonseed, safflower, soy, or sunflower oil only.

Source: These exchange lists are based on material in "Exchange Lists for Meal Planning" prepared by Committees of the American Diabetes Association, Inc., and the American Dietetic Association in cooperation with the National Institute of Arthritis, Metabolism and Digestive Diseases and the National Heart and Lung Institute, National Institutes of Health, Public Health Service, U.S. Department of Health, Education, and Welfare.

TABLE 24-11 CALORIE AND KILOJOULES PER KILOGRAM OF IDEAL BODY WEIGHT CONSIDERING ACTIVITY LEVEL AND PRESENT WEIGHT

	Sedentary		Moderate activity		High activity	
	kcal	*kJ*	*kcal*	*kJ*	*kcal*	*kJ*
Overweight	20–25	84–105	30	126	35	147
Normal	30	126	35	147	40	168
Underweight	35	147	40	168	45–50	189–210

Source: Adapted from Robert S. Goodhart and Maurice E. Shils, *Modern Nutrition in Health and Disease,* 6 ed., Lea & Febiger, Philadelphia, 1978, p. 849.

Diet Therapy

The nutritional requirements of diabetics are, in general, the same as for all individuals. Diet therapy is one of the most important factors in the management of the diabetic patient. The major aim of diet therapy for the NIDDM type of diabetic is to achieve or maintain ideal body weight; for the IDDM diabetic, the aim is to balance food intake with insulin action, while providing adequate food energy for activity and growth.

Exercise should be an integral part of diabetic management, since activity facilitates glucose entry into the cells, and therefore lowers blood sugar, as well as insulin requirements.

We will now consider in more detail some of the significant nutrients and their relationship to the diet of a diabetic patient.

Energy The decision regarding an individual's energy requirement should be based on the individual's age, height, weight, sex, activity level, and growth. A careful nutritional history should take all these factors into account. To aid in establishing an appropriate energy level some general guidelines are provided (see Table 24-11, opposite). It must be remembered that these general guidelines are to be used as an aid in planning energy levels; weight and diet should be monitored periodically with adjustments made accordingly.

Carbohydrate Recent evidence shows that as long as the total energy intake is not increased, increasing the total carbohydrate allowance does not seem to affect the insulin requirements of insulin-dependent diabetics. In the less severe, typically obese diabetic, substitution of *complex* carbohydrate (starches—breads, pasta, potato, cereal, grains) for fat does not seem to increase blood sugar or affect glucose tolerance. Furthermore, if carbohydrate is severely restricted, dietary protein and fat containing saturated fat and cholesterol will be increased to maintain the appropriate energy level of the diet. Considering the relationship between diabetes and cardiovascular disease this is not recommended. Thus, the latest recommendation for carbohydrate is that it comprise between 45 and 55 percent of the total calories. Also fiber is encouraged (see p. 564). Habitual use of simple sugars (table sugar, candy, soft drinks, etc.) is eliminated. These foods may be allowed under certain circumstances, in order to maintain the body's glucose/insulin ratio, such as prior to athletic competition or periods of vigorous exercise, or on sick days.

Protein Fifteen to twenty percent of the total food intake should be provided as protein. The diets of children and adolescents need careful supervision to ensure protein intakes of high biological value in the range of 1.5 to 2 g protein per kilogram of body weight. Patients with renal or hepatic complications may require protein restriction.

Fat Approximately 35 percent of the total food intake is recommended as fat. Polyunsaturated fat is used, and saturated fat and cholesterol are limited. (See Chap. 21.)

Food servings Once the total energy, carbohydrate, fat, and protein requirements have been determined, the amount is converted into food servings for the day, which are then spread throughout the day into 3 meals and either 2 or 3 snacks, depending on the type of management: insulin, oral hypoglycemic agents, or diet alone. With insulin therapy, the food is divided so as to match insulin activity. Current practice no longer distributes food between meals and snacks as rigidly as in the past. In the past, the total carbohydrate was calculated into very specific amounts to be consumed at certain times. The carbohydrate was divided into thirds, fifths, or sevenths at meal and snack times to match insulin activity. This often imposed hardships since it meant that a patient consumed one-half of a serving or exchange. The new system allows a more normalized meal pattern. Table 24-12 (p. 562) summarizes the calculation of a diabetic diet.

TABLE 24-12   CALCULATION OF A DIABETIC DIET

Diet calculations are based on energy needs of an overweight, sedentary diabetic weighing 72 kg.

Calories (kilojoules)

1 Determine total energy needs according to age, weight, and activity level and patient's need to lose weight. 25 kcal or 105 kJ/kg is the recommended level.

$$25 \times 72 \text{ kg} = 1800 \text{ kcal}$$
$$105 \text{ kJ} \times 72 \text{ kg} = 7560 \text{ kJ}$$

Total energy = 1800 kcal or 7560 kJ

Carbohydrate

2 Determine the total carbohydrate allowance by taking 50% of the calories or kilojoules determined above, since 50% of the energy needs may be allotted as carbohydrate in the diabetic diet.

$$1800 \text{ kcal} \times 50\% = 900 \text{ kcal of carbohydrate}$$
$$7560 \text{ kJ} \ 50\% = 3780 \text{ kJ of carbohydrate}$$

Next, determine the total grams of carbohydrate by dividing the total carbohydrate calories by 4 or dividing the total kilojoules by 16.8.

$$\frac{900 \text{ kcal}}{4} = 225 \text{ g carbohydrate}$$
$$\frac{3780 \text{ kJ}}{16.8} = 225 \text{ g carbohydrate}$$

Total carbohydrate = 225 g

Protein

3 Determine the total protein allowance by taking 15% of the calories or kilojoules determined above, since at least 15% of the total energy requirement must be allotted as protein to supply body needs.

$$1800 \text{ kcal} \times 15\% = 270 \text{ kcal of protein}$$
$$7560 \text{ kJ} \times 15\% = 1134 \text{ kJ of protein}$$

Next, determine the total grams of protein by dividing the total protein calories by 4 or dividing the total kilojoules by 17.

$$\frac{270 \text{ kcal}}{4} = 68 \text{ g protein}$$
$$\frac{1134 \text{ kJ}}{16.8} = 68 \text{ g protein}$$

Total protein = 68 g

Fat

4 Determine the total fat allowance by taking 35% of the calories or kilojoules determined above, since 35% is the level recommended to control dietary fat, yet supply energy needs.

$$1800 \text{ kcal} \times 35\% = 630 \text{ kcal of fat}$$
$$7560 \text{ kJ} \times 35\% = 2646 \text{ kJ of fat}$$

Next, determine the total grams of fat by dividing the total fat calories by 9 or dividing the total kilojoules by 38.

$$\frac{630 \text{ kcal}}{9} = 70 \text{ g fat}$$
$$\frac{2646 \text{ kJ}}{37.8} = 70 \text{ g fat}$$

Total fat = 70

Alcohol Including alcohol in the diabetic diet is at the physician's discretion. Of course, sweet mixed drinks, sweet wines, liqueurs, and aperitifs are avoided. In making the decision as to how much to include, the high caloric content of alcohol (7 kcal per g of alcohol) is a consideration. Also, since alcohol lowers blood sugar, a combination of alcohol and insulin can potentiate hypoglycemia, so alcohol when taken should be consumed with food. Alcohol with sulfonylureas oral agents can produce a harmless but disconcerting reaction (flushing, tingling of the face, etc.), and the patient should be forewarned.

Sick-day diet   On sick days, individuals are encouraged to eat in order to prevent hypoglycemia. Food is distributed throughout the day to prevent peaks and valleys of blood sugar. Sweet liquids, such as Jello or ginger ale, or soups are easy to tolerate and provide a ready source of carbohydrate. In the case of vomiting or diarrhea the patient should contact his or her physician immediately so as to avoid electrolyte imbalance and dehydration.

Travel   When traveling, food should be carried along, to circumvent delayed meals. Such portable foods as cheese and crackers or peanut butter and crackers, or any other snack providing protein plus carbohydrate, are recommended.

Special dietetic products   In food shopping, reading labels carefully provides a guide. Dietetic and diabetic foods may be costly and are often inappropriate—some "dietetic" foods are low in sodium, not sucrose. Many other "dietetic" foods may be low in sucrose but high in fat and therefore not low in calories—for example, dietetic chocolate bars.

In addition, many over-the-counter drugs contain sugar (e.g., cough syrups), and the diabetic must be taught to recognize potential sources of sugar. A sufficiently cordial relationship should exist between the individual with diabetes and the nutrition educator so that the client does not hesitate to call before buying.

New alternative sweeteners to saccharin and cyclamate are fructose and the sugar alcohols, sorbitol and xylitol.

Fructose, also known as fruit sugar or levulose, is sweeter than sucrose, and leaves no bitter aftertaste. It also causes less of a rise in blood glucose than does starch, sucrose, or glucose. In experiments replacing glucose with isocaloric amounts of fructose, diabetics were found to better utilize fructose. It has been demonstrated that children with IDDM, on a quantitative diet, can use fructose in moderate amounts without exacerbating plasma glucose.

High levels of fructose (200–500 g per day) can increase plasma triglycerides. Although some studies have not been universally confirmed, more investigation is needed. Also, after intravenous infusion of fructose, uric acid and lactate levels increase. This has not been demonstrated to occur after oral ingestion. However, it is known that fructose is rapidly metabolized in the liver to glucose and lactate. Fructose metabolism may induce lactate acidosis when hepatic clearance of peripherally produced lactate is poor.

Both sorbitol and xylitol can cause osmotic diarrhea when ingested in large amounts (30 to 50 g per day). There is no major advantage of recommending sorbitol. Xylitol shows no evidence of significantly increasing blood glucose or triglyceride levels. However, when ingested in high levels it may be associated with bladder tumors in mice. It is also toxic if administered intravenously.

No significant side effects have been demonstrated with *modest amounts of orally ingested* fructose, xylitol, or sorbitol in normal subjects and treated diabetics. However, there are no long-term studies. The possibility exists that each of these could lead to increased blood sugar in diabetics.

Education of the Individual with Diabetes

The treatment of diabetes mellitus requires diet as part of the integral treatment; thus, the nutrition education of the individual with diabetes is paramount in care.

The ability of the nutritionist to help a client to change a lifetime of eating experiences revolves around the personal meaning that the patient derives from the counseling sessions (see Chap. 10).

After diagnosis the patient must learn to cope with the threat of a long-term chronic illness and is not usually ready to hear new information, let alone integrate the information in order to make the behavioral change that is necessary. Therefore, the nutrition educator must focus first on the patient's level of need. This will vary depending upon:

Age   Education
Socioeconomic status   Culture

The nutrition educator will need to explain the following concepts during the learning program:

How food acts in the body

How food and insulin act in the body

How food and insulin act in the diabetic condition

How food, insulin, and activity are regulated in the diabetic condition

The nutrition educator should examine the patient's activity pattern to help motivate and determine an exercise program appropriate to that person's life-style (see Chap. 11).

The diabetic patient is routinely instructed as to how and when to test the urine for glucose. There are different methods for doing this, chemical and enzymatic (see Table 24-9).

The chemical methods (of which Clinitest tablets are perhaps the most widely used) are based on the fact that glucose is a reducing sugar. Copper is commonly used in the reaction—if it is reduced, there is a color change, and the amount of glucose present will determine the degree of change. Thus, these tests are quantitative. However, since other sugars within the aldehyde group are also reducing sugars, the reaction is not specific for glucose.

Testape is the popular example of the enzymatic reaction. These methods employ the enzyme glucose oxidase. Hydrogen peroxide produces the color change indicative of the presence of glucose. These methods are highly specific for glucose, but are not quantitative.

Whatever the method employed, the client should be instructed to record the results of tests, and to bring the records when making regular visits to the physician. The accuracy of the tests depends not only on the test itself, but also upon the skill of the tester.

Newer Concepts in Diabetes

Somatostatin is a polypeptide hormone that inhibits alpha-cell production of glucagon (as well as beta-cell insulin secretion) and inhibits growth hormone release. Since growth hormone has anti-insulin effects, current research is aimed at developing somatostatin into a pharmacologic agent for treating diabetics.

Research in virology has suggested several model systems in which diabetes is produced in animals via viruses. Islet cell surface antibodies have been found in serum of insulin-dependent diabetic children. The antibodies are reactive with the surface of the islet cells. It is interesting to note that insulin-dependent diabetes mellitus in children and adolescents is characterized by a dramatic decrease in glucose-induced insulin secretion and a progressive loss of endogenous insulin production that is concomitant with the disappearance of beta cells from the pancreatic islets. Epidemiologists have likewise underlined the possible link between viruses and the onset of diabetes.

Sorbitol is a sugar alcohol produced when glucose is reduced in mammalian tissues. In certain tissues (lens of the eye, liver, peripheral nerves, Schwann cells of the peripheral nerves, aorta), glucose can enter cells without the aid of insulin. Once in, it is acted on by an enzyme and converted to sorbitol. Since the sorbitol cannot leave the cell and has osmotic properties, it holds water in the cell, causing swelling and damage. Thus, sorbitol is now being considered as the cause for diabetic cataracts and a possible causative agent in diabetic neuropathy. Research is now being directed toward blocking the enzyme that allows sorbitol formation. (Dietary sorbitol is not metabolized in this fashion and has no role in cataract formation.)

Current technological and clinical research is geared toward developing methods which would provide insulin in a more continuous and need-oriented way through pancreas transplantation, islets of Langerhans transplantation, and artificial pancreas development and implantation. Artificial pancreases, in the form of insulin pumps which can be worn clipped to a belt, are currently in use. The pump steadily releases insulin via an attached needle. Work is also being conducted on cultured beta cells. Although research is not yet clinically applicable, it does offer the hope for future implementation.

Research indicates that high-fiber diets may lower blood glucose. It has long been realized that such ethnic groups as Yemenite Jews, South African Bantu, and the New Zealand Maori, whose diets are high in fiber, have a low incidence of diabetes mellitus. Moreover, when such people convert to the typically lower-fiber western diet, their incidence of diabetes mellitus increases. Generalizations are impossible, however, since conversion to western diet also generally includes conversion to western culture and its concomitant risk factors. Further, high-fiber diets may also control the caloric intake and thereby prevent obesity. There is a well-established relationship between diabetes mellitus and obesity.

A possible explanation for the blood-glucose-lowering effect lies in the fact that unabsorbable carbohydrate may limit the rise of blood glucose following a meal. Studies indicate that dietary fiber decreases the absorption of carbohydrate and peripheral insulin sensitivity or affects the release of gastrointestinal hormones which influence insulin and glucagon secretion. Some types of fiber, such as guar, slow glucose absorption. One study reported the use of guar in a diabetic diet containing 40 percent or more of the calories as carbohydrate. A reduction in glycosuria was noted. This study implies that the diabetic on a high-fiber diet may require less insulin.

Further research is required as to which type of fibrous food sources actually have a blood glucose lowering effect. Researchers experimenting with six different fiber sources conclude that the effect of fiber may be related to its composition rather than the amount consumed.

Adult Hypoglycemia

Adult hypoglycemia, defined as a plasma glucose level less than or equal to 40 mg per 100 mL, produces vague symptoms which occur several hours after meals. These include sweating, nausea, and dizziness. This reactive hypoglycemia is due to a delay in insulin secretion (as a result, the blood sugar, upon testing, is initially higher), causing insulin to be high at an inappropriate time. This is confirmed with a 5-h oral glucose tolerance test, and can be indicative of early diabetes. However, the condition also occurs after a gastrectomy, because glucose enters the intestine more rapidly, and is absorbed very quickly. In a large category of patients, symptoms are related to functional, or nonorganic, causes. A high-protein diet, low in simple carbohydrate and divided into frequent small feedings, is recommended.

BONE AND JOINT DISORDERS

Gout

As yet, the pathogenesis of gout is uncertain but the disorder is characterized by a derangement of purine metabolism. Uric acid is the end product of the metabolism of purine compounds such as nucleic acids and xanthines.

Gout, a metabolic disease with a familial tendency, is seen predominantly in men over 35 years old and occasionally in postmenopausal women. The condition is manifested by the following symptoms:

1 Hyperuricemia
2 Acute attacks of arthritis
3 Eventual degenerative and destructive changes in the joints
4 A tendency to form deposits of sodium monourate, either nodular deposits known as *tophi,* or diffuse deposits in cartilage, in tissues around joints, and around the helix of the ears

Normal serum uric acid is 2 to 6 mg per 100 mL. With gout there is an increase in serum levels to 6 to 10 mg per 100 mL; in rare cases values to 20 mg per 100 mL have been observed. High levels of uric acid are suggestive of gout but may also be attributable to renal failure, leukemia, polycythemia, multiple myeloma, or toxemia of pregnancy.

In the past it was thought that uric acid was derived solely from purines ingested in food and from the body's own tissue proteins. It is now known that metabolic precursors of urates are formed not only from endogenous and exogenous preformed purines but also from simple

TABLE 24-13 PURINE CONTENT OF FOOD

Range of purine content	Food
High (150–1000 mg/100 g)	Liver, kidneys, sweetbreads, brains, heart, mussels, anchovies, sardines, meat extract, consommé, gravies, fish roes, herring
Moderate (50–150 mg/100 g)	Meat, fowl, fish (except as noted above), other seafoods, lentils, yeast, whole-grain cereals, beans, peas, asparagus, cauliflower, mushrooms, spinach
Negligible	Vegetables, fruits, milk, cheese, eggs, refined cereals, cereal products, butter and fats (in moderation only), sugar, sweets, vegetable soups

available compounds in the body such as carbon dioxide, glycine, and ammonia, which can be synthesized into uric acid. This information makes the dietary treatment of gout less significant. However, some authorities continue to recommend diets low in purines as they feel that this influences the total metabolic pool of uric acid. Table 24-13 lists the purine content in various foods.

A high fluid intake is one dietary measure that *has* proved helpful in the treatment of gout. This increase in fluids is necessary to help eliminate uric acid, slow progressive kidney involvement, and prevent renal calculi. Coffee, tea, and chocolate contain methyl xanthines which are metabolized to methyl urates and at one time were eliminated from the diet of gouty patients. It has since been learned that these methyl urates are not deposited in the tissues and therefore the beverages are now allowed.

A high-carbohydrate diet tends to increase uric acid excretion, while a high-fat diet not only decreases excretion but actually can precipitate a gouty attack. A diet high in protein and fat is

therefore avoided. Weight control is extremely important. Although the reason has not yet been elucidated, effective weight reduction alone is likely to decrease serum urate concentration. Weight-reducing diets which cause ketosis are contraindicated since ketosis causes renal urate retention and therefore aggravates hyperuricemia. Preferably, the patient should be 10 to 15 percent below his calculated normal weight. However, sudden weight reduction and fasting can exacerbate the condition.

During an *acute* gouty attack the dietary purines should be kept to a minimum (100 mg per day) to avoid adding uric acid to the metabolic pool. A diet high in carbohydrate and low in protein and fat is recommended. Fluids should be encouraged.

The diet for the interval between attacks should be a well-balanced diet adjusted to the energy level needed to maintain the patient at his or her desired weight. Between attacks a high fluid intake, 2 qt per day, is recommended. Alcohol inclusion in the diet is controversial; it will not necessarily precipitate an attack but the usual recommendation is either to eliminate or to dilute it. Patients with gout should check with their physicians regarding use of alcohol.

Treatment of asymptomatic hyperuricemia (urate concentrations >7 mg per deciliter) includes Benemid (probenecid) a drug which promotes uric acid excretion, and sulfinpyrazone, or, for *overexcretors* (>7 mg of uric acid per deciliter of glomerular filtrate), allopurinol, which inhibits uric acid production. The use of allopurinol is controversial, since drugs which lower serum urate concentration may exacerbate gouty inflammation. However, overexcretors are more prone to renal stone formation and therefore a drug such as Benemid which promotes uric acid excretion is not desirable. When Benemid or other uriosuric agents are used, fluids plus sufficient alkalies to maintain an alkaline urine are necessary to prevent the precipitation of uric acid crystals. Alkalies such as Maalox have replaced the aklali-ash diet that was once used to maintain an alkaline urine.

Control of the inflammation which accompanies gout can be achieved by use of colchicine, indomethacin, or phenylbutazone, all of which are irritating to the gastric mucosa. To counteract this irritation, these drugs should be taken just prior to meals. Antacid therapy or bland diets are sometimes necessary. Short-term (1-week) systemic corticosteriod administration is often used for acute attacks, especially in cases where gastric ulceration contraindicates use of indomethacin or phenylbutazone.

Naproxen is a relatively new nonsteroid anti-inflammatory agent which is proving not only effective but also less irritating to the gastric mucosa than either indomethacin or phenylbutazone.

Severe gouty arthritis may necessitate the use of narcotics. Addiction is generally not a problem since narcotic use is of very short duration (first 24 h).

Research is currently geared toward developing agents which combine uricosuric activity with either anti-inflammatory characteristics or diuretic activity.

Rheumatoid Arthritis

Rheumatoid arthritis is a chronic progressive inflammatory tissue disorder of unknown etiology, resulting in stiff, sore joints, usually in the fingers, wrists, knees, ankles, or toes. The average age at onset is 35, and the incidence doubles as one nears 60. The female to male incidence rate is 3 to 1.

Negative nitrogen and calcium balance, muscle atrophy, and bone decalcification are part of the disease process. Some authorities have observed changes in carbohydrate metabolism during the active stage of the inflammatory process; however, this has not been a universal finding.

Due to a catabolic response, the patient may be underweight, and this may be further complicated by a poor food intake, especially when the disease process in the hands and the finger joints interferes with the patients' ability to feed themselves.

The anemia observed is not related to iron deficiency, but rather to a hemolytic process and as such is not amenable to iron therapy.

The dietary treatment revolves around the drugs used to control the inflammatory process, namely aspirin and, in some cases, corticosteroid therapy. The latter may necessitate a moderate sodium restriction to minimize edema. With aspirin administration, frequent small feedings are recommended to minimize gastric irritation. Aspirin should be administered after meals and in some instances a bland diet may be needed to further guard against gastric distress.

The same dietary and drug treatment is initiated with osteoarthritis.

Juvenile Arthritis

The peak age of onset in juvenile arthritis is the preschool years, and more girls are affected than boys. The clinical course of the disease is variable. Growth disturbances sometimes occur as a result of abnormal influences on the epiphyseal plate. This is an important consideration for the nutritionist monitoring diet and growth in these children. Over one-half of the children afflicted with juvenile arthritis recover completely within 1 or 2 years.

Normal nutrition, based on age, body size, and activity needs, should be considered. (Activity may be decreased substantially, thereby altering energy needs.) The child's frustration and anxiety may negatively affect food behavior, and this requires supportive management. Food may be only one area of control that the child has during an acute episode of inflammation. During this period of stress and inflammation, fever may occur, increasing basal energy needs.

STUDY QUESTIONS

1 The states of hyperthyroidism and hypothyroidism have different effect on the body's metabolism and subsequent diet therapy. Explain.

2 With corticosteroid therapy, is salt restricted? Why are frequent small meals recommended?

3 Describe the treatment approach for Cushing's syndrome and Addison's disease relating to the pathology of these conditions.

4 Differentiate between NIDDM and IDDM.

5 Describe the progressive symptomatology of diabetes from hyperglycemia to ketosis.

6 Would you recommend a low-purine diet for a client with gout?

CLINICAL STUDY 24

R. G. is a 59-year-old sedentary male executive currently undergoing his annual physical examination, which is positive for hypertension (160/100 mmHg), angina, obesity, and abnormal glucose tolerance. (His first fasting glucose was 220 mg per dL [venous plasma], and his second, 207 mg per dL.) His present height is 5 ft 10 in and his weight is 205 lb (ideal weight 154 lb).

The dietary history reveals a food intake high in cholestrol and saturated fat, and containing approximately 2800 kcal (11.76 MJ) per day. He eats frequently in restaurants, and when at home enjoys his own gourmet meals. He has 1 or 2 cocktails before his meals; however, he is not a dessert eater.

The diagnosis of NIDDM was made. He was started on Orinase and referred to the nutritionist for dietary counseling.

Clinical study questions

1 What is the major aim of therapy?

2 Calculate R. G.'s energy requirement with the proper proportions of carbohydrate, protein, and fat.

3 What life-style factors should be considered in planning his dietary regimen?

BIBLIOGRAPHY

Anderson, J. W., and K. Ward.: "Effects of a High Fiber Diet in Diabetic Patients," *Diabetes Care,* **1**(2):81, 1978.

Ballin, J. C., and P. L. White: "Fallacy and Hazard, Human Chorionic Gonadotoprin, 500 Calorie Diet and Weight Reduction," *Journal of the American Medical Association,* **230**:693, 1974.

Brunzell, J. D.: "Use of Fructose, Xylitol, or Sorbitol as a Sweetener in Diabetes Mellitus," *Diabetes Care,* **1**(4):223, 1978.

Bunn, H. F., et al.: "The Biosynthesis of Human Hemoglobin A," *The Journal of Clinical Investigation,* **57**:1652, 1976.

Cornblath, E.: "Diabetes in Childhood," *Pediatric Annals,* **4**, 1975.

"Diabetes, Epidemiology Suggests a Viral Connection," *Science,* **188**:347, 1975.

Drash, A.: "Diabetes in Childhood, a Review," *Journal of Pediatrics,* **78**:919, 1971.

Dunn, P. J., et al.: "Reproducibility of Hemoglobin A$_{1C}$ and Sensitivity to Various Degrees of Glucose Tolerance," *Annals of Internal Medicine,* **91**:390–396, 1979.

Eaton, R. P.: "Evolving Role of Glucagon in Human Diabetes Mellitus," *Diabetes,* **24**:523, 1975.

"FDA Upholds Findings of UGDP Study," *Journal of the American Medical Association,* **241**:17, 1979.

Feinstein, A. R.: "How Good Is the Statistical Evidence against Oral Hypoglycemic Agents?" *Advances in Internal Medicine,* **24**:71–95, 1979.

Goulder, T. J., and K. G. M. M. Alberti: "Dietary Fiber and Diabetes," *Diabetologia,* **15**:285–287, 1978.

Greydanus, D. F., and A. D. Hofman: "Psychological Factors in Diabetes Mellitus," *American Journal of Diseases of Children,* **133**:1061, 1979.

R. L. Jackson: "Education of the Parents of a Child with Diabetes," *Nutrition Today,* pp. 30–33, May–June 1980.

Jenkins, D. J. A., et al.: "Diabetic Diets: High in Carbohydrate Combined with High Fiber," *American Journal of Clinical Nutrition,* **33**:1729–1733, 1980.

Jirani, S. K. M.: "Does Control Influence the Growth of Diabetic Children?" *Archives of Diseases of Children,* **48**:109, 1973.

Kempe, C. H., et al. (eds.): *Current Pediatric Diagnosis and Treatment,* 3d ed., Lange Medical Publishers, Los Altos, Calif., 1974.

Koivisto, V. A.: "Fructose as a Dietary Sweetener in Diabetes Mellitus," *Diabetes Care,* **1**(4):241, 1978.

Lernmark, A., et al.: "Islet Cell Surface Antibodies in Juvenile Diabetes Mellitus," *New England Journal of Medicine,* **299**:375–380, 1978.

Meissner, C., et al.: "Antidiabetic Action of Somatostatin Assessed by Artificial Pancreas," *Diabetes,* **24**: 988, 1975.

Munoz, J. M., et al.: "Effects of Dietary Fiber on Glucose Tolerance of Normal Men," *Diabetes,* **28**:496, 1979.

National Diabetes Data Group: "Classification and Diagnosis of Diabetes Mellitus and Other Categories of Glucose Intolerance," *Diabetes,* **28**:1039, 1979.

Paxinos, R., and R. Ferguson, "Juvenile Diabetes, a Team Approach," *Journal of Human Nutrition,* **32**:294–296, 1978.

Paz-Guevara, A. T., et al.: "Juvenile Diabetes Mellitus after Forty Years," *Diabetes,* **24**:559, 1975.

Powell, G. F., and Blizzard Brasel: "Emotional Deprivation and Growth Retardation Stimulating Idiopathic Hypopituitarism," *New England Journal of Medicine,* **23**:1271, 1967.

Schmitt, B. D.: "An Argument for the Unmeasured Diet in Juvenile Diabetes Mellitus," *Clinical Pediatrics,* **14**:68, 1975.

Sestoft, L.: "Fructose and the Dietary Therapy of Diabetes Mellitus," *Diabetologia,* **17**:1, 1979.

Simkin, P. A.: "Management of Gout," *Annals of Internal Medicine,* **90**:812–816, 1979.

Silver, H. K., et al.: *Pediatrics,* 10th ed., Lange Medical Publishers, Los Altos, Calif., 1973.

"University Group Diabetes Program: V., Evaluation of Phenformin Therapy," *Diabetes,* **24**(suppl. 1), 1975.

Weininger, J., and G. M. Briggs: "Nutrition Update," *Journal of Nutrition Education,* **7**:141, 1975.

CLINICAL DISCUSSION 24

Obesity and NIDDM often go hand in hand, and often weight reduction alone will lower blood sugar and ameliorate symptoms, controlling the diabetes, not curing it. The major aim of therapy for R. G. was weight reduction. Using the criteria outlined in the chapter, his caloric and nutrient requirements approximate 1750 kcal, or 7350 kJ (70 kg $\times$ 25 kcal or 70 kg $\times$ 105kJ); and carbohydrate, 219 g; protein, 66 g; and fat, 70 g. Emphasis on a low saturated fat and low cholesterol intake along with fiber was included in dietary counseling, because of the presence of risk factors (questionable hypertension and obesity) associated with cardiovascular disease, since diabetes often affects the small and large vessels, causing atherosclerosis and circulatory complications.

R. G. was given specific advice on how to follow his diet when eating out in restaurants. His family was present to learn a total family approach and—most important—future prevention. Also, R.G. learned how to modify his gourmet recipes and how to shop, reading labels. R. G.'s physician has recommended that he limit alcohol to 1½ oz per day, which was calculated into his total calories, with no sweet mixed drinks. R. G.'s physician discontinued the Orinase when R. G. had lost 51 lb. R. G. was motivated by the fact that he wanted to discontinue this medication since he noted a flushing sensation on drinking alcohol.

Jogging was gradually instituted, with proper preconditioning under the physician's supervision. Periodic dietary follow-up was arranged.

CHAPTER 25

OVERWEIGHT AND UNDERWEIGHT CONDITIONS

Patricia A. Kreutler
Nancie Harvey Herbold
Rosanne Beatrice Howard
Peggy L. Pipes

KEY WORDS
Overweight
Obesity
Adipocyte
Prevention

INTRODUCTION

Obesity is an overriding concern, a perplexing problem of our society (see Chap. 1, Introduction). We ride to school or to the office and sit at our desks or in front of television with plenty to eat. The net result is an overweight nation imbued with anxiety about weight but doing little to prevent the problem.

The American attitude toward obesity assumes a moralistic stance, with the condition viewed as indicative of gluttony, weakness, and self-indulgence, and with thinness as a visible virtue. This puritanical, simplistic notion pervades the medical community, too, and treatment is often handicapped by it. The obese individual, especially the obese child, may be ostracized by the group and must bear the fat as a social stigma and receive the censure of all.

Society's rejection can further enhance the obese individual's use of eating as a pseudosolution to a personality problem. It is often difficult to differentiate between the psychological problems that play a role in the development of obesity and those that are a product of the obese state. Based on observations of the obese patient's ability to adjust to life stresses, Bruche has divided the population into three main groups.[1] The first group is composed of competent people who are probably heavy in accordance with their constitutional makeup, whose weight excess is not related to abnormal psychological functioning. The weight excess in this group is moderate and fairly stable; weight reduction regimens are successful or body image is accepted. In the remainder of the population, obesity is related to psychological problems. Individuals are subdivided into two groups: those with *developmental obesity,* in whom obesity is intrinsically interwoven with their whole development, which is characterized by many features of personality disturbance and disturbed patterns of family transactions; and those with *reactive obesity,* whose weight gain follows some traumatic emotional experience. In the latter two groups, overeating may serve as a defense against deeper depression. Their control over underlying anxieties may be so precarious that a "scare approach" to noncompliance with a reducing regimen can add to their difficulties, rendering them unable to maintain their fragile emotional balance and forcing them further into the obese state and deeper depression.[2]

Thus, an oversimple approach that ignores the diversity of clinical pictures presented by obese individuals can be extremely detrimental and can actually precipitate conflicts, imposing even a heavier burden than the weight. A multidisciplinary approach (doctor, nurse, nutritionist, social worker, psychologist, psychiatrist, exercise physiologist) may offer more hope for this intricate problem. However, the cure for obesity lies in its *prevention*.

Prevention of obesity calls for social acceptance of human diversity and fostering freedom and initiative in the individual. It repudiates manufactured, stereotyped ways of life and demands instead respect for human individuality.[3]

Prevention of obesity also can mean the prevention of other related diseases. Obesity is associated with diabetes, gallbladder disease, and high blood pressure. Along with other risk factors, it can contribute significantly to heart disease.

With the admonition to all future clinical practitioners of nutrition that their role is in *prevention,* this chapter in the first part explores the known causes and treatment of obesity. The middle section of this chapter examines the obese state as a clinical manifestation of Prader-Willi syndrome. This section is included because the syndrome is often misdiagnosed and the gross obesity ascribed only to environmental or social factors.

Also, obesity is a clinical manifestation of Lawrence-Moon-Biedl syndrome, Cushing syndrome, and Frolich's syndrome (hypothalamic tumor).

The last section looks at the other end of the weight spectrum, considering suggestions for the individual free from any underlying pathological condition who simply needs to gain some weight.

THE OVERWEIGHT CONDITION— THE OBESE STATE

DEFINITION

Obesity may be defined as a condition in which there is an accumulation of body fat in excessive proportion to total body mass. This concept should be contrasted with that of *overweight,* which merely indicates a weight which is greater than that assumed to be ideal or desirable, without any specific reference to body composition.

Since the body is composed of several types of tissues, including muscle, fat, and bone, each of which contributes weight to the organism, a muscular athlete may in fact be overweight yet not obese. Thus, a person who is obese is generally overweight, but someone who is overweight may or may not be obese. Most clinicians identify a person as obese, however, when he or she is 15 to 20 percent above the age-, sex-, and height-related weight norms.

ETIOLOGY

Although the overall mechanism in the development of obesity is an imbalance in energy intake versus energy expenditure, obesity is a multifactorial condition: its underlying cause is complex and not completely understood in all cases.

Much research has been undertaken to assess the importance of several factors which are thought to contribute to the imbalance, and a discussion of a few of these is in order.

Heredity

Although there are several animal strains in which obesity is an inherited trait, no such pattern has been established in humans. While it is true that obese parents often have obese children,[4] factors of life-style and attitudes toward food undoubtedly play a role in the etiology of the observed familial pattern. Some additional evidence linking obesity with genetics is provided by studies showing that identical twins, even when raised in different homes, tend to show more similar weights than do fraternal twins, even if the latter are raised together in the same environment. These types of data imply that genetic factors play a role in the development of obesity, but both their mechanisms and their relative importance are unknown. (Refer to Fig. 25-1, p. 575.)

One factor in the development of obesity that has been related to heredity is the body type *(somatotype)* passed down from parents to children. An *ectomorph* is a lean, thin person, with delicate bones and long, thin fingers; an *endomorph* is a round, "soft" individual in whom the abdominal area tends to be larger than the chest. Someone classified as a *mesomorph* has a muscular chest which is larger than the abdomen. It is very unusual for an ectomorph to become obese, and while it is not inevitable that an endomorph will be fat, the probability is quite high that this will happen unless positive steps are taken to avoid it.

Physiological and Biochemical Factors

While attempts have been made in the past to associate obesity with disturbances of the endocrine system, especially the thyroid, very few cases of obesity are caused by an underactive thyroid; moreover, hypothyroidism responds to hormone replacement therapy. Most endocrine abnormalities associated with obesity, including the hyperinsulinism observed in many patients, appear to be a consequence, rather than a cause, of the overfat condition, for they diminish or disappear following weight loss. Some researchers have suggested that the activities of certain enzymes associated with lipid metabolism are altered in some persons, but there is little concrete evidence to support this theory as a primary causative factor of obesity.

For many years there has been interest in the physiological control of hunger and satiety. Various models have been proposed to explain the signals which cause us to start and stop eating. The *glucostat* theory proposed by Mayer[5] states that a center in the hypothalamus is sensitive to the rate of glucose utilization. When food is ingested, blood glucose levels rise and glucose utilization increases; hypothalamic receptors are stimulated and send a signal to stop eating. Conversely, when glucose utilization decreases several hours after a meal, the hunger center responds and tells us to eat again.

Because the theory does not explain all the observations related to eating behavior, other models involving plasma amino acid levels, lipid stores, prostaglandins, endocrine signals, and nervous impulses have been proposed. Moreover, several studies indicate that hunger and feeding behavior are dissociated in the obese person. Schacter observed that obese subjects respond to external cues of sight, smell, and taste rather than to true feelings of hunger.[6] It is apparent that the regulation of food intake is indeed a complex phenomenon, and that its complexities are far from being understood.

A newer, somewhat speculative theory suggests that obese individuals have reduced levels of sodium-potassium-ATPase. This enzyme acts as a sodium-potassium pump, pushing these electrolytes in and out of the body's cells while burning calories and generating heat. Because of this enzyme deficiency, an individual burns fewer calories and can gain weight while consuming a moderate caloric intake. Further research is needed to determine whether there is an actual deficiency of sodium-potassium-ATPase and if this is related to the cause of the obese state or is the result of the preexisting obesity.[7]

Adipose Cell Theory

Shortly after Winick demonstrated that availability of food during growth and development affected the number and size of cells in various organs of both rats and humans,[8] Hirsch and Knittle presented evidence that both the number and size of adipose tissue cells were greater in obese than in nonobese children.[9] Studies with rats confirmed that overfeeding early in life caused hyperplasia of adipose tissue, producing an increase in the number of adipocytes which persisted throughout life.

Additional studies with obese adults indicated that the number of cells, as well as the amount of lipid contained in each cell, was increased in comparison with findings in those who were nonobese. Moreover, weight reduction decreased the amount of lipid per cell, but did not affect the number of adipose cells. Further, studies by Sims et al.[10] suggested that adult-onset obesity represents an increase in the size, but not the number, of adipocytes.

The theory that developed from these observations was that overfeeding in early life causes excessive hyperplastic growth of adipose tissue, as well as an increased lipid accumulation within each cell. According to this theory the increased cell number persists throughout life; even though weight reduction may occur later, resulting in a loss of lipid from the cells, the adipocytes remain, waiting to be refilled with fat as soon as energy intake exceeds energy output.

Although newer evidence (see Chap. 13) dispels this theory, it has helped focus attention on early intervention in the pediatric population. Several investigators questioned whether chubby infants become obese adults. Some evidence has been presented which indicates that infant obesity is correlated with obesity in childhood[11,12] and that childhood obesity predisposes to obesity in adult life.[13] A retrospective study suggested that infants' weights during the first 6 months of life correlates with their adult weights (at 20 to 30 years of age). Of those adults who were above the 90th percentile for weight as infants, 36 percent were overweight; 14 percent of the subjects who were below the 75th percentile as infants were obese as adults. Many other factors presumably were involved in this outcome, as social class, education, and parental weight were also related to adult weight.[14]

However, a prospective follow-up study from birth to age 5 of height, weight, and weight/height indices in 582 white children was carried out to determine the etiology of obesity. There were statistically significant relationships found to exist between height, weight, and ponderosity indices attained at age 5 and measurements of these indices at ages 4, 3, 2, and 1 year, at 6 months, and at birth. But approximately 70 percent of the variance in weight in ponderosity indices at age 5 could not be accounted for by measurement of weight/ponderosity during the first year of life.[15] It would appear that weight in infancy is not a predictor of adult obesity; however, obesity at age 15 seems to be a better predictor of adult obesity. Individuals overweight at this age have an 80 percent chance of becoming overweight as adults.[16] Looking for the etiology of obesity prompted nutritionists to reexamine feeding methods in relationship to obesity.

Comparative studies between breast and bottle feeding have reported that these studies showed little difference in the first 1 to 3 months. Greater weight gains were noted in the artificially fed infant from 3 to 6 months. However, weight differences are small, averaging from 200 to 500 g at the end of the first year.[17] Dine et al. did not find a difference in weight and weight/height indices between breast-fed and bottle-fed infants.[18] Another study on the effect of feeding on fat disposition in early infancy showed no significant difference in fat thickness when infants were classified by feeding methods. However, formula-fed infants, with solids started before age 2 months, had the highest mean skinfolds, which peaked at age 3 months and then decreased and became similar to those of other groups by age 5 months.[19]

Although there are unresolved questions regarding the etiology of obesity and the significance of feeding methods, obesity prevention begins at birth, and nutrition counseling regarding feeding techniques should be given during the parents' prenatal visit to the pediatrician.

Environmental and Social Factors

Several environmental factors are conducive to excessive weight gain. First and foremost is the availability of food products in our affluent society. Closely associated with this is the role of socioeconomic status in defining population groups in which obesity is common. As socioeconomic status improves, the prevalence of obesity tends to decrease.

Cultural and ethnic considerations also influence attitudes toward body size. In some cultures, being overweight is considered a sign of prosperity and contentment. The ingestion of certain types of foods, specific for a particular culture, also increases the probability of becoming obese. Another overriding attitude, seemingly unrelated to ethnic origin, is that a chubby baby is a healthy one.

Social customs also contribute to the positive energy balance that precedes weight gain. Most social occasions (weddings, funerals, holidays, or sporting events) are associated with food. In fact, it is considered rude not to offer a guest in your home something to eat or drink. This custom was perfectly acceptable, and necessary as well, when visitors arrived after a long trip; riding down the street in an automobile to visit a neighbor is hardly a trip, but the ritual of offering food as a sign of hospitality still persists.

Occupational hazards also abound in our present-day society. Business meetings over cocktails and dinner, coffee breaks, and office parties are part of our daily lives. Some students have a difficult time concentrating on homework without a snack, and study breaks may include food.

A significant change in our daily activity patterns is also responsible for the development of obesity. Not only are habits altered with age as transition is made from being a star on the high school or college athletic team to working at a predominantly "sit-down" job. Labor-saving devices have been installed in most homes and offices, the use of automobiles and public transportation has modified our mode of travel, and vertical motion can be accomplished by escalators and elevators rather than stairs. Spectator sports include a greater portion of the population than do the participatory sports.

It has been suggested that this relative lack of exercise in comparison with energy intake is the major factor contributing to the prevalence of obesity in the United States.

Regardless of its specific etiology, obesity is the result of an energy intake that exceeds energy utilization. A very fine balance between input and output must be maintained when we consider that theoretically an intake that exceeds expenditure by even 100 kcal (420 kJ) per day will result in an annual weight gain of about 10 lb (4.5 kg), since it is generally accepted that a pound of adipose tissue contains approximately 3500 kcal (14.7 MJ). Efforts at maintaining body weight at a stable level must focus on monitoring both food intake and activity patterns.

Figure 25-1 indicates some environmental (and other) factors related to the development of human obesity.

Psychological and Emotional Factors

Because food is so strongly associated with our life-styles, people sometimes tend to use it as a type of weapon. A parent who rewards a child for good behavior or a good report card with a piece of candy or chocolate cake is instilling an attitude toward food which may have far-reaching implications. Similarly, if a child's failure to eat a particular food that the parent has prepared is interpreted as "I don't love you," the child may be made to feel guilty, and may soon learn to eat in order to please others. Thus, a child can be influenced to view food as a way to manipulate, and be manipulated by, other people.

Psychological studies have not identified a particular personality type in the moderately or massively obese individual. Bruche has emphasized two traits: "the inability to recognize hunger and other bodily sensations and lack of awareness of living one's own life, as being of fundamental significance for the development of severe eating disturbances."[20] Psychological problems such as depression, anxiety, and poor self-esteem appear to be the result of the obesity—not the cause.[21] Massively obese individuals do show addictive behavior patterns. The degree of their obesity illustrates the substance abuse component of the eating disorder.[22]

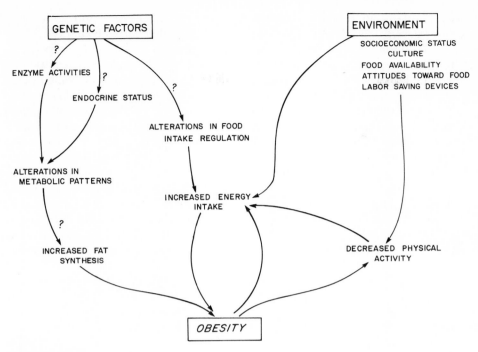

Figure 25-1
Factors related to the development of obesity.

DIAGNOSIS

There are several methods used to determine if, in fact, an overweight condition is caused by an accumulation of adipose tissue, that is, by obesity.

Physical appearance   Often the simplest and most direct way to recognize obesity is the close perusal of an individual's body, better known as the *eyeball test*. Buttons that won't button, zippers that won't zip, and steadily increasing clothes size in adults over 25 years of age indicate a weight increase that is probably caused by the accumulation of adipose tissue.

Skinfold thickness   The pinch test, in which a fold of skin and its underlying subcutaneous fat are picked up from the side of the lower chest or the back of the arm and pinched between thumb and forefinger, can also be used to assess obesity.

If the fold is greater than an inch in thickness, the individual is probably obese.

A more sophisticated and accurate pinch test has been developed, using a calibrated device called a *caliper*. This is a standardized instrument which should be used by a trained professional to ensure accurate and consistent results. Using the caliper, skinfold thickness is routinely measured at the back of the right upper arm (triceps skinfold thickness) at a point halfway between the shoulder bone and the elbow, although other sites have been used as well. The minimum skinfold thickness measurements that are indicative of obesity in Caucasian Americans are shown in the Appendix. Note that girls and women have greater values than do boys and men, and that skinfold thickness increases with age. Investigators in Sweden have defined skinfold norms for Swedish children under 3 years of age.[23] Along with skinfold measurement, arm circumference can be used to quantitate muscle, fat, and bulk. Frisancho derived from the *United States Ten-State Nutrition Survey of 1968–1970* percentiles for right upper arm circumference and triceps skinfold.[24] (See Chap. 13.)

It should be remembered that the data in the table are based on average measurements from a specific population, and also that reproducibility of measurement is extremely important yet difficult to achieve.

Height-weight tables   Charts compiled from life insurance statistics have traditionally been used in the assessment of body weight. The tables originally indicated average weights for age and height, and demonstrated an increase with age. Thus, the "recommended" or "ideal" weight increased for each age group, continuing through adulthood. We now recognize that this rate of increase is not desirable, and that average weights of an increasingly sedentary (and overweight) population are not standards consistent with overall good health. The tables are based on weights associated with the lowest mortality rates when the data were collected in 1959; they reflect the philosophy that adults should maintain their weight at a level appropriate for a 25-year-old individual. The tables (see Appendix) list a range of desirable weights for adults, allowing for differences in body frame. Unfortunately, there are no clear-cut criteria for determining whether an individual has a small, medium, or large frame; this fact imposes a limitation upon the use of these tables as an absolute guideline for an individual's desirable body weight. Nevertheless, these tables are an improvement over the original standards, and provide a rough estimate of whether a person's weight is consistent with his or her height and body frame. The Ad Hoc Committee of the New Build and Blood Pressure Study, Medical Directors of America and Society of Actuaries, is collecting data on desirable weights which will provide new guidelines.

Growth charts for children and adolescents   The presence of obesity in children, from infancy through 18 years of age, can be estimated by the use of growth charts. Rates of linear growth and weight gain are expressed in percentiles. An infant may be in the 30th percentile for length but in the 95th percentile for weight; the nutritionist should suspect that the child is being overfed, and conversation with the parents about the child's diet will probably confirm the suspicion. Similarly, feeding practices should be questioned if the child who has consistently been in the 50th percentile for weight shows a steady increase up to the 90th percentile. As with the height-weight tables used for adults, these norms do not consider factors of bone structure or body composition, but discrepancies or inconsistencies in growth patterns should be investigated.

In the past, growth charts based on data collected in Boston and Iowa about 30 years ago were used to evaluate growth patterns in children. The National Center for Health Statistics charts[25] are based on large, nationally representative samples of children, and are divided into ages 0 to 36 months, and 2 to 18 years; each age group is further subdivided by sex. These grids include weight for length and weight for stature, which aid in the assessment of obesity.

Data based on body composition   Several methods of estimating body fat content (in contrast to total body mass) are available, but because of the time and expense involved in their use, these sophisticated techniques are generally used only in a research laboratory rather than in a clinic or screening center. Determination of body density indicates the degree of fatness: since fat has a specific gravity less than that of bone or muscle (0.92 vs. 1.1), a measurement of body density (mass per unit volume) which approximates 0.92 indicates an abnormal accumulation of fat in proportion to muscle and bone. An estimation of lean body mass related to total body weight is also an indication of "fatness." Lean body mass can be measured by counting the amount of ^{40}K (a radioactive isotope of potassium) present in the nonfat cells in the body.

The best estimates of obesity are those which consider fat accumulation rather than total weight; however, many clinical situations, generally modified by time, cost, and personnel, permit only the use of tables or growth charts. If the limitations of these data are kept in mind, they are valuable to the clinician in determining whether a patient is overfat.

Diagnostic workup may include endocrine function studies.

TREATMENT

Treatment Approach

As mentioned in the introduction, a multidisciplinary approach is essential to the treatment. In order to help persons lose weight, psychological factors influencing the obese state must be identified. Weight control programs that include significant others in a person's life may help increase the success rate in treatment of obesity.[26] An example of the need to include significant

others is the slim spouse who attempts to keep a partner obese in order to maintain a feeling of superiority. This destructive pattern between husband and wife or another existing between parent and child shows the need to consider familial factors. The family meal table can be the forum for acting out neuroses. Here, food may be consumed at too rapid a pace so that individuals can get away from squabbles or food may be used as a vehicle to relieve boredom. Any successful weight control program must include consideration of all psychological factors in the complex process of weight loss and weight control.

For many, the medically oriented approach has lost appeal, and many individuals have turned to community-based programs [Weight Watchers, TOPS (which stands for Take Off Pounds Sensibly)—see Table 25-1]. Situated in neighborhood locales, these draw interest and evoke peer pressure.

TABLE 25-1 OTHER APPROACHES TO WEIGHT CONTROL

Diet	Description	Comment
Formula	Liquid formula containing carbohydrate, protein, fat, vitamins, and minerals, usually made from skim milk. Contains approximately 225 kcal (945 kJ) per 8-oz serving. Recommended intake is four 8-oz servings per day, providing 900 kcal (3780 kJ), in place of ordinary foods.	Contains no fiber, is an artificial method of eating, and is monotonous. Patients generally regain weight when they cease taking formula.
Weight groups [Weight Watchers, Diet Workshop, Take Off Pounds Sensibly (TOPS)]	Standardized energy-restricted diet is given to all participants. Weekly group meetings for encouragement and support.	Well-balanced diet but does not allow for individual differences and growth needs.
Stillman Diet		
Atkins Diet		
Mayo Clinic Diet		
Scarsdale Diet	See Chap. 16.	See Chap. 16.
Beverly Hills Diet		
Pritikin Diet		
Liquid protein		

Energy-Restricted Diets

Adults An energy-restricted diet can be planned that is nutritionally adequate and that reflects the life-style of an individual while producing a 1- to 2-lb weight loss per week. To produce a 1 lb loss of body weight per week, the individual should be in an energy deficit of 500 kcal (2100 kJ) per day. This creates a weight loss of 1 lb per week since, as stated earlier, there are 3500 kcal (14.7 MJ) (500 kcal × 7; 2100 kJ × 7) in 1 lb of body fat. The diet should accommodate cultural and religious preferences, socioeconomic level, physical activity, and age, and should meet nutrient needs for energy, protein, vitamins, and minerals. The amount of energy the adult patient must consume to achieve this weight loss can be determined by multiplying the individual's ideal body weight (in kilograms) by:

20 to 25 kcal (84 to 105 kJ) for a sedentary individual

30 kcal (126 kJ) for a moderately active individual

35 kcal (147 kJ) for a markedly active individual[27]

For example, a woman whose ideal body weight should be 55 kg and who is moderately active should consume approximately 1650 kcal (6930 kJ) (55 kg × 30 kcal or 55 kg × 126 kJ) (see Table 25-2 for sample 1600-kcal diet).

Children Like adults, each child has individual energy requirements based on body size, age, and level of activity, all of which must be considered in planning the child's weight-reducing diet. Severe restriction of food can interfere with growth potential, and a weight loss of no more than 1 lb per week is recommended for older children. An energy requirement based on height can help to provide an estimate of actual needs.[28] Through the first 2 years, the infant is given a diet based on needs per centimeter of body height. No energy deficit is promoted. The infant is given enough energy to promote growth and is allowed to grow gradually into his or her weight. The same principle applies to slightly overweight children. However, for those children who are moderately overweight or obese a caloric restriction is needed to promote a more immediate weight loss and to prevent additional distortions in body image or health problems that might occur due to an overweight condition. A child's requirement between the ages of 7 and 11 approximates 36 kcal (151.2 kJ) per inch, or 14.1 kcal (59.5 kJ) per centimeter, of body height. Once the child's energy requirement is established, 500 kcal (2100 kJ) [or 600 to 800 kcal (2500 to 3360 kJ) if inactive] can be subtracted to obtain the energy intake needed to produce a 1-lb weight loss per week.

Diet control is difficult to establish in children and requires the cooperation of all family members. The child is especially isolated when food must be restricted. Food has its own special meanings (see Chap. 11), and often a large void is caused in the child's life when the diet is imposed and special foods (cakes, candy, cookies) are removed. Activities must be planned to fill this gap. Parents must learn to establish a helping rather than a controlling relationship; they must learn to foster the control within the child rather than to control the food. They must adopt a consistent approach that utilizes some of the techniques of behavior modification and must exert patience with the child even when compliance is poor. To accomplish this approach, family therapy is often needed.

Activity is another important component of the weight control program which is often resisted by the passive, withdrawn, obese child. The child will need understanding and a gentle exercise program based on incorporating movement into the daily life-style; e.g., walking instead of riding to school, using stairs instead of elevators, playing with toys and in games that encourage body movement. Eventually, as body image improves, the child may be ready for a community- or school-based swimming program, scouting, or Little League. Recommendations must be realistic and must be based on the family's life-style.

TABLE 25-2   SAMPLE WEIGHT CONTROL DIET—1600 kcal (6720 kJ)

Food group	Servings	Carbohydrate	Protein	Fat	Energy kcal	kJ
Milk (skim)	2	24	16	—	160	672
Vegetables	3	15	6		75	315
Fruit	5	50			200	840
Breads	8	120	16		560	2352
Lean meat, fish, poultry	8		56	24	440	1848
Fat	5			25	225	945
Total					1660	7917

*Foods to avoid**

Sugar

Candy, gum

Honey

Jam, jelly

Cookies, cake, pie

Syrup

Soft drinks

Condensed milk

Fried foods, gravies

Sauces

Alcohol

Menu plan

Breakfast

8 oz	Skim milk
4 oz	Orange juice
½ cup	Bran flakes
1 slice	Whole wheat toast
1 tsp	Margarine
	Coffee

Snack

½	Grapefruit

Lunch

8 oz	Skim milk
½ cup	Tuna with 2 tsp mayonnaise
2 slices	Rye bread
	Lettuce & tomatoes
1	Peach

Snack

1	Apple

Supper

5 oz	Broiled chicken (without skin)
1 small	Potato, baked, with 1 tsp margarine
½ cup	Carrots
½ cup	String beans
1	Roll with 1 tsp margarine
½ cup	Fresh fruit cocktail
	Club soda or mineral water

Snack

4	Graham crackers
	Tea

---

*On occasion, to meet an individualized need, one or more of these foods may be planned into an energy-restricted diet.

Nutrient distribution The recommended dietary allowance for protein is 0.8 g per kilogram of ideal body weight for an adult and 1.7 g per kilogram for the school-aged child (see Appendix, Table A-1, for other age groups). This can be increased in accordance with age (for growth needs) and patient preferences without exceeding the given energy restriction.

With an energy-restricted diet, lean beef, chicken, fish, and skim milk are utilized for protein sources.

Fat provides approximately 30 percent, and carbohydrate between 45 and 50 percent, of the calories of the diet. Fat is incorporated into the diet to provide satiety but in limited amounts because of its high energy value. Carbohydrate foods are needed for proper protein utilization and to provide vitamins, minerals, and fiber. Baking and broiling are the suggested methods of food preparation.

An energy-restricted diet can usually be planned to meet vitamin and mineral requirements. However, if an individual is following a diet of 1000 kcal (4200 kJ) or less, and in energy-restricted diets for growing children, a vitamin supplement is advisable.

Total nutrient needs can be met by utilizing the food exchange system as presented under "Diabetes Mellitus" in Chap. 24. This system provides variety in the foods from the basic food groups while controlling daily intake. However, this system was not devised necessarily for weight reduction. Therefore adjustments must be made to control fat in the portion sizes. Chicken, fish, and lean meat should be stressed (see Table 25-2).

Role of Exercise

Exercise should be an adjunct of all weight-reducing programs. It increases expenditure and cardiopulmonary efficiency, tones muscles, and possibly decreases appetite in some individuals. The type and amount of exercise should be determined by the individual's previous activity patterns and current physical condition. Also, exercises that can be incorporated easily into the individual's life-style have a greater chance of success. Jogging and aerobic dancing are only two examples of accessible exercise (see Chap. 10).

Approach to Dieting by Behavioral Control

Since treatment of obesity has generally been a failure, new methods of treatment are continually being sought. Behavior modification is a technique which has been introduced into the treatment of obesity. The goal of behavior modification in this context is to change learned eating behaviors. This is accomplished by establishing an individualized program which attempts to modify eating practices (see Chap. 11).

The program starts with a description of the behavior to be controlled. For this purpose, the individual keeps daily records of the following: time of eating, place of eating, physical position when eating, social aspects of the situation, activities associated with eating, perceived degree of hunger, perceived mood, food selected, and amount consumed—both by volume and by calories.[29] Frequently, an initial weight loss will result solely from this self-monitoring process.

Antecedent conditions (also known as *discriminatory stimuli*) are environmental cues which trigger eating and must be assessed.[30,31] These antecedent conditions are also determined by food records which the patient is asked to keep for several weeks.

It must be noted that therapy does not actually begin until after the completion of these records, which are carefully scrutinized. Intervention is then based on the type of maladaptive behavior. For example, the individual who eats rapidly is instructed to put the fork down after each bite of food; for the individual who eats when bored, activities are substituted to fill the void.[32] In all behavior modification programs small changes are initially instituted and then incorporated slowly into the individual's life-style.

Reinforcement for appropriate behavior is the final component of the behavior modification program and is carried out in a number of ways. One, known as a *contingency contract,* establishes a system of rewards for the appropriate behavior. Family participation is used, especially with children, and each member is instructed on how to respond to the individual. Responses must be consistent so that changes can be incorporated into the individual's lifestyle. For long-term success, behavioral change is essential and must be associated with weight loss.[33] Ultimately, the patient should assume responsibility for his or her own behavior.[34] Self-control strategies are behavioral and cognitive techniques used to teach individuals food restraint. Clients are made to become aware of their thoughts regarding food and are taught more positive imagery as a substitute.[35]

Studies seem to indicate that there is a role for behavior modification techniques in the treatment of obesity.[36,37] Nutritionists are using behavior modification techniques. (See Chap. 11.) They are learning to conduct successful treatment groups.[38] Penick et al. compared behavior modification with group psychotherapy.[39] Therapy was conducted for 3 months with 32 obese patients. The group treated with behavior modification lost more weight than the matched control group treated with psychotherapy. These data may indicate the benefits of conducting behavior modification in a group rather than individually as had traditionally been done. The results of this study also showed that there is a range of success with behavior modification, as shown by the patients' weight losses, which ranged from minimal to maximal. However, there are few long-term studies of behavior modification programs. Those that exist do not show encouraging results.[40] But the techniques of behavior modification appear to be a tool in helping overweight individuals identify their problem behaviors. Further research is needed to develop effective weight maintenance programs.

Starvation Regimens

Starvation regimens have been used for the treatment of massive obesity. Hospitalization is usually required. During these regimens (lasting 30 days or longer) the individual is given only water (a minimum of 2 qt per day to maintain homeostasis) and a vitamin and mineral supplement (including potassium and calcium) in order to produce a state of ketosis. With starvation, the body's first physiological need is to supply the brain with adequate fuel, and all available sources of glucose are utilized. When this supply has been depleted, muscle protein and adipose tissue are metabolized to meet the body's energy requirements. Amino acids from the lean body muscle mass are deaminated and converted in the liver to glucose for use by the liver. Gradually, the body makes a metabolic adaptation to starvation, and triglycerides from adipose tissue are hydrolyzed, yielding glycerol and free fatty acids. Glycerol is converted in the liver to glucose (gluconeogenesis), but the net yield of glucose is small. The body must then rely on free fatty acids for energy. Because of the excessive rate of metabolism, these are incompletely oxidized in the liver, producing ketone bodies, water, and carbon dioxide. The ketone bodies become the major source of energy for the body, as well as for the brain, and weight loss is rapid, e.g., 1 lb per day.[41] Side effects which may accompany this type of regimen include headaches, nausea, and constipation. Biochemical alterations include elevated serum lipids and uric acid, and electrolyte abnormalities. Loss of hair, loss of muscle mass, and interference with growth in children have also been noted with starvation regimens.

The quick weight loss and reduced hunger induced by the state of ketosis make starvation regimens useful in the treatment of the massively obese patient. However, the major metabolic consequence associated with starvation is the loss of muscle protein.[42] Nitrogen is rapidly lost, initially decreasing in rate of loss during the course of the fast.[43]

Because of these side effects, the starvation regimens have been replaced by the protein-sparing modified fast in the treatment of the massively obese individual. This is discussed in the following section.

Protein-Sparing Modified Fast (PSMF)

To produce the similar large weight loss of starvation without the concomitant loss of muscle protein, investigators developed a protein-sparing modified fast. The regimen is recommended for individuals who are 30 percent or more above ideal body weight. Blackburn, one of the first investigators to use the PSMF, added protein to a starvation regime to prevent muscle loss while maintaining a state of ketosis.[44] The regimen consists of 1.5 g of protein per kilogram of ideal body weight per day in the form of animal protein (meat, fish, or chicken) which also contains approximately 1 g of potassium, one-half the potassium requirement.[45] No other food except noncaloric liquids is permitted. A multivitamin and mineral supplement including folic acid is taken daily. In addition, 5 g of sodium chloride, 25 meq of liquid potassium in the form of citrate or bicarbonate, and 800 mg of calcium are also administered daily.[46] Allopurinol is sometimes given to individuals to control ketosis-induced hyperuricemia.[47] Monitoring the individual for fluid and electrolyte imbalances, as well as for other metabolic abnormalities, is essential. During a PSMF the following biochemical changes are likely to occur:[48]

Decrease in serum insulin

Decrease in glucose concentration

Increase in free fatty acids

Increase in ketone levels

Decrease in serum cholesterol

Decrease in serum triglycerides

Decrease in total triiodothyronine

Ketonuria

Natriuresis

Kaluresis

The PSMF is not recommended for children, adolescents, women who are pregnant or lactating, or elderly people. Medical conditions that contraindicate the use of the PSMF are renal insufficiency, ischemic heart disease, congestive heart failure, liver disease, and insulin-dependent diabetes. PSMF should only be undertaken with the supervision of a physician cognizant of the side effects.

Weight loss during either a starvation regimen or a protein-sparing fast is rapid; but whether this weight loss can be maintained is questionable. Because of the frequent failure to maintain weight loss after completing a starvation regimen, more is being done to transfer the obese individual from a protein-sparing fast to an energy-restricted diet and finally to a weight maintenance plan. Behavior modification is being used in conjunction with diet to aid in weight maintenance. However, until long-term follow-up studies are done, the success of this type of treatment remains questionable.

Drugs

Because weight loss is difficult to achieve, and even more difficult to maintain, pharmaceutical agents are sometimes used to promote weight reduction. These drugs do not generally promote long-term weight maintenance and do have possible harmful side effects. *They should be used only under the supervision of a physician.* Physicians should be most discriminating in their use. Three groups of drugs are used: appetite suppressants, calorigenic agents (drugs affecting metabolism by increasing use of energy), and agents that impair intestinal absorption.

Among appetite suppressants are the classic compounds, the amphetamines. Although they cause appetite depression, their anorectic effect is relatively short-lived, and more importantly, they produce serious side effects, generally associated with their stimulatory action on the central nervous system. Among the side effects noted are addiction, insomnia, constipation, and excitability. The Food and Drug Administration has stated that amphetamines are of limited value (they often become a crutch for obese patients in their attempt to lose weight), and should be prescribed by physicians only for a short period of time and in conjunction with an energy-restricted diet.[49]

Other anorectic agents, such as phenylpropanolamine and fenfluramine, have been developed. Fenfluramine appears to exert a depressive effect on the central nervous system through the neurons that involve serotonin, producing drowsiness rather than excitability in its users. This fact will presumably reduce its potential for abuse. Studies are under way to determine the mechanism of action of fenfluramine. It appears to be an effective appetite suppressant; when it is used in conjunction with an energy-deficient diet, fenfluramine may prove to be a useful adjunct to weight reduction therapy for certain patients.

When phenylpropanolamine is used as an appetite suppressant, nasal congestants which contain the ingredient must be avoided by the individual.

Another drug, mazindol, differs from the amphetamines in suppression of appetite. It has a different action in the septal region of the brain, and has a lesser effect on blood pressure and heart rate. Also, it does not have an effect on lipid metabolism.[50]

Even though most obese people are not hypothyroid, drugs such as thyroxine and triiodothyronine affect metabolism by increasing use of energy. A weight loss does often occur; however, it is transient and the weight tends to be regained when therapy is discontinued. Severe cardiovascular effects and negative calcium and nitrogen balance have been observed in patients receiving thyroid hormones for the treatment of obesity.

Another drug used to increase the use of energy is growth hormone. It mobilizes free fatty acids without depleting nitrogen stores. However, the quantity of the hormone that is available is insufficient for adequate and conclusive testing.

Human chorionic gonadotropin (HCG) is a placental hormone that has been used in conjunction with a 500-kcal (2.1 MJ) diet for the treatment of obesity. Simeons introduced this regimen in 1954 and reported that the use of HCG reduced appetite and improved the mood of his patients.[51] However, Simeons could not dissociate the weight loss attributed to HCG from that caused by the severe dietary energy restriction.

Several studies have been carried out since Simeons' report to verify his results. Asher and Harper[52] did a double-blind study in 1973 and reported a significant weight loss in the hormone-treated group. However, Stein et al. reported that there was no statistically significant effect of HCG on weight loss over and above that related to the low-caloric diet.[53] The controversy over the effectiveness of this drug in weight reduction will undoubtedly continue. It should be remembered that hormones have been shown to be relatively ineffective in precipitating a weight loss. Their use is usually contraindicated.[54]

Drugs such as cholestyramine, diuretics, bulking agents, and belladonna are used to promote decreased absorption of ingested food or increase water loss. Their use should be discouraged, because serious fluid and electrolyte imbalances may result from their indiscrimnate use. In addition, an individual who experiments with these preparations will experience a false sense of security and accomplishment when he or she steps on the scales. Although water weight loss may have been achieved, good food habits which promote real weight loss (i.e., a reduction of adipose tissue) will not have been established. *Drugs should be used only as adjuncts to total weight reduction programs and only with certain individuals.*

For example, a study investigated the effects of combining a behavioral and pharmacological approach for the treatment of obesity. The research design established four experimental groups: routine individual treatment by a physician with the antiobesity medication fenfluramine, group behavior modification, fenfluramine use in conjunction with group behavior modification, and fenfluramine in addition to nondirective group therapy. The greatest weight loss occurred in the group whose treatment combined fenfluramine and group behavior modification.[55] The study demonstrates the positive effects of the combined treatment of an antiobesity drug and group behavior modification.

Surgery

An increasingly common approach to weight loss is intestinal bypass surgery. Because this procedure is not without risk, the careful selection of suitable patients is an important process.

The procedure should be reserved for individuals who are morbidly obese, which implies a life-threatening situation if obesity is allowed to continue, and who have been unable to lose weight by more traditional means. Weight criteria for the procedure have generally been set at more than 100 lb overweight, or double the ideal body weight. The rationale for this admittedly drastic procedure is to decrease the intestinal absorptive area so that ingested food (energy) does not gain entrance to the body.

In the original procedure, a short section of the jejunum was anastomosed to the colon, thereby bypassing the entire ileum and most of the jejunum. Extremely severe diarrhea with electrolyte depletion was an almost universal side effect. This procedure has been abandoned. One of two procedures is now generally performed. The first is called an end-to-side bypass; approximately 14 in of proximal jejunum is anastomosed to the distal ileum, leaving only 4 in of the terminal ileum above the ileocecal valve and the ascending colon. The second procedure, in which the proximal jejunum is joined to the cut end of the ileum, is called an end-to-end bypass. Either of these operations results in a 16- to 22-ft loop of intestine which is sutured closed or anastomosed to the transverse section of the colon in the respective procedures.

For most patients steady weight loss occurs for 1 or 2 years after the surgery, and then a plateau is reached. This has commonly been attributed to reactive hypertrophy of the functional bowel segment, resulting in an increase in absorptive capacity.

In addition to the observed weight loss, various clinical findings are seen; a flat oral glucose tolerance curve; steatorrhea; decreased urinary xylose; decreased serum carotene, tryglyceride, and cholesterol levels; and a decreased absorption of vitamin B_{12} (necessitating vitamin B_{12} therapy in postoperative patients).

Some of the unwanted effects of jejunoileal bypass should be mentioned. First, there is a 3 to 6 percent mortality rate associated with the surgical procedure itself. In addition, nausea and diarrhea are major problems. Negative calcium, potassium, and magnesium balances have also been reported. A serious side effect is hepatic steatosis (fat deposition in the liver). The observation that plasma amino acid patterns closely resemble those found in kwashiorkor, a condition in which fatty liver is also present, has led some clinicians to supplement the dietary intake of bypass patients with amino acids. Only limited success has been achieved, and other factors which may contribute to the pathogenesis of liver disease in these patients (accumulation of bile acids or of toxic substances produced by intestinal bacteria) have been considered.[56] Renal stones, which have been identified as calcium oxalate, are also common in bypass patients. Hyperabsorption of dietary oxalate occurs in these individuals, and has been related to intestinal and mucosal abnormalities associated with altered calcium and bile salt metabolism.

Because of the prohibitive morbidity of the jejunoileal bypass (liver failure, malnutrition, enteritis, oxalate urinary tract stones, arthritis, and osteomalacia) and the expense related to postoperative management and the symptoms of diarrhea that interfere with the quality of life, the bypass operation is no longer considered acceptable. The gastric bypass is now the surgical treatment of choice for morbid obesity. The operation involves reduction of the gastric reservoir capacity. The operation creates a gastric pouch with a capacity of 50 mL emptying into the intestine via a stoma 1.2-cm in diameter. Initially the individual is kept on a liquid diet and gradually is allowed to eat small amounts of solid food. Failure of the individual to keep to a small amount of food per feeding produces symptoms of nausea and vomiting which act as a negative reinforcement to lose weight. However, it is possible for the recalcitrant individual to gain weight by drinking high-caloric liquids such as frappes and eggnogs. Complications of the operation involve bile reflux gastritis, anastomatic leaks, stenosis, ulcerations, perforation of the proximal or distal gastric pouch, splenic injury, and dumping syndrome.[57]

A complete set of criteria for a successful candidate for gastric bypass surgery has not been agreed upon. The following seem to be most generally accepted. The candidate should be 100 lb overweight or 100 percent above ideal body weight, and should be free from esophagitis reflux and peptic ulcer diathesis.[58] There have been no consistent data to support a preoperative psychological profile of a successful candidate. The next section considers morbid obesity as part of Prader-Willi syndrome.

PRADER-WILLI SYNDROME

Peggy L. Pipes

INTRODUCTION

Prader-Willi syndrome, described by Prader, Labhart, and Willi in 1956, is a condition in which feeding difficulties such as poor sucking ability and failure to thrive in infancy are usually followed by a very rapid weight gain, resulting in obesity in early childhood.[59] The etiology of the syndrome is probably a recently discovered abnormality of chromosome 15.[60]

Other significant manifestations include hypogonadism, hypotonia, delayed motor landmarks, small hands and feet, skin problems including skin picking and easily bruised flesh, and behavior problems including temper tantrums, rage reactions, and generally destructive behavior. Intelligence ranges from severely delayed to near normal. In a survey by Holms of 76 individuals with Prader-Willi syndrome, IQ testing revealed that 12 percent were in the normal range, 29 percent in the borderline range, 41 percent mildly retarded, and 12 percent moderately retarded.[61]

Because of the hypotonia and delays in motor development, young children with the disorder tend to be inactive and, with increasing obesity, sedentary activities become preferred.

The rate of weight gain and the degree of obestiy increase with age, usually beginning as the children learn to walk and obtain their own food. Linear growth proceeds at a slow rate. Most individuals with Prader-Willi syndrome do not have an adolescent growth spurt. Most adults and adolescents with Prader-Willi are very short. Diabetes has been reported to occur commonly; however, a survey of individuals with Prader-Willi syndrome revealed an incidence of only 7 percent. Many clinicians feel that diabetes may occur less often in individuals with Prader-Willi syndrome than in the normal population with equivalent degrees of obesity.[62] Adipose tissue lipoprotein lipase levels of obese adults with Prader-Willi syndrome are generally tenfold those of normal-weight adults.[63]

Affected individuals, because of their lack of satiety awareness, usually exhibit peculiar food behavior, such as gorging and stealing food. Gorging and foraging for food are noted in a large percentage of Prader-Willi individuals. Other reported behavior problems with food include violent outbursts when food is withheld, preoccupation with food, temper tantrums, and consumption of generally unedible food products such as chicken bones, horse's vitamins, and dog food. A combination of learning problems or mental retardation along with the obesity may lead these children to have a poor self-image, manifested in tantrums, outbursts of rage, and disobedience. A successful treatment program is based on environmental control, diet, and the consideration that each child will manifest the syndrome in varying degrees and that treatment should be highly individualized. (See Fig. 25-2 on p. 589.)

ENVIRONMENTAL CONTROL

A successful program for weight control or reduction demands that all who have contact with affected individuals understand both the need to restrict energy intake and the behavioral aspect of the syndrome. The preoccupation with food that affected individuals have and their continuous effort to secure food must be viewed as a component of the syndrome and not as misbehavior. In addition, efforts to transfer the responsibility for dietary control to the individual have never been successful. Parents or caretakers must assume this responsibility, providing foods with appropriate numbers of calories, monitoring the sneaking of food, and managing any inappropriate behavior. It is important for schools, workshops, and merchants to understand that stealing food and money to buy food is common among individuals with this syndrome and that sack lunches and snacks must be locked and unavailable. The person with Prader-Willi syndrome should not enter a grocery store, enroll in cooking classes, or drop by the candy counter of the drugstore.

The family or caretakers and school or workshops must be highly motivated, willing to control the food environment by making food unavailable to these persons, and knowledgeable in, and willing to apply principles of, behavior modification. Parents, siblings, and affected individuals require support as they learn to adapt to an energy-restricted diet. Family interactions are often stressed at mealtime because of the need for constant supervision of the child with Prader-Willi syndrome. Siblings can come to resent both the attention and the fact that they cannot have certain snack foods around or that the kitchen cabinets must be locked.

An effective weight control program will require that families make food unavailable by locking refrigerators and cupboards or even putting locks on the kitchen door. It is imperative that the table be cleaned off immediately after each meal and that food remain out of reach and out of sight. The person responsible for implementation of the diet plan needs to be knowledgeable in energy values of stolen foods and should accommodate for these by making equal reductions in meal patterns.

School personnel and relatives may have difficulties in recognizing a potential problem when a child does not appear overweight. They must be included in the program to control weight. They will have to restrict the use of foods as reinforcers and carefully plan food experiences within the dietary plan for the child. Food for special occasions such as birthday parties and Halloween must be included as part of the energy intake which has been planned. Methods which have proved effective are to de-lete 50 kcal per day (210 kJ per day) from the intake for 1 or 2 weeks prior to the festivities, or to plan special low-caloric foods for these activities.

DIET

When the syndrome is diagnosed in infancy, it is possible to prevent obesity. Careful monitoring of the child's energy intakes and growth pattern can provide base-line data that can be used to design diets to prevent the very rapid rate of weight gain which usually occurs in the preschool years. If obesity is manifest then, a program to effect reduction in weight is important.

It has been suggested from carefully controlled studies which monitored food intake in relation to weight gain and linear growth that energy intake per centimeter of height is a useful reference in establishing the energy needs of children with Prader-Willi syndrome in the preadolescent years. Data from these studies have indicated that most children maintain an approximate weight and growth by consuming 10 to 11 kcal (42 to 46 kJ) per centimeter of height.[64,65] Variations in energy needs have, however, been noted among children; diets should be individually designed and adjustments in energy intakes made as children grow taller.

If attempts to prevent obesity have been unsuccessful, a goal for a slow but continuing weight loss should be established. Methods of treating obesity include a wide variety of approaches and diet plans, including an individualized low-calorie diet, protein-sparing modified fast, 1000-kcal ketogenic diet, and other hypocaloric regimens. Initial successes are often followed by regain of weight lost. Other approaches include the use of anorectic drugs, behavior therapy, bypass surgery, and a combination of several of the foregoing regimens.[66] Intakes of 8.5 kcal (36 kJ) per centimeter of height have effected losses of approximately 1 kg per month. The distribution of these calories is: fat, 20–25 percent; protein, 20–30 percent; and the remainder of the calories as carbohydrate. One study reported that early intervention with

Prader-Willi infants prevented obesity. In addition these infants, when followed to childhood, showed a mean IQ score 20 points higher than a similar group of children without early dietary intervention.[67]

Difficulties in maintaining dietary control increase as children grow older and have increased access to food. School lunch programs are often poorly monitored, and vending machines are often available with foods of questionable quality. Children often share unwanted food with their friends who have Prader-Willi syndrome. Stealing food and money to buy food increases. Children and their parents need continuing support. An interdisciplinary team approach appears to be the most effective way to manage weight control and the behavior problems associated with Prader-Willi syndrome.[68]

THE UNDERWEIGHT CONDITION

For the most part in our society, it is the overweight condition that causes the most concern, but there are also some individuals who go through life underweight when compared with growth charts or height-weight tables. These are healthy individuals who may be designated by their genes to be lean (see p. 572), or they may be very active individuals, but they are free from any pathological physical or emotional conditions that would interfere with weight increments, such as malabsorption or anorexia nervosa. They are not malnourished individuals. If these individuals are maintaining weight within their constitutional limitations, and eating appropriately for their size and activity, dietary adjustments will not alter their weight pattern.

Aside from these constitutionally lean individuals there are some individuals who are underweight because of missed meals, increased activity, or stress. If their diet is found to be inadequate, adjustments can be made in both the quality and quantity of food. High-energy-dense foods should be stressed in the diet. (Table 25-3 gives an example of a high-calorie–high-protein diet; see also Table 26-2.)

TABLE 25-3 HIGH-ENERGY HIGH-PROTEIN DIET

Approximate composition

2500 kcal (10.5 MJ)

345 g carbohydrate

110 g protein

120 g fat

Protein is increased by addition of high-caloric, high protein supplements; e.g., Sustacal

Sample menu

Breakfast

½ cup orange juice

1 slice whole wheat toast with margarine
  and jelly

1 soft-boiled egg

Tea, 1 tsp sugar

10:00 A.M. snack

8-oz milkshake

2 Uneeda biscuits, peanut butter

Lunch

½ cup cream of celery soup

Sandwich:

  2 slices whole wheat bread

  ½ cup tuna with
  mayonnaise
  lettuce & tomato

Coffee ice cream—½ cup

Vanilla wafers

Tea, ½ cup milk, 1 tsp sugar

2:00 P.M. snack

8-oz eggnog

4 arrowroot biscuits

Supper

4-oz baked meatloaf with plain gravy

Mashed potato with margarine or gravy

Baked hubbard squash with margarine

Fruited gelatin with cream

8 oz milk

Bedtime snack

Cornflakes with 1 cup milk, sliced
  peaches, and 2 tsp sugar

With infants and children whose weight problems can be attributed to a poor intake stemming from parental ignorance, poverty, abuse, or anxiety about obesity, or from the child's finicky food likes and dislikes, nutritional intervention must be holistic. Plans must be made to alter the environmental conditions interfering with the provision of adequate meals.

Adolescent boys are particularly self-conscious about being underweight. Weight is closely tied to their athletic performance and prowess. They often need assurance about the appropriateness of their height to weight ratio. Because of their increased energy demands for growth and physical exercise, extra calories may be needed to promote weight gain.

For the healthy individual who needs to gain weight, small amounts of nutrient supplements may be added to improve intakes; however, large amounts can promote diarrhea or possibly increase renal solute load (Table 25-4 lists dietary supplements). Homemade frappes and milkshakes are a more economical way to increase the energy in the diet than those products made available through drug companies. Always when using supplements or high-energy dense foods, interference with mealtime appetite should be watched.

TABLE 25-4   DIETARY SUPPLEMENTS

Brand (major ingredients)	Carbohydrate, g/L	Protein, g/L	Fat, g/L	kcal/L (kJ/L) estimate	Comments
Sustacal (liquid) (sucrose, concentrated sweet skim milk, corn syrup, soy oil, sodium and calcium caseinate, soy protein plus vitamins and minerals)	138	60	23	1000 (4200)	6 g lactose/12 fl oz 14.4 meq Na/12 fl oz may be used as a tube feeding
Meritene (liquid) (concentrated sweet skim milk, corn syrup solids vegetable oil, sodium caseinate, sucrose), vitamins, minerals	115	60	33	1000 (4200)	May be used as a tube feeding formula
Eggnog (egg, milk mixture)	129	52	30	994 (4175)	Delmark brand made with whole milk
Sustagen (powder) (powdered whole milk solids, calcium caseinate, Dextrimaltose, dextrose, vitamins, and iron)	300	105	15	1750 (7350)	3 cups Sustagen powder + 3 cups water = 1 qt (1 L) may be used as a tube feeding
Carnation Instant Breakfast (powder) (similar design to Sustagen)	140	70	36	1200 (5040)	4 packages powder, plus 1 qt whole milk
Controlyte (powder) (enzymatic hydrolysate of corn starch; polysaccharides, vegetable oil)	143	0.08	48	1008 (4234)	Concentrated source of kcal; essentially protein-free; low in electrolytes
Ensure (soy and casein isolate, corn oil, corn syrup solids, vitamins, minerals)	145	37	37	1060 (4452)	460 mosmol may be given orally (variety of flavors— orange, vanilla, cherry, strawberry, etc.) or as tube feeding; lactose-free

STUDY QUESTIONS

1 Differentiate between the terms *obesity* and *overweight*.

2 Discuss the various etiological theories proposed to explain the obese state.

3 Describe the methods of weight reduction that would be contraindicated in the treatment of obesity.

4 What type of surgical intervention may be offered to the patient who is morbidly obese?

5 What are the presently accepted treatment methods for obesity?

6 Why is control of the environment essential in planning the weight reduction diet of the child with Prader-Willi syndrome?

7 What suggestion would you offer to parents of such a child to help facilitate environmental control?

8 On the basis of the recommendations given in this section, plan a diet for Andrea (Fig. 25-2). She is 8 years old, weighs 34.4 kg, and is 129.6 cm tall.

9 Discuss when it is appropriate to use dietary supplements.

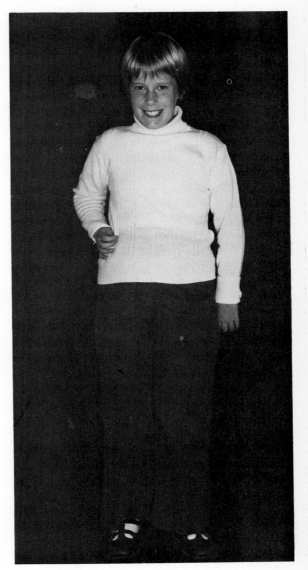

Figure 25-2
Opposite: An 8-year-old child with Prader-Willi syndrome controlled within 18 lb of the appropriate weight for her height, as a result of a positive reinforcing, controlled environment, and a total family approach.

CLINICAL STUDY 25-1

Christopher is a 7½-year-old who was brought to the school nurse by his second-grade teacher who noted that the boy was short of breath while playing during the recess period.

The nurse recorded his height at 132 cm and weight at 64.9 kg, which represented a weight gain of 4 kg since school had begun. On the suggestion of the school nurse the child was brought by his parents to the Children's Hospital Weight Control Clinic.

The history revealed a child of a normal preg-

nancy and delivery with a birth weight of 3.5 kg. Weight increments were normal until about age 4. The family history was negative for obesity. The parents were professors at a local college and extremely academically oriented. Chris's mother had returned to teaching and continued her Ph.D. program when Chris began attending preschool.

After school Chris is left in the care of a baby-sitter except for two afternoons per week when he goes to religioun classes and music lessons. He is an extremely bright boy who enjoys reading and has little time for or interest in physical activity.

On physical examination adiposity in the mammary region was noted. His abdomen was pendulous, with white and purple striae, and his penis was submerged in pubic fat. Blood pressure was 130/85 mmHg taken with a normal-size sphygmomanometer. Anthropometric data showed Christopher's height to be at the 90th percentile and his weight to be off the NCHS growth grid for 7-year-olds. He was approximately 34 kg overweight. Skinfold measurement was 30 mm (at the 95th percentile for 13-year-olds). Laboratory tests included thyroid function tests; a complete blood count; blood glucose; serum choles-

terol, potassium, chloride, sodium, pH, carbon dioxide, alkaline phosphatase, and 17-ketosteroids; urine sugar; blood urea nitrogen; and wrist x-ray for bone age determination. All tests were within normal limits.

A diet history was difficult to obtain since Chris often gets himself off to school and is left in the care of the baby-sitter after school. A diary kept by his mother showed his total food intake to approximate 1700 kcal (7140 kJ).

The diagnosis of exogenous obesity, causing slight hypertension, was made on the basis of anthropometric data, blood pressure, and normal laboratory findings. The parents' attitude was one of resistance and denial, and they repeatedly inquired about the possibility of endocrine disturbance.

Clinical study questions

1 What influences do you think have prompted the development of the child's obese state?
2 What type of program would you recommend?
3 Could this problem have been prevented? How?

REFERENCES

1 H. Bruche, *Eating Disorders: Obesity, Anorexia Nervosa and the Person Within,* Basic Books, Inc., Publishers, New York 1973, p. 124.
2 Ibid., p. 128.
3 Ibid., p. 387.
4 J. Mayer, "Obesity: Causes and Treatment," *American Journal of Nursing,* 59:1732–1736, 1959.
5 J. Mayer, *Overweight,* Prentice-Hall, Inc., Englewood Cliffs, N.J., 1968, pp. 20–21.
6 S. Schacter, "Obesity and Eating. Internal and External Cues Differently Affect the Eating Behavior of Obese and Normal Subjects," *Science,* 161:751–756, 1968.
7 M. DeLuise, G. L. Blackburn, and J. S. Flier, "Reduced Activity of Red-Cell Sodium-Potassium Pump in Human Obesity," *New England Journal of Medicine,* 299:1017–1022, October, 1980.
8 M. Winick, J. A. Brasel, and P. Rosso, "Nutrition and Cell Growth," in M. Winick (ed.), *Current Concepts in Nutrition,* vol. 1, *Nutrition and Devel-*
opment, John Wiley & Sons, Inc., New York, 1972, pp. 49–97.
9 J. Hirsch and J. L. Knittle, "Cellularity of Obese and Nonobese Human Adipose Tissue," *Federation Proceedings,* 29:1516–1521, 1970.
10 E. A. Sims, E. S. Horton, and L. B. Salans, "Inducible Metabolic Abnormalities During Development of Obesity," *Annual Review of Medicine,* 22:235–250, 1971.
11 E. E. Eid, "Follow-up Study of Physical Growth of Children Who Had Excessive Weight Gain in the First Six Months of Life," *British Medical Journal,* 2:74–76, 1970.
12 P. Asher, "Fat Babies and Fat Children," *Archives of Disease in Childhood,* 41:672–673, 1966.
13 J. K. Lloyd, O. H. Wolf, and W. S. Whelan, "Childhood Obesity: A Long-Term Study of Height and Weight," *British Medical Journal,* 2:145–148, 1961.
14 E. Charney, H. C. Goodman, M. McBride, B. Lyon, and R. Pratt, "Childhood Antecedents of Adult Obesity. Do Chubby Infants Become Obese Adults?" *New England Journal of Medicine,* 295:6–9, 1976.

15 M. S. Dine et al., "Where Do the Heaviest Children Come From? A Prospective Study of White Children From Birth to 5 Years of Age," *Pediatrics,* **63**:1–7, 1979.

16 William H. Dietz, "Treatment of Obesity in Children and Adolescents," *3rd Annual Nutrition Symposium, Dietitians in Pediatric Practice,* May 5, 1981, Children's Hospital Medical Center, Boston, Mass.

17 J. N. Himes, "Infant Feeding Practices and Obesity," *Journal of the American Dietetic Association,* **75**:122–125, 1980.

18 M. S. Dine et al., op. cit.

19 A. G. Ferris, V. Beal, M. J. Laus, and D. W. Hosmer, "The Effect of Feeding on Fat Deposition in Early Infancy," *Pediatrics,* **64**:397–401, 1979.

20 H. Bruche, op. cit., p. 50.

21 G. R. Leon, "Personality and Morbid Obesity Implications for Dietary Management through Behavior Modification," *Surgical Clinics of North America,* **56**(6): 1013, December 1979.

22 Ibid.

23 P. Karlberg, I. Engstrom, H. Lichtenstein, et al., "Development of Children in a Swedish Urban Community. A Prospective Longitudinal Study. III. Physical Growth During the First Three Years of Life," *Acta Paediatrica Scandinavica,* Supplement, **187**:48–66, 1968.

24 A. R. Frisancho, "Triceps Skin Fold and Upper Arm Muscle Size Norms for Assessment of Nutritional Status," *American Journal of Clinical Nutrition,* **27**:1052–1058, 1974.

25 National Center for Health Statistics, "NCHS Growth Charts, 1976," *Monthly Vital Statistics Report,* **25**(3), suppl. (HRA) 76-1120, Health Resources Administration, Rockville, Md., 1976.

26 J. P. Grarat, "Obesity: A Family Problem," *Obesity and Bariatric Medicine,* Viewpoint, **8**:178, November–December 1979.

27 R. Goodhart and M. Shils, *Nutrition in Health and Disease,* 5th ed., Lea and Febiger, Philadelphia, 1973, p. 849.

28 V. Beal, "Nutritional Intake," in R. W. McGammon, *Human Growth and Development,* Charles C Thomas, Publisher, Springfield, Ill., 1970, pp. 77–78.

29 H. A. Jordan, "A Behavioral Approach to the Problem of Obesity," paper presented at the Behavior Modification Workshop, Philadelphia, October 1974.

30 Ibid.

31 L. S. Levitz, "Behavior Therapy in Treating Obesity," *Journal of the American Dietetic Association,* **62**:2, 1973.

32 Ibid.

33 H. A. Jordan, op. cit.

34 R. B. Stuart and B. Davis, *Slim Chance in a Fat World: Behavioral Control of Overeating,* Research Press, Champaign, Ill., 1972.

35 G. R. Leon, "The Behavior Modification Approach to Weight Reduction," *Contemporary Nutrition,* **4**:8, 1979.

36 H. A. Jordan and L. S. Levitz, "Behavior Modification in a Self-Helf Group," *Journal of the American Dietetic Association,* **62**:27, 1973.

37 L. S. Levitz and A. J. Stundard, "A Therapeutic Coalition for Obesity: Behavior Modification and Patient Self-Help," *American Journal of Psychiatry,* **131**:4, 1974.

38 S. B. Penick et al., "Behavioral Modification in the Treatment of Obesity," *Psychosomatic Medicine,* **23**:49, 1971.

39 B. Paulson et al., "Behavior Therapy for Weight Control: Long Term Results of Two Programs with Nutritionists as Therapists," *American Journal of Clinical Nutrition,* **29**:880–888, August 1976.

40 T. G. Wilson, "Current Status of Behavioral Treatment of Obesity," *National Institutes on Drug Abuse, Research Monograph Series,* June 1979, pp. 202–223.

41 G. F. Cahill, "Physiology of Insulin in Man. The Banting Memorial Lecture 1971," *Diabetes,* **20**:785–799, 1971.

42 G. Blackburn, "Adaptation to Starvation," in *Intake: Perspectives in Clinical Nutrition,* Eaton Laboratories, Norwich, N.Y., 1973, pp. 5–6.

43 G. B. Forbes and E. J. Drenick, "Loss of Body Nitrogen on Fasting," *Journal of Clinical Nutrition,* **32**:1570, August 1979.

44 Blackburn, op. cit., pp. 3–5.

45 B. Bistrian, "Clinical Use of a Protein-Sparing Modified Fast," *Journal of the American Medical Association,* **240**(21):2299–2302, 1978.

46 Ibid.

47 M. D. Willard, H. W. Griffith, G. G. Harrison, and W. L. Roberts, "The Protein-Sparing Fast: Its Place in Office Practice," *Journal of Family Practice,* **6**(3):659–660, 1978.

48 B. Bistrian, op. cit., pp. 2299–2302.

49 U.S. Food and Drug Administration, *FDA Bulletin,* Rockville, Md., December 1972.

50 "Drug Therapy in Obesity: Part I. Round Table Discussion," *Obesity and Bariatric Medicine,* **8**: November–December 1980.

51 A. T. W. Simeons, "The Action of Chorionic Gonadotrophin in the Obese," *Lancet,* **2**:946, 1954.

52 W. L. Asher and H. W. Harper, "Effects of Human Chorionic Gonadotrophin on Weight Loss, Hunger, and Feeling of Well-Being," *American Journal of Clinical Nutrition,* **26**:211–218, 1973.

53   M. R. Stein, R. E. Julis, C. C. Peck, W. Hinshaw, J. E. Sawicki, and J. J. Deller, "Ineffectiveness of Human Chorionic Gonadotropin on Weight Reduction: A Double-Blind Study," *American Journal of Clinical Nutrition*, 29:940–948, 1976.

54   R. S. Rivlin, "Therapy of Obesity with Hormones," *New England Journal of Medicine*, 292:26–29, 1975.

55   A. J. Stunkard, "Behavioral Treatment of Obesity the Current Status," *International Journal of Obesity*, 2:237–248, 1978.

56   D. H. Lockwood, J. M. Amatruda, R. T. Moxley, T. Pozefsky, and J. K. Boitnott, "Effect of Oral Amino Acid Supplementation on Liver Disease After Jejunoileal Bypass for Morbid Obesity," *American Journal of Clinical Nutrition*, 30:58–63, 1977.

57   W. R. Jewell and J. L. McLean, "Workshop II— Comparative Assessment of Jejunoileal and Gastric Bypass," *Journal of Clinical Nutrition*, 33:525, February 1980.

58   L. J. Howard and A. I. Mendeloff, "Workshop I— For Whom Is Surgical Treatment Desirable and Undesirable?" *American Journal of Clinical Nutrition*, 33:523, February 1980.

59   V. A. Holm, "The Diagnosis of the Prader Willi Syndrome," in V. A. Holm, S. Sulzbacher, and P. L. Pipes (eds.), *The Prader Willi Syndrome*, University Park Press, Baltimore, Md., 1980.

60   G. Guanti, "A New Case of Rearrangement: Chromosone 15 Associated with Prader-Willi Syndrome," *Clinical Genetics*, 17:423–427, 1980.

61   Ibid.

62   Ibid.

63   R. S. Schwartz, J. D. Brunzell, and E. L. Bierman, "Elevated Adipose Tissue Lipoprotein Lipase in the Pathogenesis of Obesity," in V. A. Holm, S. Sulzbacher, and P. L. Pipes (eds.), *The Prader Willi Syndrome*, University Park Press, Baltimore, Md., 1980.

64   P. L. Pipes and V. A. Holmes, "Weight Control of Children with Prader-Willi Syndrome," *Journal of the American Dietetic Association*, 62:520–524, 1973.

65   V. A. Holmes and P. L. Pipes, "Food and Children with Prader-Willi Syndrome," *American Journal of Diseases of Children*, 130:1063, 1976.

66   P. L. Pipes, "Nutritional Management of Children with Prader Willi Syndrome," in V. A. Holm, S. Sulzbacher, and P. L. Pipes (eds.), *The Prader Willi Syndrome*, University Park Press, Baltimore, Md., 1980.

67   K. A. Crnic, S. Sulzbacher, J. Snow, and V. A. Holm, "Preventing Mental Retardation Associated with Gross Obesity in the Prader-Willi Syndrome," *Pediatrics*, 66:787–789, 1980.

68   P. L. Pipes, op. cit.

CLINICAL DISCUSSION 25

The increments in weight appeared to date from the mother's return to work and Chris's entrance into preschool. Examination of the family dynamics showed that Chris had been a somewhat overprotected, infantilized child whose dependency had been fostered until that time. Thus, Chris had to cope with the stress of separation and the parents' expectation that he achieve academically, which rose when he entered the first grade. He turned increasingly to food to relieve his anxiety. Another factor promoting the obese state was his extreme inactivity; he rode the bus to and from school, and read or watched television or went to sedentary types of lessons after school.

Intervention was based on the multidisciplinary team's decision that counseling which centered around family dynamics was imperative before dietary measures could be introduced. The fact that the parents' denial was so strong that it was the school nurse and teacher who initaited the referral was a significant issue. Food could not be taken away from the child without establishing the family support system that he needed. Alterations in the family's life-style to allow time for attention and activity for Chris meant that family cooperation was mandatory. In addition, the parents would have to overcome their negative and rejecting attitudes about obesity and would have to look to "the person within" Chris.

Unfortunately, this did not happen. Despite the extensive endocrine workup (laboratory analysis) the parents could not accept the diagnosis. As a result of their reaction, Chris was lost to follow-up.

If Chris had continued in the program, a 1300-kcal (5460-kJ) diet, which provided 500 kcal (2100 kJ) less than the 1800 kcal he needed on the basis of his height, would have been introduced, along with a gentle exercise program that included daily walks. With Chris's increasing physical tolerance and a stimulation of interest in activities by family example, more exercise would have been incorporated. Also, behavior modification techniques would have been simultaneously introduced as part of management.

Early recognition of Chris's problems by the parents and an open rather than a negative attitude might have prevented the problem. It is an amazing paradox that these otherwise liberal and intelligent parents could not accept the diagnosis. In this respect, much to the detriment of their child, they mirror our American hostile cultural attitude which regards even a mild degree of obesity with disdain and repulsion.

CHAPTER 26

NUTRITION IN NEUROLOGICAL DISORDERS AND IN THE CARE OF THE DISABLED

Rosanne Beatrice Howard
Linda Fetters
Dorothy M. MacDonald

KEY WORDS
Neurotransmitter
Failure to Thrive (FTT)
Anorexia Nervosa
Developmental Disability
Handicapped Adult
Primitive Oral Reflexes
Muscle Control
Muscle Tonus
Positioning
Breck Feeder
Beniflex Feeder

NUTRITION IN THE TREATMENT OF DISORDERS OF THE NERVOUS SYSTEM

Rosanne Beatrice Howard

INTRODUCTION

The nervous system organizes, integrates, monitors, and controls all of the activities of the body. Vital to body function, the system is afforded protection by bone structure, meninges, cerebrospinal fluid, and the blood-brain barrier, which prevents foreign substances from entering the cerebrospinal fluid. However, the high degree of specificity of the nervous system makes it more vulnerable to alterations in metabolism, especially to changes in levels of oxygen and glucose. The finding that minerals (calcium, magnesium, sodium) and vitamins (thiamin, pyridoxine, nicotinic acid, ascorbic acid, and vitamin B_{12}) are needed for adequate nerve cell function established the relationship between diet and the nervous system. This relationship is reinforced by research on the effects of early malnutrition on the brain (see Chap. 13) and the accumulating evidence that dietary intake of certain amino acids and other substances can have a direct effect on the synthesis and release of neurotransmitters in the brain and thus on brain function.

This chapter considers the response of the nervous system to diet and the use of diet in the treatment and rehabilitation of individuals with conditions affecting the nervous system. Later sections discuss motor control and its relationship to feeding, and present special feeding techniques for use with the handicapped individual and for the child with a cleft lip and palate.

THE NERVOUS SYSTEM

Function

The nervous system is divided anatomically into two primary components: the central and the peripheral parts. The *central nervous system* is composed of the *brain* and the *spinal cord*. The *peripheral nervous system* lies outside of the skull and the vertebral column and is composed of the spinal and the cranial nerves. The peripheral nervous system is subdivided further into the *somatic system,* which supplies the skin and skeletal muscles, and the *autonomic system,* which supplies impulses to smooth muscle, cardiac muscle, and the glands of the body, which functionally interrelate closely with the nervous system. (For example, at least two glands, the adrenal medulla and the pituitary, secrete their hormones in response to nerve stimuli.) Overall, the autonomic nervous system helps to control arterial pressure, gastrointestinal motility and secretion, urinary output, sweating, body temperature, and other body functions. In turn, the hypothalamus, one of the major areas of the brain, controls the autonomic nervous system, and also regulates body weight, fluid intake, and food intake. The role of the hypothalamus, as one of the neural centers for the control of the quantity of food intake, is considered in Chap. 25.

The nervous system is formed by two types of cells:

Neurons. The excitable, conductile units
Glia. The connective, supportive, and nutritive units

Neurons are present throughout the nervous system, with 90 percent located in the brain. It is estimated that 10 billion neurons make up the system and that the glia outnumber the neurons 10 to 1. The number of functioning units increases during development, peaking at maturity. With age, nerve cells grow old and die, and the population of neurons irrevocably declines.

The neurons are varied in size and shape but possess certain common characteristics. Each neuron contains a cell body or soma, which gives rise to one or more extensions or processes that serve to connect the cell body to other neurons and the central nervous system or to an organ. These processes are structurally and functionally of two types: the *axon,* extending from the cell body into the peripheral nerve (which conducts impulses away from the cell body), and the *dendrites,* relatively short projections of the soma serving as the receiving portions (which conduct impulses toward the cell body).

The glia cells occupy the space between neurons and are considered to have a connective, supportive, and nutritive role for the neurons they enclose. Some glia cells, known as the *oligodendrocytes,* form myelin, which makes up the sheath that may surround the axons and dendrites. (Both types of processes may develop a sheath or remain without one.) The myelin sheath is composed of layers of fat, protein, polysaccharides, water, and salt, and increases the speed of impulses along the axon or dendrite. These cells that form the myelin are particularly sensitive to a variety of diseases, which are known as the demyelinating diseases, e.g., multiple sclerosis. The major lipids in myelin are cholesterol, cerebrosides, cephalins, and sphingolipids. The lipid component of the sheath is also subject to change in those genetic disorders known as the lipidoses.

Whole neurons (cell body, axon, dendrite) may be *afferent,* conducting impulses toward the brain (as in the sensory portion of the brain), or *efferent,* conducting impulses away from the brain (as in the motor portion of the system), or they may be *internuncial* or *associative* neurons found between afferent and efferent neurons. The junction between neurons is known as the *synapse,* which is the site of impulse transmission. These areas of connection are functional, not an anatomical continuity. The passage of an impulse across a synapse is chemically mediated by substances, called *neurotransmitters,* that are present in the neurons. When the neurotransmitters are released, the neuron transmits signals across synapses or to muscle cells, or secretory cells outside the brain transmit impulses to efferent neurons within the brain. Each neuron is thought to release only a single type of neurotransmitter which either excites or inhibits the impulse, depending upon its biochemical effect on the postsynaptic neurons, or those with which it makes contact. When the impulse arrives at the axon ending, the chemical substance is released from small vesicles located in the branched ends of the axon (telodendria). Once released, the chemical diffuses across the space between the two neurons (synaptic cleft) and either depolarizes the next neuron or inhibits depolarization. The chemical is then destroyed by an enzyme or by oxidation.

About 20 to 30 chemicals are presently thought to function as neurotransmitters released by one or more sets of brain neurons, and others may be discovered. There are six compounds that are fairly well established as brain neurotransmitters: *acetylcholine; gamma-amino butyric acid;* the three catecholamines, *epineph-rine* (or *adrenaline*), *norepinephrine,* and *do-pamine;* and *serotonin.* These transmitter substances, with the exception of acetylcholine, are derived from amino acids or are amino acids themselves and as such are closely dependent on nutrient intake. Research indicates that at least three major kinds of neurotransmitters are affected by diet: acetylcholine, serotonin, and the catecholamines, such as dopamine and norepinephrine.

The Effect of Diet on Brain Function

Research by Wurtman and Fernstrom on rats has indicated that following a meal high in carbohydrate, there is an increase in the rate of synthesis of serotonin (5-hydroxytryptamine), the best studied of all the brain products.[1,2] Serotonin is produced in the body tissues (the major loci are the brain and the gastrointestinal system). In the brain all the serotonin present is confined to a group of neurons known as the raphe nuclei, whose cell bodies are located in the brainstem, and whose nerve fibers ascend into the rest of the brain and descend down through the spinal column. It has been proposed that serotonin is involved in avoidance learning, the effects of hallucinogenic drugs, sleep, sensitivity to pain, the control of food intake, and the release of pituitary hormones.

Serotonin is produced from the amino acid

tryptophan, which is carried to the brain through the bloodstream by a transport protein. Tryptophan has difficulty in competing with the other neutral amino acids for a transport protein. However, the insulin secreted by the pancreas in response to a high-carbohydrate diet assures tryptophan of a carrier protein, for it facilitates the uptake of all the neural amino acids except tryptophan, thus increasing the relative concentration of tryptophan in the blood and allowing it access to a transport protein and passage into the brain. The increased concentration of brain tryptophan then accelerates the synthesis of serotonin in the brain in response to the high-carbohydrate diet.

It is hypothesized that diet-induced changes in the concentration of serotonin in the raphe nuclei would be paralleled by changes in the amount of serotonin released into the synapses when the neurons transmit impulses. These serotoninergic neurons would therefore function as sensors, converting a signal that is circulating in the bloodstream into a statement in brain language, thereby conveying messages about peripheral metabolism. The long-term and the short-term consequences of diet changes are manifested by the plasma amino acid pattern, and also, since the serotoninergic neurons are known to be associated with a number of neuromechanisms, messages about growth, development, and stress are transmitted.

In addition to its effect on serotonin, the diet also influences the rates of synthesis of acetylcholine, produced in the brain from choline, and of the catecholamines, which are synthesized from the neutral amino acid tyrosine.

According to Growdon and Wurtman, this general principle provides a new strategy for designing treatment for nonnutritional neurologic and psychiatric diseases in which physicians may wish specifically to increase cholinergic, serotoninergic, or catecholaminergic tone. Already choline and lecithin have been used to suppress choreic movements in tardive dyskinesia and may be effective in treating some individuals with Huntington's disease and Friedreich's ataxia. Lecithin and choline are being tested in patients with dementia of the Alzheimer type with memory disturbances and in people with mood disorders such as mania.[3]

In addition, nutritional factors may play an important role in the aging process of the central nervous system by influencing brain neurotransmission or by accelerating or retarding geriatric changes in the central nervous system structure.[4]

The Effect of Emotions on Brain Function

The effect of the emotions on neurohormonal function has been subject to debate centering on two conditions with major nutritional implications: nonorganic failure to thrive, which is observed in the young child, and anorexia nervosa, which usually appears during adolescence or the young adult years.

Failure to Thrive (FTT) without Organic Reason

Growth and development are dependent on the fulfillment of the physical, emotional, and sensory needs of the child. The effects of each of these determinants are closely interrelated with one another. Deprivation of the child, whether deliberate, as with child abuse, or otherwise, as through ignorance, manifests itself in growth failure, malnutrition, and delays in motor and social development. Spitz and Wolf first noted this deleterious effect in their study of institutionalized infants.[5] In describing the anaclitic depression suffered by these children, they noted loss of appetite and weight, insomnia, greater susceptibility to infection, and gradual decline in developmental quotient. Whether the failure to thrive is related primarily to the caloric deprivation, as proposed by Whitten,[6] or is due to the effect of emotional deprivation on the pituitary, by working through the hypothalamic-pituitary axis to inhibit the secretion of growth hormone,[7] is difficult to determine.

The disorder becomes apparent somewhere between the ages of 9 and 18 months. The infant is usually withdrawn and anorexic, and may be involved in self-stimulatory behavior, including rumination. The toddler has a shallow emotional response and solemn aspect. A voracious appetite, pica, or proclivity to fluids, and a protuberant abdomen further characterize these children. Weight (and sometimes height) lies consistently below the 3d percentile for age or rapidly crosses percentiles downward.

Upon hospitalization or transfer to a different home environment, most children begin to thrive. Again, is it the food, or is it the presence of tactile, vestibular, and emotional stimulation? This underlying question has yet to be answered, but in clinical practice failure to thrive exists as a mixed entity. A treatment plan which considers all aspects—the child's nutritional, emotional, and physical needs—must be devised.

Intervention may pose a threat to parents, who fear condemnation or adverse judgment, sometimes causing them to react in a defensive or hostile manner, especially when asked about the child's daily food intake.

With hospitalization, the child's weight may make immediate increments or accrue only after a prolonged period. A regular daily caloric intake should be maintained during this period, as well as a diet based on age, with energy and protein needs related to expected height and weight. To increase the protein or energy content of the diet, formulas can be adjusted to 25 kcal/oz by changing the formula dilution (with caution, so as not to impose stress on kidneys or GI tract), adding energy supplements (see Table 23-4), or using dietary supplements (see Tables 25-4 and 26-2). With the use of supplements, care must be taken so that the child's mealtime appetite is not overwhelmed. Also these children initially may not recognize satiety and may need to have limits set on the amount of food they eat.

Many of these children had problems in the neonatal period with sucking, stooling, or sleep patterns. Recognition of these early signs and providing the parents with practical and emotional support during this period can help to establish an enduring parent-infant bond and possibly ameliorate or prevent this syndrome. Some infants are difficult to feed because of subtleties inherent in their own makeup, and parents need to be relieved of their guilt and assured that the problem is not their fault.

Infants particularly at risk for failure to thrive are those with prolonged hospitalization from birth. The setting of neonatal intensive care can prevent the parents or nurses from holding, nurturing, and stimulating the infant in an optimal manner, leading to environmental deprivation. Rumination is reported as a new complication of neonatal intensive care.[8] Early intervention consists of a variety of techniques intended to increase the infant's awareness of his or her environment and caretakers. Long-term follow-up of children with nonorganic FTT, even if successful intervention is made, indicates that they are at risk of having permanent stunting of growth, impairment of intellectual functioning, and behavioral disturbances.[9]

Anticipatory guidance directed to the period after hospital discharge helps parents to understand that feeding problems may continue because of the child's negative perceptions of food, and that time, consistency of approach, and understanding are needed on their part to work out these problems. Data suggest that stress in the household and lack of familial and social ties in the family of the child with nonorganic failure to thrive make social programming critical to ensuring nutritional well-being. Parents are often as needy as the child, and health professionals should direct care accordingly.

Anorexia Nervosa

Since the classic descriptions of Gull[10] and Lasegue[11] over 100 years ago, the attempts to explain anorexia nervosa with one psychoanalytic theory have imposed stereotyped images on a vastly complex picture. The concept that the condition was an expression of repudiation of sexuality dominated earlier clinical thinking. The modern psychoanalytical approach has turned from this symbolic concept and now focuses on the nature of the parent-child relationship from its beginning and on behavior and attitudes not directly related to food, although the preoccupations with food and weight are the characteristic manifestations of this condition.

The disorder mainly afflicts teenage girls from middle- to upper-class families who show an obsession to avoid overeating, hyperactivity, and denial of fatigue. The eating disturbance has two phases: the absence or denial of the desire for food, and uncontrollable impulses to gorge, usually without hunger awareness and followed by self-induced vomiting. Electrolyte imbalances and malnutrition resulting from the compounded effect of starvation, self-induced vomiting, and the abuse of laxatives has led to fatality in some cases.

Weight loss, amenorrhea, constipation, abdominal pain, and unusual growth of hair on the body are physical symptoms which have led some researchers to consider the syndrome primarily as a malfunction of the neuroendocrine system localized in the hypothalamus. This has led to the exploration of the role of neurotransmitters and the catecholamine, dopamine, to explain the combined changes in anorexia nervosa,[12] and to subsequent trials of antidepressants such as amitriptyline, which has been found to produce short-term success in some patients.[13] However, that a psychological origin of the illness causes the secondary physiological disturbances is the theory that presently continues to prevail.

In attempts to comprehend the behavior problems of the patient and to reconstruct the patterns of family interaction, Bruch identifies the major issue as a struggle for control and for a sense of identity, competence, and effectiveness.[14] The early history usually reveals an exceptionally healthy, cooperative, academically successful, model child. There is usually a recognizable time of onset, commensurate with an event that makes the patient feel "too fat" and prompts the self-imposed diet.

Because of distorted body images, these individuals continue to see themselves as fat. Nutritional rehabilitation of the malnourished state is a difficult task that is wholly dependent on the psychological treatment of the illness to overcome these negative perceptions and normalize food intake. The recovery period is a long and arduous process, sometimes requiring hospitalization for 6 months to a year. Management issues are complex, as these individuals are knowledgeable about food and are extremely manipulative of their energy intake and expenditure. The dietitian's role is dependent on the treatment approach used. Different modes of treatment, using psychoanalysis, behavior modification, and drugs, singly or in combinations, are employed in various centers around the country. Bruch warns that despite transient weight increases with behavior modification techniques, an approach that focuses on this treatment method without attention to the severe underlying psychological problems is potentially damaging.[15]

A new population of anorexics is young athletes.[16] These athletes, under pressure and anxious to reduce fat, starve to optimize their performance. This can lead to a pathologic degree of food and fatness aversion. Body wasting is severe enough to be diagnosed as anorexia nervosa.

A close relative to anorexia, and a possible forerunner, is a condition called *bulimarexia.* The victims alternately gorge themselves on food and then vomit. Bulimarexics are usually young women; however, it is estimated that 5 to 10 percent are men. The disorder is most likely to affect those with a food compulsion who have already lost weight. Bulimarexics are often popular, successful women whose lives center on the binge. They use food to help cope with their constant struggle to be the ideal woman. Although bulimarexics come from a variety of economic backrounds, they share common personality traits. They are attractive, intelligent individuals with great potential but a very poor self-image. They crave attention and recognition and are described as people-pleasers and perfectionists.

In an effort to become thin, bulimarexics can cause themselves irreversible physical damage such as internal bleeding, torn digestive tracts, infected salivary glands, and severe stomach cramps. Group support, individual therapy, and behavior modification is used to help bulimarexics learn to deal with the underlying anxieties causing them to binge and purge.

The Effect of Diet on Psychiatric Disorders

The use of pharmacologic doses (called orthomolecular therapy) of vitamins (e.g., niacin and vitamin C) to treat depressive anxiety and schizophrenia first gained popularity during the 1920s and 1930s, when niacin deficiency with the dementia of pellagra existed in the institutionalized mental patient and niacin therapy was the appropriate treatment for the deficiency state. Since that time there has evolved a field of orthomolecular psychiatry.[17] The practitioners of orthomolecular therapy administer large doses of vitamins to provide what they believe will be optimum concentrations for mental functioning. This treatment is based on their hypothesis that mental illness is caused by a defective enzyme that slows the rates of chemical reactions, and that the best way to overcome the condition is to increase greatly the availability of a required vitamin. Except for certain inborn errors of metabolism, there is an absence of data supporting the use of megavitamins in the treatment of psychiatric illness. An exception is the small percentage of severe alcoholics who develop Wernicke-Korsakoff syndrome. This neurological and psychiatric disorder responds to large doses of thiamin because of the somewhat increased requirement for that vitamin related to alcohol consumption. There have been no well-controlled studies to support the use of large doses of vitamins. Another treatment approach for psychiatric disorders involves the use of allergy diets and, in particular, the use of a gluten-free diet for the treatment of schizophrenia. The results are inconclusive.[18]

Although the role of diet in the treatment of mental illness awaits further elucidation, the diet of all patients suffering from psychiatric disturbances should be reviewed for adequacy, since anorexia or bizarre food preferences may be interfering with an individual's getting essential nutrients. Also, treatment medications for psychiatric disorders can inhibit certain nutrients (see the table on pp. 400–401).

The monamine oxidase inhibitors (MAOIs —e.g., pargyline, phenelzine, nialamide, tranylcypromine, and isocarboxazid) used to treat depressive, anxiety, or phobic states cause significant elevations in blood pressure when foods or beverages rich in tyramine are consumed by MAOI-treated patients.[19] The action is indirect; the combination of the food and medication releases norepinephrine and epinephrine from body storage sites, resulting in tachycardia, severe hypertension, heachaches, and nausea. The individual taking MAOIs should avoid tyramine-rich foods and beverages (see Table 26-1). Aged cheese is the most common offender; protein foods undergo putrefaction (proteolysis, whereby tyramine results from decarboxylation of tyrosine). Individuals on MAOIs should eat only fresh food or freshly prepared, frozen or canned food.

THE CHILD WITH DEVELOPMENTAL DISABILITIES

At any point in the life cycle, the brain is vulnerable to insult, but never more so than during the course of development. Problems due to gene abnormalities (e.g., hereditary diseases such as inborn errors of metabolism; see Chap. 27) or those occurring during embryogenesis which are related to sporadic preconception changes in germ cells (e.g., Down syndrome, multiple congenital anomalies) or later during pregnancy (e.g., fetal malnutrition, fetal alcohol syndrome [see Chap. 15], plasma insufficiency, toxemia, drug addiction) or at birth (e.g., prematurity, trauma, hypoglycemia, hyperbilirubinemia) or during early childhood (e.g., complications of infection, tumors, cranial trauma) may result in physical handicaps accompanied in many instances by mental retardation. The following section highlights areas that are important to the nutrition, care, and treatment of the handicapped child; however, much research is needed on which to base clinical intervention. A collaborative study between several university-affiliated training centers for developmental disabilities will soon provide some of the needed information.

Although the causes of developmental disabilities are numerous and varied, the growth and developmental milestones of childhood can act as common denominators to help parents and professionals recognize behavior apart from the condition, set appropriate goals, and develop a consistent instead of an overbenevolent approach to feeding.

Feeding these children often requires special remediation techniques (see "Feeding the Handicapped Child," and "Feeding the Child with a Cleft Lip and Palate," later in this chapter) and always requires an understanding that food to this child might not necessarily symbolize love. Because of prolonged hospitalizations, and gavage feedings or forced feedings, food may

TABLE 26-1   TYRAMINE-RICH FOODS*

Beverage	Alcoholic beverages: namely, ale, beer, chianti, sherry Caffeine sources: coffee, tea, colas, hot chocolate
Dairy	Cheese (except cottage cheese) Cheese-containng foods (pizza, macaroni and cheese) Sour cream Yogurt
Fruit, vegetable	Avocado, banana, figs, raisins Pods of broad beans (fava beans)
Meat, fish, fowl	Aged game, bologna, canned meats, pates, pepperone, pickled herring, salami, sausage
Miscellaneous	Chocolate, meat extracts (Marmite, Bovril, Offal), papaya products including meat tenderizers, raw yeast or yeast extracts (homemade yeast breads), soup cubes, soy sauce, vanilla

*Sources: Adapted from: C. L. Ravaris et al., "Use of MAOI Antidepressants," *American Family Physician,* **18**:105–111, July 1978; and *Diet Manual,* Massachusetts General Hospital, Little, Brown and Co., Boston, Mass., 1976.

possibly come to symbolize frustration or conflict to the child, an attitude around which a whole host of feeding behavior problems may develop. These must be separated from the organically based feeding problems. (see Clinical Study and Discussion 11).

Rumination is found in many severely retarded children; it involves the regurgitation of previously swallowed food and then the reswallowing of it, providing a form of self-stimulation. It is often initiated by placing the fingers in the mouth or throwing the head back with the tongue extended, causing the child to ruminate and perpetually exude a sour odor. Treatment involves programmed, brief social behavior reinforcers[20] and the thickening of feedings.

Growth

To the clinician working with an organically handicapped or mentally retarded child, the understanding of somatic growth is difficult. There is much confusion over the relationship between brain damage and growth. An anthropometric study of 678 handicapped children by Pryor and Thelander helps somewhat to elucidate an understanding of the growth deviations that can occur.[21] They found that growth was most adversely affected in children with Down syndrome that was caused by a chromosomal aberration, next in those with multiple congenital anomalies that were apparently due to prenatal environmental insults during embryogenesis, and less in those with cerebral palsy due to birth injury or severe hypoxia at birth. To elucidate growth deviations further, they propose a helpful analogy, namely a time clock. This time clock sets off a chain reaction that encompasses implantation, differentiation of tissues, growth, and development in both prenatal and postnatal life. It seems that interference with the time clock distorts growth specifically and according to when the interference occurs. Thus, the growth of a child with Down syndrome, caused by a chromosomal aberration which has occurred early on the time clock, is more adversely affected than the growth of a child with cerebral

palsy, which represents a later period after normal gestation.

In the majority of cases, the basis for poor physical growth will not be clearly known, and despite nutritional intervention children will grow within constitutional limitation. However, the clinician must not be satisfied with assuming that poor physical growth is completely due to the brain damage of the child. A detailed evaluation of the present and past food intake may provide additional clues to poor physical growth. For example, a vitamin or trace mineral (e.g., zinc) deficiency may be compromising growth in a child with a limited food intake. In this regard, severely handicapped children receiving maintenance tube feeding require careful diet supervision.

Energy Needs

Energy needs for this population of children should be determined according to body size (calories per centimeter of body height) and motor status. With regard to motor status, one study by Culley and Middleton surprisingly showed that the type of motor dysfunction did not noticeably affect the energy needs of these children except as a factor interfering in their ability to walk. Children whose motor dysfunction was severe enough to prevent ambulation required approximately 75 percent as many calories as ambulatory children of comparable height. In this study, whether the child had hypotonia, ataxia, spasticity, or choreoathetosis (see definition, p. 606), energy needs were the same per centimeter of body height and were related to the degree of ambulation.[22] A detailed food diary that is kept for a 2-week period, with the energy intake compared with the weight lost or gained, can begin to give a clue to the child's energy needs, providing the child is not edematous. Underweight and overweight are the two conditions which most demand nutritional intervention.

When it is determined that a child is underweight due to dietary inadequacy or increased energy needs brought on by the condition, calories can be increased by adding nutrient supplements to the diet (see Table 26-2; see also Tables 23-4 and 25-4). Large amounts of any one supplement are not recommended due to their effect on satiety (causing the child to refuse subsequent feedings). In addition, large amounts of a supplement can lead to symptoms of intoler- ance or, in the case of high-protein supplements such as powdered milk or evaporated milk, can impose a burden on the kidneys. Several small meals (six throughout the day) will help the handicapped child who fatigues easily.

Weight reduction should follow the same principles as outlined in Chap. 25—however,

TABLE 26-2 WAYS TO INCREASE CALORIES AND NUTRIENT INTAKE

Food	Energy	Uses	Nutrients supplied
Wheat germ	25 cal/tbsp	Cereals, baked goods, meat loaf, casseroles	Thiamin, vitamin B_6, niacin, fiber, folacin, iron
Powdered skim milk	25 cal/tbsp 95 cal/¼ cup	Beverages, meat loaf, soups	Calcium, protein, riboflavin, niacin, vitamins A and D
Corn oil	125 cal/tbsp	Vegetables, soups, casseroles	Vitamin E
Mayonnaise	65 cal/tbsp	Salads, sandwiches	Vitamin E
Evaporated milk	25 cal/tbsp	Beverages, soups, casseroles	Calcium, niacin, vitamins A and D, protein, riboflavin
Sweetened condensed milk	65 cal/tbsp	Beverages	Calcium, protein, riboflavin, niacin
Peanut butter	95 cal/tbsp	Spread	Niacin, protein, folacin, vitamin E
Egg yolk	60 cal/yolk	Meat loaf, soups, beverages, casseroles	Protein, niacin, vitamins A and E
Cream, heavy	55 cal/tbsp	Beverages, soups, casseroles	Vitamins A and E
Raisins*	25 cal/tbsp	Snack, desserts, cereals	Fiber, small amounts iron
Prunes*	70 cal/4 prunes	Snack, desserts	Fiber, iron, vitamin A
Cheeses, hard: American Swiss Cheddar	100 cal/oz	Snack, sandwiches, casseroles	Protein, calcium, vitamin A, niacin, riboflavin

*These foods tend to stick to teeth, and should be served only when teeth can be properly cleaned afterward.

Source: J. M. Borkowski and A. L. Emmerich, *Nutritional Care of the Young Child with Cerebral Palsy,* Developmental Evaluation Clinic, The Children's Hospital Medical Center, Boston, Mass., October 1980.

with the understanding that a more severe caloric restriction may be needed with a nonambulatory population to achieve weight loss and that food may be the central focus in the developmentally disabled child's life. So before imposing the dietary restrictions, other social outlets should be found, along with help from a physical therapist to increase any possible exercise.

There are certain syndromes causing developmental disabilities which affect hypothalamic control, such as Prader-Willi syndrome and Laurence-Mion-Biedl syndrome. Gross obesity is the subsequent result. The reader is referred to the section on Prader-Willi syndrome in Chap. 25.

Feeding Problems

Besides altering growth and energy needs, the handicapping condition can pose obstacles to accomplishing the developmental tasks of childhood. A child needs head support, trunk support, and sitting balance, eye-hand coordination, and the ability to grasp, hold, and release objects before feeding independence can be established. If the child's ability and readiness to progress are recognized, the handicapped child may achieve some level of feeding independence. The following areas can be commonly identified as problems for which an individualized solution must be sought:

Sitting balance

Head and neck control

Lip control

Tongue control

Sucking, swallowing, chewing, drinking

Mouth sensation (lack of mouth sensation or hypersensitivity to temperature changes or tactile stimulation)

Startle reflex (a child with cerebral palsy may respond to a loud noise with a startle reflex)

This is further discussed under "Feeding the Handicapped Child," below.

Pain and fatigue may present additional obstacles to feeding. A brief period of relaxation before meals may be helpful, and small, frequent feedings rather than large meals may impose less stress. A weak, lethargic infant who is sleeping for long periods should be awakened at appropriate intervals for feeding; otherwise, important energy needs will not be met. Initially the child might be fed earlier than other family members until he or she is ready to join the family meal without demanding too much attention. All family members should be shown the special feeding techniques so that the responsibility does not fall always to one member. Everybody concerned with feeding the child should adopt the same approach, using the *same words* at the *same time* in the *same place* with the *same utensils*. All will need the discipline to maintain a calm, friendly attitude, for overreacting to negative behavior by shouting, forcing, or cajoling only serves to reinforce the behavior.

Drugs

The use of drugs may also interfere with feeding, causing drowsiness, altering taste, interfering with appetite (amphetamines), or promoting an insatiable appetite (steroids). Drugs also affect nutritional status through their influence on nutrient absorption, gastrointestinal flora, electrolyte balance, and metabolism. Anticonvulsant drugs, which are commonly used in this population, are known to produce folate deficiency and may increase a child's need for vitamin D. Low serum folate levels and megaloblastic anemia have been associated with diphenylhydantoin therapy and also with phenobarbital and primidone.[23] Children taking these medications should be monitored through periodic complete blood counts (CBC). Rickets has been reported in mentally retarded children receiving long-term anticonvulsant therapy. Factors influencing this state are related to the number of anticonvulsants taken, the size of dosage, the child's mobility, and exposure to sunlight.[24] It is postulated that these drugs induce hepatic enzymes which degrade vitamin D.[25] Children who are receiving long-term anticonvulsant drug therapy should therefore have periodic determinations of serum calcium, phosphorus, and alkaline phosphatase. (See also the table on pp. 400–401, for other diet-drug interactions.)

Ketogenic Diets

When anticonvulsant medications prove ineffective, ketogenic diets have been used successfully in controlling intractable myoclonic and akinetic seizures in some patients.[26] A ketogenic diet is one which promotes the formation of ketones in the body (see Chap. 5) and is formulated with fat as the major energy source, with protein to meet the recommended allowances, and with carbohydrate severely restricted. Traditionally, to induce ketosis, a 3:1 ratio of fat to carbohydrate and protein was planned. Since the advent of medium-chain triglycerides (MCT), a greater ketogenic effect has been induced by providing 50 to 70 percent of the calories as MCT Oil.[27] The rapid absorption and metabolism of MCT is the explanation given for this effect.

The need for strict compliance makes this diet easier to facilitate in the very young or severely retarded child.[28] Food must be weighed or measured accurately to control the proper proportions of carbohydrate, protein, fat, and MCT Oil. Urine must be tested daily to monitor the degree of ketosis.

Additional Concerns

Increased metabolic demands from stress, fever, or underlying disease states are further nutrient considerations, along with the need to monitor fluid balance closely, a particular problem in patients with mechanical feeding difficulties or an inability to respond to thirst or to express needs. Bowel and bladder problems related to neuromuscular deficits and leading to constipation and urinary tract infections are prevalent and in many instances can be ameliorated by diet intervention. For example, a child with myelomeningocele (a congenital defect in the closure of the vertebral column) who has impaired bladder and bowel control may derive benefit from a high-fiber diet for constipation, (see Chap. 4), along with fluids and an acid-ash diet (see Chap. 23) or medications to control urinary tract infections. Vitamin-mineral supplementation is often advisable to ensure nutrition in many handicapped children, whose food intake may be unpredictable.

We now consider two conditions that are representative of the spectrum of this population of handicapped children and the types of nutritional intervention that should be offered—namely, Down syndrome and cerebral palsy. This discussion should serve as a conceptual basis for evaluating the nutritional needs of other children with handicaps or developmental disabilities. By analyzing the effect of the condition on growth, feeding ability, nutrient effectiveness, and motor activity, a nutritional care plan can be determined for every handicapped child.

Down Syndrome

Down syndrome (trisomy 21) is a chromosomal aberration involving the presence of an extra chromosome 21. (When chromosomes are examined, they are sorted and numbered from 1 to 22, plus the sex chromosomes X and Y.) In a small percentage of the population, the chromosomal disorder may be an autosomal translocation or mosaicism. Moderate to mild mental retardation, growth retardation, hypotonicity, bridged palate, and a narrow nasal passage are characteristic symptoms with feeding implications. The incidence of other congenital defects (e.g., heart defects, pyloric stenosis, tracheoesophageal fistula) is high in this population, further complicating management.

Growth deficits are marked, with the rate of gain in stature being deficient during all intervals between birth and 36 months of age, and most notably between 6 and 24 months of age, when it is as much as 24 percent lower than normal. Assessment of growth of the child with Down syndrome may be carried out with reference to charts plotting 10th to 90th percentiles based on these data.[29] Cronk has shown that 30 percent of the Down syndrome children already have excessive weight for length relations by 3 years,[30] so the use of these charts to determine ideal body weight for a child would be misleading. The charts can be used to determine how the child with Down syndrome is growing in relation to other children with the syndrome.

Hypotonicity of the muscles is a finding in all of the children; however, the degree of involvement varies considerably. Some children may have difficulty with sucking or later with chewing because of muscle weakness (usually found in the Down infant with congenital heart defects) and will need remediation techniques (see "Feeding the Handicapped Child" below), while others have no problems at all. Congenital heart disease is common in this population. Depending on the severity of the condition, the infant can experience feeding problems associated with the heart condition (respiratory distress, fatigue; see the section on congenital heart disease in Chap. 21) along with those feeding problems associated with the hypotonicity of the oral musculature.

A narrow palate also may hinder feeding as it can interfere with a proper seal for sucking and it provides an area for food to accumulate. The tongue of the child with Down syndrome is normal in size; however, it projects and appears larger because the hypotonicity affects control of the tongue muscles, and the small premaxillar area makes the tongue seem larger when protruding. Many children are mouth breathers because of a narrow nasal passage and have heavy nasal secretions, a condition to which they seem prone. Children must be trained to clear the nose of exudate and to keep the mouth closed during eating. Although tooth eruption is delayed in children with Down syndrome, food progressions can be established on the basis of developmental readiness.

The hypotonicity, which affects activity, and the growth deficits of children with Down syndrome make the incidence of obesity quite high (30 percent overweight by 3 years), and energy needs are better expressed in terms of body height (calories or kilojoules per centimeter of body height) than in terms of the recommended dietary allowances for children according to age group.[31] Parental concerns about weight can lead them to overly strict dietary control and the child to subsequent nutrient deficits. Counseling must be directed to appropriate amounts of food based on height. Also, with these children food can easily be used as a social reinforcer, and since some children do not seem to recognize their own satiety, they can quite easily be overfed.

Hypotonicity also affects muscle control of the bowel, and impaired peristalsis and constipation are frequently found in individuals with Down syndrome.

Another consistent finding in Down syndrome has been a markedly reduced serotonin level in the peripheral blood, prompting investigation to find a suitable etiological explanation. Attempts to alter this metabolic pathway by treatment with 5-hydroxytryptophan and pyridoxine have resulted in conflicting and contradictory interpretations which await further research. (It is interesting to note that serotonin, which was described earlier, is proposed to play a role in food control and that satiety is often a problem found in individuals with Down syndrome.)

A disturbance in vitamin A metabolism and an association to the frequency of respiratory and gastrointestinal[32] infection also await elucidation.

Early intervention programs with a nutritional and nursing component direct attention to normalization of the feeding experience. Parents who are overwhelmed by the birth of a child with Down syndrome need help to recognize the normal developmental aspects of feeding so that as their child achieves one developmental level, they can foster progression to the next, from baby foods to table foods to mealtime independence. Table 26-3 summarizes the guidelines used for feeding stimulation of the infant with Down syndrome between birth and 6 months in the Early Intervention Program of the Developmental Evaluation Clinic at Children's Hos-

TABLE 26-3   GUIDELINES FOR AN EARLY FEEDING STIMULATION PROGRAM*

For children with Down syndrome from birth to 6 months

Positioning	Hold the child upright, head well supported, slightly downward (never back). Bottle should be tilted so that the neck of the bottle is filled with milk.	*Stimulation (continued)*	Encourage the infant to use the hands by placing them around the bottle; as the infant develops, holding the bottle independently can be encouraged (normal skill at 9 months). When the child is ready to take over, use a small 4-oz clear plastic bottle, which will be easier for the child to manipulate.
Equipment	Nipples should be appropriate to the child. There is a range of shapes and degrees of softness to suit the child; however, nipples should remain firm. Bottles also vary from the standard 8-oz glass bottle to nursing systems such as the one put out by Playtex with a plastic pouch that can be squeezed gently during feeding to encourage intake. The type of bottle should be determined by the needs of the child.	*Baby food*	As the child begins to suck the fingers, place a small amount of strained fruit on the fingers occasionally during the feeding to let the child begin to learn that fingers come to the mouth with food. When feeding baby foods, place small amounts on the end of the baby spoon (small bowl, Teflon-coated) and insert it toward the center of the tongue with a slight downward pressure. Allow the child to swallow before presenting another mouthful. Do not rush. Bring the spoon from different sides during the feeding, encouraging the child to follow with eyes.
Stimulation	Cue into the infant's behavior and feed accordingly: 1. When the infant is hungry 2. When the infant is full Cuddling, comforting, and talking to the infant should be part of all feeding situations. As the child develops awareness, naming foods and the food color, size, and shape can help to provide meaningful stimulation.		As the child develops head control and can lateralize the tongue (move it from side to side), gradual increments in texture can begin and the cup can be introduced.

*If the infant is able, breast feeding is encouraged and intervention is given accordingly.

Source: Developmental Evaluation Clinic, Children's Hospital Medical Center, Boston, Mass.

pital Medical Center, Boston (see Fig. 26-1). One interesting observation made in the Early Intervention Program at Children's Hospital Medical Center was that parents were not able to encourage independence in feeding skills as readily as in other areas of development and appeared to be hesitant to relinquish this dependency.[33]

Pipes and Holm found that most of the nutritional and feeding problems found in the Down syndrome population were prevented or remedied by an interdisciplinary intervention program. However, while the incidence of obesity was reduced, it was not eliminated.[34]

Cerebral Palsy

The term *cerebral palsy* designates neurologic disorders created by damage to the motor centers of the brain that occurs before, during, or shortly after birth. Physical handicaps range from mild to severe and intelligence from normal to subnormal. Various types of neuromuscular problems characterize this condition, and children may have spasticity (hyperactive muscle stretch reflexes), choreoathetosis (involuntary movements), ataxia (incoordination and balance problems), or flaccidity (decreased muscle tone). The child's ability to see, hear, or speak may also be impaired.

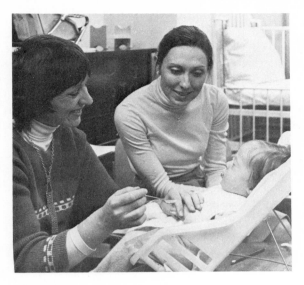

Figure 26-1
Early Intervention Program for children with Down syndrome at Children's Hospital Medical Center, Boston, Mass. Intervention program consists of pediatrics, physical therapy, psychology, speech therapy, nursing, and nutritional guidance. The nursing-nutritional component is directed toward helping parents to recognize the normal developmental aspects of feeding so that they can foster independent feeding in their child.

Because of motor involvement of the cranial nerves that control the infant's ability to suck and swallow, it is during initial feedings that neurologic deficits may first become manifest. Early intervention with remediation techniques (see "Feeding the Handicapped Child") can help facilitate feeding and prevent behavior problems from evolving around organically based ones.

Feeding difficulties due to neuromuscular impairment and persistence of primitive reflexes make nutrient deficiencies a common finding,[35-37] and demand the attention of all health professionals to help these children meet their recommended allowances for essential nutrients. Hammond et al. found that the degree of mental retardation impeding self-help skills influenced dietary intake more than the motor handicaps imposed by the cerebral palsy.[38] The degree to which the mouth area is involved has

been closely associated with poor intake, and the extent of mouth involvement and general growth have been observed to parallel one another closely.[39] Time, fatigue, and loss of food from the mouth are the implicated factors. Growth deficits are marked in these children, and athetotic children are smaller than spastic children. Berg and Isaksson reported in a survey of 23 children with cerebral palsy that all were short for their age and heavy for height. In an earlier study, Berg reported finding an abnormal body composition, with body cell mass that was reduced for height and an excess of extracellular water, and in this case inactivity and malnutrition were considered relevant.[40]

Because of body compositional differences, anthropometric measurements are difficult to interpret. In a survey of the nutritional status of 33 children with cerebral palsy at the Massachusetts Hospital School, it was concluded that skinfold standards derived from normal populations are of little use in determining nutritional status in this population because of the marked growth differences. It is noted that when using normal standards, it is assumed that changes in body fatness are proportionally reflected in triceps skinfold. However, with cerebral palsy children, the triceps skinfold may overestimate body fatness because increased skinfolds occur over the paralyzed limb. The study suggests that research on body composition is needed for the development of reliable anthropometric techniques.[41]

Energy needs should be tailored to the size of the child, with the type of motor dysfunction considered as well. Nonambulatory, spastic children are at risk of becoming overweight, especially as they approach adolescence. It is questionable whether children with athetotic motions require additional energy intake to support their constant muscular activity when their energy needs are compared with those of normal, active children. Energy expenditure in children with cerebral palsy has been found to be lower.[42] However, there is a great range of variation which must be considered in dietary planning. Since the total food intake may be small, the quality is important. Incorporating powdered milk, evaporated milk, wheat germ, and bran into foods can help to enrich the mixture, and thickening fluids slightly with yogurt or baby cereal can facilitate drinking. Fluid intake is a particular concern in this population and must be closely watched, as much fluid is dribbled from the mouth during feeding.

Another problem, constipation, is caused by decreased peristaltic activity and abnormal muscle tone. Treatment includes stool softeners, fluids, high-laxative foods (see "Constipation," in Chap. 22), and gentle abdominal massage.

Hyperkinesis and Diet

The Council on Child Health of the American Academy of Pediatrics describes the hyperkinetic child as one of normal intelligence who fails to learn at a normal rate even though given the same educational opportunities as other children with equal intelligence. In addition, the child is noted to exhibit, to some degree: (1) short attention span, (2) easy distractibility, (3) impulsive behavior, and (4) overactivity.[43] At present, the drug treatment of hyperkinesis involves the use of dextroamphetamine and methylphenidate, which are known to produce anorexia and are reported to suppress growth.[44,45]

In 1973 Feingold proposed that hyperkinesis was associated primarily with the ingestion of low-molecular-weight chemicals and suggested dietary treatment. The diet is low in salicylates and food additives and consists of homemade products and fresh meats, milk, and vegetables. Foods and beverages containing natural salicylates, food flavorings, and food colors and drugs with salicylates are avoided.[46] His findings have prompted much controversy in the lay press as well as in professional circles. The National Advisory Committee on Hyperkinesis and Food Additives of the Nutrition Foundation[47] convened in 1975 to review evidence on this subject and has since reviewed studies[48–56] in an attempt to discern the relationship between food color, flavors, and hyperactivity. They conclude that these studies refute the claim that artificial food colorings, artificial flavors,

and natural salicylates produce hyperactivity.[57] They comment that since the food additive-free diet has no apparent harmful effects and since the nonspecific (placebo) effects of this dietary treatment can be beneficial to families, they see no reason to discourage families who wish to pursue it. (Because the Nutrition Foundation was created and supported by food companies, these findings raised some suscipicion.)

Whether it is worthwhile for a family to devote the necessary time and energy to their dietary habits to create the possible effects on the hyperkinesis is a question that must be answered on an individual basis. A dietary survey of 54 children on the hyperkinesis diet showed that nutrient intakes did not change significantly while the children followed the diet and were sufficient to meet the recommended allowances during the baseline and diet periods.[58]

Another controversial approach to hyperkinesis, and also to minimal brain dysfunction (MBD) and learning disabilities, is the use of massive doses of vitamins (orthomolecular; see pp. 120, 599). Cott reported that with megavitamin therapy there was a significant decrease in hyperactivity and improved concentration.[59] However, he was not able to report any well-controlled studies. In a placebo-controlled study of the use of megavitamins for minimal brain dysfunction, there was no significant difference between the placebo and vitamin groups.[60]

THE HANDICAPPED ADULT

The handicapped adult, with limbs compromised by injury, arthritis, amputations, progressive neurologic disease (e.g., multiple sclerosis, Parkinson's disease, muscular dystrophy), or brain and spinal cord damage, faces some of the same problems in feeding as the handicapped child but in addition must learn to reintegrate the adult need for self-fulfillment and productivity into a compromised life-style. Feelings of frustration, boredom, embarrassment, anger, isolation, and exclusion may set up a host of defenses that can interfere with the rehabilitative process. The dysphagia of the stroke (cerebrovascular accident, CVA) patient makes swallowing difficult, and the often accompanying aphasia can make it impossible for the patient to communicate needs.

The need for a diet that is high in nutrient density becomes paramount in the care of the individual who can tolerate only small feedings, and vitamin-mineral supplementation is usually required. Protein is especially important in recovery from the stress of the acute phase, and fiber and fluid must be incorporated into the diet to promote peristalsis and maintain fluid balance (for the patient who cannot tolerate roughage, bran soaked in milk and mixed into foods can be a solution). Special therapeutic diets may also be used to treat the disease or condition precipitating the handicap, e.g., a low-fat, low-cholesterol diet for the patient recovering from a cerebrovascular accident. Also low-fat diets have been used with mixed success in some patients with multiple sclerosis.[61] Drug-diet interactions present complications, especially for those patients with Parkinson's disease who are being treated with levodopa. The protein in the diet should be controlled to maximize clinical benefits from the drug. Also, excessive amounts of pyridoxine taken as a vitamin supplement can interfere with the effect of levodopa.

Variations in texture should be individualized according to the patient's tolerance and degree of motor impairment. The CVA patient may more easily tolerate fluids thickened with infant cereal or strained fruit. The edentulous patient may find that dentures are loose-fitting during the recuperative phase and will require their adjustment to facilitate feeding.

Spinal cord injuries that affect bladder control make urinary tract infections a common problem. Many patients are maintained on an acid-ash diet (see Chap. 23) or on high dosages of vitamin C to acidify the urine. Prolonged immobility can lead to calcium mobilization from bones and to renal calculi, for which an acid-ash diet or a low-calcium diet may be used. Also, obesity may be an overriding problem in the handicapped adult, who may find eating the outlet for frustration or boredom.

The occupational therapist, physical therapist, and home economist become integral participants in nutritional rehabilitation as patients relearn activities of daily living. Careful selection of feeding utensils and home appliances is necessary in allowing full independence. The kitchen represents many hazards, especially to the handicapped. Simplifying tasks, and encouraging carefully planned tasks with lists to expedite the process, can help to ameliorate the frustration that is especially felt during the early stages of rehabilitation and readjustment.

Interdisciplinary Team

The development and function of the nervous system and the treatment of its disorders is dependent on nutritional status. An evaluation that acknowledges the biological and psychological characteristics of the individual and that reconciles the growth and developmental needs to the altered demands of the handicapping condition is essential. The complexities of management and the continuing aspects of care require the service of an interdisciplinary team: doctor, nurse, nutritionist, or dietitian, speech pathologist, physical therapist, occupational therapist, dentist, psychologist—working in an atmosphere of mutual respect to formulate a treatment program that addresses each individual need.

Nutritional status is dependent on feeding success, which the next section covers.

FEEDING THE HANDICAPPED CHILD

Linda Fetters

THE RELATIONSHIP OF MOTOR CONTROL AND FEEDING

The development of independent movement allows the child freedom. The development of independent movement proceeds systematically. The sequence is the same in all children; however, the *rate* and *quality* of this sequence may vary. Body (postural) control develops as the central nervous system matures and as the baby is stimulated by the environment.

Postural control develops from head to toe, and from the midline of the body toward the extremities. Control begins with the child in the horizontal position and gradually increases and improves, enabling the child to assume the upright or vertical position. Until the upright position is attained and the infant has developed skill in the use of the upper extremities, the infant must be fed by another person. This dependent feeding usually occurs with the infant in a semirecumbent position. Full support is given to the infant's body and head. In response to the acquisition of independent abilities by the infant, parents begin to remove their support. The child who is beginning to sit independently (4 to 6 months old) can be placed in a high chair for feeding rather than being cradled in the parent's arms. The infant who is developing skill in hand-to-mouth activities (beginning at 3 to 4 months) will want to self-feed, and less parental help will be necessary. This move toward independent feeding is contingent upon the acquisition of normal patterns of movement. The child must acquire *head, trunk,* and *upper extremity control* in order to make independent feeding possible.

The acquisition of postural control is in part dependent on two aspects of development: normal muscle tone and the integration of primitive reflexes. Abnormal muscle tone and the persistence of primitive reflexes are two characteristics of the child with central nervous system dysfunction that are usually associated with abnormal feeding behavior; they are now considered.

Muscle Tonus

Normal muscle tone is a prerequisite for normal movement. Muscle tone (or *tonus*) is a state of tension in the body musculature that indicates it is ready to perform its function of movement and postural control. Normal muscle tone is increased enough to permit stability and decreased enough to permit movement. Muscle tonus is controlled by the central nervous system, and abnormalities in muscle tone reflect problems with the normal neural control of tonus. In the child with central nervous system dysfunction— for example, the child with cerebral palsy— muscle tonus may be abnormally increased or decreased, or may fluctuate between these two extremes. *Hypertonic, spastic,* and *stiff* are all terms used to describe muscle tone that is abnormally increased. *Hypotonic, flaccid,* and *floppy* are terms used to describe tone that is abnormally decreased.

Normal muscle tone is important for independent feeding abilities. The state of tonus in the body affects the acquisition of independent feeding postures and arm and head movements. The child with increased tonus may not be able to bend at the hips to sit. When placed in a sitting posture, the child may not be able to control his or her head or trunk to maintain this position. If a child has decreased tone, the ability to assume and maintain a sitting posture may also be difficult or impossible. Normal tonus is also important in the oral musculature used for feeding. Tonus may be decreased, preventing jaw control and lip closure, or it may be increased, preventing movement of the tongue, lips, and jaws for chewing. Because of variability in the type of problem, the treatment should be individualized.

Primitive Reflexes

As the child grows, the central nervous system matures; during this maturation primitive reflexive responses become integrated at appropriate times so that more purposeful, voluntary activity can develop. An example of this development is the integration of the asymmetrical tonic neck reflex (ATNR). This reflexive posture, sometimes called the fencing position, is normally present in infants from birth to about 4 months of age. The posture is shown in Fig. 26-2. The arm and leg on the face side show increased extension; the opposite arm and leg show increased flexion. The normal infant's activities are not dominated by this response. Movement away from this position occurs easily

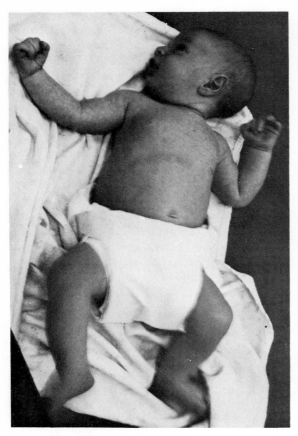

Figure 26-2
Normal asymmetrical tonic reflex posture in a 6-week-old infant. The asymmetrical tonic neck reflex is more evident in the arms than in the legs. This is never an obligatory position in the normal infant.

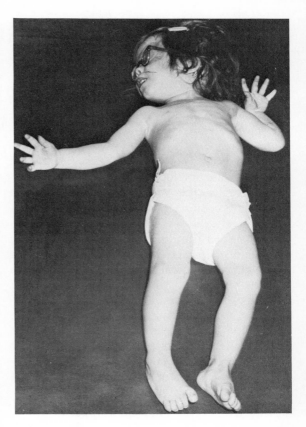

Figure 26-3
Abnormal persistence of the asymmetrical tonic neck reflex in a 3-year-old child. The retention of this reflex has interfered with the child's sitting balance and with hand-to-mouth activities.

so that the infant can suck on its fingers regardless of the position of the head. The infant with central nervous system dysfunction may be dominated by this reflex as a result of the lack of normal maturation of the central nervous system (see Fig. 26-3). The position of the infant's head may dictate the position of the limbs. The child may not be able independently to bring food to the mouth while looking at the food. The lack of normal integration of this response may prevent the child from gaining head and trunk control and may prevent the normal acquisition of arm and head movement allowing self-feeding.

Organization of Oral Reflexes for Feeding

The *suckle-swallow reflex* appears in the normal baby within the first or second day of life and remains until 3 to 5 months later.[62] It is stimulated by placing a nipple or finger into the mouth. Stimulation can be enhanced by touching the hard or soft palate. The infant will suck vigorously on the stimulant. The *rooting reflex* enables the child to find the breast or bottle. If the corners of the infant's mouth or the upper or lower lips are gently touched with a finger or nipple, the mouth will turn toward the stimulation and the head will follow. The rooting response is present from birth on, gradually becoming weaker until it disappears at around 3 months of age. In breast-fed children the rooting response may persist for a longer period.

The *biting reflex* is normally present from birth on, becoming weaker and disappearing at about 3 to 5 months. It is elicited by pressure on the gums, and consists of a phasic bite and release in response to the stimulation. This response is usually not strong. The more sustained voluntary bite develops later.

Normally, the *gag reflex* is present from birth. It becomes weaker as chewing begins.[63] The gag reflex is protective in nature and allows return of food from the back to the front of the the mouth. It can be elicited by placing a finger at the back of the oral cavity and pressing down on the tongue.

These four infantile oral reflexes—suckleswallow, rooting, biting, and gag—may be evaluated separately; however, their importance for function lies in their sequential action as the child eats.[64] The dependent infant relies on reflexive responses to find and properly ingest food. The infant performs this feeding repertoire on a background of normal respiration. The infant must be able to nose-breathe in a relaxed manner. In order to do this the infant needs an unobstructed airway from nose to lungs and the ability to coordinate breathing with swallowing. This coordination reflects the nature of control within the central nervous system.

As the primitive oral reflexes are being integrated, the infant is gaining head and trunk control, allowing an independent sitting posture. As independent sitting improves, arms become freed from their support role and the infant gains ability in upper extremity functions, including hand-to-mouth behavior. All of these sensory motor abilities indicate that the child is moving toward independence, including independent feeding.

Conclusion

The development of postural control and independent movement proceeds from head to toe, proximally to distally. The development of normal movement is contingent upon normal muscle tonus and the integration of primitive reflexive responses. The acquisition of independent postural control and movement allows the child to be independent in activities such as feeding. Just as primitive reflexes must be inhibited for independent postural control to develop, primitive oral reflexes must be integrated so that more purposeful oral reflexes may occur (see Table 26-4).

The child with central nervous system dysfunction may not be developing independent sensorimotor abilities. Abnormal muscle tone may be preventing head and trunk control, and the child may be dominated by primitive reflexive behavior in the body and oral areas, causing feeding problems. The potential problems need thorough evaluation.

EVALUATION OF A CHILD WITH A FEEDING PROBLEM

The feeding behavior of the child with central nervous system dysfunction may show abnormalities from birth. Reviewing the early histories of children with various handicapping conditions frequently reveals early feeding difficulties (e.g., poor sucking ability, taking only small amounts of liquid per feeding, prolonged feeding time, or choking and aspirating feedings). Abnormalities in early coordinated feeding behavior may be the first sign of central nervous system dysfunction. Infants with early feeding difficulties should be carefully followed in order to rule out long-term difficulties. Feeding problems may also become evident when spoon feeding and solid foods are introduced.

The evaluation of a child with a feeding problem is best accomplished with an interdisciplinary team of professionals (as described on p. 609) who are experienced in the area of feeding. Anecdotal information regarding past and present problems can be collected from the history; however, it is essential for the team to observe the child during mealtime. Evaluation at mealtime in the home or in another familiar surrounding is recommended, since fewer variables

TABLE 26-4   PRIMITIVE REFLEXES INVOLVED IN FEEDING

Reflex	Description
Moro reflex	A proprioceptive response elicited by dropping the head back suddenly; the response includes a rapid extension and abduction of the limbs, followed by flexion and adduction of the limbs
	Normal cocurrence: Birth to 4 months
	Retention produces: Total body responses to stimuli
	Interferes with: Sitting balance; hand-to-mouth activities
Asymmetrical tonic neck reflex	A proprioceptive response elicited by turning the head from side to side; increased extention is seen in the limbs on the face side and increased flexion in the opposite limbs
	Normal occurrence: Birth to 4 months
	Retention produces: Asymmetrical postures
	Interferes with: Sitting balance; hand-to-mouth activities
Hand grasp	A stimulus to the palm of the hand (from the ulnar side) elicits finger flexing and grasping of the object
	Normal occurrence: Birth to 3 or 4 months
	Retention produces: Fisted hands; difficulty in opening hands
	Interferes with: Holding utensils
Suckle-swallow	A stimulus introduced into the mouth elicits vigorous sucking followed by a swallow if liquid is present
	Normal occurrence: 1 or 2 days after birth to 3–5 months
	Retention produces: Suckling response to any oral stimuli
	Interferes with: Taking food from spoon with lips; cup drinking; chewing
Rooting	A stimulus to the oral area (corners of the mouth, upper and lower lip) causes lips, tongue, and finally head to turn toward the stimulus
	Normal occurrence: Birth to 3–5 months
	Retention produces: Asymmetrical oral response to stimuli; head turning to oral stimuli
	Interferes with: Maintaining head position for appropriate feeding
Gag	A stimulus to the posterior tongue or soft palate causes constriction of the posterior oral musculator to bring stimulating substance forward
	Normal occurrence: Birth to adulthood
	Retention produces: Increased oral sensitivity
	Interferes with: *Hyperactive gag*—Food is constantly pushed forward and out of the mouth *Hypoactive gag*—Food can passively enter the esophagus or trachea
Bite	Pressure on the gums elicits a phasic bite and release
	Normal occurrence: Birth to 3–5 months
	Retention produces: Biting all objects placed in the mouth
	Interferes with: Mouthing activities; ingesting food; more mature biting; chewing

are introduced into the feeding situation in a familiar locale.

Asking the parents about feeding does not always reveal problems because of the lack of parental objectivity. For example, the child may be ingesting a well-balanced diet, but the parents may not be aware that the texture of blenderized food is inappropriate, or that they are positioning the child with the head tipped back in order to help the food slide down passively instead of requiring active swallowing with the child positioned upright.

When observing feeding, observe the total child. Questions about the child's motor development to be answered during the observation include:

Does the child have normal muscle tone? Does the child have head and trunk control that is appropriate for age level? If the child has not achieved head and trunk control, has control been provided with the use of an appropriate chair or other support?

Are the child's movements spontaneous and in normal patterns? Can the child isolate movements of the hands to bring food or objects into the mouth?

What are the child's facial movements and expressions? Can the child isolate mouth, tongue, and jaw movements to drink, chew, and swallow?

The normal child has a relaxed face at rest, and fine facial control is exhibited during interaction with people and during feeding. The child with abnormal muscle tone may have an expressionless face because of hypotonia, or exaggerated grimacing because of hypertonia (sometimes termed the spastic grin). Isolated fine facial movements are often lacking in the child with abnormal muscle tone.

Along with general observations, the following areas must receive evaluation.

Positioning

Positioning a child properly can facilitate good feeding patterns and prevent choking, gagging, and aspiration. The flexed forward position will encourage swallowing, while the extended position (particularly if the head and neck are extended) will make swallowing very difficult and will promote gagging.

The child who has not achieved head and trunk control needs the support of an appropriate chair or should be held on the parent's lap during feeding. Feeding time is not a time for the child to struggle to keep his or her head up and trunk stable. These can be goals of therapy

at a different time, although they can be reinforced during feeding time. Support should be provided so that the child can maintain the vertical position. With certain exceptions, feeding should not take place with the child in the supine position, because in this position choking and gagging may occur, increasing the risk of aspiration. (In the event of choking or gagging, try to remove the food from the child's mouth. Avoid pushing the food further into the throat. If necessary, turn the child prone with the head hanging down so that gravity will assist in bringing the food forward into the mouth.) The child who is fed in the supine position also misses the visual experiences that can be gained in the upright position and the stimulation which the vertical position gives the body to facilitate postural control.

Oral Reflexes

The persistence of primitive oral reflexes prevents the child from developing more advanced patterns for feeding. It is not only the persistence of primitive reflexes that is abnormal; the *intensity* and *quality* of the reflexes are also frequently abnormal. The four oral reflexes should be evaluated separately, and their coordination should be functionally evaluated.

Rooting. The child with central nervous system dysfunction may show remnants of the rooting response much longer than the normal child, and as a consequence, when the mouth is stimulated, the child's head turns toward the stimulus. This will cause unwanted head movements. In some children the rooting reflex may not be normally present, e.g., in infants with severe central nervous system problems or very premature infants.

Suckle-swallow. This reflex may be retained for several years in severe cases. Stimulation in the mouth causes immediate suckling. This will prevent drinking from a cup and normal patterns of taking food from utensils such as a spoon.

Bite reflex. This is particularly persistent in the child with hypertonicity. When this reflex is retained, it is always stronger than normal. In severely handicapped children this reflex may persist for life if they have not been helped to overcome it.

Gag reflex. This reflex is often exaggerated in children with hypertonicity so that even a minimal stimulus will cause the child to gag. The reflex may be diminished or absent in the child with hypotonia, which is dangerous since it increases the risk of choking or aspirating food.

These four oral reflexes tend to be increased in the child with hypertonia and decreased or absent in the child with hypotonia.

Oral Digital Stimulation

The child's response to stimulation around the mouth must be evaluated. Stimulation can be provided by touching the inside and outside of the mouth, the tongue, and the gums with a finger. This may be done while testing oral reflexes. Muscle tone changes in response to this stimulation should be noted. Infants normally have a great deal of oral experience. The oral area is very sensitive and well utilized as the infant explores the environment. The handicapped child may have had very little or abnormal oral experience, and as a consequence the face, mouth, and lips may be overly sensitive to stimulation. The child with abnormal muscle tone may become stiff when the oral area is stimulated. Muscle tonus in the oral area will feel tight and stiff in this child, just as the rest of the body does. In contrast, the oral area of the child with hypotonia may feel flaccid, and little response to stimulation will be felt. The same responses that are elicited with oral digital stimultion may by elicited when food is placed in the child's mouth.

Jaw Control

Normally the jaws are lightly closed at rest, and in motion they can be held in any position and move freely. The handicapped child usually has poor control of the jaws. Frequently the jaws are halfway or totally open at rest. The jaws may fall open because of lack of tone, or the jaw may be pulled open and back or protruded by hypertonicity. The normal development of rotary and horizontal jaw movements may be completely absent in the child with central nervous system dysfunction.

Lip Control

The lips should be observed at rest and while the child is eating. Muscle tonus affecting lip control can be felt during oral digital stimulation. In the normal child, the lips are lightly closed at rest, and in spontaneous motion show a full range of gross and fine movements.[65] In the child with hypertonicity the lips may be tense and slightly closed at rest. When movement occurs, the lips may follow the gross movements of the jaw and lose their fine control. The child with hypotonia may show slack or parted lips and lack fine control. Good control of the soft palate will be lacking.

The lack of fine lip control will affect the child's ability to handle some foods, even if the child is fed by another person. Cleaning food from a spoon with the upper lip may be difficult or impossible. Lip closure around a cup will also be difficult, and liquid will dribble from the corners of the mouth. It is difficult to swallow normally with the lips parted or widely separated, and for some children it is impossible.

Tongue

Normally, the tongue is adaptive and flexible in its motions. It is capable of fine coordinated movements and protrudes only voluntarily.

The tongue of the child with hypertonus may be rolled (cigar-shaped) and may protrude involuntarily from the mouth. In the primitive suckle-swallow reflex, the tongue normally protrudes from the mouth and then draws liquid back into the mouth. If this primitive response is not normally inhibited with maturation of the central nervous system, tongue protrusion occurs in response to oral stimulation. As a consequence, food may be pushed out of the mouth as soon as it is introduced. The child with hypotonia may have a floppy, immobile tongue that passively protrudes from the mouth.

The child with any type of abnormal muscle

tonus may have an inflexible tongue that tends to move with the gross movements of the jaws. The abnormal pressures that the tongue exerts on the teeth, gums, and jaw, coupled with abnormal muscle tension around the oral area, may cause malformations of teeth and jaws.

Breathing

Breathing patterns should be evaluated both while the child is at rest and while active because it may be difficult for the child to coordinate relaxed breathing with ingestion of food, and the risk of aspiration may increase. Normally, breathing is regular and deep. Breathing will easily change with increased activity. The child with abnormal muscle tone may have shallow, irregular breathing patterns and frequently breathes through the mouth.

Hand-to-Mouth Activity

The newborn usually has the ability to bring the hand to the mouth for sucking activities. Reaching and voluntary grasp begins at 3 to 4 months. Reaching begins as gross flailing movements which eventually become directed and controlled. Hand and finger movements develop from gross motions to precise, fine muscular movements, with the child finally able to pick up very tiny objects with a pincer grasp by the age of 6 months.

The child with central nervous system dysfunction and resulting abnormalities in muscle tone may not be able to bring the hand to the mouth easily. The child may have a persistent, primitive hand-grasp reflex which will make handling of food and utensils difficult. Retention of the asymmetrical tonic neck reflex means that when the child attempts to bring the hand to the mouth, the head turns away.

TREATMENT OF THE CHILD WITH FEEDING PROBLEMS

A thorough evaluation of the child's feeding problem provides insight into the major problems and helps to determine the best therapeutic

intervention. A therapeutic plan should be established with the parents so that they can contribute their valuable observations and suggestions to the treatment. The techniques that are chosen and suggested to the parents must be demonstrated to them and then given a period of trial. Not all techniques result in immediate success. Specific evaluation and program planning for a child with a neurologic disorder should be accomplished by a feeding team or at least by an individual with in-depth experience and training in feeding children with special needs. Some overall guidelines can be mentioned.

Positioning

Children should be fed in an upright posture. A chair may need to be adapted or built (Fig. 26-4) to enable a child with delayed or abnormal

Figure 26-4

Proper positioning for a child with extensor hypertonicity throughout the body. Because of his extensor hypertonicity this child tends to thrust out of the chair without some adaptation of his sitting position. He is positioned with hip flexion, which will tend to reduce the extensor hypertonus. The hip flexion is maintained by securing his tray close to his body, and by placing a thick foam pad under his thighs. His feet are kept in good alignment through the use of another foam pad. The child is sitting in a symmetrical position, which is very important for him since he still exhibits an asymmetrical tonic neck reflex.

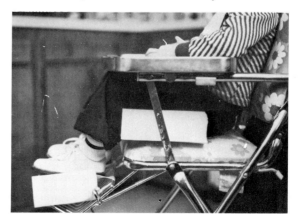

motor development to sit in the upright position. The chair should support those parts of the body that the child cannot control independently. Keeping the legs apart may add stability to the sitting posture of a child with hypotonia, and it may help to reduce hypertonicity. A well-controlled and comfortable sitting position is an important component of successful feeding. The prone position can be utilized for infants who are still sucking and for children in whom sucking should be encouraged.

Abnormal Muscle Tone

The quality and quantity of muscle tonus should be assessed by a therapist. A program intended to provide control for abnormalities in muscle tone may be designed by the therapist and may be carried out prior to feeding in order to help prepare the child for mealtime. For example, a child with extensor hypertonicity may benefit from being put on its side, with the physical therapist or parent rocking the child at the hips to encourage rotation in the trunk. This may help to inhibit hypertonicity in the total body, and as a result of the decreased extensor hypertonus the child may be able to flex the hips and assume a better sitting posture.

Feeding Environment

Mealtime can be noisy and overstimulating for a child who already may be having trouble with feeding. The child with special needs may have to be fed separately, away from the family or other people, for one meal a day. At this time the parent may work with the therapeutic plan. At other mealtimes the child with special needs may join the family or group of children to participate in the socialization that mealtime provides and to benefit from the modeling of good feeding habits by other members of the group.

It will be helpful to have all the food, utensils, and other equipment necessary for feeding the child accessible and available in one place. This will decrease the energy and time expenditure during the feeding period.

Adaptive Equipment

Various types of equipment are produced commercially to assist children with feeding. Many pieces are useful and often inexpensive. Simple adaptations of plates, cups, and utensils that are already available in the family kitchen, however, can be made by a parent at almost no cost (see Fig. 26-5, on p. 618). Each child's needs should be assessed individually, and recommendations for equipment should be made on this basis. However, some simple general suggestions may be helpful.

Wrapping a washcloth around the handle of a spoon and securing it with tape may make it easier for a child to hold if the child has a very tight grasp or hypertonicity in the upper extremities.

Securing the plate on the table with a rubber suction cup (the kind usually used to hold soap) will make it easier for the child to remove food from the plate with a utensil.

Cutting out a side piece in a paper or plastic cup will allow the child's nose to fit into the cup without forcing the child's head into an extended position, which may increase hypertonicity and also make it difficult for the child to control the head.[66]

Conclusion

In the child with central nervous system dysfunction, abnormal muscle tone and the persistence of primitive reflexes are associated with feeding problems and poor nutritional status.

An evaluation which considers the child's oral-pharyngeal motor ability and head, trunk, and arm control, along with evaluation of the home environment, utensils used, and the daily food, fluid, and drug intake, can help to alleviate the problem while affording the child the opportunity of a pleasant rather than a frustrating experience with food.

The next section—"Feeding the Child with a Cleft Lip and Palate" (p. 619)—considers another type of specialized feeding.

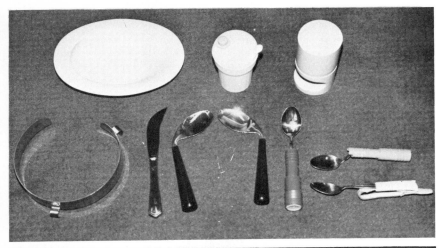

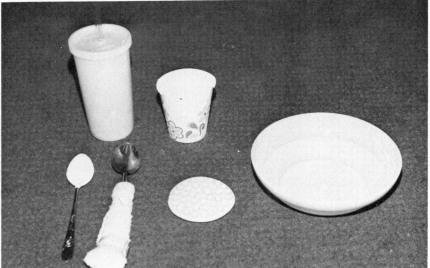

Figure 26-5

*Adaptive feeding equipment. Top: Specialized utensils. Clockwise: Shallow
Melmac bowl with sides to provide a scooping surface; plastic feeding cup with
lid, spout, and gravity device to control the flow; Melmac cup with indentation
to facilitate grasp; plate guard, attached to plate to provide a scooping surface;
curved knife to allow cutting with slight movement; right-handed and left-
handed spoons for pronation or supination difficulties; spoon with built-up handle for easier grasp; spoon with strap, placed over the back of hand to allow self-
feeding by an individual who cannot grasp a spoon; swivel spoon to help those
without the arm flexion needed to change the direction of the spoon as it reaches
the mouth. Bottom: Home adaptations and commonly available utensils for special feeding. Clockwise: Teflon-coated baby spoon for the child with persistent
bite reflex; washcloth wrapped around spoon handle and taped, for those with
a tight grasp or hypertonicity in the upper extremities; rubber suction-cup soap
holder, used to secure plates; plastic bowl with shallow sides to allow scooping;
paper cup with cut-out nose opening; Tupperware cup with cover and straw—
gentle squeezing on the sides facilitates straw drinking.*

FEEDING THE CHILD
WITH A CLEFT LIP AND PALATE*

Dorothy M. MacDonald

DEVELOPMENTAL DEFECT

The precise cause of cleft lip and cleft palate is unknown. Although heredity appears to be a factor in one-third of the cases, the exact pathogenesis is elusive. It is a developmental defect, occurring in the first trimester of pregnancy. Most researchers feel that a complex combination of factors are involved in the etiology of clefts.

A cleft lip is a split in the upper lip. Normally, the lip is formed by the union of two tabs of tissue that grow in from the sides of the face and a central tab that grows down from the tip of the nose. This occurs during the fourth to sixth week of fetal life. With a cleft lip, the maxillary and premaxillary processes forming the upper lip fail to fuse. The cleft lip may be unilateral incomplete, unilateral complete, bilateral complete, and, in rare instances, midline. These clefts vary in severity from a slight indentation to a wide-open cleft. This defect is often but not necessarily accompanied by a cleft palate (see Fig. 26-6, p. 620).

The hard or primary palate consists of the premaxilla, the maxilla, and the palatine bone. The soft or secondary palate is a fibromuscular structure that divides the nasal from the oral pharynx, and is constantly modified in shape and position by the palatal musculature. The incisive foramen, with a bilateral suture extending to the interproximal space between maxillary lateral incisor and canine, is the dividing line between the primary and secondary palate (see Fig. 26-7, p. 621).

In the seventh to twelfth week of fetal development, bone and tissue normally grow in

from the sides of the upper jaw to join in the middle. Failure of this union results in an opening between the mouth and the nose. The palatal defect varies in width and length, depending on when and where the growth process stopped. There may be a cleft of the soft palate alone or a cleft of both the soft palate and part or all of the hard palate. There may also be a cleft in one or both sides of the upper gum. The last type is usually accompanied by a cleft lip. The various types of cleft palates mentioned can all cause feeding and respiratory problems.

FEEDING APPROACH

The child born with a cleft of the lip, a cleft of the palate, or both presents a challenge to those responsible for primary care. The practitioner must be able to respond to the intake needs of the child as well as providing the family with guidance.

Parents are often overwhelmed by the birth of their handicapped infant and run the gamut of emotions from guilt, resentment, or anxiety, to depression and, in some instances, even to withdrawal. They need constant support and the opportunity to ventilate their feelings in order to provide the healthy parent-child relationship that is essential to a positive feeding experience.

It is very important to point out to the parents that most babies with clefts of the lip or palate do have feeding problems. Instead of giving assurance that might backfire and cause more anxiety, the practitioner can acknowledge the fact that these infants are difficult to feed but that for the most part, by either patient or frantic trial and error, parents do succeed, and these children thrive and return for follow-up as sturdy and robust as other children. Parents as well as hospital staff can adjust more easily to special feeding techniques if they are at ease about the eventual outcome.

Most infants with clefts are deprived of normal oral feedings. There is little documentation of the psychosocial impact on these infants, and

*The author of this section wishes to acknowledge the support of the Plastic Surgery Service of Children's Hospital Medical Center: Joseph E. Murray, M.D.; John B. Mulliken, M.D.; and George H. Gifford, M.D.

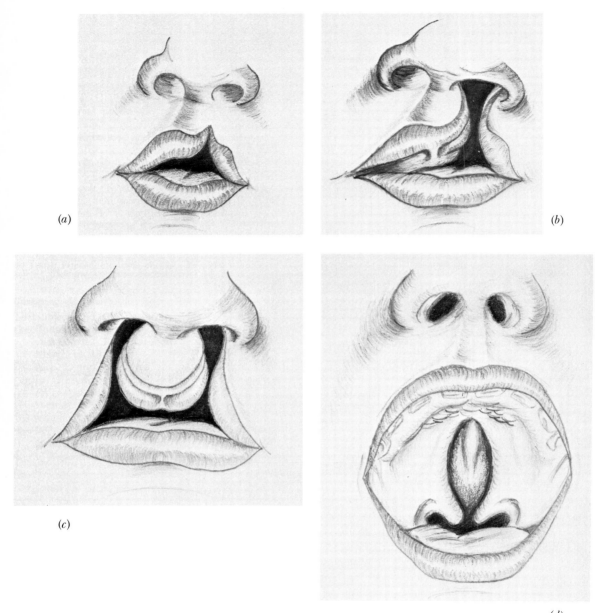

Figure 26-6
Defects of the lip and palate: (a) Unilateral incomplete cleft, (b) unilateral complete cleft, (c) bilateral complete cleft, and (d) cleft palate. (Illustration by John B. Mulliken, M.D., Plastic Surgeon, Children's Hospital Medical Center, Boston, Mass.)

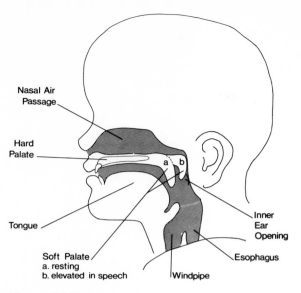

Figure 26-7
Normal physiology of the oropharynx.

(Labels in figure: Nasal Air Passage; Hard Palate; Tongue; Soft Palate a. resting b. elevated in speech; Inner Ear Opening; Esophagus; Windpipe; a b)

although a positive feeding experience helps to foster development, it is a positive parent-child relationship that is the important determinant. The approach to caring for the infant with a cleft should be to emphasize the positive (e.g., by telling the parents that the infant has beautiful eyes, is alert and responsive and nice to hold). Personal experience has shown that a supportive relationship with parents that encourages parent-child interaction (holding the infant, singing and talking to it) can help to ameliorate adjustment problems.

FEEDING TECHNIQUES

The methods of feeding an infant with a cleft vary, depending upon the philosophy of the medical center and the type of cleft.

In order to suck well, an infant must be neurologically intact, with lip and tongue control and properly formed primary and secondary palates. Normal feeding can take place because most of the sucking action employs the hard palate. Infants who have only a cleft of the soft palate can be fed normally but in a sitting-up position. Reflux of fluids through the nose sometimes happens, no matter what feeding procedure is being used; this occurs because fluids are forced through the cleft by the normal action of the tongue. If the infants were lying down, most of the feeding would enter the nose. All the other types of clefts usually require a special feeding device unless the infant is breast-fed (see below).

At Children's Hospital Medical Center in Boston,[67] the device that is primarily used is called a Breck feeder; this is a bulb-type syringe with a rubber or plastic tip on the end. Beniflex feeders (Mead Johnson) have also been used. These are soft plastic bags with a horizontal, cross-cut nipple attached. The Beniflex feeders can work well with soft palate clefts or partial clefts of the hard palate (see Fig. 26-8).

Breck Feeder Method
(Used with Clefts of Lip or Palate)

1. Prepare the infant prior to feeding; i.e., change diapers, wrap in a blanket.

2. The infant usually feeds better if its arms are restrained against the body with a special jacket or by wrapping tightly with a blanket.

Figure 26-8
Feeding equipment. Top: Beniflex feeder; bottom: Breck feeder.

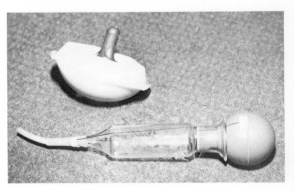

3 Prepare formula at room temperature or slightly warmer; also prepare a small amount of water.

4 Choose a comfortable chair and have equipment set up on a table where it can easily be reached.

5 Hold the infant close to you, in an upright position.

6 Fill the syringe with formula.

7 Insert the tip of the syringe in the side of the infant's mouth, with the tip resting about halfway down the tongue. (See Fig. 26-9.)

8 With one hand around the infant's head, stroke the cheek or gently move the chin up and down, which will stimulate the infant to make sucking motions.

9 The infant will probably resist these attempts and may even start to choke and gag.

10 Be patient. As the infant starts to swallow, place gentle pressure on the bulb to aid the infant in obtaining the formula.

11 Stop feeding frequently to calm the infant and to bubble (a lot of air is swallowed with this type of feeding).

12 Experiment to find where best to place the tip of the syringe on the tongue. This depends on how the infant feels most comfortable.

13 Continue the same technique until the infant has learned how to obtain nourishment.

14 When the formula is finished, rinse the syringe and give the infant a small amount of water in order to clean the mouth.

15 After feeding, continue to hold and calm the infant; also continue to bubble.

16 Place the infant on its right side or in a sitting position after feeding.

The ideal method of learning this feeding procedure is to have someone who is experienced at it demonstrate the technique.

Beniflex Feeder Method

1 Follow steps 1 through 5 as earlier.

2 Prepare the feeder as directed on the package.

3 Insert the nipple into the infant's mouth.

4 Stimulate the infant to suck by stroking the cheeks or moving the chin.

5 As the infant attempts to suck, apply gentle pressure on the feeder bag.

6 Finish feeding with a small amount of water to clean the mouth.

7 Bubble frequently.

8 Place the infant on its right side or in an upright position after feeding.

Solid foods should be introduced when the infant is the appropriate age. There is no reason why the infant cannot be taught to eat from a spoon, but if this is difficult, solids are added to

Figure 26-9
Placement of the tip of the Breck feeder. Tip of the syringe is inserted from the side of the mouth; tip rests about halfway down the tongue.

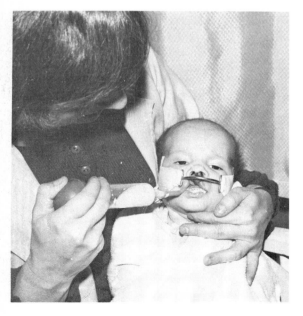

the formula feeding in order to provide the added source of nutrients.

Breast Feeding

Some mothers want to breast-feed and are often unreasonably discouraged by their physician. If the mother is knowledgeable and enthusiastic about breast feeding and realizes the inherent problems, and if the infant has the strength, breast feeding should be encouraged. It is a highly individualized process, and much care must be given to ensure adequate nutrition, since an inadequate intake is often the cause for discontinuation.

There is information available to mothers of infants with clefts from La Leche League International.[68] Included are the following guidelines:

1 Breast feeding is much easier when the breast is full.
2 Have the mother place her index finger on the top edge of the areola of the nipple and her middle finger on the bottom—this presses the nipple out. Place the nipple in the infant's mouth.
3 The infant can now "milk" the nipple.
4 Rather than sucking, the infant uses the jaws, tongue, cheeks, and gums to press the milk from the breast.
5 The infant's head should be held close to the breast during the entire feeding.
6 In counseling the mother, explain that the technique of manually extending the nipple and the "milking" motion of the infant's gums are more important than suctioning.
7 Most important, be very supportive toward the mother.

Feeding before and after Surgical Correction

Preoperative Feeding for Cleft Lip

The first repair is usually done when the infant weighs 10 lb or is 6 to 8 weeks old. The Breck feeder technique is the preferred method of feed-

ing. If solid food has been started, it is best to mix it with the formula and give it through the feeder.

Postoperative Feeding for Cleft Lip

1 Follow instructions for the Breck feeder technique.
2 Take care not to exert pressure on the suture line.
3 Give clear liquids for the first two postoperative feedings (to prevent anesthesia reaction).
4 Gradually increase feedings as tolerated by the infant.
5 Follow the formula feeding with a small amount of water (to prevent contamination of the suture line).
6 "Suture line care" must be given after each feeding to prevent infection.
7 The infant will continue to use Breck feeder for at least 1 month postoperatively, or longer if the physician so decides.

Preoperative Feeding for Cleft Palate

1 The palatal repair does not take place until the child is 12 to 14 months old.
2 The infant should be weaned from the feeder at 4 to 6 months of age. A cup and spoon should be started at this time.
3 It is often helpful to use a small cup such as a whiskey jigger. If a plain cup is too difficult, one of the infant cups on the market may be used, e.g., a Tippy-Tom cup (one that has a covered cap with a lip attached).
4 Prior to surgery it is important for the child to become accustomed to clear fluids: broths, gelatin, apple juice, water, and carbonated beverages that have been allowed to become flat. Carbonated beverages and sour fruit drinks are irritating to the nasal mucosa and should be avoided.
5 The child *must not* be taught the use of straws.

6 The child should be discouraged from putting the hands or other objects in the mouth. Using arm restraints periodically may be necessary to discourage this activity. Also, restraints are used postoperatively, so this helps the child become accustomed to them.

Postoperative Feeding for Cleft Palate

Clear fluids are offered to the child frequently for the first 5 days postoperatively. It is important to push fluids in order to prevent infection and to keep the child well hydrated. After the first 5 days the diet progresses to full fluids, which are given for the next 10 days. These fluids can consist of high-caloric, high-protein frappes, custards, blenderized diets, etc. On the second 10 days, the diet progresses to soft foods: finely mashed foods, chopped meats, strained vegetables and fruits. After 20 days of fluid and soft diet the child may resume a normal diet. Hard foods such as Zwieback, hard candy, lollipops, etc., should be avoided for at least 1 or 2 months postoperatively.

CONCLUSION

The first year of life is difficult for the child born with a cleft lip or palate. It is the health professional's responsibility to provide support and information to the parents. Frequent follow-ups through phone calls and hospital visits are imperative. Referring parents to other parents of children with a cleft also plays an important role. In Boston, there is a parents' group called Prescription Parents.

The technique used for feeding children with clefts is very complex and must be individualized to suit each child. Health professionals must exhibit the confidence and patience needed in dealing with these children in order to set a positive feeding example for parents.

STUDY QUESTIONS

1 What is the effect of the normal diet on brain neurotransmitters?

2 The effect of emotions on neurohormonal function may be related to the etiology of two clinical entities, nonorganic failure to thrive and anorexia nervosa. Explain.

3 Describe the eating disturbances that are characteristic of failure to thrive.

4 What are the considerations in feeding the handicapped child? The handicapped adult?

5 By analyzing the effect of the condition on growth, feeding ability, nutrient effectiveness, and motor activity, conceptualize a nutritional care plan for a child with Down syndrome and for a child with cerebral palsy.

6 List all the normal oral reflexes and their usual times of occurrence.

7 How does the persistence of early primitive reflexes influence the feeding behavior of the child with central nervous dysfunction?

8 What measures would you use to evaluate a feeding problem in a handicapped child?

9 What team members would you choose to participate in the feeding evaluation of a handicapped child?

10 Explain the developmental defect that is operative in cleft lip; in cleft palate.

11 Outline the feeding techniques for a child with a cleft lip and cleft palate, differentiating between the Breck feeder method and the Beniflex feeder method.

12 What are the differences in pre-and postoperative care for the child with a cleft lip and for the child with a cleft palate?

13 What type of anticipatory guidance would you give the parents of a child with a cleft?

CLINICAL STUDY 26

History

C. is a 10-month-old girl with cerebral palsy. She has hypertonicity throughout her body (spastic quadriparesis). C. has had four hospitalizations for aspiration pneumonia. Her parents have been feeding her in the supine position with her head tipped back because she had been choking, gagging, and pushing food from her mouth when she was fed in an upright position. In the supine position gravity could assist the swallowing process.

C.'s diet consisted of milk and baby cereals. All the food had a thin texture which was difficult for her to swallow. The food frequently dribbled from C.'s mouth.

Because of C.'s difficulties, parental anxiety surrounded the feeding situation, so that both the parents and the child reacted negatively to mealtime and C.'s food intake was poor. She consumed only 450 kcal (1890 kJ) per day. Her height (66 cm) and weight (6kg) fell below the 3d percentile on growth charts for infant girls. She was clearly failing to thrive.

During her last hospital admission the feeding team, consisting of a nurse, nutritionist, speech therapist, and physical therapist, was asked to evaluate C. and to make suggestions for improving her feeding, including a good position for feeding, ways to improve her ability to ingest food, and a plan for adequate calories and nutrition in her diet to ensure growth.

Main problems

C.'s overwhelming problem was her extensor hypertonicity. In addition to extensor hypertonus, increased oral sensitivity, and tongue protrusion, C. retained an asymmetrical tonic neck reflex. She responded to all stimulation by thrusting her body into an extended position with head thrown back, legs stiff, and body arched. This dominant extensor thrusting was preventing C. from developing head and trunk control, and the hypertonus was making lip closure and jaw control difficult. C. still retained remnants of a suckle-swallow reflex, and this had developed into tongue protrusion. Stimulation of any type around her mouth elicited extensor thrusting with protrusion of the tongue. The thin texture of C.'s food added to the problems caused by her hypertonicity.

Clinical study question

1 On the basis of the information in this chapter, develop a treatment plan and list goals in order of priority.

REFERENCES

1 J. D. Fernstrom and R. J. Wurtman, "Brain Serotonin Content: Increase Following Ingestion of Carbohydrate Diet," *Science*, **174**:1023–1025, 1971.

2 R. J. Wurtman and J. D. Fernstrom, "Effects of the Diet on Brain Transmitters," *Nutrition Reviews*, **32**:193–199, 1974.

3 J. H. Growdon and R. J. Wurtman, "Dietary Influences on the Synthesis of Neurotransmitters in the Brain," *Nutrition Reviews*, **37**:129–139, 1979.

4 L. D. Lytle and A. Alter, "Diet, the Central Nervous System and Aging," *Federation Proceedings*, **38**:2017, 1979.

5 R. Spitz and K. M. Wolf, "Anaclitic Depression: An Inquiry into the Genesis of Psychiatric Conditions in Early Childhood," *Psychoanalytic Study of the Child*, **2**:313, 1946.

6 C. F. Whitten, "Evidence That Growth Failure from Malnutrition Is Secondary to Undereating," *Journal of the American Medical Association*, **209**:1675, 1969.

7 G. F. Powell et al., "Emotional Deprivation and Growth Retardation Stimulating Idiopathic Hypopituitarism. II. Endocrinologic Evaluation of the Syndrome," *New England Journal of Medicine*, **276**:1279–1283, 1967.

8 T. G. Sheagren et al., "Rumination—A New Complication of Neonatal Intensive Care," *Pediatrics*, **6**:551–555, 1980.

9   P. C. English, "Failure to Thrive Without Organic Reason," *Pediatric Annals,* 7:774–781, 1978.

10 W. W. Gull, "Anorexia Nervosa," *Transactions of the Clinical Society* (London), 7:22–28, 1874.

11 C. Lasegue, "On Hysterical Anorexia," *Medical Times & Gazette,* 1873, pp. 265–266, 367–369.

12 P. Travaglini et al., "Some Aspects of Hypothalamic Pituitary Function in Patients with Anorexia Nervosa," *Acta Endocrinologica,* 81:252–262, 1976.

13 H. Needleman et al., "Amitriptyline Therapy in Patients with Anorexia," *Lancet,* 2:580, 1976.

14 H. Bruch, *Eating Disorders: Obesity, Anorexia Nervosa and the Person Within,* Basic Books, Inc., Publishers, New York, 1973, p. 251.

15 H. Bruch, "Perils of Behavior Modification in Treatment of Anorexia," *Journal of the American Medical Association,* 230:1419–1422, 1974.

16 N. J. Smith, Commentary on "Excessive Weight Loss and Food Aversion in Athletes Simulating Anorexia Nervosa," *Pediatrics,* 66:139–142, 1980.

17 D. Hawkins and L. Pauling (eds.), *Orthomolecular Psychiatry: Treatment of Schizophrenia,* W. H. Freeman and Co., San Francisco, 1973.

18 P. Ross-Smith and F. A. Jenner, "Diet (Gluten) and Schizophrenia," *Journal of Human Nutrition,* 34:107–112, 1980.

19 C. L. Ravaris et al., "Use of MAOI Antidepressants," *American Family Physician,* 18:105–111, July 1978.

20 Marc Shein, "Treatment for the Hospitalized Infantile Ruminator: Programmed Bried Social Behavior Reinforcers," *Clinical Pediatrics,* 14:719–724, 1975.

21 H. Pryor and H. Thelander, "Growth Deviations in Handicapped Children: An Anthropometric Study," *Clinical Pediatrics,* 6:501–512, 1967.

22 W. J. Culley and T. Middleton, "Caloric Requirements of Mentally Retarded Children with and without Motor Dysfunction," *Journal of Pediatrics,* 75:380–384, 1969.

23 E. H. Reynolds, "Folate Metabolism and Anticonvulsant Therapy," *Proceedings of the Royal Society of Medicine,* 67:6, 1974.

24 F. Lifshitz and N. Maclaren, "Vitamin D-dependent Rickets in Institutionalized, Mentally Retarded Children Receiving Long-Term Anticonvulsant Therapy. I. A Survey of 288 Patients," *Journal of Pediatrics,* 83:612–620, 1973.

25 K. DeLuka, R. E. Masotti, and N. W. Partington, "Altered Calcium Metabolism Due to Anticonvulsant Drugs," *Developmental Medicine and Child Neurology,* 14:318–321, 1973.

26 P. R. Huttenlocker, A. J. Wilbourn, and J. M. Signore, "Medium Chain Triglycerides as Therapy for Intractable Childhood Epilepsy," *Neurology,* 21:1097–1103, 1971.

27 J. M. Signore, "Ketogenic Diet Containing Medium-Chain-Triglycerides," *Journal of the American Dietetic Association,* 62:285–290, 1973.

28 Vera Pettaway, Children's Hospital Medical Center, Nutrition Service of Dietary Department, Boston, Mass., personal communication, 1978.

29 C. E. Cronk, "Growth of Children with Down's Syndrome: Birth to Age 3 Years," *Pediatrics,* 61:564–568, 1978.

30 Ibid.

31 W. J. Culley et al., "Caloric Intake of Children with Down's Syndrome (Mongolism)," *Journal of Pediatrics,* 60:772–775, 1965.

32 S. Palmer, "Influence of Vitamin A Nutriture on the Immune Response: Findings in Children with Down's Syndrome," *International Journal for Nutrition Research,* 48:188–216, 1978.

33 Sue Cullen, "Toward Independence in Social Development and Self-Help Skills of Young Children with Down's Syndrome. A Study Conducted in the Developmental Evaluation Clinic, Children's Hospital Medical Center, Boston, Mass." (in press).

34 P. L. Pipes and V. A. Holm, "Feeding Children with Down's Syndrome," *Journal of the American Dietetic Association,* 77:277–282, 1980.

35 S. Peeks and M. W. Lamb, "Comments on the Dietary Practices of Cerebral Palsied Children," *Journal of the American Dietetic Association,* 27:870–876, 1951.

36 A. L. Gourge and S. W. Ekvall, "Diets of Handicapped Children: Physical, Psychological and Socioeconomic Correlations," *American Journal of Mental Deficiency,* 80:149, 1975.

37 M. I. Hammond, M. N. Lewis, and E. W. Johnson, "A Nutritional Study of Cerebral Palsied children," *Journal of the American Dietetic Association,* 49:196–201, 1966.

38 Ibid.

39 D. O. Ruby and W. D. Matheny, "Comments on Growth of Cerebral Palsied Children," *Journal of the American Dietetic Association,* 40:525, 1962.

40 K. Berg and B. Isaksson, "Body Composition and Nutrition of School Children with Cerebral Palsy," *Acta Paediatrica Scandinavica,* Supplement, 204:41, 1970.

41 W. Dietz, "Nutritional Status of Children with Cerebral Palsy at the Massachusetts Hospital School" (in press), 1980.

42 K. Berg, "Nutrition of Children with Reduced Physical Exercise Due to Cerebral Palsy," *Bibliotheca Nutritio et Dieta,* 19:12, 1973.

43 Council on Child Health of the American Academy of Pediatrics, "Medications for Hyperactive Children," *Pediatrics,* 55:560, 1975.

44 D. J. Safer and R. P. Allen, "Factors Influencing the

Suppressant Effects of Two Stimulant Drugs on the Growth of Hyperactive Children," *Pediatrics,* **5**:66, 1973.

45 D. J. Safer, R. P. Allen, and E. Barr, "Growth Rebound after Termination of Stimulant Drugs," *Journal of Pediatrics,* **86**:113, 1975.

46 B. Feingold, "Food Additives and Child Development," *Hospital Practice,* **8**:11, October 1973.

47 National Advisory Committee on Hyperkinesis and Food Additives, *Report to the Nutrition Foundation,* Nutrition Foundation, New York, June 1, 1975.

48 J. P. Harley et al., *An Experimental Evaluation of Hyperactivity and Food Additives, Phase I,* private publication, University of Wisconsin, Madison, Wisconsin, 1977.

49 C. K. Conners, C. H. Goyette, D. A. Southwick, et al., "Food Additives and Hyperkinesis: A Controlled Double-Blind Experiment," *Pediatrics,* **58**:154, 1976.

50 C. H. Goyette, C. K. Conners, T. A. Petti, et al., "Effects of Artificial Colors on Hyperkinetic Children: A Double-Blind Challenge Study," *Psychopharmacology Bulletin,* **14**:39, 1978.

51 J. M. Swanson and M. Kinsbourne, "Food Dyes Impair Performance of Hyperactive Children on Laboratory Learning Test," *Science,* **207**:1485, 1980.

52 B. Weiss et al., "Behavioral Responses to Artificial Food Colors," *Science,* **297**:1487, 1980.

53 J. Mattes and R. Gittlelman-Klein, "A Crossover Study of Artificial Food Colorings in a Hyperkinetic Child, " *American Journal of Psychiatry,* **135**:987, 1978.

54 J. I. Williams, D. M. Cram, F. T. Tausig, and E. Webster, "Relative Effects of Drugs and Diet on Hyperactive Behaviors: An Experimental Study," *Pediatrics,* **61**:811, 1978.

55 F. Levy et al., "Hyperkinesis and Diet: A Double-Blind Crossover Trial with a Tartrazine Challenge," *Medical Journal of Australia,* **1**:61, 1978.

56 F. Levy and G. Hobes, "Hyperkinesis and Diet: A Replication Study," *American Journal of Psychiatry,* **135**:12, 1978.

57 National Advisory Committee on Hyperkinesis and Food Additives, *Final Report to the Nutrition Foundation,* Nutrition Foundation, New York, October 1980.

58 P. H. Harper, C. H. Goyette, and C. K. Conners, "Nutrient Intakes of Children on the Hyperkinesis Diet," *Journal of the American Dietetic Association,* **73**:515–520, 1978.

59 A. Cott, "Megavitamins: The Orthomolecular Approach to Behavioral Disorders and Learning Disabilities," *Academic Therapeutics,* **7**:245–258, 1972.

60 L. E. Arnold, J. Christopher, R. D. Huestis, and D. J. Smeltzer, "Megavitamins for Minimal Brain Dysfunction: A Placebo-Controlled Study," *Journal of the American Medical Association,* **240**:2642–2643, 1978.

61 R. L. Swank and R. D. Bourdillon, "Multiple Sclerosis: Assessment of Treatment with a Modified Low Fat Diet," *Journal of Nervous and Mental Diseases,* **131**:468–488, 1960.

62 Helen Mueller, "Facilitating Feeding and Prespeech," in P. Pearson and C. Willians (eds.), *Physical Therapy in the Development Disabilities,* Charles C Thomas, Springfield, Ill., 1972, pp. 286–288.

63 Ibid.

64 Lorraine Ogg, "Oral-Pharyngeal Development and Evaluation," *Journal of the American Physical Therapy Association,* **55**:237, 1975.

65 Helen Mueller, *Pre-Speech Evaluation and Therapy,* 16 mm black and white film with written outline, University of California, Los Angeles, Calif., 1967.

66 Nancy Finnie, *Handling the Young Cerebral Palsied Child at Home,* E. P. Dutton, New York, 1975.

67 Children's Hospital Medical Center, *Cleft Lip and Cleft Palate—Questions and Answers for Parents,* Children's Hospital Medical Center, Public Relations Department, Boston, Mass., 1976.

68 La Leche League International, Reprints: 9616 Minneapolis, Franklin Park, Ill. 60131.

CLINICAL DISCUSSION 26

The goals of treatment as outlined by the feeding team were as follows:

1 To reestablish C.'s nutritional status

2 To introduce remediation techniques in order to:
   a Inhibit extensor hypertonus
   b Facilitate postural control, beginning with head control
   c Inhibit the asymmetrical tonic neck reflex
   d Decrease oral hypersensitivity
   e Decrease tongue protrusion

3 To help provide a pleasant and successful mealtime experience for the child and her parents

In order to assist in achieving the first goal, the nutritionist designed a diet that aimed at gradually increasing C.'s intake until she was ingesting 700 kcal (2940 kJ) a day, including foods in all four basic food groups. Since children who are having difficulty with swallowing are frequently more successful with food of a thickened texture, she suggested thickening the texture of the foods by adding wheat germ, yogurt, or fortified baby cereal. A vitamin-mineral supplement with fluoride was prescribed.

The nurse began discussions with the parents about the mealtime experiences at home. She supported the family in their efforts to help C. and agreed with them that feeding a child with poor postural control and constant thrusting is extremely difficult.

In order to accomplish either of the outlined goals, the physical and speech therapists determined that the first need was to achieve inhibition of the extensor hypertonus and facilitation of head control. In addition it was necessary to decrease C.'s oral sensitivity to stimuli and facilitate oral control. The therapists felt that achieving these two goals would facilitate feeding, and that with a more successful feeding experience parental anxiety would be relieved.

Treatment

To inhibit extensor hypertonus, C. was held in a flexed posture with her head brought forward. At times she would thrust out of the position, and it was not possible to hold her. When this occurred, C. was placed in a hammock made from a bed sheet. With a person holding each end of the sheet, C. was gently rocked back and forth, gradually flexing her body. After the extensor tone was inhibited, she was placed on her side on a mat or bed. C.'s parents were shown how to rock her from this side position toward prone and supine positions while holding her at the hip. This gentle rolling encouraged rotation in C.'s trunk, which further helped to inhibit her extensor hypertonus. Once C. had been "prepared" in this way, she could maintain a sitting position more easily.

To facilitate head control, C. was held in an upright position with only partial support given to her head so that she would help in its control.

Oral stimulation and food were then given in the center of her mouth so that asymmetrical responses were not facilitated. This encouraged motor activity which would help to promote symmetry in the use of her extremities and assisted in bringing the child's extremities toward the midline of the body, thus helping to inhibit the asymmetrical tonic neck reflex.

A decrease in oral hypersensitivity may occur in response to repetitive, increasing stimulation of the oral area. The child may adapt to the sensory stimulation if it occurs in a planned sequence. C.'s parents were shown techniques of oral stimulation to be carried out before and during feeding. The techniques included stroking C.'s upper and lower lip, beginning at the center of her mouth and moving outward toward the corners of the mouth, so that four separate stroking motions occurred. The gums were then similarly stroked, again starting medially and working laterally. Once C. tolerated this type of oral stimulation (after two sessions), stimulation was given to the tongue in order to assist in reducing tongue protrusion. Pressure was applied with the theapists's finger on the front half of the tongue, starting at the lip and working back. When the spoon was introduced, the same pressure was applied to the tongue.

The treatment program was carried out before and during every mealtime. This meant organization and cooperation between the feeding team and the hospital staff responsible for her daily care. This relationship was critical to the success of treatment.

Results of Treatment

C. began feeding more successfully. She had no recurring incidences of aspiration pneumonia. At the time of discharge (2 weeks after admission), her caloric intake had increased from 450 kcal (1890 kJ) a day to 700 kcal (2940 kJ) a day, and she was beginning to eat textured food. She had gained weight (going from 6 kg to 7 kg), and her parents were becoming skilled at feeding and handling C. This made the mealtime experience pleasant.

CHAPTER 27

INBORN ERRORS OF METABOLISM

Gail Neimeth Kaplan

KEY WORDS
Gene Mutation
Heterozygote
Homozygote
Biochemical Defect
Screening
Restricted Diet

INTRODUCTION

The concept of the inborn error of metabolism was proposed by Sir Archibald Garrod in the early 1900s. He described four hereditary conditions that he believed to result from specific blocks in steps of certain metabolic processes.[1] His original proposal of inborn errors was later extended to include defects of membrane transport proteins.[2] Errors in the transport carrier proteins result in the loss of specific metabolites in the urine. Thus, both types of errors result from defects in specific proteins and cause an interruption in the metabolic sequence.

Though early in this century this concept was poorly understood or ignored, in the past few decades hundreds of metabolic errors were discovered, and the inborn error of metabolism principle became firmly established. These discoveries resulted from the development of techniques for the qualitative and quantitative determination of metabolites in the human fluids and from increased interest in biochemical causes of disease, particularly mental retardation.

Dietary treatment is effective in certain inborn errors. By limiting or eliminating the intake of the specific amino acid or carbohydrate associated with the disorder early in life, clinical symptoms can be prevented. Newborn-screening programs make it possible to begin treatment early. Clinics were established to treat inborn errors and to gather information about these disorders. As treatment techniques are new, further research is needed. This chapter will present the current understanding of inborn errors of metabolism and the appropriate treatment techniques.

BIOCHEMICAL DEFECTS OF INBORN ERRORS

The inborn errors originate in mutations of single genes which are responsible for the synthesis of specific protein products. The gene mutations result in the production of structurally altered

Note: The author acknowledges the work by Carol Hum in the first edition of this book. This chapter still contains some of her contributions.

proteins incapable of normal activity. In the inborn errors of metabolism, the gene mutation results in an altered enzyme which is not able to carry out its function as a catalyst. For the inborn errors of transport, the gene mutation results in an altered carrier protein which cannot function to reabsorb specific nutrients normally.

Inborn Errors of Metabolism

The gene mutation results in an altered enzyme that is not capable of normal catalytic activity, or in the total inhibition of the enzyme. This produces a block in all metabolic pathways which are controlled by the specific enzyme (see Fig. 27-2). The clinical complications depend upon the function of the enzyme.

In some inborn errors, there is an accumulation within the body fluids of the substrate just proximal to the enzyme block. An example is alkaptonuria, in which there is a defect in the enzyme homogentisic acid oxidase. The accumulation and deposition of homogentisic acid in the joints causes the arthritis which develops in young adults with this disorder.

In other errors, there is an accumulation of metabolites formed through minor alternative pathways proximal to the enzyme. In classical phenylketonuria, there is a defect in the enzyme

Figure 27-1
Inheritance pattern for an inborn error of metabolism. Heterozygous parents are carriers for the mutant recessive gene; they have both a mutant and a normal gene. Each offspring of these parents has a 50 percent chance of also being a carrier, while there is a 25 percent chance of being homozygous normal (not a carrier and not affected) and a 25 percent chance of being homozygous for the inborn error (an affected individual).

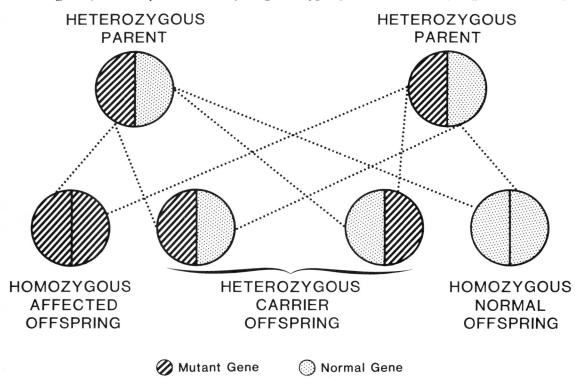

HETEROZYGOUS PARENT   HETEROZYGOUS PARENT

HOMOZYGOUS AFFECTED OFFSPRING   HETEROZYGOUS CARRIER OFFSPRING   HOMOZYGOUS NORMAL OFFSPRING

⬿ Mutant Gene   ⊙ Normal Gene

phenylalanine hydroxylase which metabolizes phenylalanine to tyrosine. When untreated, there is an accumulation of phenylalanine as well as phenylpyruvic acid, a metabolite formed from a minor pathway proximal to the enzyme defect. Severe mental retardation results if the disease is untreated, probably because of the effects of these metabolites on the brain.

A reduced production of one or more metabolites distal to the enzyme block causes the clinical manifestations in other inborn errors. In one type of albinism, there is a block between the amino acid tyrosine and the pigment melanin. This results in the lack of melanin production and a lack of pigmentation of the hair, skin, and eyes of the affected individual.

Often, an enzyme functions as part of a complex that consists of the enzyme and a coenzyme. A number of inborn errors are caused by a defect in the synthesis or transport of the coenzyme, or by such mechanisms as a poor interaction between the coenzyme and the enzyme.[3] These are often termed *vitamin-dependent* or *vitamin-responsive inborn errors* because vitamins are the precursors of the coenzyme. An example of this type of error is one form of homocystinuria, known as vitamin B_6-responsive homocystinuria. As opposed to the classical form of homocystinuria, in which there is a defect in the enzyme cystathionine synthase, here the defect is in the coenzyme of the synthase enzyme for which vitamin B_6 is a precursor.

Inborn Errors of Transport

The inborn errors of transport are a group of genetic disorders characterized by impaired intestinal and renal transport proteins or ligands, which normally function in the reabsorption of specific nutrients. The absence of the carrier protein results in the excessive loss of the substrate in the urine or feces. Hartnup disease is an inborn error of transport of the neutral amino acids (i.e., tryptophan) which results in a compromised absorption of these amino acids. Because dietary tryptophan provides half of the daily requirement of nicotinamide, this could cause a nicotinamide deficiency.

SCREENING FOR INBORN ERRORS

Genetic screening programs for infants are now widespread and can test for more than 20 inborn errors. Phenylketonuria, galactosemia, homocystinuria, maple syrup urine disease, and tyrosinemia are among the diseases which can be tested for and treated with diet therapy.

All screening programs test for phenylketonuria, the most common of these disorders. There are a number of screening programs which test for many other disorders. In the United States, phenylketonuria is the most common disorder for which screening is mandatory by individual state laws.

Cost-benefit analysis has proven PKU screening and treatment programs to be economical.[4] Cost efficiency of screening for other inborn errors has not been established. If screening tests for those disorders which occur less frequently than phenylketonuria are added to existing screening programs, the total number of infants discovered with treatable conditions may economically justify the costs.[5]

INCIDENCE

The frequency of these diseases is quite low; however, it is probably underestimated for certain conditions (i.e., organic acidurias, maple syrup urine disease) because many affected neonates die before the condition is identified. Our knowledge regarding incidence has increased during the past few years because of routine newborn screening and the establishment of national and regional registries, as well as the increased number of published surveys documenting regional incidence. As a result, it is recognized that certain conditions are more prevalent in specific regions or within certain ethnic groups. For example, in Japan phenylketonuria is quite rare, with a reported incidence of 1 in 110,000, while that reported for Northern Ireland is 1 in 6,000.[6] In Massachusetts, with a mixed population, the incidence of phenylketonuria is 1 in 15,000.[7]

INHERITANCE

The inborn errors of metabolism are inherited biochemical disorders, the majority with an autosomal recessive mode of transmission.[8] Persons carrying the mutant recessive gene are known as heterozygotes. They do not show clinical manifestations of the disorder. When both parents are heterozygous for the mutant gene, each pregnancy carries a 1 in 4 chance of the offspring being homozygous for the mutant gene, and therefore affected (see Fig. 27-1). The homozygous or affected individuals have the disorder and all the clinical manifestations.

CLINICAL MANIFESTATIONS

The pathological consequences of enzyme-deficiency diseases are attributed to the disordered pattern of metabolism and resulting biochemical imbalance. Clinical symptoms vary widely (see Table 27-1). Some defects have no clinical effect on the individual, while others may cause mental retardation and serious disease affecting several organ systems. In some, neurological damage is slowly progressive and often without

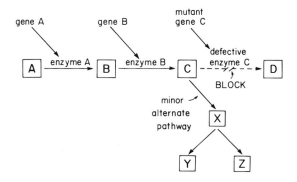

Figure 27-2
Schematic representation of an altered metabolic sequence. A genetic defect in enzyme C produces a block in the reaction that leads to accumulation of substrate C and an increased utilization of the minor alternative pathway, producing metabolites X, Y, Z.

noticeable signs in the first months of life. Still others are associated with a rapidly deteriorating neonatal course leading to early death, unless immediate treatment is instituted. Although the primary enzymatic defect is identified in many, the exact mechanism which produces the clinical manifestations is not understood.

TABLE 27-1   EXAMPLES OF INBORN ERRORS OF AMINO ACID AND CARBOHYDRATE METABOLISM

Disorder	Incidence	Biochemical defect	Biochemical analysis	
			Blood	Urine
Amino acids				
Classical phenylketonuria	1:10,000	Defective phenylalanine hydroxylase enzyme which prevents the conversion of phenylalanine, an essential amino acid, to tyrosine, another amino acid.	Increased phenylalanine.	Increased phenylacids: phenylpyruvic acid, phenylacetic acid, orthohydroxyphenylacetic acid

DIAGNOSIS

It is important to note that the majority of enzymatic defects do not have specific clinical features that indicate the presence of an inborn error of metabolism. The high morbidity and mortality in unrecognized and untreated cases of inborn errors, such as galactosemia and maple syrup urine disease, make early diagnosis essential, if clinical complications and death are to be prevented.

Thus, when unexpected symptoms or crises occur in early infancy—such as the presence of cataracts or other eye defects at birth, failure to eat, vomiting, irritability, lethargy, coma, acidosis, unusual odor, enlarged liver, or jaundice—and when they persist or do not respond to conventional treatment, the possibility of an inborn error of metabolism should be considered.[9,10] Appropriate screening tests or quantitative analysis of plasma or urine can then be made to detect signs of biochemical abnormality. The early detection of phenylketonuria, in advance of the onset of clinical symptoms, is now possible through the mass screening of newborn infants.

Symptoms warranting testing in older infants and children are delayed development, mental retardation, seizures, hematologic abnormalities, unexplained thromboses, renal defects or calculi, speech defects, failure to grow, skeletal disorders, skin lesions, fever of unknown origin, recurrent infections, unusual facies, and dark urine. In addition, those symptoms for infants that are listed above also warrant testing when present in older children.[11]

When the enzyme deficiency is detectable in amniotic fluid cells or when the presence of abnormal levels of metabolites is detectable in amniotic fluid, prenatal diagnosis of an inborn error is possible by amniocentesis. This is a special process whereby a small amount of the amniotic fluid surrounding the fetus is withdrawn and analyzed.[12]

Amniocentesis is offered to families in which a high risk for a specific inborn error has been established by the diagnosis of a disorder in an affected child. Galactosemia (see Table 27-1), maple syrup urine disease (Table 27-1), and methylmalonic aciduria are examples of inborn errors that have been detected antenatally.[13]

Clinical symptoms	Treatment	Comment
Infant appears normal at birth, followed by hyperactivity, irritability, persistent musty odor, severe mental retardation, decreased pigmentation, and eczema, if untreated.	Phenylalanine-restricted diet: no high-quality protein foods (milk, milk products, meat, fish poultry, eggs, nuts). Controlled amounts of fruits, vegetables, and grain products. Special formula, low in phenylalanine, provides protein and is supplemented with vitamins and minerals. Treatment monitored with blood phenylalanine levels, growth, and psychological data.	Phenylalanine must be provided in amounts sufficient to support growth. There are milder forms which may not require a diet, and there are variant forms which do not respond to treatment.

(Continued)

TABLE 27-1 CONTINUED

Disorder	Incidence	Biochemical defect	Biochemical analysis	
			Blood	Urine
Amino acids (continued)				
Classical homocystinuria	1:180,000	Defective cystathionine synthetase enzyme which prevents the interaction between an intermediate product of the amino acid methionine with serine to form cystathionine.	Increased methionine and homocysteine.	Increased homocysteine.
Maple syrup urine disease	1:200,000	Defective oxidative decarboxylase enzymes Keto acids of the branch chain amino acids (leucine, valine, and isoleucine) are not converted to simple acids.	Increased leucine, valine, and isoleucine and their keto acids.	Increased leucine, valine, and isoleucine and their keto acids.
Hereditary tyrosinemia (hepatorenal type)	Not determined	Defect in parahydroxy phenylpyruvic acid oxidase and perhaps other enzymes probably secondary to and as yet unknown primary defect.	Increased tyrosine and in some cases increased methionine.	Increased parahydroxy phenylpyruvic acid; generalized aminoaciduria.
Carbohydrates				
Classical galactosemia	1:100,000	Defective galactose 1-phosphate uridyl transferase. Galactose, a monosaccharide, is not converted to glucose.	Increased galactose 1-phosphate.	Increased galactose; generalized aminoaciduria.
Hereditary fructose intolerance	Over 40 cases reported	Defect in fructose 1-phosphate aldolase. Fructose, a monosaccharide, is not converted to glucose.	Increased fructose.	Increased fructose.

Clinical symptoms	Treatment	Comment
Possible mental retardation; lens dislocation; limb overgrowth; connective tissue defect leading to scoliosis, osteoporosis, vascular thrombosis; fair hair and skin.	Methionine-restricted (similar to phenylalanine-restricted) diet, supplemented with cysteine Cysteine, a product of methionine, becomes an essential amino acid when methionine is limited. Special low-methionine formula is used, and methionine levels in the blood are monitored, along with growth and psychological functioning.	There are other forms of homocystinuria. One is responsive to high doses of pyridoxine (vitamin B_6), a coenzyme of cystathionine synthetase. Another is responsive to vitamin B_{12}, a coenzyme in the remethylation reaction of homocysteine to methionine. Prenatal diagnosis by amniocentesis is possible.
Infant appears normal at birth, with symptoms showing in the first fews days. Difficulties with sucking and swallowing, irregular respiration, intermittent rigidity and flaccidity, possible grand mal seizures. Urine has the odor of maple syrup. If infant survives, mental retardation is severe if untreated.	Diet is restricted in leucine, valine, and isoleucine (similar to phenylalanine-restricted). Special formula is prepared. Blood leucine, valine and isoleucine are monitored, along with growth and psychological functioning.	There is a transient form of the disease, for which treatment is necessary only during times of illness. Prenatal diagnosis by amniocentesis is possible.
Enlargement of liver and spleen noted early in infancy; abdominal distention, liver and renal damage, vitamin D–resistant rickets.	Diet restricted in phenylalanine and tyrosine. The essential amino acid phenylalanine is a precursor of tyrosine. Methionine has also been restricted in a few individuals. A special formula is used, and blood phenylalanine, tyrosine, and methionine and growth are monitored.	Dietary treatment has not been successful in most cases. Biochemical abnormalities and renal tubular dysfunction have been corrected; however, liver disease is progressive.
Infant appears normal at birth with symptoms developing after feedings containing lactose. Symptoms include anorexia, vomiting, occasional diarrhea, lethargy, jaundice, hepatomegaly, increased susceptibility to infection. Later, cataracts and physical and mental retardation develop.	Rigid exclusion of lactose and galactose from the diet. Hydrolysis of lactose yields glucose and galactose. Diet is milk-free, free of milk products. Lactose-free formula is used. If children do not accept formula, diet will need nutrient supplementation.	Nonclassical forms include galactokinase and epimerase deficiency. The clinical features are not the same in all three forms. Prenatal diagnosis by amniocentesis is possible.
For infants, symptoms include anorexia, vomiting, failure-to-thrive, hypoglycemic convulsions, dysfunction of the liver and kidney. For older children, spontaneous hypoglycemia and vomiting occur after the ingestion of fructose.	Elimination of fructose and sucrose from the diet. Hydrolysis of sucrose yields glucose and fructose.	Differentiate from transient neonatal tyrosinemia.

TREATMENT

Early treatment is essential if mental retardation and other serious sequelae are to be prevented. The infant's rapidly developing central nervous system is particularly vulnerable to these defects in metabolism which can interfere with growth.

For several inborn errors, treatment is possible by restriction or elimination of a substrate (carbohydrate or amino acid) from the diet. Dietary treatment has been applied to a number of hereditary metabolic diseases with varying degrees of success. The control of substrate accumulation is possible when the substrate is a nutrient which the body cannot synthesize or when it is derived primarily from the diet.

For the inborn errors of amino acid metabolism, treatment consists in limiting the amino acids concerned while providing adequate amounts of protein and amino acids to support growth and tissue maintenance. Special formulas are used to provide the protein without the involved amino acids. Natural foods containing known amounts of the restricted amino acid are incorporated into the diet to supply the amount required for normal metabolism.

The treatment and its success varies with the specific inborn errors. In phenylketonuria, one amino acid, phenylalanine, is limited in the diet. Treatment is very successful. In maple syrup urine disease, the three branched amino acids are restricted and management is more difficult. The disease is not always diagnosed early enough for treatment to be effective. Tyrosinemia, another disorder, is characterized by liver disease, renal tubular dysfunction, hypertyrosinemia, and, in some cases, hypermethioninemia. The infant is treated with a diet low in phenylalanine and tyrosine or low in methionine, in addition to having restrictions on phenylalanine and tyrosine. While treatment corrects the biochemical abnormalities and the renal tubular dysfunction, the effect on the liver is generally not as favorable. Liver disease is progressive.[14] There are reported cases where the response was better,[15,16] but follow-up is

needed. Hepatoma is a significant contributor to death in tyrosinemic patients who survive beyond infancy.[17]

For those disorders caused by a defect in the coenzyme portion of the haloenzyme, treatment consists in administering large doses of the precursor vitamin for the coenzyme.

Inborn errors of carbohydrate metabolism are treated through the total elimination of the involved carbohydrate from the diet. Dietary management is less difficult for the carbohydrate disorders than for amino acid disorders, since specific disaccharides and monosaccharides are not essential nutrients. They are synthesized within the body as they are needed. Care must be taken to ensure that a balanced selection of appropriate foods is provided and that the foods are free of the involved carbohydrate as a sweetener or other ingredient.

Although the dietary management of inborn errors may appear simple in theory, the complexities of practical application must not be overlooked. In order to illustrate the broad dimensions of disease detection, therapy, and prognosis, the next section of this chapter is devoted to a discussion of phenylketonuria, an amino acid disorder, and of galactosemia, a carbohydrate disorder. These are the two inborn errors for which dietary treatment is the most successful.

PHENYLKETONURIA

Biochemical Defect

Phenylketonuria is the term used for a group of disorders. The major categories include classical, "atypical," and persistent mild hyperphenylalaninemia. In the classical form of phenylketonuria (PKU), there is a defect in the enzyme phenylalanine hyroxylase, which is necessary for the conversion of the essential amino acid, phenylalanine, to tyrosine. As a consequence, phenylalanine and its metabolites accumulate in large amounts in the blood, and phenylacids

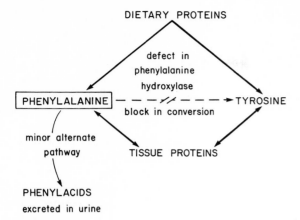

DIETARY PROTEINS

defect in
phenylalanine
hydroxylase

PHENYLALANINE — — — // — — — → TYROSINE

block in conversion

minor alternate
pathway

TISSUE PROTEINS

PHENYLACIDS
excreted in urine

Figure 27-3

The primary defect in phenylketonuria. A defect in the enzyme phenylalanine hydroxylase leads to an accumulation of the substrate phenylalanine in the blood and the excretion of its degradation products in the urine.

produced by compensatory pathways are excreted in the urine (see Fig. 27-3). In classical PKU, there is minimal function of phenylalanine hydroxylase. In "atypical" PKU and persistent mild hyperphenylalaninemia, there is slightly more of the enzyme, and therefore the levels of blood phenylalanine do not rise as high as in the classical form. Other variant forms of PKU, involving enzymes other than the hydroxylase enzyme, do exist[18], but the clinical manifestations, other than the elevation of phenylalanine, and the treatment of these variant forms are much different. These are not discussed in this section.

If abnormally elevated levels of phenylalanine and its metabolites persist, they produce deleterious effects on brain metabolism and lead to profound impairment of mental development. In addition, untreated individuals may exhibit aggressive behavior, hyperactivity, neuromuscular instability, seizures, and eczema. Blonde hair, fair complexion, and blue eyes, due to decreased pigmentation, are also common findings.

PKU Screening

The development of a simple screening test in the early 1960s made the widespread screening of newborns for PKU possible.[19] The Guthrie test is a microbiological assay for phenylalanine which can be performed on blood specimens taken from the baby's heel. Normally, the blood contains a small amount of phenylalanine, approximately 1 to 2 mg per 100 mL of plasma. However, when the infant with PKU begins formula or breast-milk feedings, the phenylalanine derived from the milk protein causes a significant rise in blood phenylalanine levels, which may reach 15 to 30 mg per 100 mL or higher, in the first week of life.

The Guthrie test, when performed in early infancy, detects the elevated levels of phenylalanine and allows for diagnosis in the interval before irreversible neurological damage takes place. However, since there are also transient states of hyperphenylalaninemia and variants of PKU that do not require dietary treatment, the results of a positive PKU Guthrie screening test must be followed by additional tests to confirm the diagnosis of PKU before diet therapy is initiated.

At present, nearly every state has laws mandating PKU screening of all newborns, while the remaining states provide voluntary screening. Current practice involves performing the test within the first week following birth, generally just before discharge from the nursery. A second determination of blood phenylalanine is recommended for all infants by 1 month of age to detect infants with PKU who had low concentrations of phenylalanine in the first few days.[20,21]

Treatment

A significant factor in determining the success of therapy is the patient's age at the time of diagnosis and initiation of therapy. The earlier treatment is begun, the better the prognosis for intellectual development. When PKU is detected in early infancy and a low-phenylalanine diet is instituted and properly maintained, mental retardation and other symptoms associated with the disease are prevented.

Normal physical and mental development occur when the diet is started within the first 2 months of life, and particularly during the first month.[22,23] As treatment is delayed, the likelihood of satisfactory mental development decreases. However, the late treatment of infants and young children may promote mental development and improve behavior. There have been a few reports of significant increases in cognitive functioning in late-diagnosed individuals.[24–26]

Phenylalanine-Restricted Diet

Phenylalanine is an essential amino acid which must be obtained from food protein since it cannot be synthesized in the body. It is required by all persons, including individuals with PKU. Phenylalanine occurs in all natural protein, making up approximately 5 percent of the total protein. The amount of phenylalanine obtained in a normal diet is far in excess of the required amount.

The basis of treatment is to provide a diet low enough in phenylalanine to maintain blood levels between 4 and 8 mg per 100 mL, while supplying enough of the amino acid protein, other nutrients, and energy to support needs for normal physical growth and health.[27] Phenylalanine requirements range from 65 to 90 mg per kilogram of body weight daily during the newborn period, to 20 to 25 mg per kilogram at 2 years.[28] Suggested protein intakes range from 4.4 g per kilogram per day in the newborn period, to 2.0 to 2.5 g per kilogram per day at 2 years of age.[29] The recommended caloric intake is 120 kcal (502.1 kJ) per kilogram per day for the newborn and 100 kcal (418.4 kJ) per kilogram per day or 1300 kcal (5.4 MJ) daily for the 2-year-old.[30]

In order to control elevations of blood phenylalanine in the child with PKU while providing an adequate amount of protein, replacement of protein is required. This is achieved through use of one of the several low-phenylalanine or phenylalanine-free protein products. Lofenalac and Phenyl-Free are the two formulas most commonly used in this country.[31] Although others have been developed, they are used primarily outside this country. Lofenalac is a casein hydrolysate from which 95 percent of the phenylalanine is removed. It is supplemented with vitamins and minerals. Lofenalac has a protein to calorie ratio of 3.3 g protein per 100 kcal (420 kJ). It was designed for infants. Phenyl-Free has a higher ratio of protein to calorie, 5 g protein per 100 kcal (420 kJ). It was designed for children 2 years of age and older.[32] Phenyl-Free is a synthetic mixture, free of phenylalanine, containing amino acids, carbohydrate, fat, vitamins, and minerals. The diet for a child on the Phenyl-Free formula includes more natural sources of food since Phenyl-Free contains no phenylalanine.

Since the formulas replace the high-quality protein sources (i.e., meat, poultry, fish, eggs), it is important that the other nutrients, particularly the trace minerals, associated with these foods be monitored. Studies have shown that the absorption of iron, zinc, and copper may be significantly less from Lofenalac than from a normal diet. Studies on Phenyl-Free are needed. The amount of magnesium supplied by both formulas is low.[33,34] Selenium, an essential nutrient also derived from the high-protein sources, is not well supplemented in most of the PKU formulas,[35] including Lofenalac and Phenyl-Free.[36] Individuals using products over a long period of time may be at risk for magnesium or selenium deficiency (see Chap. 7) as well as of the minerals already mentioned. Blood levels of these nutrients should be checked regularly. Additional supplementation may be a consideration.

The formula alone will not supply adequate amounts of phenylalanine to support growth and the maintenance of tissues. Measured amounts of natural foods that are low in protein are included in the diet to provide the amount of phenylalanine required.

In early infancy, small measured amounts of whole milk, evaporated milk, or infant formula are added to the Lofenalac to supply the infant's phenylalanine requirement. Human milk may be used instead of cow's milk if the mother desires to breast-feed. The breast milk contains about half the amount of phenylalanine contained in cow's milk. It can be given in greater quantities. The mother can either express her milk or allow the infant to breast-feed for a specific period of time, weighing the infant before and after each feeding to determine that the prescribed amount of milk is being fed.[37]

As the infant grows, milk is removed from the formula, and restricted amounts of infant foods are introduced into the diet to replace the milk phenylalanine. These foods are given in specified amounts with the aid of phenylalanine exchange lists. Each food on the list (mainly fruits, vegetables, and grains) is given in amounts that contain approximately 15 mg phenylalanine, which is considered an "equivalent." Each equivalent may be exchanged for another equivalent, allowing for variety in the diet. Also, lists of food are given with the milligrams of phenylalanine per serving size. This enables parents to add the number of milligrams eaten and keep within the prescribed amount. (See Table 27-2, below.)

Cereal and other grain products contain more phenylalanine than fruits and vegetables, so smaller quantities of the grain products make up an equivalent. Since meat, fish, poultry, and dairy products are very high in phenylalanine, they are usually excluded from the diet.

The diet is planned for the developmental progression of the infant, with introductions to food texture and self-feeding practices commensurate with those of other children (see Table 27-3, pp. 640–641).

In addition to monitoring the phenylalanine and protein in the diet along with any trace minerals that might be missing, enough calories for the child's growing body are a concern. As the child gets closer to school age, appetite and the calorie requirement increase while the requirement of phenylalanine per kilogram actually decreases. Special low-protein products (low-protein breads, pasta, cookies, baking mixes, wheat starch, egg replacer) are used to make the diet

TABLE 27-2   PHENYLALANINE CONTENT OF SELECTED FOODS

Food	Amount	Protein, g	Phenylalanine, mg	Calories
Lofenalac	1 cup	22.4	112	688
Phenyl-free	1 cup	32	—	640
Whole milk	1 cup	32	416	640
Apple, raw (2½–3″ diam)	2 med	0.6	15	170
Applesauce, canned, sweetened	1¼ cup	0.6	15	273
Applesauce, strained	10 tbsp	0.3	15	60
Bread, white, average	1 slice	1.8	99	58
Cereal, rice (infant)	1 tbsp	0.2	8	9
(oatmeal)	1 tbsp	0.3	18	9
Carrots, cooked	1 tbsp	0.1	3	3
Cheerios (General Mills)	1 tbsp	0.2	10	6
Cheese, American	1 oz	7.0	378	112
Chicken, roasted	1 oz	7.9	395	56
Graham cracker	1 sq	0.5	25	30
Green beans, cooked	1 tbsp	0.1	3	2
Orange juice, fresh	1 oz	0.2	10	14

TABLE 27-3   COMMON ISSUES IN THE MANAGEMENT OF A CHILD'S PKU DIET

Issues	Considerations
Infant refuses formula from cup upon initial attempts at weaning	This is not unusual for any child when a cup is first introduced. Try offering a cup when the child is at his or her best (well rested, not very hungry, not full). Being consistent is important. Try once daily at first.
	Because the child has only taken Lofenalac from a bottle with a lid until this time, the smell of the Lofenalac will be new and may be offensive. To prevent this, offer Lofenalac from a spoon occasionally before the weaning process.
14-month-old, fully weaned from bottle, does not drink all of the prescribed formula	Once weaning is completed, it may be necessary to decrease the total volume of the formula by using less water. At this age the child is taking solids and does not need the volume of fluid that was needed earlier to provide satiety. The body of a child this age can handle a more concentrated formula. The nutritionist should evaluate the diet to assure an adequate food and fluid intake.
20-month-old refuses to eat	Developmentally, toddlers are beginning to assert their independence, and food refusal is one of the ways of doing so. Refusal may be an attention-getting behavior for the child, a normal endeavor at this age. Offering the child a choice between two foods is a way of enabling the child to have some control. Having playtimes with the child aside from mealtimes will make the child less likely to seek attention by food refusal.
	Because the diet is quite restrictive and parents are concerned about the child taking the specified amounts of food, control issues are more likely to take place around meals. The child may sense tension if a parent is anxious about the diet. Teaching a parent how to substitute milk in the formula if a child does not eat the prescribed amount of foods can take some of the pressure off the parent.
3-year-old found eating a food not allowed on diet	It is normal for preschoolers to begin testing limits. Parents must be firm but not misleading. If children are told an unacceptable food tastes "terrible" or "it will make you sick," they are likely to find out that this is not true, and the credibility gap will be harder to mend later.
	By 3 years of age, children are capable of starting to learn "yes" and "no" foods. This knowledge can be built on as the child is able to understand more.
	The diet should be evaluated to ensure that the child is getting enough formula and food to rule out the possibility that the child is taking food because of hunger. Always be sure to have food available that the child is allowed to have.
Birthday parties in school	When the child first enters class, the teacher should be informed that the child is on a special diet and be told what foods the child can have if there is a party. There is almost always something a child can have at a party. Surprisingly, children are usually very happy to have the special treat instead of what everyone else is having. The teacher may be able to keep certain items at school (low-protein cookies, lollipops) in case the situation arises. It may be possible to obtain a list of birthdays and to be prepared for these parties by sending in a special low-protein snack for the child on those days.

TABLE 27-3 CONTINUED

Issues	*Considerations*
Lunch for the school-aged child	The child can bring lunch, including sandwiches made on special low-protein bread (or half sandwiches on regular bread if tolerance for phenylalanine is high enough), salad, fruit, and a thermos of formula. Some children do not want to take formula. They can take another beverage instead and have the formula before school and afterward with a snack.
	It is important that the parents and child in school have an open and communicative relationship so that when the child has extra food, it will not be kept a secret. Then there is the likelihood that the diet can be adjusted later in the day.

more palatable and filling. Cookbooks are available which add variety to the diet (see Table 27-4). Concentrated carbohydrates such as jellies and syrups may have to be added to maintain energy requirements. Dental hygiene and regular visits to the dentist are essential for the school-aged child.

Children should be taught from an early age which foods are appropriate for their bodies and should be encouraged to take responsibility for their own dietary management. Parents are the main teachers for their children. Some families adopt a vegetarian diet, while others prepare special recipes for their child (e.g., meatless meatballs) so that the child feels included at mealtime. The approach that best fits the family style is the approach that will work, if it is a consistent approach.

There are several teaching aids available to assist in learning (see Table 27-4). Scheduling children according to age and holding teaching sessions at a PKU clinic can help parents to learn effective teaching methods and can reinforce what the child is taught (see Fig. 27-4). It also allows the children to meet other children with PKU. Preschool children can help mix up the formula or help bake low-protein bread. They can begin learning portion sizes to lay the foundation for taking on more responsibility for their diet when, later on, they go to school. Children can keep track of the amount of equivalents they eat daily.

Monitoring Treatment

Since considerable variation exists among PKU individuals in requirements and tolerance, regular monitoring of blood phenylalanine is essential. The phenylalanine level reflects the biochemical response to dietary manipulations and the degree of dietary control. A suitable schedule for blood phenylalanine determinations is:

1 Twice weekly during the initial diet stabilization
2 Weekly in infants and toddlers
3 At 2 to 3 week intervals thereafter for the duration of the diet

The blood phenylalanine level and the rates of weight gain and growth determine when additional phenylalanine is needed in the diet. Parents are asked to bring in 3-day food diaries. The diet is monitored for phenylalanine, protein, calories, and other nutrients. Periodic checks on iron and zinc status, as well as copper, magnesium, and selenium, are made.

Inadequate intake of phenylalanine can lead to anorexia, rash, listlessness, and failure to grow. If the deficiency is not recognized and treated, it can lead to impaired intellectual function and severe illness; it can eventually be fatal.

During periods of illness and fever, blood phenylalanine levels increase; however, the general management of the child is like that of any other pediatric patient.

TABLE 27-4 TEACHING AIDS FOR PKU

Materials	Available through
For children	
What Is PKU? by Iris Crump, M.S., R.D. Coloring book explaining PKU by the analogy of different cars needing different types of gas to run well and people with PKU needing a special diet to run well.	San Diego Regional Center for the Developmentally Disabled Children's Hospital and Health Center 8001 Frost Street San Diego, Calif. 92123
Why Is Mary on a Diet? by the staff at the PKU Clinic at Children's Memorial Hospital. Storybook about a girl with PKU describing her experiences with the PKU Clinic personnel and procedures.	Children's Memorial Hospital 2300 Children's Plaza Chicago, Ill. 60614
You and PKU by Margaret Taylor and Virginia Schuett. Book explaining why people have PKU, the PKU diet, blood tests, and clinic visits.	Waisman Center on Mental Retardation and Human Development 1500 Highland Avenue Madison, Wis. 53706
Games That Teach by Carla Cox, M.S., R.D., Janie Falkenreck, M.S., R.D., and Chris Trahms, M.S., R.D. Booklet describing games to teach children about the PKU diet; Publication no. 22-50.	Washington State Department of Social and Health Services Olympia, Wash.
Phe and Me by Mary Ellen Banks. Colorful cartoon film explaining that the body needs just the right amount of "phes"; it animates foods with a lot and a little "phe" and talks about how the body responds to too much "phe" and not enough "phe."	MLK Film Productions c/o Mary Ellen Banks P.O. Box 8064 Knoxville, Tenn.
For parents	
Living With PKU by the University of Colorado Medical Center's PKU Clinic staff and parents. Booklet briefly explaining what PKU is and what the PKU diet is. Section by parents offers support to other parents around everyday living and PKU. Answers commonly asked questions about PKU.	Mead Johnson Laboratories Evansville, Ind. 47721
PKU—A Diet Guide For Parents of Children With PKU by Phyllis Acosta, Elizabeth Wenz, Graciela Shaeffler, and Richard Koch. Booklet discussing diet, preparation of Lofenalac, meal plans, developmental feeding issues, and food and social environment (i.e., school lunch, restaurants); includes diet list.	Mead Johnson Laboratories Evansville, Ind. 47721
Parents' Guide to the Child With PKU by Phyllis Acosta, Dr. PH.; Olga Boberg, B.S.; Jeanne Silberstein, B.S.; and Elizabeth Wenz, M.S. Book which explains diagnosis and inheritance, the PKU diet, and practical aspects of managing the diet throughout the childhood years; includes diet list.	Programs in Dietetics Emory University School of Medicine 2040 Ridgewood Drive NE Atlanta, Ga. 30322

TABLE 27-4   CONTINUED

Materials	Available through
Cookbooks and diet lists	
The PKU Cookbook by Elizabeth Read, R.D.; Elizabeth Wenz, M.S., R.D.; Roslyn A. Duffy, R.D.; Nancy S. Wellman, M.S., R.D.; Aissa Acosta; Phyllis B. Acosta, Dr. PH., R.D.	University of New Mexico Printing Plant Albuquerque, N. Mex.

Low Protein Cookery for Phenylketonuria by Virginia E. Schuett	Local PKU clinics, supplied by:
	    Metabolic Clinic
	    Waisman Center
	    1500 Highland Avenue
	    Madison, Wis. 53706
	(This has been funded through the March of Dimes for families of children with PKU.)
	Health professionals may purchase copies through:
	    University of Wisconsin Press
	    Box 1379
	    Madison, Wis.

Phenylalanine, Protein, and Calorie Content of Selected Foods by Melanie M. Hunt, R.D.	The Children's Hospital Research Foundation Cincinnati, Ohio 45229

Figure 27-4

Teaching sessions at a PKU clinic are a way to help parents learn effective teaching methods and to help children learn diet control.

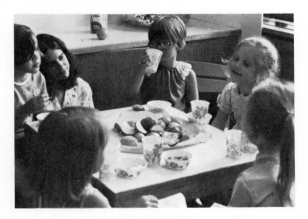

Duration of Dietary Treatment

The length of time that diet therapy should be continued is not yet determined. Many clinics have recommended terminating the diet at ages ranging from 3 to 10 years, while others have recommended continuing it indefinitely.[38] Still others suggest a "relaxed" diet beyond age 5.[39]

The results of follow-up studies on children who have terminated the diet have been equivocal. Some report reductions in IQ[40,41] while others report no changes in IQ scores.[42,43] There is a wide range of individual responses to diet termination, suggesting that perhaps some children are more vulnerable than others. There are many problems inherent in these studies, including the use of different examiners, the use of different IQ tests for on-diet and off-diet testing, the lack of control groups, the lack of comparison of subtest scores, and the lack of research correlating changes in IQ with changes in emotion or school achievement.[44] In a large, collaborative study in the United States the results have been biased because 22 percent of the parents would not accept the randomized assignments either to continue or discontinue the diet.[45]

At the current state of knowledge, it seems the prudent approach to continue the diet until it is known more conclusively when it is safe to discontinue, or to continue until we can distinguish those children who should remain on the diet from those who may safely discontinue.[46]

For those who discontinue the diet, the transition period can be stressful for both child and family. New foods that once were restricted are now allowed. The parent and child must adapt to this new experience as the parent is now in the position of encouraging formerly restricted foods and the child is exposed to the new tastes of milk and meat.

Gradual introduction of new foods helps in adjustment. First, the child is allowed any of the foods on the PKU food list without counting phenylalanine or equivalents. Next, foods of high-quality-protein value are introduced, with the exception of milk. The special formula is still included in the diet to assure adequate protein intake, as many children do not initially eat enough of the protein-rich foods. The last stage is to introduce milk and dairy products and to cut back on the special formula until it is finally eliminated from the diet. Vitamin and mineral supplementation of the diet is recommended while the child broadens his or her food acceptances.

PKU and Pregnancy

Women with PKU are at risk of having offspring with mental retardation, microcephaly, congenital heart disease, and low birth weight. It is assumed that an increased concentration of phenylalanine in the mother has a toxic effect on the fetus. It is suggested that there is a relationship between the maternal blood phenylalanine concentration and the effect on the offspring's intelligence. The risk of mental retardation is greater when the maternal blood phenylalanine is 20 mg per 100 mL or greater. Further study is needed to determine the levels of maternal blood phenylalanine which will not harm the fetus.[47]

To avoid the teratogenic effect of phenylalanine in women who wish to bear children, a phenylalanine-restricted diet during pregnancy is proposed.[48,49] The diet should begin shortly before conception. The diet is similar to that of the child with PKU; however, it provides for the nutrient demands of pregnancy. The diet includes the low-phenylalanine foods and formula. In this country, Lofenalac and Phenyl-Free formulas have been used with the few treated pregnant women.

Management issues are related to acceptance of the low-phenylalanine formula and adherence to a strict vegetarian diet. However, the pregnant mother with PKU is usually motivated to follow the diet. Another management issue is related to the composition of Lofenalac and Phenyl-Free formulas, which do not provide the proper balance of nutrients for pregnancy. These formulas provide an excess of vitamins A, D, and C and calcium and phosphorus. They do not provide the required amounts of folate, magnesium, and zinc and may require supplementation as mentioned earlier. The absorption of zinc, iron, and copper from Lofenalac is found to be poor in preliminary studies of children and raises questions about use for pregnancy.[50,51] It will be important to determine if these and other trace minerals are poorly absorbed from Phenyl-Free as well as Lofenalac. Routine determinations of those nutrients for which there is a concern is recommended.

Women on the phenylalanine-restricted diet do not require the standard prenatal vitamin and mineral supplements because of supplementation in the formula. The type of supplementation will depend on the formula used.

The maternal blood phenylalanine is monitored and kept slightly lower than that of a child with PKU. This is due to the fact that the blood level of the fetus is one and a half times greater than that of the mother.[52]

Men with PKU are not known to sire infants with congenital defects.

GALACTOSEMIA

Biochemical Defect

Galactosemia is not a singular disorder but a heterogenous group of enzyme disorders in the galactose metabolic pathway (see Fig. 27-5). The two known disorders are transferase-deficiency galactosemia, and galactokinase-deficiency galactosemia. The severest form is the transferase deficiency form, which involves the enzyme in the second step of the galactose-glucose interconversion. Galactokinase-deficiency galactosemia involves the initial step in the metabolism of galactose. A third enzyme in this pathway, epimerase, has recently been found to be deficient in certain cells; however, individuals with this deficiency are clinically normal.[53]

Other variant forms do exist, also without the clinical manifestations seen in the transferase- and galactokinase-deficiency form of galactosemia.

In the classical (transferase) form, the severest form of galactosemia, the clinical manifestations are caused by the accumulation of galactose, galactose 1-phosphate, and galactitol. Failure to thrive, vomiting, diarrhea, jaundice or hepatomegaly, and cataracts are among the early manifestations, often present within the first week of life. Later, delayed intellectual development and cirrhosis of the liver may result. In the galactokinase form, toxicity is milder, and the development of cataracts is the main clinical manifestation.[54] There is an accumulation of galactose and galactitol in this form.

Figure 27-5
Galactosemia is a heterogenous group of disorders of the galactose metabolic pathway. Transferase deficiency, galactokinase deficiency, and epimerase deficiency are three forms known to occur in humans.

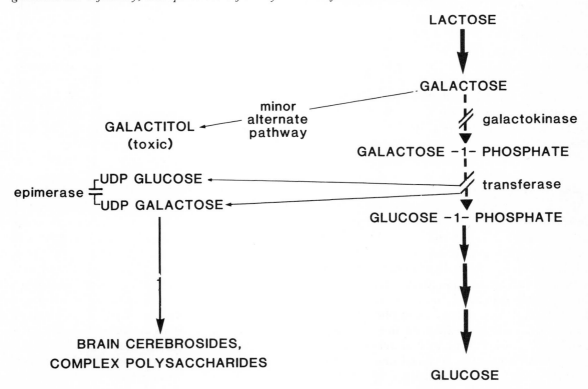

Galactose Screening

The Paigen assay for galactose[55] is commonly used in screening programs. The specimens with positive tests are then tested by the Beutler assay for transferase enzyme to distinguish which form of galactosemia is present.[56] Early death in neonates often associated with gram-negative bacteremia often occurs before the screening test can be performed. For this reason certain screening programs perform tests for galactosemia on umbilical-cord blood specimens, as well as on newborn blood specimens. Confirmatory tests are important, as abnormal results in screening may not necessarily indicate a significant disorder.[57]

Treatment

Early treatment is important if it is to be successful. A galactose-free diet is the recommended treatment. Initiation of diet will cause a regression of symptoms in those children who already manifest toxic effects. Restriction of galactose during pregnancy is recommended for those women who have had children with galactosemia.[58] Monitoring treatment for galactosemia is much less complex than monitoring treatment for PKU. Galactose, unlike phenylalanine, is not an essential nutrient. The body is able to manufacture the galactose it needs. There is no evidence that a restriction of galactose is harmful.[59]

Galactose-Free Diet

The galactose-free diet consists of eliminating all dietary sources of galactose and also lactose, because lactose is metabolized to galactose. Free galactose is very rarely found in foods; however, lactose is found in milk, milk products, and formula. It is also used as an additive in many food and medicinal products.

For infants with galactosemia, there are several milk substitutes which can be used which are essentially free of lactose. Nutramigen,[60] a casein hydrolysate with sucrose and modified tapioca starch added as the source of carbohy-

drate, is a formula commonly used. Also, Prosobee[61] and Isomil[62] are used. These formulas are prepared from soy protein isolate, with sucrose and corn syrup solids added as the carbohydrate source. A source of fat, vitamins, and minerals is added to all these products. They are considered nutritionally complete for the infant when taken in the proper amounts. As the total diet is much less restrictive than the low-phenylalanine diet, trace nutrient deficiencies are not a problem.

Introduction of strained foods, increased texture, and finger foods is begun at the same time as for a normal infant. Once solids are introduced, it is important for parents to understand which foods they must exclude and which foods are allowed. Galactose-free diet lists have been compiled (see Table 27-5).

In addition to these lists, it is very important for families to learn to read food labels. They must be aware that casein, whey, and whey solids are to be avoided, in addition to milk, butter, milk solids, milk sugar, and lactose.[63,64] Lactose is used in the manufacturing of many foods as a filler, a browning agent, a sweetening agent, a dye, and a flavor carrier. The parent or nutritionist must check with the manufacturers of baked products, colored food icings, and fondant-type candies.[65] Some dried fruits and vegetables may be processed with lactose. Cold cuts may contain lactose as a filler. The pharmaceutical industry uses lactose because it has excellent tablet-forming properties.[66] It is also used to coat the outside of pills.

In addition to milk and milk products and those products which contain lactose ingredients, peas and organ meats may contain small amounts of galactose and are also excluded. Legumes contain complex carbohydrates which contain galactose; however, it is presumed that humans do not have the enzyme necessary to break these down to galactose. It is suggested that these items be included in the diet only if the individual's blood is periodically tested.

It is important to continue using one of the galactose-free formulas beyond infancy to provide the recommended nutrients required during

TABLE 27-5 GALACTOSE-FREE DIETARY GUIDELINES

Type of food	Foods allowed	Amounts suggested/day	Foods excluded
Milk and milk products	Soy milk and soy milk formulas (Isomil, Nutramigen, Prosobee)	*Preschoolers—3 or more 6-oz servings *School-age—3 or more 8-oz servings *Adolescents—four 1-cup (8-oz) servings *Adults—2 or more 8-oz servings	Breast milk, cow milk, goat milk, or milk from any other animal source; milk-based infant formula Milk in any form: whole, skim (nonfat), low-fat, evaporated, condensed, dry milk solids, lactose, whey, casein, curds Milk-containing products such as ice cream, butter, all cheeses, cream, ice milk, sherbet, yogurt, malted milk, milk shakes, frappes, imitation or filled milks
	Nondairy creamers free of milk or milk-containing ingredients	These products cannot be substituted for the formula, because they do not provide the same nutrients; they can be used to increase the palatability of the diet	
Protein-rich foods	Plain meat, fish, poultry, eggs, kosher frankfurters, kosher cold cuts or kosher salami, nuts, nut butters	Preschoolers—two 2-oz 3- to 4-tbsp) servings School-age—two 2-oz servings Adolescents—2 or more 3-oz servings Adults—2 or more 3-oz servings	Liver, pancreas, brain; creamed or breaded meat, fish, or poultry; processed meats, fish, or poultry (cold cuts, sausage, luncheon meats, frankfurters) which may contain lactose as a filler
Fruits and vegetables	Any fresh, frozen, canned, or dried fruits and vegetables unless processed with lactose or unless on excluded list	†Preschoolers—4 or more ¼- to ½-cup servings †School-age—2 or more ⅓- to ½-cup servings †Adolescents—2 or more ½-cup servings †Adults—4 or more ½-cup servings	Fruits or vegetables processed with lactose (many dried fruits such as apricots and shredded coconut are processed this way); any creamed, breaded, or buttered vegetables; most brands of instant potatoes as they are processed with milk or lactose
	All legumes except peas may be included *if blood can be checked regularly*		Peas (contain free galactose)
Grains, cereals, pastas	Any which do not contain milk or milk products (this includes breads, cereals, crackers, cookies, macaroni, spaghetti, noodles, rice, tacos, tortillas)	‡Preschoolers—4 or more ½-cup or ½-slice servings ‡School-age—4 or more ¾-cup or 1-slice servings ‡Adolescents—4 or more 1-cup or 1-slice servings ‡Adults—4 or more 1-cup or 1-slice servings	Prepared mixes with milk or casein added; most brands of enriched white bread (contact local manufacturers for ingredients when they are not listed)

(Continued)

*If intake of the milk substitutes is low, it may be necessary to supplement diet with calcium, vitamin D, and riboflavin.
†One or more citrus fruits or high-vitamin C–containing fruits or vegetables should be included daily. A high-vitamin A–containing fruit or vegetable (orange or dark-green, leafy) should be used every other day.
‡Whole-grain or enriched products without milk or milk derivatives should be used.

TABLE 27-5   CONTINUED

Type of food	Foods allowed	Amounts suggested/day	Foods excluded
Fats	Vegetable oils (corn, soybean, safflower, cottonseed, olive, peanut); mayonnaise; any shortening, lard, margarine; salad dressings which do not contain milk or its derivatives; water-based gravies and sauces or those made with milk substitutes	As long as diet contains adequate amounts of milk substitutes and protein-rich foods, amounts of fats needed are based on individual energy needs	Butter, cream; any margarine, salad dressing, shortening, gravy, and sauces made with lactose-containing ingredients
Other foods	Water and fruit ices, gelatin, angel food cake, baked products made with lactose-free ingredients, fruit-flavored cornstarch puddings, white and brown sugar, corn syrup, molasses, honey, artificial sweeteners made with acceptable ingredients, marshmallows, sugar candies, gum (check ingredients) Jams, jellies, marmalade without lactose added Unsweetened cocoa, unsweetened cooking chocolate, semisweet chocolate, carob powder Carbonated beverages, punch base without lactose, plain chips, popcorn, catsup, mustard, pure seasonings and spices, instant coffee, plain alcoholic beverages, beer, wine	Amounts used should be determined by individual energy needs	Milk chocolate or chocolate syrup, caramels, toffee, candies made with lactose-containing ingredients, artificial sweeteners made with lactose-containing ingredients Buttered popcorn, flavored chips, or spices made with lactose; cordials, liqueurs, many premixed alcoholic drink mixes; drugs which contain lactose (check with the manufacturer)

the growing years. Often, nondairy creamers are used in place of milk. These are acceptable in terms of the galactose restriction; however, they do not contain appreciable amounts of calcium or protein. The diet must be supplemented with calcium if the child does not take formula, and protein intake must be evaluated.

Monitoring Treatment
Initially, for a child with transferase deficiency, serum is tested weekly until a normal erythrocyte galactose 1-phosphate level is reached (below 10 mg per deciliter). Monthly determinations are made in infancy, and determinations are made three to four times yearly for older children.[67] For those infants with galactokinase deficiency, an assay for galactose is performed on the same schedule. Parents are asked to bring in 3-day food records to determine adequacy of the diet. As with PKU, it is important for children with galactosemia to learn about their diet and to take some responsibility for it. Clinic visits should focus on teaching both the child and the parent.

Duration of Dietary Treatment

Diet discontinuation is a disputed area. There is evidence that an individual with galactosemia does not develop an increased ability to metabolize galactose. There have also been observations that discontinuing diet in early adolescence does not cause any of the symptoms associated with the disease.[68] Some clinics allow liberalization of diet in adolescence. Others restrict milk throughout life but allow products containing lactose as an ingredient when the child approaches adolescence in order to avoid psychological problems resulting from strict adherence.[69]

Galactosemia and Pregnancy

Women with galactosemia do not seem to be at risk for abnormal pregnancies. In the few reports in the literature, the offspring of galactosemic women were normal.[70,71]

A high incidence of ovarian failure in women with galactosemia has recently been reported.[72,73] However, further investigation is needed before the extent of this problem and its effect on fertility in these women is determined.

PUBLIC HEALTH IMPLICATIONS OF INBORN ERRORS OF METABOLISM

Despite the relatively low incidence of these inborn errors of metabolism, they are a public health concern.

Screening has spared many affected individuals of the handicapping consequences of their diseases, and has spared their families and society of the emotional and financial burdens that would have been placed on them as a result of the disorder.

Each state has the responsibility of screening and follow-up for these disorders. This includes providing treatment and formula for those families who cannot afford to pay for them.

The specially formulated products for the aminoacidopathies and special low-protein products (see section on PKU) are expensive. In 1979, the cost to feed an average 5-year-old with PKU, for example, was $1500 more a year than to feed a normal 5-year-old. The cost is even higher for some of the other inborn errors. Funding sources for formula include state Health Departments, Crippled Children's Services, county governments, Medicaid, the WIC program, family health insurances, and families of individuals using the products.[74]

In the past, the FDA classified the special formulas for the aminoacidopathies as drugs, and investigational new drug applications were required for their use. In 1972, however, the agency reclassified amino acids and amino acid-modified diets under the general class of foods for special dietary use, and in a specific category of "medical foods" to be used solely under medical supervision. This change has allowed manufacturers to develop more and better products and has lowered development cost. However, with the reclassification as foods, many third-party payers withdrew coverage, placing the burden on families. The subcommittee on Amino Acid Modified Diets of the Committee on Nutrition of the American Academy of Pediatrics has made great efforts to encourage third-party payers (e.g., private insurers) to reimburse for medical foods.[75]

In addition to its consultation with manufacturers and the FDA for purposes of improvement of products and their distribution, the aforementioned subcommittee has published a list of metabolic centers which provide consultative services, dietary treatment, and supplies on an emergency basis to physicians whose patients require them.[76]

In Canada, where the special products must be imported from the United States and Europe, the availability of the products has been enhanced by the establishment of a National Food Bank. This central treatment facility has improved importation and has controlled the distribution of the products, thus effectively preventing their misuse.[77,78]

CONCLUSION

The concept of inborn errors of metabolism was first put forth in the beginning of the nineteenth century. In recent times, as a result of advances in medical technology and clinical expertise, a number of these inherited metabolic disorders can be screened for and treated. Screening programs for certain inborn errors have been set up throughout the nation and in many other countries. Many of these disorders are treated by diet. Dietary treatment has been improved upon over the years. Synthetic formulas have been produced, and an increasing number of special food products are now available, facilitating treatment by increasing the variety of these very restrictive diets.

The field is still growing. For some of the newly discovered metabolic errors, treatment is not yet known. Treatment for maternal PKU is also an area in which we must look to the future for answers. The state of the economy will also play a role in the treatment of these conditions in terms of the availability of services, expansion of screening programs, and the provision of special formulas.

STUDY QUESTIONS

1 Why is it essential that inborn errors of metabolism be diagnosed and treated as early as possible?

2 What is the physiological change detected by the Guthrie screening test for PKU?

3 What foods would be eliminated from the diet of a child with PKU?

4 Why is it essential that a child with PKU take a special formula? Differentiate between Lofenalac and Phenyl-Free formulas.

5 What foods would be eliminated from the diet of a child with galactosemia?

CLINICAL STUDY 27

Michael is an 8-day-old infant who had a blood phenylalanine level of 20 mg per 100 mL on the Guthrie screening test for PKU. The lab reported this to his pediatrician, who immediately made plans for Michael to be brought into the regional PKU clinic.

Michael was brought to the clinic by his parents later that afternoon. A history was taken and a physical examination performed. His weight was 4.7 kg and his height 56.1 cm. Blood analysis by the amino acid analyzer, a more accurate measurement of phenylalanine, was performed. The diagnosis of PKU was confirmed. The parents were overwhelmed by the diagnosis.

The nutritionist must plan a diet for Michael and instruct the parents on formula preparation.

Clinical study questions

1 The baby begins treatment as early as possible. Explain.

2 What factors must be considered in planning the diet?

3 What teaching tools would you suggest the nutritionist use?

REFERENCES

1 A. E. Garrod, "The Croonian Lectures on Inborn Errors of Metabolism," *Lancet,* **2:**1, 1908.

2 C. R. Scriver, "Inborn Errors of Metabolism: A New Frontier of Nutrition," *Nutrition Today,* **9**(5):4, 1974.

3 C. R. Scriver, "Vitamin-Responsive Inborn Errors of Metabolism," *Metabolism,* **22**(10):1319, 1973.

4 H. L. Levy, "Cost Benefit Analysis of Newborn Screening for Metabolic Disorders," *New England Journal of Medicine,* **291:**1414, 1970.

5 H. L. Levy and J. P. Kennedy, *Genetic Screening for Inborn Errors of Metabolism,* U.S. Department of Health, Education, and Welfare Publication (HSA) 78-5124, 1975.

6 C. R. Scriver and L. E. Rosenberg, "Amino Acid Metabolism and Its Disorders," in A. L. Schaffer (ed.), *Major Problems in Clinical Paediatrics,* vol. X, W. B. Saunders Company, Philadelphia, 1973, p. 314.

7 H. L. Levy, personal communication, May 1981.

8 J. S. Thompson and M. W. Thompson, *Genetics in Medicine,* 2d ed., W. B. Saunders Company, Philadelphia, 1973, p. 435.

9 H. Ghadimi, "Diagnosis of Inborn Errors of Metabolism," *American Journal of Diseases in Childhood,* **114:**435, 1967.

10 H. K. Berry, "Screening for Genetic Disorders," *Federation Proceedings,* **34**(12):2134, 1975.

11 Ibid., p. 2134.

12 B. B. Burton, A. B. Gerbie, and H. L. Nadler, "Present Status of Intrauterine Diagnosis of Genetic Defects," *American Journal of Obstetrics and Gynecolory,* **118:**718, 1974.

13 J. B. Stanbury, J. B. Wyngaarden, and D. S. Fredrickson (eds.), *The Metabolic Basis of Inherited Diseases,* McGraw-Hill Book Company, New York, 1978, p. 21.

14 B. N. La Du and L. R. Gjessing, "Tyrosinosis and Tyrosinemia," in J. B. Stanbury et al. (eds.), op. cit., p. 262.

15 K. Tada, Y. Wada, N. Yazaki, Y. Yokoyama, H. Nakagawa, T. Yoshida, T. Sato, and T. Arakawa, "Dietary Treatment of Infantile Tyrosinemia," *Tohoku Journal of Experimental Medicine,* **95:**337, 1968.

16 K. Michals, R. Matalon, and P. W. K. Wong, "Importance of Methionine Restriction. Dietary Treatment of Tyrosinemia Type I," *Journal of the American Dietetic Association,* **73:**507, 1978.

17 A. G. Weinberg, C. E. Mize, and H. G. Worthen, "The Occurrence of Hepatoma in the Chronic Form of Hereditary Tyrosinemia," *Journal of Pediatrics,* **88:**434, 1976.

18 A. Y. Tourian and J. B. Sidbury, "Phenylketonuria," in J. B. Stanbury et al. (eds.), op. cit., p. 242.

19 R. Guthrie and A. Susi, "Simple Phenylalanine Method for Detecting Phenylketonuria in Large Populations of Newborn Infants," *Pediatrics,* **32:**338, 1963.

20 Committee for the Study of Inborn Errors of Metabolism, *Genetic Screening: Programs, Principles, and Research,* National Academy of Sciences, National Research Council, Washington, 1975, p. 293.

21 *American Academy of Pediatrics, Standards of Child Health Care,* American Academy of Pediatrics, Evanston, Ill., 1972, p. 23.

22 C. S. Shear, N. S. Wellman, and W. L. Nyhan, "Phenylketonuria: Experience with Diagnosis and Management," in William L. Nyhan (ed.), *Heritable Disorders of Amino Acid Metabolism,* John Wiley & Sons, Inc., New York, 1974, p. 143.

23 J. Dobson, R. Koch, M. Williamson, R. Spector, W. Frankenberg, M. O'Flynn, R. Warner, and F. Hudson, "Cognitive Development and Dietary Therapy in Phenylketonuric Children," *New England Journal of Medicine,* **278:**1142, 1968.

24 R. Koch, personal communication, May 1981.

25 S. Waisbren, personal communication, May 1981.

26 G. Holmgren, H. K. Blomquist, and G. Samuelson, "Positive Effect of a Late Introduced Modified Diet in an 8-Year-Old PKU Child," *Neuropaediatrie,* **10:**1, 1979.

27 J. C. Dobson, M. L. Williamson, C. Azen, and R. Koch, "Intellectual Assessment of 111 Four-Year-Old Children with Phenylketonuria," *Pediatrics,* **60:**822, 1977.

28 L. E. Holt and S. E. Snyderman, "Amino Acid Requirements of Children," in W. E. Nyhan, *Amino Acid Metabolism and Genetic Variation,* McGraw-Hill Book Company, New York, 1967, pp. 381–391.

29 P. B. Acosta, E. Wenz, and M. Williamson, "Nutrient Intake of Treated Infants with Phenylketonuria (PKU)," *American Journal of Clinical Nutrition,* **30:**198, 1977.

30 Joint FAO/WHO Ad Hoc Expert Committee, *Energy and Protein Requirements,* FAO Nutrition Meetings, Report Series No. 52, Food and Agriculture Organizations, Rome, 1971, p. 33.

31 V. Schuett and R. Gurda, *Treatment Programs for PKU in the United States: A Survey,* U.S. Department of Health, Education, and Welfare Publication No. (HSA) 79-5296, Health Services Administration, Division of Clinical Services, Rockville, Md. 20857, 1979, p. 8.

32 American Academy of Pediatrics, Committee on Nutrition, "Special Diets for Infants with Inborn Errors

of Amino Acid Metabolism," *Pediatrics,* **57**:783, 1976.

33 P. B. Acosta, "Nutrition During Pregnancy," in H. L. Levy, R. R. Lenke, and A. C. Crocker (eds.), *Proceedings of Conference on Maternal Phenylketonuria and Maternal Hyperphenylalaninemia,* December 5, 1979, U.S. Government Printing Office, Washington, in press, pp. 43–44.

34 P. B. Acosta, "Zinc and Copper Status and Linear Growth of Treated PKU Children," presented at the Collaborative Study of Children Treated for Phenylketonuria, 10th Nutritionists' Conference, March 22, 1979.

35 I. Lombeck, K. Kasperek, H. D. Harbisch, K. Becker, E. Schumann, W. Schroter, L. E. Feinendegen, and H. J. Bremer, "The Selenium State of Children. II. Selenium Content of Serum, Whole Blood, Hair and the Activity of Erythrocyte Glutathionine Peroxidase in Dietetically Treated Patients with Phenylketonuria and Maple-Syrup-Urine-Disease," *European Journal of Pediatrics,* **128**:313, 1978.

36 V. Schuett, "Selenium Status of Phenylketonuric Subjects and Clinical Implications," presented at the Collaborative Study of Children Treated for Phenylketonuria, 14th General Medical Conference, March 14, 1978.

37 A. E. Ernest, E. R. McCabe, M. R. Neifert, and M. E. O'Flynn, *Guide to Breastfeeding Infants with PKU,* U.S. Department of Health, Education, and Welfare, DHHS Publication (HSA) 79-5110, Bureau of Community Health Services, Office for Maternal and Child Health, Rockville, Md. 20857, 1980.

38 V. Schuett and R. Gurda, op. cit., p. 12.

39 I. Smith, M. F. Stevenson, O. H. Wolff, H. Schmidt, S. Grubel-Kaiser, and H. Bickel, "Effect of Stopping Low Phenylalanine Diet on Intellectual Progress of Children with Phenylketonuria," *British Medical Journal,* **2**:723, 1978.

40 Ibid.

41 B. Cabalska, N. Duczymowska, A. Koslacz-Folga, and K. Bozkowa, "Termination of Dietary Treatment in Phenylketonuria," *European Journal of Pediatrics,* **126**:253, 1978.

42 E. Koff, B. Kammerer, and S. Peuschel, "Intelligence and Phenylketonuria: Effects of Diet Termination," *Journal of Pediatrics,* **94**(2):534, 1979.

43 N. Holzman, D. Welcher, and E. D. Mellits, "Termination of Restricted Diet in Children with Phenylketonuria: A Randomized Controlled Study," *New England Journal of Medicine,* **293**(22):1121, 1975.

44 S. Waisbren and R. Schnell, "Studies on Diet Termination in PKU," presented at the Collaborative

Study of Children Treated for Phenylketonuria, 15th General Medical Conference, March 22, 1979.

45 M. Williamson, R. Koch, and S. Berlow, "Diet Discontinuation in Phenylketonuria," *Pediatrics,* **63**(5):823, 1979.

46 S. Waisbren and R. Schnell, op. cit.

47 R. R. Lenke and H. L. Levy, "Maternal Phenylketonuria and Hyperphenylalaninemia. An International Survey of the Outcome of Untreated and Treated Pregnancies," *New England Journal of Medicine,* **303**:1202, 1980.

48 S. M. Peuschel, C. Hum, and M. Andrews, "Nutritional Management of the Female with Phenylketonuria During Pregnancy," *American Journal of Clinical Nutrition,* **30**:1153, 1977.

49 P. B. Acosta, "Protocol of Diet Management of Maternal Phenylketonuria," in H. L. Levy et al. (eds.), op. cit.

50 P. B. Acosta, "Nutrition During Pregnancy" op. cit.

51 P. B. Acosta, "Zinc and Copper Status and Linear Growth of Treated PKU Children," op. cit.

52 M. Young and M. A. Prenton, "Maternal and Fetal Plasma Amino Acid Concentrations During Gestation and in Retarded Fetal Growth," *Journal of Obstetrics and Gynecology of the British Commonwealth,* **76**:333, 1969.

53 H. L. Levy and G. Hammersen, "Newborn Screening for Galactosemia and Other Galactose Metabolic Defects," *Journal of Pediatrics,* **92**(6):871, 1978.

54 S. Segal, "Disorders of Galactose Metabolism," in J. B. Stanbury et al. (eds.), op. cit., pp. 160–182.

55 K. Paigen and F. Pacheloc, unpublished data.

56 H. L. Levy and G. Hammersen, op. cit., p. 871.

57 H. L. Levy and J. P. Kennedy, op. cit.

58 S. Segal, op. cit., p. 166.

59 Ibid., p. 165.

60 Mead Johnson and Company, *Infant Formula Products, Nutrition Information,* Evansville, Ind. 47721, 1979.

61 Ibid.

62 Ross Laboratories, *Product Handbook,* Columbus, Ohio 43216, 1977.

63 R. Koch, P. Acosta, N. Ragsdale, and G. N. Donnell, "Nutrition in the Treatment of Galactosemia," *Journal of the American Dietetic Association,* **43**:216, 1963.

64 P. Cassells, J. Vermeersch, E. Wenz, and G. Donnell, *Parents' Guide to the Galactose Restricted Diet,* California Department of Health and Department of Nutrition, Maternal and Child Health Branch, University of California in Davis, 1976.

65 J. V. Reger, "New Aspects of an Old Sugar-Lactose," *Cereal Science Today,* **3**:270, 1958.

66 T. A. Nickerson, "Why Use Lactose and Its Derivatives?" *Food Technology,* **32**:40, 1978.

67 P. B. Acosta and L. J. Elsas, *Dietary Management of Inherited Metabolic Disease: Phenylketonuria, Galactosemia, Tyrosinemia, Homocystinuria, Maple Syrup Urine Disease,* ACELMU Publishers, 1939 Westminster Way, Atlanta, Ga., 1976, p. 28.

68 S. Segal, op. cit., p. 165.

69 E. Wenz and M. Mitchell, "Galactosemia," in S. Palmer and S. Ekvall (eds.), *Pediatric Nutrition in Developmental Disorders,* Charles C Thomas, Springfield, Ill., 1978, p. 260.

70 T. F. Roe, J. G. Hallatt, G. N. Donnell, and W. G. Ng, "Childbearing by a Galactosemic Woman," *Journal of Pediatrics,* **78**(6):1026, 1971.

71 S. Samuels, S. C. Sun, and S. Verasestakul, "Normal Infant Birth in White Galactosemic Woman," *Journal of the Medical Society of New Jersey,* **73**(4):309, 1976.

72 F. Kaufman, M. D. Kogut, G. N. Donnell, and R. Koch, "Ovarian Failure in Galactosemia," *Lancet,* **2**:737, 1979.

73 F. Kaufman, M. D. Kogut, G. N. Donnell, and R. Koch, "Hypergonadotropic Hypogonadism in Female patients with Galactosemia," *New England Journal of Medicine,* **304**(17):994, 1981.

74 V. Schuett and R. Gurda, op. cit., p. 11.

75 P. Justin, "Financing of Amino Acid Diets," in American Academy of Pediatrics Nutriture Committee: Amino Acid Subcommittee, *Diet Therapy for MSUD and Organic Acidurias,* Evanston, Ill., 1978.

76 American Academy of Pediatrics, Committee on Nutrition, "Special Diets For Infants with Inborn Errors of Metabolism," *Pediatrics,* **57**:783, 1976.

77 C. R. Scriver, op. cit., p. 4.

78 "Infant Screening for Inborn Errors of Metabolism," *Nutrition Today,* **9**(6):21, 1974.

CLINICAL DISCUSSION 27

It is fortunate that Michael was detected as early as 8 days of age. When the diet is begun within the first 2 months, normal physical and mental growth can be expected. Because Michael is starting on the diet at this age, good control should be established before 1 month of age.

The nutritionist first establishes the approximate amount of phenylalanine, protein, and energy needed. This is determined by the infant's age and weight. The total volume and number of ounces per feeding are determined by two things: (1) the infant's size and (2) the dilution factor of the formula.

The formula for Michael was made with 10 tablespoons Lofenalac, 3.5 oz whole milk, 1 tablespoon Karo syrup, and water added to make 24 oz. This provided 257 mg phenylalanine (54.6 mg/kg), 17.9 g protein (3.8 g/kg), and 550 kcal (117 kcal/kg). Six 4 oz. feedings were given per 24 hrs.

Michael's parents were frightened by the diagnosis. Formula instructions need to be clear and given with a demonstration and written instructions. Telephone contact on the following day is important to answer additional questions.

Ongoing follow-up will be provided by the clinic team: pediatrician, nutritionist, psychologist, and social worker. For the first month Michael will be brought once per week for clinic bloods. After this period, when his blood phenylalanine has been brought into the safe range of 4-8 mg/100 mL, his parents will send weekly bloods by taking a heel prick. The nutritionist will then make diet adjustments by adding or subtracting phenylalanine from the formula. Eventually, strained infant foods will be introduced.

CHAPTER 28

SURGERY, STRESS, BURNS, AND NUTRITIONAL CARE

Ronni Chernoff

KEY WORDS
Nutrition Support
Catabolic Response to Stress
Hospital Malnutrition
Peripheral Parenteral Nutrition
Total Parenteral Nutrition
Meal Replacements
Defined Formula Diets

INTRODUCTION

Webster's dictionary defines stress as "bodily or mental tension resulting from factors that tend to alter an existent equilibrium."[1] Stress may be caused by emotional, physical, or environmental factors; the magnitude of the stress reaction is related to the kind, duration, and complexity of the stimulus upsetting equilibrium, or homeostasis. Whatever the stimulus, stress elicits a clearly defined physiologic reaction.

Almost any type of stress, physical or emotional, will cause an immediate and marked elevation in adrenocorticotropin (ACTH), followed by a release of cortisol.[2] This is significant in that glucocorticoids' (cortisol is an example) primary action is gluconeogenesis. Gluconeogenesis is a catabolic process in which the increased formation of glucose is a result of amino acid deamination with a loss of nitrogen. Over an extended time span, this constant breakdown of protein may result in muscle wasting and weakness.[3]

Along with the hormonal response (release of ACTH and cortisol) of a rapid increase of blood glucose, the body mobilizes and hydrolyzes protein, liver glycogen, and free fatty acids from within a variety of cells.[4] In addition, heart rate will increase with the stress of fear, pain, anesthesia, muscular activity, and sensory nerve stimulation. The sympathetic nervous system transmits signals by way of another group of hormones called *catecholamines*. The effect of this hormonal discharge is the fight or flight syndrome, characterized by tachycardia (increased heart rate), pupillary dilatation, changes in skin and muscle blood flow, and an increased respiratory rate. Another result of this hormonal outpouring is the conservation of water and salt.[5]

The physiological stress that accompanies surgery, burns, trauma, pain, or infection causes these interrelated metabolic events. A major result is the initiation of a hypermetabolic state,

Note: This chapter in the first edition was written by Shirley R. Goldstein. It is revised in this edition by Ronni Chernoff.

the degree of which is dependent upon the extent and severity of the stress. Under conditions of prolonged physical stress, normal healing and immune competency are interfered with. Hypermetabolism that is not equilibrated will lead to catabolism and to progressive deterioration of protein tissue and to impairment of wound healing and immunologic response. Fever and infection will increase metabolic demands even further.[6]

Physiologic stress that causes a hypermetabolic episode demands that nutritional care be of primary importance, both during the stressful period and during convalescence. Nutritional support is a priority so as to meet increased demands and to repair incurred deficits.

The health care team member is responsible for meeting the demands of not only the physiologic response to stress but also the psychological responses which may compound the physiologic events just described.

PSYCHOLOGICAL RESPONSE TO SURGERY

People deal with psychological stress by displaying conditioned responses and behaviors that reflect their emotional defense system.[7]

Surgery, for example, poses a life-threatening experience for many. It may symbolize fear of the unknown, of possible mutilation, disfigurement, death, or pain. While some individuals may accept surgery with a degree of anxiety and fear, many exhibit symptoms of regression, depression, acute anxiety, or anger. They may deny the seriousness of their illness, and refuse to seek medical advice, or manifest their fear through frequent emotional outbursts. These patterns represent defense mechanisms with which people deal with stress and attempt to achieve emotional balance and strength.

The establishment of a trusting, helping relationship with patients by members of the health care team will help patients achieve emotional stability. An individual who requires sur-

gery is soon dependent on the health care team for his or her needs. Every patient needs reassurance as to outcome, as well as opportunities to verbalize concerns. Older patients fear physical and psychological abandonment. They frequently lose hope for the future, become depressed, and refuse to eat. In the past, burn patients were kept in special rooms, psychologically and physically removed from interaction with others. The psychological effects of long-term isolation were found to be greatly damaging.

Children especially need trusting relationships—a parent present at all times, rooming in when possible. The continuity of the parent-child unit relieves the acute anxiety of separation and enables the child to remain secure when facing surgery. Many hospitals have teaching sessions for parents and children as preparation for surgery. Surgical procedures are explained through demonstrations on dolls. The child is allowed to repeat the procedure on the doll and then care for the surrogate patient. The child is given insight into the procedure that will take place, and is better able to adjust to the surgery. The parent, when better informed and more confident, can further enhance the parent-child relationship by providing reassurance and support.

The need for psychological support and sympathetic understanding is further demonstrated when patients resume eating. A system of psychological support must be incorporated into patient care management to encourage a return to positive eating habits. Refusal to eat, use of food as a tool of manipulation, chronic complaining as an attention-getting device are all expressions of human need. Prior to surgery, diagnostic tests, pain, vomiting, anorexia, and fear often interfere with meals. Postoperatively, the patient must relearn to identify food and mealtimes as a pleasurable, nonpainful experience. With appropriate dietary management, tailored to age and need, the patient again becomes confident about food and looks forward to a positive mealtime experience.

PHYSIOLOGICAL RESPONSE TO SURGERY

As discussed in the introduction, every patient will have the same metabolic response to stress. However, the degree and duration of that response will be determined by the underlying disease state or cause for surgery, the organs involved in the surgical procedure, and the nutritional status prior to surgery.

Nutrient Stores

An individual's nutritional state is a major factor in his or her ability to withstand the stress of surgical trauma, the demands of wound healing and immunocompetency, and reattainment of health.[8] A malnourished individual, depleted of essential nutrients, is a major risk for surgery, and must, if time permits, be rehabilitated prior to surgery. Clinical signs of weight loss and hypoproteinemia characterize the at-risk patient. Weight loss, an early sign, is often the unfortunate consequence of the disease process that causes the anorexia leading to inadequate food intake. Often the hemoglobin or hematocrit levels are low as a result of insidious blood loss caused by a yet-undetected neoplasm. Preoperative attempts to renourish a patient are therefore directed at reversing these conditions to reduce surgical risk and minimize the catabolic response to the stress.

Catabolism and Hormonal Response

In response to the severe stress of surgery, burns, hemorrhage, and other traumatic events, the body directs its physiological efforts toward adaptation for survival. It attempts to compensate for the accompanying catabolic, starvationlike state by converting to metabolic pathways that will provide glucose and energy to the cells, and preserve adequate blood volume.

In addition to the responses to stress previously described, the following responses also occur:

1 The catecholamines norepinephrine and epinephrine are released into the bloodstream, where they exert a hemodynamic, metabolic effect. The outcome is:

- A *vasoconstrictive effect* on blood vessels which results in increased cardiac output, thus maintaining adequate blood pressure and volume.
- An *increased production and release of glucagon.* Its hormonal action (on the liver and adipose stores) results in increased glycogen hydrolysis and increased gluconeogenic activity (with the net result of increased glucose release) in the liver, and lipolysis of fat stores (which results in release of free fatty acids for energy needs).
- A *suppression of the peripheral action of insulin.* The alteration of the normal glucagon ratio (insulin levels are *higher* than glucagon levels during nonstressful times) results in the posttraumatic insulin resistance and mild glucose intolerance that characterize early trauma.
- A *lipolytic effect,* whereby triglycerides are hydrolyzed, releasing glycerol and free fatty acids into the bloodstream to provide another source of energy.

2 In the event of hypovolemia, the *renin-angiotensin system* is activated, resulting in increased aldosterone secretion and sodium ion retention by the kidney.

3 *Antidiuretic hormone* (ADH) is released by the pituitary. This antidiuretic effect, combined with sodium retention, serves to maintain adequate blood volume and flow, and temporarily to reduce urinary output following stress.

4 A *cortisol response* is elicited: increased ACTH is secreted by the pituitary, resulting in increased adrenal secretion of corticoste-

roids, especially cortisol. These stimulate the following gluconeogenic reactions:

- Amino acids are quickly released from muscle tissues, deaminated, and converted to glucose in the liver.
- Free fatty acids are released from fat depots.

The net catabolic result of these hormonal responses is an increased urinary nitrogen, muscle wasting, and weight loss, as the body attempts to meet its energy requirements.

(*Note:* Body weights taken during this critical phase do not reflect the true lean body mass, for depleted tissue is replaced by water and sodium.)

As injury and trauma resolve, there is a *reversal* of the above responses:

Diminution of catecholamine secretion

Return to a normal insulin to glucagon ratio in the blood

Decrease in renin secretion

Decrease in aldosterone secretion and restoration of free water diuresis

Wound Healing

Moore and Brennan describe postoperative wound healing as a phase of "convalescent anabolism," a period lasting 5 to 15 days, during which time the wound is given high biological priority for energy, amino acids, and nutrients.[9]

In the initial phase of wound healing, amino acids, energy, and vitamin C are essential. Sources of amino acids and energy are derived from gluconeogenesis. Vitamin C may be administered parenterally or orally (e.g., 500 mg orally). Vitamins and amino acids are necessary for collagen synthesis, especially the initial step in wound healing, the formation of collagen fibrils and reticulum. Vitamin C is required for the pathway in which proline is hydroxylated to hydroxyproline to form collagen.[10]

The primary stage of healing occurs during negative oral intake, again illustrating the need for sound nutritional status prior to surgery.

Although severe deficiency of vitamin A slows wound repair in animals, the mechanisms by which it works are unknown, and only in the most severe deficiency states is wound healing impaired in humans.

The B vitamins have not been shown to have any specific impact on wound healing, but in terms of overall nutritional status it is a good idea to provide injured patients with normally adequate amounts.[11]

Vitamin E has been promoted as aiding in wound healing; however, its action of suppressing wound inflammation also suppresses collagen synthesis, tending to make new repair tissue weaker. It might be better to avoid giving supplemental vitamin E during the immediate postoperative period.[12]

Trace metals such as manganese, copper, and zinc have been identified as having a role in wound healing. Zinc has been the focus of most of the research efforts, but the mechanism of its role in wound healing is still not known. Zinc is an essential cofactor in many enzyme systems (i.e., pancreatic carboxypeptidase, glutamic dehydrogenase) and concentrates in areas of rapid cell division and turnover. It seems that zinc deficiency impairs wound healing but that zinc administration only brings the ability to repair back to normal.[13]

The wound achieves tensile integrity, the point at which the wound is strong enough for suture removal, approximately 7 days after surgery.[14] Prior to this time, there are clinical signs of improvement as the stress factors are reduced. Pain is lessened; appetite increases; peristalsis returns; the ratio of insulin to glucagon is restored (blood insulin levels are again greater than levels of glucagon)—all occur with the anabolic phase of healing. The priority at this time is to provide and assure an adequate intake of protein and energy for continued protein synthesis and repletion. When there are postoperative complications or extensive surgical procedures that preclude oral feedings, nutritional support by means of a tube feeding, liquid supplements, peripheral intravenous therapy, or total parenteral nutrition may be necessary.

As a consequence of inadequate nutrition, oral or parenteral, wound healing deteriorates. The wound itself becomes a nitrogen donor to the general metabolic pool and competes for nutrients with other tissues. This state, described as "late posttraumatic starvation or nutritional failure," may result in persistent infection and failure of wounds to close and heal.[15]

Immune Response

The relationship of nutritional status to the immune response is well documented in the literature (see Chap. 19). The increased susceptibility to infection in cases of kwashiorkor or severe protein-calorie malnutrition in children has been fully cited. An increased incidence of surgical infections is also felt to be strongly related to the poor nutritional status of hospital patients.

The immune response system is the body's natural defense system. It is the reactive response of humoral (circulating antibody) and cell-mediated (lymphocytic response) mechanisms to disease and infection. Its integrity, as measured by neutrophil action, serum albumin, antibody-antigen interaction, immunoglobulin concentration, lymphocytic responses, etc., is felt to be greatly influenced by nutrition.[16-19]

Current research suggests that dietary protein, vitamin B_6, and pantothenic acid are essential in maintaining and preserving the effectiveness of the system. Vitamins A and B_{12} are also considered significant. Worthington suggests that a deficiency of these nutrients (all are vital for DNA-protein synthesis and for release of circulatory antibodies) results in an impairment of antibody synthesis.[20] Investigators support the theory that in conditions in which circulating antibody cells are reduced, the organism becomes more susceptible to disease and is hindered in its recovery from infection.

Lack of adequate protein and B_6 intake may also lead to thymus gland atrophy. Consequently, synthesis and action of lymphoid cells is greatly reduced. This is demonstrated in malnourished populations by graft rejections and delayed hypersensitivity reactions.

More important, when the nutritional status of children and malnourished hospital patients is improved by nutrition therapy, there are increased lymphocytic counts and a rise in serum immunoglobulins, both of which suggest the role of sound nutrition in preserving effective immune system responses.[21]

The immune response, the body's catabolic response to stress, and the need for specific nutrients for wound healing reinforce the need for a period of preoperative nutrition.

Evaluation of Nutrient Needs of the Surgical Patient

Nutrient needs during stress are not known, but the recommended dietary allowances (RDA) (see Appendix, Table A-1) can serve as a realistic base in planning diets for routine nonextensive surgery in well-nourished patients.

Trauma may increase these nutrient requirements well above the recommended levels of intake. An example is the escalation of vitamin C requirements during stress as compared with nonstress periods (see Table 28-1). It is estimated that in some instances of stress, such as

TABLE 28-1   VITAMIN C REQUIREMENTS* DURING NONSTRESS AND STRESS

	Nonstress	Stress (i.e., burns)
Child	45 mg	500–1500 mg
Adult	60 mg	500–1500 mg

*100 times the Recommended Dietary Allowance (see Appendix, Table A-1) may be required.

are encountered by the burn patient, 100 times the RDA may be required.

Careful clinical and dietary monitoring aids in assuring that adequate nutrient therapy is provided. Monitoring of trays at meal service by nursing and dietary personnel will provide an estimate of nutrients in oral intake.

Many individuals who require surgery are in relatively good nutritional status, depending on the cause for surgery. For this group, nutritional care plans can be implemented without complications.

On the other hand, taking care of those who are in a nutritionally debilitated preoperative state requires the efforts of the entire patient care team; the consequences of surgery in the malnourished patient are complex.[22]

Butterworth and Blackburn forcefully de-scribe the need to identify hospitalized patients who may be classified as high-risk due to the inherent malnutrition of disease, inadequate and improper diets, or hospital-induced malnutrition (known as iatrogenic malnutrition).[23] This state results when the assessment of nutritional status and appropriate nutritional management have not been planned for and implemented.[24]

These high-risk patients require aggressive, ongoing nutritional support in order to have a successful surgical and rehabilitative course. Butterworth and Blackburn advocate the need for nutritional assessment as an integral aspect of patient management, including evaluation of nutritional status by anthropometric measurements (if possible), clinical indices, biochemical parameters, and patient history[25] (Table 28-2; see also Chap. 18). All these indicators of nutri-

TABLE 28-2   SUGGESTED GUIDE FOR BLOOD VALUE DETERMINATIONS

	Deficient	Low	Normal
Hemoglobin (g/100 mL)			
Men	<12.0	12.0–13.9	>14.0
Women*	<10.0	10.0–11.9	>12.0
Children (2–5 yrs)	<10.0	10.0–10.9	>11.0
Children (6–12 yrs)	<10.0	10.0–11.4	>11.5
Serum iron (μg/100 mL)			
Men		<60	>60
Women*		<40	>40
Children (2–5 yrs)		<40	>40
Children (6–12 yrs)		<50	>50
Transferrin saturation (%)			
Men	<20		>20
Women*	<15		>15
Children (2–5 yrs)	<20		>20
Children (6–12 yrs)	<20		>20
Serum albumin (g/100 mL)			
Adults	<2.8	2.8–3.4	>3.5
Children (1–5 yrs)		<3.0	>3.0
Children (6–17 yrs)		<3.5	>3.5

*Nonpregnant, nonlactating.

Source: Adapted from D. W. Wilmore, *The Metabolic Management of the Critically Ill,* Plenum Medical Book Company, New York, 1977.

tional assessment should be reviewed at patient care conferences where individualized nutritional care plans can be formulated and thereby integrated into the patient's medical and surgical treatment.

The Malnourished Patient

The relative importance of nutritional status and its relationship to surgical outcome has been a widely researched topic in recent years.[26–29] It has been an accepted concept that malnutrition affects the hospital course of patients undergoing major surgery.[30] Malnutrition has been related to surgical morbidity and mortality, particularly in patients whose protein stores are depleted. As discussed, protein depletion will impede tissue repair; interfere with enzyme, hormone, and plasma protein synthesis; and reduce resistance to infections.[31] When patients who had depressed responses to antigen skin-testing were followed through their surgical course, significantly higher incidence of sepsis and mortality was found.[32] With the high incidence of malnutrition in surgical patients,[33] and the ability to identify high-risk surgical patients by using some basic indicators of nutritional status,[34] a clear case can be made for preoperative nutritional repletion.

PREOPERATIVE NUTRITION

The goal of preoperative nutrition therapy is physiological and nutritional repletion to enable an adult or child to meet the catabolic stress of surgery. Furthermore, a well-nourished state optimizes wound healing, increases resistance to infection, and hastens convalescence and recovery.

Goals of Preoperative Nutrition

1 *Restoration of nitrogen balance.* In the preoperative and postoperative management of the surgical patient who is protein-depleted, as well as in any case of severe trauma, especially severe burns, efforts must be made to reverse the marked nitrogen loss that occurs during the immediate postoperative period.

- The postoperative period is one of semistarvation, during which a patient is supported nutritionally by intravenous fluids and a minimal oral intake if any. This further increases nitrogen losses, depletes nitrogen stores, and prolongs convalescence.

2 *Wound healing.* Sources of nitrogen in the form of amino acids are necessary for wounds to heal properly and for tissue repair to occur. (Amino acids are essential for protein tissue synthesis, as well as for antibody, enzyme, and hormone synthesis.)

3 *Maintenance of serum protein levels.* Normal serum protein levels must be maintained, with serum albumin levels monitored closely to assure normal blood volume and concentration and to prevent edema or threat of sepsis. Weight loss and hypoproteinemia (serum albumin less than 3.5 mg per 100 mL) are indicators of diminished protein reserve.

4 *Carbohydrate stores.* Adequate carbohydrate intake is essential to maintain liver glycogen stores, necessary as reserve during anesthesia and other stress.

These preoperative goals may be met by any of the following feeding methods. These feeding methods may be used singly or in combination with one another.

Oral intake
Liquid oral supplements
Tube feedings
Intravenous therapy
Total parenteral nutrition

Preoperative Diets

An adequate calorie-protein intake with a source of high-biological-value (HBV) protein must be planned and the intake monitored.

TABLE 28-3 RECOMMENDED DAILY REQUIREMENTS FOR NEONATES AND INFANTS

Age	Energy		Protein, g/kg	Fluids, mL/kg
	kcal/kg	kJ/kg		
Newborn (0–6 months)	120	504	2–4	100–150
Infants (6 months–1 yr)	50–100	210–420	1.5–2	50

The body must meet its crucial energy requirements (preferably orally); if these requirements are not met, the body will catabolize protein reserves. To use only a high-protein regime for energy is self-defeating. The antiketogenic effect of carbohydrate and its protein-sparing action are universally recognized. Also, high-protein diets may further compromise an already stressed kidney by increasing urinary nitrogenous wastes. This may lead to osmotic diuresis and dehydration if water requirements are not increased to allow excretion of these wastes.

For practical purposes, 0.8 to 1.5 g of HBV protein per kilogram of body weight per day and 25 kcal to 50 kcal per kilogram (105 kJ to 210 kJ per kilogram) per day are recommended for adults as a reasonable plan to meet energy requirements and allow for nitrogen repletion, balance, and protein synthesis. Sufficient carbohydrate must be added to spare this protein. Table 28-3 (above) suggests daily fluid, protein, and energy requirements for neonates and infants.

For patients requiring immediate surgery, when there is no time for preoperative nutritional repletion, whole blood or plasma transfusions raise hemoglobin and hematocrit levels. The patient feels better and is more psychologically prepared for surgery.

Adequate vitamin C is necessary for wound healing. In addition, adequate vitamin K and a normal prothrombin time are needed for proper blood clotting to avoid the danger of hemorrhage.

High-Energy–High-Protein Diet

A high-energy–high-protein diet is recommended preoperatively if the patient can tolerate it. It is given in small, frequent meals and may be supplemented with between-meal snacks or beverages (see Table 28-4, p. 662, for an example of such a diet).

Restraint must be exercised because large amounts of food may defeat patients who must force themselves to eat. Consuming a small meal in its entirety is reinforcing; too large a meal may further depress an appetite which is already strained by bouts of nausea, vomiting, and anxiety.

Mealtimes should be as pleasant as possible, and not interrupted by blood tests, examinations, diagnostic procedures, or physicians' visits. This is hard to achieve in a hospital environment, but is an important goal for a patient to eat well and be rested.

Most patients accept liquids well. Feeding liquid supplements can be successful so long as supplemental feedings are not scheduled close to mealtimes.

Defined Formula Diets

Commercially available defined formula diets may present a feeding option for preoperative nutrition in the surgical patient who is having difficulty eating enough. These products may be classified as clear liquid, minimal residue, lactose-free formulas. When given in calorically adequate amounts, these formulas will provide the patient with complete nutrition.[35] They are an alternative to the clear liquid diet that is often

TABLE 28-4   HIGH-ENERGY–HIGH-PROTEIN DIET

Sample diet pattern

Breakfast
½ cup fruit juice
1 soft-cooked egg
1 slice toast
1 teaspoon margarine
coffee
2 oz milk
1 teaspoon sugar

Midmorning snack
240 mL commercial formula diet*
2 plain biscuits

Lunch
2 oz cooked meat, poultry, fish
2 crackers
1 teaspoon margarine
½ cup ice cream
2 small cookies
tea
2 oz milk

Midafternoon snack
120 mL commercial formula diet†
2 plain cookies

Dinner
3 oz cooked meat, poultry, fish
½ cup vegetables
½ cup potato, rice, noodles with 1 tsp margarine
small green salad, 1 tbsp salad dressing
½ cup fruit
tea
2 oz milk

Evening snack
½ cup commercial formula diet*
3 crackers
1 oz cheese

Approximate composition:
2600 kcal (10.9 MJ) 50 kcal/kg body weight
        (210 kJ/kg body weight)
390 g carbohydrate
100 g protein 29 g/kg body weight
 75 g fat

Nutrient levels based on a 50-kg female, 20–30 years old, with no gastrointestinal problems:
50 kcal/kg body weight
 2 g protein/kg body weight

*Values based on an average of Meritene Liquid (Doyle), Meritene & Milk (Doyle), Sustacal Liquid (Mead Johnson), Sustacal & Milk (Mead Johnson).

used in the immediate preoperative period. Even the partial incorporation of a defined formula diet as a clear liquid regimen will significantly increase nutrient density (Table 28-5). Examples of defined formula diets are compared on Table 28-6, but caution should be taken when using hyperosmolar formulas with partially or totally digested nutrients. Aside from being tolerated only in small, frequent feedings, the taste of these products is not generally accepted, and extraordinary efforts are often needed to induce patients to take adequate amounts. If a patient can be supported through the immediate pre- and postoperative phases of surgery with adequate protein, the stresses of the experience will be better tolerated.

TABLE 28-5   COMPARISON OF STANDARD CLEAR LIQUID DIET AND DEFINED FORMULA DIET

Standard	Clear liquid diet	Defined formula diet†
Volume	1800 mL	1800 mL
*Protein**	9 g	47 g
*Carbohydrate**	136 g	466 g
*Fat**	3 g	3 g
Calories (joules)*	607 (2549 kJ)	2000 (8.4 MJ)

*Approximate analysis
†Values used are for Precision LR (Doyle).

TABLE 28-6 EXAMPLES OF DEFINED FORMULA DIETS*

	Pro, g	Fat, g	CHO, g	Na, meq	K, meq†	Characteristics
Flexical (Mead Johnson)	22.4	34.0	154.0	15.2	32.0	Hydrolyzed protein with amino acids; soy oil and MCT oil; sugar and dextrins; powder to be reconstituted
Precision LR (Doyle)	23.7	1.4	223.2	27.5	20.2	Egg white solids; MCT and soy oil; maltodextrins and sugar; powder to be reconstituted
Precision HN (Doyle)	41.7	1.2	205.7	40.6	22.2	Egg white solids; MCT and soy oil; maltodextrins and sugar; powder to be reconstituted
Vipep (Cutter)	25.0	25.0	175.5	32.6	21.8	Hydrolyzed protein with amino acids; MCT and soy oil; corn syrup solids, sucrose, corn, and tapioca starches; powder to be reconstituted
Vital (Ross)	41.7	10.3	185.0	16.7	29.8	Hydrolyzed protein with amino acids; sunflower oil; glucose oligosaccharides, sucrose, cornstarch; powder to be reconstituted
Vivonex (Eaton)	20.4	1.4	230.0	37.4	30.0	Crystalline amino acids; safflower oil; glucose oligosaccharides; powder to be reconstituted
Vivonex HN (Eaton)	43.3	0.9	211.0	33.5	18.0	Crystalline amino acids; safflower oil; glucose oligosaccharides; powder to be reconstituted

*For additional information, see M. E. Shils, A. S. Bloch, and R. Chernoff, *Liquid Formulas for Oral and Tube Feeding*, 2d ed., Memorial Sloan-Kettering Cancer Center, New York, 1979.
†Values based on 1000 kcal.

NPO

The surgeon may order that the patient be given nothing by mouth (npo = nothing per os). Patients may be unable to take food orally (the preferred route) because of intractable vomiting, obstruction, pain with chewing or swallowing, fistula development, mouth sores, or coma. Preoperative repletion may be supported by the following measures:

Tube feeding with meal replacements, defined formula diets, or supplements
Peripheral parenteral nutrition
Total parenteral nutrition

These may provide a degree of support in patients with partial obstruction who now await surgical intervention, and cannot eat normally.

POSTOPERATIVE DIETARY MANAGEMENT

Postoperatively, adults and children in a well-nourished state have reserves of nutrients. This enables them to endure the short period (3 or 4 days) of semistarvation without severe physiological insult to their system. Standard intravenous therapy provides fluid and electrolyte support. Immediate postoperative management is directed at maintaining the body's fluid and electrolyte balance, preventing dehydration, and providing some calories—usually 300 to 600 kcal (1.2 to 2.5 MJ)—for energy needs until the gastrointesinal tract resumes normal functioning and the patient is able to take liquids and nourishment by mouth.

The postoperative course is a time of semistarvation. It is characterized by the catabolic response to stress that was described earlier. The net outcome of hormone release is:

Increased gluconeogenesis with mobilization of amino acids from muscle

Increased release of free fatty acids

Increased urinary nitrogen and potassium

In addition to these responses, losses of fluid, blood, and nitrogen must also be considered. There is loss of fluids and electrolytes (sodium, potassium, chloride) due to wound drainage, nasogastric suctioning, vomiting, and fever. Immediate fluid and electrolyte replacement is essential in order to prevent dehydration, especially in infants and children, who have a high body water content.

Plasma protein, especially in children, requires immediate replacement so that adequate blood volume and flow are maintained. Use of plasma or albumin, or isotonic saline, is necessary in infants in order to expand or restore blood volume. Loss of plasma poses a serious threat to infants, who have a rapid basal metabolic rate (BMR) and a large body surface area. (Adequate albumin concentration is required to ensure colloidal osmotic pressure.) Total serum protein in infants, children, and adults should be maintained at 5 g per 100 mL or higher.

Postoperative nitrogen losses can be ameliorated with an intravenous infusion of glucose, which provides energy to the brain and other vital organs and prevents ketosis (100 to 150 g of glucose is required daily to prevent ketosis).

If this period of semistarvation continues for longer than 7 to 10 days, subcutaneous fat and muscle protein will be used as sources of energy. A patient who has complications after surgery or chemotherapy or radiation therapy initiated shortly after surgery may continue to be starved if aggressive nutritional support is not instituted. It is possible to have a patient who is considered disease-free still be left in a severe state of cachexia[36] (see Fig. 28-1, opposite, and Fig. 28-2, p. 665).

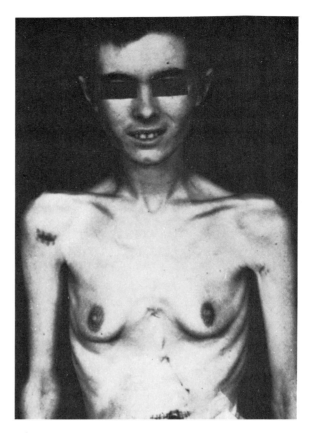

Figure 28-1
A 14-year-old female who underwent surgery and treatment for cancer and, although disease-free, became very cachectic. (Reprinted through the courtesy of M. E. Shils, M.D., Sc.D.).

It is important to plan adequate renourishment as soon as possible to avoid wasting patients' endogenous stores of calories and using protein for energy. If a patient is going to be eating in a short time (3 to 4 days), then therapeutic goals can be easily met; if there is going to be an extended period of nutritional depletion because of complications, the need for additional surgery or other treatment modalities (i.e., chemotherapy) that may interfere with the patient's ability to ingest nutrients orally, then another feeding method should be considered.

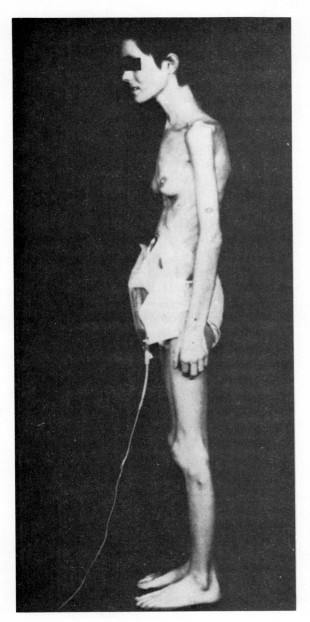

Figure 28-2
Weight loss, muscular atrophy, and severe decrease
of subcutaneous tissue can be noticed. (Reprinted through
the courtesy of M.E. Shils, M.D.,Sc.D.)

Initial Postoperative Diet

During the uncomplicated initial postoperative period intravenous therapy is employed for short-term support. It is used to restore obligatory basal fluid and electrolyte losses and to maintain homeostatic balance. Some common intravenous solutions are listed in Table 28-7 (p. 666).

Adequacy of intravenous fluid and electrolyte therapy can be assured by monitoring *urinary output* and *serum sodium and potassium levels;* when all values are within normal range, fluid and electrolyte needs are met. An example of a regimen for intravenous fluid and electrolyte replacement is given in Table 28-8 (p. 667). Careful attention to accurate intake and output (I and O) recording by the nursing staff following surgery is essential. In addition, the degree of dehydration may also be estimated by body weight losses; e.g., a 6, 8, or 10 percent weight loss reflects a comparable severity of dehydration. Daily weight records are therefore recommended because ½ L of fluid lost is equivalent to 1 lb of weight.

Fluid replacement in *infants and children* (see Table 28-9, p. 668) is required in order to provide energy support and to prevent dehydration. The energy reserve of the newborn is very small, and the BMR is high; therefore, energy deprivation and acidosis can be a very sudden and life-threatening situation. Preoperatively, 50 mL of intravenous maintenance fluid per kilogram of body weight is administered daily. Postoperatively, the nurse must carefully and closely monitor infants and young children receiving intravenous therapy, to ensure adequate urine output so as to avoid water overloading and intoxication.

Following uncomplicated procedures, there should be rapid progression to oral fluids as soon as tolerated to establish full calorie and protein intake. Glucose and water may be the first fluid tolerated. This may be followed by dilute infant formula (later, full-strength) appropriately planned for age and weight.

TABLE 28-7 SOME COMMON PARENTERAL SOLUTIONS

Component	Solution	Use	Comments
Glucose	D₅W (5% dextrose in water)	Isotonic 1 L = 50 g glucose, 170 kcal	Basal caloric requirements are 1500–2300 kcal daily. Traditional IV therapy cannot meet this requirement without overloading the body with water—2000–2500 mL/24 h = maximum allowance for fluid.
		1 g = 3.4 kcal (anhydrous glucose used)	100–150 g glucose per day will exert a protein-sparing effect, prevent starvation ketosis, and provide energy for the brain.
	D₁₀W (10% dextrose in water)	Hypertonic 1 L = 100 g glucose, 340 kcal	Use must be carefully monitored for danger of venous thrombosis.
SPA (salt-poor albumin) Plasma Dextran 40 Dextran 70 Plasmanate	Same as components	Blood volume expanders	These solutions are used to maintain adequate blood flow. Albumin is especially needed to maintain colloidal osmotic pressure.
Saline	0.9%	Isotonic (154 meq)	Replacement needs—to maintain serum Na⁺ levels at 136–145 meq/L.
Protein hydrolysates	Amigen (5% and 10%) (casein hydrolysate) Aminosol (5%) (fibrin hydrolysate) Travamin (10%) (casein hydrolysate)	Source of amino acids	Abate muscle and visceral protein catabolism (5% solutions are isotonic).
Amino acids	Aminosyn (3.5%, 5%, 7%, 10%) Freamine (8.5%) Travasol (5.5%, 8.5%) Veinamine (8%)		
Lipids	Intralipid* (10%) (soy oil emulsion) Liposyn† (10%) (safflower oil emulsion)	Concentrated source of energy (1.1 kcal/mL) 110 kcal/100 mL	Administered by peripheral vein. No "fat overloading syndrome."
	Intralipid‡ (20%) (soy oil emulsion)	2.0 kcal/mL 200 kcal/100 mL	
Whole blood	Same as components	Restoration and maintenance of adequate blood volume and flow crucial to survival	All tissues require adequate perfusion of blood as oxygenation and nourishment are necessary for their integrity.
Parenteral vitamins	C, K, B complex	Wound healing; blood clotting; carbohydrate metabolism	Multivitamin preparations may be given by mouth when a patient is able to take them.

*Contents: 10% soybean oil, 1.2% egg yolk phopholipids, 2.5% glycerol.
†Contents: 10% safflower oil, 1.2% egg phosphatides, 2.5% glycerin USP.
‡Contents: 20% soybean oil, 1.2% egg yolk phospholipids, 2.25% glycerol solution.

666

TABLE 28-8 EXAMPLE OF 24-H INTRAVENOUS THERAPY FOR ADULT REPLACEMENT NEEDS FOLLOWING ROUTINE NONEXTENSIVE SURGERY

Solution	Volume	Glucose, g	Water, mL	Sodium, meq	Potassium, meq	Comments
1 0.45% saline with D_5W*	500 mL	25	500	38.5	—	Source of sodium for routine replacement
2 D_5W* with KCl	1000 mL + 20 meq K	50	1000	—	20	125 g glucose for sparing protein and preventing ketosis Potassium given to prevent deficit (especially if there has been GI suctioning)
3 D_5W* with KCl	1000 mL + 20 meq K	50	1000	—	20	Fluid (as water) needs: Urine losses: 800–1000 mL Insensible losses: Lungs and skin 700 Sweat 600 GI losses 300
Total input	2500 mL water + 40 meq KCl	125 g†	2500	38.5	40	
Total output	2400 mL					Fluid (as water) needs: Urine losses: 800–1000 mL Insensible losses: Lungs and skin 700 Sweat 600 GI losses 300

*D_5W = 5% dextrose in water; KCl = potassium chloride; GI = gastrointestinal.
†125 g glucose equals 425 kcal (1785 kJ).

TABLE 28-9 24-H MAINTENANCE INTRAVENOUS FLUID THERAPY FOR PREMATURE, NEWBORN, AND OLDER CHILDREN

Condition and weight	Water, mL/kg	Calories, kcal/kg	Kilojoules, kJ/kg	Sodium, meq/100 kcal	Potassium, meq/100 kcal	Chloride, meq/100 kcal	Expected urine output, mL/kg
Premature	150	60	252	1–3	1–3	1–3	30 mL total in first 24h
Newborn							
First week	50–60	60	252	1–3	1–3	1–3	40–110
After first week	100–110	115–125	483–525	1–3	1–3	3	30–110
Older infants							
1–10 kg	100	100	420	1–3	1–3	3	30–110
11–20 kg	1000 mL + 50 mL/kg for wt over 10 kg	1000 kcal + 50 kcal/kg for wt over 10 kg	4200 kJ + 210 kJ/kg	—	—	—	—
20 kg and over	1500 mL + 20 mL/kg for wt over 20 kg	1500 kcal + 20 kcal/kg for wt over 20 kg	6300 kJ + 84 kJ/kg	1–3	—	—	—

Source: M. I. Rowe, "Preoperative and Postoperative Management: The Physiologic Approach," and A. G. Coram and R. M. Filler, "Total Parenteral Nutrition," in M. M. Ravitch, K. J. Welch, C. D. Benson, E. Aberdeen, and J. G. Randolph (eds.), *Pediatric Surgery*, Yearbook Medical Publishers, Inc., Chicago, 1979.

Postoperative Diets:
A Progression from Liquid to House Diet

In routine surgery in a well-nourished patient, a traditional pattern of management is followed. Intravenous fluids are supportive until a patient is able to take sufficient fluids and some nutrients by mouth; when bowel sounds return, the patient can progress to solids.

After minor surgical procedures, once the patient is fully reactive and recovered from anesthesia, often *diet as tolerated* is ordered. Consultation with the patient by dietary personnel is strongly recommended. A simple meal of tea, toast, and soup may be preferred. This illustrates the need for the dietitian, nurse, or other appropriate personnel to interact continuously with patients to determine their needs. In addition, the dietitian and the nurse can observe, evaluate, and advise diet progression based on the patient's responses and physical status. Such contact is an important exchange during a patient's hospitalization.

After more complicated surgery, the patient is kept npo, and maintained on intravenous therapy for fluid and energy support. This regimen is maintained until ambulation and peristalsis are resumed and satisfactory fluid intake and urinary output achieved. The objective in resuming oral intake as soon as possible is to prevent severe energy and protein losses. The patient at this stage is started on sips of water, or clear liquids (tea, broth, or gelatin), 30 mL, 60 mL, or 90 mL given hourly; progression is planned according to the patient's increased tolerance, signs of hunger, absence of vomiting, passage of flatus, and presence of active bowel sounds. Rapid progress is made to unrestricted intake of clear liquids (1000 to 1800 mL daily) and to full liquids—avoiding coffee and spicy broths. With children, provision of favorite juices and (if not weaned) their own bottle is important.

When diet must be related to a surgical procedure, it is planned according to the physician's request or dietitian's recommendation.

Table 28-10 (pp. 670–671) summarizes common surgical procedures and postoperative dietary management.

Careful I and O (intake-output) records must be maintained for all nutrient sources:

Foods: Solids, liquids, supplements
Intravenous fluids: D_5W, peripheral parenteral nutrition, total parenteral nutrition
Tube feedings: Defined formula diet, meal replacements

PARENTERAL AND ENTERAL SUPPORT SYSTEMS

Parenteral and enteral support systems become a choice for management of those patients whose energy and protein needs cannot be met solely by oral intake. These systems have been designed to ensure adequate protein intake for tissue synthesis and positive nitrogen balance, with resultant healing and repair. They are also used in children to prevent dehydration, provide energy, and maintain adequate blood volume. Such systems are classified as:

1 Peripheral parenteral nutrition
2 Total parenteral nutrition (TPN or IV hyperalimentation)
3 Enteral nutrition by tube

Peripheral Parenteral Nutrition

Intravenous therapy as a short-term support system has been described already. It is usually continued for approximately 4 days. As shown in Table 28-8, there is no protein administered, and only 425 kcal (1785 kJ) is provided from standard glucose solutions.

Hypertonic glucose solutions have to be administered in a central vein with a high blood flow to prevent thrombophlebitis. A peripheral vein can tolerate an infusion of a 10 percent solution before phlebitis, clotting, or swelling may occur.[37] With the introduction of intravenous isotonic fat emulsions to the United States (1977),* the possibility of using a peripheral vein for nutritional repletion became a reality.

*In the 1950s a cottonseed oil emulsion (Lipomul) was used; however, owing to its inclusion of a toxic substance that damaged erythrocytes, the product was withdrawn from the market.

TABLE 28-10 POSTOPERATIVE DIETARY MANAGEMENT

Focus	Disorder	Surgical procedure	Feeding method	Dietary modification	Comments
Head	Head injury	Burr holes	Nasogastric tube feeding	Standard tube feeding	Patient unconscious
Cranium, ear, nose, throat, eye	Tonsillitis	Tonsillectomy	By mouth	Liquids to soft foods	Not by straw
Mouth	Cataract	Removal	By mouth	As tolerated	
	Cancer	Cryosurgery	Nasogastric tube feeding or gastrostomy	Standard tube feeding	High-energy, high-protein
Jaw	Caries	Full mouth extraction	By mouth	Liquids to soft foods	Cool liquids to room temperature
	Cancer	Radical excision	Nasogastric tube feeding or gastrostomy	High-energy, high-protein	
Cheek	Fracture	Wiring and repair	By mouth	High-energy, high-protein liquids	By straw
	Tumor	Cryosurgery	Nasogastric tube feeding or gastrostomy	High-energy, high-protein	
Esophagus	Cancer	Surgical repair	Nasogastric tube feeding or gastrostomy	High-energy, high-protein	
Larynx	Cancer	Removal		Meal replacements Baby foods, liquids	
Stomach	Hiatus hernia	Repair	By mouth	Liberal bland to house diet	Liquids after meals
	Cancer; Zollinger-Ellison syndrome	Subtotal to total gastrectomy	By mouth	Blenderized diet ↑ protein, ↑ fat, moderate carbohydrate	Small frequent feedings; hypoglycemia, loss of intrinsic factor may occur
	Peptic ulcer	Pyloroplasty, subtotal Billroth gastrectomy I or II	By mouth	Anti-dumping diet ↑ protein, ↑ fat, moderate carbohydrate	

Site	Condition	Surgery	Route	Diet	Comments
Small intestine					
Duodenum	Ulcer	Resection	By mouth	As tolerated	Loss of vitamin B_{12}, water, electrolytes; ↑ lactose intolerance, fat intolerance; ↑ diarrhea, steatorrhea
Jejunum	Cancer	Resection	By mouth	As tolerated	
	Crohn's disease (regional enteritis)	Resection	By mouth	Defined formula diets	
Ileum	Regional ileitis	Resection	By mouth	Low roughage, increased as tolerated	
Colon	Cancer Ulcerative colitis	Colectomy (subtotal or total); colostomy	By mouth	Low roughage, increased as tolerated	
	Diverticulitis		By mouth	May have increased bulk, increased roughage (with physician's approval)	Bran (2 tbsp tid) may be added to diet
Rectum	Fissure Hemorrhoids	Fissurectomy Hemorrhoidectomy	By mouth	Low roughage; include laxative foods such as prune juice; increase fluids	
Heart	Stroke	Embolectomy	Nasogastric tube feeding	Baby foods as tolerated	
	Acute sclerotic heart disease—coronary arteries	CABG (coronary artery bypass graft)	By mouth	No added salt (2–4 g sodium)	Saturated fat decreased; polyunsaturates increased
Gallbladder	Cholecystitis	Cholecystectomy	By mouth	Low fat	
	Cholelithiasis	Cholecystectomy	By mouth	House diet as tolerated	Gas-forming vegetables may not be tolerated
Genitourinary	Nephrolithiasis	Nephrectomy	By mouth	Forced fluids	Calcium or uric acid may be restricted
Kidney	Cancer Fibrocystic disease	Transplantation	By mouth	Individualized according to biochemical profile	

Peripheral infusions, providing protein, calories, vitamins, and minerals, may be used successfully in patients who require preoperative nutritional support, who are receiving preoperative chemotherapy, who cannot ingest adequate calories from oral or tube feeding, or who are not good candidates for central line access due to head and neck or chest surgery, or burns in the chest and shoulder area. An example of a solution that may be administered peripherally is shown in Table 28-11.

Usually the amino acid solution and the dextrose solution, along with electrolytes and vitamins, are mixed together in one bottle and administered simultaneously with the fat emulsion in a piggyback fashion (see Fig. 28-3). It is wise to keep the lipid emulsion higher than the amino acid because its specific gravity is lower and it will run up the amino acid line if lower.[38]

Glucose-Free Parenteral Solutions

The use of glucose-free amino acid solutions has been advocated by some investigators as effective parenteral support.[39] The rationale for this approach is that glucose-free infusions serve to decrease the stimulation and release of insulin, which has an antilipolytic effect. There is then an increased mobilization of fat stores, therefore, an increased release of free fatty acids for energy needs. Gluconeogenesis and muscle catabolism

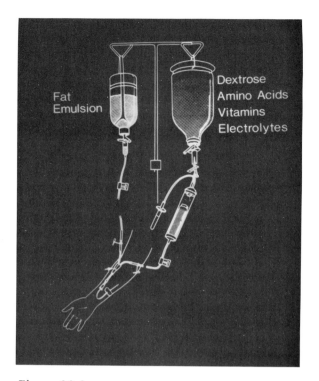

Figure 28-3
The administration of parenteral nutrition through a peripheral vein.

are no longer needed for energy requirements. Intravenous amino acids provide nitrogen for tissue repletion and synthesis and thereby diminish protein tissue catabolism. Subsequent studies showed that nitrogen balance is further enhanced by the addition of hypotonic glucose calories or fat and glycerol calories.[40]

The concept of protein-sparing parenteral solutions remains controversial and is not being widely used at present.

Total Parenteral Nutrition (TPN; IV Hyperalimentation)

Conventional intravenous therapy cannot provide the nutrition demanded by severe trauma, sepsis, and burns. Dudrick and colleagues pioneered the design and application of total parenteral nutrition (TPN).[41] This is a nutritional support system for patients whose nutritional

TABLE 28-11   EXAMPLE OF PERIPHERAL PARENTERAL NUTRITION FORMULA

Solution	Volume, mL
Amino acids (8.5%)	500
Dextrose (10%)	1000
NaCl (15%)	*
KCl (15%)	*
MgSO$_4$ (50%)	*
Ca gluconate (10%)	*
Vitamins	*
Fat emulsion (10%)	500

*As determined by physician.
Source: Adapted from M. E. Shils, "Parenteral Nutrition," in R. S. Goodhart and M. E. Shils (eds), *Modern Nutrition in Health and Disease*, Lea & Febiger, Philadelphia, 1980.

requirements cannot be met by standard intravenous, tube, or oral feedings or when use of the gastrointestinal (GI) tract is contraindicated.[42]

The infusions are designed to provide sufficient calories as hypertonic glucose (25 to 50 percent), protein as L-amino acids, and maintenance requirements for sodium, potassium, calcium, chloride, phosphorus, and vitamins (A, D, E, C, and B complex) in amounts favorable to nitrogen repletion and wound healing. Additions of vitamins K and B_{12}, folic acid, and iron are often given to the patient via another route.

TPN has been successful in providing effective nutritional support for

Short bowel syndrome[43]
Inflammatory bowel disease[44,45]
Intestinal fistulas[46]
Cardiac surgery[47]
Renal disease[48]
Cancer[49]
Pediatric surgery[50]
Burns[51]
Pediatric metabolic disease[52]
Trauma and sepsis[53]

and other problems where the patient cannot ingest enough nutrients orally or tolerate adequate volumes by tube.

TPN can be used in a variety of cases since it promotes wound healing by supplying energy, protein, vitamins, minerals, and fluid required by the injured, sick, or septic patient.

Problems Associated with TPN

There are problems that may be encountered when attempting to provide nutrition through parenterally administered solutions. Even in a normal individual an excessive rate or large total dose glucose infusion may lead to hyperglycemia, glycosuria, or hyperosmolar nonketotic dehydration and coma. Ketoacidosis may occur in diabetic patients who are not receiving adequate insulin coverage (insulin may be added to the solution and infused with the glucose).[54]

In the past, problems occurred from high levels of chloride in amino acid solutions and from excessive ammonia in protein hydrolysate solutions; however, reformulation of the available amino acid solutions has eliminated most of these problems.

Calcium and phosphorus metabolism can be upset if inadequate administration of calcium and phosphorus occurs. These minerals need to be added individually to parenteral solutions (usually as calcium gluconate and potassium phosphate). Sodium, potassium, and magnesium also need to be added to the parenteral solution to meet daily requirements based on the individual's metabolic status.[55]

Hypo- or hypervitaminosis may occur if both fat- and water-soluble vitamins are not given, or are given too enthusiastically, to a patient. All the nutrients, including trace minerals, must be provided to patients being nourished parenterally. Trace metal (zinc, iron, and copper) deficiencies have been known to occur in TPN patients.[56]

Other complications related to TPN and central line catheter insertion may include sepsis (bacterial or fungal), pneumothorax, hemothorax, thrombosis, air emboli, endocarditis, hematomas, artery or vein lacerations, or catheter misplacement (i.e., in the internal jugular vein rather than the superior vena cava).[57]

Table 28-12 gives guidelines for energy and nitrogen in TPN solution. Table 28-13 (p. 674) gives sample solutions for TPN in adults.

(Note: The cost and hazards of TPN warrant thorough investigation of other alternatives before a final decision for its use is made. TPN is indicated in long-term use in specific patients who *cannot* be managed by traditional methods. The expense of TPN therapy is 10 times the expense of a hospital meal or tube feeding.)

TABLE 28-12 SUGGESTED GUIDELINES FOR CALORIES (JOULES) AND NITROGEN IN TPN SOLUTIONS

	kcal/kg body weight	kJ/kg body weight	Nitrogen, g/kg weight
Adults	30–50	126–210	0.2
Infants	125–130	525–546	0.6–0.74

TABLE 28-13   AN EXAMPLE OF TOTAL PARENTERAL SOLUTIONS FOR ADULTS

	Volume	Concentration of nutrients per liter	Calories (joules)	Nutrient per liter
Freamine II Crystalline amino acids*	500 mL	8.5%	153 kcal (643 kJ)	42.5 g
Dextrose	500 mL	50%	850 kcal (3570 kJ)	250 g
Sodium				5 meq
Phosphate				10 meq
Osmolarity				1700–1750 mosmol
pH				6.5

The following may be added

KCl (potassium chloride)	20–40 meq/L
Magnesium sulfate	8–15 meq/L
Calcium	5–10 meq/L
Intravenous vitamins†‡	
Ascorbic acid	100 mg
Vitamin A (retinol)	3300 IU
Vitamin D	200 IU
Thiamin	3 mg
Riboflavin	3.6 mg
Vitamin B_6 (pyridoxine HCl)	4 mg
Niacinamide	40 mg
Pantothenic acid	15 mg
Vitamin E	10 IU
Biotin	60 µg
Folic acid	400 µg
Vitamin B_{12}	5 µg
or	
Berocca-C (vitamins B and C)	
Trace elements	
B_{12}, folic acid, and vitamin K may be added or given intramuscularly	

*Isolated and purified from edible soy bean hydrolysate or synthesized.
†Commercially available as MVI-12, in 2 individual vials packaged together.
‡Meets the AMA/NAG standards for intravenous vitamins.
Source: Adapted from J. H. Duke and S. J. Dudrick "Parenteral Feeding," in W. F. Ballinger et al., *Manual of Surgical Nutrition,* W. B. Saunders, Philadelphia, 1975.

Fat Emulsions

The use of fat emulsions as an aspect of TPN is gaining in application in the United States.[58] Intralipid, a soybean oil emulsion, and Liposyn, a safflower oil emulsion, are the products commercially available in this country. They are isotonic and provide 1.1 kcal (4.62 kJ) per gram. Intralipid 20 percent, providing 2 kcal/g (8.4 kJ), is now available for use for individuals who are fluid-restricted but require concentrated calories. The use of fat emulsions is necessary to prevent essential fatty acid deficiency that may result from long-term TPN. It is recommended that fat emulsions not constitute more than 60 percent of the total calories.[59] (It may still be necessary to provide sufficient glucose energy by the subclavian vein.) Adults can easily be given 1000 kcal (4.2 MJ) daily. Tables 28-14 and 28-15 show recommended infusion rates and dosages, respectively. Fat emulsions, like TPN solutions, are very expensive.

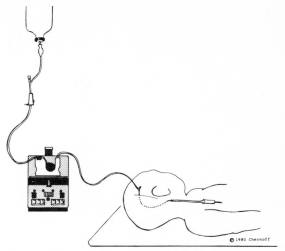

Figure 28-4
TPN being fed to an infant. The catheter is threaded from a scalp vein into the superior vena cava.

TABLE 28-14 RECOMMENDED INFUSION RATE FOR FAT EMULSIONS*

Adults: 0.5 mL/min initially, progressing to a maximum of 5 mL/min. Maximum single infusion, 500 mL; maximum total infusion, 7 L over a 14-day period.

Children: 30 mL/kg body weight delivered over a 6-h period, every other day.

*Fat emulsions may be infused simultaneously with 5% dextrose or 5% amino acid solutions. Adverse effects (fever and nausea) may be decreased with decreased dosage. Overloading syndrome (anorexia, fever, headache, sore throat, and pain) is not observed with prolonged use of fat emulsions.

TABLE 28-15 RECOMMENDED DAILY DOSAGE FOR FAT EMULSIONS

	g/kg body wt	Comments
Infants	2	May increase to maximum of 4 g/kg over several days
Adults	1.5–2.5	

Routes of Administration

TPN solutions, which are very concentrated mixtures, are delivered by insertion of a sterile catheter into a large central vein. The subclavian vein is commonly used, for at this point there is rapid blood flow into the superior vena cava. (In infants, the central vein is the route of administration.) This permits a rapid flushing and dilution of the hypertonic solution, thereby reducing the danger of thrombosis. In addition, it is important to remember that this is achieved in a volume of water that does not exceed the individual's daily fluid requirement (Fig. 28-4).

The rate of flow of the infusion must be a constant and uninterrupted flow to avoid marked fluctuations in blood glucose. A pump is always used for TPN administration. TPN pumps may be peristaltic or volumetric, but all have safety devices and alarm systems to protect patients from air embolisms, erratic drip rates, and electrical failure.

Table 28-16 gives recommendations for clinical and biochemical signs to monitor.*

*Parents and staff involved in the care of young children receiving TPN are encouraged to hold and interact with the children in attempts to normalize and foster their psychosocial development.

TABLE 28-16 CLINICAL AND BIOCHEMICAL MONITORING IN TOTAL PARENTERAL NUTRITION*

Factor	Frequency
Electrolytes (Na$^+$, K$^+$, Ca^{2+}, Cl$^-$, P)	Daily
Weight (fluid intake and output)	Daily
Vital signs	Daily
Blood urea nitrogen	Daily
Serum glucose	Daily
Urinalysis (glucose)	Daily (cover with sliding scale insulin)
Complete blood count	Weekly
Creatinine	Weekly
Magnesium	Weekly
Copper†	Weekly
Zinc†	Weekly

*Urinary and fecal nitrogen determinations will determine if positive nitrogen balance is achieved and maintained.

†Recent research indicates the need to monitor copper and zinc levels. (See C. R. Fleming et al., "Prospective Study of Serum Copper and Zinc Levels in Patients Receiving Total Parenteral Nutrition," *American Journal of Clinical Nutrition*, **29**:70, 1976.)

Additional Risks of TPN

1 *Insulin reaction.*   In response to the hypertonic glucose of TPN solutions, there is an increased secretion of insulin (as well as added parenteral insulin administration). Rebound insulin shock, or hypoglycemia, may occur if solutions are abruptly stopped. When oral feedings are to be resumed, it is also recommended that TPN solutions be tapered off.

2 *Contamination.*   Strict control in defined pharmacy areas must be assured in order to prevent bacterial contamination.

3 *Infection.*   Catheter contamination at the entry site or contaminated solutions may lead to septicemia. The patient may already be predisposed to monilial infection because

of a poor nutritional state as well as the use of broad-spectrum antibiotics.

4 *Essential fatty acid deficiency.*   Essential fatty acid deficiency may result if fat is not supplied; therefore, addition of fat emulsion to the regimen is recommended (see Table 28-14).

Tube Feedings (Enteral Alimentation)

When an individual is unable to take food orally, an alternative route may be created as a nutritional support system. Reasons why this may occur include fractures of the jaw, cancer of the mouth or esophagus, esophageal fistula of the newborn, and anorexia of long-term illness.[60] The type of feeding and the route of administration are determined by the nature of the case.

Table 28-17 lists some common tube feeding formulas. Beyond 1 kcal per milliliter (4.2 kJ per milliliter), solutions may be hypertonic or viscous as a result of the increased addition of carbohydrate sources or protein hydrolysates. When feeding is initiated, the formulas must be diluted to prevent diarrhea, which decreases nutrient intake until full-strength feeding can be achieved.

In the debilitated, the elderly, the very young, or the postoperative patient, it is judicious to proceed cautiously when planning tube feeding methods.[61] Food intake over a period of time may have been limited or decreased. Too rapid or forced feedings of large volumes of concentrated mixtures may result in vomiting or diarrhea. Mixtures containing large solute concentrations and increased levels of protein, when administered without sufficient water, may lead to osmotic diureses resulting in dehydration. These are serious setbacks to recovery that most patients can ill afford. Monitoring for symptoms of thirst, cramping, diarrhea, and urinary output is necessary.

The initial goal should be to give 1000 kcal (4.2 MJ), as a solution containing 0.5 kcal per milliliter (half strength) (2.1 kJ per milliliter), over a 24-h period without causing cramping or

TABLE 28-17   CLASSIFICATION OF COMMON TUBE FEEDINGS

Type	Examples	Comments
Blenderized	Compleat B (Doyle) Formula 2 (Cutter) Vitaneed (Organon)	Mixtures of natural foods; closest to normal diet; ready-to-serve
Milk base	Meritene (Doyle) Sustacal (Mead Johnson)*	Pleasant-tasting oral supplements; ready-to-serve
Meal replacement	Ensure (Ross) Ensure Plus (Ross)† Isocal (Mead Johnson) Magnacal (Organon)‡ Osmolite (Ross) Precision Isotonic (Doyle) Renu (Organon)	Lactose-free, tube feeding products that are made from protein isolates, oligosaccharides and starches, and fats; in adequate caloric volumes meet RDA for vitamins and minerals§; ready-to-serve
Defined formula diets	Flexical (Mead Johnson) Vipep (Cutter) Vital (Ross) Vivonex (Eaton)	Partially digested nutrients for tube feeding; hypertonic; require reconstitution

*Sustacal (Mead Johnson) is lactose-free.

†Ensure Plus (Ross) is 1.5 kcal/mL whereas all the others are 1 kcal/mL.

‡Magnacal (Organon) is 2 kcal/mL whereas all the others are 1 kcal/mL.

§For additional information, see M. E. Shils, A. S. Bloch, and R. Chernoff, *Liquid Formulas for Oral and Tube Feeding*, 2d ed., Memorial Sloan-Kettering Cancer Center, New York, 1979.

diarrhea. A gradual increase in concentration will enhance tolerance and allow for a steady progression to full-strength, full-volume formula.[62]

In addition to the formula composition (i.e., lactose levels hypertonicity) there are other causes for diarrhea: contamination, bacterial infections, use of antibiotics, too rapid a rate of administration—all are factors to be considered. Poor sanitation and handling as possible causes of contamination require close investigation when cases of diarrhea occur. However, commercially available tube feeding products are sterile and, if handled properly, will not have any bacterial growth.[63] Homemade formulas are not in general usage because the convenience, long shelf life, and low cost make commercial feedings very acceptable.

Once opened or reconstituted, feedings should be refrigerated; only a 24-h supply should be prepared and on hand, and only the amount required for the feeding should be removed and allowed to come to room temperature prior to administration.

Tube Feeding Administration

There are a number of access routes that can be used to administer tube feedings. The most common tube site is nasogastric (see Fig. 28-5). This is the most direct route for patients who cannot ingest foods normally. In recent years, access to the duodenum (see Fig. 28-6) and the jejunum (see Fig. 28-7) has been accomplished with the development of new, longer, flexible tubes. Feeding into the GI tract below the stomach has advantages in avoiding regurgitation and the possibility of aspiration. Gastric reflux can be avoided by taking advantage of both the gastro-esophageal and pyloric sphincters. Although feeding into the stomach allows the digestive process to start in the stomach, adequate digestion of intact nutrients can be accomplished

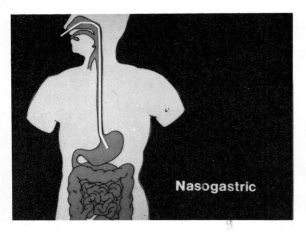

Figure 28-5
Nasogastric feeding tube placement.

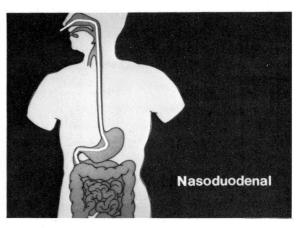

Figure 28-6
Nasoduodenal feeding tube placement.

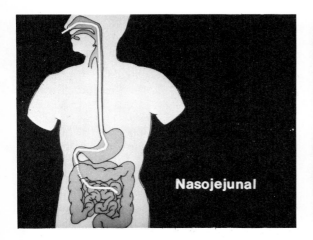

Figure 28-7
Nasojejunal feeding tube placement.

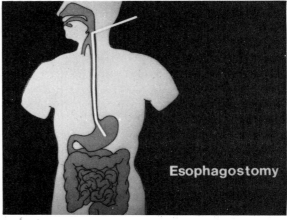

Figure 28-8
Esophagostomy feeding tube placement.

when feeding into the upper part of the small intestine.

For patients who have chewing and swallowing problems, a cervical esophagastomy (see Fig. 28-8) may be created. This provides the benefits of access to the full length of the GI tract for digestion and absorption, is easy to care for, and has a low rate of complications.

Gastrostomy (see Fig. 28-9) placement by-

passes the upper part of the GI tract and feeds directly into the stomach, which allows almost full access to digestive and absorptive processes. Long-term, in-dwelling gastrostomies are a fairly acceptable and successful method of feeding.

Jejunostomies (see Fig. 28-10) may be used for patients who have problems that forbid access to the stomach, such as gastric cancer,

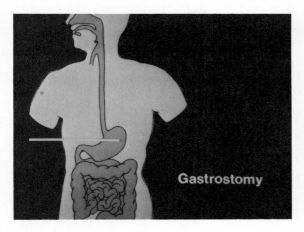

Figure 28-9
Gastrostomy feeding tube placement.

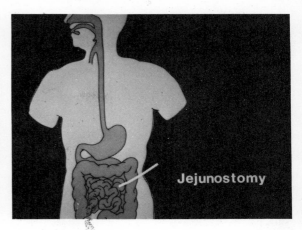

Figure 28-10
Jejunostomy feeding tube placement.

chronic nausea and vomiting, surgical intervention, or extensive peptic ulcer disease. Another mode of jejunal feeding is needle catheter jejunostomy. This method employs the use of a large-gauge needle to place a small catheter into the jejunum. When the catheter is sutured into place, this method can be used for the delivery of defined formula diets directly into the small bowel.[64]

Feeding Tubes and Equipment

One of the reasons that tube feeding has become more popular in recent years is the development of several small, soft, nonirritating tubes. These tubes are made of silicone or polyurethane compounds that range in size from 5 to 9 Fr. Many of these tubes are mercury-weighted and radiopaque so that their tip location can be checked by x-ray. Nothing should be fed into a feeding tube unless the tip location is known. Examples of tubes are the Keofeed (Hedeco Inc., California), Dobbhoff (Searle, Chicago), and Entriflex (Biosearch Medical Products, Raritan, N. J.).

Some companies have provided screw-on cap administration sets for their products. For defined formula diets that require reconstitution, there are several tube feeding bags available that will connect with most feeding tubes. Examples

are the Vivonex bag (Eaton, New York), Dobbhoff bag (Biosearch Medical Products), Keofeed bag (Hedeco, California), Kangaroo bag (Chesebrough-Pond's, Connecticut), and the Flexitainer (Ross, Ohio)

Tube Feeding Delivery Systems

Tube feedings can be administered in two ways, either intermittently or continuously. Intermittent feedings are usually given every 3 to 4 h in amounts ranging from 100 to 400 mL. It is wise to start with smaller amounts and build up to larger volumes, as tolerated by the patient. It is a good idea to check gastric residuals before each feeding to avoid regurgitation. No more than one-third of the previous feeding should be present in the stomach before a new feeding is started. Intermittent feeding may be administered by gravity drip, and each feeding should take 20 min or more.

Continuous drip feeding is recommended for the administration of defined formula diets or for patients who have a limited absorptive area. The rate of the feeding should start at 40 to 50 mL per hour, increasing as tolerated by the patient. Since it is recommended that these diets start at dilute strength, either the rate of administration or the concentration of the formula should be changed, but not both simultaneously. The administration sets previously discussed all have rate control clamps, and tube feeding pumps are now commercially available at reasonable prices.

With either method it is a good idea to keep the patient's head or upper torso elevated at least 30° while feeding, to guard against aspiration.

Tube Feeding for Infants and Children

Low-birth-weight neonates (2.5 kg) who are unable to take adequate nourishment orally because of their immaturity (i.e., an inability to suck) are supported by gavage or nasogastric tube feedings or gastrostomy feedings. In addition, supplemental intravenous glucose may be necessary for very-low-birth-weight infants (less than 1.2 kg)—administered within the first 3 to 6 h of life—in order to prevent acidosis and hypoglycemia.

Enteral feedings are planned according to gestational age, extrauterine adjustment, and clinical status. The quantity and frequency of feeding, as well as the concentration of formulas, must be based on individual tolerance. Commercial infant formulas may be used. Small quantities—9 to 15 mL—are given every 4 h, and are increased in volume, concentration, and frequency as tolerated. (For low-birth-weight infants, see Chap. 14.)

Tube Feeding for Older Infants and Young Children

Commercial infant formulas, individualized according to energy needs, may be used as tube feedings. Consideration must be given to protein, mineral, and vitamin levels, and to fluid needs, especially in those who are unable to express thirst.

The danger of solute overload (protein and electrolyte) becomes especially hazardous when the tube feeding is not followed by added water. This is mandatory in order to ensure adequate urine output (240 to 600 mL per day in young children) and to prevent dehydration.

The nurse must be alert for symptoms of vomiting, diarrhea, high fever, and delirium.

Supplementary Feedings

These preparations may be taken by mouth or given by tube. They may be milk-based, with added carbohydrate, protein, fat, minerals, and vitamins; many are designed for use as the sole source of nutritional support. They provide a sound balance of calories and protein, and are easily digested and assimilated. They are easily obtained from local pharmacies after hospital discharge.

Meal Replacement Formulas

Meal replacement formulas are lactose-free and relatively low in residue. When they are given in calorically adequate amounts, they will meet or exceed the RDA for vitamins and minerals. Although made from protein isolates, these products require intact digestive and absorptive capacity because of their complex nutrient sources.[65] These products are designed as the sole source of nutrition and may be used orally to make some of these formulas more palatable.

Defined Formula Diets

Defined formula diets are lactose-free, some are fat-free, and they leave little residue in the lower bowel. They reduce stool size, volume, and frequency, and allow the lower bowel to rest (see Table 28-6).

These preparations are designed for use as the sole source of nutrition, and are essential components of managing many surgical and medical disease states: inflammatory bowel disease (regional enteritis, ulcerative colitis), bowel fistulas, malabsorption, short-bowel syndrome, pancreatic disease, etc.[66] Other indications for use have already been mentioned: preoperatively for bowel preparation and nutritional support; they are also useful in preparation for colonic x-rays.

Defined formula diets are not at all palata-

TABLE 28-18   RECOMMENDED ADMINISTRATION OF DEFINED FORMULA DIET

Day	Strength	Volume of water	kcal/mL	kJ/mL
1	¼	1800 mL	0.25	1.05
2	½	1800 mL	0.5	2.1
3	¾	1800 mL	0.75	3.15
4	Full	1800 mL	1	4.2

ble because of their amino acid and peptide content. These formulas should be administered by tube when possible. Because the formulas are hypertonic, there is the danger of osmotic diarrhea and dehydration. The formulas should be administered in dilute concentrations in limited volumes.

If it is necessary to administer these formulas orally, patients should be advised to sip the mixture very slowly over a period of time. A recommended plan for feeding appears in Table 28-18, above.

Careful addition of water to regimens featuring defined formula diets is vital. Patients must be instructed to drink sufficient water to avoid any intolerance that may occur. Periodic clinical monitoring of blood and urine for glucose, and of blood for electrolyte levels is recommended.

Defined Formula Diets for Infants and Children

Children are very sensitive to concentrated solutions containing high solute loads. In infants, one-quarter strength solutions (0.25 kcal per milliliter, or 1.05 kJ per milliliter) are recommended as an initial course.[67] This is gradually increased over several days, according to tolerance and absence of danger signs. One-half strength is considered the limit of tolerance. Older children may be able to tolerate full-strength mixtures (1 kcal per milliliter); however, one-half strength (0.5 kcal per milliliter) is recommended as the starting level, gradually increased to the level of tolerance as the GI tract adjusts.

Transitional Feedings

Very few patients will remain on parenteral or enteral nutrition support as a permanent feeding modality. Transition from one modality to another requires careful attention. An abrupt change in nutrition support modalities may lead to weight loss during the adjustment period.

During a transitional period the nutrient levels contributed from the two feeding methods should have a constant total. The patient should be receiving adequate nutrition from the second feeding method before the first one is discontinued[68] (see Fig. 28-11).

Figure 28-11

Transitional feeding. One method of feeding should not be stopped until another is begun and there is adequate support from the new method. Patients can skip from any one method to another as long as an adaptation period is allowed.

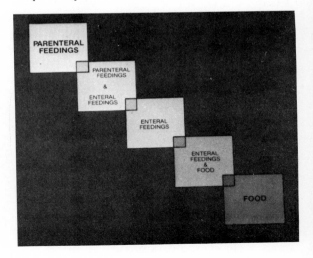

NUTRITION SUPPORT SERVICES

As with any other sophisticated modality of medical care, nutritional support—as described in this chapter, both parenteral and enteral nutrition—requires careful control and monitoring. The safest and most direct way to provide this type of care is through a team approach. The nutrition support team, or metabolic support team, is composed of several health professionals who provide specialized services depending upon their discipline. The core of the team is usually a physician, a nurse, a pharmacist, and a dietitian.

The physician serves as the overall coordinator and is responsible for writing daily orders for formulations, ordering appropriate laboratory tests, and monitoring the daily fluid and electrolyte balance of each patient. The nurse is responsible for sterile dressing changes of parenteral line insertion sites, maintaining patency of the intravenous line, monitoring fluid balance, checking feeding tube placement (and sometimes the actual placement of the tubes), data coordination of daily blood and urine tests, and daily patient condition reports. The pharmacist reviews the physician's orders for parenteral solution formulation for drug and dosage incompatibilities, compounds the solutions under sterile conditions, labels them properly, and assures prompt delivery of the solution to the patient. In some institutions, the pharmacist is responsible for the reconstitution and distribution of enteral formulas as well. The dietitian's responsibility is to interpret nutritional assessment findings and monitor the patient's changing nutritional status after therapy is instituted, to participate in establishing patient nutritional requirements, to recommend and monitor tolerance of enteral feeding solutions, and to make or suggest modifications when necessary in nutritional therapy.

Often the nutritional support team may include additional staff who fulfill other functions for the overall rehabilitation of the patient. A nutrition team may also include physical therapists, social workers, laboratory technicians, secretaries, clerks, and data processors.

As with other medical care teams, the nutrition support service meets periodically, usually once a day, for either bedside or chart rounds, to inform all the members of the team about recent developments or changes in patient status or the presentation of new referrals. A nutrition support service is a consultant service, so daily notes are recorded in patient charts to keep primary care physicians aware of the treatment of their patients who are receiving nutrition support. This approach has been very successful, and most institutions providing nutritional care as described have established a team to assure the highest quality delivery of services.

BURNS

Classification of Burns (Severity and Depth)

Degree of Severity

Burns may be classified according to severity in the following manner:

> *Small burns.* Less than 15 to 20 percent of the total body surface area (BSA) is affected.
>
> *Intermediate burns.* Twenty to 40 percent of BSA is affected.
>
> *Large* or *severe burns.* More than 40 to 50 percent of BSA is affected.

Depth of Injury

Depth of injury is classified in the following manner:

> *Full-thickness burn.* All epithelial remnants are destroyed; autografting is required.
>
> *Partial-thickness burn.* Remaining epithelium is present, which will spontaneously reepithelialize the area.

We focus on the intermediate-burn patient, bearing in mind that increased nutritional demands and requirements must be met for all cases of burn injury.

Metabolic Sequelae of Burns

The burn patient, in previous good health and sound nutritional status, now develops metabolic sequelae, which are summarized as follows:

1   There is marked metabolic response to the severe trauma of thermal injury.
    a   Increased catecholamine secretion results in increased glucagon secretion and in increased heat production (elevated basal metabolic rate) that usually lasts 6 to 8 weeks after injury.
    b   Hepatic production of glucose is elevated, leading to a hyperglycemic state.[69]

2   The loss of skin surface represents the loss of an effective defense against infections. This skin loss results in huge water losses, perhaps as high as 5 L per day;[70] in addition, much energy is expended in the process of evaporation (580 kcal per liter, or 2436 kJ per liter evaporated), so that energy requirements are well above basal needs. This emphasizes the need to close the wounds (by grafting if necessary) as soon as possible.

3   There is marked protein catabolism.
    a   Increased glucocorticoid activity results in mobilization of tissue amino acids as the need for energy becomes urgent. This is reflected in increased urinary nitrogen and potassium.
    b   There is increased loss of albumin and other plasma proteins from the oozing exudates of the open wound.

Goals of Management

The goals of management are to support the respiratory and circulatory systems, and to sustain the patient until skin cover is achieved and basal metabolic rate is normalized.[71]

Fluid and Electrolyte Replacement

Initial care is directed toward the restoration of fluid and electrolyte balance and of blood volume, in order to prevent dehydration, shock, and metabolic acidosis.

This is accomplished by means of:

Intravenous support with glucose (to prevent acidosis), electrolytes, colloids, and water is crucial.

Blood transfusions may be necessary within 24 to 36 h. The blood replacement is required because there is increased blood loss from the wound as well as depressed erythrocyte formation by the bone marrow.

Plasma or albumin may be required to support blood volume.

The formulas in Table 28-19 (p. 684) provide a guide for immediately determining the water, colloid, and electrolyte needs.

Burns in infants and children require special attention since shock and acidosis within 18 to 24 h of injury are usual. As a precaution, children are given intravenous therapy regardless of the extent of the burn injury.

Urine output is monitored hourly so as to ensure adequate fluid therapy (see Table 28-20). Oliguria may be present, but it is usually resolved within 48 h.

Children are kept npo (given nothing by mouth) for the first 48 h. After this time, the danger of vomiting has lessened, and small amounts of fluid (30 to 60 mL) may be given. The child is rapidly advanced to high-energy, high-protein liquids and then to an appropriate individualized, high-energy, high-protein diet.

Prevention of Infection

The loss of skin cover represents the loss of an effective barrier against infection. The burn wound itself is often a source of bacterial contamination. In addition, there is an early lack of resistance as the individual's defense system is depressed. Lymphadenopathy, decreased antibody response, and gamma globulin destruction often are a consequence of burn injury. All patients with full-thickness burns are given tetanus immunizations or boosters; infants and young children are given gamma globulin. Antibiotics, intravenous and topical (e.g., penicillin), are also administered.

TABLE 28-19 FORMULAS FOR CALCULATING FLUID REQUIREMENTS

Evans formula

Day 1 % BSA* burned × body weight (kg) × 1 = mL colloid
     % BSA burned × body weight (kg) × 1 = mL 5% dextrose in normal saline   } one-half given in first 8 h
     Plus maintenance fluids: 2000 mL 5% dextrose in water per day

Day 2 % BSA burned × body weight (kg) × 0.5 = mL colloid
     % BSA burned × body weight (kg) × 0.5 = mL 5% dextrose in normal saline
     Plus maintenance fluids: 2000 mL 5% dextrose in water per day

Day 3 and thereafter—intravenous fluids as indicated (burns over 50% BSA calculated as 50% burn)

Brooke Army formula

Day 1 % BSA burned × body weight (kg) × 1.5 = mL 5% dextrose in normal saline   } one-half given in first 8 h
     % BSA burned × body weight (kg) × 0.5 = mL colloid†
     Plus maintenance fluids: 2000 mL 5% dextrose in water per day

Day 2 % BSA burned × body weight (kg) × 0.75 = mL 5% dextrose in normal saline
     % BSA burned × body weight (kg) × 0.25 = mL colloid
     Plus maintenance fluids: 2000 mL 5% dextrose in water per day

Children's Hospital of Michigan formula

Day 1 % BSA burned × body weight (kg) × 2 = mL 5% dextrose in lactated Ringer's solution; two-thirds in first 8 h
     Plus maintenance fluids: 1500 mL 5% dextrose in lactated Ringer's solution per square meter BSA per day
     For burns of 40–60% BSA, add 50 meq sodium bicarbonate to each liter of fluid and reduce rate by 10%
     For burns over 60% BSA, add { 40 meq sodium bicarbonate to each liter of fluid
                            50 meq sodium chloride (12.5 mL of 15% saline) to each liter of fluid; slow rate by 20%

Day 2 Same fluids, but for burns over 40% with hyperosmolar solutions in use, monitor electrolytes at 18, 24, 30, and 36 h and q 4 h thereafter. Stop hyperosmolar solution when serum sodium rises to or above 150 meq or serum osmolarity exceeds 350 millimoles. Resume 5% dextrose in lactated Ringer's at original rate.

Day 3 and thereafter—5% dextrose in lactated Ringer's solution at a rate sufficient to maintain urinary output of 40 mL/m² BSA per hour

*BSA = body surface area.

†Because colloid is now considered ineffective during the first 24 h after a burn, some authors advocate eliminating colloid from the Brooke formula.

TABLE 28-20 GUIDE TO MONITORING HOURLY URINES IN PATIENTS WITH BURNS

Patient	Age, yr	mL/h
Infants	Under 1	5–10
Children	1–10	10–20
	Over 10	15–30
Adults		30–50

684

Burn unit To help control the spread of infection, ensure aseptic technique, and control evaporative water losses (in a 20 to 40 percent BSA burn, 1 to 2 L of water is lost through evaporation daily), special environmentally controlled burn units are used. These plastic tents have controlled humidity (20 percent) and temperature (30°C), as well as a flow of sterile air. They provide a bacteria-controlled, psychologically acceptable environment (patients are able to see their surroundings from within the transparent tent) that fosters survival.

Gastrointestinal Atony

Gastrointestinal atony or ileus may occur over a period of 24 to 36 h.[72] This is managed by nasogastric tube suction. When peristalsis resumes, the goal is to provide sufficient food to meet the great, critical energy and protein requirements. Nutritional assessment and an individualized plan of action are imperative.

The patient with a normal GI tract and no sepsis may be started on clear liquids and should rapidly progress to full liquids within 24 h after injury. Patients with large burns are usually not fed until GI mobility returns.

Nutritional Support

The body's demand for energy and protein, and the need to prevent weight loss, are paramount. Sufficient calories for energy needs and protein synthesis must be consumed or delivered by a nutritional support system—protein utilization for wound healing and prevention of hypopro-teinemia are of primary importance. The burn patient with adequate nutrient intake has greater success with the grafting procedure, has better healing at graft sites, and is less threatened by infection. Table 28-21 represents a plan for nutrient requirements.

Multivitamin preparations, especially vitamins C and B complex, along with vitamin D, are given. Iron may be required for patients who become anemic. Serum zinc levels were found to be low in burned patients. However, zinc supplementation was not felt to be necessary since adequate oral intake soon results in normalization of zinc levels.[73]

Dietary regimens As a daily dietary program for burn patients, 3000 to 5000 kcal (12.6 to 21 MJ) and 150 to 200 g of protein is not uncommon. All routes—oral, tube, and TPN—are utilized to achieve this critical goal. All possible methods must be employed, because the patient cannot take this amount of food by mouth.

1 *Oral route.* High-energy, high-protein liquids, milk shakes, and cream soups are given frequently, and are well accepted.
2 *Tube feedings.* High-nitrogen tube feedings have been successfully used.
3 *TPN.* This route requires careful supervision, but it is finding greater application. The danger of contamination and possible monilial sepsis is always present.
4 *Fat emulsions.* Use of intravenous fat has great potential in meeting energy requirements.

TABLE 28-21   RECOMMENDED NUTRITIONAL DESIGNS FOR BURN PATIENTS

	Protein		Energy	
	g/kg body weight + *g/each 1% BSA* burned*		*kcal/kg body weight* + *kcal/1% BSA* burned*	
Children (up to 12 years of age)	3 +	1	60 +	35
Adults	1 +	3	30 +	70

*BSA = body surface area.

Monitoring of nutrients by checking the tray and documenting intakes and outputs further serves to intensify the role of the dietitian and the nurse, who must set rehabilitative goals and direct the efforts made toward meeting them.

In the attempt to reach this great nutritional goal, overstimulation of the GI tract by the large volume of nutrient-rich material may occur, and hemorrhage may result; therefore, aggressive concern must be tempered with caution.

Emotional Support

In addition to technical and nutritional support, emotional support must be given. Hospitalizations are long; wound debridement is painful and discouraging. Regrafting due to failure of a graft to "take" is common. The patient requires the constant support and encouragement of all.

Severely burned children must overcome an abrupt psychological as well as physical insult to their normal development. Children may experience grief and anger over body disfigurement; skin grafting and release of disabling, painful contractures are essential. Campbell, and Holli and Oakes make several sound observations and give practical suggestions on managing and feeding burned children.[74,75]

There is a great need to encourage verbalization of feelings as well as to provide opportunities for choosing or for simple decision making on the patient's part. As best as possible and with guidance, the patient should be allowed to help plan and select a menu. Individualized diets should include popular and familiar foods, such as hot dogs, hamburgers, milk shakes, and pizza. All attempts at continuing interaction with burn patients and normalization of activities should be encouraged.

CONCLUSION

Nutrition is paramount to the recovery of the surgically stressed or burned patient and requires the team approach. For example, in managing the burn patient, the combined efforts of the burn team—the doctor, nurse, nutritionist,

respiratory therapist, social worker, etc.—must be executed judiciously, efficiently, and without delay. The toll of surgery or severe burns is great, often devastating; and rehabilitation may be long and marred by many painful episodes and setbacks.

In the team approach, the special roles of the nurse and dietitian are prominent. The dietitian is specially trained to help in establishing the patient's nutritional needs and in providing the appropriate dietary intervention. The dietitian's role is that of a translator; that is, to take those nutritional needs that are determined by assessment techniques and translate them into food with the help of the patient.[76]

The nurse with continuing patient contact can closely determine the effectiveness of the diet, monitoring the clinical signs of weight, fluid intake and output; helping with menu selection; and verbalizing the patient's requests. It should be remembered that despite all good intentions and impressive plans, if a patient will not eat, all skill and knowledge are wasted.

This chapter serves to reaffirm the need to provide human as well as nutritional support for those who must overcome and survive surgery, stress, or burns.

STUDY QUESTIONS

1 Describe the body's catabolic hormonal response to stress, surgery, and burns.

2 What are the goals of postoperative nutritional management?

3 Is is possible to maintain a patient on 5 percent dextrose in water postoperatively for an extended period of time?

4 What clinical and laboratory signs should be closely monitored in patients receiving TPN?

5 What precautions can be taken to avoid complications in patients receiving tube feedings?

6 Describe the metabolic sequelae of burns and the required nutritional support of the burn patient.

CLINICAL STUDY 28

A 23-year-old female was admitted to the hospital because of steady weight loss, cramping, and diarrhea. She had a diagnosis of Crohn's disease, made when she was 16 years old. She was hospitalized at 16 for weight loss, anemia, and dehydration associated with chronic diarrhea. Her present medications include 25 mg Azulfidine, Lomotil prn, and a low-lactose diet. Over the past 3 months she has lost 10 lb.

Her nutritional assessment showed:

Ht	5 ft 4 in
Wt	110 lb
TSF	20 mm
Arm muscle circumference	21.3 cm

Na	143 meq/L
K	4.5 meq/L
Cl	103 meq/L
Ca	10.6 mL/100 mL
P	4.2 mL/100 mL
BUN	24 mL/100 mL
Alb	3.7 g/100 mL

TLC	1800 mm^3
Serum Fe	60 µg
Hb	11.8 g/100 mL
HCT	35 percent
TIBC	165 µg
T	37.4°C
P	135/78 mmHg blood pressure
R	21

When she was admitted, she was put on a clear liquid diet, push fluids, in preparation for a barium enema, which revealed an exacerbation of her Crohn's disease and a perirectal abscess. The following care plan was established:

1 Surgical incision and drainage of the abscess

2 Increased dose of steroids and antibiotic therapy

Clinical study questions

1 What would a nutritional care plan have to include, based on her nutritional assessment?

2 How would you calculate her calorie and protein requirements?

REFERENCES

1   *Webster's New Collegiate Dictionary,* G & C Merriam Company, Springfield, Mass., 1979.

2   A. C. Guyton, *Textbook of Medical Physiology,* W. B. Saunders Company, Philadelphia, 1976.

3   A. A. Albanese and L. A. Orto, "The Proteins and Amino Acids," in R. S. Goodhart and M. E. Shils (eds.), *Modern Nutrition in Health and Disease,* Lea & Febiger, Philadelphia, 1968.

4   T. K. Hunt, "Nutritional Requirements of Repair," in W. F. Ballinger, J. A. Collins, W. R. Drucker, S. J. Dudrick, and R. Zeppa (eds.), *Manual of Surgical Nutrition,* W. B. Saunders Company, Philadelphia, 1975.

5   D. W. Wilmore, *The Metabolic Mangement of the Critically Ill,* Plenum Medical Book Company, New York, 1977.

6   M. V. Kaminski, R. P. Ruggiero, and C. B. Mills, "Nutritional Assessment: A Guide to Diagnosis and Treatment of the Hypermetabolic Patient," *Journal of the Florida Medical Association,* **66**(4):390–395, 1979.

7   W. Stahl, *Supportive Care of the Surgical Patient,* Grune and Stratton, Inc., New York, 1972.

8   C. E. Butterworth and R. L. Weinsier, "Malnutrition in Hospital Patients: Assessment and Treatment," in R. S. Goodhart and M. E. Shils (eds.), *Modern Nutrition in Health and Disease,* Lea & Febiger, Philadelphia, 1980.

9   F. D. Moore and M. F. Brennan, "Surgical Injury," in W. F. Ballinger et al. (eds.), *Manual of Surgical Nutrition,* W. B. Saunders Company, Philadelphia, 1975.

10   E. Peacock and W. Van Winkle, "Biochemistry and Environment of Wounds," in E. Peacock and W. Van Winkle (eds.), *Surgery and Biology of Wound Repair,* W. B. Saunders Company, Philadelphia, 1970.

11   T. K. Hunt, op. cit.

12   Ibid.

13   Ibid.

14   F. D. Moore and M. F. Brennan, op. cit.

15   Ibid.

16   "Cellular Immunity and Malnutrition," *Nutrition Reviews,* **30**:523, 1972.

17   D. G. Jose, "Cancer Connection with Immunity and Nutrition," *Nutrition Today,* March–April 1973, p. 4.

18   A. E. Axelrod, "Nutrition and Acquired Immunity," *Food and Nutrition News,* October–November 1974.

19   S. M. Levenson, L. V. Crowley, and E. Seifter, "Starvation," in W. F. Ballinger et al. (eds.), *Manual of Surgical Nutrition,* W. B. Saunders Company, Philadelphia, 1975.

20   B. Worthington, "Effect of Nutritional Status on Immune Phenomena," *Journal of the American Dietetic Association,* **65**:123, 1974.

21   D. K. Law, S. J. Dudrick, and N. I. Abdou, "Effects of Protein-Calorie Malnutrition on Immune Competence of the Surgical Patient," *Surgery Gynecology and Obstetrics,* **139**:257, 1974.

22   J. L. Mullen, M. H. Gertner, G. P. Buzby, G. L. Goodhart, and E. F. Rosato, "Implications of Malnutrition in the Surgical Patient," *Archives of Surgery,* **114**:121–125, 1979.

23   C. E. Butterworth, Jr., and G. L. Blackburn, "Hospital Malnutrition and How to Assess the Nutritional Status of a Patient," *Nutrition Today,* March–April 1975.

24   Ibid.

25   Ibid.

26   B. R. Bistrian, G. L. Blackburn, E. Hallowell, and R. Heddle, "Protein Status of General Surgical Patients," *Journal of the American Medical Association,* **230**:858, 1974.

27   B. R. Bistrian, G. L. Blackburn, J. Vitale, D. Cochran, and J. Naylor, "Prevalence of Malnutrition in General Medical Patients," *Journal of the American Medical Association,* **235**:1567, 1976.

28   G. L. Hill, I. Pickford, G. A. Young, C. J. Schorah, R. L. Blackett, L. Burkinshaw, J. V. Warren, and D. B. Morgan, "Malnutrition in Surgical Patients," *Lancet,* **1**:689, 1977.

29   H. D. Willcutts, "Nutritional Assessment of 1000 Surgical Patients in an Affluent Suburban Community Hospital," *Journal of Parenteral and Enteral Nutrition,* **1**:25A (abs.), 1977.

30   T. W. Hensle, "The Impact of Surgery of the Starving Patient," *Comprehensive Therapy,* **4**(10):24, 1978.

31   Ibid.

32   J. B. Pietsch, J. L. Meakins, and L. D. MacLean, "The Delayed Hypersensitivity Response: Application in Clinical Surgery," *Surgery,* **82**(3):349, 1977.

33   B. R. Bistrian, G. L. Blackburn, E. Hallowell, and R. Heddle, op. cit.

34   J. L. Mullen, G. P. Buzby, M. T. Waldman, M. H. Gertner, C. L. Hobbs, and E. F. Rosato, "Prediction of Operative Morbidity and Mortality by Preoperative Nutritional Assessment," *Surgical Forum,* **30**:80, 1979.

35   B. A. Griggs, R. Chernoff, M. C. Hoppe, and J. E. Wade, *Enteral Alimentation,* ASPEN Monograph, ASPEN National Office, Washington, 1979.

36   M. E. Shils, "Principles of Nutritional Therapy," *Cancer,* **43**:2093(Supplement), 1979.

37   S. J. Dudrick and D. W. Wilmore, "Long-term Parenteral Feeding," *Hospital Practice,* **3**(10):65, 1968.

38   M. Deitel and V. Kaminsky, "Total Nutrition by Peripheral Vein—the Lipid System," *Canadian Medical Association Journal,* **111**:152, 1974.

39   G. L. Blackburn, *Adaptation to Starvation,* Intake Perspectives in Clinical Nutrition, Eaton Laboratories, Norwich, New York, 1973.

40   M. E. Shils, and H. T. Randall, "Diet and Nutrition in the Care of the Surgical Patient," in R. S. Goodhart and M. E. Shils (eds.), *Modern Nutrition in Health and Disease,* Lea & Febiger, Philadelphia, 1980.

41   S. J. Dudrick, D. W. Wilmore, H. M. Vars, and J. E. Rhoads, "Long-term Total Parenteral Nutrition with Growth, Development and Positive Nitrogen Balance," *Surgery,* **64**:134, 1968.

42   C. R. Fleming et al., "Total Parenteral Nutrition," *Mayo Clinic Proceedings,* **31**:187, 1976.

43   C. R. Fleming, D. B. McGill, and S. Berkner, "Home Parenteral Nutrition as Primary Therapy in Patients with Extensive Crohn's Disease of the Small Bowel and Malnutrition," *Gastroenterology,* **73**(5):1077, 1977.

44   J. L. Mullen, W. C. Hargrove, S. J. Dudrick, W. T. Fitts, Jr., and E. F. Rosato, Ten Years Experience with Intravenous Hyperalimentation and Inflammatory Bowel Disease," *Annals of Surgery,* **187**(5):523, 1978.

45   R. E. Dean, M. M. Campos, and B. Barrett, "Hyperalimentation in the Management of Chronic Inflammatory Bowel Disease," *Diseases of the Colon and Rectum,* **19**(7):601, 1976.

46   M. Deitel, "Nutritional Mangement of External Gastrointestinal Fistulas," *Canadian Journal of Surgery,* **19**(6):505, 1976.

47   R. M. Abel, J. E. Fischer, M. J. Buckley, G. O. Barnett, and G. W. Austen, "Malnutrition in Cardiac Surgical Patients. Results of a Prospective, Randomized Evaluation of Early Postoperative in Parenteral Nutrition," *Archives of Surgery,* **111**(1):45, 1976.

48   R. M. Abel, "Total Parenteral Nutrition for Acute Renal Failure," *Comprehensive Therapy,* **3**(10):16, 1977.

49   E. M. Copeland, J. M. Daly, D. M. Ota, and S. J. Dudrick, "Nutrition, Cancer and Intravenous Hyperalimentation," *Cancer,* **43**:2108, 1979.

50 A. Tejani, B. Dobias, B. S. Nangia, and R. Mahad-evan, "Growth, Health and Development after Neo-natal Gut Surgery: A Long-term Follow-up," *Pediatrics,* **61**(5):685, 1978.

51 J. B. Lynch, "Current Status of Treatment of Burns," *Southern Medical Journal,* **69**(8):1085, 1976.

52 W. C. Heird and T. L. Anderson, "Nutritional Requirements and Methods of Feeding Low Birth Weight Infants," *Current Problems in Pediatrics,* **7**(8):1, 1977.

53 D. W. Wilmore, "Alimentation in Injured and Septic Patients," *Heart and Lung* **5**(5):791, 1976.

54 J. H. Duke and S. J. Dudrick, "Parenteral Feeding," in W. F. Ballinger, J. A. Collins, W. R. Drucker, S. J. Dudrick, and R. Zeppa," *Manual on Surgical Nutrition,* W. B. Saunders Company, Philadelphia, 1975.

55 Ibid.

56 M. E. Shils, op. cit.

57 J. H. Duke and S. J. Dudrick, op. cit.

58 M. Asch and E. Fonkalsrud, "Special Pediatric Considerations," in Ballinger et al., op. cit.

59 C. R. Fleming et al., "Prospective Study of Serum Copper and Zinc Levels in Patients Receiving Total Parenteral Nutrition," *American Journal of Clinical Nutrition,* **29**:70, 1976.

60 A. Gormican, "Tube Feeding," *Dietetic Currents,* April–May–June 1975.

61 J. C. Dougherty, "Influence of High Protein Diets on Renal Function," *Journal of the American Dietetic Association,* **63**:392, 1973.

62 R. Chernoff, "Enteral Feedings," *American Jouranl of Hospital Pharmacy,* **37**:65, 1980.

63 W. White, T. E. Acuff, T. K. Sykes, and R. P. Dobbie, "Bacterial Contamination of Liquid Enteral Nutrient Solution: Preliminary Report," *Journal of Parenteral and Enteral Nutrition,* **3**(6):459, 1979.

64 C. P. Page, J. A. Ryan, and R. C. Haff, "Continual Catheter Administration of an Elemental Diet," *Surgery, Gynecology, and Obstetrics,* **142**:184, 1976.

65 R. Chernoff, op. cit.

66 M. E. Shils, and H. T. Randall, op. cit.

67 M. J. Asch and E. W. Fonkalsrud, "Special Pediatric Considerations," in W. F. Ballinger et al., op. cit.

68 R. Chernoff, op. cit.

69 D. W. Wilmore, *The Metabolic Mangement of the Critically Ill,* Plenum Medical Book Company, New York, 1977.

70 Ibid.

71 B. A. Pruitt, "Postburn Hypermetabolism, and Nutrition of the Burn Patient," in W. F. Ballinger et al., op. cit.

72 B. Harpole et al., *Nutritional Mangement of Problem Patients,* Intake: Perspectives in Clinical Nutrition, Eaton Laboratories, Norwich, New York, 1975.

73 I. Cohen et al., "Hypogeusia, Anorexia and Altered Zinc Metabolism Following Thermal Burn," *Journal of the American Medical Association.* **223**:914, 1973.

74 L. Campbell, "Special Behavioral Problems of the Burned Child," *American Journal of Nursing,* **76**:220, 1976.

75 B. Holli and J. Oakes, "Feeding of the Burned Child," *Journal of the American Dietetic Association,* **67**:240, 1975.

76 R. Chernoff, "The Team Concept: The Dietitian's Responsibility," *Journal of Parental and Enteral Nutrition,* **3**(2):89, 1979.

CLINICAL DISCUSSION 28

Crohn's disease, an inflammatory disease of the bowel, is a sclerosing granulomatous disease of unknown etiology. It infiltrates all layers of the intestinal wall, with the lower terminal ileum the prime area of disease development.

In the acute phase, the disease is manifested by the presence of abscesses, fistulas, severe cramping, diarrhea, nausea, and vomiting. The patient has inadequate food intake and is unable to digest fully the food eaten. Because of the discomfort associated with meals, the patient usually reduces both solid and liquid nutrients that might be taken. For this reason the patient will show weight loss and probable dehydration. The severe stress of the disease may result in muscle proteolysis, used for energy needs. This appears as muscle wasting, weakness, and fatigue.

Extended periods of inadequate food intake and diminished protein reserves will result in hypoalbuminemia, decreased hemoglobin and hematocrit, and depressed levels of serum total iron-binding capacity. The patient becomes more likely to develop infections and anemia.

Although this patient has serum electrolyte levels within normal limits, when her laboratory values are examined more closely, it is revealed that she is quite dehydrated. If her blood volume and total body water were at normal levels, most of her serum values would be depressed. At a closer look, she is running a low-grade temperature, probably associated with her abscess, and is probably losing more than normal insensible fluid losses because of her fever. This patient shows the classic symptoms of active Crohn's disease: a recent, rapid weight loss, anemia, and infection. Preoperatively her nutritional care plan would be to rehydrate as much as possible and to provide both calorie and protein substrate to replenish losses suffered in the recent past. For this patient a recommendation might be to start on peripheral parenteral nutrition along with a low-lactose, low-residue liquid diet, a defined formula diet with low levels of fat. There is no problem with fluid overload if she takes 1800 mL of fluid by mouth and 1 L of peripheral parenteral nutrition solution. Using a defined formula diet will provide protein for nitrogen depletion, calories in easily digestible forms, and fluid. The nutrients in defined formula diets are easily digested and absorbed while low in residue and lactose-free. Proteins, calories, vitamins, and minerals available from these two methods of nutritional support will reduce this patient's catabolic state. It would most likely be recommended that this patient be given one to two units of packed cells to help correct the anemia prior to surgery. Depressed serum proteins will reverse themselves if adequate protein is fed for a long enough time. Some health professionals like to correct low serum albumins through the intravenous administration of salt-poor albumin. This is very expensive and treats the symptom, not the underlying cause of the depressed serum protein–extended dietary protein deficiency.

After surgical incision and drainage of her abscess, the patient was maintained on D_5W for 8 h immediately postoperatively. She began her preoperative regimen again on the first day after surgery, in order to continue supplying adequate calories, protein, vitamins, and minerals. By using these two methods together, the patient is encouraged to take nutrients by mouth, while receiving support intravenously. As her tolerance for oral feedings increases, a defined formula diet can be used for an additional few days until she recovers enough to eat more solid foods. This patient felt more comfortable taking a liquid diet and was discharged 10 days postoperatively on a defined formula diet and a low-lactose, low-residue meal pattern.

On her 1-month follow-up visit, she had gained back almost 5 lb, was feeling significantly stronger, and did not tire as easily. She decided to maintain herself on a low-residue, low-lactose, high-energy–high-protein diet and to discontinue the use of the defined formula diet.

Her protein and calorie requirements would be based on the weight she must gain back; they would then be recalculated for her to maintain her weight and hydration status and meet her protein requirements.

CHAPTER 29

NUTRITION AND CANCER

Nancie Harvey Herbold
Janet L. Sydness

KEY WORDS
Carcinogen
Neoplasm
Benign Tumor
Malignant Tumor
Metastasize
Cachexia
Radiation
Chemotherapy
Immunotherapy
Antineoplastic Agents

INTRODUCTION

Cancer is one of the major health problems in the United States today. Approximately one of every four individuals in the United States will develop cancer in his or her lifetime.[1] Changes have been noted over the past 20 to 30 years in the incidence of cancer for men and women. Although the overall cancer rates are higher in men than in women, the incidence of lung cancer in women has been increasing, presumably because of the greater number of women who now smoke. Stomach cancer has been steadily declining for both men and women over the past several decades. Almost 50 percent of all fatal cancers are caused by three types: lung, large intestine, and breast. Of these, cancer of the large intestine and the breast are associated with diet.

The poor nutritional status of cancer patients has long been ignored and accepted as the sequela of the disease state, and until recently the possible carcinogenic properties of our diet were not even considered. This final chapter addresses this growing area of nutritional concern as it relates to both adults and children.

THE ETIOLOGY OF CANCER: DIETARY FACTORS

Approximately 80 percent of all cancers have an environmental cause. Environmental causes include air pollution, water pollution, radiation, drugs, tobacco, alcohol, and diet. Diet comprises the largest percentage of cancer incidence due to environmental factors. The incidence of cancer related to diet is 60 percent for women and over 40 percent for men.[2] Table 29-1 provides a brief summary of the various etiological factors which may predispose an individual to the development of cancer.

Epidemiological studies have provided information regarding the relationship between food, nutrition, and cancer. For example, in Japan, where there is a low incidence of cancer of the colon, the diet is low in unsaturated fat. However, among Japanese people who immi-

TABLE 29-1   FACTORS WHICH MAY PREDISPOSE
INDIVIDUALS TO CANCER

Factor	Comment
Heredity	Some congenital and genetic abnormalities may be linked with cancer. For example, Down syndrome is associated with an increased risk of leukemia.
Familial susceptibility	There is an increased incidence of breast cancer within families which have a history of the disease.
Acquired diseases	Certain diseases such as pernicious anemia, ulcerative colitis, hepatitis, and cirrhosis are all associated with increased incidence of cancer.
Viruses	Mechanism involved and part played are still unclear.
Environment	
Tobacco and alcohol	Increased incidence of cancers of the head and neck area in individuals who smoke and drink.
Radiation	Individuals who survived the atomic explosions at Hiroshima and Nagasaki had an increased incidence of leukemia.
Drugs	Immunosuppressive drugs and estrogens are two examples of drugs which increase the incidence of cancers.
Diet	Additives such as nitrites, dyes, and artificial sweeteners can cause cancer in laboratory animals. Diets high in saturated fat and refined carbohydrates have been implicated as playing a causal role in breast cancer and cancer of the colon.

Source: Adapted from D. A. Jones, C. F. Dunbar, and M. M. Jirovec, *Medical-Surgical Nursing: A Conceptual Approach*, McGraw-Hill Book Company, New York, 1978, pp. 128–130.

grate to the United States, the incidence of cancer of the colon increases, as does the intake of saturated fat.[3] The consumption of meat has also been correlated with colon cancer. It is not known if the carcinogenic portion of the meat is the protein, the fat, or an associated factor.[4] Another theory regarding cancer of the colon relates to bile acids. The degradation of bile acids by microorganisms may produce a bile acid derivative that is a carcinogen, a cocarcinogen, or a substance which enhances cancer development of the large bowel.[5] If this hypothesis is true, a diet high in fat would stimulate bile acid production, thereby increasing the risk of cancer development.

Diets low in fiber and high in refined foods have also been associated with cancer of the colon. In primitive societies the fiber intake is high and there is little cancer of the colon, whereas in more industrialized societies the fiber intake is low and the incidence of cancer is high. There are several theories about the decreased incidence of cancer of the colon when fiber consumption is high. One theory is that fiber increases fecal bulk, thereby diluting the carcinogen contained in the feces. Another relates to transit time which decreases the carcinogen contact time with the bowel. A third hypothesis is that fiber acts similarly to a chelating agent, rendering the carcinogen unabsorbable.

Cancer of the breast is more frequently seen in women who are overweight and have a high fat intake. Overconsumption of fat may alter hormonal balance, or the metabolic by-products of fat may be carcinogenic.[6] Cancer of the mouth and esophagus has been associated with smoking and alcohol. However, individuals who do not smoke but do drink have a lesser incidence of cancer of the mouth.[7]

Food itself may be considered a possible carcinogen, or it may be considered a precursor of a carcinogen. The food may take on carcinogenic properties by virtue of its own natural organic properties which stimulate the formation of harmful compounds, or the carcinogenicity may be due to effects of processing.

Polycyclic aromatic hydrocarbons are found in cigarette smoke, barbecued food, smoked fish, ham, cooking oils, and coffee. Epidemiologic evidence shows that populations who consume a large amount of smoked fish are at high risk of developing stomach cancer.[8] Yet smokers swallow some polycyclics, and there does not seem to be a strong link between smoking and cancer of the stomach. In the United States air pollution, smoking, and industrial exposure to polycyclics seem to pose more of a problem than does food in cancer development.

Nitrosamines are formed by the combining of nitrites, which are added to food as a preservative, with amines, found in the stomach as well as in some foods, or by bacterial reduction of nitrate to nitrite. Nitrosamines, which are known carcinogens in animals, can form in the soil, during food storage or preparation, and after ingestion into the body.

Nitrites and nitrates are found naturally in small amounts in food such as carrots, spinach, beets, and water. Nitrates are used as preservatives to prevent botulism and to fix color in such foods as bacon, sausage, frankfurters, ham, and various luncheon meats. Ascorbic acid seems to have an inhibitory effect on nitrosamine formation. Therefore, drinking orange juice before consuming any of the previously mentioned foods may produce a protective benefit.[9] Many consumer advocates are attempting to prevent the use, or to decrease the amount, of nitrates being added to foods. Though nitrosamines are known to be carcinogenic in rats, there has not yet been conclusive evidence that they are directly associated with cancer in humans.

Saccharin produced cancer in rats when large amounts were implanted in their bladders. Tumors were also produced when rats were fed diets high in saccharin. This evidence, which was released by the Canadian government, prompted the U.S. Food and Drug Administration (FDA) to enact a ban on saccharin. The proposed regulations of this ban include:

1   Treatment of saccharin as a nonprescription drug.
2   Labeling that must include the warning that "saccharin may cause an increased risk of cancer and should be used only as medically indicated," i.e., by persons such as diabetics who must restrict their intake of sugar.
3   Saccharin would no longer be permitted as an ingredient in food and beverages.

As of this writing, only proposal 2 has become a regulation. The FDA must send its suggestions to Congress for a final decision. It is expected that the issue may be delayed for several years.

Since the regulation of saccharin was proposed, a study was done investigating human consumption of saccharin and its relation to cancer of the lower urinary tract. This study reported little or no increased risk of cancer of the lower urinary tract.[10]

It has been recommended that human consumption not exceed 1 g per day for an adult,[11] and that individuals consuming saccharin on a regular basis (e.g., diabetics) eliminate it from their diet periodically for 2 or 3 days so that any buildup can be metabolized and eliminated.

Aflatoxins are natural carcinogens produced by strains of *Aspergillus flavus*. This mold can be found growing on peanuts and other grains when storage humidity is high. Aflatoxins can produce liver cancer in rats. In parts of the world where environmental conditions are conducive to aspergillus growth there is an increased incidence of liver cancer. Aflatoxins are not a problem in the United States because storage conditions are controlled. Imported products are more likely to be a source of *Aspergillus flavus*. These products are monitored by the U.S. Department of Agriculture and the FDA.

DES (diethylstilbestrol) is a hormone used in animals to increase their weight, thereby improving the net meat yield. In the 1940s DES pellets were implanted in poultry to produce tender chickens. However, evidence showed that DES was carcinogenic in the mouse when given in large quantities. Since small amounts of DES could be detected in the chicken fat of implanted birds, the FDA banned its use. The FDA permitted the addition of DES to cattle feed, with the stipulation that it be removed from the feed 48 h prior to the slaughter of the animal; now this is no longer allowed.

Antioxidants such as vitamin E, selenium, BHA, and BHT have been reported to decrease incidence of chemically induced tumors.[12] The mechanism for this is unclear. One explanation is that they combine with carcinogenic free radicals, thereby rendering them ineffective.

Vegetables of the *Cruciferae* family (cabbage, brussels sprouts, broccoli) contain certain indoles which are connected with an increase in activity of aryl-hydro-C-hyroxylase (AHH). This enzyme has demonstrated a protective effect against the development of chemically induced tumors of the breast and forestomach in animals.[13]

More investigation needs to be conducted before we have definite answers about dietary factors, but in the meantime adoption of a prudent diet, calorically at a level to maintain or produce ideal body weight, low in fat, high in fiber, and with representatives from the basic food groups, is recommended.

The etiology of cancer has yet to be empirically defined. There are a number of theories about the cause of cancer; they include heredity, familial susceptibility, genetics, viruses, and environment.

PATHOPHYSIOLOGY

Before we can discuss the treatment of individuals with cancer, it is necessary to understand some of the major pathophysiological concepts associated with cancer development. Throughout the body specific cells grow and proliferate, depending upon the various tissues and organs they form. Cells of the skin and blood are constantly being reproduced to replace those that are lost or destroyed. Nerve cells, on the other hand, are not able to multiply once they have been formed. Those cells that do regenerate are under a strict control mechanism. That is, the cells only multiply enough to replace the lost or destroyed cells, thereby maintaining a cell equilibrium.

A neoplasm (new growth) or tumor is a distribution of growth characterized primarily by an excessive proliferation of cells without apparent relation to the physiological demands of the organ involved. *Neoplasm* is commonly used interchangeably with *cancer* or *malignant tumor*.

Tumors can be classified into two broad categories: benign and malignant. Benign tumors are nonspreading, localized tumors which usually do not produce serious illness. Benign tumors are caused by an increase in cell number, but the cells do not invade other tissue.[14] An example of a benign tumor is a small skin mole or a uterine fibroid. When cells multiply rapidly and invade other tissue *(metastasize)*, they are termed malignant tumors or cancers.

The spread of cancer can occur by several different means:

1   *Invasion*—growth of the tumor into the surrounding tissue
2   *Permeation*—spreading of cancerous cells via blood and lymph vessels followed by growth
3   *Metastasis*—growth of a tumor which is separate from the primary site

Table 29-2 describes the differences in behavior and appearance of benign and malignant tumors.

Malignant tumors can be classified into three general categories:

1   *Carcinomas* originate in the epithelial surfaces (skin, gastrointestinal tract, and respiratory tract).
2   *Sarcomas* develop in the supporting tissues (bone cells, blood vessels, and muscle).
3   *Hematopoietic neoplasms* originate in the blood and immune system (leukemia and Hodgkin's disease).

This classification can be further defined by the organ site and type of epithelial cell involved. For example, adenocarcinoma is a malignant tumor of the glandular epithelium.

TABLE 29-2 CHARACTERISTICS OF BENIGN AND MALIGNANT TUMORS

Behavior or appearance	Benign	Malignant
Structure and differentiation	Typical of tissue of original	Atypical
Rate of growth	Usually slow	May be rapid or very rapid
Progression	Slowly progressive (may remain stationary or regress)	Usually progressive and usually fatal if untreated
Mode of growth	Expansion	Invasive as well as permeative
Metastases	None	Frequently present
Recurrence after simple removal	Rare	Common
Vascularity	Slight	Moderate or marked
Necrosis and ulceration	Unusual	Common
Physiologic effects	Uncommon (except endocrine)	Common

Source: Adapted from S. Krey, K. Ma, and R. Palombo, *Nutrition and Cancer*, Tufts–New England Medical Center, Frances Stern Nutrition Center, Boston, Mass., 1978, p. 23.

CLINICAL SIGNS AND DIAGNOSIS

The American Cancer Society cites seven danger signals that may indicate a malignant cancer. They are:

1 Any sore that does not heal
2 A lump or thickening in the breast or elsewhere
3 Persistent indigestion or difficulty swallowing
4 Any change in a wart or mole
5 Unexplained bleeding or discharge
6 Persistent cough or hoarseness
7 Any change in bowel habits[15]

The danger signals do not necessarily indicate cancer, but they should be evaluated by a physician. If by history or physical exam the physician notes weight loss, pain, lumps, or any abnormalities in the gastrointestinal, genitourinary (GU), respiratory, or neurologic systems, a diagnostic workup is usually begun. The diagnostic workup includes a biopsy and/or exfoliative cytology (scraping to obtain cells, e.g., a Pap smear) or serological studies (antigen-antibody reactions) to help confirm the diagnosis. Biochemical studies, urinalysis, and x-rays may also add supportive information.

GENERAL SIDE EFFECTS OF CANCER AND CANCER THERAPY

Weight loss and a lack of appetite may be the first symptoms associated with cancer. The anorexia of cancer is defined as follows:

Food intake is inadequate to meet the combined needs of the host and tumor even if food intake remained constant this could result in a loss of carcass weight in a tumor bearing host.[16]

The *cachexia* (loss of carcass weight) associated with malignancy is due to the effects of anorexia, a decrease in calories (joules) consumed, and an increase in energy expenditure. Patients are frequently in an energy-deficient state and have increased basal metabolic rates. These manifestations resemble malnutrition. Generally patients are in a state of negative nitrogen balance; however, some individuals have been seen who are energy-deficient but in positive nitrogen balance. This positive nitrogen balance may be attributed to the capacity of the tumor to retain nitrogen from both dietary nitrogen and nitrogen released from tissue.

Examples of physiological changes that may be common to ... cancer patients include atrophic changes of the gastrointestinal tract and amino acid imbalances. Other metabolic and physiological changes occur seemingly as a more specific remote effect of a neoplasm and may depress appetite. Metabolic changes, such as the exothermic effect of tumor metabolism and increased glucose uptake by the liver, may mediate anorectic effects via normal sensing mechanisms. Other effects of a neoplasm, such as the development of taste abnormalities ... , may have no counterpart in normal regulation of feeding behavior. The challenge is to identify the metabolic and physiological alterations that are contributing to anorexia in each patient. If these can be adequately delineated, proper metabolic and nutritional corrections may be prescribed.[17]

Patients may develop side effects (nausea, vomiting, diarrhea) from the various modalities of treatment. Many individuals have a change in taste perception. An elevation in sweetness threshold is one of the most common abnormalities. This can be utilized to the individuals' benefit by adding extra sugar to food, thereby increasing the calories (joules). An aversion to meat is another likely complaint of cancer patients. Individuals with more advanced tumors are more likely to have changes in taste.[18] Taste acuity and meat preference will return to normal when the tumor responds to therapy.

In the following section several types of treatment are discussed—radiation, surgery, chemotherapy, immunotherapy, and bone marrow transplants—and the nutritional problems and methods of nutritional treatment associated with each type.

CANCER THERAPY

Radiation

Patients may receive radiation as a form of treatment by itself or in conjunction with chemotherapy and surgery. Radiation acts to selectively destroy abnormal cells within the body. Radiotherapy involves the use of ionizing radiation. The unit of measure for radiation exposure is roentgens (R). The amount of radiation that tissues absorb is measured by rads. The therapeutic dose of radiation for a tumor is determined by its size and type, the response to irradiation, and several other factors. The dose also takes into account the normal tissue tolerance. Tumors are classified as radiosensitive or radioresistant. Radioresistant tumors are those whose lethal dose is also toxic to normal tissue. Radiation is used as both curative and palliative therapy. Palliative treatment involves the use of smaller doses to relieve painful symptoms by shrinking the tumor mass and prolonging comfortable survival. Generally, patients are irradiated 5 days per week for approximately 4 to 6 weeks. Depending upon the site of radiation, a variety of nutritional problems may arise.

Patients receiving radiation therapy to the head and neck area, particularly radiation to the tonsillar region, palate, tongue, and nasopharynx, present numerous nutritional problems. Patients undergoing radiation to these areas frequently complain of mucositis, stomatitis, altered or unpleasant sense of taste, a loss or reduction of taste acuity, pain upon swallowing, burning sensations, dryness of the mouth, and a general lack of appetite. Taste may be altered by damage from radiation to the taste buds. Patients whose radiation field includes the salivary glands will notice a decrease in salivation and a change in the saliva composition. Saliva that is present becomes thick and viscous, making it difficult for the patient to swallow. Alcoholics, heavy smokers, patients with poor oral hygiene, and patients with chronic poor nutrition are at risk of developing mandible necrosis.

Diet therapy for the patient receiving radiation to the head and neck includes modifying the texture of the food to prevent pain on swallowing. Acid foods such as orange juice may need to be diluted or eliminated from the diet. Spices may be an irritant to the oral mucosa, as may very hot or very cold foods. For the patient with reduced salivation, moist foods, foods mixed with sauces or broths, soups, custards, and puddings may aid in swallowing and thus help to keep energy intake adequate (see Table 29-3). Some patients suffer from a decreased taste acuity. This hypogeusia can sometimes be counteracted through the use of zinc sulfate.[19]

Individuals with reduced salivation are more susceptible to dental caries; artificial saliva is available and helps to buffer acidity (see Chap. 17). In the past, these individuals would have their teeth extracted to prevent osteoradionecrosis. Today all efforts are made to preserve the patient's teeth. The nutrition educator must work with individuals to decrease sucrose and retentive sweets from the diet while maintaining adequate energy. Patients are also given, as a prophylactic measure, a 1 percent sodium fluoride gel contained in a dental tray (mouth guard) inserted into the mouth for 5 min per day.

If the individual is experiencing severe

TABLE 29-3 DIETARY SUGGESTIONS FOR PATIENTS RECEIVING RADIATION THERAPY TO THE HEAD AND NECK AREA

1 Swallowing can be made easier when liquids are taken by straw.

2 Tilting the head back when eating may make swallowing easier.

3 Avoid foods that may irritate the oral mucosa or throat, such as highly seasoned, acidic foods (citrus fruits and juices) and very hot or cold foods.

4 Use noncariogenic foods such as sugarless gum and sugarless mints to stimulate saliva production.

swallowing problems, a liquid dietary supplement or blenderized diet (see Chap. 28) may be needed, along with vitamin and mineral supplementation. High-protein milk (whole milk with added dry powdered skim milk) should be encouraged for use in eggnogs, frappes, soups, puddings, and custards. The commercially prepared supplement often proves to have an advantage over home-prepared foods, as the patient associates it with medicine and gives better compliance, resulting in a higher energy intake. Small, frequent feedings are advised for the individual who has a lack of appetite or is experiencing pain. Xylocaine, a local anesthetic, may be useful for the patient who is unable to swallow because of pain. If an individual is unable or unwilling to take anything by mouth, artificial tube feeding may be necessary (see Chap. 28). When the tumor is located at a site that would interfere with the use of a nasogastric tube, a gastrostomy may be appropriate.

Keeping the patient in positive nitrogen balance and a positive nutritional state is most important since the rate of wound healing and tissue tolerance for radiotherapy are related to the nutritional status of the patient.[20] Steiger et al. reported that in experiments with rats, well-nourished rats seemed to support tumor growth while malnourished rats did not.[21]

However, Steiger also reported that in patients, a positive nitrogen balance did not favorably alter their clinical course and that tumor growth may be exacerbated by hyperalimentation. Hyperalimentation has recently gained use in treatment of the patient who is undergoing head and neck radiation. It has been used with patients who were 10 lb below their ideal or usual body weight and whose serum albumin was less than 3.6 g per 100 mL.[22] When defined formula diets produced diarrhea or abdominal cramps, patients were given intravenous hyperalimentation of 2500 to 3000 kcal per day (10.5 to 12.6 MJ per day) until they were able to consume enough food enterally to maintain adequate nutrition. This information on the positive effects of hyperalimentation must be weighed against the possible negative effects mentioned above. Evidence shows that individuals who are well nourished will tolerate radiation therapy better and will react more favorably to chemotherapeutic agents.

Nutritional treatment is always individualized. For example, a low-roughage or a low-residue diet may be efficacious for some patients, while eliminating lactose, or a combination of these procedures, may prove beneficial for others. Adequate fluid intake is important to prevent dehydration. Electrolytes must be monitored. If diarrhea persists, the implementation of a defined formula diet (see Chap. 28) is the treatment of choice. Other side effects include nausea, vomiting, abdominal pain, and edema.

A regimen consisting of a low-residue, low-fat, gluten-free, and low-lactose diet was shown to be effective in the treatment of children who developed radiation enteritis with small bowel obstruction.[23] This regimen might also prove effective for adults. Antacids may be helpful if gastric irritation is present.

Surgery

The success of surgery for the cancer patient will depend upon the type, size, and location of the tumor as well as the individual's physical and nutritional status. There are a number of rationales for particular surgical procedures: resecting cancers, correcting obstruction, evaluating effectiveness of treatment, and debulking the cancer tumor.[24] Curative surgery is possible when the tumor is localized and can be resected entirely. Surgery can also be palliative, as in the case of an oophorectomy for some women with metastatic breast cancer.[25] Tumor regression has been aided by this type of surgery. Surgery may also be employed when there is obstruction produced by the tumor.

Individuals who receive vigorous nutritional intervention and are nutritionally repleted have a decreased surgical mortality rate, decreased postoperative infection, and improved wound healing.[26] See Table 29-4 for the nutritional complications of cancer surgery. The nutritional guidelines for cancer-surgery patients are gen-

TABLE 29-4   NUTRITIONAL COMPLICATIONS OF CANCER SURGERY

Type	Complications
Resection of oropharyngeal area	Chewing, taste, and swallowing difficulties
Esophageal resection	Vagotomy effects (gastric hypochlorohydria, gastric stasis, diarrhea, steatorrhea, fistula, malabsorption)
Gastric resection	Dumping syndrome Intrinsic factor deficiency Malabsorption (acute and chronic) Afferent loop syndrome Hypoglycemia Steatorrhea Fistula
Intestinal resection of jejunum	Decreased absorption of many nutrients
Intestinal resection of ileum	Vitamin B_{12} deficiency Conjugated bile salt loss Hyperoxaluria Fistula
Massive bowel resection	Severe malabsorption Metabolic acidosis Gastric hypersection
Ileostomy	Problems with salt and water balance Blind loop syndrome
Pancreatectomy	Maldigestion Malabsorption Diabetes mellitus Fistula
Nephrectomy, cystectomy, urethral diversion	Renal dysfunction

Source: Adapted from S. Krey, K. M. Ma, and R. Palombo, *Nutrition and Cancer*, Tufts–New England Medical Center, Frances Stern Nutrition Center, Boston, Mass., 1978, p. 422.

erally the same as those for any surgical patient (see Chap. 28).

If the individual cannot be brought to a state of positive nitrogen balance by ordinary alimentary means, other alternatives should be instituted. Nasogastric tube feedings may be useful if the patient is not in a state of catabolic stress. Then an energy intake of 30 to 35 kcal per kilogram per day with a nitrogen to calorie ratio of

1 to 300 is sufficient.[27] If the patient is in a state of severe catabolic stress, 45 to 50 kcal per kilogram per day with a nitrogen ratio of 1 to 150 is needed to achieve positive nitrogen balance.[28] Preoperative enteral alimentation should begin 14 to 21 days prior to surgery to bring the individual into a state of positive nitrogen balance and to help rebuild depleted nutrient stores. Some patients who cannot tolerate enteral feedings may benefit from preoperative hyperalimentation.[29]

The surgical procedures used for the patient with cancer of the GI tract are similar to other surgical GI procedures. The major complications of GI surgery with nutritional implication include dumping syndrome, malabsorption, and anorexia. Nutritional therapy should include small frequent feedings, restricted carbohydrates, increased protein, and liquids taken after meals. Energy intake must be sufficient to maintain the patient in a state of positive nitrogen balance. Fat may need to be restricted if malabsorption is a problem.

Chemotherapy

Chemotherapy may be the sole treatment modality or an adjunct of surgery or radiation. Chemotherapy involves the use of drugs to destroy dividing cancer cells in many phases of their cell cycle. The cell cycle has been divided into four phases: G_1, S, G_2, and M. G_1 phase is called the first growth period, S phase is the period of DNA synthesis, G_2 phase is the second growth period, and M phase is the cell division phase, or mitosis.[30] Chemotherapy interferes with some aspect of DNA or RNA synthesis, thereby causing the death of cancer cells. Cancer drugs are used in combination to affect cells during multiple phases of the cycle. Combinations of drugs are more effective than single agents in preventing the emergence of resistant tumor cells. The goal is to "achieve maximal therapeutic effect without precipitating severe toxicity."[31]

Drugs used in cancer treatment (antineoplastic agents) are cytotoxic not only to the neoplastic cells but to the normal cells as well and must be administered with great caution. Antineoplastic agents can be classified in six categories, depending upon their mode of action: alkylating agents, antimetabolites, antibiotics, alkaloids, hormones, and miscellaneous (see Table 29-5, pp. 700–701).

One of the most adverse effects of cancer chemotherapy is leukopenia (reduction in the number of leukocytes in the blood). Leukopenia increases the patient's susceptibility to infection.

Patients receiving chemotherapy are susceptible to many side effects which may alter their ability to eat. Some of the more common side effects include nausea, vomiting, mucositis (inflammation of the mucosa), ulcerations of the mouth, anorexia, and diarrhea (see Table 29-5).

Granulocytopenic patients receiving antibiotics as part of their chemotherapy may be instructed to avoid salads. Due to their changed gut flora, these patients might not be able to effectively combat pathogenic microorganisms found in salads.[32]

The astute nurse and dietitian will be familiar with these symptoms and will adjust the patient's diet accordingly. In general, soft, low-roughage, or elemental diets, as determined by individual need, may be used for the patient who is experiencing side effects from a chemotherapeutic agent. When mucositis and stomatitis are present, acid foods should be avoided. Small frequent feedings may be helpful in treating the patient who is experiencing nausea or anorexia. When fever, diarrhea, and vomiting are present, an increased fluid intake must be encouraged. Patients receiving the drug Cytoxan should have a fluid intake of 2 to 3 L per day to prevent hemorrhagic cystitis.[33] Patients respond best to chemotherapy when they are in a positive nutritional state.

Immunotherapy

Immunotherapy is a form of cancer treatment that attempts to alter the tumor to increase its antigenicity, increase the host's immune response, or both. The host may be injected with irradiated tumor cells or nonspecific immune

TABLE 29-5 SIDE EFFECTS OF COMMONLY USED ANTINEOPLASTIC AGENTS

Drug	Side effects
Antibiotics	
Dactinomycin (actinomycin D) (Cosmegen)	Stomatitis, anorexia, nausea, vomiting, diarrhea, oral ulceration
Bleomycin (Blenoxane)	Stomatitis, anorexia, nausea, vomiting, fever, oral ulceration
Daunorubicin	Nausea and vomiting, fever, stomatitis, cardiomyopathy
Adriamycin	Nausea and vomiting, anorexia, cardiac toxicity
Alkylating agents	
Cyclophosphamide (Cytoxan)	Anorexia, vomiting, nausea, hemorrhagic cystitis, hemorrhagic colitis, mucosal ulceration
Nitrogen mustard (Mustargen)	Anorexia, vomiting, nausea, diarrhea, metallic taste
Chlorambucil	Nausea and vomiting, hepatotoxicity
Antimetabolites	
Cytarabine (Cytosar)	Anorexia, nausea, vomiting, diarrhea, megaloblastic anemia; antagonist to pyrimidine
5-Fluorouracil	Stomatitis, anorexia, nausea, vomiting, diarrhea, gastrointestinal ulceration, and bleeding
6-Mercaptopurine	Stomatitis, nausea, vomiting, diarrhea, fever; antagonist to purine and pantothenic acid
Methotrexate	Stomatitis, anorexia, nausea, vomiting, diarrhea, gastrointestinal ulcerations, abnormal liver function
Ara-C	Nausea and vomiting, diarrhea, anorexia, stomatitis
Plant alkaloids	
Vinblastine (Velban)	Nausea, vomiting, constipation, diarrhea, abdominal pain, anorexia
Vincristine (Oncovin)	Constipation, diarrhea, paralytic ileus (particularly in young children), abdominal cramps, polyuria, oral ulceration
Hormones	
Estrogens Diethylstilbesterol	Reduced carbohydrate tolerance, nausea and vomiting, abdominal cramps, fluid retention, hypercalcemia
Ethinyl estradiol (Estrace)	Nausea and vomiting, abdominal cramps, bloating, edema, reduced carbohydrate tolerance, hypercalcemia
Progestin Hydroxyprogesterone caproate (Delalutin)	Minimal fluid retention, hypercalcemia
Medroxyprogesterone acetate (Provera)	Edema, change in weight increase or decrease

TABLE 29-5 CONTINUED

Drug	Side effects
Adrenocorticosteroids	
Prednisone (Deltasone)	Sodium retention, fluid retention, gastrointestinal bleeding, increased appetite
Dexamethasone (Decadron)	Sodium retention, fluid retention, potassium loss, peptic ulcer, decreased carbohydrate tolerance, negative nitrogen balance due to protein catabolism
Cortisone (Cortone acetate)	Salt and water retention, potassium loss, increased calcium excretion
Hydrocorticone (Celestone)	Same as cortisone
Miscellaneous	
5-Azacytidine	Nausea and vomiting, fever, diarrhea, stomatitis
BCNU	Nausea and vomiting, stomatitis
CCNU	Nausea and vomiting, hepatatoxicity
Cis platinum	Nausea and vomiting, anorexia, renal toxicity
Procarbazine	Nausea and vomiting, diarrhea, anorexia; amine oxidase inhibitory activity; avoid tyramine-containing foods
Quinacrine (Atabrine)	Nausea and vomiting, fever
L-Asparaginase	Nausea and vomiting, diabetes, abnormal protein/liver metabolism

Source: Data from *Physician's Desk Reference,* 35th ed., Medical Economics Company, Oradell, N.J., 1981. Children's Hospital Medical Center, Nutrition Service, Boston, Mass., 1979.

stimulants (BCG, bacterial antigens). Immunotherapy complements treatment modalities such as surgery, radiotherapy, and chemotherapy.

Immune response of the host and the tumor is a current area of investigation. Clinical trials show that augmentation of the general immune system can cause tumor destruction, and that the immune response, even under optimal experimental conditions, is not capable of dealing with large amounts of tumor.[34]

Immunotherapy is known to cause anorexia, changes in taste sensations, diarrhea, nausea, heart failure, vomiting, constipation, malabsorption, and mucosal ulcerations.[35]

Bone Marrow Transplantation

Bone marrow transplantation for individuals with acute leukemia is offered during the second or subsequent remission. A remission describes the temporary arrest of the leukemic process. The improved survival rate of children with transplants indicates that despite the risks and complications of the process, the outcome may be long-term remission.[36]

CONCLUSION

Anxiety and fear are common emotions for the individual with cancer. Side effects from the various treatments, weight and hair loss causing a poor body image, along with loss in body function and purpose in life—all can have a negative effect on an appetite already compromised by the anorexia of cancer or the therapy.

For those individuals whose prognosis is poor, an open discussion of death and dying is helpful for some. Others use denial to cope with their diagnosis. Health professionals need to be sensitive to the feelings of each individual and should provide emotional support accordingly.

Although nutrition is paramount in the care of the cancer patient, the psychological factors just mentioned often interfere with this care. The ultimate success of nutritional care depends on the clinician's ability to adjust the diet to the individual's psychological and physiological needs. It is difficult to convince a patient to eat when the prognosis may be death or to convince a parent of a child with cancer not to force-feed. The next section considers the child with cancer.

CHILDREN AND CANCER

Janet L. Sydness

Childhood cancer is a relatively rare type of disease; yet it is second only to accidents as a cause of death.[37] The incidence is 111 annually per 1 million children from birth to 14 years old in the United States.[38] The six most common sites of cancer in children are:[39]

1   Leukemia
2   Central nervous system
3   Lymphoma
4   Sympathetic nervous system
5   Soft tissue
6   Kidney

The leukemias are primary malignant diseases of the bone marrow, a blood-forming organ. They are characterized by a predominance of immature white blood cells. These abnormal white blood cells (blasts) proliferate, accumulate, and interfere with the production of normal cells. The leukemias are classified morphologically by reference to the predominant cell line involved. The two broad childhood classifications include acute lymphoblastic and acute myelogenous leukemia. Additional methods of classification include tests for immunologic cell surface markers, biochemical evaluation of the leukemia cells, and exploration of chromosomal patterns. Results of these tests form the basis of subclassification of leukemia. These classifica-

tions facilitate prediction of drug effectiveness and serve to integrate new epidemiologic and genetic information.[40]

The leukemias comprise 30 percent of childhood cancer.[41] Acute lymphoblastic leukemia (ALL) is the leukemia most common in childhood.[42] It peaks in incidence in children from 1 to 5 years of age. The outlook for children with ALL has greatly improved.[43,44] Approximately 50 percent of these children appear to be cured of their leukemia.

Central nervous system tumors rank second only to leukemia as the leading group of neoplasms in children. The most common cell types of brain tumors in children are astrocytoma, medulloblastoma, and glioma.[45] The peak age incidence in children is 5 to 9 years.[46] Increased survival has been seen in recent years with surgery and radiotherapy.[47] The role of chemotherapy in primary brain tumors is currently under investigation.

Lymphomas are the third most prevalent childhood cancer, comprising 13.6 percent of the total cancer sites; they exhibit an incidence of 15.1 per 1 million children.[48] They are divided into Hodgkin's and non-Hodgkin's lymphomas. They are primary tumors of the lymphoid tissue and most often arise in lymph nodes, spleen, tonsils, or the gastrointestinal tract. Most children with Hodgkin's lymphoma have disease limited to lymph node involvement, whereas those with non-Hodgkin's lymphoma have widespread disease.[49] Attendant with improved survival in these cases has been the recognition of late complications of treatment. These include second tumors in patients with Hodgkin's disease and problems with growth in children who receive extensive radiotherapy.[50,51]

Neuroblastoma is a solid tumor of the sympathetic nervous system occurring at a rate of 8.6 per 1 million children.[52] The age of the child at diagnosis and the stage of the neuroblastoma when discovered are critical factors in survival rate. Children contracting neuroblastoma who are less than 1 year of age have nearly an 80 percent survival rate.[53] Therapy is dictated by the stage of the disease and the age of the child and includes surgery, radiotherapy, and chemotherapy.

Attention to a classification system which describes the stage of neuroblastoma is useful in (1) assessing the cancer at various points in time, (2) directing therapeutic decisions, and (3) comparing results at various treatment centers.[54]

Soft tissue tumors (sarcomas) occur in children at a rate of 7.1 per 1 million.[55] Rhabdomyosarcoma, with many histologic variants, is the most common type of this subgroup.[56] Children under 5 years of age tend to have the embryonal type. This particular type has a favorable prognosis. Survival is estimated at 70 percent in the majority of cases where overt metastases are not present at diagnosis.[57] This tumor occurs in skeletal muscle and can be found anywhere in the body. Chemotherapy and radiotherapy are effective in achieving primary control and often eliminate the need for mutilating surgical procedures.[58]

Wilm's tumor, the most common kidney tumor in children, has an incidence of 6.8 per 1 million.[59,60] Fifteen percent of children with Wilm's tumor have congenital anomalies, the most common being aniridia, the absence of the iris, and genitourinary malformations. Multimodal therapy, including surgery, radiotherapy, and chemotherapy, has increased survival rates for all children in excess of 70 percent.[61-63] Wilm's tumor is rarely hereditary.[64,65]

NUTRITION SUPPORT IN CHILDREN WITH CANCER

Many patients have reported taste changes as a result of cancer or because of cancer treatment.[66] Experimenters on this subject have divided taste perceptions into four categories: bitter, sweet, sour, and salty.[67] Patients in Rochester General experienced an elevated taste threshold for sweet and a lowered threshold for bitter.[68] This phenomenon is consistent with our experience among pediatric oncology patients who have described a loss of taste for sweet food and an intolerance for the taste of meat. Taste changes may result in decreased food intake.

Because of illness caused by radiation and/ or chemotherapy, children may experience taste aversion when food is eaten prior to when, or at the same time as, a treatment is given. Bernstein has found that children developed a powerful, learned taste aversion to an unusually flavored, maple ice cream when it was offered before or during drug treatments which had caused past gastrointestinal illness.[69] One month after the experiment began, the treated children selected the unusually maple-flavored ice cream less often than the controls.

Neilsen's study indicated that food odors were partially responsible for food aversions.[70] Avoiding unacceptable odors may minimize this problem. Individualizing dietary management to accommodate changing taste sensations may reduce the risk of weight loss and increase food acceptance. (See Fig. 29-1.)

Figure 29-1
A sensitive nutritionist providing care and looking for the food that pleases this young cancer patient.

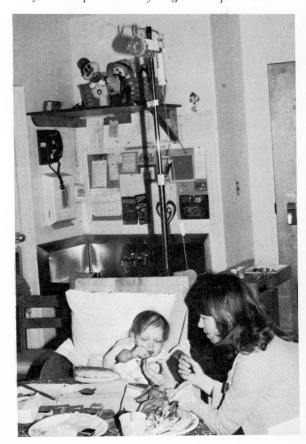

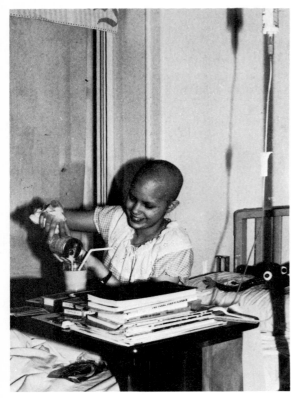

Figure 29-2
Formulas are chosen to match the child's nutritional and taste needs. Teenage cancer patient smiles as she pours.

Children not able to take enough food orally to meet nutritional requirements for growth and development require nutritional supplements. Formulas are chosen to match the child's nutritional needs. The formula choice, presentation, and route of administration should be individualized. (See Fig. 29-2.) The products most frequently tolerated are low in lactose and nearly isotonic. Children receiving cancer therapy, and eating small amounts, often require an additional protein source, vitamins, and minerals. Normally the aim is to meet the RDA for the child's age, and these are adjusted for stress. Due to stress, protein and energy requirements are increased. These increased needs reflect urinary nitrogen loss and hypermetabolism. The amount of urinary nitrogen loss and increased BMR will reflect the extent of the stress. BMR can increase by as much as 100 percent. These increased needs will remain high during recovery to replete nutrient stores. Table 29-6 (pp. 705–707) suggests diet manipulations to promote adequate nutrition. Occasionally supplements may be served as a medication to encourage compliance. Tube feedings are the alternative if the child cannot eat enough or refuses to eat and has a normally functioning GI tract.

Advances in treatment have increased survival rates in pediatric cancer patients. Total parenteral nutrition (TPN) is used as an adjunct to rigorous treatment in children experiencing prolonged anorexia, malabsorption, severe vomiting, and/or malnutrition.[71,72] When a child is nutritionally depleted, the administration of TPN solutions provides nutritional support, increases tolerance of cancer treatment, improves nutritional status prior to surgery, promotes weight gain, and instills a general sense of well-being.[73,74]

The appropriate utilization of TPN solutions in pediatric cancer patients has, however, created additional difficulties. The major difficulty (which prolongs hospitalization) involves reinstituting an adequate oral intake. A progression diet (Table 29-7, p. 708) helps increase oral intake gradually. Oral intake may be enhanced during the day if the TPN solutions are cycled. This allows the child to have a more normal routine during the day while the IV line is heparin-locked. During the night the solution rate is increased to provide needed nutrients.

TPN solutions provided at home reduce the cost of intravenous nutritional support by more than half.[75] Parents and/or guardians willing and able to take on this additional monitoring responsibility receive special instructions for TPN care. The availability of community support systems (e.g., the Visiting Nurse Association, V.N.A.), local medical services, or insurance coverage is an important factor in a parent's decision to provide TPN at home.

TABLE 29-6 DIETARY GUIDELINES FOR MANAGEMENT OF SIDE EFFECTS OF CANCER THERAPY

Side effect	Guidelines	Additional suggestions
Decreased appetite	Encourage small, frequent meals and snacks—large amounts of food at one time may appear overpowering. Concentrate on nutritious foods that are high in calories and protein and vitamins, such as enriched milk (see opposite column), frappes, eggnog, cheese, eggs, custard, ice cream, pudding, peanut butter, yogurt, cream soups, fruits and vegetables, and juices. Encourage more light to moderate exercise, when possible, to increase appetite. Experiment with ways to increase the flavor of foods such as seasonings and fruit juices. Keep favorite foods visible. Make mealtime fun and colorful. Encourage child to help in actual food preparation (to arouse interest).	Recipe for enriched milk (high calorie, high protein): 1 quart whole milk ⅔–1 cup nonfat dry milk powder Blend well. Serve cold as beverage, use in frappes and eggnog, use for cream soups and in cooking.
Nausea and vomiting	Immediately: Provide dry crackers or toast to reduce nausea. Try ice, cold, carbonated beverages to settle stomach. Wipe face with cool water, loosen tight clothes, sit in cool, well-ventilated room. For prevention: Offer plain foods that are low in fats (avoid fried foods, gravy, margarine) and aroma (smell is often heightened). Provide liquids either 1 h before or 1 h after meals, rather than with meals (to decrease amount of food in stomach). Encourage individual to eat slowly, chew foods thoroughly, and relax. Since activity may slow digestion, the individual should rest or lie down after meals. Serve foods cold or warm; avoid hot foods. Offer frequent, small meals and snacks.	Observe the individual's intake for a couple of days and encourage the greatest intake when nausea occurs least often, for example, breakfast time.

(Continued)

TABLE 29-6 CONTINUED

Side effect	Guidelines	Additional suggestions
Taste changes	Bitter and sweet tolerance changes. Serve food cold or at room temperature. Use seasonings (see opposite column) to flavor foods. Flavor milk and milk products. Try offering bland cheese. If meat products are not tolerated, select meat substitutes.	Seasoning Allow ½ tsp dried herbs = ½ tsp crushed herbs = 1 tbsp chopped herbs. Allow ¼ tsp dried herbs for each 4 servings. Do not use too many kinds of seasonings in one recipe. Crush herbs in the palm of one hand with the fingertips of the other hand before adding to a dish. This permits faster flavor release. Add herbs to uncooked food (salad dressing, fruits, juices) as long before serving as possible. Add herbs to soups and sauces toward the end of preparation and leave just long enough to lose their volatile oils (about 1 h). Heat seasoned foods carefully as certain spices (cayenne, paprika, and curry blends) scorch easily and others (caraway) become bitter if overheated.
Constipation	Increase the amount of high fiber foods in the individual's diet—raw fruit and vegetables, nuts, popcorn, bran, whole grains, and bread. If a child refuses raw fruits, try adding them to gelatin. Encourage increased fluid intake, in the form of water and juices. Hot beverages, especially, may encourage bowel movements. Encourage more light to moderate exercise, when possible.	Foods that are high in fiber may also be an irritant to sensitive intestinal tracts. Introduce these foods slowly especially when advancing a diet from full liquid → to soft → to a regular diet with fiber included.
Low resistance to infection	Individuals with very low white counts may need a diet that avoids fresh fruits and vegetables (owing to their high bacteria count). Avoid food items that would be an excellent medium for hosting bacteria—i.e., foods containing milk solids. Use cooked and processed foods.	A Reduced Bacteria Diet* may be used for patients receiving bone marrow transplantation.

*Only cooked and processed foods and sterile water allowed. Avoid fresh fruits and vegetables. Disposable dishes and utensils should be used.

TABLE 29-6 CONTINUED

Side effect	Guidelines	Additional suggestions
Sore or dry mouth and throat	Rinse mouth frequently. Offer mints or hard candy (like lemon drops) to stimulate saliva production. Use straw or tilt head back to make swallowing more comfortable. Avoid foods that are extreme in temperature (either hot or cold). Avoid tart or acid foods, such as citrus fruits, and highly seasoned and spicy foods. Offer soft and liquid foods, such as custard, ice cream, tuna salad, and scrambled egg, or soften foods by dipping them in liquid. Moisten foods with margarine, gravy, cheese sauce, and cream.	The physician or dentist will have additional information regarding meticulous dental care.
Diarrhea	Begin by providing clear liquids (apple juice, gelatin, broth, Popsicles) for 12 h. Serve warm rather than hot foods (heat increases the natural movement of the GI tract). Limit fiber and gassy foods eaten (temporarily). These include dried cooked beans, cabbage, onions, raw fruits and vegetables, whole grains, nuts, popcorn, and carbonated beverages. Offer small, frequent meals and snacks, with beverages served between meals, rather than with them. Encourage rest after meals (to reduce peristalsis). Sometimes therapy may cause temporary "lactose intolerance"—diarrhea, bloating, and abdominal cramps due to inadequate digestion of milk or milk products. If your child's diarrhea seems to be associated with milk or milk products, temporarily avoid these.	A low-lactose diet may be required. Many cheeses, because of the way they are made, contain no lactose. The following may be tolerated: Swiss, provolone, edam, blue, brick, muenster, colby, cheddar, pasteurized processed American, pasteurized processed Swiss, camembert, and mozzarella. Additionally, yogurt is usually well tolerated by most people who are lactose-intolerant.
Weight loss	Encourage more between-meal snacks. Those which are low in fat provide fewer calories, but interfere less with the next meal (if this is a problem). Examples of good snacks include: *high-energy, high-protein*—milk, custard, pudding, beverages made with enriched milk, frappes, egg nog, cheese, eggs, peanut butter, yogurt, cream soups, small sandwiches. *low fat*—jelly, honey, hard candy, fruit juices, sherbert, popsicles, gelatin, fruit, raw vegetables (low-calorie).	A good source of calories: fats, bacon, gravies, creams, salad dressing; melt butter or margarine and add to soups, hot cereals, gravies, vegetables, and most entrees without much effect on the overall flavor. Foods high in fat may contribute to nausea.

Source: Courtesy Nutrition Service, Dietary Department, Children's Hospital Medical Center, Boston, Mass. Copyright 1980.

TABLL 29-7   PROGRESSION DIET*†

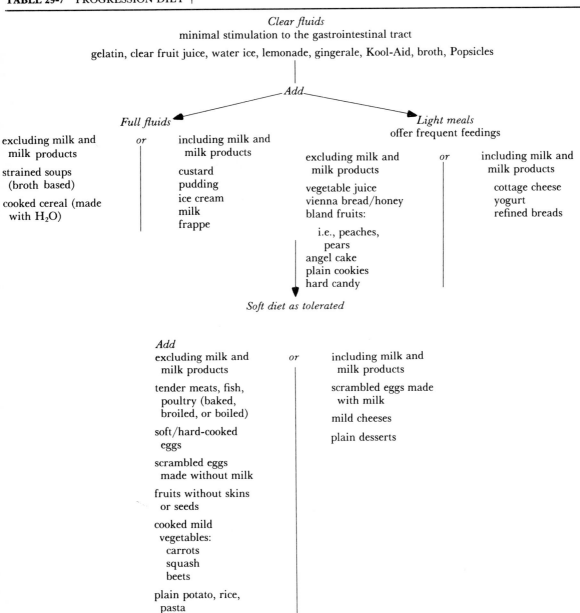

Clear fluids
minimal stimulation to the gastrointestinal tract
gelatin, clear fruit juice, water ice, lemonade, gingerale, Kool-Aid, broth, Popsicles

Add

Full fluids

excluding milk and milk products	*or*	including milk and milk products
strained soups (broth based)		custard
cooked cereal (made with H₂O)		pudding
		ice cream
		milk
		frappe

Light meals
offer frequent feedings

excluding milk and milk products	*or*	including milk and milk products
vegetable juice		cottage cheese
vienna bread/honey		yogurt
bland fruits:		refined breads
i.e., peaches, pears		
angel cake		
plain cookies		
hard candy		

Soft diet as tolerated

Add

excluding milk and milk products	*or*	including milk and milk products
tender meats, fish, poultry (baked, broiled, or boiled)		scrambled eggs made with milk
soft/hard-cooked eggs		mild cheeses
scrambled eggs made without milk		plain desserts
fruits without skins or seeds		
cooked mild vegetables: carrots squash beets		
plain potato, rice, pasta		

*This progession diet separates lactose-containing food items and lactose-free food items to facilitate appropriate instructions when individuals do not tolerate lactose. The lactose-free diet will require calcium supplementation.

†Vitamin supplementation required.

CONCLUSION

Normal eating patterns of children with cancer are disrupted during hospitalization. Children refuse to eat when they fear the additional pain of mouth sores, sore throats, and the difficulty of swallowing. The health care team should encourage the child to discuss those fears and offer him or her nonirritating fluids and foods.

Mealtime becomes a stressful time when anxious but nurturing parents force children to eat. The more the parent forces the food, the more the child refuses it. This becomes a power struggle. Children discover that their mouths are something they at least can control. This is especially true of preverbal children who are confused and angry at the hospitalization itself. To minimize conflict, the patient care plan should encourage a daily routine which offers the child choices in other areas—e.g., when to take a bath, or in which playroom activity to participate. The additional choices may reduce the child's need to try to control mealtime.

Nutritional activities which involve children in the hospital setting are an outstanding way to encourage eating—i.e., popcorn during the movies, bake-your-own dessert, prepare-your-own bag lunch, invite parents to an evening meal, food fair, birthday parties and special occasion parties, a garden picnic, make-your-own sub, etc.

Anxious parents may become overzealous in their encouragement of food items. They sometimes look to food or high doses of vitamins and minerals as "safe" solutions to the illness their child suffers during cancer treatment. They often search outside the medical community, looking for a "quick" cure. Nutrition intervention as an integral part of the management of the child's care can provide reasonable support, security, and stability in the relationships between parent, child, and the medical team.

STUDY QUESTIONS

1 Why is fiber associated with cancer of the colon?
2 Distinguish benign from malignant tumors.
3 What nutritional problems can you anticipate when a patient receives radiation to the head and neck? G.I. and G.U.?
4 What side effects are associated with chemotherapy? Radiation therapy?
5 Discuss the nutrition support in children with cancer.
6 Why do some cancer patients experience a taste change?

CLINICAL STUDY 29

M.G., a 30-month-old girl, was brought to the hospital by her parents, who were concerned about a persistent fever, loss of appetite, and bruising. The physical examination revealed a weight of 13 kg, a length of 91 cm, and weight for age, height for age, and height for weight all at the 50th percentile. Laboratory data included hematocrit of 38 percent, sodium 138 dL, potassium 4.3 dL, and calcium 9.8 dL. Her white blood count was 20,000 and blasts, 42 percent. Her bone marrow result was positive. A diagnosis of acute lymphoblastic leukemia was made. Chemotherapy was begun using the drugs prednisone, adriamycin, and vincristine.

Clinical study questions

1 *Judging from the medications that M.G. is receiving, what side effects would you anticipate and what dietary manipulations would you suggest?*
2 *What recommendation could you make which would encourage M.G. to increase her food intake?*
3 *Presently M.G. has been growing at the 50th percentile and has not been losing weight; additional energy and protein requirements for stress are not indicated. According to the RDA for protein and energy, what should M.G.'s intake be?*

REFERENCES

1   American Cancer Society, *Cancer Statistics,* Professional Education Publications, 1976, p. 4.
2   G. B. Gori, op. cit., pp. 2151–2161.
3   American Cancer Society, *Nutrition and Cancer,* Professional Education Publications, 1972, p. 5.
4   G. B. Gori, "Dietary and Nutritional Implications in the Multifactorial Etiology of Certain Prevalent Human Cancers," *Cancer,* **43**:2151–2161, 1979.
5   Ibid.
6   Ibid.
7   Ibid.
8   John Berg, "Nutrition and Cancer," *Seminars in Oncology,* **3**:17–23, 1976.
9   Ibid., p. 18.
10 A. S. Morrison and J. E. Buring, "Artificial Sweeteners and Cancer of the Lower Urinary Tract," *New England Journal of Medicine,* **302**:537–541, 1980.
11 National Academy of Sciences, *Sweeteners, Issues and Uncertainties,* Washington, 1975, p. 138.
12 G. B. Gori, op. cit., pp. 2151–2161.
13 Ibid.
14 John Cairns, *Cancer, Science and Society,* W. H. Freeman Company, San Francisco, 1978, p. 16.
15 D. A. Jones, C. F. Dunbar, and M. M. Jirovec, *Medical Surgical Nursing: A Conceptual Approach,* McGraw-Hill Book Company, New York, 1978, p. 133.
16 Council for the Analysis and Projection of the American Cancer Society, "Working Conference on Anorexia and Neoplastic Disease," *Cancer and Research,* November 1970, p. 2816.
17 W. D. DeWys, "Anorexia in Cancer Patients," *Cancer Research,* **37**:2357, 1977.
18 W. D. DeWys, "Oral Feeding in the Nutrition Management of Cancer Patients, *Cancer Research,* **37**:2429–2431, July 1977.
19 S. Dreizen et al., "Oral Complications of Cancer Radiotherapy," *Postgraduate Medicine,* **61**:85, 1977.
20 E. Copeland et al., "Intravenous Hyperalimentation in Patients with Head and Neck Cancer," *Cancer,* March 1975, p. 610.
21 E. Teiger et al., "Effects of Nutrition on Tumor Growth and Tolerance to Chemotherapy," *Journal of Surgical Research,* **18**:455–461, 1975.
22 E. Copeland and S. Dudrick, "Cancer: Nutritional Concepts," *Seminars in Oncology,* **2**:329, 1975.
23 S. S. Donaldson et al., "Radiation Enteritis in Children—A Retrospective Review of Correlational and Dietary Management," *Cancer,* **35**:1167–1178, 1975.
24 W. Bradford Patterson, "Principles of Surgical Oncology," *Clinical Oncology—A Multidisciplinary Approach,* American Cancer Society, 1978, pp. 21–28.
25 D. A. Jones, C. F. Dunbar, and M. M. Jirovec, op. cit., p. 133.
26 M. Soukop and M. C. Colman, "Nutrition Support in Patients with Malignant Disease," *Journal of Human Nutrition,* **33**:179–188, 1979.
27 S. M. Sobol et al., "Nutritional Concepts in the Management of the Head and Neck Cancer Patient," *Laryngoscope,* **89**:962–970, 1979.
28 Ibid.
29 Ibid.
30 C. A. Bingham, "The Cell Cycle and Cancer Chemotherapy," *American Journal of Nursing,* **78**:1201–1205, 1978.
31 Ibid.
32 J. S. Reminton and S. C. Schimpff, "Please Don't Eat the Salad," *New England Journal of Medicine,* **304**:433, 1981.
33 S. Hegedus and M. Pelham, "Dietetics in a Cancer Hospital," *Journal of the American Dietetic Association,* **67**:238, 1975.
34 C. F. McKhann and M. A. Tarlott, "Tumor Immunology–Tumor Antigens, Immune Responses Immunotherapy," American Cancer Society, No. 3393, 7, 1975.
35 S. S. Donaldson and R. A. Lenon, "Alterations of Nutritional Status—Impact of Chemotherapy and Radiation Therapy," *Cancer,* **43**:2036–2052, 1979.
36 E. D. Thomas, J. E. Sanders, N. Flournoy et al., "Marrow Transplantation for Patients with Acute Lymphoblastic Leukemia in Remission," *Blood,* **54**:468–476, 1979.
37 E. Silverberg, "Cancer Statistics 1981," *CA,* **31**:13–28, 1981.
38 Ibid, p. 28.
39 J. L. Young and R. W. Miller, "Incidence of Malignant Tumors in U.S. Children," *Journal of Pediatrics,* **86**:254–258, 1975.
40 A. M. Mauer, "Leukemias of Childhood," *Current Problems in Cancer,* **2**:3–46, 1977.
41 E. Silverberg, op. cit., p. 28.
42 J. L. Young and R. W. Miller, op. cit., p. 255.
43 M. E. Nesbit, W. Krivit, L. Robison, and D. Hammond, "A Follow-up Report of Longterm Survivors of Childhood Acute Lymphoblastic or Undifferentiated Leukemia," *Journal of Pediatrics,* **95**:727–730, 1979.
44 S. E. Sallan and H. J. Weinstein, "Management of Acute Lymphoblastic and Acute Myeloblastic Leukemia in Childhood," *Paediatrician,* **9**:56–67, 1980.
45 J. L. Young and R. W. Miller, op. cit., p. 255.
46 I. J. Ertel, "Brain Tumors in Children," *CA,* **30**:306–321, 1980.
47 Howard J. Weinstein, "Oncology Service, Children's Hospital Medical Center, Boston, Mass., personal communication, 1981.

48 E. Silverberg, op. cit., p. 28.

49 H. J. Weinstein and M. P. Link, "Non-Hodgkin's Lymphoma in Childhood," *Clinics in Haematology,* 8:699–716, 1979.

50 J. C. Dearth, G. S. Gilchrist, E. O. Burgert, R. L. Telander, and R. E. Cuppo, "Management of Stages I to III Hodgkin's Disease in Children," *Journal of Pediatrics,* 96:829–836, 1980.

51 R. S. Broady, "Multiple Primary Cancer Risk after Therapy for Hodgkin's Disease," *Cancer,* 40:1917–1926, 1977.

52 E. Silverberg, op. cit., p. 28.

53 T. C. Putman, D. F. Nelson, and M. Klemperer, "Pediatric Solid Tumors," *Clinical Oncology—A Multidisciplinary Approach,* American Cancer Society, Inc., pp. 259–271, 1978.

54 M. E. Nesbit, P. F. Coccia et al., "Staging in Pediatric Malignancies," *Proceedings of the National Conference on the Care of the Child with Cancer,* American Cancer Society, Inc., pp. 31–38, 1978.

55 E. Silverberg, op. cit., p. 28.

56 J. L. Young and R. W. Miller, op. cit., p. 255.

57 H. M. Maurer, "Rhabdomyosarcoma in Children and Adolescence," *Current Problems in Cancer,* 2:3–36, 1978.

58 H. M. Maurer, M. Donaldson, E. A. Gehan et al., "Multidisciplinary Approach to Management of Childhood Rhabdomyosarcoma," *National Conference on the Care of the Child with Cancer,* American Cancer Society, Inc., pp. 83–85, 1978.

59 E. Silverberg, op. cit., p. 28.

60 J. L. Young and R. W. Miller, op. cit., p. 255.

61 V. C. Canale and E. C. Muecke, "Wilm's Tumor—A Critical Review," *CA,* 24:66–77, 1974.

62 J. A. Ortega, R. Higgins, K. O. Williams et al., "Vincristine, Dactinomycin, and Cyclophosphamide (VAC) Chemotherapy for Recurrent Metastatic Wilm's Tumor in Previously Treated Children," *Journal of Pediatrics,* 96:502–504, 1980.

63 N. E. Breslow, N. F. Palmer, and L. R. Hill, "Wilm's Tumor Prognostic Factors for Patients without Metastasis at Diagnosis," *Cancer,* 41:1577–1589, 1978.

64 F. P. Li, M. A. Tucker, and J. F. Fraumeri, "Childhood Cancer in Sibs," *Journal of Pediatrics,* 88:419–423, 1976.

65 J. F. Cordero, F. P. Li, L. B. Holmes, and P. S. Gerald, "Wilm's Tumor in Five Cousins," *Pediatrics,* 66:716–719, 1980.

66 W. D. DeWys and K. Walters, "Abnormalities of Taste Sensation in Cancer Patients," *Cancer,* 36:1888–1896, 1975.

67 R. I. Henkin, P. J. Schechter, R. Hoye, and C. F. T. Mattern, "Idiopathic, Hypogeusia with Dysgeusia, Hyposmia and Dysosmia," *Journal of the American Medical Association,* 217:434–440, 1971.

68 W. D. DeWys and K. Walters, op. cit., p. 1888.

69 I. L. Bernstein, "Learned Taste Aversions in Children Receiving Chemotherapy," *Science,* 200:1302–1303, 1978.

70 S. S. Nielson, A. Theologides, and Z. M. Vickers, "Influence of Food Odors on Food Aversions and Preferences in Patients with Cancer," *American Journal of Clinical Nutrition,* 33:2253–2261, 1980.

71 K. A. Richard, A. Kirksey, R. L. Baehner et al., "Effectiveness of Enteral and Parenteral Nutrition in the Nutritional Management of Children with Wilm's Tumors," *American Journal of Clinical Nutrition,* 33:2622–2629, 1980.

72 N. Jaffe, "Nutrition and Childhood Malignancy," in Robert M. Suskind (ed.), *Textbook of Pediatric Nutrition,* Raven Press, New York, 1981.

73 R. M. Filler, W. Dietz, R. M. Suskind, and N. Jaffe, "Parenteral Feeding in the Management of Children with Cancer," *Cancer,* 43:2117–2120, 1979.

74 M. Michallet, D. Hollard, A. M. Guignier et al., "Parenteral Nutrition in Pediatrics with Leukemia and Non-Hodgkin Malignant Lymphoma under Chemotherapy," *Journal of Parenteral and Enteral Nutrition,* 3:247–254, 1979.

75 Ellen Dwyer, Nutrition Support Service, Children's Hospital Medical Center, Boston, Mass., personal communication, 1981.

CLINICAL DISCUSSION 29

Since M.G. is receiving chemotherapy that includes prednisone, adriamycin, and vincristine, with known side effects of fluid retention, cardiac toxicity, and constipation, a no-added-salt diet is recommended. This diet will help to decrease fluid retention and prevent cardiac abnormalities. Vincristine is known to cause diarrhea as well as constipation. Diet manipulations should be adjusted accordingly. An increased fluid intake may alleviate symptoms of constipation. A high-fiber diet is not recommended as it may be an irritant to the gastrointestinal tract due to inflammation of the GI mucosa. Therefore, food like prune juice is used, along with a laxative and colace when she has constipation. When diarrhea occurs, provide the child with clear liquids and progress the diet as tolerated (see Table 29-7).

Food activities which involve M.G. should be encouraged as they provide a stimulus for eating. Such activities might include allowing the child to prepare her own lunch, fixing a snack for herself and her parents, eating lunch outside. The use of the child's special cup or plate might also encourage an increased food intake. Parents should be encouraged to eat with their child in the hospital whenever possible.

M.G. should be consuming 1300 kcal (5.46 MJ) or 100 kcal per kilogram of body weight, the RDA for a 1-to 3-year-old. The protein requirement for this age is 1.8 g per kilogram of body weight or 23 g. A multivitamin supplement is recommended.

TABLES

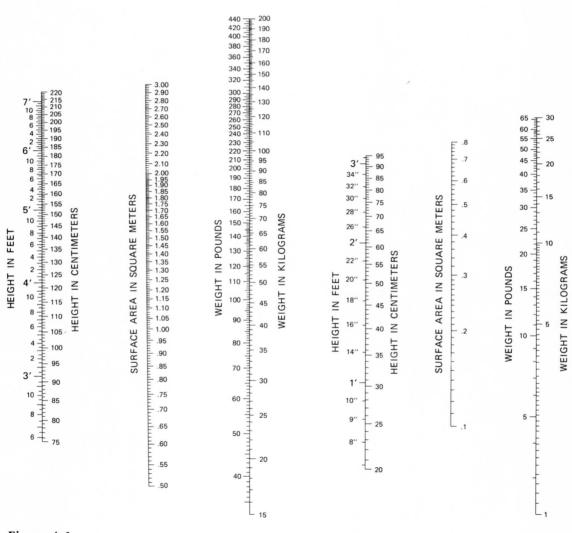

Figure A-1
Nomograms for estimating body surface area from height and body weight. The patient's body surface area is found by drawing a straight line between the point representing his or her weight and the point representing his or her height.
(From J. D. Crawford, M. E. Terry, and G. M. Rourke, *Pediatrics*, **5**:783, 1950.)

TABLE A-1 FOOD AND NUTRITION BOARD, NATIONAL ACADEMY OF SCIENCES—NATIONAL RESEARCH COUNCIL RECOMMENDED DAILY DIETARY ALLOWANCES,[a] REVISED 1980

Designed for the maintenance of good nutrition of practically all healthy people in the U.S.A.

	Age (years)	Weight (kg)	Weight (lb)	Height (cm)	Height (in)	Protein (g)	Fat-soluble vitamins Vitamin A (μg RE)[b]	Vitamin D (μg)[c]	Vitamin E (mg α-TE)[d]	Water-soluble vitamins Vitamin C (mg)	Thiamin (mg)
Infants	0.0–0.5	6	13	60	24	kg × 2.2	420	10	3	35	0.3
	0.5–1.0	9	20	71	28	kg × 2.0	400	10	4	35	0.5
Children	1–3	13	29	90	35	23	400	10	5	45	0.7
	4–6	20	44	112	44	30	500	10	6	45	0.9
	7–10	28	62	132	52	34	700	10	7	45	1.2
Males	11–14	45	99	157	62	45	1000	10	8	50	1.4
	15–18	66	145	176	69	56	1000	10	10	60	1.4
	19–22	70	154	177	70	56	1000	7.5	10	60	1.5
	23–50	70	154	178	70	56	1000	5	10	60	1.4
	51+	70	154	178	70	56	1000	5	10	60	1.2
Females	11–14	46	101	157	62	46	800	10	8	50	1.1
	15–18	55	120	163	64	46	800	10	8	60	1.1
	19–22	55	120	163	64	44	800	7.5	8	60	1.1
	23–50	55	120	163	64	44	800	5	8	60	1.0
	51+	55	120	163	64	44	800	5	8	60	1.0
Pregnant						+30	+200	+5	+2	+20	+0.4
Lactating						+20	+400	+5	+3	+40	+0.5

[a]The allowances are intended to provide for individual variations among most normal persons as they live in the United States under usual environmental stresses. Diets should be based on a variety of common foods in order to provide other nutrients for which human requirements have been less well defined. See text for detailed discussion of allowances and of nutrients not tabulated. See Table A-2 for weights and heights by individual year of age. See Table A-2 for suggested average energy intakes.

[b]Retinol equivalents. 1 retinol equivalent = 1 μg retinol or 6 μg β carotene. See text for calculation of vitamin A activity of diets as retinol equivalents.

[c]As cholecalciferol. 10 μg cholecalciferol = 400 IU of vitamin D.

[d]α-Tocopherol equivalents. 1 mg d-α tocopherol = 1 α-TE. See text for variation in allowances and calculation of vitamin E activity of the diet as α-tocopherol equivalents.

	Water-soluble vitamins (continued)				Minerals					
Riboflavin (mg)	Niacin (mg NE)[e]	Vitamin B-6 (mg)	Folacin[f] (μg)	Vitamin B-12 (μg)	Calcium (mg)	Phosphorus (mg)	Magnesium (mg)	Iron (mg)	Zinc (mg)	Iodine (μg)
0.4	6	0.3	30	0.5[g]	360	240	50	10	3	40
0.6	8	0.6	45	1.5	540	360	70	15	5	50
0.8	9	0.9	100	2.0	800	800	150	15	10	70
1.0	11	1.3	200	2.5	800	800	200	10	10	90
1.4	16	1.6	300	3.0	800	800	250	10	10	120
1.6	18	1.8	400	3.0	1200	1200	350	18	15	150
1.7	18	2.0	400	3.0	1200	1200	400	18	15	150
1.7	19	2.2	400	3.0	800	800	350	10	15	150
1.6	18	2.2	400	3.0	800	800	350	10	15	150
1.4	16	2.2	400	3.0	800	800	350	10	15	150
1.3	15	1.8	400	3.0	1200	1200	300	18	15	150
1.3	14	2.0	400	3.0	1200	1200	300	18	15	150
1.3	14	2.0	400	3.0	800	800	300	18	15	150
1.2	13	2.0	400	3.0	800	800	300	18	15	150
1.2	13	2.0	400	3.0	800	800	300	10	15	150
+0.3	+2	+0.6	+400	+1.0	+400	+400	+150	[h]	+5	+25
+0.5	+5	+0.5	+100	+1.0	+400	+400	+150	[h]	+10	+50

[e] 1 NE (niacin equivalent) is equal to 1 mg of niacin or 60 mg of dietary tryptophan.

[f] The folacin allowances refer to dietary sources as determined by *Lactobacillus casei* assay after treatment with enzymes (conjugases) to make polyglutamyl forms of the vitamin available to the test organism.

[g] The recommended dietary allowance for vitamin B-12 in infants is based on average concentration of the vitamin in human milk. The allowances after weaning are based on energy intake (as recommended by the American Academy of Pediatrics) and consideration of other factors, such as intestinal absorption; see text.

[h] The increased requirement during pregnancy cannot be met by the iron content of habitual American diets nor by the existing iron stores of many women; therefore the use of 30–60 mg of supplemental iron is recommended. Iron needs during lactation are not substantially different from those of nonpregnant women, but continued supplementation of the mother for 2–3 months after parturition is advisable in order to replenish stores depleted by pregnancy.

TABLE A-2 MEAN HEIGHTS AND WEIGHTS AND RECOMMENDED ENERGY INTAKE*

Category	Age (years)	Weight (kg)	(lb)	Height (cm)	(in)	Energy needs (with range) (kcal)		(MJ)
Infants	0.0–0.5	6	13	60	24	kg × 115	(95–145)	kg × 0.48
	0.5–1.0	9	20	71	28	kg × 105	(80–135)	kg × 0.44
Children	1–3	13	29	90	35	1300	(900–1800)	5.5
	4–6	20	44	112	44	1700	(1300–2300)	7.1
	7–10	28	62	132	52	2400	(1650–3300)	10.1
Males	11–14	45	99	157	62	2700	(2000–3700)	11.3
	15–18	66	145	176	69	2800	(2100–3900)	11.8
	19–22	70	154	177	70	2900	(2500–3300)	12.2
	23–50	70	154	178	70	2700	(2300–3100)	11.3
	51–75	70	154	178	70	2400	(2000–2800)	10.1
	76+	70	154	178	70	2050	(1650–2450)	8.6
Females	11–14	46	101	157	62	2200	(1500–3000)	9.2
	15–18	55	120	163	64	2100	(1200–3000)	8.8
	19–22	55	120	163	64	2100	(1700–2500)	8.8
	23–50	55	120	163	64	2000	(1600–2400)	8.4
	51–75	55	120	163	64	1800	(1400–2200)	7.6
	76+	55	120	163	64	1600	(1200–2000)	6.7
Pregnancy						+300		
Lactation						+500		

*The data in this table have been assembled from the observed median heights and weights of children shown in Table A-1, together with desirable weights for adults given in Table A-5. The mean heights of men (70 in) and women (64 in) between the ages of 18 and 34 years as surveyed in the U.S. population (HEW/NCHS data).

The energy allowances for the young adults are for men and women doing light work. The allowances for the two older age groups represent mean energy needs over these age spans, allowing for a 2-percent decrease in basal (resting) metabolic rate per decade and a reduction in activity of 200 kcal/day for men and women between 51 and 75 years, 500 kcal for men over 75 years, and 400 kcal for women over 75 years (see text). The customary range of daily energy output is shown in parentheses for adults and is based on a variation in energy needs of ±400 kcal at any one age (see text and Garrow, 1978), emphasizing the wide range of energy intakes appropriate for any group of people.

Energy allowances for children through age 18 are based on median energy intakes of children of these ages followed in longitudinal growth studies. The values in parentheses are 10th and 90th percentiles of energy intake, to indicate the range of energy consumption among children of these ages (see text).

Source: Food and Nutrition Board, *Recommended Daily Dietary Allowances,* Revised 1980, National Academy of Sciences, National Research Council.

TABLE A-3 ESTIMATED SAFE AND ADEQUATE DAILY DIETARY INTAKES
OF SELECTED VITAMINS AND MINERALS*

	Age (years)	Vitamins		
		Vitamin K (μg)	Biotin (μg)	Pantothenic acid (mg)
Infants	0–0.5	12	35	2
	0.5–1	10–20	50	3
Children and adolescents	1–3	15–30	65	3
	4–6	20–40	85	3–4
	7–10	30–60	120	4–5
	11+	50–100	100–200	4–7
Adults		70–140	100–200	4–7

	Age (years)	Trace elements†					
		Copper (mg)	Manganese (mg)	Fluoride (mg)	Chromium (mg)	Selenium (mg)	Molybdenum (mg)
Infants	0–0.5	0.5–0.7	0.5–0.7	0.1–0.5	0.01–0.04	0.01–0.04	0.03–0.06
	0.2–5	0.7–1.0	0.7–1.0	0.2–1.0	0.02–0.06	0.02–0.06	0.04–0.08
Children and adolescents	1–3	1.0–1.5	1.0–1.5	0.5–1.5	0.02–0.08	0.02–0.08	0.05–0.1
	4–6	1.5–2.0	1.5–2.0	1.0–2.5	0.03–0.12	0.03–0.12	0.06–0.15
	7–10	2.0–2.5	2.0–3.0	1.5–2.5	0.05–0.2	0.05–0.2	0.10–0.3
	11+	2.0–3.0	2.5–5.0	1.5–2.5	0.05–0.2	0.05–0.2	0.15–0.5
Adults		2.0–3.0	2.5–5.0	1.5–4.0	0.05–0.2	0.05–0.2	0.15–0.5

	Age (years)	Electrolytes		
		Sodium (mg)	Potassium (mg)	Chloride (mg)
Infants	0–0.5	115–350	350–925	275–700
	0.5–1	250–750	425–1275	400–1200
Children and adolescents	1–3	325–975	550–1650	500–1500
	4–6	450–1350	775–2325	700–2100
	7–10	600–1800	1000–3000	925–2775
	11+	900–2700	1525–4575	1400–4200
Adults		1100–3300	1875–5625	1700–5100

*Because there is less information on which to base allowances, these figures are not given in the main table of RDA and are provided here in the form of ranges of recommended intakes.

†Since the toxic levels for many trace elements may be only several times usual intakes, the upper levels for the trace elements given in this table should not be habitually exceeded.

Source: Food and Nutrition Board, *Recommended Daily Dietary Allowances,* Revised 1980, National Academy of Sciences, National Research Council.

TABLE A-4 ADULT HEIGHT AND WEIGHT TABLES

Desirable weights in pounds according to height and frame (in indoor clothing)

	Height (with shoes on; 1-in heels)		Small frame	Medium frame	Large frame
	ft	*in*			
Men age 25 and over	5	2	112–120	118–129	126–141
	5	3	115–123	121–133	129–144
	5	4	118–126	124–136	132–148
	5	5	121–129	127–139	135–152
	5	6	124–133	130–143	138–156
	5	7	128–137	134–147	142–161
	5	8	132–141	138–152	147–166
	5	9	136–145	142–156	151–170
	5	10	140–150	146–160	155–174
	5	11	144–154	150–165	159–179
	6	0	148–158	154–170	164–184
	6	1	152–162	158–175	168–189
	6	2	156–167	162–180	173–194
	6	3	160–171	167–185	178–199
	6	4	164–175	172–190	182–204

	Height (with shoes on; 2-in heels)		Small frame	Medium frame	Large frame
	ft	*in*			
Women age 25 and over*	4	10	92–98	96–107	104–119
	4	11	94–101	98–110	106–122
	5	0	96–104	101–113	109–125
	5	1	99–107	104–116	112–128
	5	2	102–110	107–119	115–131
	5	3	105–113	110–122	118–134
	5	4	108–116	113–126	121–138
	5	5	111–119	116–130	125–142
	5	6	114–123	120–135	129–146
	5	7	118–127	124–139	133–150
	5	8	122–131	128–143	137–154
	5	9	126–135	132–147	141–158
	5	10	130–140	136–151	145–163
	5	11	134–144	140–155	149–168
	6	0	138–148	144–159	153–173

*For girls between 18 and 25, subtract 1 lb for each year under 25.

Source: Metropolitan Life Insurance Company, New York.

TABLE A-5 AVERAGE WEIGHT OF MEN AND WOMEN AGED 18–74 YEARS, BY AGE AND HEIGHT: UNITED STATES, 1971–1974

Sex and height	Age group in years						
	18–74	18–24	25–34	35–44	45–54	55–64	65 and over
	Weight in pounds						
Men							
62 inches	140	*130	*141	*143	*147	*143	148
63 inches	147	140	151	*148	151	*147	146
64 inches	153	146	151	158	165	154	147
65 inches	155	138	155	156	161	163	155
66 inches	162	154	160	165	166	163	160
67 inches	168	157	168	173	172	168	167
68 inches	168	155	166	177	170	170	169
69 inches	173	166	176	172	178	175	172
70 inches	179	165	185	184	183	184	181
71 inches	182	176	178	188	187	187	188
72 inches	188	175	190	195	193	184	183
73 inches	195	186	195	210	196	189	*190
74 inches	197	191	191	*205	*200	*203	*194
Women							
57 inches	123	*114	*118	*125	*129	*132	130
58 inches	125	118	119	128	*133	122	133
59 inches	135	118	126	136	136	143	137
60 inches	137	123	125	135	146	142	138
61 inches	137	124	130	134	141	148	144
62 inches	138	124	135	142	140	146	146
63 inches	144	132	138	146	149	154	149
64 inches	145	133	141	148	153	151	152
65 inches	149	136	143	155	156	162	153
66 inches	150	140	146	157	155	155	162
67 inches	153	143	153	155	161	*167	173
68 inches	161	142	162	171	173	*171	168

*Estimated values obtained from linear regression equations.

Note: Examined persons were measured without shoes; clothing weight ranged from 0.20 to 0.62 lb, which was not deducted from weights shown.

Source: U.S. Department of Health, Education, and Welfare, *Vital and Health Statistics,* Data from the National Health Survey, Series 11, Number 208, *Weight by Height and Age for Adults 18–74 Years: United States 1971–1974,* Public Health Service, Office of Health Research and Technology, National Center for Health Statistics, p. 17.

TABLE A-6 SELECTED SMOOTHED PERCENTILES FOR TRICEPS SKINFOLD
OF FEMALES AGED 2-18 YEARS: UNITED STATES, 1963–1965, 1966–1970, AND
1971–1974

Age	Smoothed* percentile						
	5th	10th	25th	50th	75th	90th	95th
Female	*Triceps skinfold in millimeters*						
2.0 years	6.4	7.0	8.4	10.3	12.1	14.0	15.2
2.5 years	6.4	7.1	8.4	10.3	12.0	13.7	15.0
3.0 years	6.4	7.1	8.4	10.2	11.9	13.5	14.9
3.5 years	6.4	7.1	8.4	10.2	11.8	13.4	15.0
4.0 years	6.3	7.1	8.3	10.2	11.9	13.5	15.2
4.5 years	6.3	7.1	8.3	10.2	11.9	13.7	15.5
5.0 years	6.2	7.0	8.3	10.2	12.0	13.9	15.9
5.5 years	6.2	7.0	8.2	10.3	12.2	14.3	16.4
6.0 years	6.1	6.9	8.2	10.3	12.3	14.8	16.9
6.5 years	6.1	6.9	8.2	10.4	12.5	15.3	17.5
7.0 years	6.0	6.8	8.2	10.4	12.8	15.8	18.2
7.5 years	6.0	6.8	8.2	10.5	13.0	16.5	18.9
8.0 years	6.0	6.8	8.2	10.6	13.4	17.1	19.7
8.5 years	6.0	6.7	8.3	10.8	13.7	17.8	20.4
9.0 years	6.0	6.8	8.4	11.0	14.1	18.5	21.2
9.5 years	6.0	6.8	8.5	11.2	14.5	19.1	22.0
10.0 years	6.1	6.9	8.6	11.4	15.0	19.8	22.8
10.5 years	6.2	7.0	8.8	11.6	15.4	20.4	23.5
11.0 years	6.3	7.2	9.0	11.9	15.9	21.1	24.2
11.5 years	6.4	7.3	9.2	12.2	16.4	21.6	24.9
12.0 years	6.6	7.6	9.5	12.6	16.9	22.2	25.6
12.5 years	6.7	7.8	9.8	12.9	17.5	22.8	26.2
13.0 years	6.9	8.0	10.1	13.3	18.0	23.3	26.8
13.5 years	7.1	8.3	10.4	13.7	18.5	23.8	27.4
14.0 years	7.3	8.5	10.7	14.1	19.0	24.2	28.0
14.5 years	7.5	8.8	11.1	14.5	19.5	24.7	28.5
15.0 years	7.7	9.1	11.4	14.8	20.0	25.1	29.0
15.5 years	7.9	9.3	11.8	15.2	20.5	25.5	29.4
16.0 years	8.0	9.6	12.2	15.6	20.9	25.9	29.8
16.5 years	8.2	9.8	12.5	16.0	21.3	26.3	30.1
17.0 years	8.4	10.0	12.8	16.3	21.7	26.7	30.4
17.5 years	8.5	10.2	13.2	16.6	22.0	27.0	30.7
18.0 years	8.6	10.4	13.5	17.0	22.2	27.3	30.9

*Smoothed by cubic-spline approximation.

TABLE A-7 SELECTED SMOOTHED PERCENTILES FOR TRICEPS SKINFOLD OF MALES AGED 2–18 YEARS: UNITED STATES, 1963–1965, 1966–1970, AND 1971–1974

Age	Smoothed* percentile						
	5th	10th	25th	50th	75th	90th	95th
Male	*Triceps skinfold in millimeters*						
2.0 years	6.2	6.9	8.2	10.3	12.1	14.1	15.4
2.5 years	6.1	6.8	8.0	10.0	11.8	13.7	14.9
3.0 years	6.0	6.7	7.9	9.8	11.5	13.4	14.4
3.5 years	5.8	6.6	7.7	9.5	11.2	13.1	14.1
4.0 years	5.7	6.5	7.6	9.3	10.9	12.8	13.9
4.5 years	5.6	6.4	7.4	9.0	10.7	12.6	13.8
5.0 years	5.4	6.3	7.3	8.8	10.5	12.5	13.8
5.5 years	5.3	6.1	7.1	8.6	10.4	12.4	13.9
6.0 years	5.2	6.0	7.0	8.5	10.3	12.4	14.1
6.5 years	5.1	5.9	6.9	8.4	10.2	12.5	14.5
7.0 years	5.0	5.8	6.8	8.3	10.3	12.7	14.9
7.5 years	4.9	5.7	6.7	8.2	10.4	13.0	15.4
8.0 years	4.9	5.6	6.7	8.2	10.5	13.4	16.1
8.5 years	4.8	5.6	6.6	8.3	10.8	14.0	16.9
9.0 years	4.8	5.5	6.7	8.4	11.1	14.6	17.8
9.5 years	4.8	5.5	6.7	8.6	11.5	15.5	18.7
10.0 years	4.9	5.6	6.8	8.8	11.9	16.4	19.8
10.5 years	4.9	5.6	6.9	9.0	12.4	17.4	20.8
11.0 years	4.9	5.6	7.0	9.3	12.8	18.3	21.8
11.5 years	5.0	5.7	7.0	9.4	13.2	19.1	22.7
12.0 years	4.9	5.7	7.1	9.6	13.4	19.8	23.4
12.5 years	4.9	5.6	7.1	9.6	13.6	20.2	23.9
13.0 years	4.8	5.6	7.0	9.6	13.5	20.3	24.1
13.5 years	4.6	5.4	6.8	9.4	13.3	20.1	24.0
14.0 years	4.5	5.3	6.6	9.1	13.0	19.6	23.7
14.5 years	4.3	5.1	6.4	8.7	12.5	19.0	23.2
15.0 years	4.1	4.9	6.2	8.4	12.0	18.2	22.7
15.5 years	3.9	4.7	5.9	8.0	11.5	17.4	22.1
16.0 years	3.8	4.6	5.8	7.7	11.2	16.8	21.6
16.5 years	3.8	4.5	5.6	7.4	10.9	16.2	21.3
17.0 years	3.8	4.5	5.6	7.3	10.9	16.0	21.3
17.5 years	3.9	4.5	5.7	7.3	11.1	16.1	21.6
18.0 years	4.2	4.6	5.9	7.5	11.7	16.6	22.3

*Smoothed by cubic-spline approximation.

TABLE A-8 OBESITY STANDARDS FOR ADULT
CAUCASIAN AMERICANS

	Skinfold measurements, mm	
Age, yr	Males	Females
18	15	27
19	15	27
20	16	28
21	17	28
22	18	28
23	18	28
24	19	28
25	20	29
26	20	29
27	21	29
28	22	29
29	23	29
30–50	23	30

Source: Adapted from C. C. Seltzer and J. Mayer, "A Sample
Criterion of Obesity," *Postgraduate Medicine,* **38:**101–107,
1965.

TABLE A-9 NUTRITIONAL ASSESSMENT TOOL FOR USE WITH CHILDREN

Patient _____   Date _____

Birth date _____   Age _____

Informant _____

Presenting nutritional problem(s) _____

_____

Current concern (parental) _____

_____

Growth

Height _____ (_____%)   Head circumference _____ (_____%)

Weight _____ (_____%)   Fat-fold measure _____

Birth weight _____ lb _____ oz   Birth length _____ inches

Has weight gain since birth been: Satisfactory? _____ Slow? _____ Fluctuating? _____

Has there been recent weight: Gain? _____ Loss? _____ Neither _____

Mother's height _____ ft _____ in   Weight _____ lb

Father's height _____ ft _____ in   Weight _____ lb

As compared with siblings at the same age, patient is: Larger _____ Same size _____ Smaller _____

TABLE A-9 CONTINUED

Pertinent laboratory findings _____

Nutrition history

Has the patient taken vitamin-mineral supplements? Yes _____ No _____ Kind _____ At what age? _____

Has the patient been prescribed medication(s)? Yes _____ No _____

 Kind _____ Reason _____ At what age? _____

Indicate if there have been problems with the following:

	Patient	Family	Comment
Colic	_____	_____	_____
Spitting up	_____	_____	_____
Appetite	_____	_____	_____
Food allergies	_____	_____	_____
Diarrhea	_____	_____	_____
Constipation	_____	_____	_____
Vomiting	_____	_____	_____
Anemia	_____	_____	_____
Dehydration	_____	_____	_____
Failure to thrive	_____	_____	_____
Unusual cravings	_____	_____	_____
Overweight	_____	_____	_____
Need for special diet	_____	_____	_____

Feeding history

Who fed the child? _____

Was the child difficult to feed? Yes _____ No _____

How long did feedings take? _____

Was there any early feeding intervention? Yes _____ No _____

Was the child: Breast-fed? _____ Formula-fed? _____ Formula: _____

Was the child fed: On demand? _____ On hourly schedule? _____

At what age was the child weaned: From breast? _____ From bottle? _____

Did the child suck his/her thumb? Yes _____ No _____ Did the child use a pacifier? Yes _____ No _____

(Continued)

Feeding history (continued)

Indicate if there were early difficulties with the following:

Comment

Sucking	_____	_____
Swallowing	_____	_____
Chewing	_____	_____
Tongue control	_____	_____
Lip control	_____	_____

Developing feeding milestones

Age   Comment

Baby food introduction	_____	_____
Junior foods	_____	_____
Finger feeding	_____	_____
Cup drinking	_____	_____
Weaning	_____	_____
Whole table foods	_____	_____
Use of spoon	_____	_____
Independent feeding	_____	_____
Self-preparation of food	_____	_____

Feeding environment

Is the child fed: Alone? _____ With family? _____

Who feeds the child? _____ Others that may feed or care for the child at mealtime: _____

The child eats: Alone _____ With family _____

Does the child care for himself/herself at the table? Yes _____ No _____

Does the child serve himself/herself food? Yes _____ No _____

Does the child generally finish all food served? Yes _____ No _____

Does the child ask for second helpings? Yes _____ No _____

How long is the usual eating period? _____

Where does the child eat: Breakfast? _____ Lunch? _____ Dinner? _____

Number of persons eating together at: Breakfast _____ Lunch _____ Dinner _____

Who prepares: Breakfast? _____ Lunch? _____ Dinner? _____

TABLE A-9 CONTINUED

Feeding environment (continued)

Is the child's behavior during mealtimes: Acceptable? _____ Disruptive? _____ Dawdling? _____

   Distractible? _____

Is the rule for eating: Clean plate? _____ Taste everything? _____

   Other: _____

How many times does the family dine out during the month? _____

How often is shopping done for food? _____

How much money is spent on food each week? _____

Are food stamps used? Yes _____ No _____

Present eating habits

Child's appetite is: Excellent _____ Fair _____ Poor _____ Fluctuating _____

Has there been recent appetite: Increase? _____ Decrease? _____

When is the child most hungry? _____

Does the child know when he/she is full? Yes _____ No _____

What is the usual snacking pattern? _____

Are the child's food habits similar to those of other family members? Yes _____ No _____

Does the child get up during the night or early morning to eat or drink?

   Yes _____ No _____

Is the child's acceptance of foods: Good? _____ Fair? _____ Poor? _____ Rigidly selective? _____

What are the child's food dislikes? _____

What is the child's favorite food? _____

Dental factors

Does the child have regular dental check-ups? Yes _____ No _____

Does the child brush and floss teeth regularly? Yes _____ No _____

Is the local water supply fluoridated? Yes _____ No _____

Is a fluoride supplement taken? Yes _____ No _____ Age _____

   Kind _____

Does the child receive topical fluoride applications? Yes _____ No _____

Are sweets included as: Part of meals? _____ Snacks? _____

(*Continued*)

Present food intake

24-h recall
1- to 3-day food record
General recall of usual food pattern

Time   *Amount*   *Type of food*

Frequency of foods:

	Number of times eaten per week		
	Daily	*Occasionally*	*Seldom*
Milk	____	____	____
Cheese, ice cream	____	____	____
Cold or hot cereal	____	____	____
Sweet rolls or doughnuts	____	____	____
Sandwiches	____	____	____
Soup	____	____	____
Fruit or fruit juice	____	____	____
Peanut butter or nuts	____	____	____
Dried peas or beans	____	____	____
Meat in casseroles	____	____	____
Red meat, fish, or poultry	____	____	____
Cooked or raw vegetable	____	____	____
Potato, rice, or noodles	____	____	____
Cookies or crackers	____	____	____
Pie, cake, or brownies	____	____	____
Potato chips or corn chips	____	____	____
Candy	____	____	____
Soft drinks or Kool-Aid	____	____	____

TABLE A-9   CONTINUED

Present food intake (continued)

Does the weekend food pattern vary from the usual food intake during the week?

Yes _____ No _____ Comment _____

Comments regarding food intake: _____

_____

_____

_____

Analysis of food intake:

Total fluid _____

kcal _____ kcal/kg _____ kcal/cm _____

Protein, g _____ Protein, g/kg _____

Vitamins/minerals _____

Impressions:

Recommendations:

Summary:

Source: Developmental Evaluation Clinic, Children's Hospital Medical Center, Boston, Mass.

TABLE A-10 NUTRITIONAL ASSESSMENT TOOL FOR USE WITH ADULTS*

1. Household Dietary Questionnaire†

Name _____ Sex _____ Date of birth _____ Date _____

Address _____ Marital status _____

1. Persons fed: (give sex and age for each)
_____
_____
_____

2. Grade of school completed   3. Occupation of
   by homemaker _____   head of household _____

4. Income level $ _____   Sources of income _____

5. Where do you usually get your food supplies?
   If purchased:
      Kind of store? _____ Cash or credit? _____
      Distance to store? _____ Transportation? _____
      How often shop for food? _____ Why? _____
      If home produced, what? _____
      _____
      _____
      _____

      Do you home-preserve? _____ What? _____ How much? _____
      _____
      _____

      Other sources? _____
      _____
      _____

      Are food stamps available? _____ Do you purchase? _____
         How much do you pay? $_____ Value get? _____
      Are donated or surplus foods available? _____ Do you use? _____

6. How much did you spend for food last week? _____
   Is this the usual amount? _____

7. Do you feel you have adequate storage facilities for food? _____

8. Do you feel you have adequate cooking facilities? _____
   Kind? _____ Working oven? _____

9. Do you feel you have adequate refrigeration? _____
   Kind? _____

*From G. Christakis, "Nutritional Assessment in Health Programs," in *American Journal of Public Health,* vol. 63, November 1973, pt. 2.

†Adapted from: National Nutrition Survey, Nutrition Program; Division of Chronic Disease Program, DHEW, Atlanta, Ga. Rev. 3/69. VIII A-Dietary—Household—General Information. NCCD-3-8a (DC).

TABLE A-10 CONTINUED

2.   24-Hour Recall*

Name _____

Date and time of interview _____

Length of interview _____

Date of recall _____

Day of the week of recall _____

1-M   2-T   3-W   4-Th   5-F   6-Sat   7-Sun

"I would like you to tell me everything you (your child) ate and drank from the time you (he) got up in the morning until you (he) went to bed at night and what you (he) ate during the night. Be sure to mention everything you (he) ate or drank at home, at work (school), and away from home. Include snacks and drinks of all kinds and everything else you (he) put in your (his) mouth and swallowed. I also need to know where you (he) ate the food, and now let us begin."

What time did you (he) get up yesterday? _____

Was it the usual time? _____

What was the first time you (he) ate or had anything to drink yesterday morning? (list on the form that follows)
Where did you (he) eat? (list on form which follows)
Now tell me what you (he) had to eat and how much?
(Occasionally the interviewer will need to ask:)
   When did you (he) eat again? Or, is there anything else?
   Did you (he) have anything to eat or drink during the night?
Was intake unusual in any way? Yes _____ No _____

(If answer is yes) Why? _____

   In what way? _____

What time did you (he) go to bed last night?
Do(es) you (he) take vitamin or mineral supplements?

   Yes _____ No _____
(If answer is yes) How many per day? _____

   Per week? _____

What kind? (Insert brand name if known)

Multivitamins _____

Ascorbic acid _____

Vitamins A and D _____

Iron _____

Other _____

(Continued)

*Taken from: *Screening Children for Nutritional Status: Suggestions for Child Health Programs,* U.S. Government Printing Office, Washington, D.C., 1971.

TABLE A-10 CONTINUED

			3. Suggested Form for Recording Food Intake*			
Time	Where eaten†	Food	Type and/or preparation	Amount	Food code‡	Amount code‡

*Taken from: *Screening Children for Nutritional Status: Suggestions for Child Health Programs,* U.S. Government Printing Office, Washington, D.C. 1971, p. 13.
†Code:
  H—Home
  R—Restaurant, drug store, or lunch counter
 CL—Carried lunch from home
 CC—Child care center
 OH—Other home (friend, relative, baby sitter, etc.)
  S—School, office, plant or work
 FD—Food dispenser
 SS—Social center, e.g., Senior Citizen, etc.
‡Do not write in these spaces.

4.   Dietary Questionnaire for Adults and Adolescents*

Name _____ Sex _____ Date of birth _____

Address _____ Marital status _____ Date _____

1. Grade of school   2. Still in
   completed? _____   school? _____ 3. Occupation _____

4. Are you employed? _____ Full time? _____ Part time? _____

5. Income level $ _____ Sources of income _____

   Where appropriate:
6. Are you pregnant? _____ Stage? _____ Lactating? _____
7 If pregnant have you changed the way you eat or drink? How? _____

   On whose advice? _____

8. Where do you usually get your food supplies? _____
   If home produced, what? _____
   Do you home-preserve? What? How much? _____

   If purchased:
      Kind of store? _____   Cash or credit? _____
      Distance to store? _____   Transportation? _____
      How often shop for food? _____   Why? _____
      Are food stamps available? _____Do you purchase? _____
      How much do you pay? _____ Value get? $ _____
      Are donated or surplus foods available? _____ Do you use? _____

9. Do you feel you have adequate storage facilities for food in your home? _____

10. Do you feel you have adequate cooking facilities? _____
    Kind? _____ Working oven? _____

11. Do you feel you have adequate refrigeration? _____ Kind? _____

12. Do you eat at regular times each day? _____

13. How many days a week do you eat:
    a morning meal? _____
    a lunch or mid-day meal? _____
    an evening meal? _____

    during the evening or night? _____

14. How many days a week do you have snacks, and what do you have then?
    in mid-morning _____
    in mid-afternoon _____
    in the evening _____
    during the night _____

15. Where do you usually eat your meal?
    Morning _____ Mid-day _____ Evening _____

(Continued)

*Modified for these age groups from: *Screening Children for Nutritional Status: Suggestions for Child Health Programs,* U.S. Government Printing Office, Washington, D.C., 1971.

TABLE A-10 CONTINUED

4. Dietary Questionnaire for Adults and Adolescents (Continued)*

16. With whom do you usually eat?
    Morning _____ Mid-day _____ Evening _____

17. How many times a week do you usually eat away from home? _____

18. Would you say your appetite is Good? _____ Fair? _____ Poor? _____

19. What foods do you particularly dislike? _____

20. Are you on a special diet? _____ If yes, what kind? _____ Who prescribed? _____

21. Are there foods you don't eat for other reasons? _____

22. Do you eat anything not usually considered food (e.g., clay, dirt, starch, other)? _____
    If yes, what? _____; when? _____; how much? _____

23. Do you add salt to your food at the table? _____

24. Do you have any difficulty chewing? _____

25. How many times per week do you eat the following foods (at any meal or between meals)?
    Circle the appropriate number:
    Bacon _____ 0 1 2 3 4 5 6 7 >7, specify _____
    Tongue _____ 0 1 2 3 4 5 6 7 >7, specify _____
    Sausage _____ 0 1 2 3 4 5 6 7 >7, specify _____
    Luncheon meat _____ 0 1 2 3 4 5 6 7 >7, specify _____
    Hot dogs _____ 0 1 2 3 4 5 6 7 >7, specify _____
    Liver—chicken _____ 0 1 2 3 4 5 6 7 >7, specify _____
    Liver—other _____ 0 1 2 3 4 5 6 7 >7, specify _____
    Poultry _____ 0 1 2 3 4 5 6 7 >7, specify _____
    Salt pork _____ 0 1 2 3 4 5 6 7 >7, specify _____
    Pork or ham _____ 0 1 2 3 4 5 6 7 >7, specify _____
    Bones (neck or other) _____ 0 1 2 3 4 5 6 7 >7, specify _____
    Meat in mixtures (stew, tamales, casseroles, etc.) _____ 0 1 2 3 4 5 6 7 >7, specify _____
    Beef or veal _____ 0 1 2 3 4 5 6 7 >7, specify _____
    Other meat _____ 0 1 2 3 4 5 6 7 >7, specify _____
    Fish _____ 0 1 2 3 4 5 6 7 >7, specify _____
    Cheese and cheese dishes _____ 0 1 2 3 4 5 6 7 >7, specify _____
    Eggs _____ 0 1 2 3 4 5 6 7 >7, specify _____
    Dried beans or pea dishes _____ 0 1 2 3 4 5 6 7 >7, specify _____
    Peanut butter or nuts _____ 0 1 2 3 4 5 6 7 >7, specify _____

26. How many servings per day do you eat of the following foods? Circle the appropriate number:
    Bread (including sandwich), toast, rolls, muffins
      (1 slice or 1 piece is 1 serving) _____ 0 1 2 3 4 5 6 7 >7, specify _____
    Milk (including on cereal or other foods)
      (8 ounces is 1 serving) _____ 0 1 2 3 4 5 6 7 >7, specify _____
    Sugar, jam, jelly, syrup (1 tsp is 1 serving) ___ 0 1 2 3 4 5 6 7 >7, specify _____
    Butter or margarine (1 tsp is 1 serving) _____ 0 1 2 3 4 5 6 7 >7, specify, _____

*Modified for these age groups from: *Screening Children for Nutritional Status: Suggestions for Child Health Programs,* U.S. Government Printing Office, Washington, D.C., 1971.

TABLE A-10 CONTINUED

4. Dietary Questionnaire for Adults and Adolescents (Continued)*

27. How many times per week do you eat the following foods (at any meal or between meals)?
Circle the appropriate number:

Fruit juice _____ 0 1 2 3 4 5 6 7 >7, specify _____
Fruit _____ 0 1 2 3 4 5 6 7 >7, specify _____
Cereal—dry _____ 0 1 2 3 4 5 6 7 >7, specify _____
Cereal—cooked or instant _____ 0 1 2 3 4 5 6 7 >7, specify _____
Pancakes or waffles _____ 0 1 2 3 4 5 6 7 >7, specify _____
Potato _____ 0 1 2 3 4 5 6 7 >7, specify _____
Other cooked vegetables _____ 0 1 2 3 4 5 6 7 >7, specify _____
Raw vegetables _____ 0 1 2 3 4 5 6 7 >7, specify _____
Macaroni, spaghetti, rice, or noodles _____ 0 1 2 3 4 5 6 7 >7, specify _____
Ice cream, milk pudding, custard or cream soup _____ 0 1 2 3 4 5 6 7 >7, specify _____
Sweet rolls or doughnuts _____ 0 1 2 3 4 5 6 7 >7, specify _____
Crackers or pretzels _____ 0 1 2 3 4 5 6 7 >7, specify _____
Cookies _____ 0 1 2 3 4 5 6 7 >7, specify _____
Pie, cake or brownies _____ 0 1 2 3 4 5 6 7 >7, specify _____
Potato chips or corn chips _____ 0 1 2 3 4 5 6 7 >7, specify _____
Candy _____ 0 1 2 3 4 5 6 7 >7, specify _____
Soft drinks, Popsicles, or Kool Aid; sherbets _____ 0 1 2 3 4 5 6 7 >7, specify _____
Instant Breakfast _____ 0 1 2 3 4 5 6 7 >7, specify _____
Artificially sweetened beverage _____ 0 1 2 3 4 5 6 7 >7, specify _____
Coffee or tea _____ 0 1 2 3 4 5 6 7 >7, specify _____
Beer _____ 0 1 2 3 4 5 6 7 >7, specify _____
Wine _____ 0 1 2 3 4 5 6 7 >7, specify _____
Whiskey, vodka, rum, scotch, gin _____ 0 1 2 3 4 5 6 7 >7, specify _____

28. What specific kinds of the following foods do you eat most often?

Fruit juices _____
Fruit _____
Vegetables _____
Cheese _____
Cooked or instant cereal _____
Dry cereal _____
Milk _____
Cream or cream substitute _____
Butter or margarine _____
Salad dressings _____

*Modified for these groups from: *Screening Children for Nutritional Status: Suggestions for Child Health Programs,* U.S. Government Printing Office, Washington, D.C., 1971.

TABLE A-11   COMMON MEDICAL ABBREVIATIONS

ac	*ante cibos,* before meals	EEG	electroencephalogram
ad lib	*ad libitum,* as desired	ENT	ear, nose, and throat
ASHD	arteriosclerotic heart disease	ER or EW	emergency room or emergency ward
Ba	barium	FBS	fasting blood sugar
bid	*bis in die,* twice daily	FTT	failure to thrive
BMR	basal metabolic rate	FUO	fever of unknown origin
BP	blood pressure	Fx	fracture
BUN	blood urea nitrogen	GI	gastrointestinal
BS	blood sugar	GTT	glucose tolerance test
c̄	*cum,* with	GU	genitourinary
Ca	carcinoma	Gyn	gynecology
cath	catheter	Hct	hematocrit
CBC	complete blood count	hem	blood
CC	chief complaint	Hgb	hemoglobin
CHF	congestive heart failure	hs	*hora somni,* at bedtime
Cl	chloride	Hx	history
CNS	central nervous system	ICU	intensive care unit
CVA	cardiovascular accident	IM	intramuscular
D&C	dilatation and curettage	Imp	impression
D/C	discharge	I&O	intake and output
DOA	dead on arrival	IV	intravenous
DT	delirium tremens	IVP	intravenous pyelogram
Dx	diagnosis	K	potassium
ECG	electrocardiogram	L	liter
EDC	expected date of confinement	Lat	lateral

TABLE A-11 CONTINUED

LLQ	left lower quadrant		qh	every hour
LMP	last menstrual period		qid	4 times a day
lytes	electrolytes		qod	every other day
MI	myocardial infarction		qoh	every other hour
mL	milliliters		RBC	red blood cell
MOM	milk of magnesia		re	concerning
MS	multiple sclerosis		RHD	rheumatic heart disease
NG	nasogastric		R/O	rule out
npo	*non per os,* nothing by mouth		Rx	treatment
NTG	nitroglycerin		s̄	*sine,* without
Ob or OBS	obstetrics		SOB	shortness of breath
OPD	outpatient department		sp gr	specific gravity
OR	operating room		Staph	*Staphylococcus*
OT	occupational therapy		stat	*statim,* immediately
pc	*post cibos,* after meals		Sx	symptoms
PE	physical exam		T&A	tonsils and adenoids
PID	pelvic inflammatory disease		TB	tuberculosis
PKU	phenylketonuria		tid	*ter in die,* 3 times a day
po	*per os,* by mouth		trach	tracheostomy
pp	post prandial, after eating		URI	upper respiratory infection
prn	*pro re nata,* as needed		UTI	urinary tract infection
pt	patient		VD	venereal disease
PT	physical therapy		WBC	white blood count
PTA	prior to admission		WNL	within normal limits
qd	every day		×	times

Government food programs, United States Department of Agriculture

Food Stamp Program

With this program all individuals who meet the financial criteria can purchase food stamps or coupons that are used like money to buy food. This increases the family's food purchasing power. At the state level the program is usually run by the Department of Public Welfare.

For information, contact:

> State Public Welfare Department

School Lunch and Breakfast Program

Well balanced lunches and breakfasts are provided for school children to age 18. Special diets can be arranged.

For information, contact:

> State Director of School Lunch Program
> State Department of Education
> Local Department of Education

Child Care Food Program

A reimbursement for meals is made to child care programs for all children enrolled in nonresidential, nonschool child care programs, including summer programs.

For information, contact:

Western Regional Office:	Food and Nutrition Service United States Dept. of Agriculture 550 Kearney Street, Rm. 400 San Francisco, CA 94108
Southwest Regional Office:	Food and Nutrition Service United States Dept. of Agriculture 1100 Commerce St., Rm. 5-C-30 Dallas, TX 75242
Southeast Regional Office:	Food and Nutrition Service United States Dept. of Agriculture 1100 Spring Street, N.W. Atlanta, GA 30309
Mountain Plains Regional Office:	Food and Nutrition Service United States Dept. of Agriculture 1823 Stout Street Denver, CO 80202
Midwest Regional Office:	Food and Nutrition Service United States Dept. of Agriculture 536 Clark Street Chicago, IL 60605
New England Regional Office:	Food and Nutrition Service United States Dept. of Agriculture 34 Third Avenue Burlington, MA 01803
Mid-Atlantic Regional Office:	Food and Nutrition Service United States Dept. of Agriculture Robbinsville, NJ 08691

Government food programs, United States Department of Agriculture (continued)

Cooperative Extension Service

The extension service provides educational programs in home economics, youth development, community development and agriculture. Each local county has an extension service based at the state land grant college. Through this service nutrition information can be found.

For information, contact:

> Federal Extension Service
> Department of Agriculture
> Washington, DC 20250

> Local County Extension Service

Special Supplemental Food Program for Women, Infants, and Children (WIC)

Through this program supplemental foods (iron-fortified cereal, juices, eggs, milk, cheese, legumes, and peanut butter, and infant formula) are provided to pregnant women, women up to 6 months post partum, nursing mothers up to 1 year; children up to 5 years who qualify for financial criteria and are at nutritional risk.

For information, contact:

> Regional Office of U.S. Department of Agriculture
> (Listed above under Child Care Food Programs)

Sources of nutritional information

American Dietetic Association
430 N. Michigan Avenue
Chicago, IL 60611

American Heart Association
1329 Greenville Avenue
Dallas, TX 75231

American Home Economics Association
2010 Massachusetts Avenue, N.W.
Washington, DC 20036

American Public Health Association
1015 Eighteenth Street, N.W.
Washington, DC 20036

Center for Science in the Public Interest
1755 S. Street N.W.
Washington, DC 20009

Consumer Information
Pueblo, CO 81009

National Dairy Council
630 North River Road
Rosemont, IL 60018

United States Dept. of Agriculture
Food and Nutrition Office
Nutrition and Technical Assistance
    Division
500 12th Street S.W.
G.H.I. Building
Washington, DC 20250

National Health Systems
P.O. Box 1501
Ann Arbor, MI 48106

National Institute of Child Health
    and Human Development
U.S. Dept. of H.E.W.
Bethesda, MD 20014

Society for Nutrition Education
2140 Shattuck Ave.
Suite 110
Berkeley, CA 94704

Superintendent of Documents
U.S. Government Printing Office
Washington, DC 20402

Source: J. M. Borkowski and A. L. Emmerich, "Nutritional Care of the Young Child with Cerebral Palsy," Developmental Evaluation Clinic, The Children's Hospital Medical Center, Boston, Mass., June 1980, pp. 28–30.

TABLE A-13 COMMON METRIC EQUIVALENTS

1 U.S. fluid ounce	= 29.573 milliliter
1 U.S. liquid pint	= 0.47317 liter
1 U.S. liquid quart	= 0.94633 liter
1 U.S. gallon	= 3.78533 liter
1 U.S. dry quart	= 1.1012 liter
1 avoirdupois ounce	= 28.350 grams
1 avoirdupois pound	= 0.45359 kilogram
1 pound	= 2.2 kilograms
1 inch	= 2.54 centimeters

TABLE A-14 FOODBORNE ILLNESSES

Microorganism	Name of illness	Onset of symptoms	Symptoms	Duration	Foods susceptible
Salmonella	Salmonellosis	12 h	Cramps, fever, nausea, vomiting, diarrhea (sick people, infants, and elderly are more susceptible because of decreased resistance)	2–6 days	Poultry Eggs and egg products Milk Pork
Clostridium perfringens	Perfringens poisoning	10–20 h	Cramps, diarrhea, nausea	24 h	Meat
Staphylococcus aureus	Staphylococcus poisoning	2–8 h	Vomiting, diarrhea	1–2 days	Custards Sauces Gravies Soups Salads (chicken, tuna)
Clostridium botulinum	Botulism	12–36 h	Double vision, paralysis of respiratory muscles; can be fatal	3–8 days	Canned low-acid food Creamed soups Canned meat, mushrooms, etc.
Trichinella spiralis	Trichinosis	24–72 h	Nausea, vomiting, diarrhea, muscle pain, chest pain	Can be as long as 1 year	Pork and pork products

TABLE A-15   ADDITIVES: WHAT, WHERE, WHY THEY ARE . . .

Some additives	Where you might find them	Their functions
Purpose: To improve or maintain nutritional value *Class:* Nutrients		*Enrich:* Replace vitamins and minerals lost in processing
B vitamins: thiamin, thiamin hydrochloride, thiamin mononitrate, riboflavin, niacin, niacinamide	Flour, breads, cereals, rice, macaroni products	or
Beta carotene (source of vitamin A)	Margarine	*Fortify:* Add nutrients that may be lacking in the diet
Iodine, potassium iodide	Salt	
Iron	Grain products	
Alpha tocopherols (vitamin E)	Cereals, grain products	
Vitamin A	Milk, margarine, cereals	
Vitamin D, D_2, D_3	Milk, cereals	
Vitamin C (ascorbic acid)	Beverages, beverage mixes, processed fruit	
Purpose: To maintain product quality *Class:* Preservatives (antimicrobials)		Prevent food spoilage from bacteria, molds, fungi, and yeast; extend shelf life; or protect natural color/flavor
Ascorbic acid (vitamin C)	Fruit products, acidic foods	
Benzoic acid, sodium benzoate	Fruit products, acidic foods, margarine	
Citric acid	Acidic foods	
Lactic acid, calcium lactate	Olives, cheeses, frozen desserts, some beverages	
Parabens: butylparaben, heptylparaben, methylparaben, propylparaben	Beverages, cake-type pastries, salad dressings, relishes	
Propionic acid: calcium propionate, potassium propionate, sodium propionate	Breads and other baked goods	
Sodium diacetate	Baked goods	
Sodium erythorbate	Cured meats	
Sodium nitrate, sodium nitrite	Cured meats, fish, poultry	
Sorbic acid: calcium sorbate, potassium sorbate, sodium sorbate	Cheeses, syrups, cakes, beverages, mayonnaise, fruit products, margarine, processed meats	

(Continued)

TABLE A-15 CONTINUED

Some additives	Where you might find them	Their functions
Purpose: To maintain product quality *Class:* Preservatives (antioxidants)		Delay or prevent undesirable changes in color, flavor, or texture—enzymatic browning or discoloration due to oxidation; delay or prevent rancidity in foods with unstable oils
Ascorbic acid (vitamin C)	Processed fruits, baked goods	
BHA (butylated hydroxyanisole) BHT (butylated hydroxytoluene)	Bakery products, cereals, snack foods, fats and oils	
Citric acid	Fruits, snack foods, cereals, instant potatoes	
EDTA (ethylenediamine-tetraacetic acid)	Dressings, sauces, margarine	
Propyl gallate	Cereals, snack foods, pastries	
TBHQ (tertiary butylhydroquinone)	Snack foods, fats and oils	
Tocopherols (including vitamin E)	Oils and shortening	
Purpose: To aid in processing or preparation *Class:* Emulsifiers		Help to distribute evenly tiny particles of one liquid into another, e.g., oil and water; modify surface tension of liquid Establish a uniform dispersion or emulsion; improve homogeneity, consistency, stability, texture
Carrageenan	Chocolate milk, canned milk drinks, whipped toppings	
Lecithin	Margarine, dressings, chocolate, frozen desserts, baked goods	
Mono/diglycerides	Baked goods, peanut butter, cereals	
Polysorbate 60, 65, 80	Gelatin/pudding desserts, dressings, baked goods, nondairy creams, ice cream	
Sorbitan monostearate	Cakes, toppings, chocolate	
Dioctyl sodium sulfosuccinate	Cocoa	

TABLE A-15 CONTINUED

Some additives	Where you might find them	Their functions
Purpose: To aid in processing or preparation *Class:* Stabilizers, thickeners, texturizers		Impart body; improve consistency, texture; stabilize emulsions; affect appearance/ mouth feel of food; many are natural carbohydrates which absorb water in the food
Ammonium alginate Calcium alginate Potassium alginate Sodium alginate	Dessert-type dairy products, confections	
Carrageenan	Frozen desserts, puddings, syrups, jellies	
Cellulose derivatives	Breads, ice cream, confections, diet foods	
Flour	Sauces, gravies, canned foods	
Furcelleran	Frozen desserts, puddings, syrups	
Modified food starch	Sauces, soups, pie fillings, canned meals, snack foods	
Pectin	Jams/jellies, fruit products, frozen desserts	
Propylene glycol	Baked goods, frozen desserts, dairy spreads	
Vegetable gums: guar gum, gum arabic, gum ghatti, karaya gum, locust (carob) bean gum, tragacanth gum, larch gum (arabinogalactan)	Chewing gum, sauces, desserts, dressings, syrups, beverages, fabricated foods, cheeses, baked goods	
Purpose: To aid in processing or preparation *Class:* Leavening agents		Affect cooking results and texture; increased volume; also some flavor effects
Yeast	Breads, baked goods	
Baking powder, double-acting (sodium bicarbonate, sodium aluminum sulfate, calcium phosphate)	Quick breads, cake-type baked goods	
Baking soda (sodium bicarbonate)	Quick breads, cake-type baked goods	

(Continued)

TABLE A-15 CONTINUED

Some additives	Where you might find them	Their functions
Purpose: To aid in processing or preparation *Class:* pH control agents		Control (change/maintain) acidity or alkalinity; can affect texture, taste, wholesomeness
Acetic acid/sodium acetate	Candies, sauces, dressings, relishes	
Adipic acid	Beverage/gelatin bases, bottled drinks	
Citric acid/sodium citrate	Fruit products, candies, beverages, frozen desserts	
Fumaric acid	Dry dessert bases, confections, powdered soft drinks	
Lactic acid	Cheeses, beverages, frozen desserts	
Calcium lactate	Fruits, vegetables; dry/condensed milk	
Phosphoric acid/phosphates	Fruit products, beverages, ices/sherbets, soft drinks, oils, baked goods	
Tartaric acid/tartrates	Confections, some dairy desserts, baked goods, beverages	
Purpose: To aid in processing or preparation *Class:* Humectants		Retain moisture
Glycerine	Flaked coconut	
Glycerol monostearate	Marshmallow	
Propylene glycol	Confections, pet foods	
Sorbitol	Soft candies, gum	
Purpose: To aid in processing or preparation *Class:* Maturing and bleaching agents, dough conditioners		Accelerate the aging process (oxidation) to develop the gluten characteristics of flour; improve baking qualities
Azodicarbonamide	Cereal flour, breads	
Acetone peroxide Benzoyl peroxide Hydrogen peroxide	Flour, breads, rolls	
Calcium/potassium bromate	Breads	
Sodium stearyl fumarate	Yeast-leavened breads, instant potatoes, processed cereals	

TABLE A-15 CONTINUED

Some additives	Where you might find them	Their functions
Purpose: To aid in processing or preparation *Class:* Anti-caking agents		Help keep salts and powders free-flowing; prevent caking, lumping, or clustering of a finely powdered or crystalline substance
Calcium silicate	Table salt, baking powder, other powdered foods	
Iron ammonium citrate	Salt	
Silicon dioxide	Table salt, baking powder, other powdered foods	
Yellow prussiate of soda	Salt	
Purpose: To affect appeal characteristics *Class:* Flavor enhancers		Supplement, magnify, or modify the original taste and/or aroma of a food—*without* imparting a characteristic taste or aroma of their own
Disodium guanylate	Canned vegetables	
Disodium inosinate	Canned vegetables	
Hydrolyzed vegetable protein	Processed meats, gravy/sauce mixes, fabricated foods	
MSG (monosodium glutamate)	Oriental foods, soups, foods with animal protein	
Yeast-malt sprout extract	Gravies, sauces	
Purpose: To affect appeal characteristics *Class:* Flavors		Make foods taste better; improve natural flavor; restore flavors lost in processing
Vanilla (natural)	Baked goods	
Vanillin (synthetic)	Baked goods	
Spices and other natural seasonings and flavorings, e.g., clove, cinnamon, ginger, paprika, turmeric, anise, sage, thyme, basil	No restrictions on usage in foods— found in many products	

(Continued)

TABLE A-15 CONTINUED

Some additives	Where you might find them	Their functions
Purpose: To affect appeal characteristics Class: Natural/synthetic (N/S) colors		Increase consumer appeal and product acceptance by giving a desired, appetizing, or characteristic color; any material which imparts color when added to a food; generally *not* restricted to certain foods or food classes; may *not* be used to cover up an unwholesome food *or* be used in excessive amounts
N Annatto extract (yellow-red)	No restrictions	
N Dehydrated beets/beet powder	No restrictions	
S Ultramarine Blue	Animal feed only 0.5% by wt	
N/S Canthaxanthin (orange-red)	Limit = 30 mg/lb of food	
N Caramel (brown)	No restrictions	
N/S Beta-apo-8' carotenal (yellow-red)	Limit = 15 mg/lb of food	
N/S Beta carotene (yellow)	No restrictions	*Must* be used in accordance with FDA Good Manufacturing Practice Regulations
N Cochineal extract/carmine (red)	No restrictions	
N Toasted partially defatted cooked cottonseed flour (brown shades)	No restrictions	Synthetic color additives subject to certification; inspected and tested for impurities
S Ferrous gluconate (turns black)	Ripe olives	
N Grape skin extract (purple-red)	Beverages only	
S Iron oxide (red-brown)	Pet foods only 0.25% or less by wt	
N Fruit juice/vegetable juice	No restrictions	
N Dried algae meal (yellow)	Chicken feed only	
N Tagetes (Aztec Marigold)	Chicken feed only	
N Carrot oil (orange)	No restrictions	
N Corn endosperm (red-brown)	Chicken feed only	
N Paprika/paprika oleoresin (red-orange)	No restrictions	
N/S Riboflavin (yellow)	No restrictions	
N Saffron (orange)	No restrictions	
S Titanium dioxide (white)	Limit = 1% by wt	
N Turmeric/Turmeric oleoresins (yellow)	No restrictions	
S FD&C Blue No. 1	No restrictions	
S Citrus Red No. 2	Orange skins of mature, green, eating oranges; limit = 2 ppm	
S FD&C Red No. 3	No restrictions	
S FD&C Red No. 40	No restrictions	
S FD&C Yellow No. 5	No restrictions	

TABLE A-15 CONTINUED

Some additives	Where you might find them	Their functions
Purpose: To affect appeal characteristics *Class:* Sweeteners		Make the aroma or taste of a food more agreeable or pleasurable (i.e., sweetening)

Nutritive sweeteners
  Mannitol—sugar alcohol
  Sorbitol—sugar alcohol
	Candies, gum, confections, baked goods	

Dextrose Fructose Glucose Sucrose (table sugar)	Cereals, baked goods, candies, processed foods, processed meats	
Corn syrup/corn syrup solids Invert sugar	Cereals, baked goods, candies, processed foods, processed meats	
Nonnutritive sweeteners Saccharin	Special dietary foods, beverages	

Source: Adapted from *FDA Consumer,* HEW Publication No. (FDA) 79–2118, 79–2119, reprinted May–June 1978.

TABLE A-16 NUTRITIVE VALUES OF THE EDIBLE PART OF FOODS

Food and approximate measure		Weight, g	Food energy kcal	Food energy kJ	Protein, g	Fat (total lipids), g	Saturated (total), g	Unsaturated Oleic, g	Unsaturated Linoleic, g	Carbohydrate, g	Calcium, mg	Iron, mg	Vitamin A value, IU	Thiamin, mg	Riboflavin, mg	Niacin, mg	Ascorbic acid, mg
Milk, cream, cheese (related products)																	
Milk, cow's																	
Fluid, whole (3.5% fat)	1 cup	244	160	672	9	9	5	3	trace	12	288	0.1	350	0.08	0.42	0.1	2
Fluid, nonfat (skim)	1 cup	246	90	378	9	trace	—	—	—	13	298	0.1	10	0.10	0.44	0.2	2
Cheddar, process	1 oz	28	105	441	7	9	5	3	trace	1	219	0.3	350	trace	0.12	trace	0
Cottage, creamed	1 cup	225	240	1008	31	9	5	3	trace	7	212	0.7	380	0.07	0.56	0.2	0
Ice cream, plain, factory packed container	8 fl oz	142	295	1239	6	18	10	6	1	29	175	0.1	740	0.06	0.27	0.1	1
Yogurt, from partially skimmed milk	1 cup	246	120	504	8	4	2	1	trace	13	295	0.1	170	0.09	0.43	0.2	2
Eggs																	
Whole, without shell	1 egg	50	80	336	6	6	2	3	trace	trace	27	1.1	590	0.05	0.15	trace	0
Meat, poultry, fish, shellfish (related products)																	
Hamburger (ground beef), broiled, regular	3 oz	85	245	1029	21	17	8	8	trace	0	9	2.7	30	0.07	0.18	4.6	—
Steak, broiled, lean and fat	3 oz	85	330	1386	20	27	13	12	1	0	9	2.5	50	0.05	0.16	4.0	—
Chicken, cooked flesh only, broiled	3 oz	85	115	483	20	3	1	1	1	0	8	1.4	80	0.05	0.16	7.4	—
With bone	3.3 oz	94	155	651	25	5	1	2	1	1	9	1.3	70	0.04	0.17	11.2	—
Lamb leg roasted, lean and fat	3 oz	85	235	987	22	16	9	6	trace	0	9	1.4	—	0.13	0.23	4.7	—
Pork, fresh, trimmed to retail basis, cooked																	
Chop, thick, with bone	3.5 oz	98	260	1092	16	21	8	9	2	0	8	2.2	0	0.63	0.18	3.8	—
Bluefish, baked or broiled	3 oz	85	135	567	22	4	—	—	—	0	25	0.6	40	0.09	0.08	1.6	—
Haddock, fried	3 oz	85	140	588	17	5	1	3	—	5	34	1.0	—	0.03	0.06	2.7	2
Tuna, canned in oil	3 oz	85	170	714	24	7	—	—	—	0	7	1.6	70	0.04	0.10	10.1	—

Mature dry beans and peas, nuts, peanuts (related products)

Food	Measure																
Red beans	1 cup	256	230	966	15	1	—	—	—	42	74	4.6	trace	0.13	0.10	1.5	—
Lima beans, cooked	1 cup	192	260	1092	16	1	—	—	—	48	56	5.6	trace	0.26	0.12	1.3	trace
Cashew nuts, roasted	1 cup	135	760	3192	23	62	10	43	4	40	51	5.1	140	0.58	0.33	2.4	—
Peanut butter	1 tbsp	16	95	399	4	8	2	4	2	3	9	0.3	—	0.02	0.02	2.4	0
Peas, split, dry, cooked	1 cup	250	290	1218	20	1	—	—	—	52	28	4.2	100	0.37	0.22	2.2	—

Vegetables and vegetable products

Food	Measure																
Asparagus, canned green	6 spears	96	20	84	2	trace	—	—	—	3	18	1.8	770	0.06	0.10	0.8	14
Snap beans, green, cooked short time in small amount of water	1 cup	125	30	126	2	trace	—	—	—	7	62	0.8	680	0.08	0.11	0.6	16
Broccoli spears, cooked	1 cup	150	40	168	5	trace	—	—	—	7	132	1.2	3750	0.14	0.29	1.2	135
Carrots, cooked, diced	1 cup	145	45	189	1	trace	—	—	—	10	48	0.9	15,220	0.08	0.07	0.7	9
Peas, green, cooked	1 cup	160	115	483	9	1	—	—	—	19	37	2.9	860	0.44	0.17	3.7	33
Potato, baked, peeled after baking	1	99	90	378	3	trace	—	—	—	21	9	0.7	trace	0.10	0.04	1.7	20
Spinach, cooked	1 cup	180	40	168	5	1	—	—	—	6	167	4.0	14,580	0.13	0.25	1.0	50
Squash, winter, baked, mashed	1 cup	205	130	546	4	1	—	—	—	32	57	1.6	8610	0.10	0.27	1.4	27
Sweet potatoes, boiled, peeled after boiling	1	147	170	714	2	1	—	—	—	39	47	1.0	11,610	0.13	0.09	0.9	25
Tomato juice, canned	1 cup	242	45	189	2	trace	—	—	—	10	17	2.2	1940	0.13	0.07	1.8	39

Fruits and fruit products

Food	Measure																
Apple, raw, 2½ in diameter	1	150	70	294	trace	trace	—	—	—	18	8	0.4	50	0.04	0.02	0.1	3
Fruit cocktail, canned in heavy syrup	1 cup	256	195	819	1	1	—	—	—	50	23	1.0	360	0.04	0.03	1.1	5
Grapefruit, white, raw, medium, 4¼ in diameter	½	285	55	231	1	trace	—	—	—	14	22	0.6	10	0.05	0.02	0.2	52
Orange, raw California, naval, 2⅝ in diameter	1	180	60	252	2	trace	—	—	—	16	49	0.5	240	0.12	0.05	0.5	75
Orange juice, frozen concentrate, diluted with 3 parts water, by volume	1 cup	248	110	462	2	trace	—	—	—	27	22	0.2	500	0.21	0.03	0.8	112
Raisins, dried	1 cup	160	460	1932	4	trace	—	—	—	124	99	5.6	30	0.18	0.13	0.9	2
Strawberries, raw, capped	1 cup	149	55	231	1	1	—	—	—	13	31	1.5	90	0.04	0.10	1.0	88
Tangerine raw, medium	1	114	40	168	1	trace	—	—	—	10	34	0.3	350	0.05	0.02	0.1	26

(Continued)

TABLE A-16 CONTINUED

Food and approximate measure	Weight, g	Food energy kcal	Food energy kJ	Protein, g	Fat (total lipids), g	Fatty acids Saturated (total), g	Fatty acids Unsaturated Oleic, g	Fatty acids Unsaturated Linoleic, g	Carbohydrate, g	Calcium, mg	Iron, mg	Vitamin A value, IU	Thiamin, mg	Riboflavin, mg	Niacin, mg	Ascorbic acid, mg
Bread (related products)																
White bread, enriched	1 slice	60	252	2	1	trace	trace	trace	12	16	0.6	trace	0.06	0.04	0.5	trace
Whole-wheat bread, made with 2% nonfat dry milk	1 slice	55	231	2	1	trace	trace	trace	11	23	0.5	trace	0.06	0.03	0.7	trace
Macaroni, enriched, cooked, firm stage (8–10 min; undergoes additional cooking in a food mixture)	1 cup	190	798	6	1	—	—	—	39	14	1.4	0	0.23	0.14	1.9	0
Rice, white (fully milled or polished) cooked, common commercial	1 cup	185	777	3	trace	—	—	—	41	17	1.5	0	0.19	0.01	1.6	0
Wheat flakes, with added nutrients	1 oz	100	420	3	trace	—	—	—	23	12	1.2	0	0.18	0.04	1.4	0
Fats, oils																
Butter, pat or square (64 per pound)	1 pat	50	210	trace	6	3	2	1	trace	1	0	230	—	—	—	0
Margarine, pat or square (64 per pound)	1 pat	50	210	trace	6	1	3	1	trace	1	0	230	—	—	—	0
Corn oil	1 tbsp	125	525	0	14	1	4	7	0	0	0.	—	0	0	0	0
Mayonnaise	1 tbsp	110	462	trace	12	2	3	6	trace	3	1	40	trace	0.01	trace	—
Sugars, sweets																
Candy, fudge plain	1 oz	115	483	1	3	2	1	trace	21	22	0.3	trace	0.01	0.03	0.1	trace
Jellies	1 tbsp	55	231	trace	trace	—	—	—	14	4	0.3	trace	trace	0.01	trace	1
Sugar, cane or beet, granulated	1 tbsp	45	189	0	0	—	—	—	12	0	0	0	0	0	0	0
Beverages																
Carbonated																
Cola type	1 cup	95	399	0	0	—	—	—	24	—	—	0	0	0	0	0
Ginger ale	1 cup	70	294	0	0	—	—	—	18	—	—	0	0	0	0	0
Coffee	1 cup	2	8	trace	trace	—	—	—	trace	4	0.2	0	0	trace	0.5	0

Source: U.S. Department of Agriculture, *Nutritive Values of Food,* Home and Garden Bulletin No. 72, 1971.

TABLE A-17 NUTRIENT CONTENT OF TYPICAL FAST FOODS

Food	Wt (g)	Energy kcal	Energy kJ	Pro (g)	CHO (g)	Fat (g)	Chol (mg)	Vit A (IU)	Vit B₁ (mg)	Vit B₂ (mg)	Nia (mg)	Vit C (mg)	Ca (mg)	Fe (mg)	Na (mg)
McDonald's															
Big Mac	187	541	2218	26	39	31	75	327	0.35	0.37	8.2	2.4	175	4.3	962
Filet O' Fish	131	402	1648	15	34	23	43	152	0.28	0.28	3.9	4.2	105	1.8	709
French Fries	69	211	865	3	26	11	10	<52	0.15	0.03	2.9	11.0	10	0.5	113
Hamburger	99	257	1054	13	30	9	26	231	0.23	0.23	5.1	1.8	63	3.0	526
Quarter Pounder with Cheese	193	518	2124	31	34	29	96	683	0.35	0.59	15.1	2.9	251	4.6	1209
Cherry Pie	92	298	1222	2	33	18	14	213	0.02	0.03	0.4	1.3	12	0.4	456
Chocolate Shake	289	364	1492	11	60	9	29	318	0.12	0.89	0.8	<2.9	338	1.0	329
Pizza Hut															
Thin 'n' Crispy															
Cheese (½ 10-in pizza)	NA	450	2009	25	54	15	NA	750	0.30	0.51	5.0	<1.2	450	4.5	NA
Supreme (½ 10-in pizza)	NA	510	2091	27	51	21	NA	1250	0.38	0.68	7.0	2.4	350	7.2	NA
Thick 'n' Chewy															
Beef (topping mixture with many ingredients)	NA	620	2542	38	73	20	NA	750	0.68	0.60	8.0	<1.2	400	7.2	NA
Long John Silver's															
Breaded Oysters, 6 pc	NA	460	1886	14	58	19	NA	NA	NA	NA	NA	NA	NA	NA	NA
Chicken Planks, 4 pc	NA	458	1878	27	35	23	NA	NA	NA	NA	NA	NA	NA	NA	NA
Corn on Cob, 1 pc	NA	174	713	5	29	4	NA	NA	NA	NA	NA	NA	NA	NA	NA
Hush Puppies, 3 pc	NA	153	627	1	20	7	NA	NA	NA	NA	NA	NA	NA	NA	NA
Treasure Chest—2 pc fish, 2 peg legs	NA	467	1915	25	27	29	NA	NA	NA	NA	NA	NA	NA	NA	NA
Burger King															
Whopper	NA	606	2485	29	51	32	NA	641	0.02	0.03	5.20	13.0	37	6.0	909
Vanilla Shake	NA	332	1361	11	50	11	NA	9	0.01	0.05	0.27	tr	390	0.2	159
Hot Dog	NA	291	1193	11	23	17	NA	0	0.04	0.02	2.00	0	40	2.0	841
Burger Chef															
Double Cheeseburger	145	434	1779	24	24	26	NA	430	0.25	0.34	4.8	1	246	3.1	691
Mariner Platter	373	680	2788	32	85	24	NA	448	0.37	0.40	7.3	24	137	4.7	882

(Continued)

TABLE A-17 CONTINUED

Food	Wt (g)	Energy kcal	Energy kJ	Pro (g)	CHO (g)	Fat (g)	Chol (mg)	Vit A (IU)	Vit B₁ (mg)	Vit B₂ (mg)	Nia (mg)	Vit C (mg)	Ca (mg)	Fe (mg)	Na (mg)
Burger Chef (continued)															
Rancher Platter	316	640	2624	30	44	38	NA	367	0.30	0.37	8.7	24	57	5.1	444
Skipper's Treat	179	604	2476	21	47	37	NA	303	0.29	0.30	3.7	1	201	2.5	783
Taco Bell															
Beef Burrito	184	466	1911	30	37	21	NA	1675	0.30	0.39	7.0	15.2	83	4.6	327
Taco	83	186	763	15	14	8	NA	120	0.09	0.16	2.9	0.2	120	2.5	79
Tostada	138	179	734	9	25	6	NA	3152	0.18	0.15	0.8	9.7	191	2.3	101
Dairy Queen															
Big Brazier Deluxe	213	470	1927	28	36	24	NA	NA	0.34	0.37	9.6	<2.5	111	5.2	920
Brazier Cheese Dog	113	330	1353	15	24	19	NA	NA	NA	0.18	3.3	NA	168	1.6	NA
Brazier Chili Dog	128	330	1353	13	25	20	NA	NA	0.15	0.23	3.9	11.0	86	2.0	939
Brazier Onion Rings	85	300	1230	6	33	17	NA	tr	0.09	tr	0.4	2.4	20	0.4	NA
Banana Split	383	540	2214	10	91	15	NA	750	0.60	0.60	0.8	18.0	350	1.8	NA
Chocolate Dip Cone med	156	300	1230	7	40	13	NA	300	0.09	0.34	tr	tr	200	0.4	NA
Mr. Misty Float	404	440	2050	6	85	8	NA	120	0.12	0.17	tr	tr	200	tr	NA
Kentucky Fried Chicken															
Original Recipe Dinner (mashed potatoes and gravy, cole slaw, roll, and 3 pieces of chicken)	425	830	3403	52	56	46	285	750	0.38	0.56	15.0	27.0	150	4.5	2285
Beverages															
Whole milk, 8 oz	244	159	652	9	12	9	27	342	0.07	0.41	0.2	2.4	188	tr	122
Coca-Cola, 8 oz	246	96	394	0	24	0	NA	NA	NA	NA	NA	NA	NA	NA	20
Tab, 8 oz	237	tr	tr	0	tr	0	NA	NA	NA	NA	NA	NA	NA	NA	30
Orange juice, 6 oz	183	82	336	1	20	tr	NA	366	0.17	0.02	0.6	82.4	17	0.2	2
Chocolate milk, 8 oz	250	213	873	9	28	9	NA	330	0.08	0.40	0.3	3.0	278	0.5	118
Sprite, 8 oz	245	95	390	0	24	0	NA	NA	NA	NA	NA	NA	NA	NA	42
Coffee, 6 oz	180	2	8	tr	tr	tr	NA	0	0	tr	0.5	0	4	0.2	2
Tea, 6 oz	180	2	8	tr	NA	tr	NA	0	0	0.04	0.1	1	5	0.2	NA

Source: "Perspectives on Fast Foods," *Dietetic Currents,* September–October 1978, pp. 24–27.
Note: Nutrient composition of these foods changes continually; for up-to-date information, contact the company.

TABLE A-18   AMINO ACID CONTENT OF FOODS PER 100 g EDIBLE PORTION

Food item	Nitrogen conversion factor	Protein content, percent	Phenylalanine, mg	Isoleucine, mg	Leucine, mg	Valine, mg	Sulfur-containing			Tryptophan, mg	Threonine, mg	Lysine, mg	Tyrosine, mg	Arginine, mg	Histidine, mg
							Methionine, mg	Cystine, mg	Total, mg						
Milk, milk products															
Fluid, whole	6.38	3.5	170	223	344	240	86	31	117	49	161	272	178	128	92
Human milk	6.38	1.4	48	68	100	70	25	22	47	18	50	73	61	45	22
Isomil	6.38		105	107	153	92	29	—	29	19	69	91	—	—	53
Cheese, cheddar, processed	6.38	23.2	1244	1563	2262	1665	604	131	735	316	862	1702	1109	847	756
Eggs, whole															
Fresh or stored	6.25	12.8	739	850	1126	950	401	299	700	211	637	819	551	840	307
Meat, poultry, fish															
Hamburger, regular	6.25	16.0	658	837	1311	888	397	202	599	187	707	1398	543	1032	556
Rib roast	6.25	17.4	715	910	1425	590	432	220	652	203	768	1520	590	1122	604
Lamb leg	6.25	18.0	732	933	1394	887	432	236	668	233	824	1457	625	1172	501
Pork loin	6.25	16.4	646	842	1207	853	409	192	601	213	761	1346	585	1005	567
Chicken, fryer	6.25	20.6	811	1088	1490	1012	537	277	814	250	877	1810	725	1302	593
Haddock, raw	6.25	18.2	676	923	1374	930	530	245	775	181	789	1596	492	1025	
Legumes, dry, and nuts															
Bean, red kidney, canned	6.25	5.7	315	324	490	346	57	57	114	53	247	423	220	343	162
Peanuts	5.46	26.9	1557	1266	1872	1532	271	463	734	340	828	1099	1104	3296	749
Grains and grain products															
Bread, white, 4% milk solids	5.70	8.5	465	429	668	435	142	200	342	91	282	225	243	340	192
Rice, white or converted	5.95	7.6	382	356	655	531	137	103	240	82	298	300	347	438	128
Vegetables															
Beans, lima, canned	6.25	3.8	197	233	306	246	41	42	83	49	171	240	131	230	125

Sources:

1 M. L. Orr and B. K. Watt, *Amino Acid Content of Foods,* Home Economics Research Report No. 4, U.S. Dept. of Agriculture, Washington, D.C., 1957.

2 S. J. Fomon, *Infant Nutrition,* 2d ed., W. B. Saunders Company, Philadelphia, 1974, p. 362.

3 *Handbook of Infant Formulas,* 6th ed., J. B. Roerig Division, Charles Pfizer & Co., Inc., New York, 1969.

APPENDIX B

SPORTS MEDICINE POSITION STATEMENTS

AMERICAN COLLEGE OF SPORTS MEDICINE

**Position Statement on:
Prevention of Heat Injuries
during Distance Running***

The Purpose of this Position Statement is:

a To alert local, national and international sponsors of distance running events of the health hazards of heat injury during distance running and

b To inform said sponsors of injury preventative actions that may reduce the frequency of this type of injury.

The recommendations address only the manner in which distance running sports activities may be conducted to further reduce incidence of heat injury among normal athletes conditioned to participate in distance running. The recommendations are advisory only.

Recommendations concerning the ingested quantity and content of fluid are merely a partial preventative to heat injury. The physiology of each individual athlete varies: strict compliance with these recommendations and the current rules governing distance running may not reduce the incidence of heat injuries among those so inclined to such injury.

Based on research findings and current rules governing distance running competition, it is the position of the American College of Sports Medicine that:

1 Distance races (>16 km or 10 miles) should not be conducted when the wet bulb temperature—globe temperature exceeds 28°C (82.4°F).

2 During periods of the year, when the daylight dry bulb temperature often exceeds 27°C (80°F), distance races should be conducted before 9:00 A.M. or after 4:00 P.M.

*Reprinted with permission of the American College of Sports Medicine, *Medicine and Science in Sports*, **7**:vii, 1975.

3 It is the responsibility of the race sponsors to provide fluids which contain small amounts of sugar (less than 2.5 g glucose per 100 mL of water) and electrolytes (less than 10 meq sodium and 5 meq potassium per liter of solution).

4 Runners should be encouraged to frequently ingest fluids during competition and to consume 400–500 mL (13–17 oz) of fluid 10–15 minutes before competition.

5 Rules prohibiting the administration of fluids during the first 10 kilometers (6.2 miles) of a marathon race should be amended to permit fluid ingestion at frequent intervals along the race course. In light of the high sweat rates and body temperatures during distance running in the heat, race sponsors should provide "water stations" at 3–4 kilometer (2–2.5 mile) intervals for all races of 16 kilometers (10 miles) or more.

6 Runners should be instructed in how to recognize the early warning symptoms that precede heat injury. Recognition of symptoms, cessation of running, and proper treatment can prevent heat injury. Early warning symptoms include the following: piloerection on chest and upper arms, chilling, throbbing pressure in the head, unsteadiness, nausea, and dry skin.

7 Race sponsors should make prior arrangements with medical personnel for the care of cases of heat injury. Responsible and informed personnel should supervise each "feeding station." Organizational personnel should reserve the right to stop runners who exhibit clear signs of heat stroke or heat exhaustion.

It is the position of the American College of Sports Medicine that policies established by local, national, and international sponsors of distance running events should adhere to these guidelines. Failure to adhere to these guidelines may jeopardize the health of competitors through heat injury.

AMERICAN COLLEGE OF SPORTS MEDICINE

Position Statement on:
The Recommended Quantity and Quality of Exercise for Developing and Maintaining Fitness in Healthy Adults*

Increasing numbers of persons are becoming involved in endurance training activities, and thus, the need for guidelines for exercise prescription is apparent.

Based on the existing evidence concerning exercise prescription for healthy adults and the need for guidelines, the American College of Sports Medicine makes the following recommendations for the quantity and quality of training for developing and maintaining cardiorespiratory fitness and body composition in the healthy adult:

1 Frequency of training: 3 to 5 days per week.

2 Intensity of training: 60% to 90% of maximum heart rate reserve or, 50% to 85% of maximum oxygen uptake ($\dot{V}O_{2max}$).

3 Duration of training: 15 to 60 minutes of continuous aerobic activity. Duration is dependent on the intensity of the activity, thus lower intensity activity should be conducted over a longer period of time. Because of the importance of the "total fitness" effect and the fact that it is more readily attained in longer duration programs, and because of the potential hazards and compliance problems associated with high intensity activity, lower to moderate intensity activity of longer duration is recommended for the non-athletic adult.

4 Mode of activity: Any activity that uses large muscle groups, that can be maintained continuously, and is rhythmical and aerobic in nature, e.g., running-jogging, walking-hiking, swimming, skating, bicycling, rowing, cross-country skiing, rope skipping, and various endurance game activities.

*Medicine and Science in Sports, 10, Fall 1978. Reprinted with permission of the American College of Sports Medicine.

Rationale and Research Background

The questions, "How much exercise is enough and what type of exercise is best for developing and maintaining fitness?" are frequently asked. It is recognized that the term *physical fitness* is composed of a wide variety of variables included in the broad categories of cardiovascular-respiratory fitness, physique and structure, motor function, and many histochemical and biochemical factors. It is also recognized that the adaptative response to training is complex and includes peripheral, central, structural, and functional factors. Although many such variables and their adaptative response to training have been documented, the lack of sufficient in-depth and comparative data relative to frequency, intensity, and duration of training make them inadequate to use as comparative models. Thus, in respect to the above questions, fitness will be limited to changes in $\dot{V}O_{2max}$, total body mass, fat weight (FW), and lean body weight (LBW) factors.

Exercise prescription is based upon the frequency, intensity, and duration of training, the mode of activity (aerobic in nature, e.g., listed under No. 4 above), and the initial level of fitness. In evaluating these factors, the following observations have been derived from studies conducted with endurance training programs.

1 Improvement in $\dot{V}O_{2max}$ is directly related to frequency, intensity, and duration of training. Depending upon the quantity and quality of training, improvement in $\dot{V}O_{2max}$ ranges from 5% to 25%. Although changes in $\dot{V}O_{2max}$ greater than 25% have been shown, they are usually associated with large total body mass and FW loss, or a low initial level of fitness. Also, as a result of leg fatigue or a lack of motivation, persons with low initial fitness may have spuriously low initial $\dot{V}O_{2max}$ values.

2 The amount of improvement in $\dot{V}O_{2max}$ tends to plateau when frequency of training is increased above 3 days per week. For the non-athlete, there is not enough information available at this time to speculate on the value of added improvement found in programs that are conducted more than 5 days per week. Participation of less than two days per week does not show adequate change in $\dot{V}O_{2max}$.

3 Total body mass and FW are generally reduced with endurance training programs, while LBW remains constant or increases slightly. Programs that are conducted at least 3 days per week, of at least 20 minutes duration and of sufficient intensity and duration to expend approximately 300 kilocalories (kcal) per exercise session are suggested as a threshold level for total body mass and FW loss. An expenditure of 200 kcal per session has also been shown to be useful in weight reduction if the exercise frequency is at least 4 days per week. Programs with less participation generally show little or no change in body composition. Significant increases in $\dot{V}O_{2max}$ have been shown with 10 to 15 minutes of high intensity training thus, if total body mass and FW reduction is not a consideration, then short duration, high intensity programs may be recommended for healthy, low risk (cardiovascular disease) persons.

4 The minimal threshold level for improvement in $\dot{V}O_{2max}$ is approximately 60% of the maximum heart rate reserve (50% of $\dot{V}O_{2max}$). Maximum heart rate reserve represents the percent difference between resting and maximum heart rate, added to the resting heart rate. The technique as described by Karvonen, Kentala, and Mustala, was validated by Davis and Convertino, and represents a heart rate of approximately 130 to 135 beats/minute for young persons. As a result of the aging curve for maximum heart rate, the absolute heart rate value (threshold level) is inversely related to age, and can be as low as 110 to 120 beats/minute for older persons. Initial level of fitness is another important consideration in prescribing exercise. The person with a low fitness level can get a significant training effect with a sustained

training heart rate as low as 110 to 120 beats/minute, while persons of higher fitness levels need a higher threshold of stimulation.

5 Intensity and duration of training are interrelated with the total amount of work accomplished being an important factor in improvement in fitness. Although more comprehensive inquiry is necessary, present evidence suggests that when exercise is performed above the minimal threshold of intensity, the total amount of work accomplished is the important factor in fitness development and maintenance. That is, improvement will be similar for activities performed at a lower intensity–longer duration compared to higher intensity–shorter duration if the total energy costs of the activities are equal.

   If frequency, intensity, and duration of training are similar (total kcal expenditure), the training result appears to be independent of the mode of aerobic activity. Therefore, a variety of endurance activities, e.g., listed above, may be used to derive the same training effect.

6 In order to maintain the training effect, exercise must be continued on a regular basis. A significant reduction in working capacity occurs after 2 weeks of detraining with participants returning to near pretraining levels of fitness after 10 weeks to 8 months of detraining. Fifty percent reduction in improvement of cardiorespiratory fitness has been shown after 4–12 weeks of detraining. More investigation is necessary to evaluate the rate of increase and decrease of fitness with varying training loads and reduction in training in relation to level of fitness, age, and length of time in training. Also, more information is needed to better identify the minimal level of work necessary to maintain fitness.

7 Endurance activities that require running and jumping generally cause significantly more debilitating injuries to beginning ex-

ercisers than other non-weight-bearing activities. One study showed that beginning joggers had increased foot, leg, and knee injuries when training was performed more than 3 days per week and longer than 30 minutes duration per exercise session. Thus, caution should be taken when recommending the type of activity and exercise prescription for the beginning exerciser. Also, the increase of orthopedic injuries as related to overuse (marathon training) with chronic jogger-runners is apparent. Thus, there is a need for more inquiry into the effect that different types of activities and the quantity and quality of training has on short-term and long-term participation.

8 Most of the information concerning training described in this position statement has been conducted on men. The lack of information on women is apparent, but the available evidence indicates that women tend to adapt to endurance training in the same manner as men.

9 Age in itself does not appear to be a deterrent to endurance training. Although some earlier studies showed a lower training effect with middle-aged or elderly participants, more recent study shows the relative change in $\dot{V}O_{2max}$ to be similar to younger age groups. Although more investigation is necessary concerning the rate of improvement in $\dot{V}O_{2max}$ with age, at present it appears that elderly participants need longer periods of time to adapt to training. Earlier studies showing moderate to no improvement in $\dot{V}O_{2max}$ were conducted over a short time-span or exercise was conducted at a moderate to low kcal expenditure, thus making the interpretation of the results difficult.

   Although $\dot{V}O_{2max}$ decreases with age, and total body mass and FW increase with age, evidence suggests that this trend can be altered with endurance training. Also, 5 to 10 year follow-up studies where participants continued their training at a similar level showed maintenance of fitness. A study of older competitive runners showed decreases in $\dot{V}O_{2max}$ from the fourth to seventh decade of life, but also showed reductions in their training load. More inquiry into the relationship of long-term training (quantity and quality) for both competitors and noncompetitors and physiological function with increasing age is necessary before more definitive statements can be made.

10   An activity such as weight training should not be considered as a means of training for developing $\dot{V}O_{2max}$, but has significant value for increasing muscular strength and endurance, and LBW. Recent studies evaluating circuit weight training (weight training conducted almost continuously with moderate weights, using 10 to 15 repetitions per exercise session with 15 to 30 seconds rest between bouts of activity) showed little to no improvements in working capacity and VO_{2max}.

Despite an abundance of information available concerning the training of the human organism, the lack of standardization of testing protocols and procedures, methodology in relation to training procedures and experimental design, a preciseness in the documentation and reporting of the quantity and quality of training prescribed, make interpretation difficult. Interpretation and comparison of results are also dependent on the initial level of fitness, length of time of the training experiment, and specificity of the testing and training. For example, data from training studies using subjects with varied levels $\dot{V}O_{2max}$, total body mass, and FW have found changes to occur in relation to their initial values, i.e., the lower the intial $\dot{V}O_{2max}$ the larger the percent of improvement found, and the higher the FW the greater the reduction.

Also, data evaluating trainability with age, comparison of the different magnitudes and quantities of effort, and comparison of the trainability of men and women may have been influenced by the initial fitness levels.

In view of the fact that improvement in the fitness variables discussed in this position statement continue over many months of training, it is reasonable to believe that short-term studies conducted over a few weeks have certain limitations. Middle-aged sedentary and older participants may take several weeks to adapt to the initial rigors of training, and thus need a longer adaptation period to get the full benefit from a program. How long a training experiment should be conducted is difficult to determine, but 15 to 20 weeks may be a good minimum standard. For example, two investigations conducted with middle-aged men who jogged either 2 or 4 days per week found both groups to improve in $\dot{V}O_{2max}$. Mid-test results of the 16 and 20 week programs showed no difference between groups, while subsequent final testing found the 4 day per week group to improve significantly more. In a similar study with young college men, no differences in $\dot{V}O_{2max}$ were found among groups after 7 and 13 weeks of interval training. These latter findings and those of other investigators point to the limitations in interpreting results from investigators conducted over a short time-span.

In summary, frequency, intensity and duration of training have been found to be effective stimuli for producing a training effect. In general, the lower the stimuli, the lower the training effect, and the greater the stimuli, the greater the effect. It has also been shown that endurance training less than two days per week, less than 50% of maximum oxygen uptake, and less than 10 minutes per day is inadequate for developing and maintaining fitness for healthy adults.

INDEX

Page numbers in *italic* indicate illustrations or tables.

Abbreviations, common medical, *734–735*
Abetalipoproteinemia, 78
Absorption, 174–175, 177–179
   of calcium, 130–131
   of carbohydrate, 64–65, 178, 291
   of cholesterol, 81, 178
   of copper, 146
   of fat, 81, *82*
   of glycerides, 81
   by intestinal epithelium, *176*
   of iodine, 144
   of iron, 139, *141*
   in large intestine, 177
   of lipid, 178
   of magnesium, 137
   of manganese, 148
   of minerals, 179
   of phospholipids, 81
   of phosphorus, 135
   of protein, 177–178
   sites of, *179*
   in small intestine, 175, 177
   in stomach, 174
   of trace elements, *128*
   of vitamins, 179
   of zinc, 147–148
Acetyl CoA, 111, 182
Acetylcholine, 596
Achalasia, 464–465
Acid-base balance, 163, 503
   disturbances in, 164
Acidosis:
   metabolic, 164–165
   respiratory, 164
Acne, 280
Acromegaly, *544*
ACTH (adrenocorticotropic hormone), *83*, 541–*543*, 654
Active transport, 65, 157, 177
Activity coefficients, 106
Acute renal failure, 518–520
   causes of, 518
   diuretic phase of, 520
   nutritional considerations in, 518–520
   physiological sequelae of, *518*
   total parenteral nutrition in, 520
Acyl carrier protein, 111
Acylglycerol, 78
Addisonian crisis, 542
Addison's disease, 542
Additives, 14–15, *739–745*
Adenosine triphosphate (ATP), 50, 129–130, 135, 181, 194
Adequate diet, 13
ADH (antidiuretic hormone), *158*–159, *543*, 656
Adipose cell theory of obesity, 572–573
Adipose tissue, 64, *246–247*
Adolescence, 244
   changes during, 245
   nutrition during, 279–280, 282
   nutritional assessment levels for, *376*
   and pregnancy, 316
   protein allowances during, 45

Adrenal cortex, 158
Adrenal corticosteroids, *400, 701*
Adrenals, 540–543
Adrenocorticotropic hormone (ACTH), *83*, 541–*543*, 654
Adult hypoglycemia, 565
Adults:
  nutritional assessment levels for, *377*
  protein allowances for, 44–45
  (*See also* Older adult; *specific categories and conditions of adults*)
Aerobic exercises, 192
Aerobic metabolism, 194
Aerobics, 192
Afferent neurons, 595
Aflatoxins, 693
Agar, 62
Age:
  and basal metabolic rate, 183
  and protein needs, 203
Aging, physiological and psychological aspects of, 330–331
Agricultural Extension Service, *356*
Albumin, 420, *659*
Alcohol:
  and diabetes, 562
  and hyperlipidemia, 439
  and liver disease, 491
  and preevent meals, 206
  and pregnancy, 317
Alcoholic beverages, 19
Aldosterone, 159, 160, 504, 540
Alginates, 62
Alkalosis:
  metabolic, 165
  respiratory, 164
Alkalotic tetany, 540
Alkylating agents, side effects of, *700*
Allergens, 419–421
Allergic response and diet, 418–428
Allergy (*see* Food allergy)
Allergy diets, sources of recipes for, *427*
Allopurinol, *401*
Alpha amino acids, 40
Alpha cells, 545
Alpha-keto amino acids, 50
Alpha lipoprotein (HDL), 434
Alum, 15
Amide linkage, 77
Amino acids, 40, 50
  alpha, 40
  alpha-keto, 50
  carboxyl group of, 40, 42
  classification of, 40, 42, *181*
  essential, 43–44
  in foods, *751*
  glycogenic, *181*, 182
  inborn errors of metabolism of, *632–635*
  ketogenic, *181*, 182
  nonessential, 43–44
  placental transport of, 290

Amino acids (*Cont.*):
  sulfur in, 136
Amino group, 40
Aminopeptidase, 50
Ammonia and premature infant, 295–296
Amphetamines, 582
α-Amylase, 61
Anabolic steroids, 203
Anabolism, 50, 182, *183*
Anaerobic exercises, 192
Anaerobic metabolism, 194
Anemia:
  iron-deficiency (*see* Iron-deficiency anemia)
  microcytic hypochromic, 140
  sports, 203–204
Angina pectoris, 432, 433
Angiotensin, 159, 160, 504
Angiotensinogen, 159, 504
Anions, 156
  concentrations of, *156*
  (*See also* Chloride; Phosphorus)
Anorexia of cancer, 695
Anorexia nervosa, 214, 219, 221, 598–599
Anthropometric measurements, 186
Antibiotics, side effects of, *700*
Antibodies, 418
  and protein absorption, 177
Antibody response, 409–410
Anticoagulants, 432
Antidepressants, *400*
Antidiuretic hormone (ADH), *158*–159, *543*, 656
Antigen, 418
Antimetabolites, side effects of, *700*
Antineoplastic agents, 699
  side effects of, *700–701*
"Antisterility vitamin," 97
Aorta, 430
  coarctation of, *452*
Aortic stenosis, *452*
Apoferritin, 139
Arabinose, 59
Arachidonic acid, 75
Arm circumference, 252
Arteries, 430
  atherosclerosis of, 431–432
Arthritis:
  juvenile, 567
  rheumatoid, 567
Ascorbic acid (vitamin C), 14, 100–103, *117*
  chemistry and properties of, 100
  clinical deficiency of, 102–103
  dietary allowance and sources of, 102
  functions of, 101–102
  history and discovery of, 100
  metabolism of, 100–101
  requirements of, during nonstress and stress, *658*
  and tooth maintenance, 365

Ascorbic acid (vitamin C)(*Cont.*):
  toxicity of, 103
Aspergillus flavus, 693
Associative neurons, 595
Asymmetrical tonic neck reflex, 610–*611, 613*
Asymptomatic diabetes, 548
Atheromatous plaques, 431–432
Atherosclerosis, 431–*432*
  risk factors in, 433–*434*
Athletic performance, nutrition and, 191–207
Atkins diet, 70, *346*
ATP (adenosine triphosphate), 50, 129–130, 135, 181, 194
Attachment process, 229–230
Autonomic nervous system, 595
Autonomy, 234–235
Aversive stimuli, 219
Axons, 595
Azathioprine, *529*
Azotemia, 520–521

B-cells (bursa cells), 409
Baby foods, 263–264
  energy and protein values of, *264*
  homemade versus commercially prepared, 264–265
  sodium content of, *456*
Bacteria:
  contamination by, in total parenteral nutrition, 676
  enteric, 172–173
  in plaque, 366
Balance mechanisms:
  of chloride, 162
  of potassium, 161
  of sodium, 159–160
Banting, F. G., 545
Basal metabolic rate (BMR), 182–185
  conditions altering, *184*
Behavior:
  guiding, 220–221
  target, 219
Behavior modification, 9–10, 580
  application of, 221–222
  common concerns of, 221–222
  diet and, 218–222, 580–581
  research in, 221
Benemid (Probenecid), *401*, 566
Beniflex feeder, *621*, 622–623
Benign tumors, 694
  characteristics of, *695*
Beriberi, 103–105
  "dry," 105
  "wet," 105
Best, C. H., 545
Beta cells, 545
Beta lipoprotein (LDL), 178, 434
Beverages, 19
Beverly Hills medical diet, *346–347*
Biguanides, 556

Bile, 171
Bile salts, 81, 178
  and calcium absorption, 131
Biliary disease, tests for, *490*
Biological value (BV):
  of foods, *48*
  of protein, 46, *47*
Biotin, 111–112, 117
  chemistry and properties of, 112
  clinical deficiency of, 112
  dietary allowance and sources of, 112
  functions of, 112
  history and discovery of, 111–112
  metabolism of, 112
  sulfur in, 136
Birth size, 244
Biting reflex, 612, *613*, 614–615
Bitot's spot, 93
Blacks, food patterns of, 344
Blacktongue, 109
Bland diet, 466, 468
  progressive, *469–471*
Blood clotting, vitamin K and, 99
Blood clotting factors, 99
Blood coagulation, 130
Blood glucose levels, 65
  disease states altering, *69*
  physiological conditions altering, *69*
Blood hemoglobin, *659*
Blood plasma, lipid content of, *85–87*
Blood pressure by age group, *447*
  (*See also* Hypertension)
Blood value determinations, guide for, *659*
BMR (basal metabolic rate), 182–*184*, 185
Body composition, 185–186, 576–577
  factors affecting, 186
  measurements for estimating, 186
Body density, 186
Body fat, 250–252
Body fluid compartments, *154*
Body fluids:
  and gastrointestinal tract, 159
  and kidneys, 158–159
  and lungs and skin, 159
  and membranes, 157–158
Body growth, periods of, 242, *243*, 244–247
Body size and basal metabolic rate, 183–184
Body surface area, nomograms for estimating, *713*
Body water, 153–159
  distribution of, 153–154
  functions of, 153
  influences on, 155–159
Bone, 127, 129
Bone disease and renal failure, 514–*515*
Bone formation, 129
Bone marrow transplantation, 701
Bone mineralization and vitamin D, 95
Borderline diabetes, 548

Bottle caries syndrome, 370–371, 373
Bottle feeding, 254–255
Botulism, *738*
Bowel resection, 487
Brain function:
  diet and, 596–597
  emotions and, 597–599
Brain growth, 245–246
Bran, fiber content of, 63
Breast feeding, 254–255, 322, *323*, 324
  of child with cleft lip and palate, 623
  infant's response to, 234, 235
  technique of, 326, *328*
Breast milk, 256
  compared with infant formulas and
    cow's milk, *258–261*
Breath hydrogen test, 478
Breathing of handicapped child, 616
Breck feeder, *621–622*
  placement of, *622*
Brush border, 177
Buffer, 163
Buffer systems, *163*–164
Bulimarexia, 599
Bulk flow, 175
Burn unit, 685
Burns:
  classification of, 682
  dietary regimens for patients with, 685
  emotional support for patients with, 686
  fluid and electrolyte replacement and, 683
  fluid requirement formulas and, *684*
  full-thickness, 682
  intermediate, 682
  large, 682
  metabolic sequelae of, 683
  nutritional care and, 682–686
  partial-thickness, 682
  prevention of infection in patients with, 683, 685
  severe, 682
  small, 682
  urine monitoring of patients with, *684*
Bursa cells (B-cells), 409
Bypass surgery:
  gastric, 584–585
  intestinal, 583–584
  jejunoileal, 584

Cachexia, *664, 665*, 696
Caffeine:
  in preevent meal, 206–207
  and pregnancy, 317
Calcitonin, 131
Calcium, 127–135
  absorption and utilization of, 130–131
  circulating, 129–130
  clinical applications of, 133, 135
  dietary allowance and sources of, 132
  excretion of, 131–132

Calcium (*Cont.*):
  fecal levels of, conditions altering, *135*
  in foods, *133*
  functions of, 129–130
  magnesium and, 137
  parathyroid and, 540
  in renal calculi, 531–532
  and renal failure, 514–516
  requirements of: during lactation, 326
    for older adult, 332
    during pregnancy, 315
    for premature infant, 298–299
  serum levels of, conditions altering, *134*
  supplementation with, 132–133
  and tooth development, 364
  urinary levels of, conditions altering, *134*
  and vitamin D, 95
Calcium phosphate, 127
Calcium/phosphorus ratio, 131, 135–136
Calcium supplements, *541*
Calculi, 369, 370, 531–532
Calorie, 179
Cancer:
  ascorbic acid and, 102
  bone marrow transplantation
    treatment of, 701
  chemotherapy for (*see* Chemotherapy
    in cancer treatment)
  children and, 702–704, 709
  clinical signs and diagnosis of, 695
  of colon and breast, 85
  dietary factors and, 691–694
  etiology of, 691–694
  factors predisposing to, *692*
  immunotherapy for, 699, 701
  nutrition and, 691–709
  nutritional support in children with, 703–704
  pathophysiology of, 694
  radiation therapy for, 696–698
  side effects of, 695–696
Cancer surgery, 698–699
  nutritional complications of, *698*
Cancer therapy, 696–701
  dietary guidelines for, *705–707*
  side effects of, 696
  (*See also specific therapy*)
Capillaries, 430
Carageen, 62
Carbohydrate loading, 69, 196–198
Carbohydrate metabolism:
  hormonal control of, *67*
  inborn errors of, *634–635*
Carbohydrates, 57–71
  absorption of, 64–65, 178, 291
  catabolism of, 181
  clinical applications of, 68–70
  definition of, 57–58
  and dental caries, 69, 366, 367
  and diabetes, 561, *562*
  dietary requirements of, 67

Carbohydrates (*Cont.*):
  dietary sources of, 67–68
  digestion of, *64*
  enzymes for degradation of, *172*
  and exercise, 69, 196–198
  in foods, *68*
  functions of, 63–64
  and hyperlipidemia, 439
  and malabsorption syndrome, 70
  metabolism of, 65–66
  in preevent meals, 205
  and renal failure, 508
  in replacement fluids, 201
  requirements of, for older adult, 332
  and thyroid, 536
  use of, 63–66
  and weight reduction, 70
Carbonic acid–sodium bicarbonate
    system, 164
Carboxyl group, 40, 42
Carboxypeptidase, 50
Carcinomas, 694
  (*See also entries beginning with term:*
      Cancer)
Cardiac function and calcium, 130
Cardiovascular disease, magnesium
    and, 137
Cardiovascular function and thyroid,
    536
Cardiovascular system, 430, *431*,
    432–458
  (*See also entries beginning with term:*
      Heart)
Caries (*see* Dental caries)
Carotene, 91, 92
  in blood plasma, *85*
Carotenoids in blood plasma, *86–87*
Carrier-mediated diffusion, 177
Casal's necklace, 110
Casec, 301
Castle, William B., 114
Catabolism, 50–51, 180–182
  of carbohydrate, 181
  of fat, 182
  of nutrients, *183*
  of protein, 181–182
Catch-up growth, 241–242, 289
Catecholamines, 654, 683
  effects of, 656
Cations, *156*
  (*See also* Calcium; Magnesium;
      Potassium; Sodium)
Celiac sprue, 473–474, 476
  diet for, *475–476*
Cell cycle, 699
Cell-mediated immunity, 408–409
Cell membrane permeability, 130
Cellular membranes, phospholipids in,
    135
Cellulose, 62
Cementum, 362
Central nervous system, 594
  thyroid and, 536

Central nervous system (*Cont.*):
  tumors of, 702
Cephalins, 80
Cerebral palsy, 606–608
Cerebrocuprein, 146
Cerebrosides, 80
Cerebrovascular disease, 433
Ceruloplasmin, 146
CF (*see* Cystic fibrosis)
Chalasia, 235
Cheilosis, 106
Chemical diabetes, 548
Chemotherapy in cancer treatment, 699,
    711–712
  side effects of, *700–701*
Chief cells, 170
Child Care Food Program, *353, 736*
Childhood, 244
Childhood nephrosis, 530
Children:
  and cancer, 702–704, 709
  defined formula diets for, 681
  with developmental disabilities (*see*
      Developmental difficulties,
      children with)
  diabetes in, 549, *550*, 552, 554, 555
  energy-restricted diet for, 578
  impaired glucose tolerance in, *551*
  intravenous fluid therapy for, *668*
  malnourished, treatment of, 411
  nourishing snacks for, *279*
  nutritional assessment levels for, *375*
  nutritional support of, 703–704
  RDA of proteins for, 45
  renal failure in, *527*
  tube feeding of, 680
  (*See also specific categories of*
      children)
Chinese, food patterns of, 339–341
Chinese restaurant syndrome, 341
Chloramphenicol, 400
Chloride, 162–163
  balance mechanism of, 162
  clinical application of, 162–163
  daily intake of, *160*
  distribution of, in body, 162
  intake and dietary sources of, 162
Chloride depletion, 451
Chlorothiazides, *401*
Cholecalciferol (vitamin D$_3$), 94, 95
Cholecystitis, 494–495
Cholecystokinin, 171, 173
Cholecystolithiasis, 494
Choledocholithiasis, 494
Cholelithiasis, 494
Cholesterol, 436
  absorption of, 79, 178
  in blood plasma, *85, 86*
  digestion and absorption of, 81
  in foods, *48, 437–438*
  free, 79
  and hyperlipidemia, 436
  in nephrotic syndrome, 530

Cholesterol (*Cont.*):
  serum, 312, 442
  synthesis of, 79
Cholesterol esterase, 81, 171
Cholesterol esters, 79, *85*
Cholesterol metabolism, 77
  and ascorbic acid, 101
Cholestyramine, 96, *401*
Choline, 115
Chondrogenesis, 544
Chondroitin, 62
Chondroitin sulfate, 62
Chromium, *128*, 149
Chromosomes, 240
Chronic alcoholism, 105
Chronic diarrhea, 472
Chronic renal failure, 520–521
  diet modifications during, 521,
      522–523
  stages of, 520–521
Chylomicronemia, *440*
Chylomicrons, 81, 178, 434, *435*, 436,
      439, 441
Chyme, 171, 467
Chymotrypsin, 49
Cirrhosis, 491–493
cis configuration, 74
Citric acid cycle (Krebs cycle), 65, *180*,
      181, 182, 194
Clear liquid diet, 661, *662*
Cleft lip and palate, 620
  breast feeding of child with, 623
  feeding approach to, 619, 621
  feeding techniques with, 621–623
  postoperative feeding for, 623, 624
  preoperative feeding for, 623–624
Clofibrate, *401*
Clostridium botulinum, 738
Clostridium perfringens, 738
Coarctation of aorta, 430, *452*
Cobalt, 149
Cocoa, 19
Coenzyme A, 111
Coenzyme Q (ubiquinone), 118
Coenzyme R (biotin), 111
Coffee, 19
Cola beverages, 19
Collagen and ascorbic acid, 101
Colon (*see* Large intestine)
Colonic constipation, 488
Colostomy, 487
Colostrum, 325
Columnar epithelial cells, 170
Coma, hepatic, 493
Common cold, ascorbic acid and,
      101–102
Community nutrition, 337–*356*,
      357–358
Community resources 352–*356*,
      357–358, *736–737*
Complement system, 410
Complementary proteins, *352*
Complete proteins, 48

Conception frequency and nutritional risk during pregnancy, 316
Congenital heart defects, *452*
Congenital heart disease, 452–457
  energy supplements for children with, *454*
  feeding problems with, 456–457
  formulas for infants with, *455*
  growth curve in, *453*
Congestive heart failure, 457–458
Conjugated proteins, 40
Constipation, 487–488
  colonic, 488
  imagined, 487–488
  medications for, *488*
  during pregnancy, 321
Consumer councils, *356*
Contingency contract, 580
Continuous reinforcement, 220
Cooking methods, 24–25
Cooper, Kenneth, 192
Copper, *128*, 145–147
  absorption and excretion of, 146
  clinical application of, 146–147
  and coronary heart disease, 147
  dietary allowance and sources of, 146
  functions of, 146
  serum levels, conditions affecting, *147*
Copper deficiency, 146
Coronary artery disease, 431
Coronary heart disease:
  copper and, 147
  dietary fat and, 85
  niacin and, 110
  risk factors and, *434*
Corticosteroid therapy, 542–543
Corticosteroids, 540
Corticotropin (ACTH), *83*, 541–*543*, 654
Cortisol, 654, 656–657
Coumarin derivatives, *400*
Cow's milk:
  compared with breast milk and infant formulas, *258–261*
  "humanized," 298
Cow's milk allergy, 429
Cow's milk formula base, supplementation of, *412*
Cretinism, 145, 537
Crohn's disease, 486, 689–690
Crown of tooth, 361
Crude fiber, 63
Cultural food patterns, 3–5, 337–345
Cumulative growth, 247
Cushing's syndrome, 95, 541–542
Cysteine, 295
Cystic fibrosis (CF), 149, 478–481, 483
  modified fat diet for, *482–483*
  nutrient guidelines for children with, *481*
  pancreatic enzyme replacement in, 481, *483*
  treatment of, *480*
Cystine, 532

Cystinosis, *505*
Cystinuria, 532

Daily dietary allowances, *714–715*
Daily food guide, 29, *30–31*, 32, 37–*38*
  for pregnancy, 318, *319*
Dairy products, content of, *479*
Dam, Henrik, 99
Davis, Adele, *347*
Deamination, 50, *51*
Decanoic acid, 78
Decarboxylation, *51*
Deficiencies:
  disaccharidase, 476–478
  lactase, 477–478
  of vitamins, signs of, *116–117*
  (*See also* Clinical deficiency)
Deficiency diseases, 90
Defined formula diets, 661–*662*, *663*, 680–681
  administration of, *681*
Dehydration, 165–166, 198–200
L-Dehydroascorbic acid, 100
7-Dehydrocholesterol, 94
Dendrites, 595
Dental caries, 7, 365–369
  carbohydrate and, 69
  diet guidelines to help prevent, *368*
  fluoridation and, 145, 365, 368–369
  host-environment interaction and, *366*
  prevalence of, 367
  prevention of, 367–369
  progression of, *366*
Dental fluorosis, 368
Dental health, nutrition and, 361–371
Dental plaque, 369
Dental pulp, 361, 362
Dentin, 361–362
2-Deoxy-D-ribose, 59
Deoxyribonucleic acid (DNA), 50, 135, 240
Department of Public Health, *356*
Depletion, 383
Depletion phase, 196
DES (diethylstilbestrol), 693
Desensitization, 219
Detoxification, 136
Developmental disabilities, children with, 600–608
  energy needs in, 601–603
  feeding problems in, 603–604
  growth in, 601
Developmental obesity, 570
Dextrans, 61
Dextrins, 61
Dextrose, 59
Diabetes insipidus, *544*
Diabetes mellitus, 68, 545–565
  asymptomatic, 548
  borderline, 548
  chemical, 548
  classification of, 547–549

Diabetes mellitus (*Cont.*):
  diagnosis of, 546–547, *550–551*
  education of patient with, 563–564
  gestational, 548
  juvenile, 548
  latent, 548
  potential, 548
  and pregnancy, 321
  sequence of symptoms in, 545–546
  type I insulin-dependent (IDDM), 547–549, *550*, 552–555, 561, 563
  type II non-insulin-dependent (NIDDM), 547, 548, *550*, 555–556, 561, 569
  (*See also* Insulin)
Diabetic coma, 546
Diabetic diet, 556
  calculation of, *562*
Diabetic exchange lists, *557–560*
Dialysis, 525, 534
  peritoneal, 525
Diaphragmatic hernia, 465–466
Diarrhea, 472
  electrolyte composition of fluid loss from, *159*
  "fermentative," 477
  in tube feedings, 676–677
Diastase, 60
Diet counseling, 215–217
  for food allergy, 426–427
  helping relationship in, 215–216
  learning and, 216–*217*
Dietary adequacy, determination of, 25–29
Dietary data:
  evaluation of, 390–391
  sources of error in, 390
Dietary fiber, *63*, 71
Dietary Goals for the United States, 8
Dietary guidelines:
  for Americans, 34–*35*
Dietary management, postoperative, 663–665, 669, *670–671*
Dietary supplements, 23, *588*
Diethylstilbestrol (DES), 693
Dieting, behavioral control approach to, 580–581
Diets:
  allergic response and, 418–428
  Atkins, 70, *346*
  Beverly Hills medical, *346–347*
  bland, 466
  and brain function, 596–597
  clear liquid, 661, *662*
  culture and (*see* Cultural food patterns)
  defined formula, 661–*662*, *663*, 680–*681*
  and dental caries, 367–368
  diabetic, 556, *562*
  egg-free, 425–*426*
  elimination, 421, *422*
  energy-restricted, 578, 580

Diets (*Cont.*):
    fat-controlled, *444*
    fiber content of, *63*, 71
    galactose-free, 646, *647–648*
    gluten-free, *475–476*
    and handicapped adult, 608–609
    high-energy high-protein, *587*, 661,
        662
    hyperkinesis and, 608
    for hyperlipoproteinemia, *441*
    initial postoperative, 665
    ketogenic, 604
    during labor, 322
    liquid protein, 53, *347*
    low-cholesterol, low-saturated-fat,
        445, 446
    low-fiber, 6–7
    low-protein, *524*
    low-residue, *485*
    Mayo Clinic, *346*
    measured, 556
    milk-free, *423–424*
    modified fat, for cystic fibrosis,
        482–483
    mucusless, *347*
    phenylalanine-restricted, 638–639,
        640–641
    for Prader-Willi syndrome, 586–587
    preoperative, 660–662
    and prevention of periodontal disease,
        370
    Pritikin program, *347*
    progression, *708*
    progressive bland, for ulcer disease,
        469–471
    protein-sparing, 347
    and psychiatric disorders, 599–600
    psychology of, 211–217
    Scarsdale, 70, *346*
    sick-day, 563
    Simeon, *347*
    Sippy, 468
    sodium-restricted, *450, 451*
    Stillman, *346*
    unmeasured, 556
    weighed, 556
    weight control, sample, *579*
    wheat-free, *425*
Diffusion, 64–65, 157
    carrier-mediated, 177
    passive, 175
Digestion, 170–174
    of carbohydrate, *64*
    of cholesterol, 81
    of fat, 81
    of glycerides, 81
    neurohormonal control of, 173–*174*
    of nutrients, *183*
    of phospholipids, 81
    of protein, 49–50
Digestive enzymes, *172*
Digitalis, *401*
1,25-Dihydroxycholecalciferol, 95, 130

Dipeptidase, 50
Disaccharidase deficiencies, 70, 476–478
Disaccharides, 58, 60
Distance running, position statement on
    prevention of heat injuries during,
    752–753
Diverticula, 486
Diverticulitis, 486
Diverticulosis, 486–487
DNA (deoxyribonucleic acid), 50, 135,
    240
Dopamine, 596
Down syndrome, 604–606
    feeding stimulation program for, *606*
    growth in, 601
Drugs, 23
    among adolescents, 279
    excreted in human milk, *327*
    interfering with nutrition, 603–604
    with nutritional implications, *400–401*
    and pregnancy, 316
"Dry" beriberi, 105
Dry weight, 526
Duodenal ulcers, 467–468
Duodenum, 81
Dwarfism, pituitary, *544*

Early Intervention Program, 605–606,
    607
Eclampsia, 321–322
Economical food shopping, 20–21
    guidelines for, *21*
Ectomorph, 572
Edema, prevention of, 458
Edentulous patients, 371
Efferent neurons, 595
Egg allergy, 420
Egg-free diet, 425–*426*
Eicosatrienoic acid, 77
Eijkman, Christiaan, 103
Ejection reflex, 325
Elderly, nutritional assessment levels for,
    379–381
Elderly Feeding Program, *355*
Electrolyte balance, 503
Electrolyte therapy:
    maintenance requirements for, *165*
    principles of, 165
Electrolytes, 156, 159–165
    clinical applications of, 165–166
    gastrointestinal tract and, 159
    kidneys and, 158–159
    lungs and skin and, 159
    membranes and, 157–158
    replacement of: after burns, 683
        after surgery, 665
    in replacement fluids, 201
    safe and adequate daily dietary intake
        of, *717*
    water and, 153–166
    (*See also* Chloride; Potassium;
        Sodium)

Electroneutrality, 156
Elimination diet, 421, *422*
Embden-Meyerhof glycolytic pathway,
    65, 66, *180*, 181, 182
Emotions:
    and brain function, 597–599
    and growth, 242
Enamel, 361
Encopresis, 488–489
End-stage renal disease:
    with dialysis treatment, 525–528
    without dialysis intervention, 521,
        524–525
Endemic goiter, 538
Endocrine system, 535, *536*
    (*See also specific organs*)
Endogenous hyperlipidemia, 436
Endomorph, 572
Energy:
    and acute renal failure, 518–519
    and chronic renal failure, 521
    expenditure of, *193*
    heights and weights with intake of, *716*
    and hemodialysis, 526
    measurement of, 179–180
    needs in children with developmental
        disabilities, 601–603
    in nephrotic syndrome, 530
    and peritoneal dialysis, 525
    production of, 192–196
    and renal failure, 507
    ways to increase intake of, *602*
Energy requirements, 185, 188
    in diabetes, 561, *562*
    for ideal body weight, *560*
    during lactation, 325–326
    of older adult, 331–332
    during pregnancy, 314
    of premature infant, 296–297
Energy-restricted diets, 578, 580
Energy supplements for children with
    congenital heart disease, *454*
Enrichment, 15
Enteral feeding (alimentation), 676–680
    of premature infant, 300–301
    use of supplements in, 301
Enteral and parenteral support systems,
    669–682
Enteric bacteria, 172–173
Enteric lipases, 81
Enteritis, 486
Enterogastrone, 171
Enterohepatic cycle, 81
Enzyme activation, 130
Enzyme deficiency (*see* Inborn errors of
    metabolism)
Enzymes, digestive, *172*
Epimerase, 645
Epinephrine, 67, *83*, 596
Epithelial tissue, maintenance of, 93
Ergocalciferol (vitamin D_2), 94
Ergogenic effects, 204
Ergosterol, 94

Eruption of teeth, 362, *363*
Erythromycin, *400*
Erythropoietin, 504
Esophageal atresia, 466
Esophageal sphincter, 464–465
Esophagostomy feeding tube placement, *678*
Esophagus, 170
  diseases involving, 464–465
  normal, *465*
  special feeding considerations for, 466
  in swallowing, 464
Essential amino acids, 43–44
Essential fatty acid deficiency, 89
  and total parenteral nutrition, 676
Essential fatty acids, 75–77
Essential hypertension, 448
Ester, 77
Ester linkage, 77
Esterification, 77
Exchange lists for diabetics, *557–560*
Exchange mechanism, 163
Excretion:
  of calcium, 131–132
  of copper, 146
  of iodine, 144
  of iron, 139–140
  of magnesium, 137
  of trace elements, *128*
  of zinc, 147–148
Excretory substances, 382
Exercises:
  aerobic, 192
  anaerobic, 192
  carbohydrate and, 69
  isometric, 192
  isotonic, 192
  nutrition and, 191–207
  protein and, 53, 202–204
  types of, 192
  in weight reduction, 580
Exogenous hyperlipidemia, 436
Extension service, *737*
Extensor hypertonicity, *616*, 617, 628
Extinction, 220
Extrinsic factor, 114

FAD (flavin adenine dinucleotide), 106
Fads in food (*see* Food fads)
Failure-to-thrive infant, 231–232
Failure to thrive without organic reason, 597–598
Familial hyperbetalipoproteinemia, 442
Familial hypercholesterolemia, 442
Family structure, 7, 16–17
Fanconi's syndrome, *505*
Fast-food chains, 17–18
Fast foods, nutrient content of, *749–750*
Fast twitch fibers, 194–195
Fat absorption, 81
  mechanisms of, *82*
Fat absorption test, 81–82

Fat assimilation defects, 78
Fat-controlled diets, *444*
Fat deposition, 83–84
Fat emulsions:
  daily dosage for, *675*
  infusion rate for, *675*
  in total parenteral nutrition, 675
Fat malabsorption, 294–295
Fat metabolism, 82–*83*
  hormones affecting, 83
Fat-soluble vitamins, 90–100
Fat storage, 82
Fats, 73
  absorption of, 81, *82*
  body composition of, during development, *246*
  as body fuel store, 193
  catabolism of, 182
  clinical application of, 85
  composition of foods, *84*
  and diabetes, 561, *562*
  dietary significance and requirements of, 84–85
  digestion of, 81
  enzymes and secretions for degradation of, *172*
  in foods, *437–438*
  and hyperlipidemia, 436
  metabolism of, 82–*83*
  monosaturated, and hyperlipidemia, 439
  placental transport of, 290
  polyunsaturated, and hyperlipidemia, 439
  in preevent meals, 205–206
  and renal failure, 508
  required by older adult, 332
  saturated, and hyperlipidemia, 436
  use of, 80–84
  (*See also* Adipose tissue; Lipids; Oils)
Fats, sweets, and alcohol food group, *31*
Fatty acid derivatives, 77
Fatty acids, 74–77
  chain length of, 74
  essential, 75–77
  with glycerol, 77–79
  saturated, 74, *75*
  unsaturated, 74, 75
Federal food programs, *353–355*
Feeding:
  of child with cleft lip and palate, 619–624
  of children with developmental difficulties, 600–601
  of handicapped child, 609–617
  motor control and, 609–612
  nasogastric, 300–301
  nasojejunal, 300–301
  oral and enteral, of premature infant, 300–301
  oral reflex organization for, 611–612, *613*

Feeding (*Cont.*):
  of premature infant, 300–304
  transitional, *681*
  (*See also* Infant feeding)
Feeding behavior, postnatal environmental influences on, 228–237
Feeding difficulties with cerebral palsy, 607
Feeding environment, 617
Feeding equipment, adaptive, 617, *618*
Feeding problems, 214–215
  in children with developmental disabilities, 603–604
  evaluation of child with, 612–616
  treatment of child with, 616–617
Feeding skills, development of, *256–257*
Feeding stimulation program for children with Down syndrome, *606*
Feeding tubes, 679
"Fermentative diarrhea," 477
Ferritin, 139
Fetal alcohol syndrome, 317
Fetus, 243
Fever and basal metabolic rate, 185
Fiber:
  and cancer, 692
  crude, 63
  and diabetes, 564–565
  dietary, *63*, 71
  and diverticulosis, 486–487
Fibrocystic breast disease, 329
Filtration, 157
Fistula drainage, electrolyte composition of fluid from, *159*
Fitness, position statement on recommended exercise for developing and maintaining, 753–756
Flavin adenine dinucleotide (FAD), 106
Flavin mononucleotide (FMN), 106
Flavins, 105
Fluid replacement:
  after burns, 683
  content of solutions for, 201
  after exercise, 202
  rapid, 200–201, *202*
  after surgery, 665
  temperature of, 201–202
Fluid requirements:
  after burns, formulas for calculating, *684*
  during lactation, 326
  of premature infants, *296*
Fluids:
  and acute renal failure, 519
  body, 157–159
  and chronic renal failure, 521
  and exercise, 198–202
  and hemodialysis, 526
  and peritoneal dialysis, 525
  and preevent meal, 205
  and renal failure, 516–517

Fluids (*Cont.*):
restriction of, with congestive heart
failure, 458
Fluoride, *128*, 145, 368–369
clinical application of, 145
and dental caries, 365, 368–369
dietary allowance and sources of, 145
functions of, 145
supplemental dosage schedule of, *369*
toxicity of, 145
Fluorosis, 145
FMN (flavin mononucleotide), 106
Folacin, 112, 113
Folate, 112–113
Folic acid, 112–114, *117*
biochemical assessment of, 113
chemistry and properties of, 112
clinical deficiency of, 113–114
deficiency of, in pregnancy, 320
dietary allowance and sources of, 113
functions of, 113
history and discovery of, 112
metabolism of, 112–113
and oral health, 365
requirement of: during pregnancy,
315
by premature infants, 299–300
Food additives, 14–15
incidental, 14
intentional, 14
Food and Agriculture Organization
(FAO), 26
Food allergens, 420–421
Food allergy, 418
definition of, 418
diagnosis of, 421–423
diet counseling for, 426–427
immunological basis of, 418–419
prevention of, 427–428
sources of diet recipes for, *427*
symptoms of, *419*
treatment of, 423–426
Food aversions, 703
Food challenge, 421–422
Food composition tables for evaluating
diets, 34
Food consumption patterns, 16–19
Food and Drug Administration (FDA),
15
Food fads, 345, *346–347*
and pregnancy, 318
Food frequency, 389
Food group systems, 29–32
limitations of, 32
Food groups, *29*
fats, sweets, and alcohol, *31*
grain, *31*
during growing years, *281*
meat, *30*
milk, *30*
nutrients in, *30–31*
in prudent diet, *35*

Food groups (*Cont.*):
scoring system for, 32, *33*
vegetable and fruit, *30*
in vegetarian food guide, *351*
Food guide, daily, 29, *30–31*, 32
Food habits, 9–10
Food handling, 23–25
sanitation in, 24, *25*
Food at home, 17
Food and Nutrition Board NAC-NRC
recommended daily dietary
allowances, *714–715*
Food patterns:
of blacks, 344
Chinese, 339–341
cultural, 3–5, 337–345
Japanese, 342
Jewish, 344–345
Mexican-American, 343
nontraditional, 345–352
Puerto Rican, 342–343
Vietnamese, 341–342
Food poisoning, 24
Food preparation, handling, and
cooking methods, 23–25
Food processing, 13–16
additives, 14–15
advantages and disadvantages of, 14
nutrification, 15–16
preservation methods, 14
Food programs, federal, *353–355*
Food purchasing, 19–23
economical shopping, 20–*21*
labeling of products, 21, *22*, 23
by low-income people, 20
patterns of, 19–20
Food quality, storage to maintain, 23–24
Food record, 3- or 7-day, 390
Food Stamp Program, *353*, 356–357,
736
Food symbolism and illness, 212–214
Food technology, 6
*Food Values of Portions Commonly
Used*, 390
Food ways, *4*, 5
Foodborne illnesses, *738*
Foremilk, 325
Formulas:
for congenital heart disease infants,
455
infant, 256
Formulation, 16
Fortified foods, 15, 118, 120
Freezing, 24
Fructose, 58, 59
and diabetes, 563
Fructose intolerance, hereditary,
634–635
Fruit sugar, 59
Fruitarians, 350
Fuel factor, 180
Full-thickness burns, 682

Functional substances, 382–383
Functional tests, 383
Funk, Casimir, 5, 90, 91
Furosemide, *401*

Gag reflex, 612, *613*, 615
Galactokinase-deficiency galactosemia,
645
Galactose, 59, 645, 646, 649
Galactose-free diet, 646, 648
guidelines for, *647–648*
Galactose screening, 646
Galactosemia, *634–635*, *645*–649
biochemical defects of, 645
duration of dietary treatment for, 649
galactokinase-deficiency, 645
galactose screening for, 646
and pregnancy, 649
transferase-deficiency, 645
treatment of, 646, 648
treatment monitoring, 648
Gallbladder, 81, 171
diseases of, 494–495
Gallstones, 494
Gamma-amino butyric acid, 596
Gangliosides, 80
Garrod, Archibald, 629
Gastric acidity, 178
Gastric bypass surgery, 584–585
Gastric gland, *170*
Gastric lipase, 170
Gastric ulcers, 467–468
Gastrin, 171, 173, 467
Gastritis, 467
Gastrointestinal atony, 685
Gastrointestinal flora, 172–173
Gastrointestinal function, development
of, 290–291, 294–295
Gastrointestinal system, *169*, 462–495
Gastrostomy, 678, *679*
Gastrostomy feeding tube placement,
679
Gavage, 290, *293*, 310
Gene mutations, 629–630
Genes, 240–241
Gestational diabetes mellitus (GDM),
548
Glia, 595
Glomerular filtration rate, 312
Glomerulonephritis, 529
acute, *505*
chronic, *505*
Glossitis, 106
Glucagon, *67*, 545, 656
and fat, *83*
Glucocorticoids, 540, 541
and fat, *83*
Gluconeogenesis, 65, *66*, 182, 654
Glucose, 58–59, 63–64, 178, 182
as intravenous nutrient, 302
as metabolic substrate for muscle, 196

Glucose (*Cont.*):
   normal levels of, *552*
   placental transport of, 290
   urine tests for, *553–554*
Glucose-free parenteral solutions, 672
Glucose metabolism, *65–66*
Glucose-6-phosphatase, 195
Glucose-6-phosphate, 65
Glucostat theory, 572
Glucuronic acid, 59
Gluten, 420, 474
Gluten-free diet, *475–476*
Gluten-sensitive enteropathy (celiac
   sprue), 473–474, 476
   diet for, *475–476*
Glycerides, 77–79
   digestion and absorption of, 81
Glycerol, 82–83
   fatty acids and, 77–79
Glycogen, 61, 63–64
   utilization and storage of, 195–196
Glycogen loading, 196
Glycogenesis, *66*
Glycogenic amino acids, *181*, 182
Glycogenolysis, 65, *66*, 182
Glycolipids, 80
Glycolysis, 65, *66*, 181
Glycosidic linkage, 60
Glycosuria, 302, 545
Goiter, 144–145
   endemic, 538
   iodine-deficiency, 538
Goitrogens, 538
Gonadotropins, *543*
Gout, 565–567
Grain food group, *31*
Grave's disease, 539
Growth:
   of adipose tissue, *246–247*
   assessment of, 247–254
   background data for assessment of,
      248
   of body, periods of, 242, *243*, 244–247
   of brain, *243*, 245–246
   catch-up, 241–242
   in children with developmental
      disabilities, 601
   critical phases of, 240
   cumulative, 247
   definition of, 239
   embryonic phase of, 242
   extrinsic factors influencing, 241–242
   genes and, 240–241
   health and emotions and, 241–242
   health history for assessment of, 248
   hormones and, 241
   immigration and, 241
   information gathering for assessment
      of, 247–248
   in length, 244
   longitudinal data on, 247–248
   measurement errors in, *249*

Growth (*Cont.*):
   measurements for assessment of, 248,
      250–252
   and nutrition, 239–282
   nutrition as extrinsic factor
      influencing, 241
   postnatal, 244–247
   of premature infant, 288–289
   processes and mechanisms underlying,
      239–242
   secular trend in, 241
   socioeconomic status and, 241
   of teeth, 362, *364*
   thyroid and, 536
Growth charts, 576
   use of, 252, *253*, 254
Growth curve in congenital heart
   disease, *453*
Growth hormone (somatotropin), *67,
   543*, 544
   and fat, *83*
Growth velocity, 247
Guiding behavior, 220–221
Guthrie test, 637

Hand grasp reflex, *613*
Hand-to-mouth activity in handicapped
   child, 616
Handicapped adult, 608–609
Handicapped child, feeding of, 609–617
Hare Krishnas, *350*
HDL (high-density lipoprotein), 434,
   435, 442
Head circumference, 250
Head Start program, *356*
Health foods, 348
Heart, 430
Heart attack, 432–433
Heart defects, congenital, *452*
Heart disease:
   congenital (*see* Congenital heart
      disease)
   hypertensive, 447–451
   ischemic, 431–437
   rheumatic, 451–452
   (*See also* Coronary heart disease)
Heart failure, congestive, 457–458
Height-weight tables, 576, *718*
Hematocrit, 142
   normal values of, *144*
Hematopoietic neoplasms, 694
Heme iron, 139
Hemicellulose, 62
Hemochromatosis, 142
   idiopathic, 140
Hemodialysis, 525–528
Hemoglobin, 138–139, *659*
   copper and, 146
Hemoglobin levels, 142
   normal values of, *144*
Hemorrhoids, 489

Hemosiderin, 139
Hemosiderosis, 142
Heparin, 62
Hepatic coma, 493
Hepatitis, 490–491
Hereditary fructose intolerance, *634–635*
Hereditary tyrosinemia, *634–635*
Hernia:
   diaphragmatic, 465–466
   hiatus, *465–466*
Hexoses, 58–60
Hiatus hernia, 465–466
   mechanism of, *465*
High-biological-value protein, 660–661
High-density lipoprotein (HDL), 434,
   435, 442
High-energy high-protein diet, *587*, 661,
   662
High-energy phosphate compounds, 135
Hindmilk, 325
Hippocrates, 5
Histidine, 43
Hodgkin's lymphoma, 702
Homocystinuria, *634–635*
Hopkins, F. G., 5
Hormones, 535
   and calcium absorption, 131
   and carbohydrate metabolism, 67
   and fat metabolism, *83*
   and growth, 241
   side effects of, *700*
Household survey, 390
Human chorionic gonadotropin, 583
Human milk, 298
   drugs excreted in, *327*
Human placental lactogen, 289
"Humanized" cow's milk, 298
Humoral immunity, 409–410
Hunger, response to, 4
Hyaluronic acid, 62
Hydralazine, *401*
Hydramnios, 321
Hydrochloric acid, 170
Hydrocortisone, 67
Hydrogenation of lipids, *73*
Hydrolase, 171
Hydrolysis, 59
   of lipids, *73*
25-Hydroxycholecalciferol, 95, 96
Hyperalimentation, 697
Hyperbetalipoproteinemia, familial,
   442
Hyperbilirubinemia, 230, 328
Hypercalcemia, 96
Hypercalciuria, 133
Hypercholesterolemia, 147
   familial, 442
Hyperglycemia, 65, 545
Hyperglycemic effect, 545
Hyperhydration, 200
Hyperkalemia, 512
Hyperkinesis, 608

Hyperlipidemia, 434–439
  endogenous, 436
  exogenous, 436
  medical treatment of, 446–447
Hyperlipoproteinemias, 439–443
  diets for, *441*
  type I, 439, *440, 441*
  type II, 461
  type IIa, *440, 441,* 442
  type IIb, *440, 441, 442*
  type III, *440, 441,* 442–443
  type IV, *440, 441,* 443
  type V, *440, 441,* 443
Hypermetabolism, 452–453
Hyperoxaluria, 532
Hypertension, 447–451
  essential, 448
  labile, 447
  medications for, 449, 451
  secondary, 448
  sodium restriction for treatment of,
    448–449
  treatment of, 448–449, 451
  weight reduction for treatment of, 449
Hypertensive heart disease, 447–451
Hyperthermia, 200, 201
Hyperthyroidism, 539
Hypertonic dehydration, 165–167
Hypertonicity, 614–615
  extensor, *616,* 617
Hyperuricemia, 565
Hyperuricosuria, 532
Hypervitaminosis A, 94
Hypervitaminosis D, 96
Hypocalcemia, neonatal, 298–299
Hypocalcemic tetany, 540
Hypoglycemia, 65
  adult, 565
Hypoglycemia Foundation, *347*
Hypoglycemic effect, 545
Hypokalemia, 451, 512
Hypokalemic alkalosis, 163
Hypotension, 518
Hypothalamus, 173, 325, 543
  and water reabsorption, *158*
Hypothyroidism, 537–538
Hypotonic dehydration, 165
Hypotonicity of muscles, 605

IDDM (type I insulin-dependent diabetes
    mellitus), 547–549, *550,* 552–555,
    561, 563
Ideal body weight, energy requirements
    for, *560*
Idiopathic hemochromatosis, 140
Idiopathic steatorrhea, 473
ILDL (intermediate-low-density
    lipoprotein), *435*
Ileostomy, 487
Illness:
  disorganization of normal rhythms
    secondary to, 230–231
  food symbolism and, 212–214

Imagined constipation, 487–488
Immigration and growth, 241
Immune response:
  malnutrition and, 403–414
  and surgery, 658
Immune system during protein-calorie
    malnutrition, *410*
Immunoglobulins, 409–410, 418
Immunosuppression, nutritional
    implications of, *529*
Immunotherapy for cancer, 699, 701
Impaired glucose tolerance, 548, 551
Imuran, *529*
Inborn errors of metabolism, 629–650
  in amino acid and carbohydrate
    metabolism, *632–635*
  biochemical defects of, 629–631
  clinical manifestations of, 632
  diagnosis of, 633
  incidence of, 631
  inheritance of, *630,* 632
  public health implications of, 649
  screening for, 631
  treatment of, 636
  vitamin-dependent, 631
Inborn errors of transport, 631
Incaparina, 16
Incidental food additives, 14
Incomplete proteins, 48–49
Index of nutritional quality, 34
Infant feeding:
  acquisition of reaching in, 234
  age 0–2 months, 228–233
  age 2–4 months, 233–234
  age 4–9 months, 234–236
  age 9–16 months, 236–237
  autonomy in, 234–235
  developmental considerations in,
    227–238
  disorganization of normal rhythms in,
    230–231
  environmental and emotional
    stimulation and, 231–233
  independence in, 236–237
  quantity of intake during, 233–234
  response to breast feeding, 234
  spitting up in, 235–236
Infant formulas, 256, 262–263
  compared with breast milk and cow's
    milk, *258–261*
Infant sucking pattern, 228–229
Infants:
  defined formula diets for, 681
  development of feeding skills in,
    256–257
  failure-to-thrive, 231–232
  feeding guidelines for: during first 6
    months, *267*
    from 6–12 months, *268*
  feeding problems of, 269, *273–274*
  gastrointestinal conditions in, *489–490*
  nutrition of, 255–269
  nutritional assessment levels for, *375*
  premature (*see* Premature infants)

Infants (*Cont.*):
  recommended daily requirements for,
    45, *661*
  texture in diet of, 265
  transition to whole milk by, 265
  tube feeding for, 680
Infection:
  and malnutrition, 408
  prevention of, after burns, 683, 685
  and total parenteral nutrition, 676
Infectious hepatitis, 490
Ingestion, 168–170
Inositol, 115, 118
Institutionalized adult, dietary factors
    affecting, *333*
Insulin, 67, 545, 548, 549, 552, 564, 656
  commercially available, *553*
  and fat, *83*
  (*See also* Diabetes mellitus)
Insulin reaction, 554
  to total parenteral nutrition, 676
Intentional food additives, 14
Intermediate burns, 682
Intermediate-low-density lipoprotein
    (ILDL), *435*
Intermittent reinforcement, 220
Internuncial neurons, 595
Interviewing techniques, 387, 389
Intestinal biopsy, 474
Intestinal bypass surgery, 583–584
Intestinal mucosa, 178
Intestine (*see* Large intestine; Small
    intestine)
Intralipid, 302, 303, 310
Intrauterine malnutrition, 410–411
Intrauterine nutrition, 289–290
Intravenous alimentation, *292*
  for premature infants, 301–302
Intravenous hyperalimentation, 672–676
Intravenous nutrition products for
    premature infants, 302–*304*
Intravenous supplementation, *293*
Intravenous therapy, 669
  following surgery, *667–668*
Intrinsic factor, 114
Intrinsic substances, 382–383
Inulin, 62
Inulin clearance test, 62
Invasion, 694
Invisible fats, 73
Iodide, 536
Iodine, *128,* 144–145, 536, 538
  absorption and excretion of, 144
  clinical application of, 144–145
  dietary allowance and sources of, 144
  functions of, 144
  requirement of, during pregnancy,
    315
Iodine-deficiency goiter, 538
Iodine number of lipids, *73*
Ions, *156*
IQ scores, 643
Iron, *128,* 138–144, 204
  absorption of, 139, *141*

Iron (*Cont.*):
  ascorbic acid in absorption of, 101
  bioavailability of, 16
  clinical application of, 140, 142, 144
  dietary allowance and sources of, 140
  enrichment and fortification with, 16
  excretion of, 139–140
  function of, 138–139
  requirements of: during lactation, 326
    by older adult, 332
    during pregnancy, 315
    by premature infants, 299
  serum, *659*
  sources of, *141*
Iron-deficiency anemia, 140, 142, 152,
    265
  causes of, *141*
  in pregnancy, 318, 320
  progression of, *143*
Ischemic heart disease, 431–437
  risk factors in, 433–*434*
Islets of Langerhans, 545
Isoleucine, 43
Isometric exercises, 192
Isotonic exercises, 192

Japanese, food patterns of, 342
Jaundice, 230–231
Jaw control in handicapped child, 615
Jejunoileal bypass surgery, 500–501, 584
Jejunostomy, 678–*679*
Jejunostomy feeding tube placement,*679*
Jewish food patterns, 344–345
Joint disorders, 565–567
Joule, 179
"Junk" foods, 6
Juvenile arthritis, 567
Juvenile diabetes, 548

Kashruth, 344–345
Keratomalacia, 93
Ketogenic amino acids, *181*, 182
Ketogenic diets, 604
Ketone bodies, 82, 546
Ketonemia, 82
Ketones, placental transport of, 290
Ketonuria, 82
Ketosis, 82, 546
Kidneys:
  disorders of, *505*
  endocrine function of, 504
  failure of (*see* Renal failure)
  homeostatic functions of, 503–504
  normal functions of, 502–504
  and regulation of fluids and
    electrolytes, 158–159
Kilocalorie, 179
Kosher practice, 344–345
Krebs cycle, 65, *180*, 181, 182, 194
Kussmaul respiration, 546
Kwashiorkor, 51, 365, 405, *406*, 407
  determinants of, *407*

Labeling of products, 21, *22*, 23
  open dating, 23
  Universal Product Coding, *22*, 23
Labile hypertension, 447
Labor in childbirth, diet during, 322
Lactalbumin, 420
Lactase deficiency, 477–478
Lactation:
  calcium requirements during, 326
  energy requirements during, 325–326
  fluid requirements during, 326
  iron requirements during, 326
  nutrient needs during, 325–326
  nutrition in, 322–328
  physiology of, 324–325
  protein requirements during, 46, 326
Lactic acid, 65, 66, 194
Lacto-ovo-vegetarians, 49, 350
Lacto-vegetarians, 49, 350
Lactobacillus bulgarius, 173
Lactose, 60
  and calcium absorption, 131
  in dairy products, *479*
  and galactosemia, 646
Lactose intolerance, 341, 344
  development of, *477*
Laennec's cirrhosis, 491
Laetrile, 118
Lamina propria, 175
Large burns, 682
Large intestine (bowel):
  absorption in, 177
  diseases of, 484–489
  functions of, 484
Latent diabetes, 548
Lauric acid, 75
Lavoisier, Antoine Laurent, 5
LDL (low-density lipoprotein), 434, *435*,
    436, *440*, 442
Learning:
  observational, 218
  operant, 219–222
  stimulus-response, 218–219
Lecithin, 15, 80, 81
Letdown of milk, 325
Leucine, 43
Leukemia, 702
Levodopa, *401*
Levulose (fructose), 59
Lignin, 62
Lind, James, 5, 100
Lingual lipase, 294
Linoleic acid, 75–77, 89
Linolenic acid, 75
Lip control in handicapped child, 615
Lipases:
  enteric, 81
  lingual, 294
  pancreatic, 81
Lipemia, 302
Lipids, 72–89
  absorption of, 178
  in blood, *85–87*, 443–446
  chemical reactions of, *73*

Lipids (*Cont.*):
  classification of, *74*
  definition of, 73–74
  functions of, 72–73
  hydrogenation of, *73*
  hydrolysis of, *73*
  iodine number of, *73*
  major constituents of, 74–80
  plasma concentrations of, *435*
  rancidity of, *73*
  saponification of, *73*
  thyroid and, 536
  (*See also* Fats; Oils)
Lipogenesis, 65, 82
Lipoic acid, 118
Lipolysis, 82
Lipoproteins, 434
  alpha (HDL), 434, 435
  beta (LDL), 434
  in blood plasma, *87*
  composition of, *435*
  intermediate-low-density (ILDL), 435
  low-density (LDL), 434, *435*, 436,
    440, 442,
  normal electrophoretic band of, *436*
  plasma concentrations of, *435*
  pre-beta (VLDL), 434
  very-low-density (VLDL), 434, *435*,
    436, 439, *440*, 442, 443
Liposyn, 302
Lipotropic factor, 115
Liquid meals, 206
Liquid protein diet, 53, *347*
Liver, 65, 81, 171
  diseases of, 490–491, *492*, 493
  and fat metabolism, 83
  functions of, 490
  glycogen in, 195
  tests for diagnosis of diseases of, *490*
Lofenalac, 638, 644, 653
Low-birth-weight infant, 45, 288
  (*See also* Premature infants)
Low-calorie beverages, 19
Low-cholesterol, low-saturated-fat diet,
    445, *446*
Low-density lipoprotein (LDL), 434,
    435, 436, *440*, 442
Low-fiber diets, 6–7
Low-protein diet, menu for, *524*
Low-residue diet, *485*
Lower gastrointestinal tract, diseases of,
    6–7, 472–483
Lungs and fluid and electrolyte
    regulation, 159
Lymphomas, 702
Lysine, 43
Lysosomes, 178

McCollum, E. V., 5, 91
Macrobiotic diet, 349
Macrominerals, 126–138, *127*
Magnesium, 137–138
  absorption and excretion of, 137

Magnesium (*Cont.*):
  clinical application of, 137–138
  dietary allowance and sources of, 137
  functions of, 137
  serum levels, conditions altering, *138*
Malabsorption syndromes, 70, 473–476
Malignant tumors, 694
  characteristics of, *695*
  (*See also entries beginning with term:*
    Cancer)
Malnourished child, treatment of, 411
Malnutrition:
  and environment, 232–233
  etiology of, 403–404
  and height and weight, *405*
  and immune response, 403–414
  infection and, 408
  intrauterine, 410–411
  physical signs and causes of, 384,
    387–388
  prevention of, 413–414
  protein-calorie, 404–405
  and surgery, 660
Malnutrition grades, 404–*405*
Malt sugar, 60
Maltose, 60, 61
Manganese, *128*, 148–149
  absorption and excretion of, 148
  dietary allowance and sources of, 149
  functions of, 148
Maple syrup urine disease, *634–635*
Marasmus, 51, 405, *406*, 407
  determinants of, *407*
Mastication, 169
Maternal parity, 228–229
Mature milk, 325
Mayo Clinic diet, *346*
MCT (medium-chain triglycerides),
    78–79, 301, 441, 473, 604
Meal replacement formulas, 680
Meals:
  guidelines for preparing, *18*
  liquid, 206
  preevent, 204–207
Measured diet, 556
Meat consumption, 7
Meat factor, 139
Meat food group, *30*
Medications:
  for hypertension, 449–451
  sodium content of, *511–512*
Medium-chain triglycerides (MCT),
    78–79, 301, 441, 473, 604
Megaloblastic anemia, 115
Megavitamins, 120
Membranes and fluid and electrolyte
    distribution, 157–158
Menadione (vitamin K₃), 100
Menaquinone (vitamin K₂), 99
Menarche, 186
Menkes' steely hair syndrome, 146
Menstruation, 285–286
Mesomorph, 572

Messenger RNA, 50, 240
Metabolic acidosis, 164–165, 167
Metabolic alkalosis, 165
Metabolic rate, thyroid and, 536
Metabolic water, 154
Metastasis, 694
Methionine, 43
Methylxanthines, 329
Metric equivalents, *738*
Mexican-Americans, food patterns of,
    343
Micelles, 81, 171, 178
Microcytic hypochromic anemia, 140
Microminerals (trace elements), 126,
    127, 138–150
Microvilli, 175
Middle childhood, nutrition during,
    277, 279
Middle years, nutrition during, 328–329
Milk allergy, 420
  cow's, 429
Milk food group, *30*
Milk-free diet, 423–*424*
Milk sugar, 60
Milliosmol, 157
Mineralocorticoids, 540
Minerals, 126–150
  absorption of, 179
  and exercise, 204
  interactions of, 150
  safe and adequate daily dietary
    intakes of, *717*
  supplementation with, *412*
Molybdenum, *128*, 150
Monamine oxidase inhibitors, 600
Monosaccharides, 58–60
Monosaturated fats and hyperlipidemia,
    439
Monosodium glutamate, 341
Moro reflex, *613*
Morphogenesis, 242
Mothers, nutritional assessment levels
    for, *378*
Motor control and feeding, 609–612
Mouth, 169
  in swallowing, 463
Mucopolysaccharides, 62
Mucosa, jejunal, *176*
Mucosal function, 175
Mucosal transport, 175, 177
Mucous cells, 170–171
Mucus, 171
Mucusless diet, *347*
Multivitamin supplements, 118
  composition of, *119*
Muscle contraction, 129–130
Muscle fibers (cells):
  and energy production, 194
  glycogen in, 195–196
  types of, 194–195
Muscle tonus, 610
  abnormal, 617
Myelin sheath, 595

Myocardial infarction, 432–433
Myristic acid, 75

NAD (nicotinamide adenine
    dinucleotide), 109
NADP (nicotinamide adenine
    dinucleotide phosphate), 109
NADPH (reduced nicotinamide adenine
    dinucleotide phosphate), 109
Napoxen, 567
Nasoduodenal feeding tube placement,
    678
Nasogastric feeding, *293*, 300–301
Nasogastric feeding tube placement, *678*
Nasojejunal feeding, *293*, 300–301
Nasojejunal feeding tube placement,
    678
National Dairy Council, *356*
Natural foods, 348
Natural vitamins, 348
Nausea:
  during cancer chemotherapy, 696,
    699, *700–701*
  during pregnancy, 320
Negative reinforcers, 219
Neomycin, *400*
Neonates:
  intravenous fluid therapy for, *668*
  recommended daily requirements for,
    661
Neoplasm, 694
  (*See also entries beginning with term:*
    Cancer)
Nephrolithiasis, 531–532
Nephron, 502–*503*
Nephrosis, childhood, 530
Nephrotic syndrome, *505*, 529–530
  diet modifications in, 530
Nephrotoxins, 518
Nerve impulses, 129
Nervous system:
  autonomic, 595
  central, 594
  disorders of, 594–600
  functions of, 594–596
  peripheral, 595
  somatic, 595
Net protein utilization, 46, *47*, 48
Neuroblastoma, 702–703
Neurohormonal control of digestion,
    173–*174*
Neurohormones, 543
Neuromuscular transmission, 137
Neurons, 595
Neurotic feeding disturbances, 214
Neurotransmitter synthesis, 101
Neurotransmitters, 595
New vegetarians, *350*
Newborn:
  intravenous fluid therapy for, *668*
  recommended daily requirements for,
    661

Niacin (nicotinic acid), 108–110, *116*
  biochemical assessment of, 109
  chemistry and properties of, 109
  clinical deficiency of, 110
  dietary allowance and sources of,
      109–110
  functions of, 109
  history and discovery of, 108–109
  metabolism of, 109
  toxicity and pharmacological effects
      of, 110
Niacin deficiency, 107
Nicotinamide adenine dinucleotide
    (NAD), 109
Nicotinamide adenine dinucleotide
    phosphate (NADP), 109
  reduced (NADPH), 109
Nicotinic acid (*see* Niacin)
NIDDM (type II non-insulin-dependent
    diabetes mellitus), 547, 548, *550*,
    555–556, 561, 569
  treatment of, 556
Niemann-Pick disease, 80
Night blindness, 92
Nipple care, 326, 328
Nipple engorgement, 328
Nitrates and cancer, 693
Nitrites, 265
  and cancer, 693
Nitrogen balance, 42–43, 660
  negative, 43
  positive, 43
Nitrogen equilibrium, 43
Nitrosamines and cancer, 693
Noncellulosic polysaccharides, 62
Nonessential amino acids, 43–44
Nonorganic feeding disturbances, 214
Nontropical sprue, 473
Nonvitamins, 118
Norepinephrine, 596
Normoglycemia, 65
Nothing per os (NPO), 663
Nutrient accretion with gestational age,
    289
Nutrient content of fast foods, *749–750*
Nutrient density, 32, 34
Nutrient distribution in energy-
    restricted diet, 580
Nutrient guidelines for children with
    cystic fibrosis, *481*
Nutrient needs:
  during lactation, 325–326
  of surgical patient, 658–660
Nutrient requirements:
  of older adults, 331–333
  of premature infants, 296–300
Nutrient standards, comparison of,
    26–27
Nutrient stores and surgery, 656
Nutrients:
  body use of, 168–186
  for exercise, 196–204
  final products of, *183*

Nutrients (*Cont.*):
  restoration of, 15
  retention of, 25
  sites of absorption of, *179*
  ways to increase intake of, *602*
Nutrification, 15–16
Nutrition education, 9, *10*, 11, 217
Nutrition educator, role of, 11
Nutrition labeling, 21, *22, 23*
Nutrition support in children with
    cancer, 703–704
Nutritional assessment levels:
  for adolescents, *376*
  for adults, *377*
  for children, *375*
  for elderly, *379–381*
  for infants, *375*
  for mothers, *378*
Nutritional assessment —objective
    measurement standards, *407*
Nutritional assessment tools:
  for adults and adolescents, *728–733*
  for children, *722–727*
Nutritional care:
  of premature infants, 287–304
  surgery and, 654–682
Nutritional failure:
  causes and dietary treatment of,
      270–272
  conditions resulting in, *384*
Nutritional history, 389–390
  food frequency, 389
  household survey, 390
  3- or 7-day food record, 390
  24-hour recall, 389–390
Nutritional interview, 216
Nutritional risk during pregnancy,
    315–318
Nutritional status:
  anthropomorphic methods for, 382
  biochemical methods for, 382–384
  clinical methods for, 384, 387
  dietary methods for, 387, 389
  evaluation of, 374–381, *382*, 383–393
  laboratory evaluation of, *385–386*
  of United States population, 391–392
Nutritive Value of American Foods,
    390
Nutritive values of edible part of foods,
    746–748

Obesity, 6, 83, 570–571, 592–593
  adipose cell theory of, 572–573
  definition of, 571
  development of, *575*
  developmental, 570
  diagnosis of, 575–577
  environmental and social factors in,
      573–574
  etiology of, 571–574
  heredity and, 571–572
  and NIDDM, 569

Obesity (*Cont.*):
  physiological and biochemical factors
      of, 572
  during pregnancy, 320
  psychological and emotional factors
      in, 574
  reactive, 570
  treatment of, 576–585
  (*See also* Weight reduction)
Obesity standard for adults, *722*
Observational learning, 218
Obstetrical history and pregnancy, 316
Obstructive renal failure, 518
Octanoic acid, 78
Odontogenesis, 362
Ohsawa, George, 348
Oils, 73
  (*See also* Fats; Lipids)
Older adult:
  calcium requirements of, 332
  carbohydrate requirements of, 332
  community services for, 333–334
  energy requirements of, 331–332
  fat requirements of, 332
  iron requirements of, 332
  nutrient requirements of, 331–333
  nutrition and, 329–334
  protein requirements of, 332
  vitamin requirements of, 332–333
Oleic acid, 75
Oligodendrocytes, 595
Oliguria, 517, 518
Open dating, 23
Operant learning, 219–222
Opsin, 92
Oral contraceptives, 329
  and nutritional status, *330*
Oral digital stimulation, 615
Oral feeding of premature infant,
    300–301
Oral glucose tolerance test (OGTT),
    546–547, *550–551*
Oral health:
  nutritional influences on, 364–365
  in sick and handicapped, 371
Oral reflexes:
  organization of, for feeding, 611–612,
      613
  persistence of, 614–615
Oral tolerance test, 474
Organic feeding disturbances, 214
Organically grown food, 348
Oropharynx, normal physiology of, *621*
Orthomolecular therapy, *347*, 599
Osmosis, 157
Osmotic pressure, 157
Osteoblasts, 129
Osteoclasts, 129
Osteomalacia, 96
Osteoporosis, 96, 133, 135
Overweight (*see* Obesity)
Ovo-vegetarians, 350
Oxalate in renal calculi, 532

Oxalic acid, 131
Oxidation-reduction reactions, 136
Oxidative phosphorylation, 137
Oxytocin, 525, *543*

Paigen assay for galactose, 646
Palmitic acid, 75
Palmitoleic acid, 75
Pancreas, 81, 171, 544-565
   and cystic fibrosis, 478-479
   diseases of, 493-494
   (*See also* Diabetes mellitus)
Pancreatic cholesterol esterase, 81
Pancreatic enzyme replacement, 481,
   483
Pancreatic lipases, 81
Pancreatitis, 493-494
Pancreozymin, 171
Pangamic acid, 118
Pantothenic acid, 110-111, *117*
   chemistry and properties of, 110
   clinical deficiency of, 111
   dietary allowance and sources of,
      111
   functions of, 111
   history and discovery of, 110
   metabolism of, 111
   and oral health, 365
Parathyroid, 540
   physiology of, 540
Parathyroid hormone, 131
Parenteral nutrition:
   peripheral, 669, *672*
   total, in acute renal failure, 520
Parenteral solutions, *666*
   glucose-free, 672
Parenteral support systems, 669-682
Parietal cells, 170
Parity, high, and nutritional risk during
   pregnancy, 316
Partial-thickness burns, 682
Partial vegetarians, 350
Passive diffusion, 175
Pauling, Linus, 101, 102, 120
Pavlov, Ivan P., 218
Pectins, 62
Pellagra, 108, 110
Penicillin, *400*
Pentose phosphate shunt, 59, 65
Pentoses, 59-60
Pepsin, 49, 170
Pepsinogen, 170
Peptic ulcer, 467
Peptide, 42
Peptide bonds, 42
Perfringens poisoning, *738*
Periodontal disease, 369-370
   prevention of, 370
   progression of, *369*
Periodontal ligament, 362
Peripheral nervous system, 595

Peripheral parenteral nutrition, 669,
   672
   administration of, *672*
   formula for, *672*
Peritoneal dialysis, 525
Permanent teeth, eruption of, 362, *363*
Permeation, 694
Pernicious anemia, 114, 115
Pesco-vegetarians, 350
pH:
   and calcium absorption, 130, 131
   definition of, 163
Pharynx in swallowing, 463
Phenyl-Free formula, 638, 644
Phenylalanine, 43, 636-639, 641, 644
   in foods, *639*
   and premature infants, 295
Phenylalanine hydroxylase, 636
Phenylalanine-restricted diet, 638-641
   management of, *640-641*
Phenylketonuria (PKU), 631, *632-633*,
   636, *637*, 638-*642*, *643*, 644, 653
   biochemical defect of, 636-637
   duration of dietary treatment for,
      643-644
   and pregnancy, 644
   primary defect in, *637*
   screening, 637
   teaching aids for, *642-643*
   treatment of, 637-644
Phosphatides, 80
Phosphocreatine, 194
Phospholipids, 79-80
   in blood plasma, *85*
   digestion and absorption of, 81
Phosphorus, 135-136
   absorption and utilization of, 135
   and acute renal failure, 520
   and chronic renal failure, 521
   clinical application of, 136
   dietary allowance and sources of,
      135-136
   functions of, 135
   and hemodialysis, 526
   inorganic, 131
   in nephrotic syndrome, 530
   parathyroid and, 540
   and peritoneal dialysis, 525
   and renal failure, 514-516
   requirements of: during pregnancy,
      315
      in premature infant, 298-299
   and tooth development, 364
Phosphorylation, 135
Photosynthesis, 57
Phototherapy, 230-231, 300
Phylloquinone (vitamin K_1), 99
Physical exercise and basal metabolic
   rate, 185
Physical fitness, nutrition and, 191-207
Physiology:
   of kidneys, 502-504

Physiology (*Cont.*):
   of lactation, 324-325
   of oropharynx, *621*
   of parathyroid, 540
   of swallowing, 463-464
   of thyroid, 535-536
Phytic acid, 131
Phytosterols, 79
Pica, 214, 276
   and pregnancy, 317-318
Pinocytosis, 157-158
Pituitary, 325, 543-544
   altered function of, *544*
   hormone functions of, *543*
Pituitary dwarfism, *544*
PKU (*see* Phenylketonuria)
Placental transport, 289-290
Plant alkaloids, side effects of, *700*
Plaque, dental, 365-366, 369
Plaques, atheromatous, 431-432
Plasmalogens, 80
PMNs (polymorphonuclear leukocytes),
   409
Polycose, 301
Polycystic kidney disease, *505*
Polydipsia, 546
Polymorphonuclear leukocytes (PMNs),
   409
Polypeptide, 42
Polyphagia, 546
Polysaccharides, 58, 60-62
   derivatives of, 62
   noncellulosic, 62
   storage forms of, 60-62
   structural forms of, 61, 62
   sulfur in, 136
Polyunsaturated fats and
   hyperlipidemia, 439
Polyunsaturated fatty acids,
   requirements of, in premature
   infants, 299
Polyunsaturates/saturates (P/S) ratio, 84
Polyuria, 545-546
Ponderal index, 244
Positioning:
   of child with feeding problem,
      616-617
   for feeding, 614
Positive reinforcers, 219
Postnatal growth, 244-247
Postoperative dietary management,
   663-665, 669, *670-671*
Postoperative diets:
   initial, 665
   progression from liquid to house, 669
Postural control, 610
Potassium, 161-162
   and acute renal failure, 519-520
   balance mechanism of, 161
   and chronic renal failure, 521
   clinical application of, 161-162
   daily intake of, *160*

Potassium (*Cont.*):
 distribution of, in body, 161
 in foods, *451, 513*
 and hemodialysis, 526
 intake and dietary sources of, 161
 in nephrotic syndrome, 530
 and peritoneal dialysis, 525
 and renal failure, 512–514
Potassium conversion, 514
Potassium depletion, chronic, *505*
Potassium hyperkalemia, 519–520
Potential abnormality of glucose
  tolerance (PotAGT), 548
Potential diabetes, 548
Prader-Willi syndrome, 585–587, *589*
 diet for, 586–587
 environmental control for, 585–586
Pre-beta lipoprotein (VLDL), 434
Prealbumin, 92
Precocious puberty, *544*
Prediabetes, 548
Prednisone, *529*
Preeclampsia, 321, 322
Preevent meals, 204–207
 alcohol and, 206
 caffeine and, 206–207
 composition of, 205–206
 familiarity and acceptance of, 205
 fluids and, 207
 liquid, 206
 sample, *205*
 timing of, 204–205
Pregnancy:
 adolescence and, 316
 alcohol and, 317
 biochemical and physiological changes
  during, 311–314
 caffeine and, 317
 calcium requirements during, 315
 complications of, 318, 320–322
 constipation during, 321
 daily food guide for, 318, *319*
 diabetes and, 321
 drug addiction and, 316
 energy requirements during, 314
 folic acid requirements during, 315
 food fads and, 318
 galactosemia and, 649
 high parity as risk to, 316
 iodine requirements during, 315
 iron requirements during, 315
 low prepregnant weight and, 316
 and medical complications, 316
 nausea and vomiting during, 320
 nutrition in, 311–322
 nutritional requirements during,
  314–315
 nutritional risk during, 315–318
 and obstetrical history, 316
 phenylketonuria and, 644
 phosphorus requirements during, 315
 pica and, 317–318

Pregnancy (*Cont.*):
 protein requirements during, 45–46,
  314
 psychological conditions and, 318
 saccharin and, 319
 smoking and, 317
 sodium requirements during, 315,
  322, 336
 toxemia during, 321–322
 underweight during, 320
 vegetarians and, 318
 vitamin D requirements during, 315
 vitamin requirements during, 314–315
Premature infants:
 calcium requirements of, 298–299
 development of gastrointestinal
  function in, 290–291, 294–295
 early feeding schedule for, *294*
 energy requirements of, 296–297
 feeding of, 300–304
 feeding methods, *292–293*
 fluid requirements of, *296*
 folic acid requirements of, 299–300
 gavage of, 290, *293*, 310
 intrauterine growth of, 288
 and intrauterine nutrition, 289–290
 intravenous alimentation for, *292*,
  301–302
 intravenous fluid therapy for, *668*
 intravenous nutrition products for,
  302–304
 intravenous supplementation of, *293*
 iron requirements of, 299
 metabolic limitations of, 295–296
 nutrient requirements of, 296–300
 nutritional care of, 287–304
 oral and enteral feeding of, 300–301
 phosphorus requirements of, 298–299
 polyunsaturated fatty acid
  requirements of, 299
 postnatal growth of, 288–289
 protein requirements of, 297–298
 riboflavin requirements of, 300
 trace element requirements of, 300
 vitamin D requirements of, 298–299
 vitamin E requirements of, 98, 299
Prematurity, definition of, 288
Prenatal growth, 242–244
Preoperative diets, 660–662
Preoperative nutrition, 660–663
 diets for, 660–662
 goals of, 660
 nothing per os and, 663
Preschool child, nutrition of, 276–277
Preservation methods, 14
Preventive nutrition, 8–9
Previous abnormality of glucose
  tolerance (PrevAGT), 548
Primary structure, 42
Primary teeth, eruption and shedding
  of, 362, *363*
Primitive reflexes, 610–611, *613*

Pritikin program diet, *347*
Probenecid (Benemid), *401*, 566
Problem-oriented medical record
  system, 392–393
Progression diet, *708*
Prompting, 221
Protein availability, 46, *47*, 48
Protein-calorie malnutrition, 408–409
 classification of, 404–405
 immune system changes in, *410*
Protein catabolism, 181–182, 683
Protein complementarity, 49, *352*
Protein content:
 of dairy products, *479*
 of foods, *48*
Protein efficiency ratio, 46, *47*
Protein metabolism, 50–51
 function of cell components in, *50*
 sites of, *51*
Protein quality, 46
Protein requirements:
 for adolescents, 45
 for adults, 44–45
 for children, 45
 determinants of, 42–46
 in diabetes, 561, *562*
 and disease, 51–52
 for elderly, 46
 and exercise, 53
 for infants, 45
 during lactation, 46, 326
 for older adult, 332
 pathological conditions altering, *52*
 during pregnancy, 45–46, 312, 314
 for premature infant, 297–298
 and weight reduction, 53
Protein sparing, 64, 192–193
Protein-sparing modified fast (PSMF),
  53, *347*, 581–582
Protein supplements, 203
Protein synthesis, 50
Proteins, 39–56
 absorption of, 177–178
 and acute renal failure, 519
 in black diet, 344
 body use of, 49–51
 and calcium absorption, 131
 in Chinese diet, 340
 and chronic renal failure, 521
 classification of, 40, *41*
 classification of amino acids from
  catabolism of, *181*
 clinical application of, 51–53
 complementary, 49, *352*
 complete, 48
 conjugated, 40
 consumption of, in United States,
  39–40
 dietary significance of, 46, 48–49
 digestion of, 49–50
 digestive enzymes and secretions for
  degradation of, *172*

Proteins (*Cont.*):
  and exercise, 202–204
  functions of, 40
  future availability of, 53–54
  and hemodialysis, 526
  high-biological-value, 660–661
  incomplete, 48–49
  intravenous supplements of, 303
  in Japanese diet, 342
  in Jewish diet, 345
  liquid, 53
  in Mexican-American diet, 343
  in nephrotic syndrome, 530
  and peritoneal dialysis, 525
  in preevent meals, 206
  in Puerto Rican diet, 342
  recommended allowances of, *44*–46
  and renal failure, 506–507
  simple, 40
  structure of, 40
  thyroid and, 536
  and tooth development, 365
  in Vietnamese diet, 341
  (*See also* Amino acids)
Prothrombin, 99
Provitamin A, 92
Prudent diet, 35
PSMF (protein-sparing modified fast),
  53, *347*, 581–582
Psychiatric disorders, effect of diet on,
  599–600
Psychodietetics, 211
Psychology of diet and behavior
  modification, 211–212
Pteroylglutamic acid, 112
Puerto Ricans, food patterns of,
  342–343
Pulmonary circulation, 430, *431*
Punishment, 220
Purines in foods, *566*
Pyelonephritis, *505*
Pyridoxal phosphate, 107
Pyridoxine (vitamin B_6), 106–108, *117*
  biochemical assessment of, 107
  chemistry and properties of, 106–107
  clinical deficiency of, 108
  dietary allowance and sources of,
    107–108
  functions of, 107
  history and discovery of, 106
  metabolism of, 107
  and oral health, 365
  toxicity of, 108
Pyruvic acid, 65

Quinones, 99

Radiation therapy for cancer, 696–698
Radioallergosorbent test (RAST), 422,
  423

Rancidity of lipids, *73*
Rapid fluid replacement, 200–201
Reactive obesity, 570
Recommended Dietary Allowances
    (RDAs), 13, 22, 23, 25–28, 391
  determination of, 26
  expression of, 27
  influences on, 27–28
  interpretation and use of, 28–29
  for proteins, *44*
  for vitamins, *116–117*
  (*See also specific nutrients*)
Recommended Dietary Allowances, 9th
    ed., 127, 132
Rectal constipation, 488
Rectum, 177
Recumbent length, 248, 250
Red cell volume during pregnancy,
  311–312
Reduced nicotinamide adenine
    dinucleotide phosphate (NADPH),
    65
Reflexes:
  asymmetrical tonic neck, 610–*611, 613*
  biting, 612, *613*
  ejection, 325
  gag, 612, *613*
  hand grasp, *613*
  Moro, *613*
  oral, 611–612, *613*
  primitive, 610–611, *613*
  rooting, 611–612, *613*, 614
  suckle-swallow, 234, *256–257*, 611,
    613, 614
Regional enteritis, 486
Reinforcement, 219–220
Reinforcers, 219–220
Releasing factors, 543
Renal disorders, *505*
Renal failure (disease), 504–529
  acute (*see* Acute renal failure)
  calcium and, 514–516
  carbohydrates and fats and, 508
  chronic, 520–521, *522–523*
  end-stage, 521, 524–528
  energy and, 507
  fluid and, 516–517
  high-output phase of, 520
  nutritional considerations of, *506–517*
  obstructive, 518
  and other disease states, 517
  phosphorus and, 514–516
  potassium and, 512–514
  protein and, 506–507
  sodium and, 508–509
  supplements for, *508*
Renal osteodystrophy, 514
Renal patients, pediatric, management
  of, *527*
Renal stones (calculi), 531–532
Renal threshold, 65
Renal transplantation, 528–529

Renal tubular acidosis, *505*
Renin, 159, 160, 504
Renin-angiotensin-aldosterone system,
  159–160, 656
  and body fluids, *158*
Rennin, 49
Respiratory acidosis, 164
Respiratory alkalosis, 164
Respiratory quotient, 193
Restoration, 15
Retinal, 91–93
Retinoic acid, 91, 93
Retinol, 91–93
Retinol-binding protein, 92
Retinol equivalent (RE), 92, 93
Rewards, 219
Rhabdomyosarcoma, 703
Rheumatic fever, 451
Rheumatic heart disease, 451–452
Rheumatoid arthritis, 567
Rhodopsin, 92–93
Riboflavin (vitamin B_2), 105–106, *116*
  biochemical assessment of, 106
  chemistry and properties of, 105
  clinical deficiency of, 106
  dietary allowance and sources of, 106
  functions of, 106
  history and discovery of, 105
  metabolism of, 105
  requirements of, by premature infant,
    300
Ribonucleic acid (RNA), 135
Ribose, 59
Ribosome, 240
Rickets, 94, 96
"Rickets-preventive factor" (vitamin D),
  94
Rodale, Jerome, *347*
Rogers, Carl, 215
Rooting reflex, 611–612, *613*, 614
Rose, Mary Swartz, 6
Rumination, 214, 601
Runners, 194–198, 206–207

Saccharides, 58
Saccharin, 15
  and cancer, 693
  and pregnancy, 318
Saliva, 169
Salivary amylase, 169
Salmonella, 738
Salmonellosis, *738*
Salt tablets, 202
Sanitation in food handling, 24, *25*
Saponification, *73*
Sarcomas, 694, 703
Saturated fats:
  and cancer, 691–692
  and hyperlipidemia, 436
Saturated fatty acids, 74, 75
  naturally occurring, *76*

Saturation of fatty acids, 74, *75*
Scarsdale diet, 70, *346*
School lunch and breakfast program, *353, 736*
School years, nutrition during, 277, 279
Scurvy, 100, 102–103
Secondary hypertension, 448
Secondary reinforcers, 220
Secretin, 171, 173
Securely attached infants, 229, 230
Seizures, 78
Select Committee on Nutrition and Human Needs (U.S. Senate), 8
Selenium, 98, *128*, 149
Self-management, 221
Semivegetarians, 350
Serotonin, 596
Serum albumin, *659*
Serum albumin test, 52
Serum cholesterol, 74
   during pregnancy, 312
Serum hepatitis, 490
Serum iron, *659*
Seventh-Day Adventists, 349, 350
Severe burns, 682
Sex differences and protein needs in exercise, 203
Shaping in reinforcing behavior, 220
Sick-day diet for diabetics, 563
Sikhs, *350*
Simeon diet, *347*
Simple proteins, 40
Sippy diet, 468
β-Sitosterol, 79
Skin, and fluid and electrolyte regulation, 159
Skin test for food allergy, 422–423
Skinfold obesity standards for adults, *722*
Skinfold thickness, 250, *251*, 252, 575–576
Slow twitch fibers, 194–195
Small burns, 682
Small-for-gestational-age infants, 289
Small intestine (bowel), 171, 472
   absorption in, 175, 177
   jejunal mucosa of, *176*
Smoking:
   and cancer, 692–693
   and pregnancy, 317
Snack foods, 6
Snacks, 18–19
   guidelines for preparing, *18*
   nourishing, for children, *279*
SOAP format, 392–393
Socioeconomic status and growth, 241
Sodium, 159–160
   and acute renal failure, 519
   in baby foods, *456*
   balance mechanisms of, 159
   and chronic renal failure, 521
   clinical applications of, 160

Sodium (*Cont.*):
   and congestive heart failure, 458
   daily intake of, *160*
   distribution of, in body, 159
   and essential hypertension, 448
   in foods, *450*
   and hemodialysis, 526
   and hypertension treatment, 448–449
   in medications, *511–512*
   in nephrotic syndrome, 530
   and peritoneal dialysis, 525
   and renal failure, 508–509
   requirements of, during pregnancy, 315, 322, 336
   seasonings with low levels of, *511*
   sources with low levels of, *510*
Sodium conversion, 509
Sodium depletion, 509
Sodium-potassium-ATPase deficiency, 572
Sodium pump, 157, 177
Sodium-restricted diets, *450, 451*
Soft drinks, 19
Solutes, 155–157
Solvent drag, 175
Somatic nervous system, 595
Somatostatin, 564
Somatotropin, *543*
Somatotype, 572
Somogyi effect, 554
Sorbitol, 563, 564
Soul food, 344
Special Supplemental Feeding Program for Women, Infants, and Children (WIC), *354–355*, 357–358, *737*
Specific dynamic action of food, 185
"Spectacle eye," 111
Sphingomyelinase, 80
Sphingomyelins, 80
Spitting up, 235–236
Sports anemia, 203–204
Sports medicine, position statements on, 752–756
Sprue:
   celiac (gluten-sensitive enteropathy), 473–474, 476
   nontropical, 473
   tropical, 746
Standing height, *250*
Staphylococcus aureus, 173, *738*
Staphylococcus poisoning, *738*
Staphylococcus thermophilus, 173
Starch, 61
   hydrolysis of, 59
Starvation regimens, 581
Stearic acid, 75
Steatorrhea, 81, 82, 473
   idiopathic, 473
Steenbock, Harry, 91, 94
Stenosis, aortic, *452*
Stillman diet, *346*

Stimulation:
   during infant feeding, 228
   oral digital, 615
Stimulus-response learning, 218–219
Stomach, 170–171
   absorption in, 174
   diseases of, 466–468
   functions of, 466–467
Stool fat test, 474
Storage of food, 23–24
Stress, definition of, 654
Strokes, 433
Subscapular skinfolds, 251–252
Sucking patterns, infant, 228–229
Suckle-swallow reflex, 234, *256–257*, 611, *613*, 614
Sucrose, 60
Sufis, *350*
Sugar units, 58
Sugars, sweetness of, 60, *61*
Sulfonylureas, 556
Sulfur, 136
   dietary allowance and sources of, 136
   functions of, 136
Sunlight and vitamin D, 96
"Sunshine vitamin" (vitamin D), 94
Supersaturation phase, 196
Supplementary feedings, 680
Supplements:
   dietary, 23, *588*
   guidelines for use, *262*
   vitamin (*see* Vitamin supplements)
Surgeon General's Report on Health Promotion and Disease Prevention, 8
Surgery:
   for cancer, 698–699
   catabolism and hormonal response to, 656–657
   defined formula diets for, 680–*681*
   immune response after, 658
   initial postoperative diet for, 665
   intravenous therapy following, *667–668*
   meal replacement formulas for, 680
   nutrient stores and, 656
   nutrition after, 690
   and nutritional care, 654–682
   parenteral and enteral support systems for, 669–682
   physiological response to, 656–660
   postoperative dietary management for, 663–665, 669, *670–671*
   postoperative diets for, 669
   psychological response to, 655
   and weight reduction, 583–585
   wound healing from, 657–658
Surgical patients:
   malnourished, 660
   nutrient needs of, 658–660
Swallowing, 169
   esophageal stage of, 464

Swallowing (*Cont.*):
  oral stage of, 463
  pharyngeal stage of, 463
  physiology of, 463–464
Sweat, 198
Sweetness, 60, *61*
Synapse, 595
Synchrony, 229
  in infant feeding, 228, *229*
Systemic circulation, 430, *431*

T-lymphocytes (thymus-dependent
    lymphocytes), 408–409
Target behavior, 219
Taste buds, 168–169
  primary sets of, *169*
Taurine, 295
Tay-Sachs disease, 80
Tea, 19
Teeth, 129
  eruption of permanent, 362, *363*
  eruption and shedding of primary,
    362, *363*
  growth and development of, 362, *364*
  structure of, 361–*362*
Temperature:
  environmental and basal metabolic
    rate, 184
  of replacement fluids, 201–202
Tests:
  breath hydrogen, 478
  fat absorption, 81–82
  functional, 383
  Guthrie, 637
  inulin clearance, 62
  for liver and biliary disease, *490*
  oral glucose tolerance (OGTT),
    546–*547*
  oral tolerance, 474
  radioallergosorbent (RAST), 422, 423
  serum albumin, 52
  skin, 422–423
  stool fat, 474
  thyroid function, *537*
  total serum protein, 52
  tryptophan load, 107
  urine, for glucose, *553*–554, 564
Tetany, 130, 540
  alkalotic, 540
  hypocalcemic, 540
Tetracycline, 400
Tetralogy of Fallot, *452*
Texture:
  in infant's diet, 265
  steps to, *266*
Thiamin (vitamin B₁), 103–105, *116*
  biochemical assessment of, 104
  chemistry and properties of, 103
  clinical deficiency of, 104–105
  dietary allowance and sources of, 104

Thiamine (vitamin B₁) (*Cont.*):
  functions of, 104
  history and discovery of, 103
  metabolism of, 103–104
  and oral health, 365
  sulfur in, 136
Thiamin pyrophosphate, 104
Thiaminase, 105
Thiamine, 103
Thigh circumference, 252
3- or 7-day food record, 390
Threonine, 43
Thymus, 540
Thymus-dependent lymphocytes
    (T-lymphocytes), 408–409
Thyrocalcitonin, 536
Thyroid, 144, 535–539
  physiology of, 535–536
Thyroid function tests, *537*
Thyroid-stimulating hormone (TSH),
    144, 536
Thyrotropin, *543*
Thyroxine (T₄), *67*, 144, 279, 536, 537
  and fat, *83*
Tocopherol (*see* Vitamin E)
α-Tocopherol equivalent, 97
Tocopherols, 97
Tocotrienols, 97
Toddler, nutrition of, 274–276
Tongue in handicapped child, 615–616
Tophi, 565
Total parenteral nutrition (TPN),
    672–676
  in children with cancer, 704
  clinical and biochemical monitoring
    in, *676*
  in infant, *675*
  problems associated with, 673
  risks of, 676
Total parenteral nutrition solutions:
  administration of, 675
  for adults, *674*
  calorie and nitrogen guidelines for,
    673
  fat emulsions in, *675*
Total serum protein test, 52
Toxemia during pregnancy, 321–322
TPN (*see* Total parenteral nutrition)
Trace elements, 126, *128*
  body content of, *128*
  dietary recommendations for, *128*
  excretion of, *128*
  percent absorption of, *128*
  plasma levels of, *128*
  requirements of, for premature
    infants, 300
trans configuration, 74
Transamination, 43, 50, *51*
Transfer RNA, 240
Tranferase-deficiency galactosemia, 645
Transferrin saturation, *659*

Transient cerebral ischemic attacks,
    433
Transitional feedings, *681*
Transplantation, renal, 528–529
Transport, inborn errors of, 631
Transposition of great arteries, *452*
Treatise on Scurvy, 5
Tricarboxylic acid cycle (Krebs cycle),
    65, *180*, 181, 182, 194
Triceps skinfolds, *251*
  percentiles for, *720–721*
Trichinella spiralis, 738
Trichinosis, *738*
Triene/tetraene ratio, 77
Triglycerides, 178
  in blood plasma, *85, 86*
  formation of, *78*
  medium-chain (MCT), 78–79, 301,
    441, 473, 604
Triiodothyronine (T₃), 144, 536
Trisomy 21 (*see* Down syndrome)
Tropical sprue, 476
True catch-up, 242
Trypsin, 49
Tryptophan, 43, 109–110, 596
Tryptophan load test, 107
TSH (thyroid-stimulating hormone),
    144, 536
Tube feedings, 676–680
  administration of, 677–679
  classification of, *677*
  delivery systems for, 679–680
  for infants and children, 680
  tube placements in, *678–679*
  tubes and equipment for, 679
Tuberculosis of kidney, *505*
Tumors:
  benign, 694, *695*
  malignant, 694, *695*
  Wilm's, 703
  (*See also entries beginning with term:*
    Cancer)
24-hour recall, 389–390
Tyramine-rich food, *600*
Tyrosine, 295
Tyrosinemia, hereditary, *634–635*

Ubiquinone (coenzyme Q), 118
Ulcerative colitis, 484, 486, 499–500
Ulcers:
  duodenal, 467–468
  gastric, 467–468
  peptic, 467
  progressive bland diet for treatment
    of, *469–471*
Ultraviolet light, 94, 95
Underweight condition, 587–588
  during pregnancy, 320
United States, nutritional status of,
    391–392

U.S. Senate Select Committee on
  Nutrition and Human Needs, 8
Universal Product Coding, *22*, 23
Unmeasured diet, 556
Unsaturated fatty acids, 74, 75
  naturally occurring, *76*
Unsaturation, 74
Uremia, 521, 524–525
  diet modification for, 524–525
Uremic syndrome, 521
Uric acid, 565
  in renal calculi, 532
Urinary system, 502–532
Urinary tract infections, 530–531
Urine, 154–155
  monitoring of, after burns, *684*
Urine tests for glucose, *553–554, 564*

Vagus nerve, 173
Valine, 43
Vasopressin, *543*
Vegan diet, 56
Vegans, 49, 350
Vegetable and fruit food group, *30*
Vegetarian food guide, *351*
Vegetarianism, 349–352
Vegetarians, 350
  lacto, 49
  lacto-ovo, 49
  new, *350*
  partial, 350
  and pregnancy, 318
  traditional, 350
  Yogic, *350*
Veins, 430
Vena cava, 430
Venous pressure during pregnancy, 312
Ventricular septal defect, *452*
Very-low-density lipoprotein (VLDL),
  434, *435*, 436, 439, *440*, 442, 443
Vietnamese, food patterns of, 341–342
Viral hepatitis, 490
Viruses and diabetes, 564
Visiting Nurse Association, *356*
Visual cycle, *92–93*
Vitamin A, *116*
  in blood plasma, *85*
  chemical relationships between types
    of, *91*
  chemistry of, 91
  clinical deficiency of, 93
  dietary allowance and sources of, 93
  functions of, 92–93
  history and discovery of, 91
  metabolism of, 92
  and tooth development, 364–365
  toxicity of, 94, 124–125
  in visual cycle, *92*
Vitamin B₁ (*see* Thiamin)
Vitamin B₂ (*see* Riboflavin)

Vitamin B₆ (*see* Pyridoxine)
Vitamin B₁₂, 114–115, *117*, 149
  biochemical assessment of, 114
  chemistry and properties of, 114
  clinical deficiency of, 115
  dietary allowance and sources of,
    114–115
  functions of, 114
  history and discovery of, 114
  metabolism of, 114
  and oral health, 365
"Vitamin B₁₅" (pangamic acid), 118
"Vitamin B₁₇" (laetrile), 118
Vitamin C (*see* Ascorbic acid)
Vitamin D, 94–97, *116*
  in blood plasma, *85*
  and calcium, 130, 131
  chemistry and properties of, 94
  clinical application of, 95–96
  clinical deficiency of, 96
  dietary allowance and sources of, 96
  functions of, 95
  history and discovery of, 94
  kidney activation of, 504
  measurement of, 94
  metabolism of, 95
  and renal failure, 515
  requirements of: during pregnancy,
    315
    by premature infant, 298–299
  and tetany, 540
  and tooth development, 364
  toxicity of, 96–97
Vitamin D₂ (ergocalciferol), 94
Vitamin D₃ (cholecalciferol), 94, 95
Vitamin deficiency, primary and
  secondary, 91
Vitamin-dependent inborn errors of
  metabolism, 631
Vitamin E (tocopherol), 97–99, *116*, 333
  in blood plasma, *85*
  chemistry and properties of, 97
  clinical deficiency of, 98–99
  clinical toxicity of, 99
  dietary allowance and sources of, 98
  functions of, 97–98
  history and discovery of, 97
  measurement of, 97
  metabolism of, 97
  polyunsaturated fats and, 439
  in premature infants, 295
  requirements of, by premature
    infants, 98, 299
Vitamin H (*see* Biotin)
Vitamin K, 99–100, *116*
  administration of, to neonates, 295
  chemistry of, 99
  clinical deficiency of, 100
  dietary allowance and sources of,
    99–100
  functions of, 99

Vitamin K (*Cont.*):
  history and discovery of, 99
  measurement of, 99
  metabolism of, 99
  synthesis of, by *Staphylococcus
    aureus*, 173
  toxicity of, 100
Vitamin K₁ (phylloquinone), 99
Vitamin K₂ (menaquinone), 99
Vitamin K₃ (menadione), 100
Vitamin metabolism, effect of thyroid
  on, 536
Vitamin supplements, 118, 120, 204, *412*
  and hemodialysis, 526
  in nephrotic syndrome, 530
  and peritoneal dialysis, 525
Vitamine, 90
Vitaminlike factors, 115, 118
Vitamins, 90–115, *116–117*, 118–120
  absorption of, 179
  definition of, 90
  discovery of, 5
  and exercise, 204
  fat-soluble, 90–100
  named (*see specific vitamins*)
  natural and synthetic, 348
  requirements of: for older adults,
    332–333
    during pregnancy, 314–315
  safe and adequate daily dietary
    intakes of, *717*
  supplementation with (*see* Vitamin
    supplements)
  water-soluble, 91, 100–115
Vomiting, 464
  electrolyte composition of fluid loss
    from, *159*
  during pregnancy, 320

Wald, George, 92
"Warburg's yellow enzyme," 105
Waste excretion, 503
Water:
  and electrolytes, 153–166
  metabolic, 154
Water balance, 154–155, 503
Water content of food, *516*
Water intake, 154, *155*
Water output, 154, *155*
Water requirements, *155*
Water-soluble vitamins, 91, 100–115
Weaning, 225–226, *269*, 328, 371
Weighed diet, 556
Weight control, approaches to, *577*
Weight control diet, sample, *579*
Weight gain, 244–245
  during pregnancy, 312, *313*, 314
Weight reduction:
  carbohydrate and, 70
  drugs for, 582–583

Weight reduction (*Cont.*):
  exercise in, 580
  for hypertension treatment, 449
  protein requirements and, 53
  protein-sparing modified fast for,
    581-582
  starvation regimens for, 581
  surgery and, 583-585
  (*See also* Obesity)
Weights:
  adult, *718*
  by age and height, *719*
  dry, 526
  low prepregnant, 316
  measurement of, 250
Wernicke-Korsakoff syndrome, 599
"Wet" beriberi, 105

Wheat allergy, 420
Wheat-free diet, *425*
Wheel of Life, The (sculpture), *240*
Whey/casein ratio, 298
Whole milk, transition to, 265
Williams, R. R., 103
Wilm's tumor, 703
Wilson's disease, 146-147
Wound healing, 657-658, 660
  ascorbic acid and, 101
Wrestlers, 199-200
  weight classes for, *199*
Wrestling Rule Book, 199

Xerophthalmia, 93
Xylitol, 368, 563

Xylose, 59
Xyulose, 59

Yin and yang, 339-340, 348-349
  categorization of, *339*

Zen macrobiotics, 348-349
  diet of, *349*
Zinc, *128*, 147-148
  absorption and excretion of, 147-148
  clinical application of, 148
  dietary allowance and sources of, 148
  functions of, 147
  toxicity of, 148
  and vitamin A metabolism, 92